ENCYCLOPEDIA
OF
EPIDEMIOLOGIC METHODS

ENCYCLOPEDIA
OF
EPIDEMIOLOGIC METHODS

Editors

MITCHELL H. GAIL

National Cancer Institute, Bethesda, USA

JACQUES BENICHOU

University of Rouen Medical School, Rouen, France

John Wiley & Sons, Ltd

Chichester • New York • Weinheim • Brisbane • Singapore • Toronto

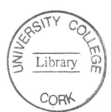

Other Wiley Editorial Offices

John Wiley & Sons, Inc., 605 Third Avenue,
New York, NY 10158-0012, USA

Wiley-VCH Verlag GmbH, Pappelallee 3,
D-69469 Weinheim, Germany

Jacaranda Wiley Ltd, 33 Park Road, Milton,
Queensland 4064, Australia

John Wiley & Sons (Asia) Pte Ltd, 2 Clementi Loop #02-01,
Jin Xing Distripark, Singapore 129809

John Wiley & Sons (Canada) Ltd, 22 Worcester Road,
Rexdale, Ontario, M9W 1L1, Canada

Library of Congress Cataloging-in-Publication Data

Encyclopedia of epidemiologic methods/editors, Mitchell H. Gail, Jacques Benichou.
        p. cm. – (The Wiley reference series in biostatistics)
    Includes bibliographical references and index.
    ISBN 0-471-86641-5 (cased : alk. paper)
        1. Epidemiology – Encyclopedias. I. Gail, Mitchell H.   II. Benichou, Jacques.   III. Series.

RA652 .E53 2000
614.4'03 – dc21

                                                        00-042285

British Library Cataloguing in Publication Data

A catalogue record for this book is available from the British Library

ISBN 0-471-86641-5

Typeset in $9\frac{1}{2}/11\frac{1}{2}$pt Times by Laser Words, Madras, India
Printed and bound in Great Britain from PostScript files by Bookcraft (Bath) Ltd
This book is printed on acid-free paper responsibly manufactured from sustainable forestry
in which at least two trees are planted for each one used for paper production.

The Wiley Reference Series in Biostatistics

Statistical methods have gained wide usage in medicine and associated health sciences. This broad discipline is generally known as "biostatistics"; the term "medical statistics" being largely synonymous. There are many introductory and advanced books on the subject, and several monographs describing the applications of statistics in particular branches of medicine and the health sciences, or using particular statistical approaches. The present Series in Biostatistics covers much of this ground, but provides an unusual and distinctive format.

The *Encyclopedia of Biostatistics*, published in 1998, is an extensive work that in six volumes and nearly 5000 pages provides a set of over 1200 articles on research design, statistical theory, and methodology relevant to the whole range of applications of biostatistics. It thus offers an unrivalled source of reference for almost any topic likely to interest a biostatistician or a health researcher concerned with the use of statistics. By its very nature, though, it does not present the most convenient format for a reader whose interest is primarily in one branch of applications, or with any particular aspect of the subject such as clinical trials or survey methodology. That is the purpose of the present Series.

Clearly, for many of these specific branches of the subject there are excellent textbooks available at both the introductory and advanced levels. We aim in this Series to take advantage of the format and material used in the *Encyclopedia of Biostatistics*, by presenting the information in separate articles, written by an international array of experts in the field and with generous selections of literature references. Many of these articles have been extracted from the *Encyclopedia of Biostatistics*, with updating of textual content and references. Others will have been written specifically for each of these volumes. Thus, the intention for each volume in this Series is to provide a useful, convenient and comprehensive resource for readers especially interested in these specific applications of biostatistics.

The Editors and contributors for each volume in the Series assume that the reader will be familiar with the basic methods and principles of statistics, such as would be covered in an introductory applied statistics course. Each volume will contain both basic and advanced statistical material related to the particular subject area of the volume, but will not systematically cover general statistical methodology. Any reader wishing to gain a fuller understanding of statistical methods will find it useful to consult the *Encyclopedia of Biostatistics*, or the wide range of books now available on statistical theory and methods.

The Series volumes adopt a uniform system of cross-referencing, with highlighting in bold type referring to articles in the *current* volume. For other topics in biostatistics, not highlighted in this way, the reader may usefully consult the *Encyclopedia of Biostatistics*.

The present *Encyclopedia of Epidemiologic Methods*, edited by Mitchell Gail and Jacques Benichou, is the first volume in the Series. We intend that later volumes will deal with clinical trials, survey methodology, statistical genetics, survival analysis, biostatistical computing, and clinical epidemiology and health service research. In addition to the hardback versions, the volumes will in due course be available on-line through the Internet.

Peter Armitage
Wallingford, UK

Theodore Colton
Boston, USA

Series Editors, 1999

Preface

This book contains extensive coverage of the statistical aspects of most areas of epidemiologic methods, as well as introductions to many areas of epidemiologic practice. A large majority of the articles have been extracted from John Wiley's *Encyclopedia of Biostatistics*, with some updating of references and coverage of more recent developments. There are, in addition, several articles written particularly for this book to cover such topics as Birth Defect Registries, Cancer Registries, Epidemiology Overview, Meta-analysis of Epidemiologic Studies, Sample Size, Sex Ratio at Birth, and Software for Design and Analysis. This entire collection of articles, written by experts, offers an excellent introduction to many topics, as well as in-depth coverage of the statistical underpinnings of contemporary epidemiologic methods. Thus, our intention with this book is to provide a useful reference tool and resource for epidemiologists, statisticians collaborating in epidemiologic research, and students of epidemiology and biostatistics. There are articles of interest to practitioners as well as to more theoretically oriented statistical readers.

This book is not intended as a textbook of epidemiology. Rather, it can serve as a complement to such texts by providing more extensive and up-to-date coverage of many specialized topics and by introducing the reader to the research literature. Used as a dictionary, it can provide concise definitions and introductions to many concepts found in textbooks.

The book contains many articles on descriptive and analytic epidemiology. For example, there are eight articles on case–control design, covering such topics as bias, general principles, hospital-based designs, nested designs, population-based designs, prevalent case designs, two-phase designs, and sequential designs. There is substantial, though less extensive, coverage of topics in allied statistical methods, such as logistic regression and survival analysis, including the Cox model. There are introductory articles for more specialized areas, including Genetic Epidemiology, Infectious Disease Epidemiology, Nutritional Epidemiology, and Occupational Epidemiology. This book does not include articles on clinical trials, as a separate volume is planned on this topic.

The articles in the book are cross-referenced to allow for more extensive exploration of a topic and to help the reader find needed definitions and related concepts. Sometimes, there is explicit reference to another article, as in "... this design (*see* **Case–Control Study, Nested**)". Sometimes bold type in the text indicates that there is a related article on this topic, but the title of the article need not be identical to the expression in bold type, as in "... exceedingly efficient to use a **nested case–control design**".

We thank the authors who contributed their material to this book. We also thank Helen Ramsey at Wiley, and Professors Peter Armitage and Ted Colton, Editors-in-Chief of the *Encyclopedia for Biostatistics*, for instigating this project and for their sound advice and help.

Mitchell Gail
Bethesda, USA

Jacques Benichou
Rouen, France

December 1999

Acronyms and Abbreviations

AC	Available case
ACME	Automated Classification of Medical Entities
ACOS	American College of Surgeons
ADL	Activities of Daily Living
AHH	Aryl hydrocarbon hydroxylase
AIDS	Acquired Immune Deficiency Syndrome
AML	Acute myeloid leukemia
ANOVA	Analysis of variance
AR	Attributable risk
ARIC	Atherosclerosis Risk in Communities
ARIMA	Autoregressive integrated moving average
ASA	American Statistical Association
ASCII	American Standard Code for Information Interchange
AZT	Zidovudine
BCDDP	Breast Cancer Detection Demonstration Project
BSE	Bovine spongiform encephalopathy
BSMS	Between subjects mean square
BUGS	Bayesian inference Using Gibbs Sampling
BWT	Birth weight
CAPI	Computer-assisted interviews in-person
CASRO	Council of American Survey Research Organizations
CATI	Computer-assisted telephone interviewing
CC	Complete case
CC	Concordance correlation
CD-ROM	Compact disk-read-only memory
CDC	Centers for Disease Control and Prevention
CDF	Cumulative distribution function
CDR	Communicable Disease Report
CDSC	Communicable Disease Surveillance Centre
Cens	Censoring indicator
CHD	Coronary heart disease
CHF	Congestive heart failure
CHS	Community Heart Study
CIOMS	Council of International Organizations of Medical Sciences
CI	Confidence interval
CJD	Creutzfeldt–Jakob disease
CL	Conditional likelihood
CMF	Comparative Mortality Figure

CM	Clinical Modification
COC	Commission on Cancer
COPD	Chronic obstructive pulmonary diseases
COVER	Cover of Vaccination Evaluated Rapidly
CPS	Cancer Prevention Study
CPS	Current Population Survey
CRIT	Critical
CSR	Center for Scientific Review
CVA	Cerebrovascular accident
CVD	Cardiovascular disease
DBCG	Danish Breast Cancer Cooperative Group
dCIS	Intraductal carcinoma *in situ*
DCO	Death Certificate Only
df	Degrees of freedom
DMV	Department of Motor Vehicles
DNA	deoxyribonucleic acid
DOS	Disk operating system
DPCP	Detectable preclinical phase
DSP	Disease Surveillance Points
DVT	Deep vein thrombosis
EAR	Excess absolute risks
EB	Empirical Bayes
EEC	European Economic Community
ELISA	Enzyme-linked immunosorbent assays
EM	Estimation–minimization
EM	Expectation-maximization
EOD	Extent of Disease
EOR	Exposure odds ratio
EPIC	European Prospective Investigation into Cancer and Nutrition
ERR	Excess relative risk
ESL	Expected significance level
EUROCAT	European Registration of Congenital Anomalies
FDA	Food and Drug Administration
FFQ	Food frequency questionnaire
FOBT	Fecal Occult Blood Test
FRSQ	Fonds de la Recherche en Santé du Quebec
FTV	Visits first trimester
GAM	Generalized additive models
GAW	Genetic Analysis Workshop
GEE	Generalized estimating equation
GHS	General Household Survey
GIS	Geographic information systems
GLM	Generalized Linear Model
GLMM	Generalized Linear Mixed Model
GOF	Goodness-of-fit

HAAS	Honolulu Asia Aging Study
HIP	Health Insurance Plan
HIV	Human immunodeficiency virus
HLA	Human leukocyte antigen
HSA	Health Service Areas
HT	Hypertension
HWE	Healthy Worker Effect
IADL	Instrumental Activities of Daily Living
IARC	International Agency for Research Against Cancer
ICC	Intraclass correlation coefficient
ICD	International Classification of Diseases
ICD-O	International Classification of Diseases for Oncology
ID	Identification code
ID	Identification Number
ID	Incidence density
IDDM	Insulin-dependent diabetes mellitus
IDR	Incidence density ratio
IEA	International Epidemiological Association
IEF	Industrial Epidemiology Forum
IHD	Ischemic heart disease
ISPE	International Society for Pharmacoepidemiology
JEM	Job-exposure matrix
LOW	Low birth weight
LQAS	Lot quality assurance sampling
LRS	Linear Risk Score
LR	Likelihood ratio
LWT	Weight in pounds at the last menstrual period
MAR	Missing at random
MCAR	Missing completely at random
MCMC	Markov chain Monte Carlo
MEDLARS	Medical Library Information Retrieval System
ME	Molecular epidemiology
MFI	Master Facility Inventory
MF/T	Multifactorial threshold
MICAR	Medical Information, Classification, and Retrieval
MISCAN	MIcrosimulation SCreening ANalysis
MI	Multiple imputation
MI	Myocardial infarction
MLE	Maximum likelihood estimator
MLR	(Maximum) likelihood ratio
ML	Maximum likelihood
MONICA	Monitoring of Cardiovascular Diseases
MOR	Mortality Odds Ratio
MOTNAC	Manual of Tumor Nomenclature and Coding
MPN	Most probable number
MRC	Medical Research Council
MRFIT	Multiple Risk Factor Intervention Trial

MRLF	Monthly Report on the Labor Force
MS	Mean square
MSBR or BRMS	"Between raters" mean square
MSBS	Between-subject mean square
MSE	Mean square error
MSGP4	Morbidity Statistics from General Practice
MTHFR	Methylenetetrahydrofolate reductase
NAACCR	North American Association of Central Cancer Registries
NAMCS	National Ambulatory Medical Care Survey
NCDB	National Cancer Data Base
NCHS	National Center for Health Statistics
NCI	National Cancer Institute
NDI	National Death Index
NHAMCS	National Hospital Ambulatory Medical Care Survey
NHANES	National Health and Nutrition Examination Surveys
NHDS	National Hospital Discharge Survey
NHIS	National Health Interview Survey
NHL	Non-Hodgkin's lymphoma
NHRDP	National Health Research and Development Programme
NHS	National Halothane Study
NHSCR	National Health Service Central Register
NICU	Neonatal intensive care units
NIH	National Institutes of Health
NLMS	National Longitudinal Mortality Study
NLTCS	National Long-Term Care Survey
NMAR	Not missing at random
NMCES	National Medical Care Expenditure Survey
NMCUES	National Medical Care Utilization and Expenditure Survey
NMES	National Medical Expenditure Survey
NND	Nearest neighbor distances
NNHS	National Nursing Home Survey
NPCR	National Program of Cancer Registries
NSABP	National Surgical Adjuvant Breast and Bowel Project
NSAID	Nonsteroidal anti-inflammatory drug
NTD	Neural tube defects
OC	Oral contraceptive
ODE	Ordinary differential equations
OMB	Office of Management and Budget
ONS	Office for National Statistics
OR	Odds ratio
OSHA	Occupational Safety and Health Administration
OV	Omitted variable
PCB	Polychlorinated biphenyls
PCNA	Proliferating cell nuclear antigen
PCR	Polymerase chain reaction
PCV	Proportion of cases vaccinated
PF	Preventable fraction

PHLS	Public Health Laboratory Service
PHS	Public Health Service
PIR	Proportional Incidence Ratio
PMR	Proportional Mortality Ratio
PO	Prevalence odds
POE	Probability of exposure
POR	Prevalence odds ratio
pps	Probability proportional to size
PPV	Proportion of the population vaccinated
PR	Prevalence ratio
PSA	Prostate Specific Antigen
PSU	Primary sampling units
PTD	Pre-term delivery
PTL	Premature labor
QALY	Quality-adjusted life-year
RACE	Race (1 = white, 2 = black, 3 = other)
RCGP	Royal College of General Practitioners
RCT	Randomized (controlled) clinical trial
RDD	Random Digit Dialing
REML	Restricted maximum likelihood
RIDDOR	Reporting of Injuries Diseases and Dangerous Occurrences Regulations
ROC	Receiver operating characteristic
RR	Relative risk
RRF	Relative risk function
RSD	Rescaled standard deviation
RSMR	Relative standardized mortality ratio
RSS	Royal Statistical Society
SAHSU	Small Area Health Statistics Unit
SBP	Systolic blood pressure
SCC	Sufficient-component cause
SEER	Surveillance, Epidemiology, and End Results
SEIR	Susceptible → Exposed → Infective → Removed
SENS	Sensitivity
SIDS	Sudden infant death syndrome
SIFTR	Service Increment for Teaching and Research
SIMEX	Simulation extrapolation
SIR	Standardized Incidence Ratio
SIR	Susceptible → infective → removed
SIS	Susceptible → infective → susceptible
SMOKE	Smoking status during pregnancy
SMOR	Standardized mortality odds ratio
SMR	Standardized Mortality Ratio
SNOMED	Systematized Nomenclature of Medicine
SNOP	Systematized Nomenclature of Pathology
SPEC	Specificity
SPMR	Standardized proportional mortality ratio
SPRT	Sequential probability ratio test

SRR	Standardized rate ratio
SRS	Simple random sampling
SSBR	Social statistics briefing room
SSBS	Sum of squares due to raters
SSE	Error sum of squares
SSE	Sum of squares due to subjects
SSN	Social Security Number
SSPE	Subacute sclerosing panencephalitis
SS	Residual sum of squares
STS	Soft-tissue sarcoma
TB	Tuberculosis
TGFα	Transforming growth factor alpha
TNM	Tumor–Node–Metastasis
TSS	Toxic shock syndrome
UDSC	Uniform Data Standards Committee
UI	Uterine irritability
UMPU	Uniformly most powerful unbiased
UNICEF	United Nations Children's Fund
UN	United Nations
USDA	US Department of Agriculture
UV	Ultraviolet
WAIFW	Who Acquires Infection From Whom
WFS	World Fertility Survey
WHO	World Health Organization
WOSCOPS	West of Scotland Coronary Prevention Study
WSMS	Within subjects mean square

Contents

Contributors

Alberman, E. *London, UK*
Andersen, P.K. *University of Copenhagen, Denmark*
Armitage, P. *University of Oxford, UK*
Axelson, O. *Linkoping University, Sweden*

Bacchetti, P. *University of California, San Francisco, USA*
Ball, F. *University of Nottingham, UK*
Balzi, D. *Centre for the Study and Prevention of Cancer, Florence, Italy*
Becker, N. *La Trobe University, Victoria, Australia*
Beckett, L.A. *Oak Park, USA*
Begg, C.W. *Memorial Sloan Kettering Cancer Centre, New York, USA*
Benichou, J. *University of Rouen Medical School, Rouen, France*
Berry, D. *Duke University, Durham, USA*
Best, N. *Imperial College of Science, Technology & Medicine, London*
Bienias, J.L. *Rush Institute for Healthy Aging, Chicago, USA*
Bithell, J. *University of Oxford, UK*
Blettner, M. *German Cancer Research Centre, Heidelberg, Germany*
Blot, W. *International Epidemiology Institute, Rockville, USA*
Breslow, N. *University of Washington, USA*
Brock, D. *Office of Epidemiology, Demography and Biometry, Bethesda, USA*
Brookmeyer, R. *Johns Hopkins University, Baltimore, USA*
Buiatti, E. *Centre for the Study and Prevention of Cancer, Florence, Italy*

Caporaso, N. *National Cancer Institute, Rockville, USA*
Carroll, R.J. *Texas A&M University, USA*
Casady, B. *Department of Labor, Washington, USA*
Chen, C.W. *US EPA, Washington, USA*
Choi, B.C.K. *Health Canada, Ottawa, Canada*

Chow, W-H. *National Cancer Institute, Bethesda, USA*
Clapp, R. *Boston University, USA*
Colton, T. *Boston University, USA*
Cook, R.J. *University of Waterloo, Canada*
Cuzick, J. *ICRF, London, UK*

Davis, P. *University of Auckland, New Zealand*
de Bock, T. *Leiden University, The Netherlands*
Dong, J. *Michigan Technical University, USA*
Dorling, D. *University of Bristol, UK*
Dunn, G. *University of Manchester, UK*

Elliott, P. *Imperial College School of Medicine, London, UK*
Elwood, J.H. *East Kent Health Authority, UK*

Farewell, V. *University College London, UK*
Farrington, C.P. *PHLS Communicable Disease Surveillance Centre, London, UK*
Felson, D.T. *Boston University, USA*
Fritz, A. *National Institutes of Health, Bethesda, USA*
Furner, S. *University of Illinois at Chicago, USA*

Gail, M.H. *National Cancer Institute, Bethesda, USA*
Gani, J. *Australian National University, Canberra, Australia*
Gastwirth, J. *George Washington University, USA*
Goldstein, H.A. *Institute of Education, London, UK*
Goldstein, R. *Brighton, USA*
Gordis, L. *Johns Hopkins University, Baltimore, USA*
Greenland, S. *Topanga, USA*
Grummer-Strawn, L. *Centers for Disease Control and Prevention, Atlanta, USA*

Hakulinen, T. *Finnish Cancer Registry, Helsinki, Finland*
Hankey, B. *National Institutes of Health, Bethesda, USA*

Hanson, J. *National Institutes of Health, Bethesda, USA*

Hartge, P. *National Cancer Institute, Rockville, USA*

Heesterbeek, H.A. *Centre for Biometry, Wageningen, The Netherlands*

Hill, H.A. *Emory University, Atlanta, USA*

Hoem, J. *Stockholm University, Sweden*

Holford, T. *Yale University School of Medicine, USA*

Hosmer, Jr, D.W. *University of Massachusetts, USA*

Inskip, H. *University of Southampton, UK*

Israel, R. *Bowie, USA*

Kendrick, S. *Scottish Health Service, Edinburgh, UK*

Keiding, N. *University of Copenhagen, Denmark*

Kleinbaum, D.G. *Emory University, Atlanta, USA*

Koch, G. *University of North Carolina, USA*

Krieger, A.M. *University of Pennsylvania, USA*

Kuha, J. *Nuffield College, Oxford, UK*

Kupper, S. *University of North Carolina, USA*

Kuritz, S.J. *Health Information Solutions, USA*

Kvis, F. *University of Illinois at Chicago, USA*

Landis, J.R. *Penn State University College of Medicine, USA*

Lang, J.M. *Boston University, USA*

Langholz, B. *University of Southern California, USA*

Lee, J. *Texas Medical Centre, USA*

Lemeshow, S. *University of Massachusetts, USA*

Lepkowki, J.M. *University of Michigan, Ann Arbor, USA*

Leufkens, H.G. *Utrecht University, The Netherlands*

Little, J. *University of Aberdeen, UK*

Little, R.J. *University of Michigan, USA*

Liu, G. *Merck Research Laboratories, Blue Bell, USA*

Lopez, A.D. *World Health Organization, Switzerland*

Lynge, E. *Danish Cancer Society, Copenhagen, Denmark*

Macfarlane, A. *Radcliffe Infirmary, Oxford, UK*

McKnight, B. *University of Washington, USA*

McLaughlin, J.K. *Johns Hopkins University, Baltimore, USA*

Meenan, R. *Boston University School of Public Health, USA*

Morgenstern, H. *UCLA School of Public Health, USA*

Neuburger, H.L. *Office for National Statistics, London, UK*

Oakley, Jr, G.P. *Emory University, Atlanta, USA*

O'Neill, R.T. *FDA, Rockville, USA*

Pak, A.W.P. *Brock University, USA*

Palmer, S. *Public Health Laboratories, Cardiff, UK*

Palmgren, J. *Rolf Nevanlinma Institute, Finland*

Pickles, A. *Institute of Psychiatry, London, UK*

Portier, C. *NIEHS-BRAP, Research Triangle Park, USA*

Prentice, R.L. *Fred Hutchinson Cancer Centre, Seattle, USA*

Preston, D. *Radiation Effects Research Foundation, Hiroshima, Japan*

Prokhorskas, R. *World Health Organization, Copenhagen, Denmark*

Renshaw, E. *University of Strathclyde, UK*

Roberts, M.G. *Wallaceville Animal Research Centre, Upper Hutt, New Zealand*

Rosenbaum, P. *Wharton School, Philadelphia, USA*

Rosenberg, L. *Boston University, USA*

Rosenberg, P. *National Cancer Institute, Bethesda, USA*

Rothman, K *Newton Executive Park, Newton Lower Falls, USA*

Samet, J. *Johns Hopkins University, Baltimore, USA*

Sasieni, P.D. *ICRF, London, UK*

Satten, G. *Centers for Disease Control and Prevention, Atlanta, USA*

Schieve, L. *Norcross, USA*

Scott, A. *University of Auckland, New Zealand*

Seber, G. *Universität Innsbruck, Austria*

Shapiro, S. *Boston University, USA*

Sharp, T.J. *University of North Carolina, USA*

Sherman, C.D. *NIEHS, Research Triangle Park, USA*

Shoukri, M. *University of Guelph, Canada*

Siemiatycki, J. *University of Quebec, Canada*

Skinner, C. *University of Southampton, UK*

Smalls, M. *Scottish Health Service, Edinburgh, UK*

Smith, L. *Australian National University, Canberra, Australia*

Spence, M.A. *UC Irvine Medical Centre, Orange, USA*

Spiegelman, D. *Harvard School of Public Health, USA*
Stevenson, C. *The Australian National University, Canberra, Australia*
Strom, B. *University of Pennsylvania, USA*
Stroup, D. *Centers for Disease Control and Prevention, Atlanta, USA*
Suissa, S. *McGill University, Montreal, Canada*
Swerdlow, A.J. *London School of Hygiene and Tropical Medicine, UK*

Tan, W-Y. *Germantown, USA*
Thacker, S.B. *Centers for Disease Control and Prevention, Atlanta, USA*
Thomas, D. *University of Southern California, USA*
Timæus, I. *Centre for Population Studies, London, UK*
Tsiatis, A.A. *University of North Carolina, USA*

Vach, W. *Universität Freiburg, Germany*
Væth, M. *Institute of Biostatistik, Arhus, Denmark*
Van Houwelingen, J.C. *Leiden University, The Netherlands*
Van Oortmarssen, G.J. *Department of Public Health, Rotterdam, The Netherlands*

Wacholder, S. *National Cancer Institute, Rockville, USA*
Wadsworth, M.E.J. *MRC National Survey of Health and Development, London, UK*
Waksberg, J. *Westat, Rockville, USA*
Wallenstein, S. *Teaneck, USA*
Walter, S. *McMaster University, Hamilton, Canada*
Wang, M-C. *Johns Hopkins University, USA*
Weinberg, C. *National Institute of Environmental Health, USA*
Wilkens, L.R. *Cancer Research Center of Hawaii, Honolulu, USA*

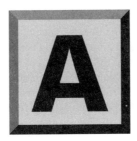

Absolute Risk

Absolute risk is defined as the probability that a disease-free individual will develop a given disease over a specified time interval given current age and individual risk factors, and in the presence of **competing risks**. In mathematical terms, the absolute risk of developing a disease of interest c_1 in the age interval $[a_1, a_2)$ in the presence of competing risks c_2 for a person of age a_1 and with initial covariates x is given by

$$\pi(a_1, a_2; x) = \frac{\int_{a_1}^{a_2} h_1(u;x) \exp\left\{-\int_0^u [h_1(v;x) + h_2(v;x)]\mathrm{d}v\right\} \mathrm{d}u}{\exp\left\{-\int_0^{a_1} [h_1(v;x) + h_2(v;x)]\mathrm{d}v\right\}},$$

(1)

where $h_1(v;x)$ and $h_2(v;x)$ are, respectively, the cause-specific **hazards** of developing c_1 and c_2 for an individual with current age v and level x of covariates X. In this formula, the numerator represents the probability of developing the disease of interest c_1 between ages a_1 and a_2 in the presence of competing risks c_2 while the denominator represents the probability of being at risk at age a_1, namely free of c_1 and c_2. This formulation underscores the conditional nature of absolute risk. However, a simpler and equivalent formulation can be obtained as

$$\pi(a_1, a_2; x) = \int_{a_1}^{a_2} h_1(u;x)$$

$$\times \exp\left\{-\int_{a_1}^{u} [h_1(v;x) + h_2(v;x)]\mathrm{d}v\right\} \mathrm{d}u.$$

(2)

The hazard $h_1(u;x)$ can be expressed as a function of both the baseline hazard $h_1(u)$ (i.e. the hazard in subjects at baseline level of covariates x) and the level x of covariates X. For instance, if the covariates X have a **multiplicative** effect on the hazard, then the multiplicative relationship $h_1(u;x) = h_1(u)rr(u;x)$ is obtained, where the multiplier $rr(u;x)$ is the relative rate, also termed the rate ratio, **incidence density ratio**, hazard ratio (the term which is used throughout this article), instantaneous relative risk or, loosely, **relative risk** (see the section "Related Quantities" below). If the covariates X have an additive effect on the hazard, then the additive relationship $h_1(u;x) = h_1(u) + d(u;x)$ is obtained, where the additive term $d(u;x)$ is the rate difference or hazard difference or incidence density difference. Upon considering such expressions, one can note that the value of absolute risk depends on both the incidence of disease in the population and the strength of the relationship between covariates and disease. One consequence is that, while the hazard ratio is often portable from one population to another (portability being more questionable for the rate difference), portability is not a property of absolute risk, as the baseline incidence rate of disease may vary widely among populations that are separated in time and location or even among subgroups of populations, possibly because of differing genetic patterns or differing exposure to unknown risk factors. Additionally, competing causes of death (competing risks) may also have different patterns among different populations which might also influence values of absolute risk.

An important consideration is that covariates X may be time-dependent, in which case one must rely on a more general formulation of (1) and (2) obtained by (i) replacing initial covariate value x in $\pi(a_1, a_2; x)$ by covariate history in interval $[a_1, a_2)$, namely $\{x(v), a_1 \leq v < a_2\}$, and (ii) by using generalized versions of cause-specific hazards, namely $h_1(v; x(v))$ and $h_2(v; x(v))$, in the right-hand terms of (1) and (2). Eqs. (1) and (2) correspond to the special case in which covariates X remain constant throughout the interval. However, unless it is possible to predict (in a probabilistic or deterministic manner) the future variation of covariates over time, estimation is based on (1) or (2) in their original form, and relies on the initial covariate value x and the assumption that it remains constant. This approach is likely to underestimate absolute risk if covariates the associated risks of which can only increase with time are considered. Such variables include, for instance, family history of breast cancer and number of previous breast biopsies for benign breast disease, which are used in estimating the absolute risk of breast cancer from the Breast Cancer Detection and Demonstration Project [47] (see the section "Estimation From Population-Based or Nested Case–Control Studies" below).

Range

Absolute risk is a probability and therefore lies between 0 and 1 and is dimensionless. A value of 0, while theoretically possible, would correspond to very special cases such as a purely genetic disease for an individual not carrying the disease gene. A value of 1 would be even more unusual and might again correspond to a genetic disease with a penetrance of 1 for a gene carrier (but, even in this case, the value should be less than 1 if competing risks cannot be ignored).

Synonyms

The term *absolute risk* or *absolute cause-specific risk* has been used by several authors, including Dupont [35], Benichou & Gail [13, 14], Benichou [11], and Langholz & Borgan [62]. However, it is not a universally accepted term. Alternative terms include risk [59], individualized risk [47], individual risk [94], crude probability [28], crude incidence [60], **cumulative incidence** [49], cumulative incidence risk [75] and absolute incidence risk [76]. It should be noted that the definition of the two latter terms [75, 76] ignores the concept of competing risks.

Interpretation and Usefulness

Absolute risk provides an individual measure of the probability of disease occurrence, and can therefore be useful in counselling. It is well suited to predicting **risk** for an individual, unlike the hazard ratio or the relative risk, which quantify the increase in the probability of disease occurence relative to subjects at the baseline level of risk factors, but do not quantify that probability itself. Moreover, individualized absolute risk estimates over specific time intervals are often more useful than general statements about risk such as "one in nine women will develop breast cancer during her lifetime" [3].

Absolute risk has been used as a tool for individual counseling in breast cancer. Indeed, a woman's decision to embark on a program of intensive surveillance with mammography or even to undergo prophylactic mastectomy depends on her awareness of the medical options, on personal preferences, and on absolute risk. A woman may have several risk factors and an elevated hazard ratio, but if her absolute risk of developing breast cancer over the next 10 years is small, she may be reassured and she may be well advised simply to embark on a program of surveillance. Conversely, she may be very concerned about her absolute risk over a longer time period, such as 30 years, and she may decide to undergo prophylactic mastectomy if her absolute risk is very high [92]. An assessment of absolute risk (and its range of uncertainty) can help the woman understand the extent of the risk and can therefore be useful in helping the woman and her doctor define an acceptable medical plan [17, 44, 47].

Absolute risk is also useful in designing trials of interventions to prevent the occurrence of a disease because the sample sizes required for these studies depend importantly on the absolute risk of developing the disease during the period of study [8]. Absolute risk has also been used to define eligibility criteria in such studies. For example, women were enrolled in a preventive trial to decide whether the drug Tamoxifen can reduce the risk of developing breast cancer. Because Tamoxifen is a potentially toxic drug and because it was to be administered to a healthy population, it was decided to restrict eligibility to women with somewhat elevated absolute risks of breast cancer. Only women over age 59 and younger women whose absolute risks were estimated to equal or exceed that of a typical 60-year-old woman were eligible to participate [8, 93].

Absolute risk can also be important in decisions affecting public health. For example, in order to estimate the absolute reduction in lung cancer incidence that might result from measures to reduce exposure to radon, one could categorize a general population into subgroups based on age, sex, smoking status, and current radon exposure levels, and then estimate the absolute reduction in lung cancer incidence, in the presence of competing risks, that would result from lowering radon levels in each subgroup [13, 42]. Such an analysis would complement estimation of population **attributable risk** and generalized impact fractions.

The concept of absolute risk is also useful in a clinical setting as a measure of the individualized probability of an adverse event, such as a recurrence or death in diseased subjects. In that context, absolute risk depends on prognostic factors of recurrence or death, rather than on factors influencing the risk of incident disease, and the time-scale of interest is usually time from diagnosis or from surgery rather than age. Absolute risk is a useful tool to help define individual patient management and, for instance, the absolute risk of recurrence in the next three years might be an important element in deciding whether to prescribe an aggressive and potentially toxic treatment regimen. Such an application is discussed in Benichou & Gail [13], who consider the absolute risk of recurrence as a function of cell type and TN staging in patients with resected lung cancer. Korn & Dorey [60] provide other examples. Note that in such a setting, 1 minus the absolute risk of recurrence differs from the standard disease-free survival probability (obtained from the disease-free interval distribution or time to recurrence distribution) in that absolute risk takes into account competing risks (deaths from other causes than the disease under study). The difference is particularly large if competing death rates are high compared to the disease-related adverse event rate, as among older people.

Properties

Two main points need to be emphasized. First, as is evident from its definition, absolute risk can only be estimated in reference to a specified time interval. One might be interested in short time spans (e.g. five years), long time spans (e.g. 30 years), or even lifetime absolute risk. Of course, absolute risk increases as the time span increases. In the clinical setting, the time span might also vary with the context and the severity of the disease.

Absolute risk can be strongly influenced by the intensity of competing risks (typically competing causes of death). Absolute risk varies inversely as a function of death rates from other causes (denoted by $h_2(v; x)$ in (1) and (2)). The same result in the clinical setting may lead to differences between 1 minus the absolute risk and the disease-free survival probability (see the section "Interpretation and Usefulness" above). Indeed, disease-free survival applies best in the situation in which no competing causes (unrelated to the disease under study) are acting to kill the patient before the occurrence of the disease or adverse event of interest [13].

Estimability

It follows from its definition that absolute risk is estimable if and only if cause-specific hazard rates for the disease (or event) of interest c_1 as well as death rates from competing causes c_2 are estimable. Therefore, absolute risk is directly estimable from **cohort** and **case–cohort studies**, but **case–control** and **cross-sectional studies** have to be complemented with follow-up data. Absolute risk is estimable from nested **case–control studies** or **population-based case–control studies**, in which the cohort or the specified population from which cases and controls are selected provides the necessary complementary information on incidence rates. While the theoretic possibility exists to complement cross-sectional studies with follow-up data, such designs do not seem to have been implemented.

An important feature of absolute risk is that it takes into account competing risks, that is the possibility for an individual to die of an unrelated disease before developing the disease (or disease-related event) of interest. Absolute risk is identifiable without any unverifiable competing risk assumptions, such as the assumption that competing risks act independently of the cause of interest because, as Prentice et al. [86] emphasize, all functions of the cause-specific hazards in (1) and (2) are estimable. Chiang [28] used the term "crude" probability to describe absolute risk, the probability of experiencing c_1 *in the presence* of competing risks c_2. This quantity is relevant for individual predictions and other applications discussed above rather than the underlying (or "net" or "latent") probability of experiencing c_1 in the absence of competing risks. One minus the standard disease-free survival represents that underlying probability of experiencing c_1 in the absence of competing risks or under the (unverifiable) assumption of independence between time to c_1 and time to c_2 (see [13], [27], [28], [43], [55], [60] and [86] for more details). The only competing risk assumption needed to estimate absolute risk concerns subjects lost to follow-up, who are assumed to be randomly selected from those at risk at the time of loss (independent noninformative censoring) [13].

Sometimes, estimates of competing hazards h_2 are based on external sources such as **vital statistics**. For instance, Gail et al. [47] developed breast cancer absolute risk estimates and used mortality rates from year 1979 for all causes except breast cancer (see also [11], [13], [14] and [60]). Although (1) and (2) allow for competing risk hazards h_2 to depend on covariate level x, it is frequently assumed that h_2 does not depend on x. It could also be assumed that h_2 depends on a set of covariates X' that are different from covariates X.

Estimation from Cohort Studies

Since all cause-specific hazards can be estimated from cohort studies, it follows that absolute risk can also be directly estimated from cohort studies. Estimation of cause-specific hazards from cohort data is a standard topic and details can be found in epidemiology or survival analysis textbooks (*see* **Survival Analysis, Overview**). However, the details of absolute risk estimation have been worked out under several models, and properties of absolute risk estimates have been studied and compared. A review is given here.

Covariate-Free Estimates of Absolute Risk

The following methods are appropriate for a homogeneous study population. They are also used to provide estimates of composite absolute risk in populations; namely, overall estimates of absolute risk that do not distinguish among levels of covariates X. Parametric and nonparametric estimators are presented.

The "density method" [59, 76, 77] estimates absolute risk $\pi(a_1, a_2)$ by the cumulative (incidence) risk given by $1 - \exp\{-\Lambda(a_1, a_2)\}$, where $\Lambda(a_1, a_2)$ is the cumulative hazard for the event of interest, c_1. This formulation ignores competing risks. The term x is omitted in Λ because an overall rather than an exposure-specific absolute risk is considered. This approach is parametric, as it relies on a piecewise exponential distribution of time to c_1, which corresponds to a piecewise constant hazard of developing c_1. It ignores competing risks, and therefore applies only in the absence of competing risks, which constitutes an important limitation.

Benichou & Gail [13] developed direct parametric estimators of absolute risk. They derived direct estimators of $\pi(a_1, a_2)$ based on (1) or (2) (still ignoring covariates X) under exponential and piecewise exponential models. Under the exponential assumption, hazards h_1 and h_2 are constant, while under the piecewise exponential assumption, hazards h_{1i} and h_{2i} are piecewise constant. The expression for $\pi(a_1, a_2)$ under the piecewise exponential assumption is given by [13]

$$
\pi(a_1, a_2) = \sum_i h_{1i}(h_{1i} + h_{2i})^{-1}
$$
$$
\times [1 - \exp\{-(h_{1i} + h_{2i})\Delta_i\}]A(i), \quad (3)
$$

with $A(i) = \prod_j \exp\{-(h_{1j} + h_{2j})\Delta_j\}$. In (3), the sum is taken over all time intervals included in $[a_1, a_2)$, i is the corresponding index, h_{1i} (respectively h_{2i}) denotes the (constant) hazard for cause c_1 (respectively c_2) in interval i, Δ_i is the width of interval i, and the product in $A(i)$ is taken over all time intervals in $[a_1, a_2)$, but the last one and indexed by j. For simplicity, a_1 and a_2 are taken to correspond to interval bounds.

Hazard rates h_{1i} can easily be estimated by d_{1i}/t_i, where d_{1i} and t_i, respectively, denote the observed number of events and **person-years** in interval i. Analogous estimates of competing hazards h_{2i} are given by d_{2i}/t_i, where d_{2i} denotes the observed number of events in interval i. Corresponding point estimates of $\pi(a_1, a_2)$ can be obtained by replacing hazards by their estimates in (3). Under the simple exponential assumption, no separate intervals are considered as the hazards h_1 and h_2 are considered constant throughout time. Eq. (3) simplifies, as the sum includes only one term and $A(i)$ equals 1. Estimates of hazards are obtained as for the piecewise exponential model with a single interval.

Unlike estimates with the density method, direct estimates of absolute risk with the exponential and piecewise exponential assumptions do not ignore competing risks, therefore providing estimates of the absolute risk of developing c_1 *in the presence* of competing risks. Moreover, as for the density method, absolute risk can be estimated for a much longer duration than the actual follow-up of individuals in the study if age is the time scale (open cohort), provided that there is no secular trend in age-specific disease incidence.

Variance estimates of the absolute risk estimate are obtained using the delta method [87], and corresponding confidence intervals follow. Details are given in Benichou & Gail [13] for the exponential and piecewise exponential models. Properties of point and variance estimators were studied by Benichou & Gail [13] for the case of a closed cohort. When the simple exponential model was correct, simulations showed no or very little **bias** in point estimates of $\pi(a_1, a_2)$, and analytic and simulation results showed that substantial gains in efficiency could be achieved with a simple exponential analysis. Simulations showed that exponential and piecewise exponential analyses yielded nearly nominal coverage with better results under the log transformation of $\pi(a_1, a_2)$. When a Weibull model with a large shape parameter of 2 was correct, simulations showed that only the piecewise exponential analysis with a sufficient number of intervals achieved little or no bias as well as good coverage, while simpler models led to serious bias and consequent failure of coverage.

The actuarial method or **life table** method [23, 33, 39, 41, 59] is an approach that shares similarities with the piecewise exponential approach, although it was derived from a less parametric viewpoint. As with the piecewise exponential approach, time is split into intervals (indexed by i in this presentation). In each time interval i, the probability for an individual at risk at the beginning of the interval to survive the interval without developing c_1 is expressed as

$$S_i = (n_i - w_i/2 - d_i)/(n_i - w_i/2), \qquad (4)$$

where n_i denotes the number of subjects in the cohort at the beginning of interval i, d_i the number of events occuring in interval i, and w_i the number of subjects either lost to follow-up or developing c_2 (competing risks) in interval i. The actuarial approach is most appropriate when grouped data are available and the actual follow-up in each interval is not known. The person-years of follow-up for subjects lost to follow-up or developing c_2 in interval i is not used but, if one assumes that the mean withdrawal time occurs at the midpoint of the interval, then the denominator in (4) can be regarded as the effective number of persons at risk of developing the disease. That is, it represents the number of disease-free persons that would be expected to produce d_i events if all persons could be followed for the entire interval [38, 59, 66]. It can be regarded as a refinement of the simple cumulative method [59, 77] that ignores quantity w_i. Absolute risk is estimated by the cumulative (incidence) risk which, from the formulation in (4), is obtained as

$$1 - \prod_i S_i. \qquad (5)$$

Since (5) ignores competing risks, the actuarial method applies in the absence of competing risks, which constitutes an important limitation, in an analogous manner as the density method. Moreover, as shown by several authors [33, 41], the actuarial method results in biased estimates of risks even in the unlikely and most favorable event (in terms of bias) of all withdrawals occurring at the interval midpoints. Alternative approaches based on different choices of the quantity to subtract from n_i (choices different from $w_i/2$) are not subject to less bias [38]. The problem can be improved best by using narrower intervals, but this is done at the expense of a larger **random error**.

Unlike the piecewise exponential models, the actuarial method does not require knowledge of follow-up time in each interval but only knowledge of the number at risk and the number of withdrawals. The piecewise exponential approach could, however, be used without knowledge of follow-up time by assigning a follow-up time of half the interval width to subjects who are lost to follow-up or who develop c_1 or c_2, in an analogous fashion as with the actuarial method [13]. The piecewise exponential approach has several advantages over the actuarial method. Bias is less of a problem with it, it takes competing risks into account, it applies naturally to open cohorts, and it extends easily to regression-based estimators (see below).

When individual follow-up times are all known, it is possible to estimate absolute risk nonparametrically as in Aalen [1], by substituting $\hat{\bar{G}}(t_1-)$, the right continuous Kaplan–Meier estimate [56] of surviving both c_1 and c_2 to time a_1 into the denominator of (1) and by replacing the numerator by $\sum \hat{\bar{G}}(t-)R^{-1}(t)$, where $R(t)$ is a left continuous process defining the number of subjects at risk just before t. The summation is over distinct times in $[a_1, a_2]$ at which events c_1 occur. The same estimator is discussed by Aalen & Johansen [2], Kay & Schumacher [57], Gray [49], Matthews [73], Keiding & Andersen [58], Benichou & Gail [13], and Korn & Dorey [60].

While nonparametric point estimates are easy to obtain, variance estimates are more complex and can be obtained in several ways. Results in Aalen [1, Theorem 2] can be used, as discussed in Benichou & Gail [13] and Korn & Dorey [60]. Alternatively, results in Aalen & Johansen [2, Theorem 4.3] can be used, as discussed by Keiding & Andersen [58]. Confidence intervals can then be obtained, based on the log transformation, as suggested by Benichou & Gail [13] and Keiding & Andersen [58], or based on results of Dorey & Korn [34], who treat the lower and upper limit differently, a procedure that they claim is advantageous under heavy censoring.

Analytic and simulation results in Benichou & Gail [13] under exponential survival distributions show that the loss of efficiency of the nonparametric method is very small compared to a detailed piecewise exponential model and that nearly nominal coverage is obtained with the log transformation as for the piecewise exponential model. In simulations under a Weibull model with a large shape parameter of 2, very little bias and near nominal coverage was observed as with the piecewise exponential model [13]. These results suggest that properties of the piecewise exponential model and the nonparametric approach agree closely. The nonparametric approach does not make any assumption on the form of the hazards, but the piecewise constant assumption can be made less stringent by increasing the number of intervals. The piecewise exponential model has the advantage of simplicity of computation, in that it uses grouped data rather than individual data. Moreover, it is well suited to open cohorts.

These approaches yield an overall composite absolute risk and ignore covariates X. In order to obtain estimates that depend on the level of covariates, the cohort can be subdivided into subcohorts, and these approaches applied to resulting subcohorts defined by levels of X. This approach yields absolute risk estimates with low precision, however, if the subcohorts are small and have few events, as can happen if several risk factors have to be considered jointly (see [47] for further discussion and illustration, and [7] and [82] for further illustration with the actuarial method and breast cancer data). In order to remedy this problem, a natural approach is to model incidence rates h_1 and h_2 through regression models.

Covariate Models

Regression-based parametric methods are a direct extension of parametric methods for composite estimates. For instance, Benichou & Gail [13] studied exponential and piecewise exponential models. Under the piecewise exponential model, it is assumed that hazards for c_1 are products of a baseline hazard in interval i and a function of the covariates, usually (but not necessarily) expressed as $\exp(\beta^T x)$. Baseline hazards as well as hazard ratio parameters β can be jointly estimated by maximizing the piecewise exponential likelihood. That likelihood is the same as that obtained by assuming that the number of events in each combination of time interval and level of X has a Poisson distribution with mean given by the product of the hazard times the corresponding number of person-years, that latter number being assumed constant [52, 61] (*see* **Poisson Regression for Survival Data in Epidemiology**). It is possible to include time by exposure **interactions** in covariates X so that the **proportional hazard** assumption is not required. Furthermore, hazards for cause c_2 are estimated separately. They are also assumed to be piecewise constant and can be assumed to depend on the set of covariates X, a different set X' if needed, or on no covariates. A point estimate of $\pi(a_1, a_2; x)$ is obtained by replacing quantities h_{1i} in (3) by quantities $h_{1i} \exp(\beta^T x)$, where h_{1i} denotes the baseline hazard in the latter expression, and by plugging in maximum likelihood estimates of the parameters. Corresponding parameter estimates for competing hazards are estimated separately and also plugged in (3). A similar approach to point estimation can be taken for other parametric models such as a simple exponential model or a Weibull model [13].

As described in Benichou & Gail [13], variance estimates can be obtained by applying the delta method [87] and relying on the observed information matrix for all parametric models. Finite sample properties were studied by Benichou & Gail [13] through simulations based on a clinical trial of lung cancer [48]. Simulations used 392 patients, an accrual period of three years, and an additional follow-up of two years. Time to c_1 was assumed to be exponentially distributed and to depend on two covariates forming six joint levels, while time to c_2 was assumed to be exponential and not to depend on any covariates. Point estimates had little bias with piecewise exponential and exponential analyses. Variance estimates were also little biased and coverage was nearly nominal with all analyses except for the level of X with the fewest patients (12 patients) in which variance estimates and corresponding coverage were too small. Loss of efficiency could be appreciable when a detailed piecewise exponential was used compared to the simple exponential model.

Finally, a semiparametric estimator of absolute risk can be obtained, as outlined in Benichou & Gail [13]. The difference with the piecewise exponential approach is that the hazard for c_1 is the product of an unspecified function of time (the baseline hazard) times a function of the covariates which is also usually of the form $\exp(\beta^T x)$ [31]. As for the piecewise exponential model, X may include time by exposure interaction and competing hazards can be assumed to depend on covariates X or X' or on no covariates (in the latter case, corresponding survival is estimated nonparametrically using the Kaplan–Meier product-limit estimator).

The expression for a semiparametric estimate of absolute risk is given in Benichou & Gail [13, formula (3.1)] and is a function of partial likelihood estimates [32] of hazard ratio parameters β and related Nelson–Aalen estimates of cumulative baseline hazards [6]. From results in Tsiatis [95] and Andersen & Gill [5] on the joint distribution of these parameter estimates, Benichou & Gail [13] derived an asymptotic variance estimator. No formal study of its finite sample properties has been undertaken.

These regression methods yield estimates of absolute risk with acceptable precision for several covariates. Regression-based methods are therefore well suited for individual prediction. Parametric or semiparametric approaches can be used. The piecewise exponential estimator seems to provide a good compromise between bias and precision, while being easy to implement both for open and closed cohorts.

Estimation from Population-Based or Nested Case–Control Studies

Case–control studies provide data on the distributions of exposure respectively in diseased subjects (cases) and nondiseased subjects (controls) for the disease under study. These data are used to estimate hazard ratios or relative risks through the estimation of odds ratios, but are not sufficient to estimate exposure-specific incidence rates (the terms "hazard" and "incidence rate" are used indiscriminately in the remainder of the text) and absolute risks. In order to do so, case–control data have to be complemented by follow-up data. Either the cases and controls are selected from a follow-up study (*see* **Case–Control Study, Nested**) that provides either grouped data or individual data with survival-type information, or they are selected from a specified population in which an effort is made to identify all **incident cases** diagnosed during a fixed time interval (*see* **Case–Control Study, Population-Based**) usually in a grouped form (number of cases and number of persons by age group). In both situations, full information on exposure is obtained only for cases and controls, but the complementary data provide information on composite incidence that can be combined with hazard ratio estimates to obtain exposure-specific incidence rates, as has long been recognized [29, 30, 68, 75, 76, 80].

The main estimation problem regards estimation of exposure- and age-specific hazards or incidence rates (age is the usual time scale in this context). Absolute risk estimates are then obtained from (1) or (2), and the delta-method [87] can be used to obtain the variance of absolute risk estimates based on the covariance matrix of incidence rate estimates. Parametric methods based on the piecewise exponential model (also termed the **Poisson regression** model) and the logistic model have been derived under a full likelihood approach, a pseudo-likelihood approach, and a hybrid approach. That latter approach will be described fully, because it has been used to obtain absolute risk estimates in practice. The former two approaches will be reviewed more briefly, because they have not yet been used to derive absolute risk estimates and fewer results are available. Finally, a semiparametric estimate of absolute risk based on partial likelihood has been proposed for nested case–control studies with time-matching of cases and controls, and will also be reviewed.

Parametric Approaches

The hybrid approach has been proposed by Gail et al. [47] as a multivariate extension of earlier work by Miettinen [75]. It relies on the possibility of estimating composite incidence rates h_{1i}^* from the population or follow-up data for each age group i or, in a more general fashion, for each stratum i defined by age and other factors observed in the follow-up or population data such as sex and region. Under a piecewise exponential assumption, the quantity h_{1i}^* is estimated by the ratio d_{1i}/t_i of the number of incident cases of disease c_1 to the number of person–years. Although information on exposure is obtained on cases and controls only, and not on the whole cohort or population, baseline incidence rates h_{1i} (for subjects at the baseline level of all exposure factors considered) can be obtained through the relationship [47, 75]:

$$h_{1i} = h_{1i}^*(1 - AR_i), \qquad (6)$$

where AR_i is the attributable risk for disease c_1 in age group i or, more generally stratum i, for all exposure factors jointly, a quantity estimable from the case–control data. Gail et al. [47] suggested using the model-based approach of Bruzzi et al. [25], that incorporates **odds ratios** from **logistic regression**, for estimating attributable risk, and obtained a point estimate for h_{1i}. Upon multiplying that estimate by the corresponding odds ratio from logistic regression, they obtained an estimate of the incidence rate for each joint age and exposure level. Finally, incidence rates for competing risks can be obtained from the follow-up or population data, provided that those rates are assumed not to be influenced by the exposure factors for c_1. The latter assumption stems from the fact that it would be impossible to estimate hazard ratios for c_2 from case–control data for disease c_1. In fact, Gail et al. [47] used external data on national US mortality rates to estimate h_{2i} and obtained absolute risk estimates from the piecewise exponential model in formula (3).

Variance estimators are complex since incidence rate estimates involve odds ratio parameters obtained through logistic regression from the case–control data and counts of incident cases from the follow-up or population data. Estimators of variances and covariances of age- and exposure-specific incidence rates have been fully worked out by Benichou & Gail [14] for simple random sampling, stratified random sampling, **frequency matching** and individual **matching** in a simple setting. The approach relies on an extension of the delta-method to implicitly related random variables [12]. It takes into account all sources of variability; namely, the variance of hazard ratio estimates and of baseline incidence rate estimates, as well as the covariance between the two. Variance estimates of absolute risk estimates are then obtained through the delta-method [87] and take into account the variance of competing hazard estimates unless they are estimated from external sources and considered fixed, as in Gail et al. [47].

The hybrid approach can be regarded as relying on two models; namely, the piecewise exponential model and the logistic model (the **conditional logistic** model for individual matching and the unconditional logistic model for the three other ways of sampling controls). The baseline incidence rates are obtained by combining follow-up (or population) data and case–control data. Benichou & Gail [14] performed simulations based on the Breast Cancer Detection Demonstration Project (BCDDP) [9], a large follow-up study of 284 780 women, from which about 3000 cases and 3000 controls were selected (case–control study within a cohort or case–control study). They used a sample size of 100 000 women in each replication and generated piecewise exponentially distributed times to breast cancer occurrence by considering four age groups and two exposure factors forming six levels. A follow-up of five years was considered, and the possibility of dying from other causes (piecewise constant competing hazards not influenced by any covariates) was taken into account. Incident cases and frequency-matched controls were selected from the follow-up data. They found a small upward bias in absolute risk estimates due to the small upward bias incurred by using odds ratios to estimate hazard ratios when the rare disease assumption is violated in the context of such a study. Complete variance estimates had very little bias and yielded confidence intervals with near nominal coverage. Coverage was improved with the logit transform. Incomplete variance estimates that took into account only the variance of hazard ratio estimates from the case–control data were too small for small values of absolute risk, because they ignored the variances of baseline incidence rate estimates, and too large for larger values of absolute risk, because they ignored the negative covariances between hazard ratio estimates and baseline incidence rate estimates.

The hybrid approach was applied to the estimation of absolute risk of breast cancer from the BCDDP data as a function of age and four risk factors [47]. Details regarding variance estimation can be found in Benichou [11], who took into account special subsampling of cases and controls. Indeed, not all incident cases were used to estimate composite hazards and not all selected cases and controls were used to estimate hazard ratios. In order to implement these results and estimate absolute risk for new subjects, tables for point estimation were given by Gail et al. [47]. Practical implementation has been greatly facilitated by the development of the computer program RISK [10] and of graphs [17] that yield point estimates and confidence intervals of the absolute risk of developing breast cancer. Absolute risk is a widely used tool in individual counseling for breast cancer [17].

A pseudo-likelihood approach and a full likelihood approach have been proposed as alternatives to the hybrid approach [15]. They also rely on the piecewise exponential (or Poisson) model or logistic model, although other parametric models could be used. They yield exposure-specific incidence rate estimates, but have not been fully developed to obtain absolute risk estimates, although this extension would be straightforward. Indeed, it would consist in (i) substituting in (1) or (2) age- and exposure-specific hazard estimates for disease c_1 and competing hazard estimates in order to obtain point estimates of absolute risk and (ii) using the delta-method [87] to derive variance estimates.

The pseudo-likelihood approach was presented by Benichou & Wacholder [15] in the context of a Poisson model (piecewise exponential model) and rests on the following principles. A full likelihood for the entire cohort or population could be written and maximized if information on exposure were available for all subjects in the population or cohort rather than just for the cases and controls. However, one can combine follow-up or population information in the form of number of events d_i and person-years t_i for each stratum i with the observed distribution of exposure in the case–control data to obtain estimates of number of events d_{1ij} and person-years t_{ij} for joint stratum level

i and exposure level j. This is simply done by multiplying quantities d_{1i} (respectively t_i) by the observed proportion of cases (respectively controls) at exposure level j in stratum i. The rare disease assumption is used to obtain person-years from the conditional distribution of exposure in controls only. Substituting these estimated quantities, one obtains a Poisson pseudo-likelihood which is then maximized to obtain maximum pseudo-likelihood estimates of incidence rate parameters (baseline incidence rates and hazard ratios for a multiplicative model). Variance estimation relies on sandwich variance estimators [64] which allow for taking into account the additional component of variability incurred by the use of estimates of quantities d_{1ij} and t_{ij}.

The full likelihood approach differs from the pseudo-likelihood approach in that a full likelihood is written as a function of the incidence rate parameters to be estimated *and* a set of nuisance parameters for the conditional distribution of exposure given the stratum in the population. Rather than using the observed conditional distributions in cases and controls as with the pseudo-likelihood approach, the nuisance parameters are estimated jointly with the incidence rate parameters by maximization of the likelihood [15]. One obtains fully efficient maximum-likelihood estimates (rather than maximum pseudo-likelihood estimates) of all parameters (incidence rate and nuisance parameters), and variance estimates of the incidence rate parameters are obtained directly from the observed information matrix. In the context of a Poisson model, this approach is faced with the potential problem of a large number of parameters if several risk factors and stratum levels are considered. Even in the simple example of Benichou & Wacholder [15], with nine strata and eight exposure levels only, 60 nuisance parameters had to be estimated. This problem can be alleviated if one is willing to consider the logistic rather than the Poisson model, as pointed out by Greenland [50]. A prospective logistic model can be applied to the case–control data and yields maximum likelihood estimates of hazard ratio parameters. Furthermore, maximum likelihood estimates of baseline incidence rates are obtained by adding to the stratum parameter estimates from the logistic model a term corresponding to the logarithm of the ratio of sampling fractions among cases and controls in the stratum [50, 85]. The covariance matrix of estimates of baseline incidence rates and hazard ratios is obtained as described in Prentice & Pyke [85].

Upon comparing the pseudo-likelihood, full likelihood and hybrid approach on population-based case-control data of bladder cancer [51], Benichou & Wacholder [15] found that the hybrid approach seemed to be less efficient for incidence rate estimation than the other two approaches, which were themselves equally efficient. This efficiency loss might be due to the following conceptual difference regarding estimation of baseline incidence rates and hazard ratios among the three approaches. With the maximum likelihood and pseudo-likelihood approaches, these quantities are jointly estimated and their negative correlations fully accounted for in variance estimates. With the hybrid approach, crude incidence rates and hazard ratios are estimated separately and then combined to obtain stratum- and exposure-specific incidence rates and, as a consequence, negative correlations between estimates of baseline incidence rates and hazard ratios are not as strong, which results in larger variances [15]. Another potential advantage of the full likelihood and pseudo-likelihood approaches is that they directly estimate hazard ratios rather than odds ratios. Furthermore, if the Poisson (but not the logistic) model is used, they can be applied to more general models of risk; for example, models with an additive form using rate difference parameters rather than hazard ratio parameters [15]. Finally, all three approaches require that cases and controls be selected at random [67] and that incident cases or at least a known proportion of them be fully identified [15].

Semiparametric Approach

The three parametric approaches described above apply to situations in which controls are not individually matched to cases. The hybrid approach can handle special cases of individual matching [14] but not time-matching, which characterizes **nested case–control studies** [24, 65, 71]. In that context, Langholz & Borgan [62] developed a semiparametric approach which can be regarded as an extension of the semi-parametric approach for cohort studies described above (see the section "Estimation from Cohort Studies" above). The context is that of a nested case–control study (case–control within a cohort), in which cases develop from a cohort, and controls are

selected from subjects still at risk. Therefore, individual follow-up times are needed and grouped data are not sufficient.

Incidence rates are expressed as the product of baseline incidence rates of an unspecified form times a function of the covariates representing the hazard ratio [31]. Hazard ratio parameter estimates are obtained from maximizing the partial likelihood of the **Cox regression model** for nested case–control data [81, 84]. Absolute risk estimates are obtained by combining partial likelihood hazard ratio parameter estimates and corresponding cumulative hazard estimates. Langholz & Borgan [62] showed that their proposed semiparametric estimate is asymptotically normal and provided a variance estimator based on results in Aalen & Johansen [2], Andersen et al. [6], and Borgan et al. [21]. Point estimates and corresponding variance estimates are based on simple sums or products of information from the case–control study, the estimated hazard ratio parameters, and the number at risk at the failure times. Competing risks can be taken into account provided that it is assumed that occurrence of c_2 is not influenced by the risk factors for occurrence of disease c_1. Finite sample properties of this approach have not been studied. A direct comparison with parametric approaches presented above is not possible because the semiparametric approach applies only to time-matched data, which the parametric approaches cannot handle. The semiparametric approach requires observation of individual follow-up time of each subject in the original cohort in order to form the risk sets for each failure time, and enable control selection. It is therefore potentially less widely applicable than the parametric approaches but makes no assumption on the baseline hazard. Finally, it has the advantage over the available parametric approaches of being able to handle continous covariates.

Special Problems

Case–Cohort and Cross-Sectional Designs

In the **case–cohort design**, information on exposure is gathered only in a subcohort of subjects randomly selected from the original cohort and among subjects who develop the disease [83]. It is therefore possible to estimate exposure-specific incidence rates and absolute risk directly from case–cohort data. However, the details of absolute risk estimation have not been worked out in the literature. **Cross-sectional studies** would need to be complemented by follow-up or population data in order to allow for incidence rate and absolute risk estimation, but such designs do not seem to have been implemented (*see* **Case–Control Study, Prevalent**).

Two-Stage Case–Control Studies

In **two-phase case–control studies** [22, 98, 99], cases and controls are selected from a cohort or a population, as in a case–control study within a cohort or a population-based case–control study. Furthermore, a nested subsample of cases and controls is selected from original cases and controls on which information is gathered on exposure factors which are more difficult to obtain, such as X-ray data or genetic markers. Several parametric approaches have been developed to allow for hazard ratio and incidence rate estimation by an extension of the pseudo-likelihood approach for two-stage case–control data [16], pseudo-conditional likelihood methods [22, 90], and weighted likelihood methods [40, 54, 88, 89]. From incidence rate estimates from these various methods, it would be easy to obtain absolute risk estimates from (1) or (2).

Continuous Risk Factors

Absolute risk can be expressed as a function of both continuous and categorical risk factors. Model-based estimation methods presented above for cohort data (see the section "Estimation from Cohort Data" above) accommodate both types of variables. For case–control data however, the situation is different. Among parametric approaches, the hybrid approach yields point estimates that apply to both types of variables, but variance estimators have been developed only for categorical covariates. The full likelihood and pseudo-likelihood approach only apply to categorical covariates. The semiparametric approach is more flexible, in that it fully allows for continuous risk factors for point and variance estimation.

Time-Dependent Risk Factors

Most estimation procedures presented above can be adapted to take into account time-dependent covariates. However, when absolute risk is used for individual prediction, estimation of absolute risk over time

interval $[a_1, a_2)$ is based on the initial value of the covariates (i.e. the value at time a_1) and assumes that it stays constant over the whole interval, unless it is possible to predict (in a probabilistic or deterministic manner) the future variation of covariates over time (see the opening text).

Secular Trend

An important feature of the estimation methods described for cohort and case–control studies is that, by combining hazard estimates from different age intervals, absolute risk can be estimated for a much longer age interval than the actual follow-up of individuals in the study. To combine these hazard estimates into a single estimate of absolute risk, one must assume that there is no secular trend in disease incidence [59, Chapter 6].

Misclassification of Exposure

Misclassification of exposure could affect the validity of absolute risk estimates, but this problem, which has been studied for estimation of other measures (e.g. odds ratio, hazard ratio, and population attributable risk; *see* **Measurement Error in Epidemiologic Studies**) has not been studied for absolute risk estimation.

Use of Two Time Scales

In some applications, it may be important to consider two time scales, such as time from entry in the cohort (e.g. time from surgery, diagnosis, or first exposure) and age. Korn & Dorey [60] give guidelines and examples for that situation.

Selection of Risk Factors and Model Misspecification

Selection of risk factors on which to base absolute risk estimation is a difficult task. Complex multivariate models containing many risk factors will usually appear to describe the variation of risk in the data used to fit the model better than simpler models. Yet the simpler models often perform as well or better in predicting risk in other populations [37]. This is because complex models fit the statistical anomalies of the given sample as well as the reproducible features, whereas the simpler models tend to reflect the reproducible features only. It might therefore be preferable to choose factors for inclusion in the model that have been previously demonstrated to be important rather than to rely solely on the current data sample to select factors for inclusion [44].

A related problem is model misspecification which can lead to severe bias in absolute risk estimates and has to be considered carefully. Model misspecification can come from an inappropriate selection of risk factors, but also from incorrectly modeling the effect of included risk factors, from selecting the wrong model for time to event distribution, or from incorrectly assuming proportional hazards. Benichou & Gail [13] illustrate the potential severity of the problem in an example which suggests that using unsaturated rather than saturated models for covariate effects can lead to a **systematic error** that is potentially larger than **random error**.

Validation

Given the potentially severe effects of model misspecification on absolute risk estimation, it is important to validate models used for absolute risk estimation. For instance, from internal validation results and two studies of external validation based on independent cohorts [20, 94] (*see* **Validation Study**), it appeared that the model developed by Gail et al. [47] to estimate absolute risk of breast cancer from the BCDDP as a function of age and four risk factors produces valid estimates of absolute risk for women in regular screening as in the BCDDP, but yields estimates that tend to be too high when applied to unscreened or sporadically screened populations [20, 44, 45, 94], as had been cautioned in the initial paper [47].

Absolute Risk and Treatment Comparison

It might be useful to use absolute risk as a means of testing for treatment effect, especially given the availability of tests for comparing k treatment groups based on absolute risk [49]. However, use of absolute risk alone may be misleading. For example, if a cancer treatment increases h_2 but leaves h_1 unaffected, absolute risk will diminish in the treated group; yet overall survival is reduced and c_1-specific survival is unchanged. Instead, one should compare overall survival and estimates of the cause-specific survival

curves in the treated and untreated groups, as is common practice. If h_2 is not affected by treatment, however, the change in absolute risk is a more realistic gauge of treatment benefit than a comparison of c_1-specific survival curves. If both h_1 and h_2 are affected, absolute risk gives useful descriptive information for summarizing the burden of recurrence in each group [13].

Overall Adjusted Absolute Risk

In order to obtain an overall measure of absolute risk at the population level, one might combine individualized estimates to obtain a direct adjusted value for the entire population by summing estimated values of absolute risk for a given level of the covariates over the distribution of the covariates in the reference population [13]. This procedure would yield a different estimate than that obtained by covariate-free estimation of absolute risk from the same population (see the section "Estimation from Cohort Studies" above). The adjusted procedure would be analogous to the methods for direct adjustment of survival curves described by Murphy & Haywood [79], Makuch [70], and Chang et al. [26], and the variance estimation methods of Gail & Byar [46] could be adapted.

Related Quantities

Attack Rate

In the investigation of a local outbreak of a **communicable disease**, a measure of interest is the absolute risk of developing the disease for the duration of the epidemic or the time during which primary cases occur. In this situation, absolute risk is often called an attack rate [59, 69].

Hazard Ratio and Relative Risk

As discussed above (see the section "Interpretation and Usefulness"), the hazard ratio, also called the relative rate, rate ratio, incidence density ratio, or instantaneous relative risk, is a useful measure in etiologic research that quantifies the strength of the relationship between exposure and disease, while absolute risk is more useful in individual prediction as a measure of the actual probability of disease for a given risk profile. Large hazard ratios may correspond to small absolute risks if the disease is rare and conversely.

Since incidence rates are a function of hazard ratios in multiplicative models, absolute risk is also a function of hazard ratios (and of baseline incidence rates) in those models. Alternatively, additive models can be used with the rate difference, also called hazard difference or incidence density difference, being the relevant parameter instead of the hazard ratio to measure the effect of covariates.

The term "relative risk" is frequently used to represent a hazard ratio or its estimator. Strictly speaking, however, relative risk refers to the ratio of absolute risks and not of incidence rates [59]. A synonym is "risk ratio" [76].

Incidence Rate

Absolute risk is a direct function of incidence rates, as is apparent from (1) and (2) that define absolute risk. As was mentioned above (see the sections "Estimability" and "Estimation" above), the problems of absolute risk estimability and estimation essentially reduce to those of incidence rate estimability and estimation.

Cumulative Risk and Cumulative Hazard

The relationships between absolute risk and cumulative risk and hazard have been defined in the section "Estimation from Cohort Studies" above.

Excess Risk

Excess risk [91], also called excess incidence [18, 69, 74], is defined as the difference between the incidence rates in the exposed and the unexposed. Like absolute risk, it takes into account the incidence of the disease in the unexposed and the strength of the association between exposure and disease. It can be expressed as the product of the baseline incidence rate times the hazard ratio minus 1, and it quantifies the difference in incidence that can be attributed to exposure at the individual level. Other terms have been used to denote this quantity; namely, "Berkson's simple difference" [96], "incidence density difference" [76], "excess prevalence" [96], and even "attributable risk" [72, 91].

Population Attributable Risk and Generalized Impact Fraction

Population **attributable risk** [63] and the generalized impact fraction [97] are measures that assess the public health consequences of an association between exposure and disease and the potential impact of prevention measures aimed at eliminating (population attributable risk) or reducing (generalized impact fraction) exposure in the population. As was mentioned above (see the section "Interpretation and Usefulness" above), absolute risk can be used to estimate the absolute reduction in incidence that would result from prevention measures in each subgroup of exposure, and can therefore be regarded as a useful complement to population attributable risk and the generalized impact fraction.

Floating Absolute Risk

The term "floating absolute risk", introduced by Easton et al. [36], refers to a concept unrelated to absolute risk, which may introduce some confusion. The purpose of those authors was to remedy the standard problem that hazard ratios are estimated in reference to a baseline group which in turn causes hazard ratio estimates for different levels of exposure to be correlated and may lead to lack of precision in hazard ratio estimates if the baseline group is small. The authors proposed a procedure to obtain hazard ratio estimates unaffected by these problems. They termed their proposed hazard ratio estimates "floating absolute risks" to indicate that their standard errors were not estimated in reference to an arbitrary baseline group.

Prospects and Conclusions

Despite the substantial development of methods for estimating absolute risk, there remain important research issues, including point and variance estimation for parametric case–control estimators when continuous risk factors are considered, the study of finite sample properties of nonparametric and semiparametric estimators and their comparison with parametric estimators, the comparison of the three main parametric approaches in case–control studies, the study of the effect of exposure misclassification on absolute risk estimation, and research issues regarding special problems (see the section "Special Problems" above).

An important issue is the development of tools to implement methods for absolute risk estimation. For instance, a graphic approach has been developed to convert relative to absolute risk [35]. Graphs [17] and a computer program [10] have been developed to estimate absolute risk of breast cancer as a function of age and four risk factors. More general programs would be worth developing.

Finally, an important challenge is to increase awareness of the proper interpretation and use of absolute risk in practice (e.g. in counseling, see [4], [17], [19], [53] and [78]), as well as of correct estimation techniques.

References

[1] Aalen, O. (1978). Nonparametric estimation of partial transition probabilities in multiple decrement models, *Annals of Statistics* **6**, 534–545.

[2] Aalen, O. & Johansen, S. (1978). An empirical transition matrix for nonhomogeneous Markov chains based on censored observations, *Scandinavian Journal of Statistics* **5**, 141–150.

[3] American Cancer Society (1992). *Cancer Facts and Figures*. ACS, Atlanta.

[4] American Society of Human Genetics Ad Hoc Committee (1994). Statement of the American Society of Human Genetics on Genetic Testing for Breast and Ovarian Cancer Predisposition, *American Journal of Human Genetics* **55**, i–iv.

[5] Andersen, P.K. & Gill, R.D. (1982). Cox's regression models for counting processes: a large-sample study, *Annals of Statistics* **4**, 1100–1120.

[6] Andersen, P.K., Borgan, Ø, Gill, R.D. & Keiding, N. (1993). *Statistical Models Based on Counting Processes*. Springer-Verlag, New York.

[7] Anderson, D.E. & Badzioch, M.D. (1985). Risk of familial breast cancer, *Cancer* **56**, 383–387.

[8] Anderson, S.J., Ahnn, S. & Duff, K. (1992). *NSABP Breast Cancer Prevention Trial Risk Assessment Program, Version 2*, University of Pittsburgh Department of Biostatistics, Pittsburgh.

[9] Baker, L.H. (1982). Breast cancer detection demonstration project: five-year summary report, *CA Cancer Journal for Clinicians* **32**, 194–225.

[10] Benichou, J. (1993). A computer program for estimating individualized probabilities of breast cancer, *Computers and Biomedical Research* **26**, 373–382.

[11] Benichou, J. (1995). A complete analysis of variability of absolute risk from a population-based case–control study on breast cancer, *Biometrical Journal* **37**, 3–24.

[12] Benichou, J. & Gail, M.H. (1989). A delta-method for implicitly defined random variables, *American Statistician* **43**, 41–44.

[13] Benichou, J. & Gail, M.H. (1990). Estimates of absolute cause-specific risk in cohort studies, *Biometrics* **46**, 813–826.

[14] Benichou, J. & Gail, M.H. (1995). Methods of inference for estimates of absolute risk derived from population-based case–control studies, *Biometrics* **51**, 182–194.

[15] Benichou, J. & Wacholder, S. (1994). A comparison of three approaches to estimate exposure-specific incidence rates from population-based case–control data, *Statistics in Medicine* **13**, 651–661.

[16] Benichou, J., Byrne, C. & Gail, M.H. (1997). An approach to estimating exposure-specific rates of breast cancer from a two-stage case–control study within a cohort, *Statistics in Medicine* **16**, 133–151.

[17] Benichou, J., Gail, M.H. & Mulvihill, J.J. (1996). Graphs to estimate an individualized risk of breast cancer, *Journal of Clinical Oncology* **14**, 103–110.

[18] Berkson, J. (1958). Smoking and lung cancer: some observations on two recent reports, *Journal of the American Statistical Association* **53**, 28–38.

[19] Biesecker, B.B., Boehnke, M., Calzone, K., Markel, D.S., Garber, J.E., Collins, F.S. & Weber, B.L. (1993). Genetic counseling for families with inherited susceptibility to breast and ovarian cancer, *Journal of the American Medical Association* **269**, 1970–1974.

[20] Bondy, M.L., Lustbader, E.D., Halabi, S., Ross, E. & Vogel, V.G. (1994). Validation of a breast cancer risk assessment model in women with a positive family history, *Journal of the National Cancer Institute* **86**, 620–625.

[21] Borgan, Ø., Goldstein, L. & Langholz, B. (1995). Methods for the analysis of sampled cohort data in the Cox proportional hazards model, *Annals of Statistics* **23**, 1749–1778.

[22] Breslow, N.E. & Cain, K.C. (1988). Logistic regression for two-stage case–control data, *Biometrika* **75**, 11–20.

[23] Breslow, N.E. & Day, N.E. (1987). *Statistical Methods in Cancer Research*, Vol. II: *The Design and Analysis of Cohort Studies*. IARC Scientific Publications 82, Lyon.

[24] Breslow, N.E., Lubin, J.H., Marek, P. & Langholz, B. (1983). Multiplicative models and cohort analysis, *Journal of the American Statistical Association* **78**, 1–12.

[25] Bruzzi, P., Green, S.B., Byar, D.P., Brinton, L.A. & Schairer, C. (1985). Estimating the population attributable risk for multiple risk factors using case–control data, *American Journal of Epidemiology* **122**, 904–914.

[26] Chang, I., Gelman, R. & Pagano, M. (1982). Corrected group prognostic curves and summary statistics, *Journal of Chronic Diseases* **35**, 669–674.

[27] Chiang, C.L. (1961). A stochastic study of the life table and its applications: III. The follow-up study with the consideration of competing risks, *Biometrics* **17**, 57–58.

[28] Chiang, C.L. (1968). *Introduction to Stochastic Processes in Biostatistics*. Wiley, New York.

[29]   Cornfield, J. (1951). A method for estimating comparative rates from clinical data: applications to cancer of the
lung, breast and cervix, *Journal of the National Cancer
Institute* **11**, 1269–1275.

[30]   Cornfield, J. (1956). A statistical problem arising from
retrospective studies, in *Proceedings of the Third Berkeley Symposium*, Vol. IV, J. Neyman, ed. University of
California Press, Monterey, pp. 133–148.

[31]   Cox, D.R. (1972). Regression models and lifetables
(with discussion), *Journal of the Royal Statistical Society, Series B* **34**, 187–220.

[32]   Cox, D.R. (1975). Partial likelihood, *Biometrika* **62**,
269–276.

[33]   Cutler, S.J. & Ederer, F. (1958). Maximum utilization
of the life table method in analyzing survival, *Journal
of Chronic Diseases* **8**, 699–712.

[34]   Dorey, F.J. & Korn, E.L. (1987). Effective sample sizes
for confidence intervals for survival probabilities, *Statistics in Medicine* **6**, 679–687.

[35]   Dupont, D.W. (1989). Converting relative risks to absolute risks: a graphical approach, *Statistics in Medicine*
8, 641–651.

[36]   Easton, D.F., Peto, J. & Babiker, A.G. (1991). Floating
absolute risk: an alternative to relative risk in survival
and case–control analysis avoiding an arbitrary reference group, *Statistics in Medicine* **10**, 1025–1035.

[37]   Efron, B. (1986). How biased is the apparent error rate
of a prediction rule?, *Journal of the American Statistical
Association* **81**, 461–470.

[38]   Elandt-Johnson, R.C. (1977). Various estimators of conditional probabilities of death in follow-up studies.
Summary of results, *Journal of Chronic Diseases* **30**,
247–256.

[39]   Elveback, L. (1958). Estimation of survivorship in
chronic disease: the "actuarial" method, *Journal of the
American Statistical Association* **53**, 420–440.

[40]   Flanders, W.D. & Greenland, S. (1991). Analytic methods for two-stage case–control studies and other stratified designs, *Statistics in Medicine* **10**, 739–747.

[41]   Fleiss, J.L., Dunner, D.L., Stallone, F. & Fieve, R.R.
(1976). The life table: a method for analyzing longitudinal studies, *Archives of General Psychiatry* **33**,
107–112.

[42]   Gail, M.H. (1975). Measuring the benefit of reduced exposure to environmental carcinogens, *Journal of Chronic Diseases* **28**, 135–147.

[43]   Gail, M.H. (1975). A review and critique of some
models used in competing risk analysis, *Biometrics* **31**,
209–222.

[44]   Gail, M.H. & Benichou, J. (1992). Assessing the risk
of breast cancer in individuals, in *Cancer Prevention*, V.T. De Vita & S.A. Rosenberg, eds. Lippincott,
Philadelphia, pp. 1–15.

[45]   Gail, M.H. & Benichou, J. (1994). Validation studies on
a model for breast cancer risk (editorial), *Journal of the
National Cancer Institute* **86**, 573–575.

[46]   Gail, M.H. & Byar, D.P. (1986). Variance calculations
for direct adjusted survival curves, with applications to

testing for no treatment effect, *Biometrical Journal* **28**,
587–599.

[47]   Gail, M.H., Brinton, L.A., Byar, D.P., Corle, D.K.,
Green, S.B., Schairer, C. & Mulvihill, J.J. (1989).
Projecting individualized probabilities of developing
breast cancer for white females who are being examined
annually, *Journal of the National Cancer Institute* **81**,
1879–1886.

[48]   Gail, M.H., Eagan, R.T., Feld, R., Ginsberg, R., God-
ell, B., Hill, L., Holmes, E.C., Lubeman, J.M., Moun-
tain, C.F., Oldham, R.K., Pearson, F.G., Wright, P.W.,
Lake, W.H., and the Lung Cancer Study Group (1984).
Prognostic factors in patients with resected stage I non-
small-cell lung cancer. A report from the Lung Cancer
Study Group, *Cancer* **54**, 1802–1813.

[49]   Gray, R.J. (1988). A class of *k*-sample tests for comparing the cumulative incidence of a competing risk,
Annals of Statistics **16**, 1141–1151.

[50]   Greenland, S. (1981). Multivariate estimation of
exposure-specific incidence from case–control studies,
Journal of Chronic Diseases **34**, 445–453.

[51]   Hartge, P., Cahill, J.J., West, D., Hauck, M., Austin, D.,
Silverman, D. & Hoover, R. (1985). Design and
methods in a multicenter case–control interview study,
American Journal of Public Health **74**, 52–56.

[52]   Holford, T.R. (1980). The analysis of rates and of
survivorship using log-linear models, *Biometrics* **36**,
299–305.

[53]   Hoskins, K.F., Stopfer, J.E., Calzone, K.A., Meraj-
ver, S.D., Rebbeck, T.R., Garber, J.E. & Weber, B.L.
(1995). Assessment and counseling for women with
a family history of breast cancer: a guide for clinicians, *Journal of the American Medical Association* **273**,
577–585.

[54]   Kalbfleisch, J.D. & Lawless, J.F. (1988). Likelihood
analysis of multi-stage models for disease incidence and
mortality, *Statistics in Medicine* **7**, 149–160.

[55]   Kalbfleisch, J.D. & Prentice, R.L. (1980). *The Statistical Analysis of Failure Time Data*. Wiley, New York.

[56]   Kaplan, E.L. & Meier, P. (1958). Nonparametric estimation from incomplete observations, *Journal of the
American Statistical Association* **53**, 457–481.

[57]   Kay, R. & Schumacher, M. (1983). Unbiased assessment of treatment effects on disease recurrence and
survival in clinical trials, *Statistics in Medicine* **2**,
41–58.

[58]   Keiding, N. & Andersen, P.K. (1989). Nonparametric
estimation of transition intensities and transition probabilities: a case study of a two-state Markov process,
Applied Statistics **38**, 319–329.

[59]   Kleinbaum, D.G., Kupper, L.L. & Morgenstern, H.
(1982). *Epidemiologic Research: Principles and Quantitative Methods*. Lifetime Learning Publications, Belmont.

[60]   Korn, E.L. & Dorey, F.J. (1992). Applications of crude
incidence curves, *Statistics in Medicine* **11**, 813–829.

16 **Absolute Risk**

[61] Laird, N. & Oliver, D. (1981). Covariance analysis of censored survival data using log-linear analysis techniques, *Journal of the American Statistical Association* **76**, 231–240.

[62] Langholz, B. & Borgan, Ø. (1997). Estimation of absolute risk from nested case–control data, *Biometrics* **53**, 767–774.

[63] Levin, M.L. (1953). The occurrence of lung cancer in man, *Acta Unio Internationalis contra Cancrum* **9**, 531–541.

[64] Liang, K.-Y. & Zeger, S.L. (1986). Longitudinal data analysis using generalized linear models, *Biometrika* **73**, 13–22.

[65] Liddell, J.C., McDonald, J.C. & Thomas, D.C. (1977). Methods of cohort analysis: appraisal by application to asbestos mining (with discussion), *Journal of the Royal Statistical Society, Series A* **140**, 469–491.

[66] Littell, A.S. (1952). Estimation of the *t*-year survival rate from follow-up studies over a limited period of time, *Human Biology* **24**, 87–116.

[67] Little, R.J.A. & Rubin, D.B. (1987). *Statistical Analysis with Missing Data.* Wiley, New York.

[68] MacMahon, B. (1962). Prenatal X-ray exposure and childhood cancer, *Journal of the National Cancer Institute* **28**, 1173–1191.

[69] MacMahon, B. & Pugh, T.F. (1970). *Epidemiology: Principles and Methods.* Little, Brown & Company, Boston.

[70] Makuch, R.W. (1982). Adjusted survival curve estimation using covariates, *Journal of Chronic Diseases* **35**, 437–443.

[71] Mantel, N. (1973). Synthetic retrospective studies and related topics, *Biometrics* **29**, 479–486.

[72] Markush, R.E. (1977). Levin's attributable risk statistic for analytic studies and vital statistics, *American Journal of Epidemiology* **105**, 401–406.

[73] Matthews, D.E. (1988). Likelihood-based confidence intervals for functions of many parameters, *Biometrika* **75**, 139–144.

[74] Mausner, J.S. & Bahn, A.K. (1974). *Epidemiology: An Introductory Text.* W.B. Saunders, Philadelphia.

[75] Miettinen, O.S. (1974). Proportion of disease caused or prevented by a given exposure, trait or intervention, *American Journal of Epidemiology* **99**, 325–332.

[76] Miettinen, O.S. (1976). Estimability and estimation in case–referent studies, *American Journal of Epidemiology* **103**, 226–235.

[77] Morgenstern, H., Kleinbaum, D.G. & Kupper, L.L. (1980). Measures of disease incidence used in epidemiologic research, *International Journal of Epidemiology* **9**, 97–104.

[78] Mulvihill, J.J., Safyer, A.W. & Bening, J.K. (1982). Prevention in familial breast cancer: counseling and prophylactic mastectomy, *Preventive Medicine* **11**, 500–511.

[79] Murphy, V.K. & Haywood, L.J. (1981). Survival analysis by sex, age group and hemotype in sickle cell disease, *Journal of Chronic Diseases* **34**, 313–319.

[80] Neutra, R.R. & Drolette, M.E. (1978). Estimating exposure-specific disease rates from case–control studies using Bayes' theorem, *American Journal of Epidemiology* **108**, 214–222.

[81] Oakes, D. (1981). Survival times: aspects of partial likelihood (with discussion), *International Statistical Review* **49**, 235–264.

[82] Ottman, R., King, M.C., Pike, M.C. & Henderson, B.E. (1983). Practical guide for estimating risk for familial breast cancer, *Lancet* **2**, 556–558.

[83] Prentice, R.L. (1986). A case–cohort design for epidemiologic cohort studies and disease prevention trials, *Biometrika* **73**, 1–11.

[84] Prentice, R.L. & Breslow, N.E. (1978). Retrospective studies and failure time models, *Biometrika* **65**, 153–158.

[85] Prentice, R.L. & Pyke, R. (1979). Logistic disease incidence models and case–control studies, *Biometrika* **66**, 403–411.

[86] Prentice, R.L., Kalbfleisch, J.D., Peterson, A.V., Flournoy, N., Farewell, V.T. & Breslow, N.E. (1978). The analysis of failure times in the presence of competing risks, *Biometrics* **34**, 541–554.

[87] Rao, C.R. (1965). *Linear Statistical Inference and Its Application.* Wiley, New York, pp. 319–322.

[88] Reilly, M. & Pepe, M.S. (1995). A mean score method for missing and auxilliary covariate data in regression models, *Biometrika* **82**, 299–314.

[89] Robins, J.M., Rotnitzky, A. & Zhao, L.P. (1994). Estimation of regression coefficients when some regressors are not always observed, *Journal of the American Statistical Association* **89**, 846–866.

[90] Schill, W., Jöckel, K-H., Drescher, K. & Timm, J. (1993). Logistic analysis in case–control studies under validation sampling, *Biometrika* **80**, 339–352.

[91] Schlesselman, J.J. (1982). *Case–Control Studies: Design, Conduct and Analysis.* Oxford University Press, New York.

[92] Schrag, D., Kuntz, K.M., Garber, J.E. & Weeks, J.C. (1997). Decision analysis – effects of prophylactic mastectomy and oophorectomy on life expectancy among women with *BRCA1* or *BRCA2* mutations, *New England Journal of Medicine* **336**, 1465–1471.

[93] Smigel, K. (1992) Breast cancer prevention trial takes off, *Journal of the National Cancer Institute* **84**, 669–670.

[94] Spiegelman, D., Colditz, G.A., Hunter, D. & Hertzmark, E. (1994). Validation of the Gail et al. model for predicting individual breast cancer risk, *Journal of the National Cancer Institute* **86**, 600–607.

[95] Tsiatis, A.A. (1981). A large-sample study of Cox's regression model, *Annals of Statistics* **9**, 93–108.

[96] Walter, S.D. (1976). The estimation and interpretation of attributable risk in health research, *Biometrics* **32**, 829–849.

[97] Walter, S.D. (1980). Prevention for multifactorial diseases, *American Journal of Epidemiology* **112**, 409–416.

[98]   Weinberg, C.R. & Wacholder, S. (1990). The design and analysis of case–control studies with biased sampling, *Biometrics* **46**, 963–975.

[99]   White, J.E. (1982). A two-stage design for the study of the relationship between a rare exposure and a rare disease, *American Journal of Epidemiology* **115**, 119–128.

JACQUES BENICHOU

Additive Model

It is common, though potentially confusing, in discussions of risks and rates to make a distinction between additive and **multiplicative risk models** (e.g. [1, Chapter 4]). Under the additive or **excess risk** (rate) model the risk is described as

$$R = R_0 + E(z), \qquad (1)$$

where R_0 is the background risk and $E(z)$ is an excess risk function associated with "exposure", z. Under the multiplicative or **relative risk model**, "exposure" is assumed to have a multiplicative effect on the rates:

$$R = R_0 \times RR(z), \qquad (2)$$

where $RR(z)$ is the **relative risk** function.

The confusion in referring to (1) and (2) as additive and multiplicative models arises because the functions used to describe the excess risk in (1) or the relative risk in (2) can include both additive and multiplicative components. In particular, the simple **excess relative risk** model $RR(z) = 1 + \beta z$ is often called an additive model. To make a clear distinction between the form of the risk function and the nature of the functions used to model the components of risk, it is best to describe (1) and (2) as excess risk and relative risk models, respectively. If this is done, then the term additive model can be used to refer to excess or relative risk models that involve additive components. With this definition of additive models, excess risk models are intrinsically additive because they always include the sum of background and excess risks, while relative risk models may be either multiplicative, e.g. $RR(z) = \exp(\beta z)$, or additive, e.g. $RR(z) = 1 + \beta z$. Thomas [4] and Breslow & Storer [2] describe general relative risk functions that include both additive and multiplicative models.

Realistic excess risk models often involve sums of multiplicative models for the background and excess risk functions. For example, in a **dose–response** analysis it might be appropriate to allow the excess risk associated with a given dose (d) to depend on sex (s) or time since exposure (t) by considering a multiplicative model for the excess risk of the form

$$E(d, s, t) = \beta_{1s} d \times t^{\theta}.$$

Preston et al. [3] describe a general class of additive models that are useful in working with either excess or relative risks.

The article on **Poisson Regression in Epidemiology** describes some specific additive models and discusses methods for parameter estimation and inference with such models.

References

[1]   Breslow, N.E. & Day, N.E. (1987). *Statistical Methods in Cancer Research*, Vol. II. *The Design and Analysis of Cohort Studies*, IARC Scientific Publication No. 82. Oxford University Press, New York.

[2]   Breslow, N.E. & Storer, B.E. (1985). General relative risk functions for case–control studies, *American Journal of Epidemiology* **122**, 149–162.

[3]   Preston, D.L., Lubin, J., Pierce, D.A. & McConney, M.E. (1993). *Epicure User's Guide*. Hirosoft International Corp., Seattle.

[4]   Thomas, D.C. (1981). General relative risk functions for survival time and matched case–control studies, *Biometrics* **37**, 673–686.

D. PRESTON

Administratively Censored *see* Biased Sampling of Cohorts in Epidemiology

Age–Period–Cohort Analysis

Age–period–cohort analysis refers to a family of statistical techniques for understanding temporal trends of an outcome, such as cancer **incidence**, in terms of three related time variables: the subject's age, the subject's date of birth (**birth cohort**), and calendar period. The fundamental ideas underlying these three perspectives of time have been understood by social scientists and public health researchers for many years. Early applications of these ideas employed innovative graphical presentations of data, but more recently investigators have also employed modeling and more formal hypothesis testing to understand better the separate contributions of each of these factors. Attempts to quantify the contributions of each factor have forced analysts to address the fact that age, period, and cohort are linearly dependent factors whose main effects cannot be uniquely and simultaneously estimated. This phenomenon is referred to as the identifiability *problem*. Available data do, however allow one to estimate the degree of curvature or departure from overall trends.

Suppose that we are interested in whether a **screening** program for breast cancer has had an impact on the **incidence rates** in a defined population. Such a program would identify cases at an earlier stage when the disease can be more effectively treated. However, shortening the time to detection would also be expected to result in a temporary rise in the calendar year (period) effect before returning to the long-term time trend. One approach we might try is to estimate the difference in the period effect before and immediately after the screening program, but we shall see that this is not an estimable quantity when we try to adjust for effects of age and year of birth. However, we can estimate a change in slope immediately before and after the program began, because this depends on curvature, and thus it is estimable. In fact, it may be reasonable to test the hypothesis that the screening program changes the slope by deflecting an ongoing trend.

Temporal Perspectives for Events

To understand the rationale for age–period–cohort analysis, as well as its inherent limitations, we first define the different time perspectives that give rise to the dynamic changes in a population, and then indicate the logical problems that arise when we try to consider all three factors simultaneously.

Definitions of Age, Period, and Cohort

Age refers to time since birth or, more generally, to time since a subject entered a study. *Period*, on the other hand, refers to the calendar date at which the outcome was determined. Finally, *cohort* identifies the calendar time when an individual was born, or entered a study; cohort thus provides an index for generational effects. The purpose of age–period–cohort analyses is to determine the separate contributions of age, period, and cohort to the outcome under consideration.

Vital statistics are often analyzed for age, period, and cohort effects. These data are readily available, and sometimes yield early hints on the etiology of a disease.

Age often influences risk of disease and socioeconomic outcomes. Hence, it would usually be essential to consider this factor in any analysis.

Period effects tend to be factors that impact all individuals under observation on a particular date, regardless of their age. For example, because everyone breathes essentially the same air, if disease incidence is affected by ambient air pollution in all age groups, and if levels of pollutants have changed over time, then we might expect to see period effects for each age group. However, not all period effects need be due to changes in causative agents. Artifacts, such as changes in medical diagnostic practice, or technology can introduce changes in disease incidence that would be manifested in the data as period effects.

Cohort effects can be attributed to factors related to the year of birth. A disease that is associated with poor nutrition in the mother might be expected to have higher incidence in cohorts born during a war or a famine. However, cohort effects may not be limited to events around the time of birth, because the cohort can also be thought of as a generational identifier. For example, cigarette smoking most commonly begins in late teens or early twenties, so that major changes in the marketing of cigarettes would affect primarily the generations who happened to be in the vulnerable age group on the date at which such marketing changes occurred. Hence, we might expect to see an effect due to cohort for diseases that are strongly associated with the smoking of cigarettes in populations that have experienced major shifts in cigarette sales.

Early analyses of period and cohort relied mainly on descriptive plots of the data. More recently, investigators have tried to formalize the study of disease trends by fitting models that include time effects, or by considering nonparametric approaches to the analysis. These attempts have forced a recognition of the inherent limitation in these analyses, namely a nonidentifiability of some model parameters.

Collinearity of Age, Period, and Cohort

Figure 1 gives a **Lexis diagram**, showing the only possible diagonal paths that may be traversed by an individual under study, and it also demonstrates the relationship among the three temporal measures under consideration. The diagonal paths represent individual cohorts, c. If an event occurs to an individual of age a in year p, then a particular cohort $c = p - a$ must be involved. Hence, $a - p + c = 0$, and these time measures are linearly dependent. This dependence leads to aliasing of parameters, i.e. a fundamental inability to identify completely the separate contributions for each of the individual time factors. We usually think of an effect due to a particular factor as the contribution from that factor if other factors are held constant. However, this concept is clearly nonsensical when the factors are functionally related, as they are here.

Interval Divisions

Population-based data are usually tabulated for the calculation of rates, by grouping age and period into

categorical intervals, as seen in Table 1. Five- or 10-year intervals are most commonly used, although for large regions these rates are often reported annually, which implies one-year intervals for period. Because the grouping results in a somewhat crude measure for age and period, there remains some ambiguity when one tries to identify a corresponding cohort. For example, if a death occurred in someone aged 50–54 in 1990–94, then that individual could have been born as early as January 1, 1935, or as late as December 31, 1945, a span of 10 years, which is twice the width of the age and period interval. In addition, the intervals are overlapping, as we can see from the fact that for the next age group, 55–59, an individual could have been born between January 1, 1940, and December 31, 1950. From the Lexis diagram shown in Figure 1 we can see the pattern of age and period intervals traversed by different cohorts. While age and period uniquely define a cohort, we have lost that uniqueness in cohort definition when time has been categorized. Hence, the same cohort may pass through different age groups during a particular period interval. The same problem arises for the third time factor, when any of the other two time factors are categorized. Tarone & Chu [37] have suggested using a finer grid when possible. For example, in their analysis of breast cancer mortality they employ two-year intervals for age and period. Nevertheless, smaller overlaps remain.

If we know the cohort for each individual, then we can obtain nonoverlapping cohort categories, along with the other two time measures, by further grouping the data along the diagonal, as shown in Figure 1 [32]. When the age and period intervals are of equal width, identical width cohort intervals can be selected so that each square is divided into two triangles along the diagonal, thus achieving the same degree of precision as age and period, and avoiding the overlap at the same time.

Graphical Displays of Temporal Trends

Graphical displays offered the first approach for analyzing the effects of age, period, and cohort. One may plot the response surface against two time axes, such as the graph showing lung cancer incidence rates for women in Connecticut plotted on the age × period plane shown in Figure 2. The vertical axis shows the natural logarithm of the rate per 100 000 person-years experience, and we shall use this outcome

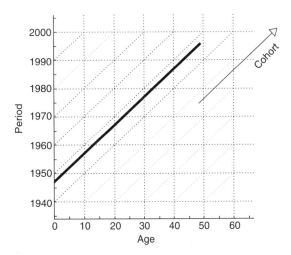

Figure 1 A Lexis diagram showing the relationship between age, period, and cohort

Table 1 Observed number of cases, denominators and rates for lung cancer incidence in Connecticut males, 1935–1984

Age	1935–44	1945–54	1955–64	1965–74	1975–84
Number of cases					
20–29	1	3	4	6	7
30–39	10	20	28	31	40
40–49	70	115	195	289	281
50–59	247	543	885	1 300	1 418
60–69	395	1 057	1 992	2 780	3 769
70–79	209	790	2 001	3 017	4 354
80–89	60	231	673	1 453	2 270
Denominators					
20–29	1 537 781	1 380 360	1 555 934	2 322 128	2 769 374
30–39	1 406 807	1 615 355	1 632 000	1 863 489	2 343 684
40–49	1 258 708	1 493 910	1 800 315	1 727 315	1 800 233
50–59	1 143 763	1 232 189	1 514 848	1 789 483	1 660 060
60–69	770 224	980 496	1 095 932	1 336 181	1 561 113
70–79	437 017	567 892	723 242	756 609	941 025
80–89	145 147	207 148	273 417	345 493	389 562
Rate × 100 000					
20–29	0.07	0.22	0.26	0.26	0.25
30–39	0.71	1.24	1.72	1.66	1.71
40–49	5.56	7.70	10.83	16.73	15.61
50–59	21.60	44.07	58.42	72.65	85.42
60–69	51.28	107.80	181.76	208.06	241.43
70–79	47.82	139.11	276.67	398.75	462.69
80–89	41.34	111.51	246.14	420.56	582.71

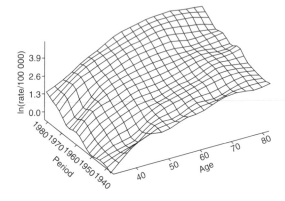

Figure 2 Natural log of the lung cancer incidence rates for Connecticut women plotted against age and period

to demonstrate each graphical method. While such graphs convey a broad picture of relationships, it is harder to extract some essential details. It is not easy, and sometimes impossible, to pick out the magnitude of the incidence in a particular surface plot. Other features are also unclear in two-dimensional representations of a three-dimensional figure, including

whether the rates are changing on one axis, at a fixed value of the other axis. This is especially difficult for the missing time axis, i.e. cohort, in this figure. Obvious alternatives to this particular graph would entail the use of the age × cohort plane or even the period × cohort plane, although the latter is not used when, as usual, there is good reason to believe that age exerts a strong effect on the response.

An alternative display projects this response surface onto the age × response plane, as shown in Figure 3. Such figures were used by Korteweg [23] and others to recognize the effect of birth cohort on disease incidence. In this graph, solid lines connect the age-specific rates for the identical periods, and broken lines for specific cohorts. Note that the age-specific rates decline at older ages for the solid lines corresponding to fixed periods. The constant cohort (broken) lines increase monotonically with age, consistent with a belief that lung cancer risk increases with age. Because it is biologically implausible that rates should decline with age, we are led to reject the age–period model and, instead, to consider age and cohort as explanatory factors for disease

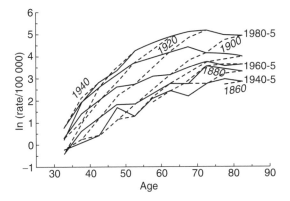

Figure 3 Natural log of the lung cancer incidence rates for Connecticut women by age (solid lines with regular font connect constant periods, broken lines with italic font connect constant cohorts)

trends. Similar reasoning was used by earlier investigators to suggest cohort as an important factor for some diseases. The cohort lines also tend to be more nearly parallel than the period lines, a feature that is especially relevant for the more formal models that can be fitted to these rates, as discussed below.

Projections of the response surface on the two remaining time axes can also be used (Figure 4). Each

line shows either the period or the cohort trend for a particular age group. Because age so dominates these trends, these graphs better highlight some of the more subtle features for period and cohort trends. If these lines are more nearly parallel for either the period or the cohort axes, then that factor offers a more parsimonious description of the age-specific rates. We use the same scale for period and cohort so that the bend in a line will have the same visual impact for either period and cohort. Otherwise, the period axis would be more spread out, thus visually diluting some of the curvatures, as we can see in a period plot of the same data in a typically proportioned graph in Figure 5. By stretching the period axis, curves begin to appear more nearly straight and more nearly parallel. Because there are generally more cohorts than periods, the period trends will tend to look straighter unless we show the axes on the same scale. Hence, to facilitate the comparison of period and cohort effects, it is important to use the same abscissal scale.

Contour plots offer yet another approach for displaying features of the response surface by projecting lines producing the same response onto the age × period plane, as shown in Figure 6. The contours represent lines of constant lung cancer incidence, and

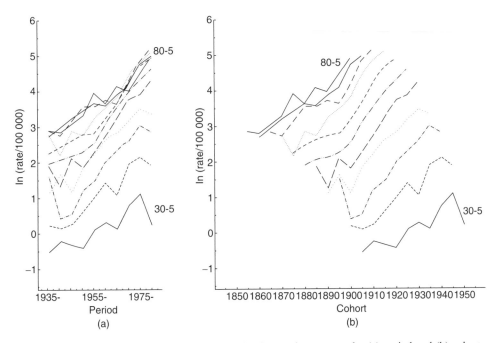

Figure 4 Natural log of the lung cancer incidence rates for Connecticut women by (a) period and (b) cohort

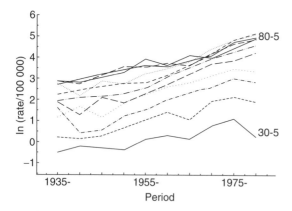

Figure 5 Natural log of the lung cancer incidence rates for Connecticut women by period

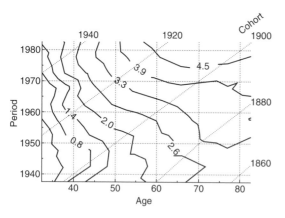

Figure 6 Contour plot for natural log of the lung cancer incidence rates for Connecticut women by age and period (cohorts are shown by the diagonal broken lines)

are labeled according to ln(incidence/100 000). Similar graphs can be produced using the age × cohort or period × cohort planes [22]. Following the lines parallel to the age (period) axis, we can tell the rate at which the surface is increasing by how rapidly we cross the contour lines. Regions where the contours are parallel to the age (period) axis do not exhibit a change in incidence with age (period). Figure 6 also shows the constant cohorts as diagonal dotted lines, and we can make similar interpretations with respect to cohort by observing whether the contours are crossed or are parallel to this axis. These graphs can be especially useful when trying to understand complex patterns, such as the contour graph for Hodgkin's disease shown in Figure 7, in which there is more than one mode.

Another refinement that can assist in the interpretation of trends is to smooth the rates before preparing the contour plot. For example, Cislaghi et al. [7] give contour plots on the age–cohort plane for observed rates, fitted rates using a polynomial regression model, and residuals that show the adequacy of the model over the entire plane. Other variations include the use of models with period effects, or spline functions, in place of polynomials.

The cohort lines shown in Figure 6 have a different scale because they are diagonals on a rectangular age × period grid. Weinkam & Sterling [40] propose the use of a triangular lattice that represents

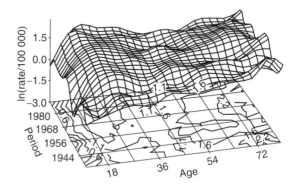

Figure 7 Surface and contour plot for the natural log of Hodgkin's disease incidence rates for Connecticut women by age and period

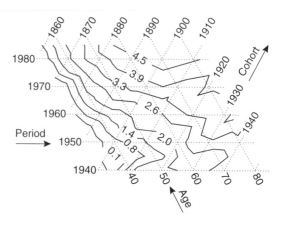

Figure 8 Contour plot for the natural log of the lung cancer incidence rates for Connecticut women on an age–period–cohort triangular lattice

the plane consisting of the locus of possible combinations of age, period, and cohort in three-dimensional age–period–cohort space. In this way they are able to present an identical scale for each time element, while at the same time using a two-dimensional time plane. This approach emphasizes that there are really only two time dimensions that underlie an age–period-cohort analysis. Figure 8 shows the contours for the lung cancer example using this approach. Interpretation of the graph is similar to that of the contour plots discussed earlier.

Modeling Temporal Effects

In this section we consider age–period–cohort analyses that arise from fitting models to data. Because of the identifiability problem that arises from the collinearity among the time factors, it is impossible to determine parameters uniquely in models based on a linear combination of age, period, and cohort factors. We discuss several proposals to overcome this difficulty.

Vital statistics are often presented as **rates**, found by taking the ratio of the number of events divided by the total person-years experience. It is common to assume that the numerator has a Poisson distribution, and that the log rate is a linear function of specified regressor variables. Models of this form belong to the class of generalized linear models, which can be readily fitted using standard statistical software (*see* **Software, Biostatistical**).

Additive Effects

To formulate a linear model for the temporal effects, we first consider the case where data have been tabulated by dividing age and period into categories of equal width. This is the most common situation in practice, and instances where the interval widths are different for age and period actually give rise to still further complications [13, 15]. Let $i(= 1, \ldots, I)$ represent the age groups, $j(= 1, \ldots, J)$ the periods and $k(= 1, \ldots, K = I + J - 1)$ the cohorts. In a typical table, i represents the row index, j the column index, and k the upper-left to lower-right diagonals, beginning with the cell in the lower-left corner of the table. These indices are also linearly dependent, $k = j - i + I$, so the issue of collinearity remains. A typical **additive model** can be given by

$$Y_{ijk} = \phi_0 + \phi_{ai} + \phi_{pj} + \phi_{ck} + \varepsilon_{ijk},$$

where Y_{ijk} represents the response (perhaps the log rate), ϕ_0 is an intercept, other parameters in the model (ϕ_{ai}, ϕ_{pj} and ϕ_{ck}) represent age, period, and cohort effects, and ε_{ijk} is a **random error**. This equation has the same general form as analysis of variance models, and additional constraints must be made. One approach is to set the parameters arbitrarily at one level to zero, $\phi_{a1} = \phi_{p1} = \phi_{c1} = 0$, say. Alternatively, we can adopt the usual constraints, $\sum_i \phi_{ai} = \sum_j \phi_{pj} = \sum_k \phi_{ck} = 0$, which will be used in the remainder of this discussion. Unfortunately, forcing the parameters to satisfy these constraints does not entirely resolve the identifiability problem; a further constraint is necessary if one is to obtain a unique set of parameter estimates. Many regression packages allow for the possibility of a linear dependence among the covariates by employing a generalized inverse when fitting a model, which results in additional arbitrary constraints. The results can differ widely depending on the constraints used in the analytical software, and the order in which the factors are assigned to the model [15].

Linear Dependencies in the Design Matrix. Parameters under the usual constraints can be determined by setting up a dummy variable design matrix. Let the age columns of the design matrix be given by

$$\mathbf{A} = (\mathbf{A}_1 \quad \mathbf{A}_2 \ldots \mathbf{A}_{I-1}),$$

where the ith column is defined as

$$A_i = \begin{cases} 1, & \text{if } i\text{th age group,} \\ -1, & \text{if } I\text{th age group,} \\ 0, & \text{otherwise,} \end{cases}$$

thus yielding the parameters ϕ_{ai}, $i = 1, \ldots, I - 1$, and $\phi_{aI} = -\sum_{i=1}^{I-1} \phi_{ai}$. The period, $\mathbf{P}$, and cohort, $\mathbf{C}$, components of the design matrix are similarly defined. Kupper et al. [24, 25] show that the columns of the overall design matrix formed by concatenating all three components satisfy

$$\sum_{i=1}^{I-1} \left[i - \frac{I+1}{2} \right] \mathbf{A}_i - \sum_{j=1}^{J-1} \left[j - \frac{J+1}{2} \right] \mathbf{P}_j$$

$$+ \sum_{k=1}^{K-1} \left[k - \frac{K+1}{2} \right] \mathbf{C}_k = 0.$$

Thus, these columns are linearly dependent. A condition for the existence of a unique set of parameter estimates in a regression model is that the design matrix be of full column rank. Hence, a model that simultaneously includes age, period, and cohort effects does not yield a unique set of estimates, which is referred to as the identifiability problem.

Partitions into Linear and Curvature Effects.
One convenient way of representing trends for a particular factor is to include the overall trend or slope and the departure from that trend, namely the curvature. This approach represents the age effects obtained under the usual constraints as

$$\phi_{ai} = \left(i - \frac{I+1}{2}\right) \times \beta_a + \gamma_{ai},$$

where β_a is the overall slope, and γ_{ai} is the curvature. Period and cohort parameters can be represented in a similar way. Holford [17] proposed using the usual least squares estimate of the slopes, which can be expressed as a linear contrast among the age parameters $\beta_a = \mathbf{C} \times \phi_a$, where the contrast vector has elements

$$C_i = \left[i - \frac{I+1}{2}\right] \times \frac{12}{I(I-1)(I+1)}$$

for equally spaced intervals. This is the first-order orthogonal polynomial contrast. We call β_a the "least squares linear component". Alternatively, Clayton & Schifflers [8] use the mean of the successive differences to represent the slope, which reduces to $(\phi_{aI} - \phi_{a1})/(I - 1)$, and thus depends only on parameters in the first and last age groups. Both of these approaches for defining slopes can also be modified by restricting the range over which the slope is determined, either by defining the contrast appropriately in the case of using least squares, or by choosing groups other than the first and last when calculating the mean differences, i.e. using $(\phi_{ai} - \phi_{ai'})/(i - i')$.

Curvature terms can be determined by taking the difference between the estimated parameters and the fitted value from a simple linear regression, i.e. the residuals. If the least squares linear component is used, then these residuals are

$$\gamma_{ai} = \phi_{ai} - \left[i - \frac{I+1}{2}\right] \times \beta_a.$$

Identifiability Problem for Parameters.   Because of the collinearity among the three temporal factors, a unique set of parameter estimates cannot be obtained without further constraints. Using different constraints can change not only the magnitude of the parameters, but the direction of trend for each time factor, thus profoundly influencing the conclusions from an analysis. The partitioning of the temporal effects into linear and curvature components provides one useful way of reducing the number of parameters involved in the collinearity, leading to a better understanding of its effect. It has been shown that the curvature parameters, such as γ_{ai}, are invariant, regardless of the parameterization or constraints on linear components [15, 33]. The same is not the case for the slopes (β_a, β_p, and β_c), which can arbitrarily take any value, $\beta. \in (-\infty, \infty)$. While each slope parameter may vary widely, all these parameters can only do so while maintaining a specific relationship among themselves. This constrained relationship suggests the use of estimable functions of the parameters, i.e. functions that do not depend on the constraints adopted to find a particular set of parameter estimates.

For an arbitrary pair of numbers, (r, s), the linear function, $r\beta_a + s\beta_p + (s - r)\beta_c$ is invariant to the particular set of parameters obtained, i.e. it is an estimable function of the slopes [15]. For example, by setting $r = s = 1$, we see that $\beta_a + \beta_p$ is estimable. Likewise, $r = 0$ and $s = 1$ demonstrate that $\beta_p + \beta_c$ is estimable, and in a similar fashion we can find other combinations of the slopes that are not affected by arbitrary constraints applied to obtain a particular set of parameters.

The completely unlimited range of values that can be arbitrarily assigned to an individual slope is certainly a serious drawback of these analyses. But through the use of estimable functions we can see that if any one slope is determined, then the other two are immediately identified as well. With this in mind, any underlying quantity representing the individual slopes can be expressed as

$$\beta_a^* = \beta_a + \nu,$$
$$\beta_p^* = \beta_p - \nu,$$
$$\beta_c^* = \beta_c + \nu,$$

where β_a, β_p, and β_c are the true slopes and ν is an indeterminant parameter. For example, if we are particularly interested in period trends, β_p, then it is disconcerting that the estimated slope might be either increasing or decreasing depending on the unknown v. However, β_a^* also depends on the same indeterminant constant, so that if it is implausible on substantive grounds for rates to decrease with age, then the values for v that make the age slope negative must be implausible for β_p^* and β_c^* as well. If one can somehow show that v lies within a particular range, then there is a corresponding range of values that must hold for the period and cohort effects as well.

We can observe the effect of nonidentifiability of the linear terms by considering a model in which we ignore the curvature components

$$Y = \mu + a \times \beta_a + p \times \beta_p + c \times \beta_c.$$

Because of the linear dependence between the time factors, we can add $0 = v \times (a - p + c)$ to the right-hand side, yielding

$$Y = \mu + a(\beta_a + v) + p(\beta_p - v) + c(\beta_c + v)$$
$$= \mu + a \times \beta_a^* + p \times \beta_p^* + c \times \beta_c^*,$$

which is the model based on parameters obtained using a particular set of constraints.

Example. To illustrate the result from fitting age–period–cohort models, consider the data on lung cancer incidence in Connecticut men shown in Table 1. An analysis of deviance for a loglinear model fitted to these incidence rates is shown in Table 2, suggesting that the model does give a good fit to the data overall, and that each of the time components is statistically significant. The adequacy of the model can be further confirmed by an analysis of the residuals. Notice that the change in the scaled deviance attributable to age has $7 - 2 = 5$ degrees of freedom (df). The additional reduction in degrees of freedom arises because a model that includes period and cohort includes terms that are completely aliased with linear age. Hence, the test for the age effect when period and cohort are included in the model is only a test of age curvature. Likewise, the contribution for each of the factors is one less than the usual degrees of freedom that result from including a categorical factor in a model.

We can observe the alternative sets of parameters from fitting the various models in Table 3. Despite the large discrepancies among these models, they each give identical fitted values. The second column was

Table 2 Summary of analysis of deviance from fitting a loglinear model to the data in Table 1

Source	df	Scaled deviance	P
Goodness of fit	15	15.99	0.3825
Age|period, cohort	5	2907.06	<0.0001
Period|age, cohort	3	118.15	<0.0001
Cohort|age, period	9	464.87	<0.0001

Table 3 Alternative parameter estimates obtained by fitting a loglinear model to the data in Table 1

	Default constraints	Mean change	Least squares
Intercept	−4.8338	−18.7566	−8.7477
$a + p$	–	1.5099	1.5433
$c + p$	–	0.3962	0.3738
Age			
20–29	−8.0544	0.0000	−0.7816
30–39	−6.1367	0.5754	−0.2449
40–49	−4.0035	1.3661	0.5073
50–59	−2.2868	1.7404	0.8429
60–69	−1.0821	1.6027	0.6665
70–79	−0.3444	0.9980	0.0233
80–89	0.0000	0.0000	−1.0134
Period			
35–44	−0.6699	0.0000	−0.1210
45–54	−0.3154	0.1871	0.0713
55–64	−0.1041	0.2309	0.1202
65–74	−0.0322	0.1352	0.0298
75–84	0.0000	0.0000	−0.1003
Cohort			
1855	−2.2875	0.0000	−0.6699
1865	−1.7225	0.3362	−0.3165
1875	−1.0593	0.7707	0.1352
1885	−0.6079	0.9933	0.3751
1895	−0.3056	1.0668	0.4658
1905	−0.2121	0.9316	0.3478
1915	−0.1045	0.8104	0.2439
1925	0.0750	0.7612	0.2118
1935	0.0654	0.5228	−0.0093
1945	0.0000	0.2287	−0.2862
1955	0.0000	0.0000	−0.4977
Scaled deviance (df = 15)	15.99	15.99	15.99

obtained by simply including age, period, and cohort in the regression model. In this instance the program set a parameter to zero when it discovered the first column of the design matrix that identified it as not being of full rank. Hence, the last two cohort effects are zero.

The third column includes linear age and cohort terms (period is not included because of the linear dependence), followed by dummy variables which constrain the first and last curvatures to be zero. The coefficients for the age and period terms correspond to net trends identified by considering the mean of successive differences, and the linear age effect estimates $\beta_a + \beta_p$, and cohort $\beta_c + \beta_p$. By dropping the curvatures we can readily see the source of the degrees of freedom for each effect, because we have applied two constraints on the components not accounted for by linear trend.

The final column shows the results of partitioning the effects into a least squares slope, and the corresponding residuals. These can be determined by: (i) simple linear regression on the parameters where the slope identifies the linear component and the residuals are the curvature; (ii) estimating a contrast using the approach described below; or (iii) forming a design matrix that is orthogonal to the linear component [21].

Approaches to Identifiability

By its very nature there cannot be a solution to the identifiability problem in the usual sense. We have already seen that alternative constraints can yield very different parameter trends, as we see from a graph of the age, period, and cohort effects in Figure 9. Notice that we can rotate the period slope 180° without affecting the fit of the model, but as we rotate period in a clockwise direction, there is a corresponding counterclockwise rotation for age and cohort. Proposals for ways to obtain a particular set of parameter estimates are necessarily arbitrary, and must be subject to critical evaluation when trying to interpret the results from an analysis. A variety of solutions have been proposed, but each has potentially serious limitations. Alternatively, we can limit our summaries to estimable functions of the parameters, thus avoiding the arbitrariness of any particular solution.

Parameter Constraints. A unique set of parameter estimates for a model of time trends is obtained

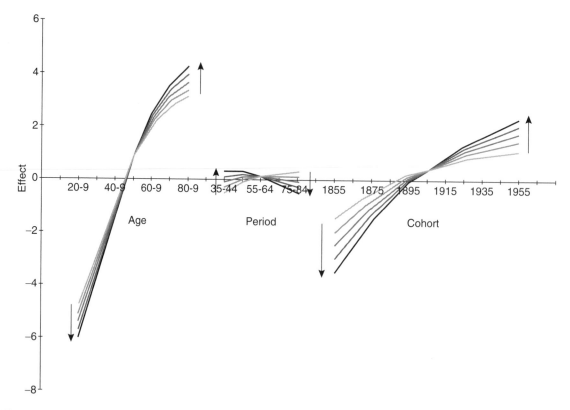

Figure 9   Age, period, and cohort effects in which the period slope takes values $-0.2(0.1)0.2$.

by setting constraints on the parameters. Sometimes these are selected arbitrarily by a regression program that makes use of a particular generalized inverse when finding maximum likelihood estimates. However, it is better for the analyst to specify the constraint and to understand the implications of that constraint.

Drop a Factor. Perhaps the simplest approach to nonidentifiability is the attempt to avoid it by not considering all three factors simultaneously. When fitting such a two-factor model, the interpretation of the results seems quite straightforward, and it may in fact be a very reasonable approach if such a model gives a good fit to the data. However, implicit in any model that drops one of the factors is that it has no effect, i.e. there is neither curvature nor a linear effect due to the factor. As we have already seen, the latter cannot be addressed from the data so that there may still be a lingering source of **bias** in the parameters – the unidentifiable constant ν – which could have influence even if the model shows a good fit to the data.

Equate Two Effects. A second approach to finding a unique set of parameters is to equate just two of the effects for one of the model factors [3, 4, 13], rather than equating all effects for one factor to zero. For instance, two adjacent period effects may be set equal to each other because there is reason to believe that no changes occurred during that epoch, e.g. $\phi_{p1} = \phi_{p2}$. A variation on this approach is an assumption that the mean of the successive differences is zero, which reduces to $\phi_{p1} = \phi_{pJ}$ in the case of period. This is actually the constraint automatically specified by some regression programs for the last factor specified for a model. This constraint is very simple to apply, and it forces the parameters to return to their original level, which can yield parameters that are similar to those obtained by setting the period slope to zero, as discussed below.

The advantage of this approach to the nonidentifiability problem is that it is quite simple to understand and apply. In addition, it does not force equality for all the effects, as is the case when one of the factors is dropped entirely from the model. Unfortunately, there is usually no more solid basis for equating two effects than reasoning such as: "There is no reason to expect a change during these years; therefore, they will be assumed to be equal." It is often true that equality

of the fourth and fifth periods is just as logical as the first and second in a particular situation, and the resulting parameter estimates can vary considerably for these equally plausible assumptions.

Minimize Euclidean Distance to Two-Factor Models. Osmond & Gardner [31] propose an approach that estimates the unidentifiable parameter, ν. Their criterion uses the Euclidean distance between the parameters from the age–period–cohort model, and a corresponding model that drops one of the factors, e.g. $\|\phi(\nu) - \phi_{(c)}\|$ in the case of a model that drops cohort. Because age plays a vital role in most responses, it is not eliminated entirely; but rather the fitted values from an age-only model are introduced as offset terms. The estimation criterion is to minimize

$$g(\nu) = \frac{\|\phi(\nu) - \phi_{(c)}\|}{\rho_c} + \frac{\|\phi(\nu) - \phi_{(p)}\|}{\rho_p}$$
$$+ \frac{\|\phi(\nu) - \phi_{(a)}\|}{\rho_a},$$

where ρ_c, ρ_p, and ρ_a are the residual mean squares from the respective models.

While this approach has the advantage of offering a unique set of model parameters, there is some question about whether the criterion is appropriate in general. At one level it seems sensible to give parameters from two-factor models with poor fit (high residual mean squares) less weight, until we recall that we can only estimate curvature in a three-factor model. A factor with a great deal of curvature will result in a relatively large residual mean square for the reduced model, thus receiving less weight according to the estimation criterion. But it is not clear why the parameter that identifies linear trend should be related to curvature, or indeed to parameters from a two-factor model that may give a poor fit to the data. Alternative underlying models for the overall trends for the time factors can give rise to the same responses, as we have seen, and this approach does not guarantee that we will find the "correct" underlying trend.

Set a Slope to Zero. An alternative to excluding a factor altogether is to assume that its slope is zero. For example, we might specify that there is no period slope, $\beta_p = 0$[15]. This approach is an immediate extension of the deletion method in that both assume that the overall slope for one factor is zero; however, this approach does not also require that all the curvature terms be set to zero. There may still be unidentifiable bias for all three slopes. Another variation on this theme is to fix the slope over a shorter span of time, rather than the entire span. For example, we might assume that there is no trend with period for the years 1940–1969, a span of three 10-year periods.

Roush et al. [34, 35] undertook a systematic study of cancer incidence using data from the Connecticut Tumor Registry. This analysis focused primarily on the curvature effects for each of the time factors, but in the summary graphs a period slope of zero was specified, $\beta_p = 0$. The rationale for this approach was that: (i) there is a strong biologic basis for an age effect on cancer, so that if only one factor is unimportant it is likely to be either period or cohort; (ii) empirical results strongly suggest that cohort has a stronger association with cancer incidence than period; and (iii) the assumption that $\beta_p = 0$ was less restrictive than ignoring the effect of period altogether.

Restrict the Range of the Slopes.   Another way to select constraints on the parameters is to employ theoretical knowledge about the underlying process with respect to one of the time factors. Wickramaratne et al. [41] analyzed the effects of age, period, and cohort on risk of major depression in five US communities. Although a specific assumption about the overall trends with period and cohort was not imposed, it seemed reasonable to assume that there was not a decreasing trend with either period or cohort, i.e. $\beta_p \geq 0$ and $\beta_c \geq 0$. Adding β_c to both sides of the first inequality, and β_p to the second gives $\beta_p + \beta_c \geq \beta_c \geq 0$ and $\beta_p + \beta_c \geq \beta_p \geq 0$. Note that the upper bounds are estimable in each case. Similarly, the age slope must satisfy the inequality $\beta_a + \beta_p \geq \beta_a \geq \beta_a - \beta_c$, which also has estimable upper and lower bounds. Using these bounds, Wickramaratne et al. [41] were able to obtain the qualitative result that there was an increasing trend in the risk of major depression in the cohort born during the years 1935–1944, even though it was not possible to obtain a point estimate for the trend.

Estimable Functions.   To avoid the adoption of arbitrary assumptions, estimable functions of the parameters offer summaries that are identical for any

particular set of model parameters. In this section we discuss several estimable functions that have been found to be useful.

Forecasting Based on Age–Period–Cohort Models. The problem of forecasting trends is one that is difficult because one must necessarily make assumptions regarding trends beyond the range of existing data, which in general cannot be verified. For example, we might assume that the trends of the past will continue into the future, an albeit strong assumption [7, 25] which may well be unwarranted in a particular instance. Nevertheless, it is an assumption that is commonly made in other contexts, and it is one that seems reasonable in the absence of contradictory information. If we make a linear extrapolation for all three time parameters, then the resulting projected rates are identifiable [16, 30]. This property can be demonstrated by using a model that only includes linear terms, remembering that more complicated models that include curvature terms present no new problems, because the curvature parameters are estimable. The resulting model for the ith age, jth period, and kth cohort is

$$Y_{ijk} = \mu + i \times \beta_a + j \times \beta_p + k \times \beta_c.$$

Following the same cohort in time by increasing the age and the period index by one unit, gives

$$Y_{i+1,j+1,k} = \mu + (i+1)\beta_a + (j+1)\beta_p + k \times \beta_c,$$

and the difference between the two rates,

$$Y_{i+1,j+1,k} - Y_{i,j,k} = \beta_a + \beta_p,$$

which is an estimable function of the slopes, as we have already seen.

Drift Based on Mean of Successive Differences.   We have already noted Clayton & Schifflers' [8, 9] suggestion of using the mean of successive differences as an estimate of overall trend for a particular factor. They also proposed the sum of the period and cohort slopes, $\beta_p + \beta_c$, as an indicator of the overall trend for the outcome during the span of time covered by the data, which they call the net drift. This is an estimable function of the model parameters, and hence it is unique. We can estimate the net drift for any set of parameter estimates by taking the contrast

$$\frac{\phi_{pJ} - \phi_{p1}}{J - 1} + \frac{\phi_{cK} - \phi_{c1}}{K - 1}.$$

Alternatively, we can estimate the drift for any range of periods and cohorts by using the contrast

$$\frac{\phi_{pj^*} - \phi_{pj}}{j^* - j} + \frac{\phi_{ck^*} - \phi_{ck}}{k^* - k}.$$

Drift Based on Slopes.   As an alternative to determining drift on the basis of the mean of first differences, we can use the sum of the least squares estimates of the slopes. This can be expressed in terms of a linear contrast among the period and cohort parameters, $\beta_p + \beta_c = (\mathbf{C}'_p | \mathbf{C}'_c) \cdot (\boldsymbol{\phi}'_p | \boldsymbol{\phi}'_c)'$, where the elements of contrast vectors are the first-order orthogonal polynomial contrasts defined previously. We accomplish this by concatenating the slope contrasts for period and cohort. The variance for the contrast can be estimated from $\mathrm{var}(\beta_p + \beta_c) = (\mathbf{C}'_p | \mathbf{C}'_c) \times \mathrm{var}(\boldsymbol{\phi}'_p | \boldsymbol{\phi}'_c)(\mathbf{C}'_p | \mathbf{C}'_c)'$.

Curvature Estimates.   While nonidentifiability of the slope for a time factor implies that we cannot identify the overall trend, there remains useful information in the curvatures or departures from linear trend which are estimable. In fact, any contrast that is orthogonal to the first-order contrast for linear trend is estimable when the equal age and period intervals are used. Hence, we can determine any aspect of the shape of the curves, including information on whether the trends are concave upward or downward.

This approach can also be applied when looking for spikes in the overall trend lines by considering second differences, such as $D_k = \phi_{c,k} - 2\phi_{c,k+1} + \phi_{c,k+2}$ in the case of cohort [8, 36]. Tango & Kurashina [36] studied such effects by comparing mortality from diabetes, ischemic heart disease, liver cirrhosis, and suicide around the Showa Era, 1925–1940. They found that men born in this era had a higher than expected risk compared with the overall trend among men born in surrounding cohorts. This particular cohort experienced nutritional deprivation in adolescence during World War II, and they contributed extensively to the rapid economic expansion during the 1960s which introduced profound changes to Japanese society.

Because of the overlapping of cohort intervals, Tango & Kurashina [36] also suggested estimating the average of second differences, $(D_k + D_{k+1})/2$.

If we think of second differences as comparing slopes between adjacent points, then a natural extension is to consider changes in slopes over longer spans of time [38]. Suppose that we wish to consider slopes for two such cohort epochs, ϕ_{c1} and ϕ_{c2}, respectively. We already know that because of the identifiability problem, we can only estimate slopes that are aliased, $\phi^*_{c1} = \phi_{c1} + \nu$ and $\phi^*_{c2} = \phi_{c2} + \nu$. However, the difference is estimable because the indeterminant constant, ν, is canceled out.

The change in slope can be estimated using a contrast matrix formed by subtracting vectors that give slopes over the corresponding epochs. For example, if $\mathbf{C}_1$ is the cohort contrast for the slope during the first epoch, and $\mathbf{C}_2$ during the second, then the change in slopes is determined by $(\mathbf{C}_1 - \mathbf{C}_2)$. To illustrate this using the 11 cohorts represented in Table 1, suppose we wish to determine whether there is a significant change in cohort trend for men born from the turn of the century until 1925, and men born in the years following 1925. The resulting contrast would be

$$(0 \quad 0 \quad 0 \quad 0 \quad 0 \quad -0.5 \quad 0 \quad 0.5 \quad 0 \quad 0 \quad 0)$$
$$- (0 \quad 0 \quad 0 \quad 0 \quad 0 \quad 0 \quad 0 \quad -0.3 \quad -0.1 \quad 0.1 \quad 0.3)$$
$$= (0 \quad 0 \quad 0 \quad 0 \quad 0 \quad -0.5 \quad 0 \quad 0.8 \quad 0.1 \quad -0.1 \quad -0.3),$$

which yields a Wald statistic of 1.39 on 1 df, and a contrast estimate of 0.172 (se = 0.149).

Autoregressive Models for Time Effects.   We have already noted the identifiability of second differences. Berzuini & Clayton [6] propose an autoregressive model for the time effects in which successive parameters are given by

$$\phi_{c,k} = 2\phi_{c,k-1} - \phi_{c,k-2} + \varepsilon_{ck}$$

in the case of cohort, with similar expressions for age and period. Each term is clearly related to the two previous parameters, along with an added random perturbation, $\varepsilon_{ck} \sim \mathrm{N}(0, \sigma^2_c)$. Berzuini & Clayton describe a Bayesian method for estimating the model parameters that employs a Markov chain Monte Carlo algorithm. One of the interesting extensions that this approach offers is Bayesian forecasting of rates, which is also an estimable function of the model parameters, as noted above. This is in contrast to the use of an autoregressive model for the cohort effect by Lee & Lin [26], who used this model to obtain a unique set of parameter estimates. As always, unique estimates for the nonestimable functions of the parameters depend on strong, unverifiable assumptions.

Design Matrices.   An alternative to the use of contrasts for parameter estimates is to construct a design matrix with linearly independent columns which will yield a set of parameter estimates that are unique. Of course, the usual approach of constructing a design matrix using dummy variables for each level of age, period, and cohort will necessarily contain a linear dependence because of the dependence among the indices noted above.

A partitioned design matrix that will partition the effects into the linear and curvature components described above can be written as

$$\mathbf{X} = [\mathbf{1}|\mathbf{A}_L|\mathbf{A}_C|\mathbf{P}_L|\mathbf{P}_C|\mathbf{C}_L|\mathbf{C}_C],$$

where each row corresponds to the rate in a particular age and period group. The columns represented by $\mathbf{A}_L$ and $\mathbf{A}_C$ are the linear and curvature components for age, and the remaining elements of the design matrix are the corresponding terms for period and cohort. Regression parameters that correspond to the components of this design matrix are given by the vector

$$\boldsymbol{\Theta} = (\phi_0|\beta_a|\gamma_a|\beta_p|\gamma_p|\beta_c|\gamma_c)'.$$

The column vector for the age slope, $\mathbf{A}_L$, may be defined as having the elements $A_{Li} = i - [I + 1]/2$ for the ith age group. For period and cohort, the slope columns, $\mathbf{P}_L$ and $\mathbf{C}_L$, are similarly defined. The linear dependence in this design matrix is readily apparent because $\mathbf{P}_L = \mathbf{A}_L + \mathbf{C}_L$. Thus, a model that includes $\mathbf{A}_L$ and $\mathbf{C}_L$ would have already effectively included $\mathbf{P}_L$. The resulting regression parameter associated with the remaining $\mathbf{A}_L$ will actually estimate the sum of the age and period slopes, $\beta_a + \beta_p$. Likewise, the $\mathbf{C}_L$ parameter would estimate $\beta_c + \beta_p$. These are two of the estimable functions of the slopes noted earlier.

Curvature elements of the design matrix are given by the remaining regressor variables that saturate the effect. If the first and last columns for age in a design matrix containing a 0–1 indicator variable for each category are dropped from the model, then we are effectively constraining $\phi_{a1} = \phi_{aI}$, which ultimately yields slopes that correspond to those obtained by

considering means of successive differences. However, if we choose to represent the curvatures using variables that are orthogonal to the linear term, then we obtain slopes that correspond to the least squares slopes.

Summary of Estimable Effects.   We now summarize the effect of the nonidentifiability problem on our ability to address questions of scientific interest. Without making strong assumptions, we cannot estimate overall changes for age, period, and cohort. This is a severe limitation because some of the most interesting scientific questions relate to whether trends are increasing or decreasing. However, there remain a number of questions that can still be addressed using quantities that are estimable, including:

1.   predicted values;
2.   slope changes or a deflection of an overall trend;
3.   temporary spikes or departures from overall trend; and
4.   net drift or combined period and cohort changes.

Interesting scientific questions can often be framed in terms of quantities that are estimable, although it may require us to conceptualize a problem in a different way. Ultimately, we want to produce valid estimates, and if we wish to do that without making strong assumptions about the model parameters, then we need to limit ourselves to estimable functions.

Nonlinear Effects.   The difficulty caused by the nonidentifiability problem has led some to consider the use of intrinsically nonlinear models. One example is the model used by Moolgavkar et al. [29]:

$$Y_{ijk} = \mu + \phi_{pj} + \phi_{ck} + \phi_{ai} \cdot \delta_j + \varepsilon_{ijk},$$

which was also considered by James & Segal [21]. In this model, ϕ_{pj} and ϕ_{ck} represent the effects due to period and cohort, respectively. The effect of age, ϕ_{ai}, is included along with a multiplicative factor involving period, δ_j, which can modify the effect of age. Even though a unique set of parameters can result from this model, the parameters can be difficult to estimate and they can be inherently unstable. A special case occurs when

$$\delta_j = 1, \quad \text{for all } j,$$

which is identical to the usual model, and in instances where this gives a good fit to data the parameters are likely to be unstable [9, 36].

Another approach that sometimes leads to nonlinear models involves the theoretical introduction of external information for one of the parameters, thus specifying its functional form. For example, Holford et al. [19] discuss the use of various forms of the **multistage carcinogenesis model** described by Armitage & Doll [1] for use in the analysis of lung cancer incidence. In this case the effect of age has the same form as a Weibull hazard

$$A(a) \propto a^\omega,$$

where the parameter ω represents the number of stages minus one. If the response represents the log hazard, then the functional form for the age effect becomes

$$\phi_{ai} = \omega \times \ln(a_i),$$

which is no longer linear in age. This and related nonlinear models for age do yield a unique set of model parameters, thus avoiding the adoption of a constraint. However, the unique set of parameters relies heavily on the success of a particular mathematical model in describing the effect of age. Even so, the parameters can be extremely unstable and difficult to estimate using the usual maximum likelihood approach. In addition, the estimates of overall trend can vary widely depending on the model chosen for the effect of age [27, 28].

Replace Temporal Variables. Underlying most studies of time trends is the idea that the effect of time is related to some factor that will affect the outcome. If this is correct, then a better analysis will include a more direct measure of the factor, rather than using time as a surrogate measure. A problem in using a model that employs information on causative agents is that we must have population data on exposure over time. Lung cancer is one instance where such a study is feasible, because we know that cigarette smoking is by far the leading cause of the disease [12, 39], and exposure information is available. Even so, there are several additional facts that must be kept in mind when developing a model, including: (i) smokers often begin in their late teens or early twenties, a fairly narrow age range, so that a change in cigarette consumption

primarily affects individuals in these age groups; (ii) there can be a long lag (over 20 years) between the time one starts to smoke until cancer is diagnosed; (iii) not everyone has the same exposure, because some consume more cigarettes, and some cigarettes pose a greater risk; (iv) there is a cumulative effect of smoking, so that individuals who consume the same number of cigarettes per day at one point in time would have different cumulative exposures if they began at different times; and (v) individuals who quit smoking have a risk intermediate between current smokers and those who never smoked [11].

The contribution to risk from beginning to smoke is clearly identifiable with birth cohort [see (i) above]. However, the introduction of filters and other manufacturing changes in cigarettes would be associated with a period effect. Other factors could have components that are identified with both cohort and period. For instance, certain generations may be more health conscious and thus able to quit smoking more readily, a cohort effect, but the overall population might also be influenced by a report from the Surgeon General or an antismoking television advertising campaign, a period effect.

Brown & Kessler [5] fitted a model to US lung cancer mortality that used US data on cigarette composition over time, which would be expected to affect primarily the period parameters. The period effect was expressed as a linear function of a measure of tar, so that the log rate became

$$Y_{ijk} = \phi_0 + \phi_{ai} + \beta X_j + \phi_{ck} + \varepsilon_{ijk},$$

where X_j is a measure of the population's tar exposure for the jth period. While estimates of the prevalence of smoking were not included in the model, the pattern in the estimated cohort effects was similar to the temporal pattern of smoking prevalence, estimated from **sample surveys** in men and women. The successful use of information on changes in cigarette composition in this particular instance does not necessarily imply that the approach will be uniformly successful. If there were a strictly linear trend in the mean tar content over time, then the X_j would be linearly dependent on I and k, resulting once again in nonidentifiability. Along similar lines, Holford et al. [20] used population information on the prevalence of smokers, ex-smokers, and mean years smoked to model incidence rates in Connecticut.

Higher-Order Models

Thus far we have only addressed models that include main effects for age, period, and cohort. We now consider work on higher-order models that allow for **interactions**, either with the time factors themselves, or with other groups. The identifiability problem continues to manifest itself in these more complex models; nevertheless, it is possible to address some substantive questions.

Interactions with Temporal Factors.   Each of the models considered above assumes that the effect of a time factor is not modified by the level of the others, i.e. there are no interactions. Part of the problem with considering interactions between these temporal variables arises because in any two-factor model the incorporation of an interaction results in a saturated model. For example, if we only consider age and period the model becomes

$$Y_{ij} = \mu + \phi_{ai} + \phi_{pj} + \phi_{ap,ij} + \varepsilon_{ij},$$

where ϕ_{ai} and ϕ_{pj} are the main effects for age and period, and $\phi_{ap,ij}$ is the interaction. Comparing this model with the age–period–cohort model, we can see that the only difference between the two is that the first model includes a cohort effect, ϕ_{ck}, and the second an age–period interaction, $\phi_{ap,ij}$. Because the interactions saturate the model that only includes main effects due to age and period, we can think of the cohort effect as a particular type of age–period interaction [25]. In a similar way we can describe the period effect as a particular type of age–cohort interaction or the age effect as a particular type of period–cohort interaction, both of which are saturated models. Fienberg & Mason [14] have studied polynomial models for the three time factors, and have indicated which interactions can be identified. The interpretation of interactions in higher-order polynomial models is difficult under the best of circumstances, without complicating things still further with the nonidentifiability problem. Hence, considerable care is needed when introducing interactions into these models.

An alternative to polynomial interactions among temporal factors is simply to split times as, for example, in the comparison of cohort trends in breast cancer among women younger and older than 50 [18]. In one study this division was used because of a suggestion that breast cancer trends may differ between pre- and postmenopausal women [2]. In this instance the model may be written as

$$\log \lambda_{ijk} = \begin{cases} \mu + \phi_{ai} + \phi_{pj} + \phi_{ck} + \phi_{ac,k} + \varepsilon_{ijk}, \\ \quad \text{if } i < i_0, \\ \mu + \phi_{ai} + \phi_{pj} + \phi_{ck} - \phi_{ac,k} + \varepsilon_{ijk}, \\ \quad \text{if } i \geq i_0, \end{cases}$$

where $\phi_{ac,k}$ represents the difference from the mean log rate, and i_0 is the age category where the split is made. This type of interaction would cause no additional difficulties if we were only considering an age–period model, but another complication does arise when cohort is involved. If we follow the cohort diagonals in a typical table of rates, we see that by changing the row or age group at which the interaction occurs, we are at the same time changing the set of cohorts involved in making inferences about the interaction.

Interactions with Nontemporal Factors.   Non-identifiability also affects our ability to compare trends among groups by testing for interactions with the temporal variables. Once again it is convenient to partition the trends into linear and curvature components and, as before, only the linear terms are affected by the identifiability problem. We can express the differences between two groups by

$$(\beta_{a1}^* - \beta_{a2}^*) = (\beta_{a1} - \beta_{a2}) + (v_1 - v_2),$$
$$(\beta_{p1}^* - \beta_{p2}^*) = (\beta_{p1} = \beta_{p2}) - (v_1 - v_2),$$
$$(\beta_{c1}^* - \beta_{c2}^*) = (\beta_{c1} - \beta_{c2}) + (v_1 - v_2),$$

which are clearly aliased. In some circumstances we may be able to assume that the trends for one of the factors are identical for the groups. For example, we may be willing to assume that the age effect reflects an underlying biological process that is the same for all populations, i.e. $\beta_{a1} - \beta_{a2} = 0$. Hence, equating the two age linear trends identifies $v_1 - v_2$, and thus the remaining slope differences.

To illustrate how this result can be used in practice, consider the comparison of lung cancer trends for men and women in Connecticut. We can force the age trends to be equivalent for males and females by fitting a model that includes A, P, C, S, S·P and S·C, where S represents sex and where a dot indicates interaction terms. However, we might question whether it is reasonable to equate the age trends, because there is a variety of biological factors that might result in differences between men and women, including the possible effects of hormonal changes resulting from the menopause. Hence, we may have to settle for comparing the estimable interactions, such as those with curvature trends or drift. Equating age effects may be more reasonable when comparing rates for the same gender among different geographic regions [10]. However, Clayton & Schifflers [9] indicate that there is still the danger of regional differences in age-specific exposure to risk factors which can affect the age parameters.

Polynomials and Splines.   In the analyses above, the time factors are treated as categoric, which allows for complete curvature flexibility for the trends. However, in some instances the variances for the individual responses may be large, such as the case when rates are based on small numbers of cases. In these circumstances it may be desirable to smooth the curvature, either by representing the effects by polynomials or by using spline functions. For age, these can represented by

$$\phi_{ai} = \left(i - \frac{I+1}{2}\right)\beta_a + X_{a2i}\beta_{a2} + \cdots$$
$$+ X_{api} \times \beta_{ap},$$

where X_{api} represents a regressor variable for a pth-order polynomial or a particular term in a spline function. The usual representation of these regressor variables is highly collinear with the first-order linear term, $i - (I+1)/2$. Thus, the identifiability problem can result in parameters that are difficult to interpret, unless an effort is made to identify the separate components of trend using the principles discussed above.

We can partition the effects into least squares linear components and the remaining curvature by defining regressor variables that are orthogonal to the linear components of trend. In the case of polynomials, this can be accomplished by employing orthogonal polynomials, which give rise to underlying slope parameters that can be interpreted in much the same way as in the models described earlier. Likewise, alternative representations of curvature, such as spline functions, can be constructed by defining variables that are orthogonal to the linear term. This can be accomplished for age by using

$$\mathbf{X}_a^* = \mathbf{X}_a - \mathbf{L}_a(\mathbf{L}_a' \times \mathbf{L}_a)^{-1} \times \mathbf{L}_a' \times \mathbf{X}_a,$$

where $\mathbf{L}_a$ is a vector of linear regressors, $\mathbf{X}_a$ is a matrix or regressor variable, and $\mathbf{X}_a^*$ is the matrix or regressor variable that is orthogonal to $\mathbf{L}_a$. A similar method can be applied to the period and cohort effects. An example of this method is shown in an analysis of thyroid cancer incidence in Connecticut [42].

Nonparametric Methods

A nonparametric approach to the analysis of period and cohort trends has been developed by Tarone & Chu [37]. To address the question of a cohort effect, age-specific rates are compared between adjacent cohorts and the total number of decreases is used to construct a permutation test. The null hypothesis is that there is no trend with cohort, and the mean and variance of the number of decreases expected out of n comparisons between successive cohorts in the same age group are $n/2$ and $(n+2)/12$ respectively. In a typical rectangular age–period matrix of rates, not all cohorts are represented by the same number of age groups. For example, in the data shown in Table 1 only one age group can be compared for the 1855 and 1955 cohorts, but four each can be made for the four cohorts from 1885 to 1915. The expected number of decreases is

$$(1 + 2 + 3 + 4 \times 4 + 3 + 2 + 1)/2 = 14,$$

and the sum of the corresponding variances is 4. Only three decreases are observed in the table, yielding the test statistic $z = (3 - 14)/4 = -2.75$, which may be compared with a standard normal deviate. In this case we can conclude that the rates are not constant across the cohorts.

A similar analysis can be conducted across periods, which results in the same observed and expected numbers of decreases; only the total variance has changed. In the example from Table 1, four comparisons are made in each of seven age groups, resulting in a total variance of $7 \times (4 + 2)/12 = 3.5$, instead of 4.

Additional refinements offered by Tarone & Chu [37] include the consideration of blocks of cohorts for analysis to address the possibility that cohort effects may only be important during certain epochs and not others. This raises the issue of multiple comparisons that must be taken into account when trying to interpret the results. They also suggest comparing the results of analyses obtained by forming blocks of cohorts with blocks of periods to determine whether one factor predominates in the overall direction of the trends.

References

[1]   Armitage, P. & Doll, R. (1954). The age distribution of cancer and a multi-stage theory of carcinogenesis, *British Journal of Cancer* **8**, 1–12.

[2]   Avila, M.H. & Walker, A.M. (1987). Age dependence of cohort phenomena in breast cancer mortality in the United States, *American Journal of Epidemiology* **126**, 377–384.

[3]   Barrett, J.C. (1973). Age, time, and cohort factors in mortality from cancer of the cervix, *Journal of Hygiene (Cambridge)* **71**, 253–259.

[4]   Barrett, J.C. (1978). The redundancy factor method and bladder cancer mortality, *Journal of Epidemiology and Community Health* **32**, 314–316.

[5]   Brown, C.C. & Kessler, L.G. (1988). Projections of lung cancer mortality in the United States: 1985–2025, *Journal of the National Cancer Institute* **80**, 43–51.

[6]   Berzuini, C. & Clayton, D. (1994). Bayesian analysis of survival on multiple time scales, *Statistics in Medicine* **13**, 823–838.

[7]   Cislaghi, C., Negri, E., La Vecchia, C. & Levi, F. (1988). The application of trend surface models to the analysis of time factors in Swiss cancer mortality, *Sozial-und Präventivmedizin* **33**, 259–373.

[8]   Clayton, D. & Schifflers, E. (1987). Models for temporal variation in cancer rates. I: age–period and age–cohort models, *Statistics in Medicine* **6**, 449–467.

[9]   Clayton, D. & Schifflers, E. (1987). Models for temporal variation in cancer rates. II: age–period–cohort models, *Statistics in Medicine* **6**, 469–481.

[10] Day, N.E. & Charnay, B. (1982). Time trends, cohort effects, and aging as influence on cancer incidence, in *Trends in Cancer Incidence*, K. Magnus, ed. Hemisphere, Washington, pp. 51–65.

[11] Doll, R. (1971). The age distribution of cancer: implications for models of carcinogenesis, *Journal of the Royal Society, Series A* **134**, 133–166.

[12] Doll, R. & Peto, R. (1981). The causes of cancer, *Journal of the National Cancer Institute* **66**, 1192–1308.

[13] Fienberg, S.E. & Mason, W.M. (1978). Identification and estimation of age–period–cohort models in the analysis of discrete archival data, in *Sociological Methodology 1979*, K.F. Schuessler, ed. Jossey-Bass, San Francisco, pp. 1–67.

[14] Fienberg, S.E. & Mason, W.M. (1985). Specification and implementation of age, period and cohort models, in *Cohort Analysis in Social Research*, W.M. Mason & S.E. Fienberg, eds. Springer-Verlag, New York, pp. 45–88

[15] Holford, T.R. (1983). The estimation of age, period and cohort effects for vital rates, *Biometrics* **39**, 311–324.

[16] Holford, T.R. (1985). An alternative approach to statistical age–period–cohort analysis, *Journal of Clinical Epidemiology* **38**, 831–836.

[17] Holford, T.R. (1991). Understanding the effects of age, period, and cohort on incidence and mortality rates, *Annual Reviews of Public Health* **12**, 425–457.

[18] Holford, T.R., Roush, G.C. & McKay, L.A. (1991). Trends in female breast cancer in Connecticut and the United States, *Journal of Clinical Epidemiology* **44**, 29–39.

[19] Holford, T.R., Zhang, Z. & McKay, L.A. (1994). Estimating age, period and cohort effects using the multistage model for cancer, *Statistics in Medicine* **13**, 23–41.

[20] Holford, T.R., Zhang, Z., Zheng, T. & McKay, L.A. (1996). A model for the effect of cigarette smoking on lung cancer incidence in Connecticut, *Statistics in Medicine* **15**, 565–580.

[21] James, I.R. & Segal, M.R. (1982). On a method of mortality analysis incorporating age-year interaction, with application to prostate cancer mortality, *Biometrics* **38**, 433–443.

[22] Jolley, D. & Giles, G.G. (1992). Visualizing age–period–cohort trend surfaces: a synoptic approach, *International Journal of Epidemiology* **21**, 178–182.

[23] Korteweg, R. (1951). The age curve in lung cancer, *British Journal of Cancer* **5**, 21–27.

[24] Kupper, L.L., Janis, J.M., Karmous, A. & Greenberg, B.G. (1985). Statistical age–period–cohort analysis: a review and critique, *Journal of Chronic Diseases* **38**, 811–830.

[25] Kupper, L.L., Janis, J.M. Salama, I.A. Yoshizawa, C.N. & Greenberg, B.G. (1983). Age–period–cohort analysis: an illustration of the problems in assessing interaction in one observation per cell data, *Communications in Statistics – Theory and Methods* **12**, 2779–2807.

[26] Lee, W.C. & Lin, R.S. (1996). Autoregressive age–period–cohort models, *Statistics in Medicine* **15**, 273–281.

[27] Moolgavkar, S.H. & Venzon, D.J. (1979). A stochastic two-stage model for cancer risk assessment. I. The hazard function and the probability of tumor, *Mathematical Biosciences* **47**, 55–77.

[28] Moolgavkar, S.H. & Knudson, A.G. (1981). Mutation and cancer: a model for human carcinogenesis, *Journal of the National Cancer Institute* **66**, 1037–1052.

[29] Moolgavkar, S.H., Stevens, R.G. and Lee, J.A.H. (1979). Effect of age on incidence of breast cancer in females, *Journal of the National Cancer Institute* **62**, 493–501.

[30] Osmond, C. (1985). Using age, period and cohort models to estimate future mortality rates, *International Journal of Epidemiology* **14**, 124–129.

[31] Osmond, C. & Gardner, M.J. (1982). Age, period and cohort models applied to cancer mortality rates, *Statistics in Medicine* **1**, 245–259.

[32] Robertson, C. & Boyle, P. (1986). Age, period, and cohort models: the use of individual records, *Statistics in Medicine* **5**, 527–538.

[33] Rogers, W.L. (1982). Estimable functions of age, period, and cohort effects, *American Sociology Review* **47**, 774–796.

[34] Roush, G.C., Schymura, M.J., Holford, T.R., White, C. & Flannery, J.T. (1985). Time period compared to birth cohort in Connecticut incidence rates for twenty-five malignant neoplasms, *Journal of the National Cancer Institute* **74**, 779–788.

[35] Roush, G.C., Holford, T.R., Schymura, M.J. & White, C. (1987). *Cancer Risk and Incidence Trends, The Connecticut Perspective*. Hemisphere, New York.

[36] Tango, T. & Kurashina, S. (1987). Age, period and cohort analysis of trends in mortality from major diseases in Japan, 1955 to 1979: peculiarity of the cohort born in the early Showa Era, *Statistics in Medicine* **6**, 709–726.

[37] Tarone, R.E. & Chu, K.C. (1992). Implications of birth cohort patterns in interpreting trends in breast cancer rates, *Journal of the National Cancer Institute* **84**, 1402–1410.

[38] Tarone, R.E. & Chu, K.C. (1996). Evaluation of birth cohort patterns in population disease rates, *American Journal of Epidemiology* **143**, 85–91.

[39] US Public Health Service (1979). *Smoking and Health: A Report of the Surgeon General*. US Department of Health, Education and Welfare, Public Health Service, Washington.

[40] Weinkam, J.J. & Sterling, T.D. (1991). A graphical approach to the interpretation of age-period-cohort data, *Epidemiology* **2**, 133–137.

[41] Wickramaratne, P.J., Weissman, M.M. Leaf, P.J. & Holford, T.R. (1989). Age, period and cohort effects on the risk of major depression: results from five United States communities, *Journal of Clinical Epidemiology* **42**, 333–343.

[42] Zheng, T., Holford, T.R. Chen, Y., Ma, J.Z., Flannery, J., Liu, W., Russi, M. & Boyle, P. (1996). Time trend and age–period–cohort effects on incidence of thyroid cancer in Connecticut, *International Journal of Cancer* **67**, 504–509.

THEODORE R. HOLFORD

Agreement, Measurement of

Reliability of measurements taken by clinicians or diagnostic devices is fundamental to ensure efficient delivery of health care. Consequently, clinicians and health professionals are becoming more aware of the need for evaluating the extent to which measurements are error-free and the degree to which clinical scores might deviate from the truth. Specifically, the recorded ratings or findings made during clinical appraisal need to be consistent, whether recorded by the same clinician on different occasions or by different clinicians within a short period of time. The consistency of the ratings reflect agreement, which is a distinct type of association. A clearly defined measure of agreement describes how consistent one clinician's rating of a patient is with what other clinicians have reported (interclinician reliability), or how consistently a clinician rates a patient over a number of occasions (intraclinician reliability). High agreement is indicative of how reproducible the results might be at different times or at other laboratories [9].

Investigators often have some latitude on the choice of how to measure the characteristics of interest in assessing agreement between raters. One practical aspect of this decision may relate to the implications of measuring the characteristic on a continuous or categorical scale. For categorical measurements, or when the levels of a continuous characteristic are categorized, the **kappa** coefficient and its variants seem to be appropriate tools to measure agreement among raters. The kappa coefficient gives an estimate of the proportion of agreement above chance [12]. For interval or continuous scale measurements, we estimate interclinician reliability with the "intraclass correlation coefficient" (ICC).

In this paper we review some of the well-known indices of agreement, the conceptual and statistical issues related to their estimation, and interpretation for both categorical and interval scale measurements.

Cohen's Kappa and Darroch's Measure of Category Distinguishability

Let n subjects be classified into c nominal scale categories $1, \ldots, c$ by two clinicians using a single rating protocol, and let π_{jk} be the joint probability that the first clinician classifies a subject as j and the second clinician classifies the subject as k. Let $\pi_{j.} = \sum_k \pi_{jk}$, and $\pi_{.k} = \sum_j \pi_{jk}$. There are two questions that need to be addressed; the first is related to the interclinician **bias**, or the difference between two sets of marginal probabilities $\pi_{j.}$ and $\pi_{.j}$, while the second is related to the magnitude of $\sum \pi_{jj}$, or the extent of agreement of the two clinicians about individual subjects or objects.

Cohen [12] proposed that a coefficient of agreement be defined by

$$
\kappa = \frac{\sum_{j=1}^{c}(\pi_{jj} - \pi_{j.}\pi_{.j})}{1 - \sum_{j=1}^{c}\pi_{j.}\pi_{.j}} \tag{1}
$$

as a measure of agreement between two raters or clinicians. Cohen's justification was that the sum of the diagonal probabilities, $\pi_0 = \sum \pi_{jj}$, is the percentage of agreement between the two raters. Since $\pi_e = \sum \pi_{j.}\pi_{.j}$ is the probability of random or chance agreement, it should be subtracted from π_0. The division by $1 - \pi_e$ results in a coefficient whose maximum value is 1, which is attained when $\pi_{jk} = 0$, $j \neq k$. An estimate of κ is obtained by substituting n_{jk}/n for π_{jk}, where n_{jk} is the observed frequency for the j, kth cell.

The definition of κ given in (1) is suitable for $c \times c$ tables with nominal response categories. For ordinal response, Cohen [13] introduced the weighted kappa, κ_w, to allow each cell j, k to be weighted according to the degree of agreement between the jth and kth categories. Assigning weights $0 \leq d_{jk} \leq 1$ to the j, k cell with $d_{jj} = 1$, Cohen's weighted kappa is

$$
\kappa_w = \frac{\sum_{j=1}^{c}\sum_{k=1}^{c}d_{jk}(\pi_{jk} - \pi_{j.}\pi_{.k})}{1 - \sum_{j=1}^{c}\sum_{k=1}^{c}d_{jk}\pi_{j.}\pi_{.k}}. \tag{2}
$$

The large sampling distribution of the estimated κ_w has been investigated by Everitt [24] and Fleiss et al. [35]. The equivalence of κ_w to the ICC was shown by Fleiss & Cicchetti [32], Fleiss & Cohen [33], Krippendorff [46], and Schouten [61, 62].

In many circumstances the categories into which subjects are classified do not have clear objective definitions. As a result, clinicians may interpret the category definitions differently and the categories may not be completely distinguishable from each other, even by the same clinician. Darroch & McCloud [16] defined the degree of distinguishability from the joint classification probabilities for two clinicians. They

derived an average measure of degree of distinguishability, δ, as

$$
\delta = 2\sum_{j<k}\frac{\pi_{jj}\pi_{kk} - \pi_{jk}\pi_{kj}}{\pi_{jj}\pi_{kk}}\Bigg/ c(c-1). \tag{3}
$$

We estimate δ by substituting n_{jk}/n for π_{jk}.

Aickin's Alpha for Nominal Responses

It is evident from the definition of κ that it represents a fraction of subjects not classified in some category by chance; that is, they are classified for reasons other than chance. Aickin [2] attempted to make the notion of "agreement for cause" concrete by introducing another measure of agreement termed "α-measure", later referred to as Aickin's α. He based his argument on the idea that subjects to be classified are drawn from a population which is a mixture of two subpopulations. The first subpopulation consists of subjects which are difficult to classify, so that agreement between the two raters will be by chance alone. The second subpopulation consists of subjects that are easy to classify, so the raters will always agree (agreement for cause). The proposed parameter α is defined as the fraction of the entire population that consists of items that are classified identically for cause rather than by chance.

Interestingly, a case for Aickin's α can be made from reviewing the literature on the reliability of clinical methods. Koran [43] reported a study by Conn et al. [14] on physicians' agreement in diagnosing varices by esophagoscopy. In that study, two "experienced endoscopists" examined 39 male cirrhotic patients for esophageal varices during the same esophagoscopic examination. When the physicians disagreed, the one not reporting varices usually reported prominent mucosal folds, with which varices may be confused. The authors noted that "most diagnostic difficulties occur in the patients in whom esophageal varices are small". Clearly, the more prominent a sign, the easier it should be to recognize. One may argue, then, that in the population of male cirrhotic patients, the fraction with prominent signs is α (those which are easy to classify), while $1 - \alpha$ have less prominent signs and therefore are difficult to diagnose.

According to Aickin's setup, let $\pi_r(j)$ and $\pi_c(j)$, $j = 1, 2, \ldots, c$, be any two probability distributions on the classification categories. The joint distribution π_{jk}, governing the classification of a subject by the first clinician in category j, and the second clinician in category k, is defined by

$$\pi_{jk} = (1 - \alpha)\pi_r(j)\pi_c(k) + \alpha s^{-1}d_{jk}\pi_r(j)\pi_c(k), \tag{4}$$

where $d_{jk} = 1$ if a row classification of j and column classification of k are considered to be in agreement; $d_{jk} = 0$ otherwise, and $s = \sum d_{jk}\pi_r(j)\pi_c(k)$.

This can be seen as a mixture of two discrete distributions. The first occurs with probability $1 - \alpha$, and is a distribution under which the two classifications are independent with marginal probabilities $\pi_r(j)$ and $\pi_c(k)$ for the two raters. The second which occurs with probability α is a distribution under which there can only be perfect agreement. In this manner the parameter α acquires its meaning as the fraction of the population that produces "agreement for cause" between the two clinicians. A consequence of (4) is

$$\alpha = \frac{\sum_{jk} d_{jk}\pi_{jk} - \sum_{jk} d_{jk}\pi_r(j)\pi_c(k)}{1 - \sum_{jk} d_{jk}\pi_r(j)\pi_c(k)}. \tag{5}$$

This shows that the parameter α follows the pattern of kappa-like statistics given in (1). The fundamental difference lies in the fact that $\pi_r(j)$ and $\pi_c(k)$ are not marginal table probabilities, but rather the marginal probabilities of the subpopulation of difficult-to-classify patients.

The above model contains $2(c - 1)$ marginal probabilities and the α parameter (total of $2c - 1$ parameters). Since the saturated model contains $c^2 - 1$ parameters, the number of degrees of freedom are $(c^2 - 1) - (2c - 1) = c(c - 2)$. For model fitting by maximum likelihood with application to cancer registry data (*see* **Disease Registers**), see Aickin [2].

Monotonic Agreement

Other measures of agreement for ordinal data, which do not involve any assumptions concerning the exact size of the interval between pairs of ordinal classes, are Kendall's τ [42] and Goodman and Kruskal's γ [37]. These two statistics measure monotonic agreement. The basic building blocks of most ordinal measures are the concepts of concordant and discordant pairs of observations. For example, select two subjects at random from the $c \times c$ table and let X_l and Y_l represent the lth subject's score by the first and the second rater; X_m and Y_m stand for the corresponding score for the mth subject. A pair is said to be concordant if one of the two subjects is higher (or lower) on both X and Y than the other person. Specifically, if $X_l > X_m$ and $Y_l > Y_m$, or $X_l < X_m$ and $Y_l < Y_m$, then the pair $(X_l, Y_l)(X_m, Y_m)$ is concordant. The simplest way to calculate the total number of concordant pairs, N_C, is to multiply each cell frequency, n_{jk}, by the total number of subjects falling in cells lying to the right and below it and then summing the results. If, on the other hand, $X_l > X_m$ and $Y_l < Y_m$, or $X_l < X_m$ and $Y_l > Y_m$, then the pair is discordant. The total number of discordant pairs in a table, N_D, is obtained by multiplying each cell frequency, n_{jk}, by the total number of subjects in the cells lying to the left and below it, and then summing the results. If there are tied observations, they are given the average of the ranks they would have received if there had been no ties. The formula for τ is

$$\tau = \frac{N_C - N_D}{\left\{\left[\binom{n}{2} - T_1\right]\left[\binom{n}{2} - T_2\right]\right\}^{1/2}}, \tag{6}$$

where $T_1 = \frac{1}{2}\sum_{j=1}^c n_{j\cdot}(n_{j\cdot} - 1)$, $n_{j\cdot}$ being the number of tied observations on the jth group of ties of rater 1, and $T_2 = \frac{1}{2}\sum_{j=1}^c n_{\cdot j}(n_{\cdot j} - 1)$, $n_{\cdot j}$ being the number of tied observations in the jth group of ties of rater 2.

Binary Responses: Agreement in the 2 × 2 Table

One of the most familiar and extensively studied types of cross-classification in medical research is the 2×2 table, as shown in Table 1.

In addition to the simplicity of computing measures of agreement in such tables, many such measures reduce to functions of the cross-product ratio, $\Phi = \pi_{11}\pi_{22}/\pi_{12}\pi_{21}$, which is the most widely known measure of association in epidemiologic studies.

Recall that a crude measure of agreement is $\pi_0 = \pi_{11} + \pi_{22}$, which is estimated by $\hat{\pi}_0 = (n_{11} + n_{22})/n$. This measure is equivalent to Dunn & Everitt's [22] "matching coefficient of numerical

Table 1 Classification probabilities into two categories by two raters

		Clinician 1		
		Disease	No disease	
Clinician 2	Disease	π_{11}	π_{12}	$\pi_{1.}$
	No disease	π_{21}	π_{22}	$\pi_{2.}$
		$\pi_{.1}$	$\pi_{.2}$	

taxonomy". If the clinicians are diagnosing a rare condition, the fact that they agree on the absence of the condition (the frequency, n_{22}) may be considered uninformative. A better measure of agreement in this case is estimated by

$$s = \frac{n_{11}}{n_{11} + n_{12} + n_{21}}. \tag{7}$$

This is the Jaccard coefficient of numerical taxonomy [20, 22]. Before we discuss other indices of agreement for binary data, we show the relationship between association and agreement. Such a relationship is harder to demonstrate when the number of categories is larger than two.

First, the Pearson product moment correlation in a 2×2 table is

$$\rho = \frac{\pi_{11}\pi_{22} - \pi_{12}\pi_{21}}{(\pi_{1.}\pi_{2.}\pi_{.1}\pi_{.2})^{1/2}}, \tag{8}$$

and its sample estimate is

$$\hat{\rho} = \frac{n_{11}n_{22} - n_{12}n_{21}}{(n_{1.}n_{2.}n_{.1}n_{.2})^{1/2}}. \tag{9}$$

The value of ρ varies between -1.0 and 1.0. It equals zero if the two sets of ratings are independent. From Eq. (8), $\rho = 1.0$ if $\pi_{12} = \pi_{21} = 0$, and $\rho = -1.0$ if $\pi_{11} = \pi_{22} = 0$. In this sense, the correlation coefficient gives both the direction and strength of association.

If we standardize the 2×2 table so that both row and column marginal totals are $(1/2, 1/2)$ while the cross-product ratio ϕ remains unchanged, the adjusted cell probabilities are

$$\pi_{11}^* = \pi_{22}^* = \frac{1}{2}\left(\frac{\phi^{1/2}}{\phi^{1/2} + 1}\right)$$

and

$$\pi_{12}^* = \pi_{21}^* = \frac{1}{2}\left(\frac{1}{\phi^{1/2} + 1}\right)$$

[7, p. 379]. It can be shown that

$$\rho = \frac{\phi - 1}{(\phi^{1/2} + 1)^2}.$$

Another well-known measure of association is Yule's Q. It is defined as

$$Q = \frac{\pi_{11}\pi_{22} - \pi_{12}\pi_{21}}{\pi_{11}\pi_{22} + \pi_{12}\pi_{21}} = \frac{\phi - 1}{\phi + 1}. \tag{10}$$

Clearly, the cell probabilities in Table 1 can be reparameterized and rewritten as functions of any of the above measures of association. In terms of ρ we have

$$\pi_{11} = \pi_{1.}\pi_{.1} + \rho\omega,$$

$$\pi_{22} = \pi_{2.}\pi_{.2} + \rho\omega,$$

$$\pi_{12} = \pi_{1.}\pi_{.2} - \rho\omega, \tag{11}$$

and

$$\pi_{21} = \pi_{.1}\pi_{2.} - \rho\omega,$$

where $\omega = (\pi_{1.}\pi_{2.}\pi_{.1}\pi_{.2})^{1/2}$. Shoukri et al. [66] showed that Cohen's kappa can be written as

$$\kappa = \frac{2\rho\omega}{\pi_{1.}\pi_{.2} + \pi_{.1}\pi_{2.}} \tag{12}$$

$$= \frac{2(\pi_{11}\pi_{22} - \pi_{12}\pi_{21})}{\pi_{1.}\pi_{.2} + \pi_{.1}\pi_{2.}}. \tag{13}$$

Note that, when the two raters are unbiased relative to each other, i.e. $\pi_{1.} = \pi_{.1}$, then $\kappa = \rho$. It is also noted that perfect association ($\rho = 1$) does not generally imply perfect agreement (unless $\pi_{1.} = \pi_{.1}$).

Rogot & Goldberg [59] proposed another index of agreement based on the conditional probabilities $\pi_{11}/\pi_{1.}$, $\pi_{11}/\pi_{.1}$, $\pi_{22}/\pi_{2.}$, $\pi_{22}/\pi_{.2}$. Their proposed index is

$$A_1 = \frac{1}{4}\left[\frac{\pi_{11}}{\pi_{1.}} + \frac{\pi_{11}}{\pi_{.1}} + \frac{\pi_{22}}{\pi_{2.}} + \frac{\pi_{22}}{\pi_{.2}}\right]. \tag{14}$$

The chance expected value of A_1 was shown by Fleiss [28] to be $1/2$. Hence, their chance corrected measure is

$$M(A_1) = \frac{A_1 - 1/2}{1 - 1/2} = \frac{2(\pi_{11}\pi_{22} - \pi_{12}\pi_{21})}{\left(\frac{1}{\pi_{1.}\pi_{2.}} + \frac{1}{\pi_{.1}\pi_{.2}}\right)}.$$

Recently, Hirji & Rosove [40] argued that an ideal measure of agreement should have the following characteristics:

1. In the case of perfect agreement, it should yield a standard value, usually 1.
2. In the case of perfect disagreement, it should also yield a standard value, of -1.
3. When the two raters are independent, it should return a value of 0.

They proposed an index of agreement that satisfies the above characteristics. They defined λ_i such that

$$1 + \lambda_i = \frac{\pi_{ii}}{\pi_{i.}} + \frac{\pi_{ii}}{\pi_{.i}}. \quad (15)$$

Clearly, $1 + \lambda_1$ is the sum of the conditional probabilities of agreement given that the first rater classifies a patient as diseased and the conditional probability of agreement given that the second rater classifies the patient as diseased, and λ_2 has a complementary interpretation. Note that $-1 \leq \lambda_i \leq 1$. Hirji & Rosove [40] defined an overall measure of agreement, λ, as

$$\lambda = \frac{\lambda_1 + \lambda_2}{2}$$
$$= 2A_1 - 1. \quad (16)$$

It is easy to see that the chance corrected value of λ is 0, and that it satisfies the above three characteristics. The maximum likelihood estimate of λ is obtained by replacing π_{ii} by n_{ii}/n. Hirji & Rosove [40] extended their index of agreement to the case of multiple categories.

Armitage et al. [3] proposed, as another index of agreement, the standard deviation of the subject's total scores, where a subject scores 2 if both raters judged them positive, 1 if one observer judged a subject positive and the other negative, and 0 if both observers judged a subject negative. Their index of agreement is easily shown to be

$$SD^2 = \pi_{11} + \pi_{22} - (\pi_{11} - \pi_{22})^2. \quad (17)$$

Fleiss [28] noted that the above measure is inadequate since it does not have the range of values required by the traditional index. He suggested rescaling SD^2 to become

$$RSD^2 = \frac{\pi_{11} + \pi_{22} - (\pi_{11} - \pi_{22})^2}{1 - \left(\frac{\pi_{1.} + \pi_{.1}}{2} - \frac{\pi_{2.} + \pi_{.2}}{2}\right)^2}, \quad (18)$$

which will have the desired range of variation. In fact, $RSD^2 = 1$ if $\pi_{12} = \pi_{21} = 0$ and $RSD^2 = 0$ if $\pi_{11} =$

Table 2 2×2 table with marginal homogeneity

		Clinician 1		
		Disease	No disease	
Clinician 2	Disease	π_{11}	π_{12}	π
	No disease	π_{21}	π_{22}	$1 - \pi$
		π	$1 - \pi$	

$\pi_{22} = 0$. As before, a consistent estimator of the rescaled standard deviation (RSD) can be obtained by replacing π_{ij} by n_{ij}/n.

Under marginal homogeneity ($\pi_{1.} = \pi_{.1} = \pi$), or when the raters are deemed unbiased relative to each other (as in test–retest reliability studies), Table 1 can be rewritten as Table 2.

Thus, (11) becomes

$$\pi_{11}(\kappa) = \pi^2 + \kappa\pi(1 - \pi),$$
$$\pi_{22}(\kappa) = (1 - \pi^2) + \kappa\pi(1 - \pi), \quad (19)$$

and

$$\pi_{12}(\kappa) = \pi_{21}(\kappa) = \pi(1 - \pi)(1 - \kappa).$$

The maximum likelihood estimates of π and κ are given, respectively, as

$$\hat{\pi} = \frac{2n_{11} + n_{12} + n_{21}}{n} \quad (20)$$

and

$$\hat{\kappa} = \frac{4(n_{11}n_{22} - n_{12}n_{21}) - (n_{12} - n_{21})^2}{(2n_{11} + n_{12} + n_{21})(2n_{22} + n_{12} + n_{21})}. \quad (21)$$

This estimator of κ is identical to the estimator of an intraclass correlation coefficient for 0–1 data [72, pp. 294–296; 9], and was proposed by Scott [63] as a measure of agreement between two clinicians when their underlying base rates are the same (i.e. marginal homogeneity). Bloch & Kraemer [9] derived a $\sin^{-1}$ transformation to stabilize the variance of $\hat{\kappa}$. Calculations of confidence intervals are eased using such a transformation.

The observed frequencies n_{11}, n_{12}, and n_{22} follow a multinomial distribution conditional on $n = n_{11} + n_{12} + n_{21} + n_{22}$, with estimated probabilities $\hat{\pi}_{11}(\kappa)$, $\hat{\pi}_{12}(\kappa)$, and $\hat{\pi}_{22}(\kappa)$, where we obtain $\hat{\pi}_{ij}(\kappa)$

by replacing π by $\hat{\pi}$ in (20). It follows that

$$
\chi_G^2 = \frac{[n_{11} - n\hat{\pi}_{11}(\kappa)]^2}{n\hat{\pi}_{11}(\kappa)} + \frac{[n_{12} - n\hat{\pi}_{12}(\kappa)]^2}{n\hat{\pi}_{12}(\kappa)}
$$

$$
+ \frac{[n_{22} - n\hat{\pi}_{22}(\kappa)]^2}{n\hat{\pi}_{22}(\kappa)} \tag{22}
$$

has a limiting chi-square distribution with one degree of freedom.

Donner & Eliasziw [19] obtained corresponding two-sided confidence limits on κ by finding the admissible roots $(\hat{\kappa}_L, \hat{\kappa}_U)$ to the equation $\chi_G^2 = \chi_{(1,1-\alpha)}^2$, which is cubic in $\hat{\kappa}$, where $\chi_{(1,1-\alpha)}^2$ is the $100(1-\alpha)$ percentile point of the chi-square distribution with one degree of freedom. They provided explicit expressions for $\hat{\kappa}_L$ and $\hat{\kappa}_U$; this method of estimation was referred to as the goodness-of-fit (GOF) method.

The simulation study conducted by Donner & Eliasziw [18] showed that the coverage levels associated with the GOF procedure are close to nominal over a wide range of parameter values (π, κ) in samples having as few as 25 subjects.

Some Remarks on the Use of Kappa

The purpose of this Section is to bring to the reader's attention some of the conceptual issues that arise when the kappa coefficient is used as an index of quality of measurements for a binary variable. Some of these issues have received attention; we mention, among others, Carey & Gottesman [11], Spitznagel & Helzer [69], Feinstein & Cicchetti [25, 26], and Thompson & Walter [70, 71].

Since the device by which subjects can be correctly classified may not be available, then neither of the two raters is a valid indicator of the true state of the subject to be classified. However, the magnitude of the simple index of chance corrected agreement between the two raters may provide a valid interpretation of the true state of a subject. Thompson & Walter [70] showed that the kappa coefficient depends not only on the **sensitivity** and **specificity** of the two raters, but also on the true **prevalence** of the condition. They showed that, under the assumption that the classification errors are conditionally independent (an assumption that may hold if the two raters have a different biological basis for classifying subjects),

kappa is given by

$$
\text{kappa} = \frac{2\pi(1-\pi)(1-\theta_1-\eta_1)(1-\theta_2-\eta_2)}{p_1(1-p_2)+p_2(1-p_1)}, \tag{23}
$$

where π is the true proportion having the condition, $\theta_i = 1 - \textit{specificity}$ for the ith rater, $\eta_i = 1 - \textit{sensitivity}$ for the ith rater, and $p_i = \pi(1 - \eta_i) + (1 - \pi)\theta_i$ is the proportion classified as having the condition according to the ith rater $(i = 1, 2)$. The strong dependence of kappa on the true prevalence π complicates its interpretation as an index of agreement. Thompson & Walter [70] stated that it is not appropriate to compare two or more kappa values when the true prevalences of the conditions compared may differ. For further discussion on misinterpretation and misuse of kappa, we refer the reader to Bloch & Kraemer [9], Thompson & Walter [71], and Maclure & Willett [52]. Other issues related to modeling of kappa can be found in recent reviews by Kraemer [45] and Agresti [1].

Agreement of Multiple Raters Per Subject

In the previous section we discussed indices of agreement for present/absent characteristics as measured by two raters. Here we discuss the issue of agreement when more than two raters classify groups of subjects for dichotomous data. We distinguish between two situations: (i) when the subjects are evaluated by the same group of clinicians. This situation occurs in practice when a group of clinicians are presented with samples of slides, X-rays, or radiograms, and based on some clearly identified protocol each item is classified as having/not having the characteristic; (ii) when subjects are classified by different (possibly unequal) numbers of raters. For example [34], the subjects may be hospitalized mental patients, the studied condition may be the presence or absence of some psychological disorder, and the raters may be those psychiatry residents, out of a much larger pool, who happen to be on call when a patient is newly admitted. Not only may the particular residents responsible for one patient be different from those responsible for another, but different numbers of residents may provide diagnoses on different patients.

Let Y_{ij} represent the assessment of the ith subject by the jth rater, $(i = 1, \ldots, n; j = 1, \ldots, k)$, with $Y_{ij} = 1$ if the ith subject is judged by the jth rater to have the condition, and 0 otherwise. Let Y_i. represent the total number of raters who judged the ith subject to have the condition, and let $y._j$ represent the total number of subjects the jth rater judges to have the condition. Finally, let $Y_{..}$ represent the total number of subjects for which the condition is judged to be present.

Since the raters differ in their sensitivities and specificities, it may be of interest to test whether these differences are statistically significant. This test is equivalent to testing the equality of the observed marginal probabilities. The appropriate test of marginal homogeneity for binary data is the use of Cochran's Q statistic [27; 20, pp. 141–142].

If we make the a priori assumption of no rater bias, then an estimate of the reliability kappa can be obtained from the analysis of variance (ANOVA) just as if the results were interval scores. From the ANOVA table a variance components estimate of reliability is

$$\hat{\rho}_{1\omega} = \frac{\text{MSBS} - \text{MSE}}{\text{MSBS} + (k-1)\text{MSE}}, \quad (24)$$

where MSBS is the between-subject mean square, MSE is the mean square error, and k is the number of raters. For a reasonably large number of subjects, $\hat{\rho}_{1\omega}$ is approximately equivalent to

$$R_1 = \frac{\text{SSBS} - (\text{SSBR} + \text{SSE})}{\text{SSBS} + \text{SSBR} + \text{SSE}}, \quad (25)$$

where SSBR is the sum of squares due to raters, SSBS is the sum of squares due to subjects, and SSE is the error sum of squares. Fleiss [28] demonstrated that, for $k = 2$, R_1 in (25) is mathematically identical to $\hat{\kappa}$ in (21). Therefore the assumption of marginal homogeneity in the calculation of chance-corrected kappa is equivalent to that of ignoring rater bias using the one-way ANOVA model for derivation of the variance component estimate of the intraclass reliability coefficient. If one were not prepared to assume the lack of rater bias, then the appropriate model would either be a two-way random effects ANOVA, or a two-way mixed model [20, p. 146]. For the random effects model, the appropriate intraclass correlation can be estimated by

$$\hat{\rho}_{2\omega R} = \frac{\hat{\sigma}_g^2}{\hat{\sigma}_g^2 + \hat{\sigma}_c^2 + \hat{\sigma}_e^2}, \quad (26)$$

where

$$\hat{\sigma}_g^2 = \frac{\text{MSBS} - \text{MSE}}{k},$$

$$\hat{\sigma}_c^2 = \frac{\text{MSBR} - \text{MSE}}{n},$$

$$\hat{\sigma}_e^2 = \text{MSE},$$

and MSBR is the "between raters" mean square. $\hat{\sigma}_g^2$, $\hat{\sigma}_c^2$, and $\hat{\sigma}_e^2$, are, respectively, the variance component estimates for subjects, raters, and error. Fleiss [28] demonstrated that (26) is approximately the same as

$$R_2 = \frac{\text{SSBS} - \text{SSE}}{\text{SSBS} + \text{SSE} + 2\text{SSBR}}. \quad (27)$$

For $k = 2$, R_2 is mathematically equivalent to the estimated value of kappa in (13), i.e.

$$R_2 = \hat{\kappa} = \frac{2(n_{11}n_{22} - n_{12}n_{21})}{n_1.n._2 + n._1 n_2.}. \quad (28)$$

In the second situation, when subjects are assigned different numbers of patients, Fleiss & Cuzick [34] extended the definition of the estimate of kappa to

$$\hat{\kappa} = 1 - \frac{1}{n(\bar{k}-1)\hat{\pi}(1-\hat{\pi})} \sum_{i=1}^{n} \frac{R_i(k_i - R_i)}{k_i}, \quad (29)$$

where

$$\bar{k} = \frac{1}{n}\sum_{i=1}^{n} k_i, \quad R_i = \sum_{j=1}^{k_i} y_{ij} \quad \text{and} \quad \hat{\pi} = \frac{1}{n\bar{k}}\sum_{i=1}^{n} R_i.$$

They also showed that $\hat{\kappa}$ is asymptotically (as $n \to \infty$) equivalent to the estimated intraclass coefficient

$$\hat{\kappa} = \frac{\text{MSBS} - \text{MSE}}{\text{MSBS} + (k_0 - 1)\text{MSE}}, \quad (30)$$

where

$$k_0 = \frac{1}{n-1}\left[\sum k_i - \frac{\sum k_i^2}{\sum k_i}\right]$$

(see Fleiss [30]).

Another estimate of the reliability kappa was constructed by Mak [53], and was given as

$$\tilde{\kappa} = 1 - \frac{2}{n(n-1)}$$

$$\times \left[\sum_i \frac{R_i}{k_i}\sum_i \frac{k_i - R_i}{k_i} - \sum \frac{R_i(k_i - R_i)}{k_i^2}\right]. \quad (31)$$

When all the k_i are equal, the estimators $\hat{\kappa}$ of (30) and $\tilde{\kappa}$ are asymptotically equivalent as $n \to \infty$.

Agreement of Multiple Readings with Unanimous and Majority Rules

In this Section we discuss agreement from a different direction. If a single observation per subject does not produce a satisfactory value for kappa, then a sufficient number of repeated observations on each subject may produce a score close to the consensus score. Kraemer [44] has shown that, if there are k independent raters, then the reliability of the proportion of positive ratings is

$$R \simeq \frac{k\hat{\kappa}}{1 + k\hat{\kappa}}, \qquad (32)$$

where $\hat{\kappa}$ is the estimated kappa when each subject is measured once by each rater.

Lachenbruch [47] introduced a sequential strategy for the use of the k tests. The tests are assumed to be given in a fixed order: the second test is applied after the results of the first are known, the third test is applied after the results of the second are known, and so on. We may consider one of two rules for the combination of the individual test results. To declare a subject as positive, the unanimity rule requires that all of the individual tests yield positive results. The majority rule requires that the majority of the individual tests yield positive results (which means an odd number of diagnostic tests being administered).

For example, if we have three diagnostic tests which are given in a fixed order, the unanimity rule implies that the negative individuals give the results $(-)$, $(+-)$, $(++-)$, while the positives are $(+++)$. Assuming, for simplicity, that each of the three tests has the same specificity (SPEC) η and also the same sensitivity (SENS) θ, then the specificity of the unanimous rule is given by

$$\text{SPEC} = 1 - (1 - \eta)^3,$$

and its sensitivity is

$$\text{SENS} = \theta^3.$$

Clearly, SENS $< \theta$, while SPEC $> \eta$.

The above derivations are based on the assumption that θ and η are constant across subjects. Lachenbruch [47] considers cases when this assumption is relaxed.

Note also that the above derivations are dependent on the assumption of independence of the diagnostic tests. Lui [51] assessed the effect of the intraclass correlation ρ under the unanimity rule. When $\rho = 1$, the multiple reading procedure will yield the same sensitivity and specificity as those of a single reading. For small values of ρ, SENS $< \theta$ and SPEC $> \eta$, as stated above.

Interval Scale Agreements

In the first part of this review we were concerned with measures of agreement for categorical responses. Categories may be nominal, ordinal, or the result of categorizing a continuous variable. The advantage of such categorization makes the index of agreement easier to comprehend and interpret; a disadvantage is the dependence of the value of the index of agreement on the number of categories. Hermann & Kliebsch [39] demonstrated that quadratically weighted kappa coefficients tend to increase with the number of categories. Their findings contrast with findings by MacLure & Willett [52] for unweighted kappa coefficients, which decrease with the number of categories.

In the second part of this article, we discuss agreement for inherently continuous measurement, whereby categorization may not be advantageous. For example, if two trained nurses measure the weight of an infant to the nearest milligram, experience shows us that the two measurements will usually not be identical, and that differences of 10–20 g are not uncommon. Differences may, in part, be due to the effect of the rater and in part due to **measurement error**. Dunn [21] reported that it is not uncommon among clinical psychologists, for example, to use linear regression to associate the two sets of measurements, which is not appropriate when the two rating devices commit measurement error. Moreover, product–moment correlation coefficients are measures of association and should not be used as indices of agreement.

In his recent review, Dunn [21] classified reliability studies into two types. The first involves the comparison of two or more raters (or measuring instruments) and the second explicitly examines the sources of variability in measurements. The distinction between the two is not always clear-cut.

The simplest design used to assess the reliability or the agreement between sets of scores is the one-way random effects model. Suppose that we have n

patients and we would like to take several measurements by a single device. How can we assess the consistency of the set of measurements taken from each patient? The one-way model stipulates that

$$Y_{ij} = \mu + s_i + e_{ij}, \qquad (33)$$

where Y_{ij} is the jth measurement taken on the ith subject, μ is the bias, s_i is the subject effect, and e_{ij} is a random measurement error, assumed independent of s_i, where $s_i \sim N(0, \sigma_s^2)$ and $e_{ij} \sim N(0, \sigma_e^2)$.

The reliability estimate of R is defined as

$$R = \frac{\hat{\sigma}_s^2}{\hat{\sigma}_s^2 + \hat{\sigma}_e^2} \qquad (34)$$

(see [23], [54], [31], and [4]). Here, $\hat{\sigma}_s^2$ and $\hat{\sigma}_e^2$ are the estimates of the corresponding variance components and are obtained from the one-way random effects ANOVA. This reliability estimate is the familiar estimate of the ICC (Snedecor & Cochran [68]). It is clear, then, that a precise estimate of R depends on the precision of estimating σ_s^2 and σ_e^2. It is noted by Dunn [21] that R is not a fixed characteristic of a measuring device–it changes with the population of subjects being sampled. This is analogous to the effect of prevalence on the kappa statistic. However, the estimate is useful as an indicator of how a particular device will perform in a particular clinical setting. As can be seen from the definition of the ICC estimate in (34), low ICC occurs when the variation between subjects is low relative to that within subjects. This means that, in a typical reliability study it is desirable to have low differences between readings for a given subject and large differences between subjects. Large between-subject differences usually reflect the condition where the raters are given the chance to test their skills with a full range of a measurement scale. Normal subjects, or subjects with predefined severity, are examples of a narrow range study where raters' reliability is a test only of agreement on the absence of the condition or a subsection of the disease scale, and not a test of the instrument on the full range (see [5]).

Rater Comparison

Two Raters

Bland & Altman [8] described the following clinical experiment. Data on cardiac stroke volume or blood pressure using direct measurement without adverse

effects are difficult to obtain. The true values remain unknown. Instead, indirect methods are used, and a new method has to be evaluated by comparison with an established technique. If the new method agrees sufficiently well with the old, then the old may be replaced. When the two methods are compared, neither provides an unequivocally correct measurement. We need to assess the degree of agreement.

Bland & Altman [8] recommended plotting the difference between the two measurements $(Y_{i1} - Y_{i2})$ against their mean $(Y_{i1} + Y_{i2})/2$. This plot can be useful in detecting systematic bias, outliers, and whether the variance of the measurements is related to the mean.

Alternatively, we can simply plot Y_{i1} against Y_{i2}. We would like to see, within tolerable error, that the measurements fall on a 45° line through the origin. Lin [49] provided several graphs demonstrating how the Pearson correlation coefficient fails to detect any departure from the 45° line. For example, if the measurement taken by rater 2(Y_{i2}) has systematic bias relative to rater 1, i.e. $Y_{i1} = Y_{i2} - c$, where c is a fixed constant, then Pearson's correlation will attain its maximum value of 1 while there is little or no agreement between Y_{i1} and Y_{i2}. The least squares approach may fail to detect departure from the intercept equal to 0 and slope equal to 1 (see [48; 65, p. 37].

Based on a random sample of n subjects, where the ith subject provides the pairs of measurements (Y_{i1}, Y_{i2}) taken by the two raters, Lin [49] constructed a measure of agreement between readings which he called "concordance correlation" (CC). Assuming that $(Y_{i1}, Y_{i2}), i = 1, 2, \ldots, n$, have a bivariate normal distribution with means μ_1, μ_2 and covariance matrix

$$\begin{bmatrix} \sigma_1^2 & \rho\sigma_1\sigma_2 \\ \rho\sigma_1\sigma_2 & \sigma_2^2 \end{bmatrix}, \qquad (35)$$

where ρ is Pearson's correlation, then the concordance correlation is defined as

$$\rho_c = \frac{2\rho\sigma_1\sigma_2}{\sigma_1^2 + \sigma_2^2 + (\mu_1 - \mu_2)^2}. \qquad (36)$$

Let $\beta_1 = \rho\sigma_1/\sigma_2$ and $\beta_0 = \mu_1 - \beta_1\mu_2$. Then,

$$\rho_c = \frac{2\beta_1\sigma_2^2}{(\sigma_1^2 + \sigma_2^2) + [(\beta_0 - 0) + (\beta_1 - 1)\mu_2]^2}, \qquad (37)$$

and thus the sample estimate of ρ_c is

$$\hat{\rho}_c = \frac{2s_{12}}{s_1^2 + s_2^2 + (\bar{y}_1 - \bar{y}_2)^2}. \qquad (38)$$

The concordance correlation has the following properties:

1. $-1 \leq -|\rho| \leq \rho_c \leq |\rho| < 1$
2. $\rho_c = 0$ if and only if $\rho = 0$
3. $\rho_c = \rho$ if and only if $\sigma_1 = \sigma_2, \mu_1 = \mu_2$
4. $\rho_c = \pm 1$ if and only if $\rho = \pm 1, \sigma_1 = \sigma_2, \mu_1 = \mu_2$.

It is also clear from (36) that the magnitude of ρ_c is inversely related to the bias $= |\mu_1 - \mu_2|$.

As an alternative procedure for assessing agreement between the two raters, Bradley & Blackwood [10] suggested regressing $Y_i = (Y_{i1} - Y_{i2})$ on $X_i = (Y_{i1} + Y_{i2})/2$. A simultaneous test of $\mu_1 = \mu_2$ and $\sigma_1^2 = \sigma_2^2$ is conducted using the F statistic,

$$F(2, n-2) = \frac{\sum Y_i^2 - \text{SSReg}}{2\text{MSReg}},$$

where SSReg and MSReg are the residual sum of squares and the mean square with $n - 2$ degrees of freedom, respectively, from the regression of Y on X.

Suppose now, as in Bland & Altman [8], that each of the two raters or methods provides two replicates, as in Table 3.

Let

$$x_{ij} = \mu + s_i + \xi_{ij} \qquad (39)$$

and

$$y_{ij} = \mu + s_i + \eta_{ij}, \quad i = 1, 2, \ldots, n; j = 1, 2. \qquad (40)$$

Table 3 Comparing two raters with two replicates per subject

Rater	Subject			
	1	2	$\ldots$	n
1	x_{11}	x_{21}		x_{n1}
	x_{12}	x_{22}		x_{n2}
2	y_{11}	y_{21}		y_{n1}
	y_{12}	y_{22}		y_{n2}

It is assumed that $s_i \sim N(0, \sigma_s^2), \xi_{ij} \sim N(0, \sigma_\xi^2)$, and $\eta_{ij} \sim N(0, \sigma_\eta^2)$, and that s_i, ξ_{ij}, and η_{ij} are mutually independent. As can be seen, the relative bias between the two raters, μ, is assumed constant. The above equations represent regression models where both variables are measured with error.

Dunn [21] suggested that the analysis starts with estimating the within-subjects mean squares by fitting two separate one-way ANOVAs – one for each rater. The estimated reliabilities are

$$R = \frac{\text{BSMS} - \text{WSMS}}{\text{BSMS} + \text{WSMS}} \qquad (41)$$

(see [31]), where BSMS is the between subjects mean square and WSMS the corresponding within subjects mean square.

Let $x_i^* = (x_{i1} + x_{i2})/2$ and $y_i^* = (y_{i1} + y_{i2})/2$. Grubbs [38] showed that the maximum likelihood estimates of σ_s^2, σ_ξ^2, and σ_η^2 are given, respectively, as $\hat{\sigma}_s^2 = s_{xy}, \hat{\sigma}_\xi^2 = 2(s_{xx} - s_{xy})$, and $\hat{\sigma}_\eta^2 = 2(s_{yy} - s_{xy})$, where $(n-1)s_{ab} = \sum_{i=1}^n (a_i - \bar{a})(b_i - \bar{b})$ and $\bar{a} = 1/n \sum_{i=1}^n a_i$.

The null hypothesis that the two raters are equally precise ($H_0 : \sigma_\xi^2 = \sigma_\eta^2$) can be tested using a result due to Shukla [67], who showed that H_0 is rejected whenever $t_0 = r[(n-2)/(1-r^2)]^{1/2}$ exceeds $|t_{n-2,\alpha/2}|$, where $t_{\alpha/2}$ is the cutoff point in the t-table at $100(1 - \alpha/2)\%$ confidence and $n - 2$ degrees of freedom, and r is Pearson's correlation between u_i and v_i, $u_i = x_i^* + y_i^*$, $v_i = x_i^* - y_i^*$. Approximate $100(1 - \alpha)\%$ confidence limits on the relative precision $q = \sigma_\xi^2/\sigma_\eta^2$ are

$$q_U = \frac{b + \sqrt{c}}{a - \sqrt{c}}, \qquad q_L = \frac{b - \sqrt{c}}{a + \sqrt{c}},$$

with $a = \hat{\sigma}_\eta^2/2$, $b = \hat{\sigma}_\xi^2/2$, and $c = [t_{\alpha/2}^2 (s_{ss}s_{yy} - s_{xy}^2)]/(n-2)$.

Regression models with errors in variables, or structural equations to assess reliability of two raters, have received considerable attention from many researchers. For example, we refer the reader to Kelly [41], Linnett [50], Nix & Dunston [56], and the earlier work of Deming [17].

Example

Table 4 provides measurements derived from an experiment in microbiology. The primary aim was

Table 4 Logarithm of the number of colonies of *E. coli* 157:H7 in samples taken from 12 beef carcasses

Test (subsample)		1	2	3	4	5	6	7	8	9	10	11	12
Standard	1	2.356	2.149	2.452	2.255	2.694	2.43	2.322	2.322	2.491	2.322	2.322	2.491
	2	2.384	2.263	2.417	2.299	2.684	2.44	2.491	2.041	2.322	2.322	2.491	2.785
New test	1	2.283	2.061	2.322	2.162	2.068	2.322	2.491	2.041	2.322	2.491	2.041	2.785
	2	2.265	1.987	2.316	2.127	2.111	2.28	2.491	2.041	2.041	2.71	2.322	2.322

to determine the number of colonies of the *E. coli* 0157:H7 pathogen in contaminated fecal samples collected from 12 beef carcasses. For a given faecal sample, the number of colonies was determined by a new test (Petrifilm HEC) and by a "standard test" in two subsamples; results are recorded as the logarithm of the number of colonies (Table 4). The first two rows correspond to the repeated determinations based on the use of the standard test, and the second two rows correspond to the repeated determinations of the new test. (These data were kindly provided by Dr Christine Power from the Ontario Veterinary College, Guelph, Ontario.)

We begin the analysis by first investigating the repeatability of each of the two tests separately. Following the recommendations of Bland & Altman [8], we plotted the difference between the two against their sum (Figure 1).

Dunn [21] pointed out that the graph can be extremely useful in (i) allowing us to detect systematic bias and (ii) looking for outliers. The regression of the difference on the sum shows that observation #5 has a large standardized residual. We subsequently produced a one-way ANOVA to obtain estimates of the corresponding test–retest reliabilities using the

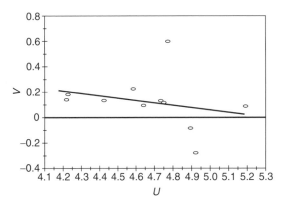

Figure 1 Plot of the difference, *V*, vs. the sum, *U*, with regression line imposed

Table 5 ANOVA of the logarithm of the number of colonies for the standard test and the new test

(a) Standard test (intraclass correlation = 0.61)

Source of variation	Sum of squares	df	Mean square
Cow	0.500	11	0.045
Residual	0.134	12	0.011
Total	0.634	23	

(b) New test (intraclass correlation = 0.62)

Source of variation	Sum of squares	df	Mean square
Cow	0.837	11	0.076
Residual	0.215	12	0.018
Total	1.052	23	

intraclass correlation (41). The results are given in Table 5.

As can be seen, the two tests have equivalent test–retest reliability estimates. The models (39) and (40) assume that the relative biases of the two estimates are constant. This allows us to estimate the error variances using the Grubbs [38] method. If X represents the mean of the standard test log counts, and Y the mean of the new test log counts, then $\hat{\sigma}_s^2 = 0.010$, $\hat{\sigma}_{\xi}^2 = 0.026$, and $\hat{\sigma}_{\eta}^2 = 0.057$. It appears that the standard test is almost twice as precise as the new test.

We now proceed to test the significance of the difference $(\sigma_{\xi}^2 - \sigma_{\eta}^2)$. Using the results of Shukla [67], we have $s_{xx} = 0.023$, $s_{yy} = 0.038$, and $s_{xy} = 0.010$. The Pearson correlation between $U = X + Y$ and $V = X - Y$ is $r = -0.27$ and $t_0 = -0.87$. We are unable to detect a significant difference between σ_{ξ}^2 and σ_{η}^2. This may be because the sample size was insufficient.

Multiple Raters

The simplest reliability study involves having each member of a sample of *n* subjects rated once by each member of a sample of k raters. Raters might be considered as fixed, or as a random sample drawn from a potentially larger population of raters. If raters are assumed fixed, the estimate of reliability can be obtained from the two-way mixed effects ANOVA model,

$$Y_{ij} = \mu + s_i + r_j + e_{ij}, \qquad (42)$$

where Y_{ij} is the score of the jth rater on the ith patient, μ is the bias, $s_i \sim N(0, \sigma_s^2)$, $e_{ij} \sim N(0, \sigma_e^2)$, and the $r_i, \ldots, r_k$ are the raters effects such that $\sum r_j = 0$. Both s_i and e_{ij} are independent. From Fleiss [31], the appropriate reliability estimate is

$$R_f = \frac{n(\text{BSMS} - \text{WSMS})}{\begin{aligned}&n(\text{BSMS}) + (k-1)\text{BRMS}\\&+(k-1)(n-1)\text{WSMS}\end{aligned}}. \qquad (43)$$

The components of (43) are as defined in (41), with BRMS as the between-raters mean square. If raters are assumed random, then the added assumptions that $r_j \sim N(0, \sigma_r^2)$ and that r_j, s_i, and e_{ij} are mutually independent give an estimate of reliability identical to $\hat{\rho}_{2\omega R}$ in (26); simplified, this becomes

$$R_r = \frac{n(\text{BSMS} - \text{WSMS})}{n(\text{BSMS}) + k(\text{BRMS}) + (nk - n - k)\text{WSMS}}. \qquad (44)$$

Remarks

It is evident that estimation of indices of agreement for interval scale measurements is tied to estimation of variance components. The total variance is decomposed into subjects effect, raters effect (if raters are considered random), and the error component. The traditional ANOVA, either one-way or two-way, is used when the data are balanced and/or complete (no missing data). For unbalanced data, one may use the maximum likelihood (ML) and restricted maximum likelihood (REML) [57, 64]. The advantage of ML or REML methods is that we obtain estimates of the standard errors of the estimates. Depending on the nature of the study, more complex designs other than the ANOVA may be used. Bassin et al. [6] used crossover designs for method comparisons. Other designs such as balanced incomplete block designs [27, 29] and hierarchical designs [36] can be used for nested reliability studies.

Table 6 Summary of basic formulas

Parameter	Interpretation
Eq. (1)	Cohen's kappa – nominal-scale measure of agreement between two raters
Eq. (2)	Cohen's weighted kappa – used as an ordinal scale measure of agreement between two raters
Eq. (3)	Darroch & McCloud measure of category distinguishability
Eq. (14)	Rogot & Goldberg index of agreement
Eq. (18)	Armitage et al. index of disagreement
Eq. (24)	Intraclass kappa – obtained from the one-way random effects model under the assumption of no interrater bias
Eq. (26)	Reliability kappa – obtained from the two-way random effects model accounting for rater's effect
Eq. (36)	Concordance correlation – measures the departure from the 45° line

We emphasize that there is no single procedure which can be used to assess raters' reliability agreement. Bartko [5] pointed out that procedures for exploring agreement should be based upon the nature of the study and the purposes of various agreement measures. Table 6 summarizes the basic formulas mentioned in this article.

Computer Programs

Cyr & Francis [15] provided a menu-driven PASCAL program to compute Cohen's kappa and weighted kappa using the two types of weights, d_{jk}.

$$\text{(i) } d_{jk} = 1 - \frac{(j-k)^2}{(c-1)^2}, \quad \text{(ii) } d_{jk} = 1 - \frac{|j-k|}{c-1},$$

and other user-defined weights.

The SAS software (*see* **Software, Biostatistical**) [60] has a number of procedures referred to as "PROC" statements. PROC FREQ provides estimates of a variety of measures of association in $c \times c$ contingency tables, including an unweighted estimate of kappa. As an illustration, using Dunn's [20, p. 24] data, PROC FREQ in SAS provides the following estimates of kappa: unweighted Cohen's kappa ($= 0.21$) and weighted kappa ($= 0.58$), using the weights as described in (ii) above. Alternately, Cyr & Francis's, [15] program which uses the quadratic weights in (i), gives 0.80 as an estimate of weighted kappa. For multiple raters and the 0–1 category, estimates of kappa, in (24), (26), and (30), are obtainable using PROC ANOVA or PROC GLM in SAS. The SAS procedures provide the appropriate sum of squares and the corresponding mean squares to calculate reliability kappa estimates. It is also possible to use StatXact [55] to calculate Cohen's kappa or a weighted kappa statistic.

Estimates of variance components from the balanced one-way random effects, two-way random effects, and mixed effects models can be obtained using either PROC ANOVA with the RANDOM statement or PROC VARCOMP in SAS. For more complex designs with multiple levels of nesting and crossing, PROC MIXED in SAS may be used to estimate the components of variance. For unbalanced data or when some data points are missing, Robinson's [58] REML program can be used to obtain estimates of variance components and hence the intraclass correlations. With little programming experience in SAS, PROC UNIVARIATE, PROC CORR, and PROC REG are quite easy to implement and may be used to calculate the concordance correlation and Bradley & Blackwood [10] statistics.

References

[1] Agresti, A. (1992). Modelling patterns of agreement and disagreement, *Statistical Methods in Medical Research* **1**, 201–218.

[2] Aickin, M. (1990). Maximum likelihood estimation of agreement in the constant predictive probability model and its relation to Cohen's kappa, *Biometrics* **46**, 293–302.

[3] Armitage, P., Blendis, L.M. & Smyllie, H.C. (1966). The measurement of observer disagreement in the recording of signs, *Journal of the Royal Statistical Society, Series A* **129**, 98–109.

[4] Bartko, J.J. (1966). The intraclass correlation coefficient as a measure of reliability, *Psychological Reports* **19**, 3–11.

[5] Bartko, J.J. (1994). General Methodology II–Measures of agreement: a single procedure, *Statistics in Medicine* **13**, 737–745.

[6] Bassin, L., Borghi, C., Costa, F.V., Strocchi, E., Mussi, A., & Ambrossioni, E. (1985). Comparison of three devices for measuring blood pressure, *Statistics in Medicine* **4**, 361–368.

[7] Bishop, Y.M.M., Feinberg, S.E. & Holland, P.W. (1975). *Discrete Multivariate Analysis: Theory and Practice*. MIT Press, Cambridge, Mass.

[8] Bland, M. & Altman, D.G. (1986). Statistical methods for assessing agreement between two methods of clinical measurement, *Lancet* **1**, 307–310.

[9] Bloch, D.A. & Kraemer, H. (1989). 2X2 kappa coefficient: measure of agreement or association, *Biometrics* **45**, 269–287.

[10] Bradley, E.L. & Blackwood, L.G. (1989). Comparing paired data: a simultaneous test of means and variances, *American Statistician* **43**, 234–235.

[11] Carey, G. & Gottesman, H. (1978). Reliability and validity in binary ratings: areas of common understanding in diagnosis and symptom ratings, *Archives of General Psychiatry* **35**, 1454–1459.

[12] Cohen, J. (1960). A coefficient of agreement for nominal scales, *Educational and Psychological Measurements* **20**, 37–46.

[13] Cohen, J. (1968). Weighted kappa: nominal scale agreement with provisions for scaled disagreement or partial credit, *Psychological Bulletin* **70**, 213–220.

[14] Conn, H.O., Smith, H.W. & Brodoff, M. (1965). Observer variation in the endoscopic diagnosis of esophageal varices: a prospective investigation of the diagnostic validity of esophagoscopy, *New England Journal of Medicine* **272**, 830–834.

[15] Cyr, L. & Francis, K. (1992). Measures of clinical agreement for nominal and categorical data: the kappa coefficient, *Comparative Biological Medicine* **22**, 239–246.

[16] Darroch, J.N. & McCloud, P. (1986). Category distinguishability and observer agreement, *Australian Journal of Statistics* **28**, 371–388.

[17] Deming, W.E. (1943). *Statistical Adjustment of Data*. Wiley, New York.

[18] Donner, A. & Eliasziw, M. (1987). Sample size requirements for reliability studies, *Statistics in Medicine* **6**, 441–448.

[19] Donner, A. & Eliasziw, M. (1992). A goodness of fit approach to inference procedures for the kappa statistics: confidence interval construction, significance testing and sample size estimation, *Statistics in Medicine* **11**, 1511–1519.

[20] Dunn, G. (1989). *Design and Analysis of Reliability Studies: The Statistical Evaluation of Measurement Errors*. Oxford University Press, New York.

[21] Dunn, G. (1992). Design and analysis of reliability studies, *Statistical Methods in Medical Research* **1**, 123–157.

[22] Dunn, G. & Everitt, B.S. (1982). *An Introduction to Mathematical Taxonomy*. Cambridge University Press, Cambridge.

[23] Ebel, R. (1951). Estimation of the reliability of ratings, *Psychometrika* **16**, 407–423.

[24] Everitt, B.S. (1968). Moments of the statistics kappa and weighted kappa, *British Journal of Mathematical and Statistical Psychology* **21**, 97–103.

[25] Feinstein, A.R. & Cicchetti, D.V. (1990). High agreement but low kappa: I. The problems of two paradoxes, *Journal of Clinical Epidemiology* **43**, 543–549.

[26] Feinstein, A.R. & Cicchetti, D.V. (1990). High agreement but low kappa: II. Resolving the paradoxes, *Journal of Clinical Epidemiology* **43**, 551–558.

[27] Fleiss, J.L. (1965). Estimating the accuracy of dichotomous judgements, *Psychometrika* **30**, 469–479.

[28] Fleiss, J.L. (1975). Measuring agreement between two judges on the presence or absence of a trait, *Biometrics* **31**, 651–659.

[29] Fleiss, J.L. (1981). Balanced incomplete blocks designs for interrater reliability studies, *Applied Psychological Measurements* **5**, 105–112.

[30] Fleiss, J.L. (1981). *Statistical Methods for Rates and Proportions*, 2nd Ed. Wiley, New York.

[31] Fleiss, J.L. (1986). *The Design and Analysis of Clinical Experiments*. Wiley, New York.

[32] Fleiss, J.L. & Cicchetti, D.V. (1978). Inference about weighted kappa in the non-null case, *Applied Psychological Measurements* **2**, 113–117.

[33] Fleiss, J.L. & Cohen, J. (1973). The equivalence of weighted kappa and intraclass correlation coefficient as measures of reliability, *Educational and Psychological Measurements* **33**, 613–619.

[34] Fleiss, J.L. & Cuzick, J. (1979). The reliability of dichotomous judgement: unequal number of judges per subject, *Applied Psychological Measurement* **3**, 537–542.

[35] Fleiss, J.L., Cohen, J. & Everitt, B.S. (1969). Large sample standard errors of kappa and weighted kappa, *Psychological Bulletin* **72**, 323–327.

[36] Goldsmith, C.H. & Gaylor, D.W. (1970). Three stage nested designs for estimating variance components, *Technometrics* **12**, 487–498.

[37] Goodman, L.A. & Kruskal, W.H. (1954). Measures of association for cross classifications, *Journal of the American Statistical Association* **49**, 732–764.

[38] Grubbs, F.E. (1948). On estimating precision of measuring instruments and product variability, *Journal of the American Statistical Association* **43**, 243–264.

[39] Hermann, B. & Kliebsch, U. (1996). Dependence of weighted kappa coefficient on the number of categories, *Epidemiology* **7**, 199–202.

[40] Hirji, K. & Rosove, M. (1990). A note on interrater agreement, *Statistics in Medicine* **9**, 835–839.

[41] Kelly, G.E. (1985). Use of the structural equations model in assessing the reliability of a new measurement technique, *Applied Statistics* **34**, 258–263.

[42] Kendall, M.G. (1938). A new measure of rank correlation, *Biometrika* **30**, 81.

[43] Koran, L.M. (1975). The reliability of clinical methods, data and judgement, *New England Journal of Medicine* **293**, 642–646, 695–701.

[44] Kraemer, H.C. (1979). Ramification of a population model for κ as a coefficient of reliability, *Psychometrika* **44**, 461–472.

[45] Kraemer, H.C. (1992). Measurement of reliability for categorical data in medical research, *Statistical Methods in Medical Research* **1**, 183–199.

[46] Krippendorf, K. (1970). Bivariate agreement coefficients for reliability of data, in *Sociological Methodology*, F. Borgatta & G.W. Bohrnstedt, eds. Jossey-Bass, San Francisco, pp. 139–150.

[47] Lachenbruch, P.A. (1988). Multiple reading procedures: the performance of diagnostic tests, *Statistics in Medicine* **7**, 549–557.

[48] Leugrans, S. (1980). Evaluating laboratory measurement techniques, in *Biostatistics Case-Book*, R. Miller, B. Efron, B. Brown & L. Moses, eds. Wiley, New York, pp. 190–219.

[49] Lin, L.I. (1989). A concordance correlation coefficient to evaluate reproducibility, *Biometrics* **45**, 255–268.

[50] Linnet, K. (1990). Estimation of the linear relationship between the measurements of two methods with proportional errors, *Statistics in Medicine* **9**, 1463–1473.

[51] Lui, K.J. (1992). A note on the effect of the intraclass correlation in the multiple reading procedure with a unanimity rule, *Statistics in Medicine* **11**, 209–218.

[52] Maclure, M. & Willett, W.C. (1987). Misinterpretation and misuse of the kappa coefficient, *American Journal of Epidemiology* **126**, 161–169.

[53] Mak, T.K. (1988). Analyzing intraclass correlation for dichotomous variables, *Applied Statistics* **37**, 344–352.

[54] Maxwell, A.E. & Pilliner, A.E.G. (1968). Deriving coefficients of reliability and agreement for ratings, *British Journal of Mathematical and Statistical Psychology* **21**, 105–116.

[55] Mehta, C. & Patel, N. (1995). *StatXact 3 for Windows; User Manual*. Cytel Software Corporation, Cambridge, Mass., Chapter 23.

[56] Nix, A.B.J. & Dunston, F.D.J. (1991). Maximum likelihood techniques applied to method comparison studies, *Statistics in Medicine* **10**, 981–988.

[57] Robinson, D.L. (1987). Estimation and use of variance components, *Statistician* **36**, 3–14.

[58] Robinson, D.L. (1987). *REML User Manual*. Scottish Agricultural Statistical Service, Edinburgh.

[59] Rogot, E. & Goldberg, I.D. (1966). A proposed index for measuring agreement in test-retest studies, *Journal of Chronic Diseases* **19**, 991–1006.

[60] SAS Institute, Inc. (1992). *SAS Release 6.07.* SAS Institute Inc., Cary.

[61] Schouten, H.J.A. (1985). Statistical Measurement of Interrater Agreement, Ph.D. Doctoral Dissertation. Erasmus University, Rotterdam.

[62] Schouten, H.J.A. (1986). Nominal scale agreement among obsevers, *Psychometrika* **51**, 453–466.

[63] Scott, W.A. (1955). Reliability of content analysis: The case of nominal scale coding, *Public Opinion Quarterly* **19**, 321–325.

[64] Searle, S.R. (1987). *Linear Models for Unbalanced Data*. Wiley, New York.

[65] Shoukri, M.M. & Edge, V.L. (1996). *Statistical Methods for Health Sciences*. CRC Press, Boca Raton.

[66] Shoukri, M.M., Martin, S.W. & Mian, I.U.H. (1995). Maximum likelihood estimation of the kappa coefficient from models of matched binary responses, *Statistics in Medicine* **14**, 83–99.

[67] Shukla, G.K. (1973). Some exact tests on hypothesis about Grubbs estimators, *Biometrics* **29**, 373–377.

[68] Snedecor, G.W. & Cochran, W.G. (1980). *Statistical Methods*, 7th Ed. Iowa State University, Ames.
[69] Spitznagel, E.L. & Helzer, J.E. (1985). A proposed solution to the base rate problem in the kappa statistics, *Archives of General Psychiatry* **42**, 725–728.
[70] Thompson, W.D. & Walter, S.D. (1988). A reappraisal of the kappa coefficient, *Journal of Clinical Epidemiology* **41**, 949–958.
[71] Thompson, W.D. & Walter, S.D. (1988). Kappa and the concept of independent errors, *Journal of Clinical Epidemiology* **41**, 969–970.
[72] Winer, B.J. (1971). *Statistical Principles in Experimental Design*. McGraw-Hill, New York.

(*See also* **Reliability Study**)

M.M. SHOUKRI

Aickin's Alpha *see* Agreement, Measurement of

Analytic Epidemiology

Analytic epidemiology denotes epidemiologic studies, such as **cohort studies**, **cross-sectional studies**, and **case–control studies**, that obtain individual-level information on the association between disease status and exposures of interest. Such analytic studies often include individual-level information on potential **confounders** and **effect modifiers**. Usually such studies are designed to evaluate predetermined hypotheses concerning possible causal relationships between exposure and risk of disease (*see* **Causation**). Analytic epidemiology is distinguished from **descriptive epidemiology**, which focuses on quantifying trends and rates of disease in populations and on **ecologic studies** that attempt to correlate rates of disease in populations with average levels of exposure in such populations. Descriptive studies are often used to generate etiologic hypotheses that are tested in subsequent analytic studies.

M.H. GAIL

Antagonism *see* Synergy of Exposure Effects

Areal Data *see* Geographical Analysis

Asymptotic Validity *see* Measurement Error in Epidemiologic Studies

Attack Rate *see* Absolute Risk

Attenuation *see* Measurement Error in Epidemiologic Studies

Attributable Fraction in Exposed

The attributable fraction in the exposed (AF_E) is defined as the proportion of disease cases that can be attributed to an exposure factor among the exposed subjects only [2–5]. It can be formally written as

$$AF_E = [\Pr(D|E) - \Pr(D|\bar{E})]/\Pr(D|E), \quad (1)$$

where $\Pr(D|E)$ is the probability of disease in the exposed individuals, E, and $\Pr(D|\bar{E})$ is the hypothetical probability of disease in the same subjects but with all exposure eliminated. It is also called the **attributable risk** (AR) among the exposed [1, 3] and can be rewritten as

$$AF_E = (RR - 1)/RR, \quad (2)$$

a one-to-one increasing function of the **relative risk** (RR). It can be seen to equal the attributable risk in the special case of an exposure present in all subjects in the population (exposure **prevalence** of 1).

When the exposure factor under study is a risk factor ($RR > 1$), it follows from the above definition that AF_E lies between 0 and 1, and it is usually expressed as a percentage. AF_E increases with the strength of the association between exposure and disease measured by the relative risk and tends to 1 for an infinitely high relative risk. AF_E is equal to zero when there is no association between exposure and disease ($RR = 1$). Negative values of AF_E correspond to a protective exposure ($RR < 1$), in which case AF_E is not a meaningful measure.

While AF_E has some usefulness in measuring the disease-producing impact of an association between exposure and disease, it is much less useful than the attributable risk and does not share the same public health interpretation. This is because it is only a one-to-one transformation of relative risk. It does not take the prevalence of exposure into account, and, for instance, it can be high even if the prevalence of exposure is low in the population. Moreover, while AR estimates for several risk factors can be compared meaningfully to assess the relative importance of these risk factors at the population level, such is not the case with AF_E estimates. Indeed, each AF_E estimate refers to a different group which is specific to the risk factor under consideration (subjects exposed to that risk factor). However, one advantage of AF_E over attributable risk is that, since it does not depend on the prevalence of exposure, portability from one population to another is less problematic than with attributable risk and depends only on the portability of relative risk.

Issues of estimability and estimation of AF_E are the same as those for relative risk. AF_E can be estimated from the main types of epidemiologic studies (**cohort, case–control, cross-sectional, case–cohort**). Point estimates are obtained from point estimates of relative risk (**odds ratio** in case–control studies). Variance estimates can be obtained from variance estimates of relative risk (odds ratio in case–control studies) through the delta-method [6], which yields:

$$\mathrm{var}(\widehat{AF}_E) = \mathrm{var}(\widehat{RR})/RR^4, \qquad (3)$$

where $\widehat{RR}$ denotes a point estimate of relative risk (odds ratio in case–control studies), and $\widehat{AF}_E$ denotes a point estimate of AF_E.

References

[1]   Benichou, J. (1991). Methods of adjustment for estimating the attributable risk in case–control studies: a review, *Statistics in Medicine* **10**, 1753–1773.

[2]   Cole, P. & MacMahon, B. (1971). Attributable risk percent in case–control studies, *British Journal of Preventive and Social Medicine* **25**, 242–244.

[3]   Levin, M.L. (1953). The occurrence of lung cancer in man, *Acta Unio Internationalis Contra Cancrum* **9**, 531–541.

[4]   MacMahon, B. & Pugh, T.F. (1970). *Epidemiology: Principles and Methods*. Little, Brown & Company, Boston.

[5]   Micttinen, O.S. (1974). Proportion of disease caused or prevented by a given exposure, trait or intervention, *American Journal of Epidemiology* **99**, 325–332.

[6]   Rao, C.R. (1965). *Linear Statistical Inference and Its Application*. Wiley, New York, pp. 319–322.

JACQUES BENICHOU

Attributable Risk

The attributable risk (AR), first introduced by Levin [45], is a widely used measure to assess the public health consequences of an association between an exposure factor and a disease. It is defined as the proportion of disease cases that can be attributed to exposure and can be formally written as:

$$AR = [\mathrm{Pr}(D) - \mathrm{Pr}(D|\overline{E})]/\mathrm{Pr}(D), \qquad (1)$$

where $\mathrm{Pr}(D)$ is the probability of disease in the population, which may have some exposed (E) and some unexposed ($\overline{E}$) individuals, and $\mathrm{Pr}(D|\overline{E})$ is the hypothetical probability of disease in the same population but with all exposure eliminated.

The AR takes into account both the strength of the association between exposure and disease and the **prevalence** of exposure in the population. This can be seen, for instance, through rewriting AR from (1), using Bayes' theorem, as [15, 53]:

$$AR = [P(E)(RR - 1)]/[1 + P(E)(RR - 1)], \qquad (2)$$

a function of the prevalence of exposure, $P(E)$, and the **relative risk** (RR). Therefore, while the relative risk is mainly used to establish an association in etiologic research, AR has a public health interpretation as a measure of preventable disease. A high relative risk can correspond to a low or high AR depending on the prevalence of exposure, which leads to widely different public health consequences. One implication is that, while the relative risk is often portable from one population to another, as the strength of the association between disease and exposure might vary little among populations, portability is not a property of AR, as the prevalence of exposure may vary widely among populations that are separated in time or location.

Range

When the exposure factor under study is a risk factor (relative risk > 1), it follows from the above definition that AR lies between 0 and 1, and is, therefore, very often expressed as a percentage. AR increases both with the strength of the association between exposure and disease measured by the relative risk, and with the prevalence of exposure in the population. A prevalence of 1 (or 100%) yields a value of AR equal to $(RR - 1)/RR$, and AR tends to 1 for an infinitely high relative risk provided the prevalence is greater than 0.

AR is equal to zero when either there is no association between exposure and disease ($RR = 1$) or no subject is exposed in the population.

Finally, negative values of AR are obtained for a protective exposure (relative risk < 1). In this case, AR varies between 0 and $-\infty$ and AR is not a meaningful measure. Either one must consider reversing the coding of exposure to go back to the situation of a positive AR or one must consider a different parameter; namely, the prevented fraction (*see* the section "Related Quantities" below).

Synonyms

Numerous terms have been used in the literature instead of attributable risk. Attributable risk was the term originally introduced by Levin [45], but it is not a universally accepted term because (i) the word "risk" may be misleading as AR does not represent a risk in the usual sense and (ii) it may not allow a clear enough distinction from the more restrictive concept of attributable risk (or fraction) in the exposed (*see* **Attributable Fraction in Exposed** and the section "Related Quantities" below). Most common alternative terms are population attributable risk [47] and population attributable risk percent [15], etiologic fraction and fraction of etiology [53], and attributable fraction [33, 43, 58]. Up to 16 terms

have been used to denote attributable risk in the literature [26].

Interpretation and Usefulness

AR is used to assess the potential impact of prevention programs aimed at eliminating exposure from the population. It is often thought of as the fraction of disease that could be eliminated if exposure could be totally removed from the population.

However, this interpretation can be misleading because, for it to be strictly correct, the three following conditions have to be met. First, estimation of AR has to be unbiased (see the section "Estimation" below). Secondly, the exposure factor has to be causal rather than merely associated with the disease (*see* **Causation**). Thirdly, elimination of the risk factor has to be without having any effect on the distribution of other risk factors. Indeed, as it might be difficult to alter the level of exposure to one factor independently of other risk factors, the resulting change in disease load might be different from the AR estimate [77]. For these reasons, various authors elect to use weaker definitions of AR, such as the proportion of disease that can be related or linked, rather than attributed, to exposure [53].

Other problems in interpreting AR values in preventive terms are discussed in two papers by Rockhill et al. [64, 65]. They include the lack of practical usefulness of AR when one considers either very prevalent risk factors or unmodifiable risk factors such as family history or age at menarche for breast cancer.

Despite these limitations, AR can serve as a useful guide in assessing and comparing various prevention strategies. It should be noted that authors have estimated AR in situations where causality was far from being established, and the association between exposure and disease still tentative and controversial. For instance, Alavanja et al. [2] estimated the risk of lung cancer attributable to elevated saturated fat intake in a population of nonsmoking women in the state of Missouri. They interpreted their estimate as quantifying the potential impact of eliminating elevated saturated fat exposure were it later proven to be causally related to lung cancer. This use of AR is somewhat controversial, the more so when the association is not well established, and it needs, therefore, to be presented with proper qualification.

Estimation of AR can usefully be complemented by applying the AR estimate to the **incidence rate** of the disease in the population to see not just what proportion of disease, but how many cases per unit of time are attributable to exposure. Moreover, multiplying an estimate of $1 - AR$ times an estimate of the incidence rate in the population yields an estimate of the incidence rate in the unexposed (baseline incidence rate), which can be useful in a perspective of etiologic research. For instance, Silverman et al. [69], estimated the risk of pancreatic cancer attributable to alcohol in white and black men separately in the United States. They found that the substantial difference in incidence rates between black and white men (16.0 vs. 12.8 per 100 000 person-years, a 25% higher rate in black men) could be explained in part by the higher AR for alcohol among black men, since the race difference among the unexposed (i.e. having removed the contribution of alcohol) was reduced by almost half (14.2 vs. 12.5 per 100 000 person-years, a 14% higher rate in black men). The higher AR estimate among black men was itself related to both a higher relative risk estimate for elevated alcohol consumption and a higher prevalence of that exposure among black men.

Finally, AR can be considered for not just one, but several, risk factors in combination. One can be interested in the potential effect on disease load of removing these risk factors from the population. Alternatively, one might interpret an AR estimate for all known risk factors as a gauge of what is known about the disease etiology, and its complement to 1 as a gauge of what remains unexplained by known risk factors. For instance, Madigan et al. [48] estimated at 41% the AR of breast cancer for well-established risk factors; namely, later age at first birth, nulliparity, family history of breast cancer in a first-degree relative and higher socioeconomic status. They argued in favor of more etiologic research to find new risk factors, whether genetic, hormonal, or biological, to account for the remaining 59% of unexplained breast cancer cases. In fact, most authors in that field have come to similar conclusions and the AR figure of 50% or less is a useful indicator and reminder of the need for new research directions in breast cancer etiology.

Properties

Two basic properties of AR need to be emphasized. First, AR values greatly depend on the definition of the reference level for exposure (unexposed or baseline level). A larger proportion of subjects exposed corresponds to a more stringent definition of the reference level and, as one keeps depleting the reference category from subjects with higher levels of risk, AR values and estimates keep rising. This property has a major impact on AR estimates as was illustrated by Benichou [5] and Wacholder et al. [74]. For instance, Benichou [5] found that the AR estimate of esophageal cancer for an alcohol consumption greater or equal to 80 g/day (reference level of 0–79 g/day) was 38% in the Ille-et-Vilaine part of France [73], and increased dramatically to 70% for an alcohol consumption greater or equal to 40 g/day (more restrictive reference level of 0–39 g/day). This property plays a role whenever studying a continuous exposure with a continuous gradient of risk and when there is no obvious choice of threshold. Therefore, AR estimates must be reported with reference to a clearly defined baseline level in order to be interpreted validly. In the previous example, one notes that the interpretation in preventive terms would differ for the two AR estimates. One would conclude that 70% (respectively 38%) of all esophageal cancers in Ille-et-Vilaine can be attributed to an alcohol consumption of at least 40 g/day (respectively 80 g/day) and could potentially be prevented by reducing alcohol consumption to less than 40 g/day (respectively 80 g/day).

The second main property is distributivity. If several categories of exposure are considered instead of just one, then the sum of the category-specific ARs (see the section "Special Problems" below) equals the AR calculated from combining those categories into a single exposed category, regardless of the number and the divisions of the categories that are formed [5, 74, 77], provided the reference category remains the same. This property applies strictly to unadjusted AR estimates and to adjusted AR estimates calculated on the basis of a saturated model (see below) [5]. In other situations, it applies approximately [74]. For instance, Wacholder et al. [74] used data on malignant mesothelioma [70], and obtained an unadjusted AR estimate equal to 82% for a nontrivial (moderately low, medium, or high) likelihood of exposure to asbestos, identical to the sum of the respective category-specific AR estimates of 13%, 6%, and 64% for moderately low, medium, and high likelihoods of exposure. Thus, if an overall AR estimate for exposure is the focus of interest, there is no need to break the exposed category into several mutually exclusive categories, even in the presence of a gradient of risk with increasing exposure.

Estimability

AR can be estimated from the main types of epidemiologic studies, namely **cohort, case–control, cross-sectional**, and **case–cohort studies**. It can be seen immediately that all quantities in (1) are estimable from all four types of studies except case–control studies. For case–control studies, one has to consider (2) and estimate $P(E)$ from the proportion exposed in the controls, making the rare-disease assumption also involved in estimating odds ratios rather than relative risks. Alternatively, one can rewrite (1) using Bayes' theorem in yet another manner as

$$AR = \Pr(E|D)(RR - 1)/RR. \qquad (3)$$

In (3), the quantity $\Pr(E|D)$ can be directly estimated from the diseased individuals (cases) and RR can be estimated from the **odds ratio**. Therefore, AR is estimable from case–control studies as well.

Often, cohort studies are based on groups with a different prevalence of exposure than the general population. This renders AR estimates obtained from cohort studies less applicable to the general population and might explain why AR is seldom estimated from cohort studies.

Estimation

Since Levin [45] first introduced AR, there has been a very active research in AR estimation and numerous developments have appeared, particularly in recent years. Case–control studies have been the most explored. The outline given here applies to cohort, case–control and cross-sectional studies, unless stated otherwise. While AR is estimable from case–cohort studies, no study of AR estimation methods seems to have been published, and case–cohort studies will be considered separately (see the section "Special Problems" below).

Unadjusted Estimation

From the three types of studies considered, it is easy to obtain unadjusted (crude) AR estimates, either from (2) or (3). No other factor than the exposure of interest is considered, and the data are limited to exposure and disease state. For instance, one obtains the following estimate both from (2) and (3) in case–control studies:

$$AR = (n_1 m_0 - m_1 n_0)/m_0 n, \qquad (4)$$

where n_0 and n_1 respectively denote the numbers of unexposed and exposed cases ($n_0 + n_1 = n$) and m_0 and m_1 the numbers of unexposed and exposed controls ($m_0 + m_1 = m$).

Variance estimates can be obtained from the delta-method [61] by considering the following distributions. In case–control studies, the quantities n_1 and m_1 have independent binomial distributions with respective indexes n and m considered as fixed (exposure is random conditional on disease status). In cohort studies, the quantities n_0 and n_1 have binomial distributions with respective fixed indexes $n_0 + m_0$ and $n_1 + m_1$ considered as fixed (disease status is random conditional on exposure). In cross-sectional studies, one has to consider the full (unrestricted) multinomial model in which all four quantities n_0, n_1, m_0, and m_1 come from a common multinomial distribution with index $n + m$ considered as fixed (exposure and disease status are random).

Once a variance estimate is obtained, a standard confidence interval for AR can be constructed based on the asymptotic normal distribution of AR. Alternatively, Walter [76] suggested using the interval based on the log transformed variable $\log(1 - AR)$, and Leung & Kupper [44] based the interval on the logit-transformed variable $\log[AR/(1 - AR)]$. Whittemore [80] noted that the log-transformation yields a wider interval than the standard interval for $AR > 0$. Leung & Kupper [44] showed that the interval based on the logit transform is narrower than the standard interval for values of AR strictly between 0.21 and 0.79, whereas the reverse holds outside this range for positive values of AR. While the coverage probabilities of these intervals have been studied in some specific situations and partial comparisons have been made, no general study has been performed to determine their relative merits in terms of coverage probability.

Unadjusted estimates of AR are, in general, biased, because they fail to take into account other risk factors that **confound** the association between exposure and disease. The problem is analogous to estimation of relative risks or odds ratios, and has been studied by several authors [53, 77–81]. It is one of inconsistency rather than small-sample **bias**. Walter [78] showed that, if X_1 and X_2 are two binary exposure factors and if one is interested in estimating an AR for X_1, then the following applies. The crude AR estimate is unbiased if and only if at least one of the following two conditions is true:

1. X_1 and X_2 are independently distributed in the population, that is:

$$\Pr(X_1 = 0, X_2 = 0)\Pr(X_1 = 1, X_2 = 1)$$
$$= \Pr(X_1 = 0, X_2 = 1)\Pr(X_1 = 1, X_2 = 0),$$

where level 0 denotes the absence of exposure and 1 the exposed category.
2. Exposure to X_2 alone does not increase disease risk; that is:

$$\Pr(D|X_1 = 0, X_2 = 1) = \Pr(D|X_1 = 0, X_2 = 0).$$

Therefore, if X_2 acts as a true confounder of the association between exposure X_1 and the disease, then the crude estimate of AR is inconsistent, as is a crude estimate of relative risk or odds ratio. When neither condition 1 nor 2 is true, the direction of the bias can be determined. If X_2 alone increases risk, then the bias is positive (AR is overestimated) if X_1 and X_2 are positively correlated, and negative if they are negatively correlated [78]. When considering several factors $X_j (j = 2, \ldots, J)$, conditions 1 and 2 can be extended to a set of $2(J - 1)$ analogous sufficient conditions concerning factors X_1 and $X_j (j = 2, \ldots, J)$ as shown by Walter [78].

Adjusted Estimation – Inconsistent Approaches

Let us first note that two simple adjusted estimation approaches discussed in the literature are inconsistent. The first approach ever proposed to obtain adjusted AR estimates, based on decomposing AR into exposure and confounding effects [77], was shown to be inconsistent [27] and, accordingly, bias was exhibited in simulations for the crossover design [26, 27]. The approach based on using (2) and plugging in an adjusted relative risk estimate (odds ratio estimate in case–control studies), along with an estimate of $P(E)$, has also been advocated [15, 55], but it too has been shown to yield inconsistent estimates [28, 32] of AR, and, accordingly, bias was exhibited in

simulations for the crossover design (i.e. under the unrestricted multinomial model) [26, 27].

Two adjusted approaches based on **stratification**, the **Mantel–Haenszel** approach and the weighted-sum approach, yield valid estimates.

Adjusted Estimation – The Mantel–Haenszel Approach

The Mantel–Haenszel (MH) approach has been developed by Greenland [29] and Kuritz & Landis [38, 39]. It allows adjustment for one or more polychotomous factors forming J joint levels or strata. It is based on the formulation of AR as a function of the relative risk (odds ratio in case–control studies) and the prevalence of exposure in diseased individuals, as given by (3). One plugs in an estimate of $\Pr(E|D)$ (given by the observed proportion of cases exposed) and an estimate of the common adjusted relative risk (odds ratio in case–control studies). The MH estimate of the common odds ratio [49] can be used in case–control studies, while MH-type estimates of the common relative risk [36, 72] can be used in cohort or cross-sectional studies.

Other choices than the MH estimator of odds ratio or MH-type estimators of relative risk are possible, and this approach could be more generally termed the common relative risk (odds ratio in case–control studies) approach. Other choices have been suggested, such as an internally standardized mortality ratio [53] (*see* **Standardization Methods**) or the maximum likelihood estimator from **logistic regression** [29]. MH-type estimators combine properties of lack of (or very small) bias even for sparse data (e.g. individually matched case–control data), good efficiency except in extreme circumstances [10–12, 42], and the existence of consistent variance estimators even for sparse data ("dually-consistent" variance estimators) [29, 63].

While point estimation with the MH approach is simple, variance estimation is more complex. Variance estimators can be obtained either through applications of the delta method [38, 39] or by relying on asymptotic properties of first derivatives of log likelihood functions [29]. Finite sample properties were studied by simulations under the assumption of a common odds ratio or relative risk. It was found that bias in estimating AR was negligible in case–control studies with simple random sampling [38], stratified random sampling [29] and individual **matching** [39], as well as in cross-sectional studies [26, 27]. Variance estimates were also unbiased and coverage probabilities close to nominal for those various designs.

The crucial assumption in the MH approach is that of a common or homogeneous relative risk or odds ratio, which amounts to a lack of **interaction** between the adjustment factor(s) and the exposure factor (no **effect modification**). If interaction is present, the MH estimator of AR is inconsistent, which was illustrated in simulations for the crossover design [26, 27]. Greenland [29] proposed a modification of the MH approach, consisting in defining H levels out of the original J levels formed by adjustment factors. The H levels are defined so that, within each of them, the odds ratio or relative risk can be considered as homogeneous and is estimated separately. This constitutes a possible solution although (i) the definition of the H levels, which is critical to this modified approach, is somewhat arbitrary in view of the low power of tests to detect interaction, and (ii) finite sample properties of this modified approach might not be as favorable as the original MH approach and bias might arise as with the weighted-sum approach (see below). Indeed, this modified approach is a hybrid approach, being intermediate between the MH and weighted-sum approaches.

Adjusted Estimation – The Weighted-Sum Approach

This approach allows adjustment for one or more polychotomous factors forming J levels or strata. AR is written as a weighted sum of the ARs over strata, namely [77, 80, 81]:

$$AR = \sum_j w_j AR_j, \tag{5}$$

where AR_j and w_j are respectively the AR specific to level j and the corresponding weight. Setting w_j as the proportion of diseased individuals (cases) in level j yields an asymptotically unbiased estimator of AR, which can be seen to be a maximum-likelihood estimator [76, 80]. This choice of weights defines the "case-load method". An alternative choice of weights, called "precision-weighting" is given by setting w_j as the inverse variance of the AR estimate in level j over the sum of inverse variances over all levels [25]. It can be shown to be an inconsistent estimator of AR except in special circumstances [27].

The weighted-sum approach does not require the assumption of a common relative risk or odds ratio. The odds ratios or relative risks are estimated separately for each level j. No restrictions are placed on them, which corresponds to a saturated model. Thus, the weighted-sum approach not only accounts for confounding but also for interaction. It is interesting to note that, under the assumption of a common relative risk or odds ratio, the weighted-sum approach yields the same expression for AR as the MH approach [5].

Point estimates are easy to obtain for the various types of designs. Variance estimates can be obtained from specializing the distributions described above (see the subsection "Unadjusted Estimation" above) for each level j and applying the delta-method [61]. They have been worked out for case–control designs [80], cross-sectional designs [27] and cohort designs [48].

Unlike the MH approach, small-sample bias is an issue with the weighted-sum approach, at least for case–control designs. Negative bias was found in simulations of case–control studies for **frequency matching** and simple random sampling of the controls, under the assumption of a common odds ratio and with case-load weighting [38, 80]. This bias was substantial for sparse data and a high prevalence of exposure in controls. Precision-weighting yielded a positive bias of similar magnitude [38]. The strong negative (or positive) bias renders the approach inappropriate for individual matching [38, 80]. A tendency towards conservative variance estimates and confidence intervals was also observed [38, 80]. For crossover designs, however, the results were much more favorable, as no severe small-sample bias was found in simulations, whether or not a common relative risk was considered [26, 27].

Model-Based Adjusted Estimation

The MH approach rests on the assumption of a common relative risk or odds ratio and yields biased estimates in the case of interaction between exposure and adjustment factors. The weighted-sum approach does not impose any structure on the relative risk or odds ratio and its variation with levels of adjustment factors, but is plagued by problems of small sample bias, particularly for case–control designs. A natural alternative has been to develop adjustment procedures based on regression models in order to take advantage of their flexible and unified approach to efficient parameter estimation and hypothesis testing.

Walter [77] first suggested this route, and others have followed [22, 71]. Greenland [29] proposed a modification of the MH approach for case–control studies, consisting in substituting a maximum-likelihood estimate of the odds ratio from conditional logistic regression rather than the MH estimate of odds ratio in (3), and he worked out the corresponding variance estimate for AR. This modification could be applied to other designs but retains the constraint of a homogeneous odds ratio.

The full generality and flexibility of the regression approach was first exploited by Bruzzi et al. [14] who expressed AR as:

$$AR = 1 - \sum_j \sum_i \rho_{ij}/RR_{i|j}. \qquad (6)$$

In this formula, the first sum is taken over all J levels formed by polychotomous adjustment factors, and the second sum is taken over all exposure levels (usually one unexposed level and one exposed level). The quantity ρ_{ij} represents the proportion of diseased individuals (cases) with respective levels i and j of exposure and adjustment factors, while $RR_{i|j}$ represents the relative risk for level i of exposure given level j of adjustment factors. An informal proof of (6) can be found in Bruzzi et al. [14] and a more formal one in Benichou [5].

The model-based approach based on (6) is very general in several respects. First, while it was derived by Bruzzi et al. [14] for case–control studies, it can be used as well for cohort and cross-sectional studies. For all three designs, an estimate is obtained by replacing ρ_{ij} by the observed proportion among diseased individuals, and by replacing $RR_{i|j}$ by a maximum likelihood estimate obtained from a regression model. In case–control studies, an estimate of the odds ratio from unconditional or conditional logistic regression can be used; in cross-sectional studies, an estimate of the relative risk from unconditional logistic regression can be used; in cohort studies, an estimate of the relative risk from unconditional logistic regression or from **Poisson regression** can be used. Models with additive forms have also been proposed [17].

Secondly, since estimates of odds ratio and relative risk are obtained from regression models, this approach provides a unified framework for testing hypotheses and selecting models. In particular,

interaction terms can be introduced in the model, tested and retained or not, depending on the result of the test. This approach allows control for confounding and interaction and essentially parallels the estimation of the relative risk or odds ratio. Parsimony can be balanced against bias and the "best" model selected. More elaborate models (e.g. models with interaction terms) protect against inconsistency but can lead to small-sample bias and larger **random error**, while more parsimonious models have the reverse properties.

Thirdly, the model-based approach is general in that it includes the crude and other adjusted approaches as special cases [5]. The unadjusted approach corresponds to models with exposure only. The MH approach corresponds to models with exposure and confounding, but no interaction terms between exposure and confounding factors. The weighted-sum approach corresponds to fully saturated models with all interaction terms. Intermediate models are possible; for instance, models allowing for interaction between exposure and one confounder only, or models in which the main effects of some confounders are not modeled in a saturated way.

While point estimates are easy to obtain, variance estimates are complex because they involve covariances between quantities ρ_{ij} and $RR_{i'|j'}$ that are related implicitly (rather than explicitly) through score equations. Benichou & Gail [8] worked out a variance estimator for all types of case–control studies (with simple random sampling, stratified random sampling, frequency-matching and individual matching of the controls), using an extension of the delta method to implicitly related random variables [7]. Basu & Landis [3] used a similar approach for cohort and cross-sectional designs. In case–control studies, simulations showed little or no bias in most situations [8]. However, as the data became sparse, negative bias was observed with the unconditional logistic model [8]. This could be remedied by the use of more parsimonious models when appropriate or the use of conditional logistic regression. Use of the latter approach, however, remains a research issue, as variance estimates have been derived for conditional logistic regression only for the situation of individual matching. Finally, variance estimates were unbiased and coverage probabilities close to nominal for all types of case–control studies in the aforementioned simulations [8].

Greenland & Drescher [31] have made the point that Bruzzi et al.'s estimator of AR is not exactly a maximum likelihood estimator, and have proposed a modified approach in order to obtain a maximum likelihood estimator. The proposed modification consists in using a model-based estimate of quantities ρ_{ij} rather than estimating these quantities from the corresponding observed quantities. They developed point and variance estimators for case–control designs under the unconditional logistic model, and for cohort designs under the unconditional logistic model and the Poisson model. In case–control studies, their approach can be seen as a generalization of Drescher & Schill's approach [24]. Variance estimators rely on the delta-method [61] rather than on the implicit delta-method [7] as for Bruzzi et al.'s estimator.

The two model-based approaches are identical for fully saturated models, in which case they also coincide with the weighted-sum approach. More generally, provided that the model is not misspecified, the two approaches are practically equivalent, as was illustrated by simulations for the case–control design [31]. Point and variance estimators differed only trivially between the two approaches, with mean differences equal to less than 0.001 and correlations in excess of 0.999. In simulations of the cohort design for Greenland & Drescher's modified model-based approach, some downward bias was found, in a similar way to what had been observed for Bruzzi et al.'s model-based approach for case–control designs [8], and variance estimates appeared to be without substantial bias [31].

In practice, the two model-based approaches seem, therefore, to differ very little. The maximum likelihood approach might be more efficient for small samples, although no difference was observed in simulations of the case–control design even for samples of 100 cases and 100 controls. The maximum likelihood approach might be less robust to model misspecification, however, as it relies more heavily on the model for the relative risk or odds ratio. In one circumstance, the distinction between the two approaches is unequivocal. The modified approach does not apply to the conditional logistic model, and if that model is to be used (notably, in case–control studies with individual matching), Bruzzi et al.'s original approach is the only possible choice.

Special Problems

Case–Cohort Design

In the case–cohort design, information on exposure is gathered only in a subcohort of subjects randomly selected from the original cohort and among subjects who develop the disease [60]. Case–cohort data contain information on the prevalence of exposure and allow estimation of the relative risk. Therefore, AR is estimable from case–cohort data, and all estimation methods presented above could, in principle, be used to estimate AR. However, the details have not been worked out in the literature and variance estimators may prove complex to derive.

Risk Factor with Multiple Levels of Exposure

It has been seen above that, because of the distributive property (see the section "Properties" above), it is sufficient to consider one overall exposed level to estimate AR. However, several levels of exposure are worth considering when estimates of AR at specified levels are of interest.

The concept of partial or level-specific AR corresponds to the proportion of disease cases that can be attributed to a specified level of exposure, and may have important policy implications for screening groups at highest risk of disease, for instance [21, 53, 77]. All estimation methods described above can be extended to produce such AR estimates. In particular, Denman & Schlesselman [21] have developed unadjusted estimates for case–control designs. The model-based approach lends itself naturally to this problem, as (6) need only be slightly modified (all RR are set equal to 1 in it, except those for the exposure level of interest). Use of the model-based approach is illustrated in Coughlin et al. [16] who considered the esophageal cancer case–control data mentioned above (see the section "Properties" above) and showed that the AR for "moderate" drinkers (40–79 g/day) was higher than that for heavy drinkers (120+ g/day) (27% vs. 22%), suggesting that prevention policies targeting "moderate" drinkers might be potentially more effective than those aimed at heavy drinkers in that population.

Finally, AR estimates have been developed for a continuous exposure [8], but their main interest is not for AR estimation but, rather, for the estimation of a related quantity; namely, the generalized impact fraction (see below).

Multiple Risk Factors

When there are several risk factors at play, it is useful to estimate AR for each risk factor separately as well as an overall AR for all risk factors jointly. Contrary to some investigators' intuition, the sum of AR estimates for each risk factor does not equal the overall AR except in special circumstances. Walter [79] showed that the equality holds for two risk factors if and only if either no subject is exposed to both risk factors or the effect of the two risk factors on disease incidence is additive. This generalizes into a set of *J* sufficient conditions when more than two factors forming *J* levels are taken into account [79]. Another important result is that, if the risk factors are statistically independent and their joint effect on disease incidence is **multiplicative** (i.e. no interaction on a multiplicative scale is present), then the complement to 1 of the overall AR is equal to the product of the complements to 1 of the separate ARs [14, 53, 77].

Finally, it has been recommended to consider a single exposed level defined by exposure to at least one risk factor, and a reference level defined by exposure to no risk factor, in order to estimate the overall AR for several risk factors [5, 74]. However, this procedure, while appealingly simple, can lead to a very small reference level and thus a very unstable AR estimate. For this reason, some authors prefer to use the model-based approach (6) and retain one parameter for each exposure factor in an overall relative risk or odds ratio model to obtain a more stable AR estimate [20, 40].

Misclassification of Exposure

The effects of **misclassification** of exposure have been studied by several authors [35, 74, 79]. AR has a "canceling feature" [79] in that misclassification may result in compensatory effects. For example, if misclassification of exposure is **nondifferential**, reduced **specificity** of exposure classification (marked by the presence of false positive subjects in terms of exposure) biases the odds ratio or relative risk towards the null (*see* **Bias Toward the Null**), but exposure prevalence increases, so that the net result is an absence of

bias. However, still for nondifferential misclassification, reduced **sensitivity** (marked by the presence of false negative subjects in terms of exposure) biases AR estimates towards the null. Hsieh & Walter [35] gave a formal proof of this result and Wacholder et al. [74] a heuristic proof based on the distributive property of AR. Moreover, this downward bias increases with the prevalence of exposure.

Thus, in order to minimize bias in estimating AR, a sensitive classification scheme is an appropriate strategy, even when specificity is exceedingly low. In other words, the estimate of AR is unbiased as long as all exposed individuals are classified as exposed, regardless of the proportion of unexposed subjects who are misclassified nondifferentially as exposed. This is illustrated by Wacholder et al. [74] with case–control data on mesothelioma and asbestos exposure (see the section "Properties" above). As exposure to asbestos is hard to prove, there are categories with "moderately low" or "medium" probability of exposure in their example. They recommend to consider these subjects as exposed in order to obtain a perfectly sensitive classification. However, there is a price to pay when high sensitivity is obtained at the expense of reduced specificity. Precision decreases (the variance of the AR estimate increases) when the definition of exposure encompasses levels of exposure that have the same risk of disease as the unexposed [74]. Therefore, there might be a tradeoff between bias and precision.

If misclassification is differential with diseased subjects (cases) being falsely classified as exposed more often that nondiseased subjects (controls), then the estimate of AR, as well as of relative risk or odds ratio, will be biased upward [74].

Finally, it should be noted that Hsieh studied the effect of disease status misclassification ("outcome misclassification") on AR estimation, and defined conditions under which bias occurs in this less common situation [34].

Use of AR to Determine Sample Size

Browner & Newman [13] derived formulas for sample size determination in case–control studies that are based on AR instead of odds ratio. Upon comparing sample size and power estimates based on the detection of a given AR with conventional estimates based on the detection of a given odds ratio, they found the following results. For a rare dichotomous exposure, case–control studies having little power to detect a small odds ratio may still have adequate power to detect a small AR. However, even relatively large case–control studies may have inadequate power to detect a small AR when the exposure is common. Such sample size calculations may be useful when the public health importance of an association is of primary interest, as further discussed by Coughlin et al. [16] and Adams et al. [1].

Ordinal Data

Basu & Landis [4] considered the situation where the disease classification is not dichotomous (diseased, nondiseased) but includes more than two ordered categories (e.g. none, mild, moderate, severe) and the exposure factor has at least two ordinal levels (e.g. none, low, medium, high exposure). They extended the concept of AR to that special case in order to quantify the potential extent of disease reduction in the target population relative to each increasing level of the ordinal disease classification, which could be realized if the exposure factor were eliminated. They developed model-based estimates based on a cumulative logit model, assuming a proportional odds structure for cohort, case–control and cross-sectional designs, and obtained corresponding variance estimates based on the delta method for implicitly related random variables [7].

Recurrent Disease Events

Pichlmeier & Gefeller [59] extended the concept of AR to diseases that may recur, such as some skin diseases (e.g. urticaria, psoriasis) or chronic diseases like asthma, epilepsy, or multiple sclerosis. They defined the "recurrent attributable risk" as the proportion of disease events (first occurrence plus recurrences) that can be attributed to an exposure factor. This concept is of interest for risk factors that also act as prognostic factors of recurrences. Point estimators were derived for cohort, case–control and cross-sectional designs based on the unadjusted, weighted-sum and MH approaches. Corresponding approximate variance estimators were developed using the delta method [61].

Oja et al. [57] further considered this problem. They developed adjusted AR point estimates and corresponding standard error estimates for cohort studies based on standard as well as autoregressive logistic models. They presented an application of their methods to data on middle ear infection. They found that the AR for type of day care (a time-dependent risk factor) was more precisely estimated with the autoregressive model, since this model allows one to capture the time-dependency of risk factors.

Conceptual Problems

The public health interpretation of AR refers to the proportion of cases that are excess cases, i.e. that would not have occurred if exposure had not occurred. Greenland & Robins [33, 62] identified a different concept. From a biologic or legal perspective, one might refer to cases for which exposure played an etiologic role, i.e. cases for which exposure was a contributory cause of the outcome. They argued for the distinction between "excess fraction" and "etiologic fraction" to refer to the standard and new concept, respectively. While the "excess fraction" can be estimated under the usual conditions for validity of an epidemiologic study (e.g. lack of biases), estimation of the etiologic fraction requires nonidentifiable biologic assumptions about exposure action and interactions [62]. It is true, however, that the interpretation of the excess fraction also depends on considerations of causality, as discussed in the section "Interpretation and Usefulness" above.

Related Quantities

AR in Exposed

The attributable risk in the exposed or **attributable fraction in the exposed** (AF_E) is defined as the proportion of disease cases that can be attributed to an exposure factor among the exposed subjects only [15, 45, 47, 53]. It can be formally written as:

$$AF_E = [\Pr(D|E) - \Pr(D|\overline{E})]/\Pr(D|E), \qquad (7)$$

where $\Pr(D|E)$ is the probability of disease in the exposed individuals (E) and $\Pr(D|\overline{E})$ is the hypothetical probability of disease in the same subjects but with all exposure eliminated.

Excess Incidence

Excess incidence δ is defined as the difference between the incidence rate in the exposed and the incidence rate in the unexposed, or $\delta = \lambda_1 - \lambda_0$ [9,

47, 51]. It takes into account the incidence of the disease in the unexposed and the strength of the association between exposure and disease, as it can be rewritten as $\delta = \lambda_0 (RR - 1)$. It can be seen to equal the numerator of the AR in the exposed (7) if the latter is expressed in terms of incidence rates rather than probabilities. Its main interest lies, however, at the individual, rather than the population, level. It quantifies the difference in incidence that can be attributed to exposure for an individual. Other terms have been used to denote this quantity; namely, **"excess risk"** [66], "Berkson's simple difference" [77], "incidence density difference" [54], "excess prevalence" [77], or even "attributable risk" [50, 66], which may have introduced some confusion. Moreover, it should not be confused with the concept of "excess fraction" [33, 62] (see above). Estimation of δ pertains to estimation of incidence rates.

Prevented Fraction

When considering a protective exposure or intervention, an intuitively appealing alternative to AR is the prevented fraction (PF). The prevented fraction measures the impact of an association between a protective exposure and disease at the population level. It is sometimes called the **preventable fraction**, although this term may have a different meaning. It is defined as the proportion of disease cases averted by a protective exposure or intervention [53]. It can be written formally as:

$$PF = [\Pr(D|\overline{E}) - \Pr(D)]/\Pr(D|\overline{E}), \qquad (8)$$

where $\Pr(D)$ is the probability of disease in the population, which may have some exposed (E) and some unexposed ($\overline{E}$) individuals, and $\Pr(D|\overline{E})$ is the hypothetical probability of disease in the same population but with all (protective) exposure eliminated. Another formulation of PF is the proportion of cases prevented by the (protective) factor or intervention among the totality of cases that would have developed in the absence of the factor or intervention [53], which is why the denominator in (8) is the hypothetical probability of disease in the population *in the absence of the protective factor.*

Generalized Impact Fraction

The generalized impact fraction (or generalized attributable fraction) was introduced by Walter [78]

and Morgenstern & Bursic [56] as a measure that generalizes AR. It is defined as the fractional reduction of disease that would result from changing the current distribution of exposure in the population to some modified distribution; namely, $[\Pr(D) - \Pr^*(D)]/\Pr(D)$, where $\Pr(D)$ and $\Pr^*(D)$, respectively, denote the probability of disease under the current distribution of exposure and under the modified distribution of exposure. AR corresponds to the special case in which the modified distribution puts unit mass on the lowest risk configuration and can be used to assess interventions aimed at eliminating exposure. A level-specific AR corresponds to the special case where the modified distribution of exposure differs from the current distribution in that subjects at the specified level of exposure are brought to the lowest risk configuration and can be used to assess interventions aimed at eliminating exposure in that specified group only. The generalized impact fraction is a general measure that can be used to assess various interventions, targeting all subjects or subjects at specified levels, and aimed at modifying the exposure distribution (reducing exposure), but not necessarily eliminating exposure.

It has been used, for instance, by Lubin & Boice [46] who considered the impact on lung cancer of a modification in the distribution of radon exposure consisting in truncating the current distribution at various thresholds. Wahrendorf [75] used this concept to examine the impact of various changes in dietary habits on colo-rectal and stomach cancers.

Methods to estimate the generalized impact fraction are similar to methods for estimating AR. However, unlike for AR, it might be useful to retain the continuous nature of risk factors to define the modification of the distribution considered (for instance, a shift in the distribution), and extensions of methods for estimating AR for continuous factors [8] are useful. Drescher & Becher [23] proposed extending the model-based approaches of Bruzzi et al. [14] and Greenland & Drescher [31] to estimate the generalized impact fraction in case–control studies and considered categorical as well as continuous exposure factors.

Probability of Causation – Assigned Share

Cox [18, 19] proposed a method of partitioning the increase in disease risk among several risk factors for subjects jointly exposed to them. The part corresponding to each factor is called the assigned share or probability of causation [6, 18, 19, 41, 67, 68]. It is useful in a legal context to assign shares of responsibility to risk factors in tort liability cases but does not have a population interpretation, unlike AR [6]. The assigned share enjoys the additive property that the sum of separate assigned shares for two (or more) factors is equal to the joint assigned share for these factors [19].

Prospects and Conclusion

Although most important issues about AR estimation have been settled, research is still needed on specific points, such as the use of resampling methods to estimate variance and confidence intervals [30, 37], the development of model-based estimates based on conditional logistic regression for stratified or frequency-matched, case–control studies [8], improvements of the weighted-sum approach in case–control studies, or the development of AR estimators for case–cohort designs and complex survey designs (e.g. cluster sampling). Research is also needed for issues regarding quantities related to AR (see above), special problems (see above), and for software development [52] (*see* **Software, Biostatistical**).

The biggest challenge at this point, however, might be the need to encourage the proper use and interpretation of AR in practice and to make investigators aware of correct estimation techniques.

References

[1]　Adams, M.J., Khoury, M.J. & James, L.M. (1989). The use of attributable fractions in the design and interpretation of epidemiologic studies, *Journal of Clinical Epidemiology* **42**, 659–662.

[2]　Alavanja, M.C.R., Brownson R.C., Benichou, J., Swanson, C. & Boice, J.D. (1995). Attributable risk of lung cancer in lifetime nonsmokers and long-term ex-smokers (Missouri, USA), *Cancer Causes and Control* **6**, 209–216.

[3]　Basu, S. & Landis, J.R. (1995). Model-based estimation of population attributable risk under cross-sectional sampling, *American Journal of Epidemiology* **142**, 1338–1343.

[4]　Basu, S. & Landis, J.R. (1993). Model-based estimates of population attributable risk for ordinal data, Personal communication.

[5]　Benichou, J. (1991). Methods of adjustment for estimating the attributable risk in case–control studies: a review, *Statistics in Medicine* **10**, 1753–1773.

[6]　Benichou, J. (1993). Re: "Methods of adjustment for estimating the attributable risk in case–control studies: a review" (letter), *Statistics in Medicine* **12**, 94–96.

[7]　Benichou, J. & Gail, M.H. (1989). A delta-method for implicitly defined random variables, *American Statistician* **43**, 41–44.

[8]　Benichou, J. & Gail, M.H. (1990). Variance calculations and confidence intervals for estimates of the attributable risk based on logistic models, *Biometrics* **46**, 991–1003.

[9]　Berkson, J. (1958). Smoking and lung cancer. Some observations on two recent reports, *Journal of the American Statistical Association* **53**, 28–38.

[10]　Birch, M.W. (1964). The detection of partial associations, I: the 2 × 2 case, *Journal of the Royal Statistical Society, Series B* **27**, 313–324.

[11]　Breslow, N.E. (1981). Odds ratio estimators when the data are sparse, *Biometrika* **68**, 73–84.

[12]　Breslow, N.E. & Day, N.E. (1980). *Statistical Methods in Cancer Research. Vol. 1: The Analysis of Case-Control Studies.* Scientific Publications No. 32, International Agency for Research on Cancer, Lyon.

[13]　Browner, W.S. & Newman, T.B. (1989). Sample size and power based on the population attributable fraction, *American Journal of Public Health* **79**, 1289–1294.

[14]　Bruzzi, P., Green S.B., Byar, D.P., Brinton, L.A. & Schairer, C. (1985). Estimating the population attributable risk for multiple risk factors using case–control data, *American Journal of Epidemiology* **122**, 904–914.

[15]　Cole, P. & MacMahon, B. (1971). Attributable risk percent in case–control studies, *British Journal of Preventive and Social Medicine* **25**, 242–244.

[16]　Coughlin, S.S., Benichou, J. & Weed, D.L. (1994). Attributable risk estimation in case–control studies, *Epidemiologic Reviews* **16**, 51–64.

[17]　Coughlin, S.S., Nass, C.C., Pickle, L.W., Trock, B. & Bunin, G. (1991). Regression methods for estimating attributable risk in population-based case–control studies: a comparison of additive and multiplicative models, *American Journal of Epidemiology* **133**, 305–313.

[18]　Cox, L.A. (1984). Probability of causation and the attributable proportion of risk, *Risk Analysis* **4**, 221–230.

[19]　Cox, L.A. (1985). A new measure of attributable risk for public health applications, *Management Science* **7**, 800–813.

[20]　D'Avanzo, B., La Vecchia C., Negri, E., Decarli, A. & Benichou, J. (1995). Attributable risks for bladder cancer in Northern Italy, *Annals of Epidemiology* **5**, 427–431.

[21]　Denman, D.W. & Schlesselman, J.J. (1983). Interval estimation of the attributable risk for multiple exposure levels in case–control studies, *Biometrics* **39**, 185–192.

[22]　Deubner, D.C., Wilkinson, W.E., Helms, M.J., Tyroler, H.A. & Hames, C.G. (1980). Logistic model estimation of death attributable to risk factors for

cardiovascular disease in Evans County, Georgia, *American Journal of Epidemiology* **112**, 135–143.

[23] Drescher, K. & Becher, H. (1997). Estimating the generalized attributable fraction from case–control data, *Biometrics* **53**, 1170–1176.

[24] Drescher, K. & Schill, W. (1991). Attributable risk estimation from case–control data via logistic regression, *Biometrics* **47**, 1247–1256.

[25] Ejigou, A. (1979). Estimation of attributable risk in the presence of confounding, *Biometrical Journal* **21**, 155–165.

[26] Gefeller, O. (1990). A simulation study on adjusted attributable risk estimators, *Statistica Applicata* **2**, 323–331.

[27] Gefeller, O. (1992). Comparison of adjusted attributable risk estimators, *Statistics in Medicine* **11**, 2083–2091.

[28] Greenland, S. (1984). Bias in methods for deriving standardized mortality ratio and attributable fraction estimates, *Statistics in Medicine* **3**, 131–141.

[29] Greenland, S. (1987). Variance estimators for attributable fraction estimates, consistent in both large strata and sparse data, *Statistics in Medicine* **6**, 701–708.

[30] Greenland, S. (1992). The bootstrap method for standard errors and confidence intervals of the adjusted attributable risk (letter), *Epidemiology* **3**, 271.

[31] Greenland, S. & Drescher, K. (1993). Maximum-likelihood estimation of the attributable fraction from logistic models, *Biometrics* **49**, 865–872.

[32] Greenland, S. & Morgenstern, H. (1983). Morgenstern corrects a conceptual error (letter), *American Journal of Public Health* **73**, 703–704.

[33] Greenland, S. & Robins, J.M. (1988). Conceptual problems in the definition and interpretation of attributable fractions, *American Journal of Epidemiology* **128**, 1185–1197.

[34] Hsieh, C.C. (1991). The effect of non-differential outcome misclassification on estimates of the attributable and prevented fraction, *Statistics in Medicine* **10**, 361–373.

[35] Hsieh, C.C. & Walter, S.D. (1988). The effect of non-differential misclassification on estimates of the attributable and prevented fraction, *Statistics in Medicine* **7**, 1073–1085.

[36] Kleinbaum, D.G., Kupper, L.L. & Morgenstern, H. (1982). *Epidemiologic Research: Principles and Quantitative Methods*. Lifetime Learning Publications, Belmont.

[37] Kooperberg, C. & Petitti, D.B. (1991). Using logistic regression to estimate the adjusted attributable risk of low birthweight in an unmatched case–control study, *Epidemiology* **2**, 363–366.

[38] Kuritz, S.J. & Landis, J.R. (1988). Summary attributable risk estimation from unmatched case–control data, *Statistics in Medicine* **7**, 507–517.

[39] Kuritz, S.J. & Landis, J.R. (1988). Attributable risk estimation from matched case–control data, *Biometrics* **44**, 355–367.

[40] La Vecchia C., D'Avanzo, B., Negri, E., Decarli, A. & Benichou, J. (1995). Attributable risks for stomach cancer in Northern Italy, *International Journal of Cancer* **60**, 748–752.

[41] Lagakos, S.W. & Mosteller, F. (1986). Assigned shares in compensation for radiation-related cancers (with discussion), *Risk Analysis* **6**, 345–380.

[42] Landis, J.R., Heyman, E.R. & Koch, G.G. (1978). Average partial association in three-way contingency tables: a review and discussion of alternative tests, *International Statistical Review* **46**, 237–254.

[43] Last, J.M. (1983). *A Dictionary of Epidemiology*. Oxford University Press, New York.

[44] Leung, H.K. & Kupper, L.L. (1981). Comparison of confidence intervals for attributable risk, *Biometrics* **37**, 293–302.

[45] Levin, M.L. (1953). The occurrence of lung cancer in man, *Acta Unio Internationalis contra Cancrum* **9**, 531–541.

[46] Lubin, J.H. & Boice, J.D. Jr (1989). Estimating Rn-induced lung cancer in the United States, *Health Physics* **57**, 417–427.

[47] MacMahon, B. & Pugh, T.F. (1970). *Epidemiology: Principles and Methods*. Little, Brown, & Company, Boston.

[48] Madigan, M.P., Ziegler, R.G., Benichou, J., Byrne, C. & Hoover, R.N. (1995). Proportion of breast cancer cases in the United States explained by well-established risk factors, *Journal of the National Cancer Institute* **87**, 1681–1685.

[49] Mantel, N. & Haenszel, W. (1959). Statistical aspects of the analysis of data from retrospective studies of disease, *Journal of the National Cancer Institute* **22**, 719–748.

[50] Markush, R.E. (1977). Levin's attributable risk statistic for analytic studies and vital statistics, *American Journal of Epidemiology* **105**, 401–406.

[51] Mausner, J.S. & Bahn, A.K. (1974). *Epidemiology: An Introductory Text*. W.B. Saunders, Philadelphia.

[52] Mezzetti, M., Ferraroni, M., Decarli, A., La Vecchia, C. & Benichou, J. (1996). Software for attributable risk and confidence interval estimation in case–control studies, *Computers and Biomedical Research* **29**, 63–75.

[53] Miettinen, O.S. (1974). Proportion of disease caused or prevented by a given exposure, trait or intervention, *American Journal of Epidemiology* **99**, 325–332.

[54] Miettinen, O.S. (1976). Estimability and estimation in case–referent studies, *American Journal of Epidemiology* **103**, 226–235.

[55] Morgenstern, H. (1982). Uses of ecologic analysis in epidemiological research, *American Journal of Public Health* **72**, 1336–1344.

[56] Morgenstern, H. & Bursic, E.S. (1982). A method for using epidemiologic data to estimate the potential impact of an intervention on the health status of a target population, *Journal of Community Health* **7**, 292–309.

[57] Oja, H., Alho, O.P. & Laara, E. (1996). Model-based estimation of the excess fraction (attributable fraction):

day care and middle ear infection, *Statistics in Medicine* **15**, 1519–1534.

[58] Ouellet, B.L., Romeder, J.M. & Lance, J.M. (1979). Premature mortality attributable to smoking and hazardous drinking in Canada, *American Journal of Epidemiology* **109**, 451–463.

[59] Pichlmeier, U. & Gefeller, O. (1997). Conceptual aspects of attributable risk in the case of recurrent disease events, *Statistics in Medicine* **16**, 1107–1120.

[60] Prentice, R.L. (1986). A case-cohort design for epidemiologic cohort studies and disease prevention trials, *Biometrika* **73**, 1–11.

[61] Rao, C.R. (1965). *Linear Statistical Inference and Its Application*. Wiley, New York, pp. 319–322.

[62] Robins, J.M. & Greenland, S. (1989). Estimability and estimation of excess and etiologic fractions, *Statistics in Medicine* **8**, 845–859.

[63] Robins, J.M., Breslow, N.E. & Greenland, S. (1986). Estimators of the Mantel–Haenszel variance consistent in both sparse-data and large-strata limiting models, *Biometrics* **42**, 311–323.

[64] Rockhill, B., Newman, B. & Weinberg, C. (1998). Use and misuse of population attributable fractions, *American Journal of Public Health* **88**, 15–19.

[65] Rockhill, B., Weinberg, C. & Newman, B. (1998). Population attributable fraction estimation for established breast cancer risk factors: considering the issues of high prevalence and unmodifiability, *American Journal of Epidemiology* **147**, 826–833.

[66] Schlesselman, J.J. (1982). *Case–Control Studies. Design, Conduct and Analysis*. Oxford University Press, New York.

[67] Seiler, F.A. (1986) Attributable risk, probability of causation, assigned shares, and uncertainty, *Environment International* **12**, 635–641.

[68] Seiler, F.A. & Scott, B.R. (1987) Mixture of toxic agents and attributable risk calculations, *Risk Analysis* **7**, 81–90.

[69] Silverman, D.T., Brown, L.M., Hoover, R.N., Schiffman, M., Lillemoe, K.D., Schoenberg, J.B., Swanson, G.M., Hayes, R.B., Greenberg, R.S., Benichou, J., Schwartz, A.G., Liff, J.F. & Pottern, L.M. (1995). Alcohol and pancreatic cancer in Blacks and Whites in the United States, *Cancer Research* **55**, 4809–4905.

[70] Spirtas, R., Heineman, E.F., Bernstein, L., Beebe, G.W., Keehn, R.J., Stark, A.S., Harlow, B.L. & Benichou, J. (1994). Malignant melanoma: attributable risk of asbestos exposure, *Occupational and Environmental Medicine* **51**, 804–811.

[71] Sturmans, F., Mulder, P.G.H. & Walkenburg, H.A. (1977). Estimation of the possible effect of interventive measures in the area of ischemic heart diseases by the attributable risk percentage, *American Journal of Epidemiology* **105**, 281–289.

[72] Tarone, R.E. (1981). On summary estimators of relative risk, *Journal of Chronic Diseases* **34**, 463–468.

[73] Tuyns, A.J., Pequignot, J. & Jensen, O.M. (1977). Le cancer de l'oesophage en Ille-et-Vilaine en fonction des niveaux de consommation d'alcool et de tabac, *Bulletin of Cancer* **64**, 45–60.

[74] Wacholder, S., Benichou, J., Heineman, E.F., Hartge, P. & Hoover, R.N. (1994). Attributable risk: advantages of a broad definition of exposure, *American Journal of Epidemiology* **140**, 303–309.

[75] Wahrendorf, J. (1987). An estimate of the proportion of colo-rectal and stomach cancers which might be prevented by certain changes in dietary habits, *International Journal of Cancer* **40**, 625–628.

[76] Walter, S.D. (1975). The distribution of Levin's measure of attributable risk, *Biometrika* **62**, 371–374.

[77] Walter, S.D. (1976). The estimation and interpretation of attributable risk in health research, *Biometrics* **32**, 829–849.

[78] Walter, S.D. (1980). Prevention for multifactorial diseases, *American Journal of Epidemiology* **112**, 409–416.

[79] Walter, S.D. (1983). Effects of interaction, confounding and observational error on attributable risk estimation, *American Journal of Epidemiology* **117**, 598–604.

[80] Whittemore, A.S. (1982). Statistical methods for estimating attributable risk from retrospective data, *Statistics in Medicine* **1**, 229–243.

[81] Whittemore, A.S. (1983). Estimating attributable risk from case–control studies, *American Journal of Epidemiology* **117**, 76–85.

JACQUES BENICHOU

Average Age of Infection *see* Communicable Diseases

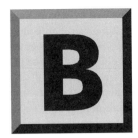

Back-Calculation

Back-calculation – also called back-projection – estimates past infection rates of an epidemic infectious disease by working backward from observed disease **incidence** using knowledge of the **incubation period** between infection and disease. Although potentially applicable to various diseases, it was first proposed [15, 16] to study the acquired immune deficiency syndrome (AIDS) epidemic and has mainly been applied in this area. Performance of back-calculation requires a technical framework for defining and maximizing a likelihood to obtain estimated infection rates, detailed information about key inputs such as incubation and reporting completeness assumptions, and a strategy for assessing uncertainty in the key inputs and resulting uncertainty in back-calculated estimates.

The Basic Method

Suppose that we have n nonoverlapping intervals, (T_{j-1}, T_j), $j = 1, \ldots, n$; let Y_j be the number of persons developing disease in the jth interval, and assume that no infections occurred before time T_0. In practice, these intervals will often be calendar months or quarters. For example, AIDS incidence in the US is reported as the number of new diagnoses each month. Thus, a discrete-time formulation is realistic for practical applications, and we will employ such notation here, assuming a monthly time scale. Back-calculation is based on the following convolution equation:

$$E(Y_j) = \sum_{i=1}^{j} \theta_i, D_{ij}, \quad j = 1, \ldots, n, \qquad (1)$$

where θ_i is the expected number of new infections in month i and D_{ij} is the probability of developing disease in month j given infection in month i; that is, the probability that the incubation time is equal to $j - i$ given infection in month i. Back-calculation is thus a deconvolution method. Given a set of observed values $\mathbf{y} = (y_1, \ldots, y_n)$, it uses known D_{ij} to find a θ likely to have produced $\mathbf{y}$ via (1).

Eq. (1) only specifies the first moment of the Y_j, so implementation of the strategy requires additional specifics. A simple approach is to assume that the Y_j are independent with Poisson error structure. This follows from an assumption that infections arise according to a nonhomogeneous Poisson process. In our discrete-time framework, this means that the number of infections in month i is Poisson with expectation θ_i and the numbers of infections in different months are independent. This assumption produces a log likelihood (up to a constant) of

$$l(\mathbf{y}|\theta) = \sum_{j=1}^{n} \left[y_j \log \left(\sum_{i=1}^{j} \theta_i D_{ij} \right) - \sum_{i=1}^{j} \theta_i D_{ij} \right], \tag{2}$$

which can be maximized to obtain an estimate of θ. To avoid ill-posedness [48], some structure must be imposed on θ. For example, a parametric model might specify that $\theta_i = f_\beta(i)$, where β is a (small) vector of parameters and f is a family of functions indexed by β. Projected values of Y_k for $k > n$ (yet to be observed) can be obtained from (1) using estimates $\hat{\theta}_j$, with $\hat{\theta}_j$ obtained by extrapolation for $n < j \le k$.

Finding parameters that maximize the likelihood (2) may be possible using general numerical approaches such as the Newton–Raphson method, depending on the complexity of the structure imposed on θ. Using an expectation-maximization (EM) algorithm, however, can greatly simplify the computations. Consider the complete data $\{x_{ij}\}$, where x_{ij} is the number of persons infected in month i and diagnosed in month j. Under the assumptions leading to (2), these counts are independent Poisson with means $\theta_i D_{ij}$. The complete-data log likelihood is therefore (up to a constant)

$$\sum_{i=1}^{n} \left[x_i \log(\theta_i) - \theta_i \sum_{j=i}^{n} D_{ij} \right], \qquad (3)$$

where $x_i = \sum_{j=i}^{n} x_{ij}$. This is a linear function of x_i, so its expected value can be calculated using the formula [30]

$$E(x_i | \mathbf{y}, \theta) = \sum_{j=i}^{n} y_j \frac{\theta_i D_{ij}}{\sum_{k=1}^{j} \theta_k D_{kj}}. \qquad (4)$$

The EM algorithm begins with an initial guess for the parameters that determine θ, calculates the expected value of (3) using (4) (the E-step), and finds the new values of the parameters that maximize (3) (the M-step). The E- and M-steps are iterated until the parameter estimates converge. The simple forms of (3) and (4) make this approach computationally easy.

Inputs

Back-calculation requires a known incubation distribution (the D_{ij}) and accurate data on incidence of disease. In addition, a realistic model for infection patterns must be specified.

Incubation

The estimate of the infection pattern θ depends crucially on the assumed incubation distribution [6, 8, 58]. Accurate estimates, however, may be difficult to obtain. Estimation of distributions of incubation times from human immunodeficiency virus (HIV)

infection to AIDS diagnosis illustrates many potential problems in obtaining accurate D_{ij}. These include inherent limitations in available data, heterogeneity of distributions in different populations, and changes over time (nonstationarity).

Data Sources. Inherent limitations arise because HIV infection is usually not immediately detected, and observed incubation times are therefore only available for special groups whose times of HIV infection can be determined retrospectively. These include persons whose HIV infection can be traced to a particular blood transfusion and those whose time of infection can be bracketed by antibody testing of stored specimens from various times in the past. These special groups may not be representative of the wider population for which back-calculation is to be performed. In addition, the data from these sources may suffer from right-truncation [38, 39, 42] or double-censoring [8, 27]. Such data require specialized statistical analysis and convey less information than fully observed data. An extreme form of double-censoring is present for **prevalent** cases – those already infected at the time that they were recruited into a cohort study and followed for development of AIDS. Such subjects are known to have been infected at some time between the start of the epidemic and their time of recruitment (an interval-censored starting time), and their time of AIDS may be right-censored. An additional difficulty is that persons who had already developed AIDS may have been excluded from recruitment. Thus, methods for left-truncated data must be used. Prevalent cohort participants are much more numerous than those with infection times that are more narrowly bracketed by a positive HIV antibody test preceded by a negative one, so investigators have attempted to utilize data from prevalent subjects by imputing infection times using laboratory markers that change with length of infection [36, 47] and by other methods [5, 41, 59].

Heterogeneity. Back-calculation is usually applied to entire populations defined by region of residence and possibly by risk behaviors, but data on incubation times come from highly selected, small groups of persons with known infection times. This would not be a problem if all populations and all the groups shared the same incubation distribution, or if all differences could be accurately explained and quantified in terms of readily measured characteristics such as age. This, however, does not appear to be the case. Direct comparison of data from different sources has shown statistically significant differences between different groups [12], including groups of gay men of similar ages who differ on other characteristics [7, 8, 60, 65]. This heterogeneity adds considerable uncertainty about what incubation distribution to use for a particular population, especially understudied populations such as women or intravenous drug users.

Nonstationarity. Estimation would be simplified if the D_{ij} all depended only on the elapsed time, $j - i$; that is, if the incubation distribution were stationary. In general, however, the chance of developing disease may be nonstationary and also depend on the time of infection, i, or on the current time, j. For example, diagnosis of AIDS may depend on several factors that change over time, including availability and effectiveness of preventive treatments, changes in the official case definition of AIDS [21, 22, 24], changes in care-seeking patterns, and possible evolution of the virus toward more or less virulence. Such phenomena place even greater demands on limited data. A widely used approach has been to assume that no factor other than treatment has caused nonstationarity, and to use data on effectiveness of treatment and usage rates of treatment over time to modify stationary incubation estimates [13]. This results in models in which persons infected more recently have longer incubation times. A more direct approach is to examine the special groups discussed above who have approximately known infection dates, and to use standard **survival analysis** methods to estimate the effect of infection date or calendar time (a time-dependent covariate) on development of AIDS. This estimates the net effect of all factors that may be changing over time. Several such studies have found that incubation times remained constant or actually shortened in the late 1980s and early 1990s compared with earlier in the epidemic [12, 29, 35, 62]. This suggests that other factors, such as more aggressive care seeking or evolution of the virus, accelerated diagnosis of AIDS more than it was slowed by beneficial treatment effects. A dramatic source of nonstationarity in the US is the expansion in 1993 of conditions officially qualifying as an AIDS diagnosis [24]. This had such a large and sudden impact that accurate estimates of the affected D_{ij} may not be obtainable. In addition, introduction of potent protease inhibitors and increased

use of combination antiretroviral therapy starting in the mid-1990s will also influence incubation times.

Incidence

In practice, true disease incidence is not observed exactly because of imperfections in the surveillance system. Incompleteness of the observed incidence arises from reporting delays and from underreporting; that is, cases who are never reported. This incompleteness must be corrected before back-calculation is applied. In addition, the incidence series may contain short-term perturbations, such as seasonal patterns, that can be adjusted out to make long-term trends clearer and to improve the accuracy of back-calculation.

Reporting Delay. Because there is often a lag between diagnosis of disease and the time that it is recorded and tabulated, recent incidence is incomplete. This typically causes a downturn in recent incidence that would severely distort back-calculation results if left uncorrected. The usual strategy is to estimate for each month j a completeness factor, R_j, the proportion of true incidence that has been reported. If y_j^* denotes observed incidence, one can apply back-calculation to corrected counts $y_j = y_j^*/R_j$. (Alternatively, the R_j can be incorporated directly into the back-calculation procedure [6].) A common practice is to exclude counts that are so recent that they are estimated to be less than 50% complete. If surveillance provides both date of disease and date of report, incompleteness due to reporting delay can be estimated if one assumes a maximum possible length of delay [25]. This requires specialized methods [14, 39, 50] because of the severe right-truncation caused by the fact that the only cases available for analysis are those with short enough delays to have been already reported. In addition, dependence of delays on case characteristics and changes in delay patterns over time can be estimated. Estimates of changes over time can be strongly influenced by irrelevant shifts in the patterns of very short delays, so modifications to avoid this lead to better estimates [1]. In the US, the 1993 change in the AIDS case definition apparently had a strong impact on reporting, even of cases meeting the earlier definition [4].

Underreporting. In addition to delays in reporting, there also may be cases that are never reported. Such underreporting of AIDS cases has been investigated to a limited extent by cross matching reported AIDS cases to cases identified by other means, notably **death certificates** that list HIV under cause of death [19, 31]. The proportion of cases found by other means that are not also in the **surveillance** system provides an estimate of the underreporting rate. (More sophisticated capture–recapture methods have not been widely used.) Studies of underreporting require use of personal identifiers, and so are usually carried out at a local level. They also usually apply to a specific time period. Consequently, extensive systematic data on underreporting is typically not available for the population under consideration, and assuming constant underreporting of between 10% and 20% is a common practice. Such assumptions must be combined with estimated incompleteness due to reporting delay to obtain R_j that reflect both sources of incompleteness.

Short-term Patterns.   Season can influence the incidence of some infectious diseases, notably AIDS, and incidence of AIDS in a particular month is also influenced by how many workdays it includes [2]. The lengths of calendar months also vary by 10%. These short-term influences increase month-to-month variability and can degrade back-calculation results. Performance can be improved by estimating these effects and adjusting them out of the incidence series to be used [2, 3].

Infection Model

As noted above, some structure must be imposed on θ to allow stable estimation. Both parametric and nonparametric approaches have been used. Parametric approaches include smooth families indexed by two or three parameters [26, 58, 63], as well as step functions with four or five steps, within which infection rates are assumed to be constant [16, 55]. Although these step models are not plausible, they are flexible, and have been made more so by modifications to allow adaptive selection of cutpoints between steps [56]. Nonparametric approaches do not directly parameterize θ but obtain smooth estimates by either adding a smoothing step after the M-step of the EM algorithm [11], or by using penalized maximum likelihood [6] or ridge regression [49]. Some methods combine aspects of the parametric and nonparametric approaches [13, 32].

Sensitivity Analyses

Asymptotic standard errors for estimated infection rates and future incidence projections can be obtained from the observed information matrix for θ or by bootstrap methods, but this captures only a small part of the real uncertainty. Possible errors in the inputs to back-calculation cause much greater uncertainty in the results. Sensitivity analyses that employ a wide variety of inputs (consistent with available data on incubation and incidence) can serve to more realistically illustrate the plausible range of possibilities. (Bayesian methods that incorporate priors for the various inputs could offer a more formal assessment of uncertainty [20, 58], but these have not been widely used.) If the range of plausible inputs is large, as in the case of HIV and AIDS, exhaustive exploration of possible uncertainty may be difficult. Sensitivity analyses for back-calculation from AIDS incidence have generally considered from two to five possible incubation distributions [6, 54, 63], and often not considered uncertainty in the incidence series. An additional difficulty when uncertainties in the inputs are wide is that back-calculated results from some inputs may contradict what is known (at least qualitatively) from other sources, such as cross-sectional prevalence surveys or cohort studies. Simply dropping the offending inputs from the sensitivity analyses, however, is not adequate, because the remaining set of possibilities will be too narrow, even if the original set was adequate. This is because there is a continuum of plausible possibilities between the eliminated and retained possibilities, some of which are consistent with the outside information. When inputs that are a priori plausible produce implausible results, formal methods to combine back-calculation with the outside data [17] should be considered, as should the possibility that back-calculation cannot meaningfully improve on what is known directly from the outside data.

Incubation

The assumed incubation distribution strongly influences estimated infection rates. This is apparent from the forms of (1) and (2), where the incubation terms D_{ij} and the θ_i always appear multiplied together. Different plausible AIDS incubation distributions can lead to estimates of cumulative HIV infections in the US that differ by factors of two or more, while providing nearly identical fits to the observed AIDS incidence data [6, 8]. This implies that errors in the D_{ij} will not be detectable in the back-calculation process itself, because their influence will be masked by compensating errors in the estimate of θ and no lack of fit will be apparent. This and the sources of uncertainty noted above underscore the need for careful sensitivity analysis of incubation assumptions. Nonstationarity in the incubation distribution can also influence back-calculated estimates. For example, a slowdown in incidence will be attributed to an earlier decline in infections if a stationary incubation is assumed, but could also be explained by recent lengthening of incubation times.

Disease Incidence

Assumptions about reporting delay and underreporting can strongly influence projections. Differing reasonable assumptions about underreporting and late reporting of AIDS cases diagnosed through 1991 in the US resulted in two-year projections that differed by 20% or more [1], and additional uncertainty about very late reporting increases this difference to at least 30% [3, 25]. In addition, one can see from (1) that underreporting has a direct impact on the estimate of θ. For example, assuming constant 80% reporting instead of 90% reporting would increase all of the imputed y_j by about 13% (0.9/0.8), resulting in a corresponding proportional increase in all of the estimated θ_i.

Refinements

A wide variety of technical refinements, extensions, and modifications of back-calculation have been studied. Notable among these are methods for: incorporating results of HIV **prevalence** surveys [17]; allowing for dependence in the HIV infection process [9]; estimating overdispersion in a quasi-likelihood approach [17, 43]; utilizing data on HIV tests [45, 52]; using age at time of AIDS to back-calculate age-specific HIV incidence [10, 53]; nonparametric modeling of infection rates, including data-driven choices of smoothness parameters [6, 32, 44]; incorporating knowledge of the size of the susceptible population [61]. Because of the considerable uncertainty about crucial inputs, however, these refinements may not be able meaningfully to improve the accuracy of back-calculation.

Limitations

A key limitation of back-calculation is the need for accurate inputs, as noted above. Because uncertainty in the results comes mainly from uncertainty about these inputs, estimates of pure statistical uncertainty are misleading. Two additional limitations of the method are that it provides little information about recent infection rates and that projections can be overly sensitive to recent incidence.

Back-calculation is primarily useful with epidemic infectious diseases for which there is a substantial lag between infection and disease. If a disease is in a steady state or if disease rapidly follows infection, then infection rates can be adequately ascertained directly from disease incidence. Because of this focus, there will be little direct information about recent infection rates and back-calculated estimates of θ_j for j close to n will be determined mainly by implicit extrapolation, from either the parametric model of θ or the form of the smoothness assumption. For example, because few persons develop AIDS within two years following HIV infection, back-calculation from AIDS incidence provides little information about infection rates in the last two years.

Projections from back-calculation can be overly sensitive to counts near the end of the incidence series. This is particularly true for AIDS if seasonal patterns are not adjusted out of the incidence series [3]. For example, anomalously high AIDS incidence in the US in the first half of 1987 caused projections from back-calculations to be too high, which was interpreted as evidence for a treatment-induced downturn in incidence [28]. The projections would have been more accurate if deseasonalized incidence had been used, and would have been much better if a more robust projection method had been used. Two- or three-year projections based on incidence through the end of 1986 also would have been fairly accurate [3].

Alternatives

A simple alternative for projecting future incidence is empirical extrapolation [34, 40, 46, 64]. This can be reasonably accurate [3], but provides no information about infection rates and has no ability to anticipate changes in trajectory. Measurement of infections in cross-sectional surveys and cohorts followed over time provides direct information on prevalence and incidence of infections. Such studies are most useful when performed anonymously on specimens collected for other purposes [33, 51], because this can eliminate the potentially serious problem of **nonresponse bias** [23]. In **cohort studies** of incidence, serious dropout bias can result from the fact that higher-risk subjects may be more likely to fail to return for follow-up testing. Markers of recent infection can be used to estimate current incidence without relying on follow-up and to correct dropout bias [18], provided that the initial sample is representative and that the average duration of the marker is known. One can deduce the shape of the infection density from the mix of laboratory markers, such as CD4 counts, in one or more cross-sectional surveys of infected individuals [57]. This requires a representative sample of infected persons and detailed knowledge of how the marker evolves over time since infection, which may be more difficult to obtain than the incubation information required by back-calculation [37]. Mathematical epidemic modeling is used mainly to further qualitative understanding, and typically requires too detailed input to provide useful quantitative results (*see* **Epidemic Models, Deterministic**; **Epidemic Models, Stochastic**).

References

[1]   Bacchetti, P. (1994). The impact of lengthening AIDS reporting delays and uncertainty about underreporting on incidence trends and projections, *Journal of Acquired Immune Deficiency Syndromes* **7**, 860–865.

[2]   Bacchetti, P. (1994). Seasonal and other short-term influences on United States AIDS incidence, *Statistics in Medicine* **13**, 1921–1931.

[3]   Bacchetti, P. (1995). Historical assessment of some specific methods for projecting the AIDS epidemic, *American Journal of Epidemiology* **141**, 776–781.

[4]   Bacchetti P. (1996). Reporting delay of deaths with AIDS in the United States, *Journal of Acquired Immune Deficiency Syndromes and Human Retrovirology* **13**, 363–367.

[5]   Bacchetti, P. & Jewell, N.P. (1991). Nonparametric estimation of the incubation period of AIDS based on a prevalent cohort with unknown infection times, *Biometrics* **47**, 947–960.

[6]   Bacchetti, P., Segal, M.R. & Jewell, N.P. (1993). Back-calculation of HIV infection rates, *Statistical Science* **8**, 82–119.

[7]   Bacchetti, P., Koblin, B.A., van Griensven, G.J.P. & Hessol, N.A. (1996). Determinants of HIV disease progression among homosexual men, *American Journal of Epidemiology* **143**, 526.

[8]   Bacchetti, P., Segal, M.R., Hessol, N.A. & Jewell, N.P. (1993). Differing AIDS incubation periods and their impacts on reconstructing HIV epidemics and projecting AIDS incidence, *Proceedings of the National Academy of Sciences* **90**, 2194–2196.

[9]   Becker, N.G. & Chao, X. (1994). Dependent HIV incidences in back-projection of AIDS incidence data, *Statistics in Medicine* **13**, 1945–1958.

[10]   Becker, N.G. & Marschner, I.C. (1993). A method for estimating the age-specific relative risk of HIV infection for AIDS incidence data, *Biometrika* **80**, 165–178.

[11]   Becker, N.G., Watson, L.F. & Carlin, J.B. (1991). A method of nonparametric back-projection and its application to AIDS data, *Statistics in Medicine* **10**, 1527–1542.

[12]   Biggar, J. (1990). AIDS incubation in 1891 HIV seroconverters from different exposure groups, *AIDS* **4**, 1059–1066.

[13]   Brookmeyer, R. (1991). Reconstruction and future trends of the AIDS epidemic in the United States, *Science* **253**, 37–42.

[14]   Brookmeyer, R. & Damiano, A. (1989). Statistical methods for short-term projections of AIDS incidence, *Statistics in Medicine* **8**, 23–34.

[15]   Brookmeyer, R. & Gail, M.H. (1986). Minimum size of the acquired immunodeficiency syndrome (AIDS) epidemic in the United States, *Lancet* **2**, 1320–1322.

[16]   Brookmeyer, R. & Gail, M.H. (1988). A method for obtaining short term predictions and lower bounds on the size of the AIDS epidemic, *Journal of the American Statistical Association* **83**, 301–308.

[17]   Brookmeyer, R. & Liao, J. (1990). Statistical modelling of the AIDS epidemic for forecasting health care needs, *Biometrics* **46**, 1151–1163.

[18]   Brookmeyer, R., Quinn, T., Shepherd, M., Mehendale, S., Rodrigues, J. & Bollinger, R. (1995). The AIDS epidemic in India: a new method for estimating current human immunodeficiency virus (HIV) incidence rates, *American Journal of Epidemiology* **142**, 709–713.

[19]   Buehler, J.W., Berkelman, R.L. & Stehr-Green, J.K. (1992). The completeness of AIDS surveillance, *Journal of Acquired Immune Deficiency Syndromes* **5**, 257–264.

[20]   Carlin, J.B. & Gelman, A. (1993). Comment: assessing uncertainty in backprojection, *Statistical Science* **8**, 104–106.

[21]   Centers for Disease Control (1985). Revision of the case definition of acquired immune deficiency syndrome for national reporting–United States, *Morbidity and Mortality Weekly Reports* **34**, 373–375.

[22]   Centers for Disease Control (1987). Revision of the CDC surveillance case definition for acquired immunodeficiency syndrome, *Morbidity and Mortality Weekly Reports* **36**, 3S–15S.

[23] Centers for Disease Control (1991). Pilot study of a household survey to determine HIV seroprevalence, *Morbidity and Mortality Weekly Reports* **40**, 1–5.

[24] Centers for Disease Control and Prevention (1992). 1993 revised classification system for HIV infection and expanded surveillance case definition for AIDS among adolescents and adults, *Morbidity and Mortality Weekly Reports* **41** (No. RR-17), 1–18.

[25] Cooley, P.C., Hamill, D.N., Meyers, L.E. & Liner, E.C. (1993). The assumption of no long reporting delays may result in underestimates of US AIDS incidence, *AIDS* **7**, 1379–1381.

[26] Day, N.E., Gore, S.M., McGee, M.A. & South, M. (1989). Predictions of the AIDS epidemic in the UK: the use of the back projection method, *Philosophical Transactions of the Royal Society of London, Series B* **325**, 123–134.

[27] DeGruttola, V. & Lagakos, S.W. (1989). Analysis of doubly-censored survival data, with application to AIDS, *Biometrics* **45**, 1–11.

[28] Gail, M.H., Rosenberg, P.S. & Goedert, J.J. (1990). Therapy may explain recent deficits in AIDS incidence, *Journal of Acquired Immune Deficiency Syndromes* **3**, 296–306.

[29] Gauvreau, K., DeGruttola, V. & Pagano, M. (1994). The effect of covariates on the induction time of AIDS using improved imputation of exact seroconversion times, *Statistics in Medicine* **13**, 2021–2030.

[30] Green, P.J. (1990). On use of the EM algorithm for penalized likelihood estimation, *Journal of the Royal Statistical Society, Series B* **52**, 443–452.

[31] Greenberg, A.E., Hindin, R., Nicholas, A.G., Bryan, E.L. & Thomas, P.A. (1993). The completeness of AIDS case reporting in New York City, *Journal of the American Medical Association* **269**, 2995–3001.

[32] Greenland, S. (1996). Historical HIV incidence modelling in regional subgroups: use of flexible discrete models with penalized splines based on prior curves, *Statistics in Medicine* **15**, 513–525.

[33] Gwinn, M., Pappaioanou, M., George, J.R., Hannon, W.H., Wasser, S.C., Redus, M.A., Hoff, R., Grady, G.F., Willoughby, A., Novello, A.C., Petersen, L.R., Dondero, T.J., Jr & Curran, J.W. (1991). Prevalence of HIV infection in childbearing women in the United States. Surveillance using newborn blood samples, *Journal of the American Medical Association* **265**, 1704–1708.

[34] Healy, M.J.R. & Tillet, H.E. (1988). Short-term extrapolation of the AIDS epidemic, *Journal of the Royal Statistical Society, Series A* **151**, 50–65.

[35] Hessol, N.A., Koblin, B.A., van Griensven, G.J.P., Bacchetti, P., Liu, J.Y., Stevens, C.E., Coutinho, R.A., Buchbinder, S.P. & Katz, M.H. (1994). Progression of human immunodeficiency virus type 1 (HIV-1) infection among homosexual men in hepatitis B vaccine trial cohorts in Amsterdam, New York City, and San Francisco 1978–1991, *American Journal of Epidemiology* **139**, 1077–1087.

[36] Hoover, D.R., Taylor, J.M.G., Kingsley, L., Chmiel, J.S., Munoz, A., He, Y. & Saah, A. (1994). The effectiveness of interventions on incubation of AIDS as measured by secular increases within a population, *Statistics in Medicine* **13**, 2127–2139.

[37] Jewell, N.P. & Kalbfleisch, J.D. (1992). Marker models in survival analysis and applications to issues associated with AIDS, in *AIDS Epidemiology: Methodological Issues*, N.P. Jewell, K. Dietz & V.T. Farewell, eds. Birkhauser, Boston.

[38] Kalbfleisch, J.D. & Lawless, J.F. (1988). Estimating the incubation period for AIDS patients, *Nature* **333**, 504–505.

[39] Kalbfleisch, J.D. & Lawless, J.F. (1989). Inference based on retrospective ascertainment: an analysis of the data on transfusion-related AIDS, *Journal of the American Statistical Association* **84**, 360–372.

[40] Karon, J.M., Devine, O.J. & Morgan, W.M. (1989). Predicting AIDS incidence by extrapolating from recent trends, in *Mathematical and Statistical Approaches to AIDS Epidemiology*, C. Castillo-Chavez, ed. Springer-Verlag, New York, pp. 58–88.

[41] Kuo, J.-M., Taylor, J.M.G. & Detels, R. (1991). Estimating the AIDS incubation period from a prevalent cohort, *American Journal of Epidemiology* **133**, 1050–1057.

[42] Lagakos, S.W., Barraj, L.M. & DeGruttola, V. (1988). Nonparametric analysis of truncated survival data with applications to AIDS, *Biometrika* **75**, 515–523.

[43] Lawless, J.F. & Sun, J. (1992). A comprehensive back-calculation framework for the estimation and prediction of AIDS cases, in *AIDS Epidemiology: Methodological Issues*, N.P. Jewell, K. Dietz & V.T. Farewell, eds. Birkhauser, Boston.

[44] Liao, J. & Brookmeyer, R. (1995). An empirical Bayes approach to smoothing in backcalculation of HIV infection rates, *Biometrics* **51**, 579–588.

[45] Marschner, I.C. (1994). Using time of first positive HIV test and other auxiliary data in back-projection of AIDS incidence, *Statistics in Medicine* **13**, 1959–1974.

[46] Morgan, W.M. & Curran, J.W. (1986). Acquired immunodeficiency syndrome: current and future trends, *Public Health Reports* **101**, 459–465.

[47] Munoz, A., Wang, M.-C., Bass, S., Taylor, J.M.G., Kingsley, L.A., Chmiel, J.S. & Polk, B.F. (1989). Acquired immunodeficiency syndrome (AIDS)-free time after human immunodeficiency virus type 1 (HIV-1) seroconversion in homosexual men, *American Journal of Epidemiology* **130**, 530–539.

[48] O'Sullivan, F. (1986). A statistical perspective on ill-posed inverse problems, *Statistical Science* **1**, 502–527.

[49] Pagano, M., DeGruttola, V., MaWhinney, S. & Tu, X.M. (1992). The HIV epidemic in New York City: statistical methods for projecting AIDS incidence and prevalence, in *AIDS Epidemiology: Methodological Issues*, N.P. Jewell, K. Dietz & V.T. Farewell, eds. Birkhauser, Boston.

[50] Pagano, M., Tu, X.M., DeGruttola, V. & MaWhinney, S. (1994). Regression analysis of censored and truncated data: estimating reporting-delay distributions and AIDS incidence from surveillance data, *Biometrics* **50**, 1203–1214.

[51] Pappaioanou, M., Dondero, T.J., Peterson, L.R., Onorato, I.M., Sanchez, C.D. & Curran, J.W. (1990). The family of HIV seroprevalence surveys: objectives, methods, and uses of sentinel surveillance for HIV in the United States, *Public Health Reports* **105**, 113–119.

[52] Raab, G.M., Fielding, K.L. & Allardice, G. (1994). Incorporating HIV test data into forecasts of the AIDS epidemic in Scotland, *Statistics in Medicine* **13**, 2009–2020.

[53] Rosenberg, P.S. (1994). Backcalculation models of age-specific HIV incidence rates, *Statistics in Medicine* **13**, 1975–1990.

[54] Rosenberg, P.S. (1995). Scope of the AIDS epidemic in the United States, *Science* **270**, 1372–1375.

[55] Rosenberg, P.S. & Gail, M.H. (1990). Uncertainty in estimates of HIV prevalence derived by backcalculation, *Annals of Epidemiology* **1**, 105–115.

[56] Rosenberg, P.S. & Gail, M.H. (1991). Backcalculation of flexible linear models of the human immunodeficiency virus infection curve, *Applied Statistics* **40**, 269–282.

[57] Satten, G.A. & Longini, I.M. (1994). Estimation of incidence of HIV infection using cross-sectional marker surveys, *Biometrics* **50**, 675–688.

[58] Taylor, J.M.G. (1989). Models for the HIV infection and AIDS epidemic in the United States, *Statistics in Medicine* **8**, 45–58.

[59] Taylor, J.M.G., Kuo, J-M. & Detels, R. (1991). Is the incubation period of AIDS lengthening?, *Journal of Acquired Immune Deficiency Syndromes* **4**, 69–75.

[60] van Griensven, G.J.P., Veugelers, P.J., Page-Shafer, K.A., Kaldor, J.M. & Schechter, M.T. (1996). Determinants of HIV disease progression among homosexual men, *American Journal of Epidemiology* **143**, 525.

[61] Verdecchia, A. & Mariotto, A.B. (1995). A back-calculation method to estimate the age and period HIV infection intensity, considering the susceptible population, *Statistics in Medicine* **14**, 1513–1530.

[62] Veugelers, P.J., Page, K.A., Tindall, B., Schechter, M.T., Moss, A.R., Winkelstein, W.W., Jr., Cooper, D.A., Craib, K.J.P., Charlebois, E., Coutinho, R.A. & van Griensven, G.J.P. (1994). Determinants of HIV disease progression among homosexual men registered in the Tricontinental Seroconverter Study, *American Journal of Epidemiology* **140**, 747–758.

[63] Wilson, S.R., Fazekas de St. Groth, C. & Solomon, P.J. (1992). Sensitivity analyses for the backcalculation method of AIDS projections, *Journal of Acquired Immune Deficiency Syndromes* **5**, 523–527.

[64] Zeger, S.L., See, L.-C. & Diggle, P.J. (1989). Statistical methods for monitoring the AIDS epidemic, *Statistics in Medicine* **8**, 3–21.

[65] Zwahlen, M., Vlahov, D. & Hoover, D.R. (1996). Determinants of HIV disease progression among homosexual men, *American Journal of Epidemiology* **143**, 523–525.

Bibliography

In addition to the above references, see the following for readable discussions of many topics related to back-calculation as applied to the AIDS epidemic:

Brookmeyer, R. & Gail, M.H. (1994). *AIDS Epidemiology: A Quantitative Approach*. Oxford University Press, New York.

PETER BACCHETTI

Balancing Scores *see* Confounder Summary Score

Baseline Hazard; Baseline Survival Function *see* Cox Regression Model

Berkson Error Model *see* Measurement Error in Epidemiologic Studies

Berkson's Fallacy

Berkson's fallacy, also referred to as Berkson's bias or Berkson's paradox, was first described in 1946 by Joseph Berkson, a physician in the Division of Biometry and Medical Statistics at Mayo Clinic. Berkson demonstrated mathematically that an association reported from a **hospital-based case–control study** can be distorted if cases and controls experience differential hospital admission rates with respect to the suspected causal factor [1].

His hypothetical example involved the association between two medical conditions – cholecystitis (the suspected causal factor) and diabetes (the outcome of interest). Assuming a hospital-based study, he defined controls as persons with a third condition, refractive errors, not thought to be correlated with cholecystitis. Calculations were based on the following assumptions: (i) the incidence of cholecystitis does not vary between diabetics and persons with refractive errors in the general population (i.e. **relative risk** and **odds ratio** close to 1.0); (ii) hospital admission rates *do* vary between diabetics and persons with refractive errors (5% and 20%, respectively); (iii) persons with cholecystitis experience a 15% probability of hospitalization; and (iv) the probabilities of hospitalization for the three conditions – diabetes, refractive errors, cholecystitis – behave independently and combine together according to the laws of probability. Using these conditions, a hospitalized subset was defined from Berkson's fabricated general population (Tables 1 and 2). Comparison of these

two populations reveals that the association between cholecystitis and diabetes apparent in the hospitalized data (odds ratio of 1.89 calculated from data in Table 2) is not indicative of the "true" association (or lack of it) in the general population (odds ratio of 0.90 calculated from data in Table 1).

Berkson's bias remained theoretical and was largely disregarded by epidemiologists [3] until 1978 when Roberts et al. provided the first empirical support using data from household surveys of health care utilization [2]. They examined associations between several medical conditions and documented significant differences between community- and hospital-based risk estimates. These **biases** occurred in both directions.

Berkson's original representation of the admission rate bias was based on a conservative assumption of independence for disease-specific admission rates [1]. In practice, however, a given medical condition may exacerbate a second condition, increasing the probability of differential hospitalization rates. Additionally, other circumstances such as the

Table 1 Cholecystitis and diabetes, hypothetical general population[a]

	Cholecystitis	Not cholecystitis	Total
Diabetes[b]	3 000	97 000	100 000
Refractive errors (not diabetic)	29 700	960 300	990 000
Total	32 700	1 057 300	1 090 000
Cholecystitis in diabetic group			3%
Cholecystitis in control group (refractive errors)			3%
Difference			0%

[a]Adapted from [1].
[b]10 000 of the 100 000 cases of diabetes also have refractive errors (300 cases with cholecystitis and 9700 cases without cholecystitis); the refractive errors control group contains no known cases of diabetes.

Table 2 Cholecystitis and diabetes, hypothetical hospital population[a]

	Cholecystitis	Not cholecystitis	Total
Diabetes	626	6 693	7 319
Refractive errors (not diabetic)	9 504	192 060	201 564
Total	10 130	198 753	208 883
Cholecystitis in diabetic group			8.55%
Cholecystitis in control group (refractive errors)			4.72%
Difference			+3.83%

Hospital admission rates for cholecystitis = 0.15, diabetes = 0.05, refractive error = 0.20.
[a]Adapted from [1].

manifestation and severity of symptoms, treatment regimen of choice, and specialization of certain hospitals (or physicians practicing within certain hospitals) in treating given medical conditions, may further increase the disparity between case and control admission rates.

Berkson's fallacy has been primarily described for a certain subset of analyses in which the association of interest is between two medical conditions. It is conceivable that a similar bias might impact **case–control studies** considering a nonmedical explanatory variable, if: (i) the explanatory variable is represented disproportionately in a hospital setting; and (ii) cases and controls experience differential hospital admission rates. Berkson gives a hypothetical example of a study of occupation as an explanatory variable for heart disease in which one occupation group is more likely to present to a hospital for heart disease treatment than another.

Finally, Berkson's bias may have applications beyond the hospital setting. For example, a study of drug use and violent crime in a prison population, using nonviolent criminals as the control group, might result in a different risk estimate than the same study performed in a community-based population.

It is not possible to correct for admission rate bias during analysis. Berkson's bias, like other biases, is a design issue that needs consideration prior to initiating a case–control study drawing participants from a select segment of the general population.

References

[1]   Berkson, J. (1946). Limitation of the application of fourfold tables to hospital data, *Biometrics Bulletin* **2**, 47–53.
[2]   Roberts, R.S., Spitzer, W.O., Delmore, T. & Sackett, D.L. (1978). An empirical demonstration of Berkson's bias, *Journal of Chronic Diseases* **31**, 119–128.
[3]   Sartwell, P.E. (1974). Retrospective studies: a review for the clinician, *Annals of Internal Medicine* **81**, 381–386.

LAURA A. SCHIEVE

Bernoulli Sampling *see* Case–Control Study, Two-Phase

Bias

Bias is the expected deviation of an estimate from the true quantity to be estimated. If an estimator $\hat{\theta}$ of a parameter θ has expectation $\theta + b$, the quantity b is called the bias. If $\hat{\theta}$ converges to $\theta + b$ as the sample size increases, then $\hat{\theta}$ is said to have asymptotic bias b. Some biases result from the small sample properties of the estimator used and vanish asymptotically. Most biases that result from **systematic error**, however, such as **selection biases** or biases in measuring outcomes, persist as the sample size increases. Indeed, increasing the sample size does not eliminate such biases but only leads to more precise biased estimates.

(*See also* **Bias in Case–Control Studies**; **Bias in Cohort Studies**; **Bias in Observational Studies**; **Bias, Overview**)

M.H. GAIL

Bias, Nondifferential

When comparing exposed with unexposed groups, unbiased estimates of exposure effect may result if the same (nondifferential) **biases** affect each exposure group. Nondifferential bias is bias that affects each exposure (or treatment) group in such a way that the resulting exposure effect measure remains unbiased. For example, suppose that 10% of the exposed group and 5% of the unexposed group develop cancer in a given time period, corresponding to a true **relative risk** of 10%/5% = 2.0. Suppose, however, that follow-up procedures fail to detect 20% of incident cancers in each group, resulting in apparent cancer risks of 8% and 4%, respectively. Despite the fact that each of these **risks** is biased, the relative risk, 8%/4% = 2.0, is unbiased. Thus, with respect to relative risk, these biases are nondifferential. If, instead, the chosen measure of exposure effect was the risk difference, 10% − 5% = 5%, these same errors would yield a biased estimate of 8% − 4% = 4%. Thus, an error process may induce nondifferential bias with respect to one effect measure but differential bias with respect to another measure.

Nondifferential bias results from a **nondifferential error** process. In the previous example, the underestimates, 8% and 4%, depended only on the corresponding true values, 10% and 5%, respectively, and not on the exposure group, because the error process missed 20% of incident cancers, regardless of exposure group. Thus, the error was nondifferential.

(*See also* **Misclassification Error**)

M.H. GAIL

Bias, Overview

Bias is defined as the "deviation of results or inferences from the truth, or processes leading to such deviation" [11]. In other words, it is the extent to which the expected value of an estimator differs from a population parameter. Bias refers to **systematic errors** that decrease the validity of estimates, and does not refer to **random errors** that decrease the precision of estimates. Unlike random error, bias cannot be eliminated or reduced by an increase in sample size.

Bias can occur as a result of flaws in the following stages of research [16]:

1. literature review,
2. study design,
3. study execution,
4. data collection,
5. analysis,
6. interpretation of results, and
7. publication.

Literature Review Bias

Literature review bias (syn. reading-up bias) refers to errors in reading-up on the field [16]. Examples include:

Foreign language exclusion bias: literature reviews and meta-analyses that ignore publications in foreign languages [5].

Literature search bias: caused by lack of a computerized literature search, incomplete search due to poor choice of keywords and search strategies, or failure to include unpublished reports or hard-to-reach journals through interlibrary loans.

One-sided reference bias: investigators may restrict their references to only those studies that support their position [16].

Rhetoric bias: authors may use the art of writing to convince the reader without appealing to scientific fact or reason [16].

Design Bias

Design bias refers to errors occurring as a result of faulty design of a study [11]. This can arise from faulty selection of subjects, noncomparable groups chosen for comparison, or inappropriate sample size.

Selection Bias

Selection bias is a distortion in the estimate of effect resulting from the manner in which subjects are selected for the study population. Bias in selection can arise: (i) if the sampling frame is defective, (ii) if the sampling process is nonrandom, or (iii) if some sections of the **target population** are excluded (noncoverage bias) [13].

Sampling frame bias. This type of bias arises when the sampling frame that serves as the basis for selection does not cover the population adequately, completely, or accurately [13]. Examples include:

Ascertainment bias: arising from the kind of patients (e.g. slightly ill, moderately ill, acutely ill) that the individual observer is seeing, or from the diagnostic process which may be determined by the culture, customs, or individual disposition of the health care provider [11]. (See also diagnostic access bias.)

Berkson bias (*see* **Berkson's Fallacy**) (syn. admission rate bias, hospital admission bias): caused by selective factors that lead hospital cases and controls in a case–control study to be systematically different from one another [1, 6].

Centripetal bias: the reputations of certain clinicians and institutions cause individuals with specific disorders or exposures to gravitate toward them [16].

Diagnostic access bias: patients may not be identified because they have no access to diagnostic process due to culture or other reasons. (See also ascertainment bias, hospital access bias.)

Diagnostic purity bias: when "pure" diagnostic groups exclude comorbidity, they may become nonrepresentative [16].

Hospital access bias: patients may not be identified because they are not sick enough to require hospital care, or because they are excluded from hospitals as a result of distance or cost considerations. (See also ascertainment bias, diagnostic access bias, referral filter bias.)

Migrator bias: migrants may differ systematically from those who stay home [16].

Neyman bias (syn. attrition bias, prevalence–incidence bias, selective survival bias; *see* **Bias from Survival in Prevalent Case–Control Studies**): caused by excluding those who die before the study starts because the exposure increases mortality risk [6, 14].

Telephone sampling bias: if **telephone sampling** is used to select a sample of individuals, then persons living in households without telephones would be systematically excluded from the study population, although they would be included in the target population.

Nonrandom sampling bias.   This type of bias arises if the sampling is done by a nonrandom method, so that the selection is consciously or unconsciously influenced by human choice [13]. Examples include:

Autopsy series bias: resulting from the fact that autopsies represent a nonrandom sample of all deaths [11].

Detection bias (syn. selective surveillance bias, verification bias): caused by errors in methods of ascertainment, diagnosis, or verification of cases in an epidemiologic investigation, for example verification of diagnosis by laboratory tests in hospital cases, but not in cases outside the hospital [6, 11]. (See also diagnostic work-up bias, unmasking bias.)

Diagnostic work-up bias (syn. sequential-ordering bias): arises if the results of a diagnostic or screening test affect the decision to order the "gold standard" procedure that provides the most definitive result about the disease [15], for example those who have a negative screening test are systematically excluded from the gold standard procedure [3]. (See also detection bias, unmasking bias.)

Door-to-door solicitation bias: subjects obtained by door knocking are more likely to be the elderly, unemployed, and less active individuals who tend to stay at home.

Previous opinion bias: the tactics and results of a previous diagnostic process on a patient, if known, may affect the tactics and results of a subsequent diagnostic process on the same patient [16]. (See also diagnostic work-up bias.)

Referral filter bias: as a group of patients are referred from primary to secondary to tertiary care, the concentration of rare causes, multiple diagnoses, and severe cases may increase [16]. (See also hospital access bias.)

Sampling bias: caused by the use of nonprobability sampling methods that do not ensure that all members of the population have a known chance of selection in the sample [11].

Self-selection bias (syn. self-referral bias): subjects contact the investigators on their own initiative in response to publicity about the investigation.

Unmasking bias (syn. signal detection bias): an innocent exposure may become suspect if, rather than causing a disease, it causes a sign or symptom which leads to a search for the disease [16]. (See also detection bias, diagnostic work-up bias.)

Noncoverage bias.   This type of bias arises if some sections of the population are impossible to find or refuse to cooperate [13]. Examples include:

Early-comer bias (syn. latecomer bias): "early-comers" from a specified sample may exhibit exposures or outcomes which differ from those of "latecomers" [6], for example early-comers in a study tend to be healthier, and less likely to smoke [16]. (See also response bias.)

Illegal immigrant bias: when census data are used to calculate death rates, bias is caused by illegal immigrants who appear in the numerator (based on death records) but not in the denominator (based on census data).

Loss to follow-up bias: caused by differences in characteristics between those subjects who remain in a cohort study and those who are lost to follow-up [6] (*see* **Bias from Loss to Follow-Up**).

Response bias (syn. nonrespondent bias, volunteer bias): caused by differences in characteristics between those who choose or volunteer to participate in a study and those who do not [11] (*see* **Bias from Nonresponse**). An example is the forecast of the US presidential election in a 1936 survey of 10 million individuals that went wrong because the response rate was only 20%, and the respondents presumably came from a higher social class than the general electorate [13]. (See also early-comer bias.)

Withdrawal bias: caused by differences in the characteristics of those subjects who choose to withdraw and those who choose to remain [11, 16].

Noncomparability Bias

Noncomparability bias occurs if the groups chosen for comparison are not comparable. Examples include:

Ecological bias (syn. **ecologic fallacy**): the associations observed between variables at the group level on the basis of ecological data may not be the same as the associations that exist at the individual level.

Healthy Worker Effect (HWE): an observed decrease in mortality in workers when compared with the general population [4] (*see* **Occupational Epidemiology**). This is a type of membership bias [6].

Lead-time bias (syn. zero time shift bias): occurs when follow-up of two groups does not begin at strictly comparable times, for example when one group has been diagnosed earlier in the natural history of the disease than the other group owing to the use of a screening procedure [11].

Length bias: caused by the selection of a disproportionate number of long-duration cases (cases who survive longest) in one group and not in the other. An example is when prevalent cases, rather than incident cases, are included in a case–control study [11].

Membership bias: membership in a group (e.g. workers, joggers) may imply a degree of health which differs systematically from that of the general population because the general population is composed of both healthy and ill individuals [6, 16].

Mimicry bias: an innocent exposure may become suspect if, rather than causing a disease, it causes a benign disorder which resembles the disease [16].

Nonsimultaneous comparison bias (syn. noncontemporaneous control bias): secular changes in definitions, exposures, diagnoses, diseases, and treatments may render noncontemporaneous controls noncomparable [16], for example use of historical controls [11].

Sample Size Bias

Samples that are too small may not show effects even when they are present; samples that are too large may show tiny effects of little or no practical significance [16]. Another name for sample size bias is wrong sample size bias.

Study Execution Bias

Study execution bias refers to errors in executing the experimental maneuver (or exposure) [16]. Examples include:

Bogus control bias: when patients who are allocated to an experimental maneuver die or sicken before or during its administration and are omitted or reallocated to the control group, the experimental maneuver will appear spuriously superior [16].

Contamination bias: when members of the control group in an experiment inadvertently receive the experimental maneuver, the differences in outcomes between experimental and control patients may be systematically reduced [16] (*see* **Bias Toward the Null**).

Compliance bias: in experiments requiring patient adherence to therapy, issues of efficacy become **confounded** with those of compliance, for example when high-risk coronary patients quit exercise programs [16].

Data Collection Bias

Data collection bias (syn. information bias, **measurement error**, **misclassification** bias, observational bias) refers to a flaw in measuring exposure or outcome that results in differential quality or accuracy of information between compared groups [11] (*see* **Bias, Nondifferential**). Bias in data collection can arise from (i) defective measuring instruments, (ii) wrong data source, (iii) errors of the observer, (iv) errors of the subjects, and (v) errors during data handling.

Instrument Bias

Instrument bias (syn: instrument error) refers to defects in the measuring instruments [16]. This may be due to faulty calibration, inaccurate measuring instruments, contaminated reagents, incorrect dilution or mixing of reagents, etc. [11]. Examples include:

Case definition bias: definition of cases, for example based on different versions of **International Classification of Diseases** (ICD) codes, or first-ever cases vs. recurrent cases, may change over time or across regions, resulting in inaccurate trends and geographic comparisons [12]. (See also diagnostic vogue bias.)

Diagnostic vogue bias: the same illness may receive different diagnostic labels at different points in space or time, for example the British term "bronchitis" vs. North American "emphysema") [16]. (See also case definition bias.)

Forced choice bias: questions that provide inadequate choices, for example only "yes" and "no", and without other choices like "do not know" or "yes but do not know type", may force respondents to choose from the limited choices. (See also scale format bias.)

Framing bias: preference depends on the manner in which the choices are presented, for example telling a prospective candidate for surgery that an operation has a 5% mortality, vs. 95% survival rate.

Insensitive measure bias: when outcome measures are incapable of detecting clinically significant changes or differences, type II errors occur [16].

Juxtaposed scale bias (syn. questionnaire format bias): juxtaposed scales, a type of self-report response scale which asks respondents to give multiple responses to one item, may elicit different responses than when separate scales are used [9].

Laboratory data bias: data based on laboratory test results are subject to errors of the laboratory test including faulty calibration of the instruments, contaminated or incorrect amounts of reagents, etc.

Questionnaire bias: leading questions or other flaws in the questionnaire may result in a differential quality of information between compared groups [6].

Scale format bias: even vs. odd number of categories in the scale for the respondents to choose from can produce different results, for example (Agree) 1–2–3 (Disagree) tends to obtain neutral answers, i.e. 2, while (Agree) 1–2–3–4 (Disagree) tends to force respondents to take sides. (See also forced choice bias.)

Sensitive question bias: sensitive questions such as personal or household incomes, sexual orientation, or marital status, may induce inaccurate answers.

Stage bias: method for determining stage of disease of patients may vary across the groups being compared, across geographic areas, or through time, leading to spurious comparison of stage-adjusted survival rates [8].

Unacceptability bias: measurements which hurt, embarrass or invade privacy may be systematically refused or evaded [16].

Underlying/contributing cause of death bias: results of data analysis will be different depending on whether the underlying or the contributing cause of death as recorded on the death certificates is used (*see* **Cause of Death, Underlying and Multiple**; **Death Certification**).

Voluntary reporting bias: voluntary reporting system vs. mandatory reporting system can generate differences in the quality and completeness of routine data.

Data Source Bias

Data source bias refers to wrong, inadequate, or impossible source or type of data. Examples include:

Competing death bias: some causes of death (e.g. cancers) are associated with older age, while others (e.g. infectious diseases) are associated with younger age. Therefore in places where infectious diseases are prevalent, the cancer rates will be underestimated owing to competing causes of death from infectious diseases (*see* **Competing Risks**).

Family history bias: positive family history is not an accurate indicator of familial aggregation of a disease and the influence of genetic factors, because it is a function of the number of relatives and the age distribution of relatives [10].

Hospital discharge bias: hospital discharge data do not reflect hospital admission data since they are affected by length of hospital stay, and therefore do not provide accurate information for disease incidence.

Spatial bias: many environmental data used for health applications, for example geographic information systems (GIS), derive from point measurements at monitoring or survey stations. Unfortunately, many environmental monitoring networks are too sparse spatially and biased towards high pollution sites, generating an inaccurate pollution surface [2].

Observer Bias

Observer bias is due to differences among observers (interobserver variation) or to variations in readings by the same observer on separate occasions (intraobserver variation) [11]. Examples include:

Diagnostic suspicion bias (syn. diagnostic bias): a knowledge of the subject's prior exposure to a putative cause (e.g. ethnicity, drug use, cigarette smoking) may influence both the intensity and the outcome of the diagnostic process [6, 16].

Exposure suspicion bias: a knowledge of the subject's disease status may influence both the intensity and outcome of a search for exposure to the putative cause [6, 16].

Expectation bias: observers may systematically err in measuring and recording observations so that they concur with prior expectations, for example house officers tend to report "normal" fetal heart rates [16].

Interviewer bias: caused by interviewers' subconscious or even conscious gathering of selective data [11], for example questions about specific exposures may be asked several times of cases but only once of controls [16]. Can result from interinterviewer or intrainterviewer errors [6].

Therapeutic personality bias: when treatment is not blind, the therapist's convictions about efficacy may systematically influence both outcomes and their measurement (e.g. desire for positive results) [16].

Subject Bias

Subject bias (syn. "observee" bias) refers to the inaccuracy of the data provided by the subjects (respondents, "observees") at the time of data collection. Examples include:

Apprehension bias: certain measures (e.g. pulse, blood pressure) may alter systematically from their usual levels when the subject is apprehensive (e.g. blood pressure may change during medical interviews) [16].

Attention bias (syn. Hawthorne effect): study subjects may systematically alter their behavior when they know they are being observed [16].

Culture bias: subjects' responses may differ because of culture differences, for example some ethnic groups, because of their cultural background, do not want to share publicly their pain or problems such as unemployment, marital troubles, youth crime, and parental difficulties.

End adversion bias: subjects usually avoid end of scales in their answers, try to be conservative, and wish to be in the middle.

Faking bad bias (syn. hello–goodbye effect): subjects try to appear sick in order to qualify for support. Also, subjects try to seem sick before, and very well after, the treatment.

Faking good bias (syn. social desirability bias): socially undesirable answers tend to be underreported.

(See also unacceptable disease bias, unacceptable exposure bias.)

Family information bias: the family history and other historical information may vary markedly depending upon whether the individual in the family providing the information is a case or a control, for example different family histories of arthritis may be obtained from affected and unaffected siblings [16].

Interview setting bias: whether interviews are conducted at home, in a hospital, the respondent's workplace, or the researcher's office may affect subjects' responses.

Obsequiousness bias: subjects may systematically alter questionnaire responses in the direction they perceive desired by the investigator [16].

Positive satisfaction bias (syn. positive skew bias): subjects tend to give positive answers, typically when answering satisfaction questions.

Proxy respondent bias (syn. surrogate data bias): for deceased cases or surviving cases (e.g. brain tumors) whose ability to recall details is defective, soliciting information from proxies (e.g. spouse or family members) may result in differential data accuracy.

Recall bias: caused by differences in accuracy or completeness of recall to memory of prior events or experiences [6], for example mothers whose children have had leukemia are more likely than mothers of healthy children to remember details of diagnostic X-ray examinations to which these children were exposed *in utero* [11].

Reporting bias (syn. self-report response bias): selective suppression or revealing of information such as past history of sexually transmitted disease [11]. (See also unacceptable disease bias, unacceptable exposure bias, sensitive question bias.)

Response fatigue bias: questionnaires that are too long can induce fatigue among respondents and result in uniform and inaccurate answers.

Unacceptable disease bias: socially unacceptable disorders (e.g. sexually transmitted diseases, suicide, mental illness) tend to be underreported [11]. (See also reporting bias, faking good bias.)

Unacceptable exposure bias: socially unacceptable exposures (e.g. smoking, drug abuse) tend to be underreported. (See also reporting bias, faking good bias.)

Underlying cause bias (syn. rumination bias): cases may ruminate about possible causes for their illness and thus exhibit different recall or prior exposures than controls [16]. (See also recall bias.)

Yes-saying bias: some subjects tend to say "yes" to all questions.

Data Handling Bias

Data handling bias refers to the manner in which data are handled. Examples include:

Data capture error: errors in the acquisition of the data in digital form, normally by manual encoding (coding error), digitizing (data entry error), scanning, or electronic transfer from pre-existing data bases [2]. (See also data entry bias.)

Data entry bias: difference in data entry practices may cause unreal observed differences in geographic variations in incidence rates [17]. (See also data capture error.)

Data merging error: incorrect merging of data from different databases, for example erroneous merging and failure to merge as a result of illegible handwriting on the routine forms, different dates of service recorded in different databases, etc. (See also record linkage bias.)

Digit preference bias (syn. end-digit preference bias): in converting analog to digital data, observers may record some terminal digits with an unusual frequency [16], for example rounding off may be to the nearest whole number, even number, multiple of 5 or 10, or, when time units like a week are involved, 7, 14, etc. [11].

Record linkage bias: computerized **record linkage** is based on a probabilistic process based on identifiers. Some identifiers, e.g. some surnames, may have a poor record linkage weight, causing linkage problems, and therefore tend to exclude subjects having those identifiers.

Analysis Bias

Analysis bias results from errors in analyzing the data. It can arise from (i) lack of adequate control of **confounding** factors, (ii) inappropriate analysis strategies, and (iii) *post hoc* analysis of the data set.

Confounding Bias

Confounding bias occurs when the estimate of the effect of the exposure of interest is distorted because it is mixed with the effect of a confounding (extraneous) factor. A confounding factor must be a risk factor for the disease, be associated with the exposure under study, and not be an intermediate step in the causal path between the exposure and the disease [6]. Examples include:

Latency bias: failure to adjust for the **latent period** in the analysis of cancer or other chronic disease data.

Multiple exposure bias: failure to adjust for multiple exposures.

Nonrandom sampling bias: when a study sample is selected by nonrandom (nonprobability) sampling, failure to account for variable sampling fractions in the analysis may introduce a bias, for example weighting by the strata population sizes is needed for a disproportionate stratified sample.

Standard population bias: choice of standard population will affect estimation of standardized rates (a weighted average of the category-specific rates) (*see* **Standardization Methods**).

Spectrum bias (syn. case mix bias): heterogeneous groups of patients with different proportions of mild and severe cases can lead to different estimates of **screening** performance indicators [15].

Analysis Strategy Bias

Analysis strategy bias (syn. analysis method bias) refers to problems in the analysis strategies. Examples include:

Distribution assumption bias: wrong assumption of sampling distribution in the analysis, for example time variables follow lognormal distribution rather than normal distribution, and therefore geometric mean time rather than mean time should be used [7].

Enquiry unit bias: choice of unit of enquiry may affect analysis results, for example with the school as the unit of enquiry, half the high schools offered no physics, but when the student becomes the unit of enquiry, only 2% of all high school students attended schools that offered no physics, since the small schools do not teach physics.

Estimator bias: the difference between the expected value of an estimator of a parameter and the true value of this parameter [11], for example **odds ratio** always overestimates **relative risk**).

Missing data handling bias: how **missing data** are handled, for example treated as a missing case vs.

interpreted as a "no" answer, will lead to different results.

Outlier handling bias: arising from a failure to discard an unusual value occurring in a small sample, or due to exclusion of unusual values that should be included [11]. The latter is also called tidying-up bias (the exclusion of outliers or other untidy results which cannot be justified on statistical grounds) [16].

Overmatching bias: matching on a nonconfounding variable that is associated with the exposure but not the disease can lead to conservative estimates in a matched case–control study [6].

Scale degradation bias: the degradation and collapsing of measurement scales tend to obscure differences between groups under comparison [16].

Post Hoc *Analysis Bias*

Post hoc analysis bias refers to the misleading results caused by *post hoc* questions, data dredging, and subgroup analysis. Examples include:

Data dredging bias: when data are reviewed for all possible associations without prior hypothesis, the results are suitable for hypothesis-generating activities only [16].

Post hoc *significance bias*: when decision levels or "tails" for type I and type II errors are selected after the data have been examined, conclusions may be biased [16].

Repeated peeks bias: repeated peeks at accumulating data in a randomized trial are not independent, and may lead to inappropriate termination [16].

Interpretation Bias

Interpretation bias arises from inference and speculation, for example failure of the investigator to consider every interpretation consistent with the facts and to assess the credentials of each, and mishandling of cases that constitute exceptions to some general conclusion [11]. Examples include:

Assumption bias (syn. conceptual bias): arising from faulty logic or premises or mistaken beliefs on the part of the investigator, for example having correctly deduced the mode of transmission of cholera, John Snow falsely concluded that yellow fever was transmitted by similar means [11].

Cognitive dissonance bias: the belief in a given mechanism may increase rather than decrease in the face of contradictory evidence [16].

Correlation bias: equating correlation with causation leads to errors of both kinds [16].

Generalization bias (syn. lack of external validity): generalizing study results to people outside the study population may produce bias, for example generalizing findings in men to women (*see* **Validity and Generalizability in Epidemiologic Studies**).

Magnitude bias: when interpreting a finding, the selection of a scale of measurement may markedly affect the interpretation, for example $1 000 000 may also be 0.0003% of the national budget [16].

Significance bias: the confusion of statistical significance, on the one hand, with biologic or clinical or health care significance, on the other hand, may lead to fruitless studies and useless conclusions [16].

Underexhaustion bias: the failure to exhaust the hypothesis space may lead to erroneous interpretations [16].

Publication Bias

Publication bias refers to an editorial predilection for publishing particular findings, e.g. positive results, which can distort the general belief about what has been demonstrated in a particular situation [11]. Examples include:

All's well literature bias: scientific or professional societies may publish reports or editorials which omit or play down controversies or disparate results [16].

Positive results bias: authors are more likely to submit, and editors accept, positive than null results [16].

Hot topic bias (syn. hot stuff bias): when a topic is hot, investigators and editors are tempted to publish additional results, no matter how preliminary or shaky [16].

References

[1] Berkson, J. (1946). Limitations of the application of fourfold table analysis to hospital data, *Biometrics Bulletin* **2**, 47–53.

[2] Briggs, D.J. & Elliott, P. (1995). The use of geographical information systems in studies on environment and health, *World Health Statistics Quarterly* **48**, 85–94.

[3] Choi, B.C.K. (1992). Sensitivity and specificity of a single diagnostic test in the presence of work-up bias, *Journal of Clinical Epidemiology* **45**, 581–586.

[4] Choi, B.C.K. (1992). Definition, sources, magnitude, effect modifiers, and strategies of reduction of the healthy worker effect, *Journal of Occupational Medicine* **34**, 979–988.

[5]   Choi, B.C.K. (1996). Occupational cancer in develop-ing countries, *American Journal of Epidemiology* **144**, 1089.

[6]   Choi, B.C.K. & Noseworthy, A.L. (1992). Classifica-tion, direction, and prevention of bias in epidemio-logic research, *Journal of Occupational Medicine* **34**, 265–271.

[7]   Choi, B.C.K., Pak, A.W.P. & Purdham, J.T. (1990). Effects of mailing strategies on response rate, response time, and cost in a questionnaire study among nurses, *Epidemiology* **1**, 72–74.

[8]   Farrow, D.C., Hunt, W.C. & Samet, J.M. (1995). Biased comparisons of lung cancer survival across geographic areas: effects of stage bias, *Epidemiology* **6**, 558–560.

[9]   Hunt, D.M., Magruder, S. & Bolon, D.S. (1995). Ques-tionnaire format bias: when are juxtaposed scales appro-priate. A call for further research, *Psychological Reports* **77**, 931–941.

[10] Khoury, M.J. & Flanders, W.D. (1995). Bias in using family history as a risk factor in case–control studies of disease, *Epidemiology* **6**, 511–519.

[11] Last, J.M. (1988). *A Dictionary of Epidemiology*, 2nd Ed. Oxford University Press, New York.

[12] May, D.S. & Kittner, S.J. (1994). Use of medicare claims data to estimate national trends in stroke inci-dence, 1985–1991, *Stroke* **25**, 2343–2347.

[13] Moser, C.A. & Kalton, G. (1971). *Survey Methods in Social Investigation*. Gower, Brookfield.

[14] Neyman, J. (1955). Statistics – servant of all sciences, *Science* **122**, 401.

[15] Ransohoff, D.F. & Feinstein, A.R. (1978). Problems of spectrum and bias in evaluating the efficacy of diagnostic tests, *New England Journal of Medicine* **299**, 926–930.

[16] Sackett, D.L. (1979). Bias in analytic research, *Journal of Chronic Diseases* **32**, 51–63.

[17] Sarti, C. (1993). Geographic variation in the incidence of nonfatal stroke in Finland: are the observed differ-ences real?, *Stroke* **24**, 787–791.

(*See also* **Bias in Case–Control Studies**; **Bias in Cohort Studies**; **Bias in Observational Studies**)

BERNARD C.K. CHOI & ANITA W.P. PAK

Bias from Exposure Effects on Controls

In population-based case–control studies, controls are selected at random from the source (or "base")

population (*see* **Case–Control Study, Population-Based**). In hospital-based case–control studies, cases in the hospital with a disease of interest are compared with controls in the hospital who have other diseases (*see* **Case–Control Study, Hospital-Based**). In hospital-based case–control studies, the exposure **odds ratio** comparing cases with controls may be a **biased** estimate of the **relative risk** of disease in the underlying source population if the risks of the control diseases are themselves associated with the exposure under study. For example, in a pioneering hospital-based case–control study of the risk of lung cancer from smoking, Doll & Hill [2] included subjects with bronchitis among the controls. Because the risk of bronchitis is now known to be increased by smoking, we can infer that estimates of the relative risk of lung cancer from smoking were biased downward by the inclusion of such controls. A quantitative treatment of such bias is given by Breslow & Day [1, pp. 153–154].

References

[1]   Breslow, N.E. & Day, N.E. (1987). *Statistical Methods in Cancer Research*, Vol. 2: *The Design and Analysis of Cohort Studies*. International Agency for Research on Cancer, Lyon.

[2]   Doll, R. & Hill, A.B. (1952). A study of the aetiology of carcinoma of the lung, *British Medical Journal* **2**, 1271–1286.

(*See also* **Bias in Case–Control Studies**)

M.H. GAIL

Bias from Loss to Follow-Up

Loss to follow-up **bias** results when subjects lost from a cohort (*see* **Cohort Study**) have different health response distributions from subjects who remain in follow-up. For example, if sicker patients are lost from a cohort during follow-up, the estimated sur-vival distribution (*see* **Survival Analysis, Overview**) will be biased upward. As another example, if a cohort of subjects with the human immunodeficiency virus (HIV) are being followed in a natural history study to track decreases in T-helper lymphocyte (CD4+ lymphocyte) levels, and if the subjects with low CD4+ lymphocyte levels are dropped from the study in order to begin treatment, then the CD4+ lymphocyte levels in those remaining on study will be upwardly biased. If loss to follow-up bias is greater in an exposed cohort than in an unexposed cohort, the estimates of exposure effects will be biased, but if the same degree of loss to follow-up bias operates in both cohorts, **nondifferential error** will result, and estimated exposure effects may be unbiased or nearly unbiased.

(*See also* **Bias from Nonresponse**; **Bias in Cohort Studies**; **Bias in Observational Studies**; **Bias, Overview**; **Missing Data in Epidemiologic Studies**)

M.H. GAIL

Bias from Nonresponse

Nonresponse **bias** results when some members of the intended **study population** fail to provide required data (the nonresponders), and when those who respond are not representative of the entire study population (*see* **Nonresponse**). In comparative studies, such as studies comparing exposed and unexposed **cohorts**, nonresponse bias may severely distort estimates of **exposure effect** if the degree of nonresponse bias differs in the exposed and unexposed groups, resulting in differential nonresponse bias. If the degree of nonresponse bias is the same in the exposed and unexposed groups, then the nonresponse bias is said to be nondifferential, and the bias in the estimate of exposure effect may be minimal, or even zero, depending on which measure of exposure effect is used.

(*See also* **Bias in Case–Control Studies**; **Bias in Cohort Studies**; **Bias in Observational Studies**; **Bias, Overview**; **Validity and Generalizability in Epidemiologic Studies**)

M.H. GAIL

Bias from Survival in Prevalent Case–Control Studies

In a prevalent case–control study, the exposures of prevalent cases sampled from among living cases are compared with the exposures of living noncases (*see* **Case–Control Study, Prevalent**). Because an exposure that causes disease may also influence the probability that an incident case will survive long enough to be sampled from the population of prevalent cases, exposure **odds ratios** from prevalent case–control studies may yield **biased** estimates of the odds ratio of etiologic interest that relates exposure to the risk of incident disease.

(*See also* **Bias, Overview Biased Sampling of Cohorts in Epidemiology**)

M.H. GAIL

Bias in Case–Control Studies

In recent years, the concept of a *study base* [5, 10, 26, 28] as the source from which any analytical epidemiologic study is derived has gained widespread acceptance [25]. Under this concept, **case–control** and **cohort studies** represent alternative approaches to sampling and information gathering from a definable population/time experience, and the **biases** that arise are a consequence of doing so inappropriately. A common earlier view [11] was that case–control studies are uniquely susceptible to bias because they "look back" from the outcome to the exposure, whereas cohort studies "look forward". For that reason, it has sometimes been claimed that case–control studies are intrinsically more susceptible to bias than cohort studies. Today, it is better recognized that while certain biases occur more commonly when using one or the other approach, others affect them equally, and the problems are not fundamentally different.

The unifying concept of a single study base might be expected in its turn to lead to unified definitions of bias, applicable both to case–control and cohort studies, and attempts to create such definitions have been made [18, 42]. But the matter is complex, and thus far none has gained wide currency. In this article, we use the existing terminology as applied to case–control studies [3, 25].

Bias is present in a case–control study if there is systematic distortion in the data that leads to an **odds ratio** estimate that is different from the true odds ratio in the study base. Because the bias is systematic, large sample sizes do not eliminate it; indeed, the only effect of enlarging sample sizes is to produce biased estimates that are more precise. Bias may arise as a consequence of **systematic errors** in the selection of cases or controls, or errors in the recording of exposure data, or because of **confounding**. When there is **nondifferential** misclassification of exposure data among cases and controls, the usual effect is to bias odds ratio estimates towards unity (*see* **Bias Toward the Null**); if such misclassification is substantial, so may be the bias. Failure to adjust for confounding may distort odds ratio estimates towards or away from unity and, again, the bias may be substantial. The reader interested in a discussion of nondifferential misclassification is referred to the articles **Misclassification Error** and **Measurement Error in Epidemiologic Studies**. Here, we focus on two remaining sources of distortion, **selection bias** and information bias. The term information bias is sometimes used to denote both nondifferential and differential misclassification of exposure [36]; here, we use it to denote only differential misclassification (*see* **Differential Error**).

Selection Bias

Selection bias exists when cases or controls are selected in a way that is not representative of the respective exposure distributions in the study base.

Specification of the Study Base

A fundamental step in the avoidance of selection bias is to ensure that the cases and controls are drawn from the same study base. Otherwise, if the **prevalence** of exposure is different in the different bases, bias is unavoidable. A primary study base is one in which

the population/time experience, including the cases that occur, can be specified (e.g. new cases of acute myeloid leukemia (AML) occurring in the population of Massachusetts from 1990 to 1994). In a **population-based case–control study**, all cases are identified and selected; alternatively, a representative sample (e.g. a random sample) is selected. In either instance, a properly specified **control** series consists of noncases sampled from the same study base. When the base is well defined, and all cases are identifiable, it is possible in principle to sample them using methods that are unbiased. In practice, however, problems such as **nonresponse** may nonetheless lead to bias, as discussed below.

Sometimes it may not be possible to specify a primary base, as happens when a series of cases is selected without full insight into the population/time experience from which they are drawn (e.g. new cases of AML diagnosed in one hematology laboratory from 1990 to 1994). The secondary study base may then be conceived of as that population/time experience from which any person would have been selected as a case had he (or she) developed the disease under study. The proper selection of **controls** requires that they be sampled from that hypothetical secondary study base. Operationally, such controls are often sampled from the same source as the cases (in this example, the control series could perhaps comprise a sample of persons with normal blood counts, recorded in the same laboratory). In other words, certain selection characteristics of the cases determine the secondary study base, which cannot otherwise be specified. Since it is not possible to identify members of a secondary base explicitly, it is necessary to rely on judgment and experience in order to select controls likely to be representative of the exposure in the hypothetical base.

It is worth illustrating how incorrect specification of a secondary study base may give rise to selection bias. Consider a hypothetical study of radon exposure and lung cancer, carried out in one hospital. The hospital has a large thoracic surgery department and selectively admits lung cancer cases from an entire city, in some areas of which household radon levels are high, while in other areas they are low. The hospital admits patients with conditions other than lung cancer only from an immediately adjacent area, in which household radon levels are high. In this example, the cases and controls have not been selected from the same study base, the exposure rates in the different bases are different, and the data are biased. The bias could only be overcome if the case series were to be restricted to those resident in the same area as the controls – in which case the comparison groups are now drawn from the same study base.

Selection Bias due to Nonresponse

Assuming the study base is correctly specified, selection bias may nevertheless arise if there is differential sampling or identification of cases and controls. A common way in which differential sampling may occur is if there are substantial losses in the enrollment of cases or controls originally deemed eligible for inclusion (nonresponse). In a population-based case–control study, all cases, or a representative sample of those that occur in the study base, are included. Alternatively, in a study with a secondary base, the cases should be representative of those occurring in that base (e.g. a single hospital). In each instance, potentially eligible controls should constitute a representative sample of all noncases in the same base. In practice, however, it is virtually inevitable that some of the cases or controls initially specified as eligible will not be enrolled (e.g. because of failure to trace subjects, refusal to participate, severe illness, or death). If, either among the cases or the controls, the exposure rate is systematically different among those who are and are not enrolled, there is selection bias due to nonresponse.

Bias due to nonresponse is negligible if close to 100% of the cases and controls scheduled for sampling are successfully enrolled. Some studies come close to meeting that objective. Other studies do not, and the greater the proportion unenrolled, the greater must be the concern about possible selection bias. Hospital-based case–control studies tend to have higher response rates than population-based studies, especially if it is necessary to collect biological samples.

In the face of high nonresponse rates, some limited reassurance about the absence of material selection bias may be gained when it can be shown that distributions of known characteristics (such as age, sex, or residence) are similar among enrolled and unenrolled subjects. That reassurance may be unjustified, however, if the compared variables are not themselves correlates of the exposure.

Sensitivity analyses are sometimes used in an attempt to cope with high nonresponse rates [15].

Varying assumptions are made about possible exposure rates among unenrolled subjects, and their effects upon the magnitude of any given association are then assessed. Clearly, however, the assumptions may be incorrect, and that possibility limits the interpretability of the data. In general, the more the attrition, the greater is the potential for bias. To limit this source of bias, there is simply no substitute for high enrollment rates.

Selection Bias in the Identification of
Study Subjects

Selection bias may also arise if cases or controls are identified in a way that is not independent of the exposure (*see* **Detection Bias**). To illustrate how the biased identification of cases may occur, consider a hypothetical example in which each of two women has a tender and swollen leg due to deep vein thrombosis (DVT); one woman takes oral contraceptives (OCs – a known cause [40]), the other does not. The OC taker is aware that she is at risk of DVT, and so consults her physician, who correctly makes the diagnosis and admits her to a hospital; the nonuser stays home, undiagnosed; both women recover. Even though the diagnosis, when made, is correct, the case identification is incomplete, and exposure-dependent: a case–control study that enrolls cases of DVT, regardless of whether it is population-based or derived from a secondary study base, would overestimate the association with OC use, because knowledge of the exposure increases the likelihood that exposed cases would be included in the study.

This type of selection bias may take many forms, as can be illustrated further by the following examples. In a study of breast cancer risk in relation to female hormone use, "screening" or "detection" bias may arise if hormone users are more commonly subjected to mammography than nonusers (e.g. because of concern about possible breast cancer risk). As a result, users are more commonly diagnosed than nonusers as having breast cancer that might not otherwise have become clinically apparent for many years [39].

There are instances in which the biases brought about by **screening** may not be at all subtle. It has been estimated, for example, that over 60% of men over the age of 60 years have asymptomatic prostatic cancer [12]. It is now possible to detect cases that would otherwise have remained asymptomatic for many years, and perhaps for life, by means of a new test (the prostate-specific antigen test [41]). Any association of prostatic cancer with a correlate of the likelihood of undergoing such a test (e.g. high socioeconomic status) would likely be biased. That bias may be reduced, or perhaps avoided, in a study restricted to cases that must inevitably come to diagnosis, regardless of screening, because of symptoms that oblige them to seek medical care, such as hematuria or bone pain due to metastases. As a general rule, studies that enroll cases (or controls) from screening programs run a substantial risk of selection bias [4, 29].

A similar bias arises when registries that selectively record exposed cases are used as sources for case enrollment (see **Disease Registers**). Perhaps the best-known example of this type was the American Registry of Blood Dyscrasias [48], which was initiated in the mid-1950s and maintained for over a decade following reports of an association of aplastic anemia with the use of the antimicrobial drug, chloramphenicol [44]. Exposed cases were far more likely than nonexposed cases to be reported. There is little doubt that chloramphenicol does indeed increase the risk of aplastic anemia, but it is now clear that the association was overestimated [19]. This example illustrates how important it is to ensure that *all* cases within any specified study base, whether primary or secondary, should have the same chance of being identified and included in a case–control study, regardless of exposure status. It also illustrates the limited interpretability of **case series** reported to regulatory agencies, or to medical journals, without reference to the background occurrence of nonexposed cases – or, indeed, without reference to the exposure prevalence among suitably selected controls.

Biased identification of cases may also occur when a cluster of exposed cases gives rise to a hypothesis, and then the same cluster is included in an independent study mounted to confirm the hypothesis. Thus, if a cluster of cases of leukemia occurs in the vicinity of a nuclear power plant [1], it would be inappropriate to include that cluster in an independent study designed to test the hypothesis that leukemia is associated with proximity to a nuclear power plant.

Bias due to the Selection of Nonrepresentative Controls from a Secondary Study Base

Hospitalized patients continue to constitute the most commonly selected controls in case–control research

[22, 25, 45–47], and the potential problems posed by their selection serve well to illustrate the biases that may arise when controls are selected from a hypothetical secondary study base.

Particular attention must be paid to ensure that hospitalized patients selected for inclusion as controls have been admitted for diseases that are independent of the exposure under study. An illustration of how bias may occur if this is not done is the classical study by Doll & Hill of smoking and lung cancer [7], in which the control series included patients with chronic bronchitis, a disease not appreciated at the time to be tobacco-related [8, 9]. The magnitude of the association with lung cancer was somewhat underestimated for that reason. The association was nevertheless identified, because most of the control diagnoses were independent of smoking status, and because smoking was more strongly associated with lung cancer than with chronic bronchitis.

Despite the risk of biases of this type, hospital-based studies have remained a mainstay of case–control research. When well conducted, such studies have continued to document important and valid associations (e.g. OCs and myocardial infarction [34]). There are several reasons. Interview data are usually less biased among hospital controls (see the section "Information Bias" below), and hospital-based studies are usually easier to conduct than studies that enroll community controls: response rates are usually higher, and when needed, high success rates in obtaining blood or tissue samples can be achieved. Perhaps the most important reason, however, is that there is today a better appreciation of the steps that should be taken to ensure that the selection of hospital controls is unbiased.

In formal terms, the selection of hospital controls is unbiased if the control diagnoses that are selected for inclusion are representative of the exposure distribution in the hypothetical secondary base. In practice, there is usually no reason why such controls cannot be identified if only those persons are selected whose reason for hospital admission (the *primary* diagnosis) is independent of the exposure under study. Those admitted for conditions that are not independent of the exposure should be excluded. When in doubt, one should opt for *exclusion*: what matters is that the selection of those subjects that are *included* should be valid. Clearly, the valid selection of hospital controls calls for experience and judgment. If that judgment is called into question, the interpretation of hospital-based case–control data can sometimes be controversial.

Hospitalized patients, whether cases or controls, commonly have more than one diagnosis, and it is important to note that *secondary* diagnoses are irrelevant to the selection of controls, unless the *secondary* diagnoses have also influenced the selection of the cases (which is unusual). For example, in a study of the risk of myocardial infarction (MI) in relation to OC use [34], cases admitted for a *primary* diagnosis of MI who had a *secondary* diagnosis of diabetes mellitus (a condition that is inversely associated with OC use) were not excluded; correspondingly, controls admitted with *primary* diagnoses unrelated to OC use, such as trauma, but with a *secondary* diagnosis of diabetes, were also not excluded. Instead, potential confounding due to diabetes was controlled in the analysis. If, however, we conceive of a hypothetical study in which patients admitted for MI are excluded if they are also diabetic, then controls admitted for trauma who also happen to be diabetic should also be excluded.

As a general rule, persons whose primary diagnoses are acute conditions for which admission is obligatory (e.g. trauma; appendicitis) meet the requirement of independence, as may persons with other conditions (e.g. elective admission for cataract surgery). However, it is always necessary to consider the particular hypothesis under study, and to use informed judgment. For example, consider a study of the risk of ovarian cancer in relation to OC use [35]: among women hospitalized for trauma, the reason for admission is likely to be independent of the exposure; such women would be eligible as controls. However, if the example is changed to a study of breast cancer risk in relation to alcohol intake [33]), trauma would not be a suitable control diagnosis because its occurrence may not be independent of the exposure.

Reassurance that the identification of hospital controls is unbiased may be gained if the exposure rates among major diagnostic categories (e.g. trauma, acute infections, orthopedic conditions) are uniform: in that circumstance, bias is only possible if the selection of an entire control series is biased, and biased to the same degree for each diagnostic category. However, the confident demonstration of uniformity requires that the categories be large enough to ensure that the rates in each of them are reasonably precise.

As an alternative, it has been suggested [25] that a hospital control series should include as wide a range of diagnoses as possible. If it can be assumed that most of them will be independent of the exposure, then any bias, if present, will be diluted. This latter option is seldom acceptable unless there are good grounds to be reasonably sure that by far the overwhelming majority of the individual diagnoses that led to admission are, indeed, independent of the exposure. This is rarely the case. For this reason, the selection of a random sample of an entire hospital population, without any regard for diagnostic eligibility, can seldom be defended.

Despite the generally distinguished record of hospital-based case–control studies, some epidemiologists have argued that hospital controls are almost always unrepresentative of exposure in the population at large [43, 49]. That argument ignores the premise that when the cases represent a secondary study base (as is usual in hospital-based studies), the only valid control series may be patients admitted to the same hospitals as the cases.

One theoretical drawback to the sampling of hospital controls is that the judgment that the included conditions are independent of the exposure is an assumption, and one that is not needed when selecting controls in a **population-based study**. In addition, there is evidence to suggest that certain exposures differ for in-hospital and out-of-hospital populations [25, 45–47]. That evidence, however, has been derived from studies that did not take into account the specific eligibility of each control diagnosis in the context of the specific hypothesis under study – an essential step in the proper selection of hospital controls. Nevertheless, there may be circumstances when the exposure under study (e.g. alcohol [33]) influences admission across such a wide range of diagnoses that it may be difficult or impossible to select a valid series of hospital controls.

Bias due to the Nonrepresentative Selection of Controls from a Primary Study Base

Selection bias may arise in analogous ways when population-based controls are chosen [45–47]. For example, if the sampling scheme is based on incomplete coverage of the base population (e.g. a motor vehicle owners' registry, or **random digit dialing**), it may underrepresent people of low socioeconomic status (because they do not have cars or telephones). Similarly, the selection of other controls, such as friends of the cases, or classmates, may give rise to other problems. For example, nonexposed friends of an exposed case may tend selectively to participate in a study because they would like to help. As with hospital controls, it remains important to use judgment in ensuring that population-based controls, however selected, are representative of the study base.

In an idealized example of a **population-based case–control study** with a 100% response rate among the sampled cases and among controls, confidence in the validity of the findings would be greater than for an otherwise identical study in which hospital controls are selected because no unverifiable assumptions about representativeness are required. In practice, however, that theoretical advantage is commonly not achieved because response rates among population controls tend to be considerably lower than among hospital controls, and lower still when it is necessary to obtain biological samples.

Partly in order to circumvent the problem of low response rates in the selection of population controls, random digit dialing [16, 25, 46] has been advocated as one way to obtain high participation rates, at least in societies with almost universal telephone coverage. This method had its origins in market research and opinion polls, and its application in epidemiologic research enjoyed some early success. However, with the passage of time, answering machines, voice mail, call forwarding, and an increasingly hostile attitude in society to what are perceived to be invasions of privacy, have lowered response rates, and sometimes even rendered such rates unmeasurable (because the presence or absence in the household of a potentially eligible control could not be determined) [13]. Despite these difficulties, however, adequate participation rates can sometimes be achieved if the interviewers are carefully trained and care is taken with the wording of invitations to participate.

Selection Bias in Nested Case–Control Studies

In recent years **nested case–control studies** have come to play an increasingly important role in case–control methodology. In a nested case–control study, the cases are members of a cohort who develop a given condition, and the controls are a sample of noncases selected from the same cohort, and followed for the same length of time. There are several advantages to this approach: the cases and controls are unambiguously representative of the same study base; if the follow-up has been successful nonresponse

rates are low; and information bias (see below) is avoided, since exposure status is usually determined before the subject qualifies as a case. A further advantage is that it may be easier to obtain biological specimens from people who are already collaborating in a study. All of these advantages were demonstrated in a study [31] that documented an increased risk of stomach cancer in relation to antecedent *Helicobacter pylori* infection, as determined from immunological assays of frozen serum specimens that had been collected and stored an average of 14 years earlier. As a general rule, however, a major disadvantage to the conduct of nested case–control studies is that it may not be possible to assemble sufficient cases, unless the follow-up study is massive.

Information Bias

Information bias exists when cases or controls report their exposures differently, or when the information is solicited differently (as noted above, in this article, bias due to nondifferential misclassification of exposure is excluded from the definition). The likelihood that information bias will occur is greatest when the study subject, or those responsible for collecting the data, know the hypothesis.

Differential reporting (**recall bias**) may occur if cases aware of the hypothesis tend to report their exposures more fully than controls, with resultant overestimation of the odds ratio. For this bias to occur, it is not necessary to assume that cases may report exposures that did not actually take place (although they may overestimate duration or dosage). Even if the controls share knowledge of the hypothesis with the cases, if they are healthier they may have less reason to probe their memories. For example, one study of breast cancer risk in relation to OC use [24] specifically informed participants of the hypothesis, thus rendering recall bias all but unavoidable (this is also an example of biased solicitation of information – see below). Cases may also be prompted to recall their exposures more completely if their memories (but not those of the controls) have already been "primed" by repeated questioning from their medical attendants about the putative cause before they are interviewed by the study personnel.

A lack of awareness of the hypothesis reduces the likelihood of information bias, but it does not necessarily eliminate it. Hospitalized cases, for example, because of the setting in which the questions are asked, may remember their exposures better than population controls interviewed at home. For this reason, the interviewing of controls in a hospital setting may reduce the likelihood of information bias. Similarly, without any specific hypothesis in mind, patients with cancer, or mothers who have given birth to children with birth defects, may be more inclined than controls to probe their memories for possible "causes", even if such "causes" have not specifically been hypothesized.

These examples illustrate how cases might report their exposures more fully than controls. Sometimes, however, the reverse may occur. In a hypothetical study of trauma in relation to alcohol intake, for example, the cases might understate their consumption relative to controls if they are embarrassed at having contributed to their own illness.

Much the same considerations that apply to recall bias on the part of the study subjects may also apply when those responsible for the data collection are aware of the hypothesis, and it is not uncommon for such awareness to coexist both among the subjects and the study personnel, as in the OC/breast cancer example [24] mentioned above. Or, to give another example, in a further study of the same question [30], women with breast cancer were interviewed face-to-face by a single male physician, while the controls were subjected to telephone interviews, conducted by two female interviewers. The biased solicitation of exposure information may be quite subtle: the inflection of an interviewer's voice, the "body language", the use of open-ended questions, or the way in which they are worded may all influence the respondent's answers.

It is sometimes argued that the presence of **dose–response** or duration–response effects constitutes evidence against information bias. This argument may have merit inasmuch as long-duration exposures, and perhaps high doses, are less likely to be misremembered than short-duration exposures or low doses. The countervailing argument, however, is that cases may tend systematically to overreport, and controls to underreport, duration or dosage. Thus, apparent duration or dosage gradients cannot necessarily be taken as evidence against information bias.

Occasionally, it is possible to avoid or minimize information bias. To give some examples: in a study of breast cancer risk in relation to use of the anti-hypertensive drug reserpine [20], women were questioned before their breast lumps were biopsied: the cases were those with breast cancer, and the controls were women given a diagnosis of benign breast disease. (But it should be noted that selection bias may have been present if reserpine increased the risk of benign breast disease – an instance in which the control diagnosis would not be independent of the exposure.) In a study of spermicide use at the time of conception in relation to Down's syndrome [23], pregnant women were questioned about exposure before they underwent an amniocentesis: the cases were fetuses with trisomy 21, the controls were fetuses with normal chromosome counts. And in a study of uterine cancer in relation to conjugated estrogen use [50], medical records were examined for prescriptions after all information on case or control status was masked: the biased recording of the exposure information was thus avoided.

Information bias can sometimes be assessed by the independent evaluation of exposure, using information from other sources. For example, some interview-based case–control studies have suggested that induced abortion increases the risk of breast cancer [6]. Information bias could account for the association if women with breast cancer more fully report such a sensitive exposure than do control women [32]. Evidence that this may be so is suggested by the results of a recent Danish cohort study [27] based on national registry data. An increased risk was ruled out, and in that study there was no information bias [17], since the data on abortion status were recorded before the breast cancer outcomes were observed. Indeed, this example serves to illustrate how cohort studies can avoid information bias.

Unfortunately, as illustrated by the abortion/breast cancer example, the circumstances in which information bias can confidently be ruled out in case–control studies tend to be the exception rather than the rule. Usually, even if the investigator judges information bias to be minimal, it may not be possible to demonstrate that this is so. It is necessary to resort to the next best alternative, which is to design studies in which the potential for information bias is reduced as much as possible: for example, by concealment of the hypothesis from the study subjects, and the interviewers – or, if that is not possible, by avoiding mention of the hypothesis; by the use of highly structured and unambiguous questions; memory prompts (e.g. photographs of OCs) to maximize recall; the administration of questionnaires as soon as possible, before there is a substantial opportunity for memory loss; and the rigorous training of interviewers.

Even with optimal study design, the question of whether information bias is, or is not, sufficient to invalidate an association is ultimately a matter of judgment. For example, in a study documenting an increased risk of sinonasal cancer among workers exposed to wood dust [21], we may judge that occupational exposure is likely to be equally well remembered by cases and controls. Alternatively, we may judge that information bias is likely, as with the example of breast cancer risk in relation to a history of induced abortion [6, 32].

Conclusions

In this article, we have described two types of systematic bias (confounding, of course, is a third). Yet, in the past, the view has sometimes been taken that there are many more types of bias, each of them sufficiently different to require separate classification, that may affect observational studies: Sackett [37] described more than 35 (*see* **Bias, Overview**). However, all the specific biases that have been reported can readily be classified as instances of selection bias and information bias. For example, **Berkson's fallacy** [2], the proposition that the selection of hospitalized cases may be biased if admission for the condition under study is dependent on the coexistence of another condition, is a form of selection bias.

Systematic bias due to confounding has not been considered in this article. But it is important to mention that selection bias or information bias may affect not only the recording of exposures, but also the recording of confounders. Indeed, both the differential and the nondifferential recording of a confounder can lead to residual confounding, with a bias that can act in either direction [14, 38].

Information bias is sometimes mentioned as the Achilles' heel of case–control methodology. One of the major advantages of follow-up studies, relative to case–control studies, is that exposures are usually measured before the health outcomes occur, thus reducing or eliminating the likelihood of information bias. However, that advantage may be offset by

biases that sometimes affect cohort studies, such as high nonresponse rates on follow-up, with differential losses according to exposure status. Another potential disadvantage is that changes in exposure status over time may be missed in cohort studies, unless the recording of the variables at issue is updated frequently (*see* **Bias in Cohort Studies**). And to complete the picture, certain biases (e.g. confounding, selection bias due to knowledge of exposure, or due to selective screening according to exposure status) may affect both approaches. In short, neither the case–control nor the cohort approach can circumvent all sources of bias, and they should, instead, be thought of as complementary strategies, each with certain strengths and certain weaknesses.

Since bias cannot be entirely eliminated in **observational studies**, concern about whether its existence is sufficient to invalidate any given association may be reduced if, in any study, the magnitude of the effect, relative to the magnitude of the plausible biases that may exist, is considerable. By contrast, the possibility of bias limits the interpretability of small associations. Concern about validity may also be reduced when a variety of well-conducted studies based on different epidemiologic methods, and some of them based on nonepidemiologic methods, converge on the same large and relatively invariant association – an obvious example being lung cancer and smoking, for which the validity of a causal connection (*see* **Causation**; **Hill's Criteria for Causality**) has long been beyond dispute.

Finally, one strength of the case–control approach can also be considered a major weakness: the ease with which case–control studies can sometimes be done, relative to cohort studies, means that the method can also more easily be abused. Case–control studies should be carried out by experienced investigators who are aware of their limitations, and they should be designed to anticipate and cope with potential sources of bias. When this has been done, there can be no doubt that they have made a major contribution to medical knowledge and to public health.

References

[1]   Beral, V. (1990). Childhood leukemia near nuclear plants in the United Kingdom: the evolution of a systematic approach to studying rare disease in small geographic areas, *American Journal of Epidemiology* **132**, Supplement, S63–S68.

[2] Berkson, J. (1976). Limitations of the application of fourfold table analysis to hospital data, *Biometrics Bulletin* **2**, 47–53.

[3] Breslow, N.E. & Day, N.E. (1980). *Statistical Methods in Cancer Research*, Vol. I. *The Analysis of Case–Control Studies*, IARC Scientific Publication No. 32. International Agency for Research on Cancer (IARC), Lyon.

[4] Cole, P. & Morrison, A.S. (1980). Basic issues in population screening for cancer, *Journal of the National Cancer Institute* **64**, 1263–1272.

[5] Cornfield, J. & Haenszel, W. (1960). Some aspects of retrospective studies, *Journal of Chronic Diseases* **11**, 523–524.

[6] Daling, J.R., Malone, K.E., Voigt, L.F., White, E. & Weiss, N.S. (1994). Risk of breast cancer among young women: relationship to induced abortion, *Journal of the National Cancer Institute* **86**, 1584–1592.

[7] Doll, R. & Hill, A.B. (1952). A study of the aetiology of carcinoma of the lung, *British Medical Journal* **2**, 1271–1286.

[8] Doll, R. & Hill, A.B. (1964). Mortality in relation to smoking: ten years' observation of British doctors, *British Medical Journal* **1**, 1399–1410, 1460–1467.

[9] Doll, R. & Peto, R. (1976). Mortality in relation to smoking: 20 years' observations on male British doctors, *British Medical Journal* **ii**, 1525–1536.

[10] Dorn, H.F. (1959). Some problems arising in prospective and retrospective studies of the etiology of disease, *New England Journal of Medicine* **261**, 571–579.

[11] Feinstein, A.R. (1975). The epidemiologic trohoc, the ablative risk ratio, and retrospective research, *Journal of Clinical Pharmacology and Therapy* **14**, 291–306.

[12] Gittes, R.F. (1991). Carcinoma of the prostate, *New England Journal of Medicine* **324**, 236–245.

[13] Greenberg, E.R. (1990). Random digit dialing for control selection. A review and a caution on its use in studies of childhood cancer, *American Journal of Epidemiology* **131**, 1–5.

[14] Greenland, S. (1980). The effect of misclassification in the presence of covariates, *American Journal of Epidemiology* **112**, 564–569.

[15] Greenland, S. (1996). Basic methods for sensitivity analysis of biases, *International Journal of Epidemiology* **25**, 1107–1116.

[16] Hartge, E.R., Brinton, L.A., Rosenthal, J.F., Cahill, J.I., Hoover, R.N. & Waksberg, J. (1984). Random digit dialing in selecting a population-based control group, *American Journal of Epidemiology* **120**, 825–833.

[17] Hartge, P. (1997). Abortion, breast cancer, and epidemiology (Editorial), *New England Journal of Medicine* **336**, 127–128.

[18] Kass, P.H. (1992). Converging toward a "Unified Field Theory" of epidemiology (Editorial), *Epidemiology* **3**, 473–474.

[19] Kaufman, D.W., Kelly, J.P., Levy, M. & Shapiro, S. (1991). *The Drug Etiology of Agranulocytosis and Aplastic Anemia*. Oxford University Press, Oxford.

[20] Kewitz, H.J., Jesdinsky, H., Schröter, P. & Lindtner, E. (1977). Reserpine and breast cancer in women in Germany, *European Journal of Clinical Pharmacology* **2**, 79–83.

[21] Leclerc, A., Martinez Cortes, M., Gerin, G., Luce, D. & Brugere, J. (1994). Sinonasal cancer and wood dust exposure: results from a case–control study, *American Journal of Epidemiology* **140**, 340–349.

[22] Linet, M.S. & Brookmeyer, R. (1987). Use of cancer controls in case–control cancer studies, *American Journal of Epidemiology* **125**, 1–11.

[23] Louik, C., Mitchell, A., Werler, M., Hanson, J. & Shapiro, S. (1987). Maternal exposure to spermicides in relation to certain birth defects, *New England Journal of Medicine* **317**, 474–478.

[24] Lund, E., Meirik, O., Adami, H.O., Bergstrom, R., Christoffersen, T. & Bergsjo, P. (1989). Oral contraceptive use and premenopausal breast cancer in Sweden and Norway: possible effects of a different pattern of use, *International Journal of Epidemiology* **18**, 527–532.

[25] MacMahon, B. & Trichopoulos, D. (1996). *Epidemiology. Principles and Methods*. Little, Brown & Company, Boston.

[26] Mantel, N. & Haenszel, W. (1959). Statistical aspects of the analysis of data from retrospective studies of disease, *Journal of the National Cancer Institute* **22**, 719–748.

[27] Melbye, M., Wohlfahrt, J., Olsen, J.H., Frisch, M., Westergaard, T., Helweg-Larsen, K. & Andersen, P.K. (1997). Induced abortion and the risk of breast cancer, *New England Journal of Medicine* **336**, 81–85.

[28] Miettinen, O.S. (1985). *Theoretical Epidemiology: Principles of Occurrence Research in Medicine*. Wiley, New York.

[29] Morrison, A.S. (1985). *Screening in Chronic Disease*, 2nd Ed. Oxford University Press, Oxford.

[30] Olsson, H., Moller, T.R. & Ranstam, J. (1989). Early oral contraceptive use and breast cancer among premenopausal women: final report from a study in southern Sweden, *Journal of the National Cancer Institute* **81**, 1000–1004.

[31] Parsonnet, J., Friedman, G.D., Vandersteen, D.P., Chang, Y., Vogelman, J.H., Orentreich, N. & Sibley, R.K. (1991). *Helicobacter pylori* infection and the risk of gastric carcinoma, *New England Journal of Medicine* **325**, 1127–1131.

[32] Rosenberg, L. (1994). Induced abortion and breast cancer: more scientific data are needed (Editorial), *Journal of the National Cancer Institute* **86**, 1569–1570.

[33] Rosenberg, L., Metzger, L.S. & Palmer, J.R. (1993). Epidemiology of breast cancer. Alcohol consumption and the risk of breast cancer: a review of the evidence, *Epidemiology Review* **15**, 133–144.

[34] Rosenberg, L., Palmer, J.R., Lesko, S.M. & Shapiro, S. (1990). Oral contraceptive use and the risk of myocardial infarction, *American Journal of Epidemiology* **131**, 1009–1016.

[35] Rosenberg, L., Shapiro, S., Slone, D., Kaufman, D.W., Helmrich, S., Miettinen, O.S., Stolley, P., Rosenshein, N.B., Schottenfeld, D. & Engle, R.L. (1982). Epithelial ovarian cancer and combination oral contraceptives, *Journal of the American Medical Association* **247**, 3210–3212.

[36] Rothman, K.J. (1986). *Modern Epidemiology*. Little, Brown & Company, Boston.

[37] Sackett, D.L. (1979). Bias in analytic research, *Journal of Chronic Diseases* **32**, 51–63.

[38] Shapiro, S., Castellana, J.V. & Sprafka, J.M. (1996). Alcohol-containing mouthwashes and oropharyngeal cancer: a spurious association due to underascertainment of confounders?, *American Journal of Epidemiology* **144**, 1091–1095.

[39] Skegg, D.C.G. (1988). Potential for bias in case–control studies of oral contraceptives and breast cancer, *American Journal of Epidemiology* **127**, 205–212.

[40] Stadel, B.V. (1981). Oral contraceptives and cardiovascular disease, *New England Journal of Medicine* **305**, 612–618.

[41] Stamey, T.A., Yang, N., Hay, A.R., McNeal, J., Freiha, F.S. & Redwine, E. (1987). Prostate-specific antigen as a serum marker for adenocarcinoma of the prostate, *New England Journal of Medicine* **317**, 909–916.

[42] Steineck, G. & Ahlbom, A. (1992). A definition of bias founded on the concept of the study base, *Epidemiology* **3**, 477–482.

[43] Swan, S.H., Shaw, G.M. & Schulman, J. (1992). Reporting and selection bias in case–control studies of congenital malformations, *Epidemiology* **3**, 356–363.

[44] Volini, I.F., Greenspan, I., Ehrlich, I., Gonner, J.A., Felfenfeld, O. & Schwartz, S.R. (1950). Hemopoietic changes during administration of chloramphenicol, *Journal of the American Medical Association* **42**, 1333–1335.

[45] Wacholder, S., McLaughlin, J.K., Silverman, D.T. & Mandel, J.S. (1992). Selection of controls in case–control studies. I. Principles, *American Journal of Epidemiology* **135**, 1019–1028.

[46] Wacholder, S., Silverman, D.T., McLaughlin, J.K. & Mandel, J.S. (1992). Selection of controls in case–control studies. II. Types of controls, *American Journal of Epidemiology* **135**, 1029–1041.

[47] Wacholder, S., Silverman, D.T., McLaughlin, J.K. & Mandel, J.S. (1992). Selection of controls in case–control studies. III. Design options *American Journal of Epidemiology* **135**, 1042–1050.

[48] Welch, H., Lewis, C.N. & Kerlan, I. (1954). Blood dyscrasias, a nationwide survey, *Antibiotics and Chemotherapy* **4**, 607.

[49] West, D.W., Sehaman, K.L., Lyon, J.L., Robison, L.M. & Allred, R. (1984). Differences in risk estimation from a hospital and a population-based case–control study, *International Journal of Epidemiology* **13**, 235–239.

[50] Ziel, H.K. & Finkle, W.D. (1975). Increased risk of endometrial carcinoma among users of conjugated estrogens, *New England Journal of Medicine* **293**, 1167–1170.

(*See also* **Prevalence–Incidence Bias**)

SAMUEL SHAPIRO & LYNN ROSENBERG

Bias in Cohort Studies

An epidemiologic **cohort** (or follow-up) study is typically performed by: (i) identifying a group of subjects who are at risk for a disease or condition of interest; (ii) determining the exposure status of each individual; and (iii) observing the subjects over time for the occurrence of the health outcome(s) under investigation. While this approach is advantageous in that it ensures that the temporal relationship between exposure and outcome is unambiguous, cohort studies are susceptible to the same kinds of **bias** (i.e. **selection, misclassification**, and **confounding**) as are other types of study design (*see* **Bias in Observational Studies Bias, Overview**).

Selection bias occurs when the study population available for analysis is not representative of the (theoretical) cohort of all eligible participants. This may result from biased sampling of the eligible cohort and/or selective losses from the study population during follow-up (*see* **Biased Sampling of Cohorts in Epidemiology**). The common attribute of all sources of selection bias is that the effect estimated from the available study population is meaningfully different from the one that would have been obtained had all subjects theoretically eligible to participate been included in the analysis. A potential source of nonrepresentative sampling is self-selection, whereby subjects who become aware of a study volunteer themselves for participation. If such volunteers have a different probability of developing the outcome of interest compared with the group of all eligible subjects [1, 4], then the result may be a biased estimate of effect. A related concept is the "healthy worker effect," based on the observation that people in the workforce have lower mortality rates than members of the general population [2, 4]. Studies that utilize workers must take this situation into account in order to avoid biased results (*see* **Occupational Epidemiology**).

Other important potential sources of selection bias in cohort studies include losses to follow-up and **nonresponse** during data collection (*see* **Cohort Study**; **Missing Data in Epidemiologic Studies**). However, bias is created only if data are missing disproportionately from one or more cells of the 2×2 table that relates a dichotomous exposure to a dichotomous outcome. Follow-up on a given subject may be incomplete for a variety of reasons. The subject may choose to withdraw his or her consent and no longer participate in the study. More commonly, the investigator simply loses contact with the subject, and thus cannot know with confidence whether he or she experienced the outcome of interest during the relevant follow-up period. When the outcome of interest is time to an event (e.g. death, diagnosis of disease, relapse, etc.), those individuals who do not experience the event during the study period are said to be censored. An assumption that is generally made with regard to such studies is that subjects who are censored at a given time have similar risks compared with those not censored at that time, i.e. that the censoring is "noninformative". If this assumption is violated, then bias results. Biased sampling may also occur if the probability that one is selected into the study sample depends upon whether he or she experiences the event of interest during a prescribed time window.

A final example of selection bias is illustrated by the "prevalent" cohort study. In such a study, subjects who already have a disease or other health condition are enrolled and then followed over time for events such as disease progression, relapse, or death. The goal is to obtain information about the natural history of the disease; however, problems of interpretation arise if the time since disease diagnosis remains unknown and is not uniform across subjects. Such difficulties must be weighed against the effort and costs required to assemble a cohort of newly diagnosed subjects, as would be done with the analogous "incident" cohort study.

Another type of bias to which cohort studies are susceptible is misclassification bias, a distortion in effect estimation that occurs when measurement errors result in incorrect classification of the exposure and/or disease status of study participants (*see* **Measurement Error in Epidemiologic Studies**). Such misclassification errors may be differential or nondifferential. When errors made in classifying subjects along one axis (i.e. exposure or disease) are independent of the subject's status on the other axis, the misclassification is said to be **nondifferential**. If the magnitude of the error along one axis varies

according to the category of the other axis (e.g. disease status is misclassified more frequently among the unexposed), then differential misclassification has occurred [4]. This distinction is of value, since, for dichotomous exposure and disease variables, nondifferential misclassification leads consistently to an underestimation of the magnitude of the association (**bias toward the null**). In contrast, bias from differential misclassification can be in any direction.

Classification errors arise from a variety of sources, including imprecise measurement tools, mistaken or missed diagnoses, and conscious or unconscious inaccuracies in self-reported disease and/or exposure information. An inaccurate diagnostic tool could lead to either over- or underascertainment of cases, causing disease misclassification that may be either differential or nondifferential with respect to exposure status. A potential source of differential disease misclassification is **detection bias**, whereby exposed subjects are followed more closely than their unexposed counterparts and are thus less likely to have unrecognized subclinical disease. The behavior of study personnel can also affect the accuracy of the data being collected. For example, an interviewer who is aware of both the study hypothesis and the exposure status of study participants may be more thorough in his or her questioning of exposed subjects regarding signs and symptoms indicative of the outcome of interest. Such **interviewer bias** is another potential source of differential misclassification and could thus lead to invalid study results.

The final category of bias which may affect cohort studies is **confounding**. Confounding operates similarly in all types of study designs, occurring when the effect of the exposure of interest is mixed up with that of one or more "extraneous" variables. The result can be over- or underestimation of the true effect of the exposure, the magnitude of the bias depending upon the nature of the relationships among the confounder(s), the exposure, and the disease. Confounding can be addressed in the design stage of a study – using randomization, restriction or matching – or in the analysis stage by employing stratified analysis (*see* **Stratification**) or applying a mathematical modeling technique [3] (*see* **Matching**; **Matched Analysis**).

References

[1]   Criqui, M.H., Austin, M. & Barrett-Connor, E. (1979). The effect of non-response on risk rations in a

cardiovascular disease study, *Journal of Chronic Diseases* **32**, 633–638.

[2]   Fox, A.J. & Collier, P.F. (1976). Low mortality rates in industrial cohort studies due to selection for work and survival in the industry, *British Journal of Preventive and Social Medicine* **30**, 225–230.

[3]   Kleinbaum, D.G., Kupper, L.L. & Morganstern, H. (1982). *Epidemiologic Research*. Van Nostrand Reinhold, New York.

[4]   Rothman, K.J. (1986). *Modern Epidemiology*. Little, Brown & Company, Boston.

HOLLY A. HILL & DAVID G. KLEINBAUM

Bias in Observational Studies

Bias can be defined as any **systematic error** (in contrast to sampling error) that results in inaccurate estimation of the effect of an exposure on an outcome. Such errors may occur in the design and/or analysis phase of an epidemiologic study and may result in either over- or underestimation of the true effect. Since bias is due to systematic rather than **random error**, the magnitude of the bias is not affected by sample size. Studies that produce effect estimates free of bias are said to be internally valid. An estimate which is internally valid may or may not be considered externally valid as well; the contrast between internal and external validity is discussed below. Although many sources of bias have been identified [14, 20, 21, 23], biases can generally be classified into one of three categories: **selection bias**, information bias, and **confounding** [14].

Selection Bias

Selection bias refers to a distortion in the estimate of effect resulting from (i) the manner in which subjects are selected for the study population and/or (ii) selective losses from the study population prior to data analysis. There are many sources of selection bias, and more than one source can contribute to bias in a given study. The common attribute of all sources of selection bias is that the effect estimated from the available study population is meaningfully different from the one that would have been obtained

had all subjects theoretically eligible to participate been included in the analysis. Selection bias can occur under any type of study design; however, it is of special concern in the design and conduct of **case–control studies** because the outcome has already occurred prior to selection of study subjects.

Sources of Selection Bias

In **cohort** (follow-up) **studies**, two important potential sources of selection bias include losses to follow-up and **nonresponse** during data collection (*see* **Bias in Cohort Studies**; **Missing Data in Epidemiologic Studies**). Both situations result in missing exposure and/or outcome information at the time of analysis for some eligible subjects. This creates the potential for selection bias, depending upon whether information is missing disproportionately from one or more cells of the 2×2 table that relates a dichotomous exposure to a dichotomous outcome (Table 1). Because the degree of bias relates to the amount of missing data in a cell relative to each of the other cells, selection bias may occur even with a fairly high overall response rate and/or very little loss to follow-up. For example, a cohort study might be conducted in which 90% of all subjects originally assembled into the cohort remain available for analysis at the end of the study (i.e. 10% of subjects were lost to follow-up). If the losses to follow-up are concentrated among the exposed subjects who ultimately developed the disease, the true **relative risk** could be underestimated by a substantial amount. Conversely, there may be no selection bias despite small response rates and/or large follow-up losses in each exposure category. If only 20% of all eligible subjects choose to participate in a study, but this 20% represents a true random sample of all potential participants, the resulting estimate of relative risk will be unbiased. In fact, even an assumption this stringent is not required. As long as, within each exposure category, the likelihood of being selected into the study (and available for analysis) is the same for subjects who develop the disease and subjects who do not, the risk for each

Table 1 2×2 table

	Exposed	Unexposed
Diseased	*a*	*b*
Nondiseased	*c*	*d*

exposure group (and thus the relative risk) can be estimated without bias.

The validity of any effect estimated from case–control data depends in part upon the appropriate choice of a comparison (**control**) group. The purpose of the controls is to estimate the **prevalence** of the exposure(s) of interest in the population from which the cases emerged. Any control group that yields over- or underestimates of this prevalence produces biased study results, unless there are compensating biases in the case sample. In terms of the 2×2 table (Table 1), selection bias results from an imbalance in the probability of being selected into the study (or remaining for the analysis) across the four cells. For example, **detection** (also called diagnostic or unmasking) **bias** [12, 21] can result from closer follow-up or more intense scrutiny of exposed vs. unexposed subjects. The detection of a higher proportion of subclinical outcomes among the exposed leads to an overrepresentation of exposed cases in a case–control study. Hospital-based case–control studies are subject to unique types of selection bias as a result of factors associated with admission to the hospital (*see* **Case–Control Study, Hospital-Based**). For example, **Berkson's fallacy** (bias) [3] results when an individual with two or more medical conditions is more likely to be hospitalized than someone with only one of the conditions. Thus, in a study utilizing hospital cases, there could be an apparent association between two conditions that does not exist in the general population. More generally, exposed cases may have a different chance of entering the hospital than nonexposed cases. Likewise, exposed and unexposed participants with control diseases may have different chances of hospital admission. These selection effects can bias the estimates of exposure effect [23]. Therefore, the choice of an appropriate control group can be difficult in a hospital-based case–control study. If the conditions for which controls have been hospitalized are associated with the exposure under study, then bias will result (*see* **Bias in Case–Control Studies**).

Certain types of selection bias may operate in either cohort or case–control studies. Among these is self-selection (or volunteer) bias, whereby subjects self-refer for participation in a study. Especially if the study hypothesis has been publicized, people who volunteer to become involved may differ in important ways from the group of all potentially eligible participants [5, 20]. Self-selection can also occur

prior to the initiation of a study. For example, it has been observed that active workers experience lower mortality than the general population, presumably because one must maintain a certain degree of health in order to remain a part of the workforce [8, 20]. Studies utilizing workers as subjects must therefore account for this "healthy worker effect" by choosing an appropriate comparison group to avoid the risk of drawing invalid conclusions (*see* **Occupational Epidemiology**).

A final illustration of selection bias involves the use of prevalence data to draw conclusions about incidence, for example in a **cross-sectional study** or a case–control study employing prevalent cases (*see* **Case–Control Study, Prevalent**). The problem, commonly referred to as selective survival, arises when persons with the disease of interest are unavailable to participate in a study because they have died prior to the study's initiation. If exposure status happens to be over- or underrepresented in the survivors, then the use of prevalence data to estimate incidence-based effect estimates can lead to biased results (*see* **Bias from Survival in Prevalent Case–Control Studies**).

Addressing Selection Bias

Efforts to avoid or minimize selection bias should be emphasized over attempts to correct for it in the analysis stage. As implied above, one of the most important ways of achieving this goal is through the careful choice of an appropriate comparison group, i.e. the controls should be representative of the population from which the cases emerged. It has been recommended that researchers conducting case–control studies use two or more control groups, as a means of drawing some conclusions about the likelihood of selection bias [16, 17]. If the effect estimate remains the same regardless of which control group is utilized, then this offers some degree of reassurance that selection bias has been avoided (although the possibility remains that all estimates are equally biased). If the estimated effects differ, then one is left with the decision of which control group is the most suitable. Other strategies for minimizing the potential for selection bias include efforts to achieve high response and follow-up rates and to assure equal opportunity for disease detection among exposed and unexposed subjects. Case–control studies using incident cases (including

nested case–control studies) are preferable to those using prevalent cases or to hospital-based studies.

The degree to which selection bias can be corrected after the collection of data depends on whether reliable estimates of the underlying selection or loss probabilities can be determined [14]. Since these probabilities are rarely known with accuracy, a suggested strategy is to consider a range of values of these parameters to assess the magnitude and direction of the bias that may be operating in a given study.

Information Bias

Information bias refers to a distortion in effect estimation that occurs when measurement of either the exposure or the disease is systematically inaccurate. This presentation focuses on "**misclassification bias**", the term used when such **measurement errors** result in incorrect classification of the exposure and/or disease status of study participants. It is useful to distinguish two types of misclassification – nondifferential and differential – since the distinction has implications for the direction and overall impact of the bias. If the misclassification is **nondifferential**, the errors made in classifying subjects along one axis (i.e. exposure or disease) are independent of their status with regard to the other axis. Differential misclassification occurs when such classification errors along one axis are not independent of the other axis [20]. For example, if a certain proportion of exposed subjects are mistakenly designated as unexposed, but the probability of misclassifying exposure is the same among diseased and nondiseased, then the result is nondifferential misclassification of exposure. If a certain proportion of diseased subjects are mistakenly designated as nondiseased, and the proportion misclassified varies by exposure status, then this represents differential misclassification of disease. In the case of the simple 2×2 table, nondifferential misclassification leads consistently to an underestimation of the magnitude of association between exposure and disease. Since the biased estimate is in the direction of no exposure–disease association, this phenomenon is termed **bias toward the null**. The situation becomes more complex when polytomous rather than dichotomous exposure variables are employed. In this circumstance, it is possible for

nondifferential misclassification to result in bias away from the null [6]. Bias from differential misclassification can be in any direction. Therefore, depending upon the situation, differential misclassification can result in an underestimation (bias toward the null) or an overestimation (bias away from the null) of the magnitude of an association. The biased and unbiased effect estimates can even be on opposite sides of the null value ("crossover bias").

It should be borne in mind that misclassification of both exposure and disease can occur in the same study and that errors can be made simultaneously in both directions (e.g. some truly diseased subjects are mistakenly classified as nondiseased while some truly nondiseased are mistakenly classified as diseased). Misclassification probabilities are often expressed in terms of **sensitivity** and **specificity**, terms that are more frequently used in discussions of **screening** or diagnostic test accuracy [9, 14].

Sources of Information (Misclassification) Bias

Classification errors can occur in any type of study and may be due to imprecise measurement (of exposure and/or disease), mistaken or missed diagnoses, conscious or unconscious inaccuracies in self-reported information, or any other factor that causes a subject to be placed into the wrong cell of the 2×2 table (Table 1). For example, if subjects are followed over time for the occurrence of a disease, some may develop subclinical disease which goes unrecognized by the investigators. Such subjects would be misclassified as nondiseased. If exposed subjects are under greater scrutiny than the unexposed, then they may be less likely to have undiagnosed subclinical disease. This implies that **detection bias**, described above as a type of selection bias for case–control studies, can lead to differential misclassification in a follow-up study. With an inaccurate diagnostic tool, overascertainment of cases is also possible, and could be either differential or nondifferential with respect to exposure status.

Another potential source of misclassification has to do with the quality of information provided by study subjects. It can probably be assumed that some degree of misclassification is inevitable when subjects are asked to report exposures or to provide other aspects of their medical histories. **Recall bias**, which induces differential misclassification, occurs when the accuracy of self-reported information varies across comparison groups [1]. For example, people who have recently been diagnosed with an illness may be seeking an explanation and therefore could be more motivated to recall past exposures than are those unaffected by the illness. This could lead to an underestimate of exposure prevalence among controls compared to cases, causing the **odds ratio** to be artificially inflated. Recall bias is a potential problem in any case–control study in which subjects are asked to recall previous exposures. Recall bias would be unlikely to affect cohort studies because exposure information is usually based on exposure status at baseline. Misclassification is also likely if it becomes necessary to gather data from surrogate respondents, depending upon the nature of the information requested and the level of detail required. Another potential source of inaccuracy has been termed "social desirability bias", which results from subjects' natural reluctance to report exposures and/or behaviors that are deemed socially unacceptable [24].

Those who are conducting the study can also have an impact on the degree and type of misclassification that occur during data collection. Knowledge of the study hypothesis and the comparison group to which a subject belongs could influence the behavior of personnel responsible for conducting interviews. For example, in a case–control study of the potential association between oral contraceptive use and development of venous thrombosis, subjects known to have experienced a venous thrombosis might be probed more deeply than controls for a history of oral contraceptive use. A similar situation might arise in a cohort study if an interviewer were more thorough in his or her questioning of exposed vs. unexposed subjects regarding signs and symptoms indicative of the outcome of interest. Such **interviewer bias** is a potential source of differential misclassification and could thus lead to invalid study results.

Addressing Information (Misclassification) Bias

Although there is always likely to be some degree of inaccuracy in measuring both exposures and outcomes, steps can be taken to minimize classification errors and reduce the probability that such errors will be differential (see below). Since nondifferential misclassification is more predictable in its impact and tends to result in underestimation of effects, it has generally been considered to be less of a threat

than differential misclassification [20]. It should be noted that if a study finds a significant relationship between an exposure and an outcome, it is illogical to dismiss the study results on the grounds that nondifferential misclassification is present, since the effect estimate obtained in the absence of such misclassification would only be stronger.

One strategy for addressing misclassification bias is to ensure that all study participants are subject to the same follow-up procedures and standardized diagnostic criteria. To the extent possible, both the study personnel responsible for data collection and the study subjects should be blinded as to the main hypothesis under investigation. Interviewers must follow standardized protocols and, if practical, should remain unaware of the comparison group (i.e. case/control or exposed/unexposed) to which study participants from whom they gather information belong. Acceptance of surrogate responses may not be appropriate for information that is subjective, highly personal, time-specific, or otherwise difficult to obtain from someone other than the subject him- or herself.

After data collection, correction for misclassification depends on the availability of information on probabilities of misclassification (e.g. sensitivity and specificity estimates) for variables that have been misclassified. Several authors have offered correction procedures: Barron [2] and Copeland et al. [4] provide correction formulae for 2×2 tables that assume nondifferential misclassification. These formulas were extended to allow for differential misclassification by Kleinbaum et al. [14] and to arbitrary multiway cross-classifications by Korn [15]. Greenland & Kleinbaum [10] provide correction formulae for matched data. Espeland & Hui [7] use log-linear models and maximum likelihood estimation to incorporate estimates of nondifferential misclassification probabilities gathered either by resampling the study population, sampling a separate population, or a priori assumption. Reade-Christopher & Kupper [19] use **logistic regression** to correct for nondifferential misclassification of exposure with a priori assumptions about misclassification probabilities. Also, recent work by Satten & Kupper [22] provides odds ratio regression methods when we have available only the probability of exposure (POE) for each study subject, and where these POE values are assumed to be known without error.

Correction for misclassification bias often requires information from a **validation study**, which may not be available. If such data are not available, then the best approach to evaluating the results of a study is to assess the probable magnitude and direction of suspected misclassification errors and discuss the likely impact of such errors on the estimated effect. Formulas used for correction for misclassification are useful for this purpose.

Confounding

Confounding is a type of bias that occurs when the effect of the exposure of interest is mixed up with that of one or more "extraneous" variables. This can result in an observed exposure–disease relationship being attributed exclusively to the exposure of interest, when in reality the relationship is due, either wholly or in part, to the effect of another variable or variables (i.e. **confounders**). Confounding can also create the appearance of an exposure–disease relationship when in fact none exists. The amount of bias introduced can be large or small, depending upon the nature of the relationships among the confounder(s), the exposure, and the disease. Confounding can lead to an over- or underestimation of the true effect and can also result in an estimated effect that is on the opposite side of the null from its true value.

Sources of Confounding

There is essentially only one source of confounding – the presence of certain key relationships between an extraneous variable and both the exposure and the disease. The first requirement is that the extraneous variable be a risk factor for the disease, i.e. that it is either causally related to the disease or is a correlate of a causal factor [14, 20] (*see* **Causation**). More specifically, the status of a confounder as a risk factor for the disease must be independent of its association with the exposure of interest; therefore, it must be a risk factor among the unexposed. The second criterion is that the confounder be associated with the exposure of interest. Theoretically, this relationship should hold in the source population that produces the cases of disease [18]. Practically speaking, it is generally assessed among all subjects in a follow-up study and among the controls in a case–control study. A final criterion is that the confounder should not be an "intervening variable" in the causal pathway between exposure and disease. In other words, if an extraneous variable were actually a measure of some type of biological alteration caused by the exposure, which in turn went on to cause the disease, then such a variable would not fulfill the criteria for a confounder but would simply be a mediator between exposure and disease.

In addition to the theoretical considerations described above, there is also a data-based criterion for assessing confounding. The crude measure is considered to be confounded "in the data" if it differs meaningfully in value from the "adjusted" estimate of effect that removes the influence of the extraneous variables being assessed as possible confounders. This "data-based" criterion is also referred to as the "**collapsibility**" criterion [11]. The absence of data-based confounding implies that the strata considered when controlling for a potential confounder can be collapsed (or pooled) without introducing bias.

Addressing Confounding

Although applicable only to experimental rather than observational studies, one technique for decreasing the likelihood of confounding is randomization. If the exposure of interest is allocated randomly to study subjects, then the probability that the exposure will be associated with a potential confounder is greatly reduced. Importantly, this benefit is gained for previously unidentified (and unobserved) potential confounders as well as for those suspected potential confounders that are measured. Restriction is another means of avoiding an unwanted relationship between the exposure and an extraneous variable. For example, if gender is a risk factor for the outcome of interest, and there is concern that gender will be unequally distributed between exposure groups, then restricting the study to either males or females will eliminate the possibility of confounding by this variable. However, the advantage of this approach must be weighed against the potential threat to generalizability (external validity, see below) that may result. Another strategy for addressing confounding is the practice of **matching**, whereby the comparison group is selected to be similar to the index group with regard to key variables that are suspected confounders. Although confounding can be controlled in unmatched designs, the primary statistical advantage of matching is that it can make control of confounding more efficient (i.e. increase the precision of an adjusted estimate) [14, 20].

In contrast to the other types of bias, viable options also exist for addressing confounding in the analysis phase of a study. If only one potential confounder is identified, then the simplest approach is to perform a stratified analysis (*see* **Stratification**), calculating a separate effect estimate for subjects in each category of the potential confounder (e.g. separate estimates for males and females, smokers and nonsmokers, etc.). If the estimates are similar across categories (i.e. there is no **interaction**), then they can be combined into a single adjusted estimate which removes the influence of the potential confounder (*see* **Mantel–Haenszel Methods Matched Analysis**). When several potential confounders are identified, the assessment of confounding is complicated, requiring simultaneous control of several variables as well as determination of which subset of potential confounders is most appropriate for simultaneous control [14]. The "gold standard" (i.e. most valid subset) to which all subsets should be compared contains the entire set of potential confounders. The use of stratified analysis is not a viable option when there is even a moderate number of potential confounders, since the number of strata becomes too large and individual strata may contain few or no subjects. An alternative approach uses a mathematical modeling procedure (e.g. **logistic regression**), and requires determining whether the estimated measure of effect changes meaningfully when potential confounders are deleted from the model [13, 14]. The term "meaningfully" implies a decision that does not involve statistical testing, but rather the consideration of biologic and/or clinical experience about the importance of a change in the effect measure. Variables identified as nonconfounders from this approach may be dropped from the model provided their deletion leads to a gain in precision (i.e. narrower confidence interval). In the absence of interaction, the assessment of confounding simplifies to monitoring changes in the estimated coefficient of the exposure variable. However, if there is interaction, then the assessment is more subjective because the collective change in several coefficients must be monitored. Consequently, when interaction is present, we recommend keeping all potential confounders in the model. Note, furthermore, that whether stratified analysis or mathematical modeling is used, misclassification of confounders can lead to incomplete or incorrect control of confounding [9]. Also, the use of regression modeling for control of confounding may yield misleading results if incorrect assumptions are made about the form and characteristics of the model being fit. Important characteristics to consider include the specific variables (e.g. "risk factors") chosen for control, the quantitative form that such variables should take in the model, the interaction effects to be evaluated, and the measurement scale (e.g. **additive** or **multiplicative**) used to assess interaction effects (*see* **Effect Modification**; **Relative Risk Modeling**).

Internal vs. External Validity

The discussion to this point has centered upon the issue of internal validity, or lack of bias. One may also be interested in assessing the external validity of an estimated effect (*see* **Validity and Generalizability in Epidemiologic Studies**). The distinction between internal and external validity has to do with the population about which inferences are to be made [14]. An internally valid effect estimate is one that correctly describes the association between exposure and outcome in the **target population**, i.e. the collection of individuals upon which the study was designed to focus and about whom one is able to draw direct conclusions. This is the group that has been sampled, though not necessarily in a random fashion. By contrast, external validity, or generalizability, refers to the making of inferences to an external population beyond the restricted interest of the particular study from which the effect is estimated. Assessing external validity involves making a judgment regarding whether the results of a study can be extended to apply to individuals who are dissimilar in some aspects (e.g. age, race, occupation) compared with those upon whom the study was focused.

References

[1]   Austin, H., Hill, H.A., Flanders, W.D. & Greenberg, R.S. (1994). Limitations in the application of case–control methodology, *Epidemiologic Reviews* **16**, 65–76.

[2]   Barron, B.A. (1977). The effects of misclassification on the estimation of relative risk, *Biometrics* **33**, 414–418.

[3]   Berkson, J. (1946). Limitations of the application of fourfold table analysis to hospital data, *Biometrics Bulletin* **2**, 47–53.

[4]   Copeland, K.T, Checkoway, H., McMichael, A.J., & Holbrook, R.H. (1977). Bias due to misclassification in the estimation of relative risk, *American Journal of Epidemiology* **105**, 488–495.

[5]   Criqui, M.H., Austin, M. & Barrett-Connor, E. (1979). The effect of non-response on risk ratios in a cardiovascular disease study, *Journal of Chronic Diseases* **32**, 633–638.

[6]   Dosemeci, M., Wacholder, S. & Lubin, J.H. (1990). Does nondifferential misclassification of exposure always bias a true effect toward the null value?, *American Journal of Epidemiology* **132**, 746–748.

[7]   Espeland, M.A. & Hui, S.L. (1987). A general approach to analyzing epidemiologic data that contain misclassification errors, *Biometrics* **43**, 1001–1012.

[8]   Fox, A.J. & Collier, P.F. (1976). Low mortality rates in industrial cohort studies due to selection for work and survival in the industry, *British Journal of Preventive and Social Medicine* **30**, 225–230.

[9]   Greenland, S. (1980). The effect of misclassification in the presence of covariates, *American Journal of Epidemiology* **112**, 564–569.

[10]   Greenland, S. & Kleinbaum, D.G. (1983). Correcting for misclassification in two-way tables and matched-pair studies, *International Journal of Epidemiology* **12**, 93–97.

[11]   Greenland, S. & Robins, J.M. (1986). Identifiability, exchangeability, and epidemiological confounding, *International Journal of Epidemiology* **15**, 412–418.

[12]   Horwitz, R.I. & Feinstein, A.R. (1978). Alternate analytic methods for case–control studies of estrogens and endometrial cancer, *New England Journal of Medicine* **299**, 1089–1094.

[13]   Kleinbaum, D.G. (1994). *Logistic Regression: A Self-Learning Text*. Springer-Verlag, New York.

[14]   Kleinbaum, D.G., Kupper, L.L. & Morganstern, H. (1982). *Epidemiologic Research*. Van Nostrand Reinhold, New York.

[15]   Korn, E.L. (1981). Hierarchical log-linear models not preserved by classification error, *Journal of the American Statistical Association* **76**, 110–112.

[16]   Lilienfeld, A.M. & Lilienfeld, D.E. (1980). *Foundations of Epidemiology*. Oxford University Press, New York.

[17]   MacMahon B. & Pugh, T.F. (1970). *Epidemiology – Principles and Methods*. Little, Brown & Company, Boston.

[18]   Miettinen, O.S. & Cook, E.F. (1981). Confounding: Essence and detection, *American Journal of Epidemiology* **114**, 593–603.

[19]   Reade-Christopher, S.J. & Kupper, L.L. (1991). Effects of exposure misclassification on regression analyses of epidemiologic follow-up study data, *Biometrics* **47**, 535–548.

[20]   Rothman, K.J. (1986). *Modern Epidemiology*. Little, Brown & Company, Boston.

[21]   Sackett, D.L. (1979). Bias in analytic research, *Journal of Chronic Diseases* **32**, 51–63.

[22]   Satten, G.A. & Kupper, L.L. (1993). Inferences about exposure–disease associations using probability-of-exposure information, *Journal of the American Statistical Association* **88**, 200–208.

[23]   Schlesselman, J.J. (1982). *Case–Control Studies*. Oxford University Press, New York.

[24]   Wynder, E.L. (1994). Investigator bias and interviewer bias: The problem of reporting systematic error in epidemiology, *Journal of Clinical Epidemiology* **47**, 825–827.

HOLLY A. HILL & DAVID G. KLEINBAUM

Bias Toward the Null

Bias toward the null usually refers to an effect of **nondifferential errors** in exposure measurements that reduces the apparent effect of the exposure on the dependent variable, which might be a health outcome. For linear regressions, bias toward the null is called attenuation (*see* **Measurement Error in Epidemiologic Studies**). Attenuation (or bias toward the null) does not change the sign of the coefficient of exposure in the regression, but it reduces the absolute magnitude toward zero. Similar effects are found for estimates of log relative odds in **logistic regression** and for **odds ratios** in 2×2 tables (*see* **Bias in Observational Studies**; **Misclassification Error**). The odds ratios are biased toward, but not beyond, unity. There are, however, more complex situations in which nondifferential error can induce a bias away from the null and thus exaggerate an apparent exposure effect or induce a bias that reverses the direction of an apparent exposure effect, as mentioned in the articles cited above.

Bias toward the null can also result from other sources of bias, such as **confounding** and **selection bias**.

M.H. GAIL

Biased Sampling of Cohorts in Epidemiology

The epidemiologic **cohort study** involves a sample of individuals followed over time. Individuals are monitored to ascertain the incidence of various endpoints such as the incidence of disease, infection, or death. The goal is to estimate the absolute **incidence rates** of the event or to identify covariates called risk factors that modify this risk. Individuals may also be monitored for changes in various markers of health status such as blood pressure measurements in prospective studies of cardiovascular disease, or CD4+ T cell counts or viral load measurements in natural history studies of acquired immune deficiency syndrome (AIDS). Usually cohort studies are prospective because subjects are monitored following establishment of the cohort. In a **historical cohort study**, however, earlier records are used to define membership in the cohort and to determine subsequent changes in health status.

Traditional approaches to the analysis of epidemiologic cohort studies include **person-years** analyses for rare events [1], **survival analyses** for more general time-to-event data [9], and longitudinal data analysis for repeated marker data [14]. While classical statistical methodologies routinely address sampling variation, other more systematic sources of error and **bias** that can overwhelm sampling variation are sometimes ignored. For example, **selection bias** resulting from biased sampling of the cohort either at enrollment or during the course of follow-up can seriously distort incidence and **relative risk** estimates. The objective of this article is to review how these different forms of sampling bias arise and how they can affect the results of studies. Other biases that result from **confounding** and measurement errors are discussed in other articles (*see* **Measurement Error in Epidemiologic Studies**; **Bias in Observational Studies**; **Bias in Cohort Studies**).

Self-Selection into the Study

Cohort studies may involve a sample of self-selected volunteers. In some circumstances, the self-selection into cohorts may be an important source of bias. Individuals may be solicited to participate in a cohort study through questionnaires and invitations, and those who respond and choose to participate may differ from those who do not participate with respect to known and unknown disease risk factors. For example, the Framingham Study, a long-term cohort study of heart disease initiated about 1950, issued an invitation to every town resident in the age range 20–70 to join the study. A lower death rate was subsequently observed among those individuals who chose

to participate compared with nonparticipants [20]. One explanation for the mortality difference was that nonparticipants may be selectively frailer because study participation required a clinic visit. Although one might expect the differences in mortality rates to diminish over time, the Framingham Study found higher mortality rates among nonparticipants at both two and five years after study invitation. In another example involving a cohort study of British physicians, lower mortality rates were observed among physicians who replied to an initial questionnaire compared with those physicians who did not respond [1, 15]. In a population-based **cross-sectional study** of cardiovascular disease, less cardiovascular disease was found among respondents compared with nonrespondents [10]. In the above examples, less disease was observed among the study participants or responders. However, it is also possible to observe more disease among respondents. For example, the Centers for Disease Control investigated leukemia incidence among individuals near the Smoky Atomic Test in Nevada [7, 35]. Among the 18% of subjects who were self-referred and contacted the investigators, because of publicity about the study, there were four leukemia cases. Among the remaining 82% of subjects who were traced by investigators, there were also four leukemia cases. These data suggest that those individuals with disease were more likely to respond voluntarily and to participate in the study.

Self-selection is a potentially important source of bias particularly if the main comparison is with an external **control** group. For example, if the mortality rates of a self-selected group of smokers were compared with general population mortality rates, then the effect of smoking could be masked if the study participants were healthier than the general population. However, if the main comparison is with an internal control group, then self-selection may not be a source of bias. For example, among those who self-selected into the study, the mortality rates of smokers could be compared with those of nonsmokers. If the assumption is that the effect of self-selection was comparable for both smokers and nonsmokers, then the relative risk of smoking based on the self-selected group may be unbiased. However, the absolute mortality rates of the self-selected groups of smokers and nonsmokers may be a biased estimate of the rates in the general population. There is, however, no guarantee that the relative risks are unbiased because self-selection may act differentially on the exposure groups. Both empirical and theoretical investigations of the impact of self-selection on relative risks have been performed [11, 21, 29].

A related bias is the healthy worker effect (*see* **Occupational Epidemiology**). The healthy worker effect occurs in cohort studies of occupational risks [1, 34]. For example, a cohort study may be conducted to evaluate the health effects associated with working in a particular occupational setting. The mortality rates among those individuals who are employed in the occupation might be compared with an external control group. However, employed individuals may have a lower mortality rate than the general population that is also made up of unemployed. Indeed, individuals may leave employment upon the onset of severe life-threatening diseases. Internal control groups help to correct the bias from the healthy worker effect, where an exposed group of employees is compared with an unexposed group of employees. For example, workers exposed to carbon disulfide were compared with workers in the paper industry as well as with the general Finnish population [23, 28]. Although the exposed workers had the highest coronary heart disease mortality rates, the rates among both exposed and unexposed workers in the paper industry were considerably lower than the rates in the general population.

Follow-Up Bias

Cohort studies typically follow individuals until an event occurs. However, there is often incomplete follow-up; that is, an individual may have follow-up data only up to time t and there is no information on the status of the individual beyond t. In that case, all that is known is that the individual did not have an event prior to time t. Such observations are right censored. There are different reasons for censoring. One reason may be because the cohort study is ending and the investigators wish to analyze the data. In this case we say the individual is administratively censored. We say the individual is lost to follow-up if the individual is right censored because of all other reasons including the patient has moved away or the individual no longer wishes to participate in the study.

Most statistical methods for the analysis of follow-up data from cohort studies assume that individuals censored at some time t have similar risks as individuals not censored at t. This is noninformative censoring [30]. Generally, the assumption of noninformative censoring is plausible for administrative censoring because the reason for the censoring was external from the individual. If the assumption of noninformative censoring is violated, then we say there is follow-up bias. If the individuals lost to follow-up are at lower risk than those who remain under follow-up, then the event rates will be overestimated. For example, those individuals who are particularly healthy may move away from the study area. Alternatively, if the individuals lost to follow-up are at higher risk of an event than those who remain under follow-up, then the event rates will be underestimated. For example, the frailer individuals may be too weak to attend clinic visits, and are thus the ones lost to follow-up. Of particular concern are studies where the event of interest is a particular cause of death, and individuals who die of other causes are considered censored [17] (*see* **Competing Risks**). The assumption of noninformative censoring may be violated if there is dependence between the cause of death of interest and another cause of death. This can occur if an unknown risk factor is associated with both causes of death. The dependence can be either positive or negative. For example, positive dependence arises between coronary heart disease and some types of cancer if smoking, which is a risk factor for both, is ignored. Alternatively, negative dependence may arise if alcohol consumption is ignored because alcohol may increase risk for some cancers but decrease risk for coronary heart disease [36].

Unfortunately, the assumption that censoring is noninformative cannot usually be verified from observable data [38]. One way to evaluate the sensitivity of the Kaplan–Meier estimate to the assumption is to create bounds assuming perfect positive and negative dependence between the censoring and survival times [33]. The lower bound of the estimated survival curve is obtained by assuming that censored observations experience the event immediately after being censored. The upper bound is obtained by assuming censored observations never experience the event. Dependent censoring cannot only bias survival curve estimation but can also reverse the effect of a true risk factor and make it appear protective [36].

One approach to control the bias introduced by informative censoring is to attempt to identify a variable (covariate) such that in a given level or stratum of the variable, censoring is noninformative. Such a variable would be associated both with the risks of disease and the risk of loss to follow-up. The statistical analysis must then account for this covariate using either regression or stratified analyses (*see* **Stratification**). Similar problems arise in longitudinal data analysis where dropouts are informative as opposed to completely random [14]. Some approaches for modeling the dropout process in longitudinal data analysis have been proposed that allow the probability of dropout at time t to depend on the history of measurements up to time t [13].

Truncation

Truncation is a potentially important source of bias in cohort studies with nonstandard sampling. Generally, truncation occurs if the probability that an individual is sampled for follow-up depends on the individual's event time. There are different forms of truncation. Left truncation arises if the individual comes under observation only if the individual's event (survival) time exceeds a known time, which we call the truncation time. Right truncation arises if the individual is included in the cohort only if the individual's event time is less than a known (truncation) time. Left truncation is discussed in more detail in this section, and an example of right truncation is discussed in detail in a later section of this article.

As a simple example of left truncation, consider a study whose objective is to identify prognostic factors for survival among patients with a particular disease. Now suppose only individuals with the disease who are *alive* at calendar time C are eligible for sampling into the study. Under this sampling design only individuals with survival times $t_i \geq C - u_i$, where u_i is the calendar time of diagnosis of disease have the opportunity to be included in the cohort. Individuals with shorter survival times are selectively excluded. Unless special adjustments are made for the left truncated data, standard statistical analyses can be seriously biased. For example, suppose the standard nonparametric Kaplan–Meier (product–limit) estimate is calculated based on the data (t_i, δ_i), where t_i is the event time for uncensored individuals or the last follow-up time for censored individuals and δ_i is a right censoring indicator that indicates if the individual had an event at time t_i (in which case, $\delta_1 = 1$)

or was censored at time t_i (in which case $\delta_i = 0$). The Kaplan–Meier estimate of the survival function, $S(t)$ (probability of surviving beyond time t) is

$$\hat{S}(t) = \prod_{\{t_i \leq t\}} \left(\frac{n_i - d_i}{n_i} \right),$$

where n_i is the number at risk at t_i, i.e. the number of individuals with survival times greater or equal to t_i who have not been previously censored, and d_i are the numbers of (uncensored) events that occurred at t_i. Under usual sampling (i.e. a random sample of individuals are chosen for the cohort), the standard Kaplan–Meier estimate is a consistent estimate of the survival curve [2]. However, if the data are left truncated, then the standard Kaplan–Meier estimate of the survival curve will overestimate the true survival curve. The intuition for this bias is as follows. If we look at all individuals diagnosed with disease at time u_i, only those with long survival ($t_i \geq C - u_i$) are included in the data set, and this selection results in an overestimation of survival probabilities.

The correct Kaplan–Meier analysis that accounts for left truncation requires a different definition of the risk set. The correct definition of the risk set at time t to account for left truncation includes only those individuals who have neither had an event nor been censored prior to t and *who are under active follow-up at time t.* That is to say we require for an individual to be included in the risk set at time t that (i) the individual has not had an event or been censored prior to time t and (ii) $u_i + t \geq C$. The Kaplan–Meier estimator based on this definition of risk sets has been called the truncation product–limit estimator, and its theoretical properties have been studied by Tsai et al. [37]. Implicit in the truncation product–limit estimator is the assumption that risks (hazards) of the event depend only on follow-up time and depend neither on calendar time of disease diagnosis nor calendar time of study enrollment. These stationarity assumptions are discussed in [39].

Parametric estimation of survival curves from left truncated data also requires modification of traditional methods. The key idea is that the contributions from each individual to the likelihood function must be *conditional* on the sampling criteria. Specifically, because individuals are required to be alive at calendar time C, we can account for left truncation by conditioning on the event that an individual's survival time is at least $C - u_i$. Then the likelihood function for estimating the parameters in a survival distribution $S(t)$ with density $f(t)$ from data (t_i, δ_i, u_i) for N individuals is

$$\prod_{i=1}^{N} \left[\frac{f(t_i)}{S(C - u_i)} \right]^{\delta_i} \left[\frac{S(t_i)}{S(C - u_i)} \right]^{1-\delta_i} .$$

The usual naive likelihood function that did not account for left truncation would not include the denominator terms $S(C - u_i)$ in the above likelihood function.

Special care is also needed in computing incidence rates when the data are left truncated. The incidence rate is usually calculated as the ratio of the number of events divided by the total person time of follow-up. This estimator of incidence is justified if the hazard of the event is constant over time. A source of confusion in the calculation of total person time is the amount of person time contributed by left truncated individuals. A naive analysis might allocate person time equal to t_i for all individuals, even if left truncated. However, that would lead to an underestimation of event incidence rates because events that occurred before C are not included in the calculation, but person time of the left truncated individuals is included. The correct analysis that accounts for left truncation has individuals contribute person time only during the period that they are actually under observation [1, 3]. Thus, in our example, a left truncated individual contributes person time accrued only after enrollment at calendar time C, that is, the contribution is $t_i - (C - u_i)$.

Special care is also needed in applying the **proportional hazards model** to left truncated data. The model formalizes the relative risk concept for studies of time to response and generalizes it to the regression setting. The model assumes that the time-specific incidence **(hazard) rate** in an exposed population is proportional to the incidence rate in an unexposed population. For a covariate with two levels the model is

$$\lambda_1(t) = \theta \lambda_0(t), \qquad (1)$$

where $\lambda_1(t)$ and $\lambda_0(t)$ are the hazard rates at time t among those with and without the risk factor, respectively, and the parameter θ is the hazard ratio (or relative risk). An important question is: What is the time scale t on which the proportional hazards model (1) is defined? The most appropriate time scale is the one that needs the most careful control to obtain valid comparisons between the treatment groups. Often the time scale is follow-up time, i.e. t is the time the individual has been under active follow-up. Sometimes, however, there is a more natural time scale whose origin is defined by some initiating event [39]. For example, in studies of chronic disease incidence, the most appropriate time scale might be chronological age. In a prognostic factor study for survival among patients with a disease, the origin of the time scale might be the time of disease diagnosis. In this last example, if the time scale refers to time since diagnosis (as opposed to follow-up time) special care is needed in constructing the risk sets of the partial likelihood analysis when the data are left truncated. A naive proportional hazards analysis that defined risk sets in the standard way (i.e. all individuals with event times greater than or equal to t_i and not previously censored) can yield biased estimates of the relative risk. For example, suppose the cohort study recruits individuals alive with disease at calendar time $C = 1995$. The covariate of interest is disease diagnosed before 1990 ($X = 0$) or after 1990 ($X = 1$). Even if there were no differences in the hazards of death by calendar year of diagnosis ($\theta = 1$), the naive proportional hazards analysis would give $\theta > 1$ (aside from sampling variation). This is because all individuals diagnosed before 1990 ($X = 0$) who have survival times that are less than five years would not have an opportunity to be sampled and included in the cohort. However, among all individuals diagnosed after 1990 ($X = 1$), at least some of the individuals with survival times less than five years could have an opportunity to be sampled. The correct proportional hazards analysis of left truncated data requires an adjusted definition of risk sets similar to the adjustments described previously for Kaplan–Meier estimation. Basically, individuals should be included in risk sets only if they are under active follow-up at that time.

Truncation in Retrospective Studies

Some studies have selected individuals for enrollment based on the occurrence of the primary event of interest, and then studied these cases retrospectively to ascertain their survival time in order to estimate survival curves. The key feature of this type of design is that only individuals who have an event are eligible for inclusion in the study. For example, the first study of the **incubation period** of AIDS involved only a sample of AIDS cases who developed AIDS from a blood transfusion [32]. These patients were identified and selected for study *because they developed AIDS*. These patients were then studied retrospectively to determine the dates of transfusion with infected blood. Thus, the incubation period was determined as the time between blood transfusion and AIDS diagnosis. Another example of a retrospective study with truncation involved the selection of pediatric AIDS patients whose only known risk was maternal transmission; the dates of infection were assumed to be the dates of birth. In this case the incubation period is the time between birth and AIDS diagnosis. These are examples of retrospective studies with *right* truncated data in which individuals with long incubation periods are selectively excluded because they may not yet have had an event at the time of sampling (i.e. the time that individuals are selected for inclusion in the study).

There are also examples of **retrospective studies** with *left* truncated data. For example, a study was conducted to estimate the interval between first exposure to the human immunodeficiency virus (HIV) and the development of detectable HIV antibodies (seroconversion); this interval is called the preantibody phase [41]. This study selected only those individuals who seroconverted late in calendar time (in the late 1980s). Sera samples from these individuals had been stored and were tested by polymerase chain reaction (PCR) to ascertain the time of first exposure to HIV. However, these individuals are a biased sample and over-represent the longer preantibody durations because individuals with short preantibody duration would have been more likely to seroconvert earlier in calendar time and thus not be included in the study [40, 42].

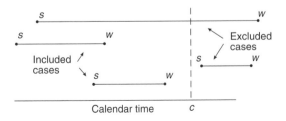

Figure 1 Schematic illustration of a retrospective study of cases (transfusion-associated AIDS) with right truncated data. Only cases diagnosed before calendar time of sampling (C) are included (i.e. $w_i < C$): s = infection date; w = AIDS diagnosis date; c = case ascertainment date

The remainder of this section considers the analysis of retrospective studies with right truncated data. The methods and issues are illustrated with the study of incubation periods of transfusion associated AIDS described previously. Figure 1 illustrates the sampling scheme: all (AIDS) cases diagnosed before some calendar time C are sampled. The figure illustrates the main problems with the analysis and interpretation of this type of data. First, since the data involve only individuals who have experienced events (AIDS diagnoses), without strong parametric assumptions, they can provide no information about the prospective probability that an infected individual eventually develops the disease. Secondly, the sampling scheme tends to over-represent individuals with shorter incubation periods. The data are right truncated because individuals with very long incubation periods are selectively excluded. The data consist of the calendar dates of infection s_i and the calendar dates of diagnosis w_i. The time to event (incubation period) is $u_i = w_i - s_i$. The criterion for inclusion in the data set is that $u_i \leq T_i$, where $T_i = C - s_i$ is called the truncation time. As illustrated in Figure 1, individuals with longer incubation periods tend to be selectively excluded because such individuals are less likely to have developed the endpoint (AIDS) at the time of ascertainment. Failure to account for such **length-biased** sampling will cause the incubation time to be underestimated.

Both nonparametric and parametric statistical procedures have been proposed for estimating the distribution function of the times to event from such data. Nonparametrically, the best that can be done is to estimate the distribution function conditional on the time to event being less than the maximum truncation time. The maximum truncation time T^* refers to the longest event time that could possibly be observed under this sampling procedure. There are simple computational approaches for calculating the nonparametric estimate of $F^*(t)$, which is the cumulative probability that an incubation period is less than t conditional on it being less than T^*. This is based on expressing F^* as the product of conditional probabilities as follows [26, 31]. Let $t_1, t_2, \ldots, t_n$ be the ordered observed event times. In the AIDS example, these are the incubation times. The nonparametric estimate $\hat{F}^*(t)$ of $F^*(t)$ is

$$\hat{F}^*(t_s) = \prod_{j=s+1}^{n} \left(1 - \frac{d_j}{m_j}\right), \quad s = 1, \ldots, n-1,$$

(2)

and $\hat{F}^*(t_n) = 1.0$, where d_j is the number of individuals with event times exactly equal to t_j, and m_j are the numbers of individuals with truncation times greater than or equal to t_j (i.e. $T_i = C - s_i \geq t_i$) and whose event times are less than or equal to t_j. The estimate (2) is a step function with jumps at observed incubation times; $\hat{F}^*$ reaches the value 1.0 at the largest observed event time. The estimate $\hat{F}^*$ accounts for the length-biased sampling that arises from right truncation. A naive estimate that was based simply on the proportion of event times less than t would grossly overestimate the true distribution function $F(t)$ and would suggest that event times are shorter than they really are.

Parametric approaches can also be used to analyze retrospective studies with right truncated data. While some parametric assumptions may permit estimation not only of the conditional distribution F^* but also the unconditional distribution F, the resulting estimates of F are extremely imprecise and depend strongly on parametric assumptions. This is because parametric approaches do not circumvent the main weakness in the data; it is not possible to observe event times greater than the maximum truncation time. Several likelihood functions have been proposed for the parametric analysis of retrospective data on cases with right truncation [5, 26]. The differences in the various likelihood functions that have been proposed arise from using different conditioning events. At a minimum, the likelihood function must condition on having an event prior to the case ascertainment time C. In addition, some of the proposed likelihood functions condition on the time origins (dates of infection s_i).

Prevalent Cohort Studies

Prevalent cohort studies are used to study the natural history of disease [6]. The prevalent cohort study consists of a sample of individuals who have a condition or disease at the time of enrollment in the study. These individuals are then followed over time to monitor endpoints such as disease progression or death. In some situations the durations of time the individuals have been prevalent with the disease or condition prior to enrollment are known. For example, Cnaan & Ryan [8] considered survival analysis of a registry of sarcoma patients seen at certain institutions that included some patients who were initially diagnosed elsewhere. These data are left truncated because the patients diagnosed at other institutions must have survived long enough to be included in the sample. The methods for left truncated data outlined in the previous section are required to account adequately for the sampling scheme [8].

A more serious complexity arises in the analysis and interpretation of prevalent cohort studies if the durations of time the individuals have been prevalent with the disease or condition prior to enrollment is unknown. This section is concerned with the issues in the analysis and interpretation of prevalent cohort data when the prior durations are unknown.

An example of a prevalent cohort concerns a study of HIV infected individuals with the objective to estimate rates of progression to AIDS and to identify covariates that modify these rates. In this example, individuals who are alive and previously infected with HIV are eligible for enrollment. These individuals are then followed for the onset of disease progression (AIDS). The main complexity is that the previous calendar times of infection are unknown. Figure 2 gives a schematic illustration of the prevalent cohort study. There are three time scales: calendar time (s), the time from infection (u), and follow-up time (t). A prevalent sample of individuals who are HIV infected and alive is taken at calendar time Y. The main advantage of the prevalent cohort study is that it can be performed more rapidly than can traditional cohort studies of individuals with incident (new) HIV infection. The traditional cohort study requires a sample of newly infected individuals and there could be considerable expense and effort entailed to identify such a sample. However, a number of important problems arise in the interpretation and analysis of a prevalent cohort that do not arise with a series of newly infected (incident) individuals because the duration of time a person has been infected prior to the beginning of follow-up is not known.

This section outlines the biases and problems of interpretation in prevalent cohorts. Although the prevalent cohort is discussed using the HIV/AIDS example described above, the conclusions, of course, apply to many other settings: for example, a study among prevalent carriers of hepatitis B surface antigen in order to identify modifiers of risk for hepatocellular carcinoma. The unifying feature is that there is an initiating event of a disease (e.g. infection) that

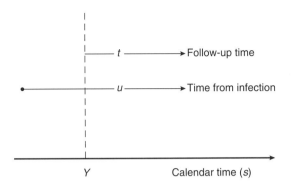

Figure 2 Schematic illustration of the prevalent cohort study

defines the natural biological time scale, and individuals who are prevalent with the condition are then enrolled. This results in left truncated data but, unfortunately, one cannot analyze prevalent cohorts using methods for left truncated data because the truncation times are unknown.

Suppose analyses are performed on the time scale of the observed follow-up time (t) instead of the desired, but unobservable, natural time scale (u) such as time from infection. Specifically, how do estimates derived from prevalent cohorts of the probability of an event within t years of follow-up, $F_p(t) = 1 - S_p(t)$, relate to $F(t)$ which is the probability of an event within t years of infection? The proportion of persons in a prevalent cohort who develop disease within t years of follow-up, $F_p(t)$, does not in general approximate $F(t)$. Only if the hazard function on the natural time scale $\lambda(u)$ is constant (an exponential distribution for F) do the two coincide. This follows from the lack of memory property of an exponential distribution, which implies that a newly infected individual will progress to the event at the same rate as an individual who has been alive for some time. However, if the hazard $\lambda(u)$ is monotonically increasing, then individuals in the prevalent cohort will be at greater risk of an event than are newly infected individuals. That is to say, the cumulative probability of an event within t years of follow-up of a prevalent cohort is larger than that based on t years of follow-up of an incident (newly infected) cohort $[F_p(t) > F(t)]$. The direction of the bias is reversed for a decreasing hazard. No general statements can be made about the direction of the bias for nonmonotonic hazard functions. Regardless of the shape of the

hazard, $F_p(t)$ is a lower bound on the ultimate proportion of individuals who will have an event, $F(\infty)$. Brookmeyer & Gail [4] derived exact expressions for the distribution function on the observed follow-up time scale, $F_p(t)$, in terms of the probability density of infection times among cohort members and the true distribution function F. The magnitude of the biases depend both on the hazard function, $\lambda(t)$, and the density of calendar times of prior infection (the initiating event) among those individuals in the prevalent cohort. For example, the bias would be small if the prevalent cohort is assembled near the beginning of the epidemic, in which case the backward recurrence times (or the times from infection to the onset of follow-up) would be short (see **Back-Calculation**).

The prevalent cohort study is a rapid and convenient approach to identify cofactors and markers of disease progression. However, because the onset date is unknown, there are biases that result from using follow-up time instead of time from infection. The most important bias associated with identifying cofactors from prevalent cohorts is called *onset confounding* [4, 6]. This occurs when the unknown calendar date of infection is associated both with the risk of disease and the cofactor under study. A subgroup may appear at higher risk of progression to disease simply because they were infected earlier than another subgroup. For example, individuals in one geographic region may exhibit a higher progression rate to disease than other individuals. This finding could be an artifact if individuals in one city were infected earlier in calendar time, and the hazard function $\lambda(t)$ is increasing. The requirement to insure no onset confounding is that the probability densities of infection times among individuals infected before calendar time Y is the same in the two subgroups. Onset confounding can be controlled by stratification on factors such as geographic region. Stratification on a covariate is useful provided we are not interested in determining whether the covariate itself is a cofactor of disease progression.

Unfortunately, even if a covariate has no direct effect on the probability density of infection times among members of the prevalent cohort so that there is no onset confounding, relative risk estimates obtained from prevalent cohorts may still be biased. To see this, assume that a cofactor with two levels obeys the following simple proportional hazards model:

$$\lambda_1(u) = \theta\lambda_0(u),$$

where $\lambda_1(u)$ and $\lambda_0(u)$ are the disease incidence rates at time u among those with and without the factor, respectively, and θ is the ratio of the hazards. In this model, the underlying primary time scale is the natural but unobservable scale u, time since first infection. If this model holds, but a proportional hazards analysis is performed based on follow-up time, then tests of the null hypothesis $H_0 : \theta = 1$ will be valid provided there is no confounding. However, estimates of θ based on the incorrect assumption of proportional hazards on the observed follow-up time scale will usually be biased for θ. The term *differential length biased sampling* is used to refer to this bias, which results from differences in the distributions of prior durations of infection (backward recurrence times) between the two prevalent subgroups [4]. Differential length-biased sampling may bias the relative risk from a prevalent cohort, and the direction of the bias depends on whether the hazard function is increasing or decreasing, as discussed below.

If the hazard function is increasing, then relative risk estimates obtained from follow-up on a prevalent cohort will be biased toward unity. A theoretical proof is given in [4] but an intuitive justification is as follows. Infected persons with a risk factor are at higher risk of disease than infected persons without the risk factor. Persons sampled for the prevalent cohort who are in the low-risk group will tend to have longer prior durations of infection than persons in the high-risk group. This is because high-risk persons infected many years earlier are more likely to have developed disease and thus be excluded from the prevalent cohort. Since low-risk persons tend to have been infected for a longer time, their disease is further advanced [with an increasing hazard $\lambda_0(u)$] and therefore the disparity in risk of disease between two groups is reduced, biasing the relative risk toward 1. Analogously, if the hazard function $\lambda_0(u)$ is decreasing, then the relative risk will be biased away from 1. Fortunately, the magnitude of differential length-biased sampling phenomena is never enough to reverse the conclusion, that is to push the relative risk to the other side of 1. Furthermore, there are two situations when the effect of differential length bias could be expected to be negligible: (i) if there is little dispersion in the infection dates (in which case all backward recurrence times are nearly identical) and (ii) if the

hazard $\lambda_0(u)$ is small so that only a small proportion of those infected before the initiation of the prevalent cohort study develop disease before the end of follow-up and are selectively excluded (see [4] for a more formal statement of the conditions when the bias from differential length biased sampling is small).

Other types of biases in prevalent cohorts arise in the analysis of the time-dependent covariate, that is the variable whose value changes over time u. There are two types of time-dependent covariates, "external" and "internal" [27]. The main distinction is that internal time-dependent covariates reflect the health of the individual (markers) while external time-dependent covariates are applied externally, such as a random assignment to a treatment group. For example, consider an external time-dependent variable which takes effect at some point after the onset of follow-up. An example might be a treatment given to some members of a prevalent cohort. If the treatment is assigned randomly, then the condition for no onset confounding is satisfied. Unfortunately, even without onset confounding, relative risk estimates of the treatment effects will still be biased [4]. Specifically, assume that the effect of the treatment is to multiply the hazard by θ, that is consider a proportional hazards model with a time-dependent covariate $x(u)$, where $x(u)$ is 0 before initiation of treatment and 1 thereafter:

$$\lambda_1(u) = \theta^{x(u)}\lambda_0(u). \qquad (3)$$

Then, the relative risk estimate of θ based on the proportional hazards analysis with a time-dependent covariate on the follow-up time scale t will yield an estimate of θ that is biased toward unity, regardless of whether the hazard function is strictly increasing or decreasing. This bias results because the analysis controls for follow-up time t when in fact the analysis should control for the unknown time from infection u. The result that the risk estimates are biased toward unity is seen intuitively from the following argument. Suppose, without loss of generality, that $\theta > 1$. Then the effect of the variable $x(u)$ is to accelerate disease, especially among frail individuals. If the hazard is increasing, then the frail individuals are those that have been infected for a longer time. Therefore the individuals with $x(u) = 1$ tend to be selectively depleted from the frail individuals, and the net effect is to decrease the disparity in risk between those with $x(u) = 1$ and those with $x(u) = 0$. This bias has been called *frailty selection*. A similar argument holds if the hazard is decreasing. In either case, the effect of frailty selection is to bias the relative risk toward unity.

Internal time-dependent covariates, also known as *markers*, present different issues. Markers track the progression of disease and change value over the course of follow-up. Markers change in response to disease progression and may convey information about the duration of infection. For example, persons with abnormal marker levels are likely to have been infected longer than persons with normal levels. Suppose the proportional hazards model (3) holds. In model (3) the parameter θ reflects the disease–marker association controlling for duration of infection; that is θ quantifies the prognostic information in the marker over and above the prognostic information in the duration of infection. Unfortunately, in prevalent cohort studies of markers that are performed on the follow-up time scale, estimates of θ in model (3) as well as hypothesis tests of $\theta = 1$ may not be valid and are not comparable with results obtained from an incident cohort. Furthermore, no general statements can be made about the direction of the biases because both frailty selection and onset confounding are operating. For example, a high relative risk associated with an elevated marker may reflect the fact that individuals with the elevated marker have been infected longer.

The various biases associated with prevalent cohorts are summarized in Table 1. Because of these biases, prevalent cohort studies pose serious limitations for studying the disease–marker association of model (3). Prospective studies of an incident cohort are required to disentangle the role of markers and duration of infection on disease risk. Nevertheless, prevalent cohort studies of markers may serve other important purposes. For example, baseline values of markers measured at enrollment ($t = 0$) are useful for prognostic purposes. Survival analyses and proportional hazards analyses on the scale of time since enrollment address the prognostic information in the baseline marker over and above time since enrollment. This is useful for counseling individuals, and for deciding on a course of treatment. These analyses answer the question: "What prognostic information does the baseline marker value provide in addition to *time since enrollment*?" The question "What prognostic information does the baseline marker value provide in addition to *time since infection*?" cannot be answered from such studies and analyses. Nonetheless, such analyses are useful, because the dates of infection are usually unknown in clinical practice; such analyses thus provide important prognostic information for advising patients from similar prevalent cohorts about risk. Such studies may also identify important variables for stratification and adjustment in controlled clinical trials of individuals with prevalent infection.

Table 1 Bias of relative risk estimate, θ^*, from a prevalent cohort study compared with relative risk estimate, θ, obtained from an incident cohort study[a] (adapted from [6])

		Effect of bias			
		Increasing hazard		Decreasing hazard	
Type of factor	Source of bias	$\theta > 1$[b]	$\theta = 1$	$\theta > 1$[b]	$\theta = 1$
Fixed cofactor affects risk of infection nonmultiplicatively	Onset confounding	No reliable inference from prevalent cohort			
Fixed cofactor unrelated to or acts multiplicatively on risk of infection	Differential length-biased sampling	Biased toward 1 $(1 < \theta^* \leq \theta)$	Unbiased $(\theta^* = 1)$	Biased away from 1 $(\theta^* \geq \theta)$	Unbiased $(\theta^* = 1)$
Time-dependent cofactor which takes effect after enrollment	Frailty selection	Biased toward 1 $(1 \leq \theta^* \leq \theta)$	Unbiased $(\theta^* = 1)$	Biased toward 1 $(1 \leq \theta^* \leq \theta)$	Unbiased $(\theta^* = 1)$
Marker	Onset confounding and frailty selection	No general statements about direction of bias			

[a]θ^* and θ are the large sample expected values of the relative risks obtained from prevalent and incident cohorts, respectively.
[b]Analogous results hold for $\theta < 1$.

Selection and Regression Towards the Mean

Cohort studies are sometimes performed among the individuals at highest risk of disease. For example, a double blind trial of clofibrate in the primary prevention of ischemic heart disease randomized men who were in the upper third of the distribution of serum cholesterol values [22]. In the Hypertension Detection and Follow-up Program Cooperative Group Study [24], individuals with elevated blood pressure at initial screening were enrolled for follow-up. In these examples, the individuals selected were sampled for inclusion in the study because measurements on a variable at initial screening were extreme. In some instances this selection process can be a source for bias because of regression toward the mean.

Regression towards the mean refers to the phenomenon that if a variable is extreme on the first measurement, then later measurements may tend to be closer to the center of the distribution [12]. Regression towards the mean was first described by Sir Francis Galton who found that offspring of tall parents tended to be shorter than their parents while offspring of short parents tended to be taller. Galton called this regression toward mediocrity [18].

As a simple example, consider a study to evaluate a treatment to lower blood pressure. Individuals are screened for blood pressure and those in the highest decile are enrolled in the cohort study and given the treatment. Some of those extremely high measurements at initial screening will decline at the follow-up measurement not because of the efficacy of the treatment but because the initial extreme high measurements were statistical flukes. A naive analysis could lead one to conclude incorrectly that the decline in mean blood pressure is evidence that the treatment is effective. In this example it was especially important to account for regression towards the mean because the study design was a before–after comparison without a control group. Regression towards the mean can lead one to conclude incorrectly that not only are there treatment effects, but there are also treatment–covariate interactions. For example, several studies of serum cholesterol lowering diets, such as the National Diet Heart Study, have reported that individuals with initially high serum cholesterol levels experience greater reductions than individuals with initially low cholesterol levels [16].

The effect of regression towards the mean can be formalized [12, 19]. Suppose the only individuals enrolled in a cohort study are those whose initial screening measurement, y_1, are greater than a prespecified value, k. A second measurement, y_2, is taken on follow-up. Suppose y_1 and y_2 are each normally distributed with mean μ and variance σ^2. Then

$$\mathrm{E}(y_1|y_1 > k) - \mathrm{E}(y_2)|y_1 > k) = c\sigma(1 - \rho), \quad (4)$$

where c is a positive constant that depends on k, μ and σ, and ρ is the correlation coefficient between y_1 and y_2. Thus, even though there is no difference in expected measurements at baseline and follow-up in the entire population [$\mathrm{E}(y_1) = \mathrm{E}(y_2) = \mu$], there is an expected decline in the two measurements in the *sampled cohort* because of the selection criterion ($y_1 > k$). The effect of regression towards the mean becomes greater as ρ approaches 0. There is no regression towards the mean if $\rho = 1$.

One approach for accounting for regression towards the mean is to have a suitable control group. For example, if individuals are randomized to either a treated or control group, then both groups could be expected to have the same amount of regression towards the mean, and any significant differences between groups could be attributed to real treatment effects. If a control group is not available, then corrections can be made for the regression towards the mean [12, 25]. The basic idea of these corrections is based on (4) and uses either external or internal estimates of the parameters of the equation.

Various suggestions have been made for improvements in study design to minimize regression towards the mean. For example, the initial selection criteria could be based on the mean $\bar{y}_1$ of n measurements rather than on only a single measurement y_1. Then, only individuals with $\bar{y}_1 > k$ are sampled for inclusion in the cohort. It can be shown that $\mathrm{E}(\bar{y}_1 - y_2|\bar{y}_1 > k)$ goes to 0 as n gets large [12]. Thus, the effect of regression towards the mean can be reduced by using the average of a number of initial measurements as the basis of the selection criteria. Another proposed approach is to use an initial measurement as the basis for selecting individuals into the study. However, then a second initial measurement is taken on the selected sample, and it is this second measurement that is used as the baseline measure to calculate change from the subsequent follow-up measurement. Under this scheme there will be no regression towards the mean if the observations are equicorrelated [12, 16].

References

[1]   Breslow, N.E. & Day, N.E. (1987). *Statistical Methods in Cancer Research*. Vol. 2: *The Design and Analysis of Cohort Studies*. International Agency for Research on Cancer, Lyon.

[2]   Breslow, N.E. & Crowley, J. (1974). A large sample study of the life table and product limit estimates under random censorship, *Annals of Statistics* **2**, 437–453.

[3]   Brookmeyer, R. (1987). Time and latency considerations in the quantitative assessment of risk, in *Epidemiology and Health Risk Assessment*, L. Gordis, ed. Oxford University Press, Oxford, pp. 178–188.

[4]   Brookmeyer, R. & Gail, M.H. (1987). Biases in prevalent cohorts, *Biometrics* **43**, 739–749.

[5]   Brookmeyer, R. & Gail, M.H. (1994). *AIDS Epidemiology: A Quantitative Approach*. Oxford University Press, Oxford

[6]   Brookmeyer, R., Gail, M.H. & Polk, B.F. (1987). The prevalent cohort study and the acquired immunodeficiency syndrome, *American Journal of Epidemiology* **126**, 14–24.

[7]   Caldwell, G.G., Kelley, D.B. & Heath, C.W., Jr (1980). Leukemia among participants in military maneuvers at a nuclear bomb test: a preliminary report, *Journal of the American Medical Association* **244**, 1575–1578.

[8]   Cnaan, A. & Ryan, L. (1989). Survival analysis in natural history studies of disease, *Statistics in Medicine* **8**, 1255–1268.

[9]   Cox, D.R. & Oakes, S.D. (1984). *Analysis of Survival Data*. Chapman & Hall, London.

[10] Criqui, M.H., Barrett-Connor, E. & Austin, M. (1978). Differences between respondents and nonrespondents in a population based cardiovascular disease study, *American Journal of Epidemiology* **108**, 367–372.

[11] Criqui, M.H., Austin, M. & Barrett-Connor, E. (1979). The effect of nonresponse on risk ratios in a cardiovascular disease study, *Journal of Chronic Diseases* **32**, 633–638.

[12] Davis, C.E. (1976). The effect of regression to the mean in epidemiological and clinical studies, *American Journal of Epidemiology* **104**, 493–498.

[13] Diggle, P.J. & Kenward, M.G. (1994). Informative dropouts in longitudinal data analysis (with discussion), *Applied Statistics* **43**, 49–93.

[14] Diggle, P.J. et al. (1994). *Analysis of Longitudinal Data*. Oxford University Press, New York.

[15] Doll, R. & Hill, A.B. (1954). The mortality of British doctors in relation to their smoking habits. A preliminary report, *British Medical Journal* **ii**, 1451–1455.

[16] Ederer, F. (1972). Serum cholesterol: effects of diet and regression toward the mean, *Journal of Chronic Disease* **25**, 277–289.

[17] Gail, M.H. (1975). A review and critiques of some models in competing risk analysis, *Biometrics* **35**, 209–222.

[18] Galton, F. (1985). Regression towards mediocrity in hereditary stature, *Journal of the Anthropology Institute* **15**, 246–263.

[19] Gardner, M.J. & Heady, J.A. (1973). Some effects of within person variability in epidemiological studies, *Journal of Chronic Diseases* **26**, 781–795.

[20] Gordon, T.F.E., Moore, F.E., Shurtleff, D. & Dawber, T.R. (1959). Some epidemiologic problems in the long-term study of cardiovascular disease. Observations on the Framingham Study, *Journal of Chronic Diseases* **10**, 186–206.

[21] Greenland, S. (1977). Response and follow-up bias in cohort studies, *American Journal of Epidemiology* **106**, 184–187.

[22] Heady, J.A. (1973). A cooperative trial in the primary prevention of ischemic heart disease using clofibrate, design methods and progress, *Bulletin of the World Health Organization* **48**, 243–256.

[23] Hernberg, S.M., Nurminen, M. & Tolonen, N. (1973). Excess mortality from coronary heart disease in viscose rayon workers, *Work Environmental Health* **10**, 93–98.

[24] Hypertension Detection and Follow-up Program Cooperative Group (1977). Blood pressure studies in 14 communities, *Journal of the American Medical Association* **237**, 2385–2391.

[25] James, K.E. (1973). Regression toward the mean in uncontrolled clinical studies, *Biometrics* **29**, 121–130.

[26] Kalbfleisch, J.D. & Lawless, J.F. (1989). Inference based on retrospective ascertainment: an analysis of data on transfusion related AIDS, *Journal of the American Statistical Association* **84**, 360–372.

[27] Kalbfleisch, J.D. & Prentice, R.L. (1980). *The Statistical Analysis of Failure Time Data*. Wiley, New York

[28] Kelsey, J.L. & Thompson, W.D. (1986). *Methods in Observational Epidemiology*. Oxford University Press, Oxford.

[29] Kleinbaum, D.G., Morgenstern, H. & Kupper, L.L. (1981). Selection in epidemiologic studies, *American Journal of Epidemiology* **113**, 452–463.

[30] Lagakos, S.W. (1979). General right censoring and its impact on the analysis of survival data, *Biometrics* **35**, 139–156.

[31] Lagakos, S.W., Barraj, L.M. & DeGruttola, V. (1988). Nonparametric analysis of truncated survival data with application to AIDS, *Biometrika* **75**, 515–523.

[32] Lui, K.-J. Lawrence, D.N., Morgan, W.M., Peterman, T.A., Haverkos, H.W. & Bregman, D.J. (1986). A model based approach for estimating the mean incubation period of transfusion-associated acquired immunodeficiency syndrome, *Proceedings of the National Academy of Sciences* **83**, 3051–3055.

[33] Peterson, A. (1976). Bounds for a joint distribution function with fixed subdistribution functions. Applications to competing risks, *Proceedings of the National Academy of Sciences* **73**, 11–13.

[34] Robbins, J.M. (1986). A new approach to causal inference in mortality studies with a sustained exposure period–applications to control of the healthy workers effect, *Mathematical Modelling* **7**, 1393–1512.

[35] Rothman, K.J. (1986). *Modern Epidemiology*. Little, Brown, & Company, Boston.

[36] Slud, E. & Byar, D. (1988). How dependent causes of death can make risk factors appear protective, *Biometrics* **44**, 265–269.

[37] Tsai, W.Y., Jewell, N.P. & Wang, M.C. (1987). A note on the product–limit estimator under right censoring and left truncation, *Biometrika* **74**, 883–886.

[38] Tsiatis, A. (1975). A nonidentifiability aspect of the problem of competing risks, *Proceedings of the National Academy of Sciences* **72**, 20–22.

[39] Wang, M.C., Brookmeyer, R. & Jewell, N.P. (1993). Statistical models for prevalent cohort data, *Biometrics* **49**, 1–11.

[40] Winkelstein, W., Royce, R.A. & Sheppard, H.W. (1990). Median incubation time for human immunodeficiency virus (HIV) (letter), *Annals of Internal Medicine* **112**, 797.

[41] Wolinsky, S.M., Rinaldo, C.R. & Phair, J. (1990). Response to letter, *Annals of Internal Medicine* **112**, 797–798.

[42] Wolinksy, S.M., Rinaldo, C.R. & Kwok, S. (1989). Human immunodeficiency virus type 1 (HIV-1) infection a median of 18 months before a diagnostic Western Blot, *Annals of Internal Medicine* **111**, 961–972.

(*See also* **Cross-Sectional Study**; **Incidence–Prevalence Relationships**; **Length Bias**)

RON BROOKMEYER

Birth Cohort Studies

Birth cohort studies are those which begin at or before the birth of their subjects, and continue to study the same individuals at later ages, on more than one occasion. They are a type of observational study in which "there is no randomization to exposure classes nor is there any attempt to manipulate the exposure" [10]. They vary in population size from large studies that aim to be nationally representative [12, 24, 33], to those that are area based and with populations of 1000 or more subjects [1, 8, 11, 14, 16, 19, 21, 26, 27, 29, 36]. Currently new, nationally representative birth cohort studies are being started in Denmark and Canada.

Although historical birth cohorts have been imaginatively used in epidemiology [3, 17] they are not discussed here.

Study Population

Selection

Prospective and historical birth cohort studies usually select their populations using time and/or geographical sampling frames. Three British birth cohort studies, which began at the birth of their subjects, each used a sampling frame of all births occurring in one week [12, 24, 33]. The oldest study followed up a class-stratified sample of all the single and legitimate births that occurred during a week, in 1946, and the two later studies followed up all births from the chosen week in 1958 and in 1970. The Avon longitudinal study of all births occurring in one English county used a year's births as a sampling frame, and recruited at antenatal clinics during that period, in order to collect data on risk exposure during pregnancy [14].

Population Size

In a birth cohort study the size of population must be selected at the outset, which may be far in time from some intended outcome measures. Definition of the outcome measures, their age-related incidence, and expected sample attrition at different future times can be used to calculate sample size. Large samples offer the opportunity to study relatively rare occurrences, but not without penalty. Inevitably, sample size is associated with frequency of data collection and with data quality. Large samples are more costly in terms of data collection and subjects can be so costly to contact that time intervals between data collections become long, and undue reliance has then to be given to subjects' recall of events and experiences occurring since the previous data collection.

Contact Maintenance

Contact maintenance is a constant task in a large birth cohort study. Annual contact is the ideal, so that changes of name and address can be kept up to date. In return, information on the study's work helps to maintain the subjects' interest. The two older British studies achieve these ends by means of a birthday card, which is an advantage of the time-based sampling frame. Each also sends an annual description of current work, and an annual request for information on address and name changes.

The tracing of lost contacts is relatively easy during the preschool and school years, when health and education systems may offer assistance, but in the subjects' adult lives investigators have to rely on information given by parents (rapport developed with parents during the school years is of value in these later years), and on agreements with others to forward letters to subjects.

Attrition and Representativeness

None of the British national studies found attrition and its effects on representativeness a serious problem during the preschool and school years, because of the help received from health and education authorities. But, whereas during the childhood and school years of the 1946 national birth cohort study – for instance, data collection was achieved from between 85% (lowest) and 96% (highest) of the live study population resident in Britain – the comparable adult range of response was from 67% to 85% (highest) [33].

Loss of sample members through failure to maintain contact is usually higher in those with the lowest educational attainment or interest in education, those living in the poorest socioeconomic circumstances, those who are single in adult life, and in the mentally ill, but not in those with serious physical illness [35].

Loss of sample members through death can, in Britain, be checked with the National Health Service register, on which study members in the two earlier birth cohorts are "flagged" so that death certification is notified to the study. In other countries similar methods of checking against files of the deceased may be possible (*see* **Death Indexes**).

Attrition in birth cohort studies through emigration, refusal, and loss of contact distort the representation of the study population. Distortion is caused also by inward migration. The 1946 birth cohort, for example, represented at age 43 years the native born, legitimate population, but not those who had been illegitimately born (4% of those born in the chosen week), nor the 5% of the British population of the same age as cohort members at 43 years who (in 1989) were not native born. The 1958 cohort augmented the population selected at birth by including

in data collections at ages 7, 11, and 16 years all the children born in the sampled week, even if they had not been included in the original study of births.

Topics of Study

Unique Assets of Prospective Studies from Birth

Two groups of assets of birth cohort studies are conferred by their design. The first is an advantage of having information on individual developmental time passing, and the second is associated with the individual's experience of historical time.

First are assets conferred by prospective data collection. This method provides information on the sequence of events, which is essential to the understanding of causation, and of risk and protective factors. It also provides information which cannot be gained on all cohort members, or even at all in retrospect, or from records – for example, cognitive scores, and information on attitudes, hopes and aspirations, growth, and behavior. This includes information on individuals' physical and mental change over time, and exposure to illness risk. Birth cohorts that are general population samples can provide viable denominator as well as numerator information, and therefore the relative and absolute risks, the effects of differential mortality, and the heterogeneity of outcomes of the hypothesized risk can all be calculated with some accuracy.

The second asset of birth cohort studies conferred by their design is that their populations have passed through known historical times. Thus, for example, the earliest British birth cohort was born at a time of high likelihood of parental smoking, lived the first eight years of life in circumstances of wartime food rationing and the first two years without a national health service, experienced selective entry to secondary schools, and lived all of the infant and childhood years before the Clean Air Act greatly reduced atmospheric pollution. The later-born cohorts, by contrast, lived in less austere times, with increasing awareness of the risks of smoking, less atmospheric pollution from coal burning, and comprehensive education. Members of each cohort came to the historical high period of unemployment, which began in the 1980s, at different career stages. Members of the 1946 cohort lived through the early postwar polio epidemics, and mothers of the 1958 cohort were pregnant during the influenza epidemic in the winter of

1957–1958. These differences of experience can be used to investigate the effects of different kinds of risk and exposure to risk. For example, a study of schizophrenia in the 1958 cohort confirmed that exposure to influenza in pregnancy was associated with raised risk of schizophrenia in offspring [6]. Comparative studies of perinatal mortality in the three British cohorts have been used to examine the effects of changes in obstetric care over the 24 year period [5], and these studies of maternity and childbirth were why the national cohort studies began.

Effects of Historical Time on Topics of Study

Although birth cohort studies are necessarily science-led, they are also inevitably products of their time. This is seen in the population size, which has been conditioned in the past by available information technology and in the selection of data collected, as well as in the initial decision to begin the studies, as already described.

In retrospect, in a long running study it is easy to see what appear later to be omissions in data collection. For example, in the 1946 birth cohort no information was collected during the early years on parental smoking, because the recognition of its damaging effects came almost a decade after the study began. Similarly, in the same study the data on child health collected by school nurses followed the pattern of the current school medical examinations; with hindsight, information on biological function, such as blood pressure and respiratory function, would have been invaluable.

Some kinds of information were perceived as important in the early years of the 1946 cohort, but there were no suitable research instruments for their collection. The importance of postweaning nutrition in childhood, for instance, although recognized, was very little studied in any of the British birth cohorts. None of the British studies has information on the parents' relationships with one another during the child's early years, because it was thought to be impossible to assess at earlier times, and later because available instruments were too time-consuming. In consequence, whilst each has been able to study the associations of parental divorce and separation with the child's health and well-being, it has not been possible to compare the apparent effects of divorce with those of living in harmonious and disharmonious family circumstances.

Not only is the choice of variables and measurement instruments a product of the time, so also is the general direction of the studies [27]. Current scientific and political expediency are vital forces that shape long-running studies. The 1946 cohort continued to be viable in the children's first five years because of current questioning of the value of home visiting undertaken by nurses involved in maternal and child welfare: the study was able to show the good effects of such a service [33]. During the cohort's school years, the effectiveness of the selective process for entry to secondary school (at age 11 years) was questioned. By having measures of cognitive attainment taken at age 8 years, three years before the selection process, the 1946 study was able to show that the method of selection was, as had been feared, biased in favor of the middle-class child. Furthermore, the study showed that the origins of this problem lay not simply with the selection process itself, but also in child–parent–teacher relationships from the earliest times at school, and in parent attitudes to education [7, 33]. Similarly, the 1958 cohort was well-placed to undertake studies of primary school education for the contemporary government enquiry into education in primary schools [13, 23]. In more recent times, the 1958 study has been ideally placed to investigate the effects of unemployment and preexisting circumstances on mental and physical health and on the acquisition of social capital in early adulthood, since cohort members were in their early years of work when the national rise in unemployment began [20]. The 1946 study is now contributing to understanding the processes of aging, and is well-placed to do so, not only because of its lifetime data, but also because this population represents the beginning of the boom years in the population of the elderly.

Previous and Later Generations

The two older British birth cohorts have some information on the parents of study members, particularly their educational attainment, occupation, marital status and stability, concern for the study child's education, and cause of death, as well as some information about health. This has made it possible to study social mobility, the effects of parental ill health on the life of the study child, and intergenerational differences in religious and political adherence, as well as the effect of some important aspects of family of origin, and cohort members' educational attainment [25, 34].

The first two British cohorts also have information on the offspring of cohort members. The 1946 study interviewed mothers of all first children born to male and female cohort members between ages 19 and 25 years. Information on these second-generation children was collected at the end of the preschool period, at age 4 years, and again at 8 years, because the purpose of the study was to explore further the finding in the previous generation that parental concern for education was strongly associated with attainment scores [32, 33]. The 1958 study, on the other hand, interviewed a randomly selected one in three of the cohort members who were parents at age 33 years about all their children ($n \simeq 4000$), to compare differences in a wide range of aspects of childhood in two generations.

Now that the 1946 cohort members are in middle life, questions have been included at the interview at 43 years about their relationships with, and (where necessary) care of, their elderly parents, who were by that time aged 71 years, on average [34].

Although these studies of the two generations adjacent to cohort members are useful for the study of intergenerational relationships, their populations cannot be regarded as representative of those generations.

Forward Planning

Forward planning is difficult in a long-term prospective study because the variables selected for current data collection will be used for two purposes. They will be used as outcome measures in relation to data collected at earlier times. They will also become precursor variables used to test hypotheses about risk. It is therefore necessary, in planning data collections, to consider the needs of future hypothesis testing. For example, planning midlife data collection in the 1946 cohort has had to include consideration of requirements for testing hypotheses about health in later life. For instance, current hypotheses about skeletal fractures and repair in old age implicate smoking, diet, and exercise in midlife, and so information on these health-related habits will be collected. The risk is that by the time the cohort reaches old age, hypotheses will change, and new ideas will develop. Although that is an inevitable problem, in practice, for biological questions, measures of current function and its change over time, and the preservation of blood samples, provide a range of data possibilities for future

use. In general, once a future biological, psychological, or social outcome has been defined, then, the demands of current hypotheses having been taken into account, the most detailed possible measures available should be taken to make future accurate assessments of change, and not to constrain future analyses.

In retrospect, it is clear that the 1946 study has been fortunate. Investigations of midlife cognitive function, for example, have been able to use data on this topic collected in childhood, adolescence, and early adulthood for the study of educational attainment. Similarly, information on birth weight and infant growth and development, originally collected to study social variation in physical development, has proved to be of unanticipated value in the study of midlife blood pressure and respiratory function, and of schizophrenia.

Other Sources of Data

In addition to cohort members themselves, and in childhood their parents, birth cohort studies have found it invaluable to collect information from other sources, for four reasons.

First, confirmatory information can usefully be collected, with permission, for example, from hospital records and educational certification bodies. Secondly, information can be collected to provide another view of the circumstance. For instance, in the 1946 study, teachers' comments added considerably to the information given by cohort members and by parents. Thirdly, information from other sources, including census data, can provide information on an area basis about exposure to such things as atmospheric pollution and the nature of water supplies, as well as local rates of unemployment, educational attainment, and socioeconomic structure. The fourth kind of information concerns the current social and scientific context. In a long-running prospective study it is difficult to know in retrospect the political and scientific pressures and social concerns of the day that affected the direction that the study took. They are difficult to ascertain years later, because histories of the period are usually concerned with political pressure and events rather than social and scientific histories, although there are notable exceptions. In trying to account for earlier choice of subjects, measures, and direction of analyses, a study logbook is needed to supplement such other sources as reports of funding bodies, government enquiries, and commissions.

Analysis

Coding

The effects of historical time in a long-running study can also be problematic in terms of how information is coded and stored. Classifications of illnesses and socioeconomic position change over time, and it is often necessary to recode information already coded, and to retain two or more sets of classifications both to study change over time and to be comparable with current work in other studies.

Concepts of Analysis

Now that birth cohorts, historical cohorts, and other forms of longitudinal studies have been collecting data for 50 years and more, the long-term nature of these investigations has brought a life-span perspective to analysis [15, 22, 31]. This has generated new ideas about the nature of psychological and biological aging, and raised the question of the role and measurement of adaptation with age [2]. So far, this has been largely a matter of psychological study, but questions about variation in biological vulnerability in relation to age are now being discussed in view of the data available from prospective and historical studies that encompass many years of life [3].

The most commonly used approach to analysis in birth cohort and other long-term investigations is concerned with variables, and the most commonly used method is linear regression. More recently, structural equations models have also been used to handle interactions between variables that measure function or environment [9]. Alternatively, a person-oriented, as compared with a variable-oriented, approach has been advocated [4, 18]. This method compares individuals' profiles of characteristics determined by analysis of clusters or patterns. Magnusson and Bergman [18] illustrate this approach in comparison with variable-based analysis, which in a study of precursors of crime and aggression would show how

each of a number of single aspects of individual functioning – aggressiveness, hyperactivity, low school motivation, poor peer relations – is significantly related to various aspects of adult maladjustment. ...Applying the pattern approach to this research area, the focus instead becomes: what typical patterns or configurations of adjustment problems of this kind actually exist in childhood; how are

major adjustment problem areas in adult age interconnected; and what are the relationships between typical problem patterns in childhood and typical problem patterns in adulthood?

This account of the nature of birth cohort studies cannot describe all aspects, nor refer to every study. Broader summaries and reviews are given by Sontag [30], Mednick et al. [19], Schneider & Edelstein [28], and Young et al. [37].

References

[1]   Alison, L.H., Counsell, A.M., Geddis, D.C. & Sanders, D.M. (1993). First report from the Plunket National Child Health Study: smoking during pregnancy in New Zealand, *Paediatric and Perinatal Epidemiology* **7**, 318–333.

[2]   Baltes, P.B. & Baltes, M.M. eds (1990). *Successful Aging*. Cambridge University Press, Cambridge.

[3]   Barker, D.J.P. (1991). Fetal and infant origins of adult disease, *British Medical Journal*.

[4]   Block, J. (1971). *Lives Through Time*. Bancroft, Berkeley.

[5]   Chamberlain, R., Chamberlain, G., Howlett, B. & Claireaux, A. (1975). *British Births 1970*, Vols 1 and 2. Heinemann, London.

[6]   Done, D.J., Crow, T.J., Johnstone, E.C. & Sacker, A. (1994). Childhood antecedents of schizophrenia and affective illness: social adjustment at ages 7 and 11 years, *British Medical Journal* **309**, 699–703.

[7]   Douglas, J.W.B. (1964). *The Home and the School*. McGibbon and Kee, London, pp. 119–128.

[8]   Dragonas, T., Golding, J., Ignatyeva, R. & Prokhorskas, R., eds (1996). *Pregnancy in the 90s*. Sansom, Bristol.

[9]   Dunn, G., Everitt, B. & Pickles, A. (1993). *Modelling Covariances and Latent Variables Using EQS*. Chapman & Hall, London.

[10]   Feinleib, M., Breslow, N.E. & Detels, R. (1991). Cohort studies, in *The Oxford Textbook of Public Health*, W.W. Holland, R. Detels & R.G. Knox, eds. Oxford University Press, Oxford, pp. 145–159.

[11]   Fergusson, D.M., Horwood, L.J., Shannon, F.T. & Lawton, J.M. (1989). The Christchurch Child Development Study: a review of epidemiological findings, *Paediatric and Perinatal Epidemiology* **3**, 302–325.

[12]   Ferri, E., ed. (1993). *Life at 33*. National Children's Bureau, London.

[13]   Fogelman, K., ed. (1983). *Growing Up in Great Britain*. Macmillan, London, pp. 231–326.

[14]   Golding, J. (1989). European longitudinal study of pregnancy and childhood, *Paediatric and Perinatal Epidemiology* **3**, 460–469.

[15]   Goldstein, H. (1979). *The Design and Analysis of Longitudinal Studies*. Academic Press, London.

[16] Kolvin, I., Miller, F.J.W., Scott, D.M., Gatzanis, S.R.M. & Fleeting, M. (1990). *Continuities of Deprivation? The Newcastle 1000 Family Study*. Avebury, Aldershot.

[17] Lumey, L.H., Ravelli, A.C.J., Wiessing, L.G., Koppe, J.G., Treffers, P.E. & Stein, Z.A. (1993). The Dutch famine birth cohort study, *Paediatric and Perinatal Epidemiology* **7**, 354–367.

[18] Magnusson, D. & Bergman, L.R. (1990). In *Straight and Devious Pathways from Childhood to Adulthood*, L.N. Robins & M. Rutter, eds. Cambridge University Press, Cambridge, pp. 101–115.

[19] Mednick, S.A., Baert, A.E. & Bachmann, B.P., eds. (1981). *Prospective Longitudinal Research*. Oxford University Press, Oxford.

[20] Montgomery, S., Bartley, M., Cook, D. & Wadsworth, M.E.J. (1996). Health and social precursors of unemployment in young men, *Journal of Epidemiology and Community Health* **50**, 415–422.

[21] Olsen, P., Laara, E., Rantakallio, P., Jarvellin, M.-R., Sarpola, A. & Hartikainen, A.-L. (1995). Epidemiology of preterm delivery in two birth cohorts with an interval of 20 years, *American Journal of Epidemiology* **142**, 1184–1193.

[22] Plewis, I. (1985). *Analysing Change*. Wiley, Chichester.

[23] Plowden Report (1967). *Children and Their Primary Schools*, Vol. 2. HMSO, London, pp. 401–543.

[24] Power, C. (1992). A review of child health in the 1958 birth cohort, *Paediatric and Perinatal Epidemiology* **6**, 81–110.

[25] Power, C., Manor, O. & Fox, J. (1991). *Health and Class: The Early Years*. Chapman & Hall, London.

[26] Rantakallio, P. (1988). The longitudinal study of the North Finland birth cohort of 1966, *Paediatric and Perinatal Epidemiology* **2**, 59–88.

[27] Roche, A. (1992). *Growth, Maturation and Body Composition: the Fels longitudinal study, 1929–1991*. Cambridge University Press, Cambridge, p. 199.

[28] Schneider, W. & Edelstein, W. eds (1990). *Inventory of European Longitudinal Studies in the Behavioural and Medical Sciences*. Max-Planck Institute, Berlin.

[29] Silva, P. (1990). The Dunedin Multidisciplinary Health and Development Study: a 15 year longitudinal study, *Paediatric and Perinatal Epidemiology* **4**, 76–107.

[30] Sontag, L.W. (1971). The history of longitudinal research, *Child Development* **42**, 987–1002.

[31] Sugarman, L. (1993). *Life-Span Development*. Routledge, London.

[32] Wadsworth, M.E.J. (1986). Effects of parenting style and preschool experience on children's verbal attainment, *Early Childhood Research Quarterly* **1**, 237–248.

[33] Wadsworth, M.E.J. (1991) *The Imprint of Time*. Oxford University Press, Oxford.

[34] Wadsworth, M.E.J. (1996). Social and historical influences on parent–child relations in midlife, in *The Parental Experience in Midlife*, C. Ryff & M.M. Seltzer, eds. Chicago University Press, Chicago, pp. 169–212.

[35] Wadsworth, M.E.J., Mann, S.L., Rodgers, B., Kuh, D.L., Hilder, W.S. & Yusuf, E.J. (1992). Loss and representativeness in a 43 year follow up of a national birth cohort, *Journal of Epidemiology and Public Health* **46**, 300–304.

[36] Yach, D., Cameron, N., Padayadhee, N., Wagstaff, L., Richter, L. & Fonn, S. (1991). Birth to ten: child health in South Africa in the 1990s. Rationale and methods of a birth cohort study, *Paediatric and Perinatal Epidemiology* **5**, 211–233.

[37] Young, C.H., Savola, L.K. & Phelps, E. (1991). *Inventory of Longitudinal Studies in the Social Sciences*. Sage, London.

M.E.J. WADSWORTH

Birth Defects Registries

Birth defects registries can be used to determine the newborn prevalence of birth defects and they can provide cases for studies [3]. Both of these functions are important foundations for the prevention of birth defects.

A birth defects registry is an organized database containing information on individuals born with specified congenital disorders, ascertained from a defined source. Birth defects are a heterogeneous group of conditions, present at birth, and not generally considered to include injuries suffered in and around the birth process. In the US, the March of Dimes Birth Defects Foundation defines a birth defect as "an abnormality of structure, function or body metabolism (inborn error of body chemistry) present at birth that results in physical or mental disability, or is fatal" [9].

There are more than 4000 known types of birth defects. These include conditions ranging from congenital malformations of unknown etiology, to genetic conditions due to abnormal genes or chromosomes, to conditions due to damage to the developing fetus related to prenatal maternal exposure to hazardous environmental agents. Thus, this term includes a range of disorders such as cleft lip and palate, heart malformations, clubfoot, Down syndrome, phenylketonuria (PKU), fragile X-linked mental retardation, fetal alcohol syndrome and the thalidomide syndrome. Not all of these conditions are necessarily medically or cosmetically significant. Some "minor" defects, such as small birthmarks or skin tags, are of no significant consequence.

Causes of Birth Defects

Birth defects may be caused by genetic or environmental factors (including drugs and chemicals, infectious agents, physical agents, and maternal health or nutritional factors) acting singly or in combination. The causes of more than half of all birth defects are unknown at present. Collectively, birth defects are a major cause of disability and morbidity, and in the US, represent the leading cause of infant mortality.

Information in Birth Defects Registries

Birth defects registries systematically collect information such as identifiers and demographic information, description of the defects present, family history, history of the pregnancy (including prenatal exposures), and other information potentially related to risk factors. This information may be gathered from vital records, hospital or clinic records, or other sources of case ascertainment. Registries that rely upon records collected for other purposes (e.g. birth certificates) are sometimes referred to as using "passive" methods of ascertainment, while those that use multiple sources and collect information from patient records are said to use "active" ascertainment. Information stored in birth defects registries is typically stored as both paper files and in electronic systems, often using a relational database. Considerable effort is expended to ensure data security, as well as the confidentiality and privacy of the individuals and families who are participants in the registry.

Usually, information collected is restricted to a defined age range such as the neonatal period or the first year of life. Indeed, since many defects are not identified before neonatal hospital discharge, the longer the ascertainment period used, the higher the frequency of children identified with birth defects in a particular birth cohort. Systems actively ascertaining cases throughout the first year of life typically find that 3.5%–5% of infants have such conditions.

Birth defects registries generally collect cases from a defined population, such as that in a specified geographic area. When they do, the registry can use birth certificate data collected for governmental purposes on all babies as the denominator. Thus, it becomes possible to determine the newborn prevalence of birth defects in this geographic area. Such population-based registries also permit case–control studies. Many countries have national registries. These programs share information through an International Clearinghouse for Birth Defects Monitoring Programs [4]. This organization has contributed to standardized terminology and methods and has helped in the organization of international collaborative research efforts. Non population-based registries can provide cases for studies that do not need a population base. Such collections of patients have been particularly useful for studies seeking to identify the gene responsible for a single gene cause of a birth defect.

Uses of Birth Defects Registries

Registries that are population-based permit the rates of birth defects to be determined. Such rates can be monitored to look for changes that would suggest a newly introduced environmental/drug agent. It has been argued that had there been registries established prior to the thalidomide epidemic, the cause may have been determined sooner than it was. On a more positive note, when there is the possibility to prevent birth defects like rubella and folic-acid-preventable spina bifida and anencephaly, monitoring the trends can determine the effectiveness of prevention programs. There is currently great interest to determine whether or not the folic acid fortification plan in the US will provide full protection from folic-acid-preventable birth defects.

Given that we do not know the causes of the birth defects in the majority of infants born with them, a major function of birth defects registries has been to supply cases for studies seeking to find the causes of birth defects. The most common kind of epidemiologic study seeking to find causes is the **case–control study**. In these studies the exposures and family history of cases are compared with those of controls selected from the same population from which the case is drawn.

One notable example of such a study is the one from France that found that cases of spina bifida were much more likely to have been exposed to valproic acid than controls. This study led rapidly to a health warning in the US [6]. Another useful example is provided by the Atlanta Case–Control Study conducted by the US Centers for Disease Control and Prevention (CDC). This study provided the opportunity to examine possible associations between many kinds of birth defects and many drug and environmental exposures.

The protective association between regular multi-vitamin consumption and the reduction in spina bifida and anencephaly shown in Atlanta and other observational studies, provided critical data for public health policy [8]. These studies led to a recommendation by the US Public Health Service (PHS) that women of reproductive age consume 400 µg of synthetic folic acid daily, rather than the 4000 µg that was used in the randomized controlled trial [2,7]. Because data on so many exposures were collected, there remain data yet to be analyzed that may provide insight to other etiologies of these and other birth defects [5].

Recently, investigators have sought to improve the search for causes of birth defects by using both molecular markers of exposure and outcomes [10]. With the genome project soon to provide data on all genes, investigators will have even more powerful tools to try to understand the interplay between environmental and genetic risk factors in the cause of birth defects. Thus, registries are a rich resource for clinical and family studies, for health outcomes and services research, and for public health planning and programming [1].

Authority for Operation of Birth Defects Registries

Birth defects registries are generally established and operated under the authority of public health agencies. In the US, authority for such public health surveillance programs is generally the responsibility of the states. As a consequence, there are specific statutes authorizing such a registry or surveillance system, and there is considerable variation in specific goals, methods of financing, operational policies, and scope of disorders covered. Furthermore, other state and federal policies (e.g. health information and privacy policies) affect the type and circumstances under which research can proceed.

References

[1] Adams, M.M., Greenberg, F., Khoury, M.J., Marks, J.S. & Oakley, G.P. Jr (1985). Survival of infants with spina bifida – Atlanta, 1972–1979, *American Journal of Diseases of Childhood* **139**, 518–523.

[2] Centers for Disease Control and Prevention (1992). Recommendations for the use of folic acid to reduce the number of cases of spina bifida and other neural tube defects, *Morbidity and Mortality Weekly Reports* **41**, 1–7.

[3] Edmonds, L.D., Layde, P.M., James, L.M., Flynt, J.W. Jr, Erickson, J.D. & Oakley, G.P. Jr (1981). Congenital malformations surveillance: two American systems, *International Journal of Epidemiology* **10**, 247–252.

[4] Erickson, J.D. (1991). The International Clearinghouse for Birth Defects Monitoring Systems: past, present, and future, *International Journal of Risk and Safety Medicine* **2**, 239–248.

[5] Erickson, J.D. (1991). Risk factors for birth defects: data from the Atlanta birth defects case–control study, *Teratology* **43**, 41–51.

[6] Lammer, E.J., Sever, L.E. & Oakley, G.P. Jr (1987). Teratogen update: valproic acid, *Teratology* **35**, 465–473.

[7] MRC Vitamin Study Research Group (1991). Prevention of neural tube defects: results of the Medical Research Council Vitamin Study, *Lancet* **338**, 131–137.

[8] Mulinare, J., Cordero, J.F., Erickson, J.D. & Berry, R.J. (1988). Periconceptional use of multivitamins and the occurrence of neural tube defects, *Journal of the American Medical Association* **260**, 3141–3145.

[9] Petrini, J., ed. (1997). *March of Dimes Birth Defects Foundation StatBook*. March of Dimes Birth Defects Foundation, White Plains, p. 259.

[10] Shaw, G.M., Wasserman, C.R., Murray, J.C. & Lammer, E.J. (1998). Infant TGF-alpha genotype, orofacial clefts, and maternal periconceptional multivitamin use, *Cleft Palate-Craniofacial Journal* **35**, 366–370.

JAMES W. HANSON & GODFREY P. OAKLEY, Jr

(*See also* **Cancer Registries**; **Infant and Perinatal Mortality**; **Teratology**)

BMDP *see* Software, Biostatistical

Burden of Disease

"Burden of disease" is the name given to a concept dealing with a range of medical statistics. It aims to give a comprehensive picture of how different diseases impact on society. Some analysts use this concept to allocate health care and research resources. Because it covers a range of impacts of disease on society, the burden is often referred to in the plural, a practice followed in this article.

"Burdens of disease" aims to give an account of the dimensions of damage inflicted by ill health on society. The main burdens covered are mortality, morbidity, and resources costs of care and treatment. Applications were developed first in the US, but examples here are based on experience in the UK. The main interest is in how the burdens of different diseases compare. It aims to answer questions like: Is heart disease a bigger killer than cancer? Which diseases afflict women especially? Which diseases impose greatest cost on healthcare services? Table 1 is taken from the latest UK table of burdens of disease [4] and summarizes the main results. Answering such questions raises a host of problems. Some of them arise from one of the burdens and some arise from attempts to bring them all together.

Mortality

What do we mean when we say that one disease is a bigger killer than another? Looking simply at unadjusted death rates will not capture the flavor of the question. Since all must die, the simple causing of death does not impose a burden on society. It is premature death that is the burden. One commonly adopted solution is to look at deaths below a certain age. Choosing the age is not simple. If it is set very low, then it will focus attention on a very narrow range of causes of death such as sudden infant death syndrome (SIDS), accidents, etc. Set too high and it loses any focus on policy issues. Over the age of, say, one hundred, the precise cause of death is of less interest than the survival thus far. Recent presentations have looked not at simple death rates, but weighted them by the years below a certain age. Thus SIDS deaths are given a high weight because they are seen as destroying almost a whole lifespan. While the usual presentation focuses on life-years lost, there is no reason in principle why both crude and weighted death rates should not be used. They reflect different concerns. Even though inevitable, the event of death is always painful to survivors and fearful to the dying. The curtailing of life is an additional loss. A further difficulty is whether the life-years lost calculation should use different age standards for men and women, to reflect their different **life expectancy**.

Compared with other burdens, the data difficulties of mortality statistics are relatively few. In many developed countries the measurement has become simpler with the recording of several **causes of death** on death

certificates. There remain problems with causes like acquired immune deficiency syndrome (AIDS) and suicides, where there will be a *bias* against recording such conditions on death certificates.

Morbidity

Data on morbidity tend to come from three main sources: administrative records associated with welfare benefits, surveys of physicians, and household surveys. In the UK these are represented by sickness benefit records, the morbidity survey of general practitioners, and surveys like the Disability Survey and the Health Survey. The first dataset records total days of certificated sickness absence. The second source records the patient consulting rate for a given condition. Household surveys will, in principle, obtain a direct measure of the number of people suffering from a given condition at a particular point in time, and so come closest to a measure of the extent to which the population at a given moment is suffering from ill health. While certificated sickness measures the same thing in principle, it suffers, besides the problems associated with administrative sources like policy change, from the problem that only those otherwise in work will be recorded. It therefore omits most of the population who are ill, the old, and many of the chronically sick. The number of people consulting primary physicians gives a useful indication of something between incidence and prevalence of disease, but requires additional weighting to give a useful picture of the burden of morbidity. Chronic conditions clearly impose a greater burden than short-lived conditions, so this measure of prevalence has to be adjusted by some estimates of average duration.

Another weighting that is required is an adjustment for severity. A frequently used measure is the quality-adjusted life-year (QALY). The implied days of sickness are weighted by the degree of suffering caused. A variety of scales have been developed such as the Euroqol [5], and estimates of discomfort and disability impact have been attached to different conditions.

While statistics on certificated sickness days may be of limited value in obtaining an overall picture of such suffering, they provide valuable subsidiary information on the burden imposed on the economy from not having workers available, on those who

Table 1 Twenty leading causes of mortality, patients consulting in general practice, and expenditure by ICD-9 subchapter. England except MSGP = England and Wales, GHS = Great Britain [4]

Rank	Mortality (1991)	Patients consulting in general practice[a] by cause[b] (1991/92) (%)	by cause	Rate per 1000	NHS hospital expenditure (1992/93)	(%)	NHS primary care expenditure[c] (1992/93)	(%)	Community health and social care for adults net expenditure (1992/93)	(%)
1	Ischemic heart disease	26.2	Acute respiratory infections	242.0	Injury and poisoning	5.8	Mouth disease[e]	26.0	Learning disability	12.5
2	Stroke	12.1	Skin diseases	159.6	Learning disability	5.2	Acute respiratory infection	7.7	Stroke	7.1
3	Lung cancer	6.0	Infectious diseases other than TB	156.2	Symptoms	4.3	Eye disorders[d]	6.3	Other arthropathies	6.5
4	Pneumonia	5.0	Injury and poisoning	139.0	Stroke	4.2	Symptoms	5.7	Eye disorders	5.2
5	Chronic obstructive pulmonary diseases (COPD)	4.8	Symptoms	138.7	Schizophrenia	4.0	Injury and poisoning	3.8	Dementia	5.2
6	Colorectal cancer	3.0	Preventive medicine	138.0	Normal delivery	3.1	Infections other than TB	3.0	Neuroses	3.8
7	Arteries	2.8	Screening	121.0	Dementia	2.7	Skin diseases	3.0	Ear disorders	3.7
8	Cancer of other sites	2.7	Ear disorders	101.2	Ischemic heart disease	2.4	Heart failure	2.7	Rheumatism	3.7
9	Female breast cancer	2.4	Family planning	72.8	Other pregnancy	2.3	Preventive medicine	2.2	Prevention	3.5
10	Other heart	2.0	Other neuroses, etc.	64.9	Procedures and aftercare	2.3	Osteoarthritis	2.1	Alcohol, drugs, etc.	3.1
11	Dementia	1.7	Eye disorders	63.7	Skin diseases	2.0	Screening	2.0	Multiple sclerosis	2.7
12	Prostatic cancer	1.5	Social and social marital	61.3	Arteries and veins	2.0	Ear disorders	2.0	Other CNS and disorders of the PNS	2.7
13	Stomach cancer	1.5	Other back diseases	59.1	Other nonorganic psychoses	1.9	COPD	2.0	Osteoarthritis	2.3
14	Diabetes	1.4	Dorsopathies	59.1	Other neuroses, etc	1.9	Hypertension	1.8	Rheumatoid arthritis	2.1
15	Urinary cancer	1.3	Female genital tract	57.4	Female genital tract	1.9	Ischemic heart disease	1.8	Pregnancy	1.8
16	Pancreatic cancer	1.1	Sprains and strains	55.0	Social and social marital, etc.	1.8	Other urinary	1.6	Old age	1.7
17	Suicide and unknown motive	1.0	Rheumatism	49.0	Heart failure	1.6	Stroke	1.5	Other heart disease	1.6
18	Genito-urinary cancers female	1.0	Upper respiratory tract diseases	43.0	Pneumonia	1.6	Intestines and peritoneum	1.4	Schizophrenia	1.6
19	Other systemic cancers	1.0	Asthma	42.5	Eye disorders	1.5	Asthma	1.4	Epilepsy	1.6
20	Heart failure	1.0	Hypertension	41.9	Other respiratory	1.4	Other back disorders	1.2	Symptoms	1.6
	Total leading causes	79.5				53.7		79.1		73.8
	All other causes	20.5				35.4[f]		20.9		26.2[g]

Sources: Mortality: OPCS 1991.
Patient consultations: Morbidity Statistics from General Practice (MSGP4) 1991–92.
Expenditure: MSGP4, HES and Programme Budget.

[a] Patient consulting rates are based on consultations with general practitioners and practice nurses.
[b] 78% of patients consult their GP at least once per annum. If a patient consults for more than one cause, they will be recorded once for each cause. Therefore, rates should not be added as there will be an element of double counting.
[c] NHS Primary care expenditure excluding pharmaceutical expenditure.
[d] Primary care expenditure relating to eye disorders include all costs attributable to General Optical Services.
[e] Primary care expenditure relating to mouth disease include all costs attributable to General Dental Services.
[f] Includes expenditure on day patients in hospitals, Accident and Emergency, Teaching Hospital Uplift (SIFTR) and "other" hospital expenditure.
[g] Includes unallocated expenditure.

depend on the income they might otherwise have earned, and on the agencies that pay benefit.

Resource Costs

Societies devote considerable resources both to curing disease and to remedying some of its consequences. In most industrial countries much of this burden falls on the state, while in some there is considerable private finance of health insurance. However financed, these represent a use of resources which could otherwise perform some other useful function. Simplest to measure in most health services are the number of beds devoted to different conditions, and the average cost of bed occupancy. Slightly more difficult is out-patient (ambulatory) care, where records of conditions seem to be less systematically maintained. Where morbidity data are based on surveys of primary carers, these sources can also be used to estimate the cost burden of primary care. Here, of course, it is the consultation rate rather than the number of patients consulting which is relevant. Separate estimates are often required for dental care.

The disease classification of pharmaceuticals requires a certain amount of judgment to align with conditions. Classification becomes progressively more difficult with care which requires support against disability rather than curative interventions where the recording of causes of such conditions may be limited.

As well as pecuniary burdens borne both by the public and private sectors, there are nonpecuniary burdens – particularly in terms of caring. While such burdens are less often recorded in official compilations of burdens of disease, there are sources of such information in general and in dedicated household surveys.

There is conceptual difficulty with measuring the resource burden. It reflects what is considered appropriate by current medical practice. There is an implied but incorrect assumption that the scale of resources devoted to different conditions is such as to bring every sufferer back to a similar kind of condition. This is clearly far from the case. One of the conditions that imposes the heaviest burden on in-patient care is stroke, although it is unclear that the scale of those resources reflect the effectiveness of the interventions, compared, with, say, interventions in heart disease. The cost burdens therefore reflect a combination of prevalence and medical practice. If it were decided that more care should be devoted to mental illness, say, then there would be a perceived rise in burden, which might be accompanied by an unrecorded abatement in the severity of morbidity.

Uses and Abuses

In a 1996 publication the UK Department of Health presents burdens in a range of different categories [4]. There is no attempt to combine these into one overall indicator of burden. This was not the practice adopted in the first attempt by Black & Pole [1]. They combined all burdens together using implicit weights reflecting both the severity of disease relative to full health and death, and an implied pecuniary value of death. While it is always open to users to make such combinations using their own assumptions, the attribution of a money value to life is seen as too controversial to form the basis of a statistical publication.

Black & Pole, and many of those who have followed them, have seen burdens of disease as of potential value in decisions on where to direct preventive or curative resources and research which might develop them. While the epidemiologic mapping contained in burdens of disease provides an essential component of any system for making such allocations, it must be combined with indicators of the effectiveness of interventions. There is no point in throwing a large amount of resources at a disease, however burdensome, if it makes no difference to that burden.

Indicators of cost effectiveness are now available for a range – albeit still a fairly limited range – of conditions [4]. The technique for effective resource allocation depends on a combination of burdens of disease statistics and cost-effectiveness information. In practice nearly all interventions vary in their effectiveness depending both on the condition of the sufferer, the general circumstances, and the quality of the medical practitioner. An effective allocation of interventions will depend on the scale of the condition and the extent to which further intervention is likely to be effective in reducing the burden. It turns out that making such an allocation is relatively complicated. One scheme for doing so is described in Neuburger & Fraser [2].

Another potential use of burdens is to indicate the burden of a particular risk factor. Thus it would be possible to show the burden of smoking or car exhaust fumes by weighting together appropriate fractions of the burden of those disease associated with such risk factors. In terms of policy these could then be compared with interventions which might be taken to abate them.

Conclusion

Burdens of disease provides a valuable framework for compiling a range of data on different diseases. Used with care it can provide an invaluable tool for the development of health policy.

References

[1] Black, D.A. & Pole, J.D. (1975). Priorities in biomedical research; indices of burden, *British Journal of Social and Preventative Medicine* **29**, 222–227.

[2] Neuburger, H. & Fraser, N. (1993). *Economic Policy Analysis; A Rights Based Approach*. Aldershot, UK.

[3] UK Department of Health (1994). *Register of Cost-Effectiveness Studies*. Department of Health, London.

[4] UK Department of Health (1996). *Burdens of Disease: A Discussion Document*. Department of Health, London.

[5] Williams, A. (1995). *Measurement and Valuation of Health: A Chronicle*. Centre for Health Economics Discussion Paper 136, University of York, York.

H. NEUBURGER

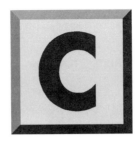

Calibration Sample *see* Prevalence of Disease, Estimation from Screening Data

Caliper Matching *see* Matching

Cancer Registries

History of Cancer Surveillance

Early forms of cancer surveillance involved registering cancers diagnosed in a population of interest for the purpose of providing accurate statistics on the morbidity and prevalence of cancer. The first attempts to do this were in the early 1700s in London, in Hamburg in 1900, and subsequently in the Netherlands, Spain, Portugal, Hungary, Sweden, Denmark, and Iceland during the period 1902–1908. These efforts were unsuccessful because doctors often refused to fill out the questionnaires needed to document each diagnosed cancer [27].

The first successful attempt at cancer registration took place in Mecklenberg in 1937. The data recorded on each cancer included the name of the patient, which facilitated the elimination of multiple records on the same case. Also, registration cards were sent to all medical practitioners, hospitals, and pathological institutes and there was telephone follow-up for the purpose of obtaining complete ascertainment as well as complete data on each case. Subsequently, similar surveys were conducted in Saxony-Anhalt, Saarland, and Vienna in 1939, but were soon discontinued because of political developments [27].

In the US, the first attempt to register cancers was initiated by the American College of Surgeons (ACOS) in 1921, and involved only malignancies of the bone [2]. Registration was expanded in the next decade to include other malignancies. The first cancer morbidity survey was conducted in 1937–38 in 10 metropolitan areas by the National Cancer Institute (NCI), and subsequent surveys were conducted in 1947–48 and 1969–71. In principle, all cancers diagnosed in residents of these areas during a one-year period were registered during each of the three time periods. A problem with surveys of this type was that the fate of cancer patients was not known. The lack of information on the survival of cancer patients indicated the need for alternative approaches to cancer registration.

In 1971, the National Cancer Act, announced as the "War on Cancer", called for the NCI to "collect, analyze, and disseminate all data useful in the prevention, diagnosis, and treatment of cancer. . .". This legislation led to the creation of the Surveillance, Epidemiology, and End Results (SEER) Program which was based at the NCI.

Case ascertainment for the SEER Program began on January 1, 1973, in several geographic areas of the US and its territories. Those areas that have participated in the program since 1975 include the states of Connecticut, Iowa, New Mexico, Utah, and

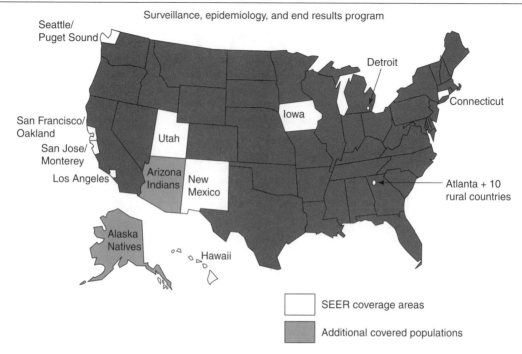

Figure 1   Map of US indicating areas and populations covered by the SEER Program

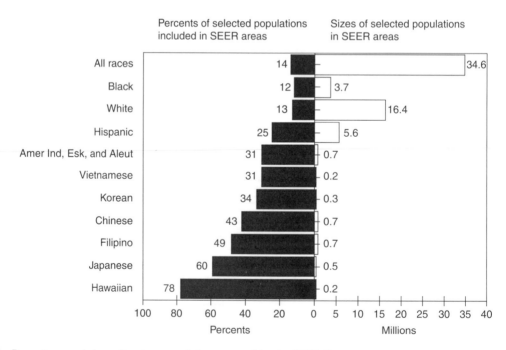

Figure 2   Percentages and sizes of various populations covered by the SEER Program

Hawaii, and the metropolitan areas of Detroit, San Francisco/Oakland, Seattle, and Atlanta. Subsequent additions to the program included 10 predominantly black rural counties in Georgia in 1978, and American Indians residing in Arizona in 1980. In 1992, the program was further expanded to increase coverage of minority populations, especially Hispanics. The two new areas added were Los Angeles County, and four counties in the San Jose/Monterey area south of San Francisco. Alaskan natives in Alaska have been added to those populations covered by SEER. The SEER Program currently includes population-based data from about 14% of the US population and is reasonably representative of subsets of the different racial/ethnic groups residing in the US. Figure 1 provides a map of the SEER areas and Figure 2 gives the percentages and sizes of various populations included in geographic areas covered by SEER [13].

The SEER database contains records on more than two million cancers and is growing at the rate of more than 160 000 records per year. Other data resources used by the SEER Program include cancer mortality data by county for the total US, obtained from the National Center for Health Statistics (NCHS). To provide for the calculation of incidence and mortality rates, population estimates are obtained through an interagency agreement with the Census Bureau.

Other organizations are also involved in cancer surveillance activities in the US. The North American Association of Central Cancer Registries (NAACCR) was organized in 1987 as an umbrella organization for cancer registries, governmental agencies, professional organizations, and private groups in North America interested in enhancing the quality and use of cancer registry data. Most population-based cancer registries in the US and Canada are members. The mission of NAACCR is to support and coordinate the development, enhancement, and application of cancer registration techniques in population-based groups, so that data of high quality and completeness may be used for epidemiologic research, public health programs, and patient care to reduce the burden of cancer in North America.

The American College of Surgeons Commission on Cancer and the American Cancer Society jointly founded the National Cancer Data Base (NCDB), which is a nationwide oncology outcomes database that includes data from over 1500 hospitals in 50 states, and is in its tenth year of operation. This database can be used to study patterns of care and factors associated with patient outcome, and patient care evaluation studies are periodically carried out in participating cancer registries [25]. Uses of this database focus on clinical surveillance of people with cancer, and cannot be used to calculate incidence rates.

Current Cancer Registration Practices

Cancer registration is the process of collecting data about patients with malignant diseases. The data collected identify the demographics of the patient with the disease, the type of cancer, how it is treated and the outcome of the patient. The data collected reside in a cancer registry, a term which can mean simply the database or data system that manages and analyzes the information or the data system and all of the associated systems and personnel who perform cancer surveillance and cancer control. Cancer registries serve several purposes.

A *hospital-based cancer registry* is a cancer data base maintained in a health care facility to collect pertinent information on all cancer patients who use the services of that facility for diagnosis, staging, and treatment. The service area for a hospital-based registry varies from facility to facility, depending on the types of specialty treatment it offers, the types of third-party payors it attracts, and a number of other factors. As a result, the number of potential patients in the facility's customer base can only be estimated. A hospital-based cancer registry can calculate frequency of cases and measure outcomes for the patients it monitors. A hospital-based cancer registry cannot calculate incidence rates because the denominator population is not known.

A *population-based cancer registry* is a centralized cancer database covering a known population, usually residents of a defined geographic area, such as a county or state. Because the population denominator can be counted or estimated by a census, a population-based registry can calculate incidence rates. Population-based registries are the principal source of cancer surveillance data.

Population-based registries must gather information on cancer patients from a variety of sources, including registries in hospital and other healthcare facilities, physician offices, pathology laboratories, and facilities outside the defined geographic area to which residents travel for cancer diagnosis and treatment. Population-based registries can be of two types: (1) those that report incidence only (the first report of a new cancer) or (2) multipurpose registries that collect data on incidence and subsequent outcomes.

A population-based registry is one type of *central registry*. A central registry collects data from a variety of sources but it may not be population-based. For example, a provider of cancer registry software may maintain a pooled database of all the cancer cases submitted by its customers, or a hospital corporation may pool the cases from all facilities it owns. In each of these cases, it is not possible to determine an appropriate denominator, so these central registries are not population-based.

Registry Operations

The four main aspects of registry operations are: case ascertainment, abstracting and coding, follow-up or mortality follow-back, and quality control. Data collection procedures will also be reviewed.

Case Ascertainment

Case ascertainment, also called casefinding, is the process of identifying patients with malignant disease who meet the criteria for inclusion in the registry. Because cancer surveillance requires monitoring of cancer incidence and mortality, case ascertainment must identify all cases of the disease in a defined population, regardless of where the cancer patient encounters the healthcare system; including hospitals, independent treatment centers, clinics, pathology laboratories, physician offices, and nursing homes. For practical purposes, the principal source of cancer information is the hospital health information or medical record, which includes all contacts with the hospital inpatient, outpatient and clinic. The medical record contains reports of diagnostic and staging procedures, physical examination, operations and other treatments. In addition, consultation reports from outside pathology departments and physicians are usually retained as part of the medical record. Medical records are maintained as legal documents in most facilities where patients are treated; the exception is the pathology laboratory.

Most cancer patients come to a hospital at some point in their disease process, usually for a biopsy or treatment; thus, hospital medical records are an important source of casefinding. In hospitals, medical records are coded and indexed by disease and procedure so that patient records can be retrieved for analysis. The database containing these codes is one of the principal sources of case ascertainment in a healthcare facility. Specific codes for cancer diagnosis and treatment permit retrieval of records pertaining to reportable neoplasms that must be included in the registry.

A neoplasm is a "new growth" or tumor that develops somewhere in the body. The term neoplasm refers to either benign or malignant (having the potential to spread from the site of origin and ultimately kill the patient) tumors. A *reportable neoplasm* is a tumor that meets the inclusion criteria for a registry. Reportable neoplasms are well defined in the *International Classification of Diseases for Oncology*, a coded nomenclature published by the World Health Organization (WHO). This coding system defines each type of tumor and its behavior: benign, uncertain malignant potential, *in situ*, invasive, or metastatic. The reportable neoplasms collected by all general-purpose cancer registries are those that are malignant (*in situ* or invasive). Metastatic tumors (malignancy growing in a site at a distance from the organ in which it started) are not reported individually; rather, metastases are reported as progression of the tumor at the site of origin. Occasionally a central registry will require that another type of tumor be reported, such as benign brain tumors, which cannot spread but do have the potential to be lethal, and tumors of uncertain malignant potential, such as carcinoids of the appendix. On the other hand, a few cancers are very common and are associated with such a good prognosis that it is generally not necessary to monitor their outcomes, such as basal cell and squamous cell carcinomas of the skin and carcinoma *in situ* of the cervix.

All the inclusion and exclusion guidelines for case ascertainment are compiled into a *reportable list*, which the data collector uses to identify cases to be abstracted for the registry.

Abstracting and Coding

Abstracting is the process of deriving and recording pertinent data about each reportable case. The resulting document, the *abstract*, is an abridgement or summary of what happened to the patient, and may be in paper or electronic form. Data items include demographics of the patient, a description of the disease (site of origin, type of malignancy), stage at diagnosis (documentation of how far the cancer had spread when it was diagnosed), treatment, and the course of the disease from the time it was diagnosed. Parts of the abstract are encoded, such as site and type of cancer, stage, and treatment. In addition to the standard data items, some registries collect information on items of special interest, such as smoking history, family history of cancer, or co-morbid conditions.

The abstracting process is exacting and highly technical, requiring great attention to detail. The aim of abstracting is to collect the data about each cancer case as accurately as possible (high correlation between source document and abstract) and as consistently as possible for similar cases (all cases following the same rules). Abstracting rules and guidelines have been developed to cover nearly every situation, but human interpretation of both the facts of the case and the rules of abstracting can sometimes cause problems, and there is always the danger of incorrect data entry. As a result, a series of edits have been developed and included in most cancer registry database systems.

There are several types of edits, including range checks and logic checks. The simplest edits are range checks or allowable codes. Logic checks are a type of inter-item edit where the program looks at two or more data fields to ensure that they make sense together. For example, an error message should be generated when "sex" is male and "primary site" is cervix. Inter-item edits can be quite complex, such as looking at a morphologic diagnosis code as noninvasive, the corresponding stage at diagnosis coded as *in situ*, the method of diagnostic confirmation coded as histologic, and the sites of distant metastasis fields that should be left blank. Computer edits such as these are the first line of defense against inaccurate data. Other editing mechanisms and preventive measures such as training and standardization of procedures are described in the following sections on data collection and quality control.

An additional function of population-based central registries is case consolidation or case matching. Because the registry receives reports from many sources, it is necessary to identify multiple reports on the same patient so that the case is not counted more than once. Case consolidation involves not only various computer algorithms but human review as well. For example, Hospital A might send in a report on Ric Smith with a birth date of 11-19-35 and a

diagnosis of sigmoid colon cancer, and Hospital B might send in a report on Frederic Smith with a birthdate of 11-18-35 or 11-19-36 and a diagnosis of rectal cancer. The registry must decide whether these reports are about the same patient, and, furthermore, whether they are about the same cancer. Without a case consolidation operation in the registry, the numerator (newly diagnosed cases) of the incidence rate may be inflated.

Data Collection Procedures

When data collection for the SEER Program began in 1973, it was imperative that data be collected uniformly and systematically in all participating areas. As a result, the SEER Program published a series of manuals providing specific rules for case inclusion and staging. The most recent of these is the *SEER Program Code Manual, 3rd Ed.* [20]. Since its inception, the SEER Program has been a leader in documentation of data collection rules, training of data collectors, and quality assurance of the data collected. Many central registries in the US follow SEER rules even though they are not funded by the National Cancer Institute.

In addition to these coding guidelines developed in the US, an international body established definitions of what was considered to be cancer. The WHO has been publishing revisions of the International Classification of Diseases (ICD) on a decennial basis since 1893. Originally developed to code mortality, ICD has been modified to code all types of diseases and conditions, and the current edition, ICD-9-CM (Ninth Revision, Clinical Modification) is the coding standard for health care facilities and reimbursement through federal Medicare programs [26]. The next edition, ICD-10, is in use in vital statistics offices to code death certificates [30]. As the WHO began development of the ninth revision in the early 1970s, clinicians expressed a desire for a more complete coding system for neoplasms, one that would describe both where the tumor started (topography) and what the tumor was (morphology). ICD contained a coded list of anatomic sites for the topography, and another coding system, the *Systematized Nomenclature of Pathology* (SNOP), published by the College of American Pathologists, contained the codes for cell types or morphology [4]. SNOP was a functional descendant of the *Manual of Tumor Nomenclature and Coding* (MOTNAC), published in 1951 and revised in 1968 by the American

Cancer Society. The WHO used the topography code structure from ICD-9 and selected the code structure from SNOP for the morphology codes. The first edition of the *International Classification of Diseases for Oncology* (ICD-O) was published in 1976 by the WHO [28]. A second edition using the alphanumeric topography codes from ICD-10 was published in 1990 and implemented in the US in 1992 [29]. A third edition of ICD-O is scheduled for publication in 2000. The College of American Pathologists maintains the descendant of SNOP, called the *Systematized Nomenclature of Medicine* (SNOMED) [5,6], now in its fourth generation as SNOMED RT (Reference Terminology) [24]. By international treaty, the neoplasm sections of SNOMED and ICD-O are identical, although the topography codes differ between the two coding systems.

US cancer organizations collected data for specific purposes; the American College of Surgeons for quality management of patient care, and the SEER Program for incidence, survival, and mortality statistics. For many years there was no effort on the part of these organizations to collaborate on the development of data-collection rules. An example of the resulting problems relates to the collection of data pertaining to stage of disease at diagnosis. There are currently four major staging systems in use in the US: Tumor–Node–Metastasis (TNM), a product of the International Union Against Cancer and the American Joint Committee on Cancer [1]; SEER Extent of Disease (EOD) [19]; Summary Staging [16] and SEER Historic Stage (local–regional–distant) [18]. These staging systems are not comparable for a number of cancers.

The American College of Surgeons Commission on Cancer (COC) uses TNM as the standard for coding stage of disease for hospitals participating in its approvals program. The SEER Program uses EOD as its data-collection standard and some versions of TNM can be derived from it [19], and SEER historic stage as its reporting standard which can be derived from EOD [18]. The National Program of Cancer Registries (NPCR) uses Summary Stage as its standard [16]. As a consequence, a registry approved by the American College of Surgeons COC in a state receiving NPCR funds and an area where SEER data is collected must stage each case using three different systems, each having their own codes, timing rules, and inclusion/exclusion criteria. Efforts are in progress to define a single data set for staging and a single set of

rules [10], but these efforts are far from fruition, much less implementation, data collection and analysis.

In the early 1980s, the SEER Program and the American College of Surgeons COC began meeting to resolve differences in data fields, such as field lengths, definitions, and code structures. The 1988 publications of the COC's *Data Acquisition Manual* [7] and *The SEER Program Code Manual*, 2nd Ed. [17] were in substantial agreement.

In 1987, the population-based central registries in the US and Canada formed an "organization of organizations" to share information on coding practices, registry operations, standards and other factors that affect the accuracy and reliability of published cancer information. One of the first activities of the NAACCR was to establish the Uniform Data Standards Committee (UDSC). The UDSC formalized the standardization efforts begun by SEER and the COC. This committee, consisting of representatives from all the standard-setting organizations, central registries, data collectors, registry software vendors, and other users of registry data, serves as a forum for identifying and resolving problems in data collection. The committee compiled all the rules regarding data collection and identified areas of discrepancy, publishing four volumes of standards in 1994: *I. Data Exchange Standards and Record Description*; *II. Data Standards and Data Dictionary*; *III. Standards for Completeness, Quality, Analysis and Management of Data*; and *IV. Standard Data Edits*.

Adherence to coding rules established by the UDSC and the NAACCR in general is voluntary. However, in the current practice of cancer registration in the US and Canada, all revisions to existing data fields, coding guidelines and data-collection rules, as well as proposed new data fields, data record layouts, and other enhancements, are discussed and voted upon by the members of the UDSC. An implementation date for approved changes is widely published so that software vendors can make changes in sufficient time to meet the needs of cases diagnosed after the implementation date, and the standard setters can publish necessary revisions to their data-collection manuals.

Outcome Measurements and Quality Control

As noted previously, a population-based cancer registry can be either incidence-only or multipurpose. If the registry is incidence-only, then the registry does no outcomes assessments. Outcomes measurement is the current vernacular for describing the results of treatment and the disease process in terms of survival rates and mortality. Outcomes processes include follow-up and mortality follow-back, two specific additional operations performed by multipurpose central registries. Follow-up is long-term surveillance of cancer patients. Once a patient is treated and rehabilitated, he or she resumes a relatively normal life, but monitoring for disease recurrence or sequelae of treatment must continue for the patient's lifetime. Follow-up is the process of contacting someone – either the patient directly or the patient's physician – to obtain current information on the status of the cancer. Ideal follow-up information includes a recent date of last contact, vital status (alive or dead), and disease status (free of disease, recurrent disease, a subsequent primary cancer, additional treatment, etc.). Most registries prefer to contact the patient's physician for this information as it will be more accurate, technical, and specific than that received from the patient. However, response rates are generally good when patients are contacted directly. Either type of direct contact is called *active follow-up*.

If a registry chooses not to contact the patient, follow-up information less complete than the ideal can be obtained by linking the cancer registry database with other governmental databases, such as voter registration, local tax rolls, and Department of Motor Vehicles (DMV) drivers' license renewal files. Little can be determined from these linkages other than the patient's vital status, and that might only be at the last point of contact with the agency. For example, DMV would only have a record of the last time the patient renewed his driver's license (possibly several years previously) or reported a change of address. This indirect method of obtaining the vital status of the patient is called *passive follow-up*. Another method of obtaining follow-up is linkage to Social Security Administration death lists and to the National Death Index; this linkage will update only deceased patients, however.

Tracing a patient who no longer regularly visits a physician for his disease is both an art and a science. Confidentiality guidelines must be observed when information is requested about any patient, but the higher the percentage of complete follow-up, the more reliable are estimates of survival rates. The SEER standard for complete follow-up is to have current information (within the past 15 months) on at least 95% of all cases.

Occasionally a patient with cancer will be missed in the case ascertainment process and not be abstracted into the registry database. Missing a case lowers the incidence rate for that particular cancer; thus high standards of case completeness are important for accurate and reliable cancer data. If a previously unreported cancer patient dies, a cancer diagnosis on the death certificate may be the first and only report of the cancer case. It is good policy for a registry to follow-back a Death Certificate Only (DCO) case to see where it was missed in the casefinding process. Follow-back is the process of contacting physicians and facilities noted on the death certificate to review their medical records to determine any earlier diagnosis or treatment of the cancer. In many instances the case was simply missed, so the abstract is processed as a late report and reporting-source procedures are investigated. In other instances the death certificate diagnosis is the only identification of the case. These cases are tagged as DCO in the database, and usually very little information is known about them. A registry monitors its percentage of DCOs as part of its quality control processes.

Quality control encompasses all registry activities that monitor and resolve data problems. Quality control usually deals with facts and data items. On the other hand, quality improvement or quality management usually deals with procedures and processes. Quality control is performed on all aspects of registry operations. Standards have been established for case completeness, database completeness, accuracy and reliability of data, and timely reporting of cases to the registry. The purpose of quality control is to determine whether these standards are being met.

Quality has been defined as "fitness for use". Analysis of data which are not fit for use can result in incorrect conclusions and inappropriate cancer control and cancer surveillance activities. The principal components of data quality are accuracy, completeness and timeliness [9].

Completeness has at least two aspects: completeness of the database and completeness of the data in each record. Completeness of the database means that all cases in the population under investigation have been included for the specified time period. Without a complete database, incidence rates and relative frequencies may be inaccurate. Completeness of the database is a function of thorough case ascertainment, described above. Completeness is assessed by several techniques, including re-casefinding studies, projections of the number of cases reported in previous years, and the ratio of incidence to mortality for all cancers combined and for selected cancers. The SEER Program's target rate for database completeness is 98% complete reporting for a diagnosis year at the time the data are first submitted (14 months after the end of the diagnosis year).

Completeness of the data is a function of abstracting. This means that all data have been reported and there are no omissions, unnecessary blanks, or fields coded as unknown that should have been completed. It is possible to have a data field considered complete because there are no blanks, but unusable because the data are coded as unreportable or unknown. However, a data collector must find a balance between tracking down every last data item for 100% completeness, and coding unknown if the data are not easily obtained.

Timeliness is a corollary to completeness. It is presumed that every case may eventually be found, but the issue is how long to wait before using the data. There is a tradeoff between having potentially incomplete data available for use quickly, and having complete data available after so long a wait that the data are no longer current or useful. To meet the needs of most (if not all) data users, it is necessary to set a cut-off date and assess completeness at that time. Thus, timeliness is determined by setting a final date for data submission, and ensuring that all records have been submitted by that date.

Accuracy is the quality measure that establishes the reputation for a registry. Accuracy is necessary in all parts of registry operations. Accurate incidence rates neither overcount nor undercount the number of cases in the population. Accurate abstracting ensures that results are appropriate for research. Accurate follow-up permits survival rates and other outcomes to be measured correctly.

The SEER Program performs quality control studies annually that are designed to provide quantitative assessments of accuracy and completeness of the data collected by the various participating registries. Some findings from these studies have been published [31]. In the near future, findings from all quality control studies designed to provide estimates of completeness and accuracy both at the registry level and for all registries combined will be available on the Internet at http://www-seer.ims.nci.nih.gov/

Current Cancer Surveillance Activities

The discussion here will focus on the activities of the NCI, since it has been in the forefront of cancer surveillance activities for more than 60 years. As previously mentioned, other organizations are involved in cancer surveillance; however, an attempt will not be made to associate specific activities with specific organizations. At this time it is not clear how cancer surveillance responsibilities in the US will ultimately be divided, as that is currently being negotiated by the parties involved. However, it is reasonable to assume that the NCI will continue to play a major role in all aspects of cancer surveillance.

The fundamental tool of cancer surveillance is the population-based cancer registry. The establishment of the SEER Program in 1972 was the beginning of a new era in cancer surveillance in the US. Beginning in 1973, the continuous registration of all cancers diagnosed in residents of geographic areas initially covered by SEER allowed the calculation of incidence rates for calendar years beginning in 1973. Follow-up to determine vital status for all cancer patients in SEER areas, including the coding of cause of death, allowed the calculation of survival rates as the SEER database matured.

A question frequently raised is: How representative are the SEER areas of the total US population? To address this question, it is necessary to define "representativeness" in this context. It is certainly desirable to be able to derive cancer rates from SEER areas that approximate those for the total US by age, sex, and racial/ethnic group. But it is probably more important to be able to establish that the trends in cancer rates in SEER areas approximate those for the total US. SEER rates have been assumed to be reasonably representative of those from the total US. However, in the future, cancer rates in SEER areas will be modeled using ecologic data available from the census in order to refine national estimates.

Cancer mortality data for the total US have been used to examine the representativeness of trends in SEER areas versus those for the total US. This was done by systemically comparing trends in cancer mortality for selected cancer sites in SEER areas with those for the total US. It was concluded that,

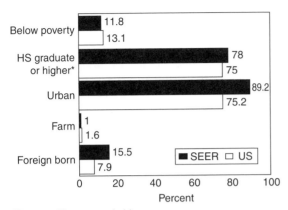

*Persons 25 years and older.

Figure 3 Comparison of selected ecologic variables from the 1990 census for the total population in SEER areas versus the total US population

with few exceptions, mortality trends for selected cancers in SEER areas were representative of those for the total US [11]. Therefore, it seems reasonable to assume that trends in SEER incidence rates approximate those for the total US. Further information on the representativeness of SEER areas is given in Figure 3, which compares selected ecologic data from the 1990 census in SEER areas with that for the total US.

A variety of reports are available on cancer rates in SEER areas, the most recent of which includes data for the time period 1973–1996 [21]. There are also reports on cancer incidence rates published by the NAACCR which include data from SEER registries plus other US and Canadian registries that have been found to have data of high quality. The most recent NAACCR publication is for the time period 1992–1996 [3].

The scope of cancer surveillance has broadened considerably since the early attempts at cancer registration. Current cancer surveillance activities include: developing and reporting estimates of cancer incidence, prevalence, and mortality on a periodic basis for the total US; monitoring annual cancer incidence trends to identify unusual changes in specific forms of cancer occurring in population subgroups defined by geographic, demographic, and social characteristics and providing insight into their etiology; and providing continuing information on changes over time in the extent of disease at diagnosis, trends in therapy, and associated changes in patient survival. Of

particular importance is the inclusion of sufficient numbers of various racial/ethnic populations, and other populations defined by a variety of measures including access to medical care, urban versus rural, and measures of poverty and socioeconomic status. Such research can benefit cancer prevention and control activities, and identify areas where improvements in treatment may be needed. Other uses of incidence, prevalence and survival data include identifying cancer sites showing unusual rates of increase or decrease that would warrant special etiologic investigation (e.g. non-Hodgkin's lymphoma increases associated with the acquired immune deficiency syndrome (AIDS) epidemic); helping health policy-makers set priorities for spending on research and for allocating resources among etiologic, prevention, diagnosis, treatment and control areas; and informing the general public and Congress on the extent and trends in the cancer burden. These data also have direct clinical relevance for advising individual patients. For example, age- and race-specific SEER data were used (together with other data on specific risk factors) to help develop a model for projecting the chance that a woman with particular risk factors would develop breast cancer in a given time period [8].

Other important research components to cancer surveillance include promoting studies designed to identify cancer risk factors amenable to cancer control interventions. These studies may pertain to the environment, occupation, socioeconomic status, tobacco, diet, screening practices, patterns of care, and determinants of the length and quality of patient survival. Other areas of investigation include planning, conducting, and supporting research related to evaluating patterns and trends in cancer rates and cancer-related risk factors. Also studied are health behaviors, cost of care, patient outcomes, health services as part of an attempt to determine the influence of such factors at the individual, societal, and systems level on patterns and trends in the various measures of cancer burden. Also included in this activity are identifying, improving and developing databases and methods for cancer-related surveillance research; maintaining, updating, and disseminating these databases and methods; and promoting and facilitating their use among investigators within the extramural research community and federal agencies. No attempt will be made to document all of these activities; however, information about them can be obtained from the following Internet sites: `http://www-dccps.ims.nci.nih.gov/arp/` and `http://www-dccps.ims.nci.nih.gov/srab/surveillance/survdesc.html`

The SEER contracts are primarily with cancer research organizations affiliated with universities. Thus, they provide an infrastructure for conducting analytic epidemiologic studies on a variety of emerging issues in cancer prevention and control which can be used by the NCI. The ability to do special studies was established in the early 1990s. The workscopes of SEER contracts were modified to include the capabilities of interviewing patients, conducting surveys of the covered populations, obtaining biological materials from patients and survey respondents, conducting methodologic research which utilizes cancer registry data, and establishing tissue banks. Standard competitive procurement procedures within the SEER framework have been used to plan and fund studies on a wide range of topics that have included identification of risk factors, quality of life, statistical modeling, etiology of trends in cancer rates, and operational issues pertaining to data collection and reporting. No attempt will be made to document the findings from these studies here, but they have resulted in a large number of peer-reviewed publications in scientific journals on a variety of issues pertaining to etiology, cancer control, quality of life, and registry operations [13].

There have also been significant efforts to involve the general research community in cancer surveillance activities. This has been done by distributing to cancer researchers public use files that include SEER data. The files are made available on CD-ROM and include more than two million individual records of cancers registered in SEER areas from 1973 to the most recent year for which complete data are available, population data, and documentation of all files. Also included is SEER*Stat which is a free Windows-based computer program developed by the SEER Program to calculate incidence rates, frequencies, trends, and survival rates. Another program, called SEER*Prep, allows registries outside of the SEER Program to put their data into SEER*Stat, greatly facilitating analysis of their data. Currently, about 1500 SEER public use files are distributed annually, and a number of non-SEER registries are using the SEER*Stat software via SEER*Prep. More information about this software

can be obtained on the Internet at: `http://www-seer.ims.nci.nih.gov/scientific systems/SEERStat/`

Recent developments in statistical methodology pertaining to the analysis of trends in age-adjusted rates deserve mention, since the analysis of trends is a fundamental activity of cancer surveillance. The first is the use of join point regression using log linear or linear models to describe trends in age-adjusted rates [14]. Models of this type assess the statistical significance of recent changes in trends as well as describe the trends over the period for which they are fit. Figure 4 presents a fit of a log linear join point regression model to the age-adjusted (1970 US Standard) mortality rates for all cancers combined for the total US for the total population and by sex. Annual percent changes and join points are given to describe the trends.

A second methodology of interest partitions a trend based on fitting linear regression models [12]. For example, it is possible to derive the relative contributions of various individual cancers or groups of cancers to an increasing or decreasing trend in the age-adjusted rate for all cancers combined. This type of analysis provides useful information about the impact of targeted interventions on the overall trend in age-adjusted rates for a group of diseases of interest. Figure 5 presents a partition of the most recent cancer mortality decrease for the total population and by sex based on rates adjusted to the 1970 US Standard. The contributions of cancers for which interventions have been introduced into the general population are given. Thus, it is possible to quantify the contributions of cancers of the lung, oral cavity, colon and rectum, female breast, cervix, and prostate to the decreasing trend.

The Future of Cancer Surveillance

Medical practices have led to a new role for cancer surveillance. In theory, prevention, screening, and treatment interventions are tested for efficacy by randomized controlled trials. If such trials demonstrate that an intervention is efficacious, then it is introduced into the general population. An important role for cancer surveillance is to make an assessment of the impact of the intervention in the population by analyzing trends in incidence, survival, or mortality rates as appropriate. This paradigm has been violated

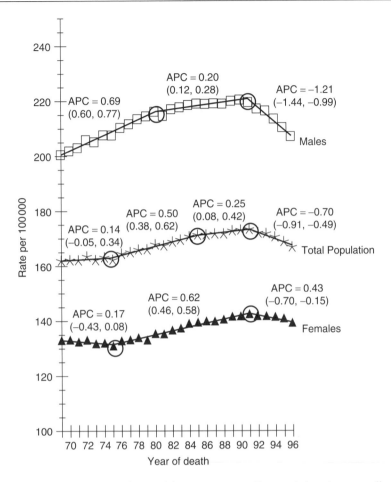

Figure 4 Fits of log linear join point regression models to cancer mortality trends based on age-adjusted rates (1970 US Standard) for the total population of the US and by sex. The linear segments are indicated by a solid line, and the join points are circled. The observed points are also given

in some cases in the past, particularly in the development of new screening tests where new tests have been introduced into the general population before establishing their efficacy in regard to reducing mortality. A prime example is the Prostate Specific Antigen (PSA) test for detecting prostate cancer [15]. The use of Spiral CT for diagnosing lung cancer may be a second example [23]. This practice has resulted in the use of surveillance data to not only establish some measure of the impact of the introduction of such a new test on population cancer rates, but to also make some assessment of its efficacy. If such practices continue, it will likely result in the establishment of more sophisticated surveillance systems directed toward accommodating this expanded role.

Cancer surveillance activities at the NCI have been reviewed by a committee of researchers from within and outside the Institute [22]. Recommendations for future directions have been made in a number of areas. The first priority is to expand the scope of surveillance research through additional data collection and methods development. Specific activities will include collection of data on patterns of care, health status, and quality of life, as well as cohort studies of newly diagnosed cancer patients for the purpose of documenting levels and trends in these parameters; collection of risk factor and screening data in defined populations, particularly those covered by high quality cancer registration; development of research methods to measure the dimensions of the cancer burden

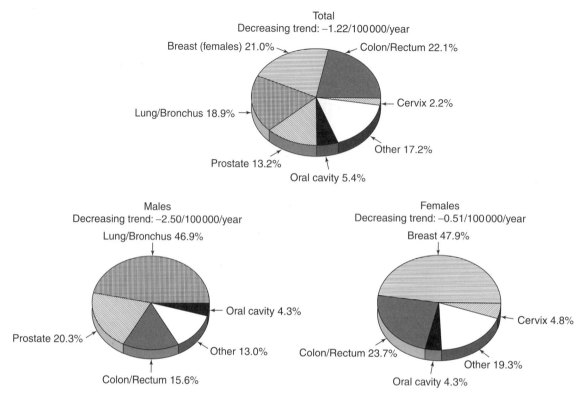

Figure 5 Partition of the cancer mortality trend from 1991 to 1996 based on fits of a linear regression model to the age-adjusted rates (1970 US Standard) for the total US population and by sex

and factors affecting the burden, as well as methods to explain patterns and trends in cancer rates; and exploration of the feasibility and utility of employing geographic information systems for geocoding surveillance data and reporting geographic relationships among screening measures, risk factors (including environmental exposures), and improved cancer outcomes.

A second area of focus is to expand the scope of surveillance to improve the representativeness of cancer burden estimates. Specific activities will include expanding SEER population coverage to improve representation of ethnic minority and underserved populations including rural African Americans, Hispanics from Caribbean countries, American Indians, residents of Appalachia and other rural areas, especially those of lower socioeconomic classes; developing methods for improving national estimates of the cancer burden; and working with other organizations involved in cancer surveillance to develop a national cancer surveillance plan.

A third area to be addressed is the production and dissemination of a national report card on the cancer burden. Specific activities will include the collection, analysis, and dissemination of data on important cancer outcomes and trends in risk factors, screening, and treatment to be incorporated into a national cancer report card; and the development of improved methods for disseminating information via the report card and other NCI communications.

The fourth area to be addressed is the support of molecular and genetics research for surveillance. Specific activities will include the development of valid tools to assess family history of cancer which will provide for the collection of data on the population prevalence of familial cancers; and the investigation of the feasibility of expanding population-based molecular and genetic biomarker studies within the Cancer Surveillance Research Program.

The final area to receive attention is the development of a training strategy for individuals interested in cancer surveillance research. Specifically, training pertaining to the needs of surveillance sciences will be developed along with a plan to incorporate surveillance training as a priority in mechanisms for training cancer prevention and control scientists. Much more detail is provided in the Cancer Surveillance Research Implementation Plan [22] which can be obtained at http://camp.nci.nih.gov/dccps/

Thus, in addition to their basic goals of supplying timely information on trends in site-specific cancer incidence, prevalence, and survival, cancer surveillance programs are evolving to provide improved quantitative benchmarks to document the impact of research advances in cancer prevention, detection, and treatment, and to identify problems that can be addressed through cancer prevention and control efforts.

References

[1] American Joint Committee on Cancer (1997). *AJCC Cancer Staging Manual*, 5th Ed. Lippincott-Raven, Philadelphia.

[2] Brennan, M.F., Clive, R.E. & Winchester D.P. (1994). The COC: its roots and destiny, *American College of Surgeons Bulletin* **79**, 14–21.

[3] Chen, V.W., Wu, X.C. & Andrews, P.A., eds. (1999). *Cancer Incidence in North America, 1991–1995; Volume One: Incidence.* North American Association of Central Cancer Registries, Sacramento.

[4] College of American Pathologists (1965). *Systematized Nomenclature of Pathology.* Chicago.

[5] College of American Pathologists (1977). *Systematized Nomenclature of Medicine.* Two Vols., R.A. Cote, ed., Skokie.

[6] College of American Pathologists (1993). *The Systematized Nomenclature of Human and Veterinary Medicine: SNOMED International*, R.A. Cote, D.J. Rothwell, J.L. Palotay, R.S. Beckett & L. Brocher, eds. Northfield.

[7] Commission on Cancer of the American College of Surgeons (1988). *Data Acquisition Manual.* American College of Surgeons, Chicago.

[8] Costantino, J.P., Gail, M.H., Pee, D., Anderson, S., Redmond, C.K., Benichou, J. & Wieand, H.S. (1999). Validation studies for models projecting the risk of invasive and total breast cancer incidence, *Journal of the National Cancer Institute* **91**, 1541–1548.

[9] Department of Health and Human Services (1985). *Quality Control for Cancer Registries.* Public Health Service, National Institutes of Health, Bethesda. Out of print.

[10] Edge, S., Fritz, A., Clutter, G.G., Page, D.L., Watkins, S., Blankenship, C., Douglas, L. & Fleming, I. (1999). A unified cancer stage data collection system: preliminary report from the Collaborative Stage Task Force/American Joint Committee on Cancer, *Journal of Registry Management* **26**, 57–61.

[11] Frey, C.M., McMillen, M., Cowan, C.D., Horm, J.W. & Kessler, L.G. (1992). Representativeness of the Surveillance, Epidemiology, and End Results Program data: Recent trends in cancer mortality rates, *Journal of the National Cancer Institute* **84**: 872–877.

[12] Hankey, B.F., Ries, L.A., Kosary, C.L., Feuer, E.J., Merrill, R.M. & Edwards, B.E. (1999). Partitioning linear trends in age-adjusted rates, *Cancer Causes and Control*.

[13] Hankey, B.F., Ries, L.A.G. & Edwards, B.K. (1999). The SEER Program: a national resource, *Cancer Epidemiology, Biomarkers, and Prevention*.

[14] Kim, H.J., Fay, M.P., Feuer, E.J. & Midthune, D.N. (1999). Permutation tests for joinpoint regression with applications to cancer rates, *Statistics in Medicine*.

[15] Mandelson, M.T., Wagner, E.H. & Thompson, R.S. (1995). PSA screening: a public health dilemma, *Annual Reviews Public Health* **16**, 283–306.

[16] National Cancer Institute (1986). *Summary Staging Guide, NIH Publication No. 86-2313.* National Institutes of Health, Baltimore. Hard copy available at: http://www-seer.ims.nci.nih.gov/cgi-bin/pubs/order1.pl.

[17] National Cancer Institute (1992). *The SEER Program Code Manual*, 2nd Ed., *NIH Publication No. 94-1999.* National Institutes of Health, Baltimore. Hard copy available at: http://www-seer.ims.nci.nih.gov/cgi-bin/pubs/order1.pl.

[18] National Cancer Institute (1993). *Comparative Staging Guide for Cancer: Major Cancer Sites*, Version 1.1., *NIH Publication No. 93-3640.* National Institutes of Health, Baltimore. Hard copy available at: http://www-seer.ims.nci.nih.gov/cgi-bin/pubs/order1.pl.

[19] National Cancer Institute (1998). *Extent of Disease 1998, Codes and Coding Instructions*, 3rd Ed., *NIH Publication No. 98-1999.* National Institutes of Health, Baltimore.

[20] National Cancer Institute (1998). *The SEER Program Code Manual,* 3rd Ed., *NIH Publication No. 98-2313.* National Institute of Health, Baltimore.

[21] National Cancer Institute (1999). *SEER Cancer Statistics Review, 1973–1996.* National Institutes of Health, Bethesda.

[22] National Cancer Institute (1999). *Cancer Surveillance Research Implementation Plan.* Surveillance Implementation Group, National Institutes of Health, Bethesda.

[23] Sone, S., Takishima, S., Li, F., Yang, Z., Honda, T., Maruama, Y., Hasegawa, M., Yamanda, T., Kubo, K. & Asakura, K. (1998). Mass screening for lung cancer with mobile spiral computed tomography scanner, *Lancet* **351**, 1242–1245.

[24] Spackman, K.A., Campbell, K.E. & Cote, R.A. (1997). SNOMED RT: a reference terminology for health care. AMIA Fall Symposium.

[25] Steele, G.D. Jr., Winchester, D.P. & Menck, H.R. (1994). The National Cancer Data Base. A mechanism for assessment of patient care, *Cancer* **73**, 499–504.

[26] US Public Health Service (1991). *International Classification of Diseases, Clinical Modification.* 9th rev., 4th Ed.

[27] Wagner, G. (1985). In *The Role of The Registry in Cancer Control*, D.M. Parkin, G. Wagner & C.S. Muir, eds., IARC Scientific Publications, No. 66. International Agency for Research on Cancer, Lyon.

[28] World Health Organization (1976). *International Classification of Diseases for Oncology*, 1st Ed. WHO, Geneva.

[29] World Health Organization (1990). *International Classification of Diseases for Oncology*, 2nd Ed., C. Percy, V. Van Holten & C. Muir, eds. WHO, Geneva.

[30] World Health Organization (1992). *International Statistical Classification of Diseases and Related Health Problems*, 10th rev., 3 Volumes. WHO, Geneva.

[31] Zippin, C., Lum, D. & Hankey, B.F. (1995). Completeness of hospital cancer case reporting from the SEER Program of the National Cancer Institute, *Cancer* **76**, 2343–2350.

(*See also* **Vital Statistics, Overview**)

B. HANKEY & APRIL FRITZ

Carrier-Borne Epidemic *see* Epidemic Models, Stochastic

Cartograms *see* Mapping Disease Patterns

Case Fatality

The concept of case fatality refers to patients with a common defined index disease or other medical problem, not to healthy people. Case fatality indicates how serious a disease condition is in causing death to the patients, usually within a defined period of time. It is common to hear about case fatality without reference to the time period of follow-up of the patients, but this should be avoided for reasons of ambiguity. There can, nevertheless, be applications in which the follow-up time may be virtually zero as, for example, with heart attacks or automobile accidents.

Technically, case fatality is expressed as the proportion of the number of patients dying in the follow-up interval out of all patients under observation. This concept is useful only under a fairly complete follow-up, where the proportion of persons lost to follow-up or otherwise withdrawn alive is small. Moreover, **competing risks** of death can, in addition to the index disease, cause deaths among the patients. If the follow-up period is short, deaths due to competing risks unrelated to the index disease may be uncommon, and the case fatality indeed reflects the seriousness of the disease in an adequate way.

Conceptually, case fatality may be seen as a complement to survival. Thus, the methods of **survival analysis** can be employed in assessing case fatality. For example, the proportion of survivors after a one-year follow-up among patients diagnosed in Finland in 1967–1974 with cancer of the tongue was 64%. The case fatality within the first year was thus 36%.

The models in survival analysis generally are based on assumptions concerning the risk of dying for the patients. Thus, it would also be natural to express case fatality in terms of fatality or lethality rate of the disease by defining any death or death due to index disease as the main outcome event in survival analysis. This rate is the incidence of death or death due to disease and as a rate is calculated as the number of outcome events in the follow-up period divided by the appropriate person-time denominator (*see* **Person-Years At Risk**). Although this may sound theoretically appealing, a conversion to a proportion-type measure produces a quantity with an easier numerical interpretation for clinical medicine.

T. HAKULINEN

Case Series, Case Reports

A case report refers to a description of a person with a particular disease, and a case series refers to a series of case reports, often representing all cases with the given disease in a defined time period in a particular practice, clinic, or geographic area. Case reports are used by clinicians to describe responses to treatment, among other things. Epidemiologists may rely on case reports to find clues to disease etiology.

Case reports can be very informative for rare diseases. Such reports identified chimney sweeping as a risk factor for scrotal cancer [1] in 1775, and many modes of transmission of the human immunodeficiency virus were identified in the early 1980s from case reports of the Acquired Immune Deficiency Syndrome (AIDS). For more reliable inferences, however, it is usually necessary to compare rates of exposure in cases with rates of exposure in disease-free controls to develop etiologic evidence (*see* **Case–Control Study**).

Reference

[1]   Potts, P. (1775). Cancer scroti, in *Chirurgical Observations*. Hawes, Clarke & Collins, London, pp. 63–68.

M.H. GAIL

Case–Cohort Study

The case–cohort design is a method of sampling from an assembled epidemiologic **cohort study** or clinical trial in which a random sample of the cohort, called the *subcohort*, is used as a comparison group for all cases that occur in the cohort. This design is generally used when such a cohort can be followed for disease outcomes but it is too expensive to collect and process covariate information on all study subjects. Though it may be used in other settings, it is especially advantageous for studies in which covariate information collected at entry to the study is "banked" for the entire cohort but is expensive to retrieve or process (see examples below) and multiple disease stages or outcomes are of interest. In such circumstances, the work of covariate processing for subcohort members can proceed at the beginning of the study. As time passes and cases of disease occur, information for these cases can be processed in batches. Since the subcohort data are prepared early on and are not dependent on the occurrence of cases, statistical analyses can proceed at regular intervals after the processing of the cases. Furthermore, staffing needs are quite predictable. Motivated by the case–base sampling method for simple binary outcome data [9, 15], Prentice described the design and a pseudo-likelihood method of analysis (see below) for the case–cohort design.

Design

The basic components of a case–cohort study are the *subcohort*, a sample of subjects in the cohort, and *nonsubcohort cases*, subjects that have had an event and are not included in the subcohort. The subcohort provides information on the **person-time** experience of a random sample of subjects from the cohort or random samples from within strata (*see* **Stratification**) of a **confounding** factor. In the latter situation, differing sampling fractions could be used to align better the person-time distribution of the subcohort with that of the cases. Methods for sampling the subcohort include sampling a fixed number without replacement [17] and sampling based on independent Bernoulli "coin flips" [24]. The latter may be advantageous when subjects are entered into the study prospectively; the subcohort may then be formed concurrently rather than waiting until accrual into the cohort has ended [21, 24]. Simple case–cohort studies are the same as case–base studies for simple binary outcome data. But, in general, portions of a subject's time on study might be sampled. For example, the subcohort might be "refreshed" by sampling from those remaining on study after a period of time [17, 26]. These subjects would contribute person-time only from that time forward. While the subcohort may be selected based on covariates, a key feature of the case–cohort design is that the subcohort is chosen without regard to failure status; methods that rely on failure status in the sampling of the comparison group are **case–control studies**.

Examples

Study of Lung Cancer Mortality in Aluminum Production Workers in Quebec, Canada.   Armstrong et al. [1] describe the results of a case–cohort study selected from among 16 297 men who had worked at least one year in manual jobs at a large aluminum production plant between 1950 and 1988. This study greatly expands on an earlier cohort mortality study of the plant, which found a suggestion of increased rates of lung cancer in jobs with high exposures to coal tar pitch [7]. Through a variety of methods, 338 lung cancer deaths were identified. To avoid the expense associated with tracing subjects and abstraction of work records for the entire cohort, a case–cohort study was undertaken. To improve study efficiency a subcohort of 1138 subjects was randomly sampled from within year-of-birth strata with sampling fractions varying to yield a similar distribution to that of cases. This was accommodated in the analysis by stratification by these year-of-birth categories. The random sampling of subcohort members resulted in the inclusion of 205 cases in the subcohort. Work and smoking histories were abstracted for the subcohort and the additional 133 nonsubcohort cases. Cumulative exposure to coal tar pitch volatiles was estimated by linking worker job histories to measurements of chemical levels made in the plant using a **"job-exposure matrix"**. The analyses confirmed the lung cancer–coal pitch association observed in the earlier study and effectively ruled out confounding by smoking.

Women's Health Trial.   To assess the potential health benefits of a low fat diet, a randomized trial of women assigned to low fat intervention and control groups has been undertaken. Of particular interest is the effect of this intervention on the risk of breast cancer. The study, as described in Self et al. [21], includes a cohort of 32 000 women between ages 45 and 69 whose percent calories from fat is greater than the median and who have at least one of a list of known risk factors for breast cancer. The study will involve 20 clinics across the US for a period of 10 years of follow-up. At two-year intervals, each participant will fill out four-day food records and food frequency questionnaires and blood will be drawn and stored. While evaluation of the intervention will be based on the full cohort, questions that require abstraction and coding of the questionnaires and blood lipid analyses are being addressed in a case–cohort study with a 10% sample serving as the subcohort. It was calculated that, relative to the entire cohort, this sample avoids about 80% of the cost of the analyses requiring these data with only a modest reduction of efficiency. The subcohort can also be used for making other comparisons between intervention and control groups. For example, the case–cohort sample could be used to investigate the joint relationship of blood hormone and nutrient levels and dietary intakes to breast cancer risk. Also, questions relating to other outcomes, such as cardiovascular disease, could be explored using the same subcohort as the comparison group, although additional data processing would be required for cases that occur outside the subcohort.

Statistical Analysis

Several methods have been developed to analyze case–cohort samples. Essentially, each of the methods available for the analysis of complete cohort data has an analog for the case–cohort sample. For point estimation of rate ratio parameters, the likelihood for full cohort data applied to the case–cohort data yields a valid estimator. However, estimation of the variance of point estimates, or tests of hypotheses, requires adjustment to the standard full cohort variance estimators, as these will be too small. For likelihood-based methods, case–cohort sampling induces a covariance between score terms so that the variance of the score is given by $\Sigma + \Delta$, where Σ is the full cohort score variance and Δ is the sum of the covariances between the score terms. Since the subgroup used to compute the score terms has less variability than the full cohort, this covariance is positive. This leads to a larger variance for the parameter estimates, taking into account the subcohort sampling variability [12, 17, 20, 26]. Estimation of **absolute rates or risk** requires incorporation of the subcohort sampling fraction (or fractions) into the estimator.

Pseudo-Likelihoods for Proportional Hazards Models

Assume the underlying model for disease rates has a **multiplicative** form:

$$\lambda[t, z(t); \beta_0] = \lambda_0(t)r[z(t); \beta_0],$$

where $r[z(t); \beta_0]$ is the rate ratio of disease for an individual with covariates $z(t)$ at time t and $r(0; \beta) = 1$, so $\lambda_0(t)$ is the rate of disease in subjects with $z = 0$. The pseudo-likelihood approach described by Prentice [17] parallels the partial likelihood approach to the analysis of full cohort data. We start with the full cohort situation and then return to the analysis of the case–cohort sample. The partial likelihood approach is illustrated in Figure 1 for a small hypothetical **cohort study** of 15 subjects. Each horizontal line represents one subject. A subject enters the study at some *entry time*, is *at risk*, denoted by the horizontal line, over some time period, and exits the study at some *exit time*. A subject may contract or die from the disease of interest, and thus be a *failure* (represented by "•" in Figure 1 or be censored, i.e. be alive at the end of the study, died never having had the disease of interest, or be lost to follow-up. At

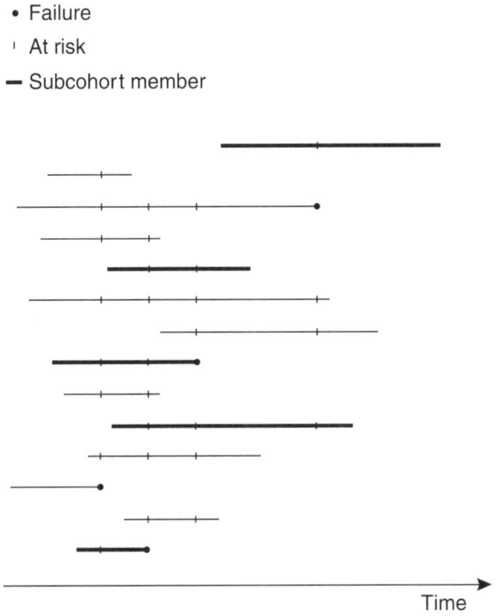

• Failure
ı At risk
— Subcohort member

Figure 1 Prentice pseudo-likelihood approach to the analysis of case–cohort data. Pseudo-likelihood contributions are conditional probabilities based on the case and the subcohort members at risk at the failure time

each failure time a *risk set* is formed that includes the *case*; namely, the failure at that failure time, and all *controls*, namely, any other cohort members who are at risk at the failure time (these are denoted by a "|" in Figure 1). The partial likelihood for full cohort data is based on the conditional probabilities that the case failed given that one of the subjects in the risk set failed at that time. With r_k the rate ratio and Y_k the "at risk" indicator for subject k at the failure time, and r_{case} the rate ratio associated with the case, the full cohort partial likelihood is

$$\prod_{\text{failure times}} \frac{r_{\text{case}}}{\sum_{\text{case and all controls}} Y_k r_k}.$$

Now in a case–cohort sample, covariate information is obtained for the subcohort and all nonsubcohort failures and only these subjects can contribute to the analysis. Prentice's pseudo-likelihood approach is illustrated in Figure 1 in which subcohort members are denoted by a thick horizontal line. For each failure, a *sampled risk set* is formed by the case and the controls who are in the subcohort (those with thick lines and a "|" at the failure time). As

the figure indicates, subcohort members contribute to the analysis over their entire time on study, but the nonsubcohort failures contribute only at their failure times. Analogous to the full cohort partial likelihood, a pseudo-likelihood contribution is based on the conditional probability that the case fails given that someone fails among those in the sampled risk set. The pseudo-likelihood is then the product of such conditional probabilities over failure times:

$$\prod_{\text{failure times}} \frac{r_{\text{case}}}{\sum_{\text{case and subcohort controls}} Y_k r_k}, \quad (1)$$

where the sum in the denominator is over the subcohort members when the case is in the subcohort and over the subcohort and nonsubcohort case when the case is not in the subcohort. This "likelihood" has the property that the expected value of the score is zero at β_0 but, as discussed above, the inverse information does not estimate the variance of the maximum pseudo-likelihood estimator. Prentice provided an estimator of the covariance Δ from the covariance between each pair of score terms, conditional on whether or not the failure occurring later in time was in the subcohort [17]. This is a rather complicated expression and only one software package has implemented it (Epicure, Hirosoft International Corp., Seattle, WA). Development of other methods of variance estimation has been an area of much research. These include "large sample" [20], bootstrap [27], "empirical" [4, 19], and influence function based [2, 14] methods. Alternative pseudo-likelihoods of a similar form have been proposed. These involve differential weightings of the r_k terms based on the sampling fractions of the associated with subject k [2, 8, 20].

Absolute Risk Estimation

Estimation of the cumulative baseline hazard and related quantities parallel the nonparametric estimators based on the Nelson–Aalen estimator for full cohort data. Since the subcohort is a random sample from the full cohort, a natural estimator of the cumulative baseline hazard $\int_0^t \lambda_0(u)\,\mathrm{d}u$ is given by summing contributions for failure times up to t of the form:

$$\frac{1}{1/f \sum_{\text{subcohort}} r_k(\hat{\beta})},$$

where f is the proportion of the cohort in the subcohort [17, 20]. Again, adjustment of the cohort variance estimator is required.

Other Estimation Methods

Methods for estimating standardized mortality ratios (*see* **Standardization Methods**) with a case–cohort sample have been described [25]. These involve "boosting up" the subcohort person-time in each age–year–exposure group "cell" by the inverse sampling fraction. Methods of variance adjustment are also discussed. When disease is rare and there is little censoring, methods of analysis for case–base studies with simple binary outcome data [15] will approximate the failure time analyses (e.g. [6], [18] and [23]).

Asymptotic Properties and Efficiency

Self & Prentice [20] give conditions for the consistency and asymptotic normality of the Prentice pseudo-likelihood for simple (stratified) case–cohort sampling. They show that the asymptotic variance of the maximum pseudo-likelihood estimator of relative risk parameters has the form $\Sigma^{-1} + \Sigma^{-1} \Delta \Sigma^{-1}$, where Σ is the full cohort variance of the score, and they provide a formula for the asymptotic sampling-induced covariance Δ. This covariance depends on the censoring distribution even when $\beta_0 = 0$, so that efficiencies relative to the full cohort analysis must take the censoring distribution into account. Assuming a cohort with complete follow-up over a fixed observation period, an exponential relative risk model for a single binary covariate, a subcohort that is a simple $100\alpha\%$ random sample of the cohort, and probability of failure during the observation period of d, they calculate the asymptotic relative efficiency as

$$\left\{ 1 + 2 \frac{1-\alpha}{\alpha} \left[1 + \frac{1-d}{d} \log(1-d) \right] \right\}^{-1}.$$

Wacholder et al. [26] provide an alternative approach to large-sample variance and efficiency calculations. Their method is adapted for use when the cohort is assembled so that entry and exit times and failure status are known for all cohort members, but covariate information is not. Furthermore the method assumes that $\beta_0 = 0$ and that the underlying censoring distribution does not depend on covariates. Variance

formulas are given for simple random sampling of the subcohort and when the subcohort is "augmented" by adding subjects to the subcohort at one later time in the study.

Comparison with Nested Case–Control Sampling

Nested case–control and case–cohort methods are the two main approaches to sampling from assembled cohort studies. The former takes a retrospective point of view by sampling time-matched controls after the outcome (failure) occurs. In contrast, case–cohort sampling is prospective and unmatched in the sense that the comparison group, the subcohort, is picked without regard to failure status. Considerations for choosing between the designs have been the subject of some interest [5, 11, 13, 16, 17, 22, 24]. We summarize some of these considerations below.

Prospective Studies

If the study is **retrospective** and has been assembled, the major consideration in choosing between sampling designs is the statistical efficiency for the proposed analyses and the information to be collected on the sample, as this will translate quite directly into cost. If the study is prospective in that the study group will be assembled as time passes and outcomes occur in the future, the decision about which design to choose will depend on whether it is advantageous to have a comparison group early on in the study or whether it is better to wait until near the end. If the sample is to be chosen at the beginning, or concurrent with accrual into a prospective study, the case–cohort study has a number of advantages. First, as discussed above, processing of covariate information for the subcohort may proceed early on in the study during the accrual period. During the follow-up period, data for cases arising outside the subcohort could be processed in batches at various times. A nested case–control study requires waiting until cases occur and controls are selected for them, delaying the processing of covariate information until later in the study than would be required in the case–cohort design. Thus, the case–cohort study can potentially be completed sooner than the nested case–control study. Secondly, although subcohort members should not be treated differently from cases occurring outside the subcohort, the subcohort can serve as a sample for assessing compliance, or quality control, as the study proceeds. However, a nested case–control sample may be advantageous if it is important that processing of information be "blinded" to case-comparison group status. Since case–control covariate information can be processed simultaneously, potential information bias can be avoided. This is not always possible with a case–cohort sample when subcohort data are processed early in the study.

Statistical Efficiency

Comparison of statistical efficiency for studying a single outcome has been a topic of much research. It has been conjectured that the case–cohort design should be more efficient than the nested case–control design. This belief has been based on a comparison of the contribution of a failure to the pseudo-likelihood (1) with that of the corresponding nested case–control contribution. The former uses all subcohort members at risk at the failure time, whereas the latter uses only the controls selected for that case, usually resulting in the case–cohort having many more "controls per case". In fact, analytic and empirical efficiency comparisons indicate that in most situations encountered in practice, nested case–control sampling will be more efficient than the case–cohort, although often not by a large amount [11, 12, 24, 26]. The reason for the lower-than-anticipated relative efficiency is that the large number of controls per case in the case–cohort sample, which by itself increases efficiency, is offset by the sampling-induced positive correlation in score terms (see above), which lowers efficiency. The nested case–control design has relatively few controls per case, but there is no sampling-induced correlation between score terms [12].

Multiple Disease Outcomes

Since the subcohort is chosen without regard to failure status, it may serve as the comparison group for multiple disease outcomes. This would seem to be a great advantage over the nested case–control design, since controls are selected for specific cases. In fact, there are few published studies that exploit this feature of the design. Nevertheless, the most cost-effective use of the case–cohort design would

seem to be to study a single set of explanatory factors and multiple outcomes. Thus, it seems likely that the case–cohort design may have application in clinical investigations in which researchers are often interested in multiple-event outcomes such as relapse, local and distant recurrence, and death as a function of a single set of treatment and prognostic factors. If, for instance, the prognostic factors involve expensive laboratory work, a case–cohort sample would be a natural way to reduce costs associated with the laboratory work, but still allow a full analysis of multiple endpoints. Using the same comparison group will result in correlation between estimates of the same parameter for different endpoints. Appropriate adjustments to test statistics for comparing these estimates is a topic that requires study.

Matching

Often, it is desirable to match (*see* **Matching**) comparison subjects closely on certain factors, either to control for **confounding** or so that information of comparable quality may be obtained. For instance, it is common to compare a case with controls close in year of birth to adjust for secular trends in behavior. Fine matching, and matching based on time-dependent factors is accommodated in a natural way in a nested case–control sample. Matching may only be done crudely for case–cohort sampling and must be based on factors available at the time the subcohort is sampled.

Analysis Flexibility

The nested case–control design is inherently associated with methods for analysis of cohort data based on semiparametric **proportional hazards** models. Estimation of rate ratio parameters is based on partial likelihood methods and estimation of absolute-risk-related quantities is based on the Nelson–Aalen estimator of the **cumulative hazard**. (One interesting exception to the restriction to proportional hazards models is estimation of excess risks using the Aalen linear model [3].) The case–cohort design is not associated with any particular model or method of analysis. Thus, in theory, "Poisson likelihood" or "grouped time" case–base analysis approaches, as well as the risk-set-based pseudo-likelihood (1), may be used for parameter estimation. In particular, parameters in nonproportional hazards models may be estimated using **Poisson regression**. These possibilities have not been explored in the literature and represent an area for further research. For a subcohort that is a simple random sample, changing time scales and analysis stratification variables poses no difficulties in the analysis. Since the nested case–control sample is bound to the risk set defined by the time scale and stratification variables used in matching controls to failures, these must be fixed in the analysis. However, inference from case–cohort samples is complicated by the need to adjust standard errors and test statistics for the sampling-induced covariance.

Computation

Standard conditional logistic regression software, for the analysis of matched case–control data, may be used to analyze rate ratio parameters from nested case–control studies (*see* **Software, Biostatistical**). Furthermore, if the numbers of subjects in the risk sets are known, absolute risk estimators and standard errors are relatively simple to compute [10]. Since the latter are based on standard nonparametric cumulative hazard and survival estimators, standard software for the analysis of full cohort data may be "tricked" into computing the nested case–control estimators. For case–cohort samples, standard **Cox regression** software may be used to estimate parameters but, as discussed above, special software is needed to estimate corresponding variances.

References

[1] Armstrong, B., Tremblay, C., Baris, D. & Gilles, T. (1994). Lung cancer mortality and polynuclear aromatic hydrocarbons: a case–cohort study of aluminum production workers in Arvida, Quebec, Canada, *American Journal of Epidemiology* **139**, 250–262.

[2] Barlow, W.E. (1994). Robust variance estimation for the case–cohort design, *Biometrics* **50**, 1064–1072.

[3] Borgan, Ø. & Langholz, B. (1997). Estimation of excess risk from case–control data using Aalen's linear regression model, *Biometrics* **53**, 690–697.

[4] Edwardes, M.D. (1995). Re: Risk ratio and rate ratio estimation in case–cohort designs: hypertension and cardiovascular mortality, *Statistics in Medicine* **14**, 1609–1610.

[5] Ernster, V.L. (1994). Nested case–control studies, *Preventive Medicine* **23**, 587–590.

[6] Flanders, W.D., Dersimonian, R. & Rhodes, P. (1990). Estimation of risk ratios in case–base studies with competing risks, *Statistics in Medicine* **9**, 423–435.

[7] Gibbs, G.W. (1985). Mortality of aluminum reduction plant workers, 1950 through 1977, *Journal of Occupational Medicine* **27**, 761–770.

[8] Kalbfleisch, J.D. & Lawless, J.F. (1988). Likelihood analysis of multi-state models for disease incidence and mortality, *Statistics in Medicine* **7**, 149–160.

[9] Kupper, L.L., McMichael, A.J. & Spirtas, R. (1975). A hybrid epidemiologic study design useful in estimating relative risk, *Journal of the American Statistical Association* **70**, 524–528.

[10] Langholz, B. & Borgan, Ø. (1997). Estimation of absolute risk from nested case–control data, *Biometrics* **53**, 767–774.

[11] Langholz, B. & Thomas, D.C. (1990). Nested case–control and case–cohort methods of sampling from a cohort: a critical comparison, *American Journal of Epidemiology* **131**, 169–176.

[12] Langholz, B. & Thomas, D.C. (1991). Efficiency of cohort sampling designs: some surprising results, *Biometrics* **47**, 1563–1571.

[13] Langholz, B., Thomas, D.C., Witte, J.S. & Peters, R.K. (1995). Re: Thompson et al. a population based case–cohort evaluation of the efficacy of mammography screening for breast cancer, *American Journal of Epidemiology* **142**, 448–449.

[14] Lin, D.Y. & Ying, Z. (1993). Cox regression with incomplete covariate measurements, *Journal of the American Statistical Association* **88**, 1341–1349.

[15] Miettinen, O.S. (1982). Design options in epidemiology research: an update, *Scandinavian Journal of Work, Environment, and Health* **8**, Supplement 1, 1295–1311.

[16] Moulton, L.H., Wolff, M.C., Brenneman, G. & Santosham, M. (1995). Case–cohort analysis of case-coverage studies of vaccine effectiveness, *American Journal of Epidemiology* **142**, 1000–1006.

[17] Prentice, R.L. (1986). A case–cohort design for epidemiologic cohort studies and disease prevention trials, *Biometrika* **73**, 1–11.

[18] Sato, T. (1992). Maximum likelihood estimation of the risk ratio in case–cohort studies, *Biometrics* **48**, 1215–1221.

[19] Schouten, E.G., Dekker, J.M., Kok, F.J., Le Cessie, S., van Houwelingen, H.C., Pool, J. & Vandenbrouke, J.P. (1993). Risk ratio and rate ratio estimation in case–cohort designs: hypertension and cardiovascular mortality, *Statistics in Medicine* **12**, 1733–1745.

[20] Self, S.G. & Prentice, R.L. (1988). Asymptotic distribution theory and efficiency results for case–cohort studies, *Annals of Statistics* **16**, 64–81.

[21] Self, S., Prentice, R., Iverson, D., Henderson, M., Thompson, D., Byar, D., Insull, W., Gorbach, S.L., Clifford, C., Goldman, S., Urban, N., Sheppard, L. & Greenwald, P. (1988). Statistical design of the women's health trial, *Controlled Clinical Trials* **9**, 119–136.

[22] Thompson, R.S., Barlow, W.E., Taplin, S.H., Grothaus, L., Immanuel, V., Salazar, A. & Wagner, E.H. (1994). A population-based case–cohort evaluation of the efficacy of mammographic screening for breast cancer, *American Journal of Epidemiology* **140**, 889–901.

[23] van den Brandt, P.A., Goldbohm, R.A. & van't Veer, P. (1995). Alcohol and breast cancer: results from the Netherlands cohort study, *American Journal of Epidemiology* **141**, 907–915.

[24] Wacholder, S. (1991). Practical considerations in choosing between the case–cohort and nested case–control designs, *Epidemiology* **2**, 155–158.

[25] Wacholder, S. & Boivin, J.-F. (1987). External comparisons with the case–cohort design, *American Journal of Epidemiology* **126**, 1198–1209.

[26] Wacholder, S., Gail, M.H. & Pee, D. (1991). Selecting an efficient design for assessing exposure–disease relationships in an assembled cohort, *Biometrics* **47**, 63–76.

[27] Wacholder, S., Gail, M.H., Pee, D. & Brookmeyer, R. (1989). Alternative variance and efficiency calculations for the case–cohort design, *Biometrika* **76**, 117–123.

BRYAN LANGHOLZ

Case–Control Study

The case–control design provides a framework for studying the relationship between possible risk factors and a disease by collecting information about exposure from those with disease but only from a fraction of the individuals under study who do not develop disease. When the disease is rare, this approach offers a major gain in efficiency relative to the full **cohort study**, in which an investigator seeks information on exposure for everyone. The savings compensate handsomely for the loss in the precision of estimates of parameters describing the relationship between exposure and disease that could have been obtained from studying everyone. In fact, the reduction in precision often is marginal. By collecting data on exposure about *cases*, the subjects who have developed disease, and **controls**, specially selected subjects without disease, the case–control design also compresses the time needed to complete the study. In a classic case–control study, Doll & Hill [10] recruited 649 male lung cancer cases and 649 male controls during an 18-month period in London. They were able to show a clear increase in **risk** with increasing daily cigarette consumption in this case–control study. By contrast, in a cohort study of an equal number of men at the very highest risk – that is, very heavy smokers above age 70 – one would expect to find only a handful of lung cancer cases within 1.5 years, not nearly enough to draw convincing conclusions about the relationship between smoking and lung cancer.

A hypothetic example illustrates the extent of the savings. In Table 1 are displayed the results of a cohort study of 1 000 000 individuals who are followed for disease for one year; 10% of them are exposed.

The expected results from a case–control study in which all 56 of the cases from this cohort are studied are displayed in Table 2. Expected cell counts are also shown in Table 2. For example, the expected number exposed among the 56 studied controls is calculated as $56 \times (99\,984/999\,944) = 5.6$.

The estimate of the **odds ratio** for disease, $(16/40)/(99\,984/899\,960)$ in Table 1, equals the estimate of the exposure odds ratio in Table 2, $(16/40)/(5.6/50.4)$. Both odds ratios equal 3.6004, and approximate the risk ratio (*see* **Relative Risk**) $(16/100\,000)/(40/900\,000) = 3.60$ to four significant digits. Thus, the study of 112 individuals would give the same estimate as the study of 1 000 000, apart from random variation. While the 95% confidence interval (CI) for the odds ratio from the case–control study, (1.3–10.3), is substantially wider than the CI (2.0–6.4) from the full cohort study, using $5 \times 56 = 280$ controls instead of only 56 would narrow the CI for the case–control study to (1.8–7.2), which is notably closer to that of the full

Table 1 Hypothetical full cohort study

	Diseased	Nondiseased	Total	Relative risk[a]	Relative odds[b]
Exposed	16	99 984	100 000	3.60	3.60
Unexposed	40	899 960	900 000	1.00	1.00

[a]Relative risk = $(16/100\,000)/(40/900\,000)$.
[b]Relative odds = $(16/99\,984)/(40/899\,960)$.

Table 2 Expected values from case–control study in same setting as Table 1

	Diseased (cases)	Nondiseased (controls)	Relative odds
Exposed	16	5.6	3.60
Unexposed	40	50.4	1.00
Total	56	56	

cohort study. This minor loss of precision is a small price to pay for the savings in exposure assessment costs and in time that may make feasible a study that would otherwise be too expensive.

In principle, although not always in practice, all case–control studies yield an unbiased estimate of the odds ratio and other functions of the odds. Most are designed so that the odds ratio directly estimates the relative risk or the incidence-rate ratio. However, only **population-based case–control studies** that yield estimates of overall disease risk or rate in the population permit estimation of exposure-specific **incidence rates** and thus of all parameters that could be estimated from studying the entire cohort.

Along with these considerable design strengths, the case–control study has several weaknesses. Incomplete or inaccurate ascertainment of outcome and improper selection of controls can cause **selection bias**. Retrospective assessment of exposure history can lead to **nondifferential** and **differential** measurement error and **biased** estimates of exposure effects. As in any nonexperimental or **observational study, confounding** can distort the estimates of effect from a case–control study (*see* **Bias in Case–Control Studies**; **Bias in Observational Studies**; **Bias, Overview**; **Measurement Error in Epidemiologic Studies**; **Misclassification Error**).

The Range of Case–Control Studies

A MEDLINE search for papers published since 1992 found over 1500 entries per year mentioning case–control or one of its cognates, usually case–referent. The case–control study is a fundamental tool of epidemiology with broad application in areas as diverse as the etiology of cancer and birth defects, the effectiveness of vaccination and **screening** for disease, and the causes of automobile accidents.

Case–control studies vary greatly in scope, sources of data, and complexity. At one extreme are investigations of an outbreak, which may include fewer than ten cases (*see* **Communicable Diseases**). These studies often encompass a wide-ranging, open-ended examination of many exposures and host characteristics of the cases. Often, the selection of controls can precisely correspond to the source of cases because there is a roster of the source population (for example, in a hospital outbreak) or a convenient collection of willing participants. At the other extreme are multicenter, multiyear, highly focused studies of tens of thousands of cases and controls. These are not common, because of their high cost. More typical are studies of a few hundred cases and an equal number of controls selected without a roster, but with an algorithm intended to represent the population from which the cases arose. These intermediate-sized studies provide a practical approach when the relative risk is expected to be around 2 or greater and the exposure is reasonably common (10% or more).

Weaknesses of the Case–Control Approach

Case–control studies, like **cross-sectional** and observational cohort studies, suffer from the common drawbacks of all nonexperimental, or observational, research, stemming from the investigator's lack of control in assigning exposure. Foremost is the absence of randomization as a tool for reducing confounding. An observational study will not be as reliable as a clinical trial for investigating questions such as the effectiveness of a new treatment or screening program.

Even though a case–control study has no intrinsic shortcomings compared exposuto a nonexperimental full cohort study that collects information on everyone in the same setting, the case–control design has often been disparaged as fundamentally weaker than the full cohort study. Several conceptual, statistical, and practical reasons explain this negative attitude. Many early observers saw the case–control study as a "backward cohort study", with inference made from effect to cause. It was not obvious how to translate a difference in exposure between cases and controls into a parameter describing prospective risk until Cornfield in 1951

[7] showed theoretically that the exposure odds ratio from a case–control study approximates the disease risk ratio from a case–control study when the outcome is rare. Selection bias can arise from poor study design or poor implementation in choosing cases and controls. Retrospective ascertainment of information about exposure and confounders may yield inaccurate data leading to bias. These issues are discussed in detail later in this article.

Another apparent weakness of the case–control approach is that ordinarily it yields relative but not absolute measures of the effect of exposure on disease. It is possible, however, to estimate exposure-specific **absolute risk** and risk differences when the crude risk of disease is known in the study population [1, 7, 10, 30].

Case–Control Study as a Missing-Data Problem

A population-based case–control study can be regarded as a cohort study with many nondiseased subjects missing at random [30]. This view of the case–control study helps to resolve many conceptual issues. It reveals when and how a broader class of parameters, including absolute risk and risk difference, can be estimated. It clarifies the requirements for proper control selection (*see* **Missing Data in Epidemiologic Studies**; **Missing Data**).

Consider a population-based case–control study to examine the effect of an exposure on the risk of developing disease. In the ideal study, the investigator is able to identify all cohort members newly diagnosed with disease during a specified follow-up period. These people with disease, or a random subset, become the cases in the study. Controls are a random sample of the noncases. The investigators obtain information on exposure that preceded the time of onset of disease from these cases and controls. Exposure information for those noncases who never develop disease during the study period will be *missing at random* if the investigator determines whose exposure will be collected, based only on disease status, which is known for individuals during the specified time. Thus, the case–control study is a missing-data problem, albeit with two unusual features: the "missingness" is a planned maneuver rather

than an uncontrollable accident, and the ratio of missing to observed data can be extraordinarily high.

Under these assumptions, the cases and controls will have the same exposure distribution as the diseased and nondiseased, respectively, in the cohort, and the investigator can estimate from the case–control data all of the parameters estimable from the full cohort study. Indeed, under these assumptions, there are no intrinsic weaknesses to the case–control design. This outlook recognizes the prospective nature of the study, allows estimation of all parameters available from the full cohort, including absolute risk and risk difference, and demonstrates why the controls selected should have the same exposure distribution as other nondiseased individuals in the study population [30]. The inference from the missing data approach is identical to standard case–control inference in this setting [30].

Case–Control Studies to Estimate a Hazard Ratio

In the idealization described above, risk is described as the probability of developing disease during a fixed interval. If the study aims to estimate functions of **hazard rates** of disease, or numbers of new events per unit of person–time (*see* **Person-Years At Risk**), the time element must be incorporated more precisely. For instance, in the standard **proportional hazards** analysis of the full cohort study designed to estimate the hazard ratio, the partial likelihood compares the exposure of a case to that of the members of the *risk set*; namely, all other members of the cohort who are at risk at the time of the event that defines when the cohort member became a case.

In the **nested case–control study** that would be undertaken in the same cohort, as first described by Thomas [27], exposure from only a few randomly selected members of each risk set is collected and used in a time-matched case–control analysis, an analog to partial likelihood. Again, except for the use of fewer individuals, there is no intrinsic difference between the full cohort and nested case–control analyses. All noncases in the risk set should be eligible and equally likely to be sampled as controls, even those who were previously selected as controls or who later develop disease [15]. Sampling at event times should be mutually independent in the nested study.

The **case–cohort design**, first described by Prentice [21], is a useful alternative with several practical advantages. The controls are selected as a single sample or *subcohort* from the entire cohort, including cases. While the sampling is not time-matched, in the analysis the likelihood at each event time uses the exposures of the case and of the subcohort members who are in the risk set at the event time. The fact that the subcohort is a random sample of the cohort leads to more flexibility in the analysis and allows the same controls to be used for analyses of several endpoints.

Design

There are three interlocking steps in planning the design of a case–control study:

1. Investigators must decide whether a cohort or case–control study is appropriate.
2. Investigators must determine who will be cases and controls in the study and how to assess exposure.
3. Investigators must decide on all the specific details to be included in the study protocol.

Full Cohort vs. Case–Control?

The first decision required in planning a case–control study is to determine whether the case–control design is more appropriate than a full cohort design [29]. The reasons for preferring a case–control study to the full cohort study are almost always practical, revolving around feasibility, economy, speed, and the need to study multiple exposures or their joint effects. On the other hand, a prospective cohort study sometimes affords an opportunity to collect more reliable exposure information, and can be used to study multiple health outcomes simultaneously. It can offer slightly more statistical precision. Finally, justifiably or not, the cohort study has more credibility.

Lower Cost vs. Higher Statistical Efficiency. Studying fewer subjects reduces the cost but also lowers the precision of the estimate of effect. When the disease is rare, the impact will be very modest, as the above example demonstrates. The variance estimate of the log-odds ratio estimate from two-by-two tables of the form in Table 1 or Table 2 is the sum of the reciprocals of the cell entries, so the size of the smallest cell in the two-by-two table is the factor limiting precision. When exposure is rare, this smallest cell almost always will be the number of exposed cases. This quantity is the same in the full cohort or in the case–control study performed in the same setting. Thus, the relative efficiency of the case–control study with k controls per case is $k/(k+1)$ compared to the full cohort [28]. The choice of design often boils down to whether to look for cases among the exposed (as in a cohort study) or exposed among cases (as in the case–control approach).

The clearest advantage for the case–control study occurs when the outcome of interest is rare and the exposure of interest is common. As the percentage of individuals experiencing the outcome during the follow-up period increases, the efficiency advantage of the case–control design diminishes. As the exposure of interest becomes rare, the ability of the case–control study to estimate an effect diminishes and a cohort design that ensures that individuals with the rare exposure will be followed for disease may become more advantageous.

Data Quality.   Exposure assessment is the Achilles heel of the case–control study. If information collected retrospectively about exposure is of lower quality than concurrent data, more *nondifferential* **misclassification** or error, and consequently, attenuation of estimates of effect, almost inevitably ensue. Worse still, exposure information that is self-reported is susceptible to *differential* error or misclassification, namely different error patterns in cases and controls.

The resulting bias can work to exaggerate, attenuate, or reverse the direction of an effect. While differential error from interviews has been difficult to establish conclusively in particular situations, it seems realistic to assume that the accuracy and thoroughness of reports from cases, who are touched by the research question and whose lifestyle may be affected by the disease, will be greater than for controls. The effect of differential error is often called report or **recall bias**. Some nutritional epidemiologists are extremely skeptical of dietary data collected from cases and controls retrospectively, for fear of differential misclassification. By contrast, when previously written records are the source of exposure information, the errors are no different from those in a full cohort study. So a retrospective or even a prospective full cohort study would not automatically have higher data quality. Correspondingly, collection of reliable information on outcomes in all members of a cohort or a case–control study is also a challenge, especially for softer endpoints, such as infertility.

Other Scientific Issues.   Apart from considerations of efficiency, reflecting the rarity of disease and exposure, other considerations come into play. When confounding poses a major problem for a study, accurate **confounder** assessment may dictate one design or the other. The need to study multiple exposures magnifies the advantage of the case–control design, while a cohort study allows additional outcomes to be included in the study with little increase in cost. Some well-established cohorts [37] have demonstrated that results on the relationships between multiple exposures and multiple exposures from a full cohort study can justify its substantially greater cost relative to a single case–control study.

Credibility.   While most researchers and journals now appreciate the case–control design, some still consider case–control studies automatically suspect [11]. While this attitude is becoming less widespread, it may affect how one's work is accepted.

Choice of Setting

The specific setting for the study must be chosen within constraints imposed by logistics, convenience, and cost. Investigators must also consider the key factors that determine the quality of a case–control study in a particular location. How complete and accurate will the case ascertainment be? How rapidly will investigators receive reports of cases, thereby reducing the influence of the postdiagnosis period, such as effects of treatment, and the number of fatal or debilitated cases who might be excluded or whose exposure information may need to be collected from a proxy, such as a spouse or child? Is there a roster or sampling frame, possibly from electoral lists or a health insurance plan, from which to select suitable controls? Are written records available to evaluate exposure, thereby reducing the possibility of differential misclassification? Are participants likely to give reliable information on exposure or confounders, including perhaps family medical history, prescription drug use, or highly personal questions about sexual history or a previous abortion? Are participation

rates likely to be high? (*see* **Nonresponse**). Will participants be amenable to a procedure needed for the study, such as blood drawing for assessing a biomarker? What is the rate of occurrence of events and how will it affect the amount of time needed in the field? Is there enough heterogeneity of exposure to reduce the cost of a study and the number of subjects needed to achieve a specified precision?

Case–control studies can be oriented toward measuring the effect of exposure on disease **prevalence, cumulative hazard**, or **incidence rate**. Thus, the temporal perspective must be considered. Ought the study be limited to future cases, or can previously diagnosed individuals be used? Using only those cases that are newly diagnosed (**incident cases**) generally works to improve case ascertainment and participation, reduce reliance on proxy respondents for deceased or disabled cases and simplify control selection, but is slower and more costly. One subtly different definition of cases produces an estimate of cumulative risk rather than **incidence density ratio**; namely, when cases are all subjects who developed disease throughout the duration of follow-up of a population. Finally, diseases with poorly defined onset and long duration call for prevalence studies, with the definition of cases correspondingly changed to subjects who have the disease at the specified point in time, regardless of when they first developed it (*see* **Case–Control Study, Prevalent**).

Case and Control Selection

Case and control selection must be defined together because they are intrinsically linked. Miettinen's [20] concept of the *study base* helps to clarify this connection. The study base at a given time consists of those individuals who would become cases in the study if they developed disease at that time. When the study base is well-defined, the study is called a *primary-base* study or a *population-based case–control* study; cases are simply those members of the study base who experience the outcome and controls can be a random sample from the base. In this situation, it is possible to determine whether any individual is in or out of the study base at a given time and whether that individual is eligible to be a case or control in the study. The problem is making sure that all cases in the base come to the attention of the study investigators. The alternative starts with a set of cases, perhaps chosen for convenience, as in a *hospital-based case–control* study of lung cancer diagnosed at a single hospital during a single year. In these *secondary-base* studies, the study base is poorly defined because it is not always clear whether an individual who did not develop disease would have been a case in the hypothetic circumstance of development of disease. With no way to know whether a potential control would have come to the study hospital upon development of disease, random sampling for control selection is impossible. Thus, these secondary-base controls must be *assumed* to be an approximation to a hypothetic random sample that could characterize the study base. So in the primary base study, the difficulty is finding the cases, while, in the secondary base study, the difficulty is ensuring an appropriate set of controls.

Case Selection.   In the idealized case–control study, all subjects with disease in the study base (or a random sample of them) become cases. In reality, some cases do not come to the attention of the investigators, some individuals are falsely called cases when in fact they do not meet the diagnostic criteria, and some eligible cases refuse to participate. In a study of male infertility, factors that lead to someone to regard lack of children as a problem might appear as risk factors because of differential case ascertainment [31]. Inaccurate and incomplete case ascertainment can create selection bias as well as reduce precision. When there is ambiguity as to whether someone truly developed disease, as in the absence of a definitive pathology report, the standard practice of excluding the case is not harmless, if those lacking information have different exposure distributions than those with the information, perhaps because they are seen at a hospital in a poorer area [29].

Principles of Control Selection.   There are three principles that underlie control selection: *study-base, comparable-accuracy*, and *deconfounding* [31]. The essence of the study-base principle is that controls can be used to characterize the distribution of exposure in the study base from which the cases arise. The comparable-accuracy principle calls for equal reliability in the information obtained from cases and controls so that there is no *differential* misclassification. Thus, a study of drug use during pregnancy as a risk factor for a specific type of birth defect might call for

a control group of children who experienced a comparably serious outcome at birth so that the mothers of cases and controls would be equally likely to recall exposure during pregnancy accurately. The deconfounding principle allows elimination of confounding through control selection, such as through matching or stratified sampling, to be a consideration in control selection. These principles may conflict with one another and may have strong negative impacts on efficiency. They should not be regarded as absolute, but rather as points to consider in choosing a control group.

Controls for Studies with a Roster.   In fortuitous situations, the investigator can use a roster listing all individuals and the period when they are in the study base. Investigators can then sample at random from the roster to satisfy the study-base criterion.

Controls for Primary-base Studies without a Roster.   When a roster is not available and cannot be created from electoral or town residence lists, it is impossible to generate a random sample directly. A commonly used approach when there is no roster is random digit dialing (RDD) [34], an efficient way to generate a near-random sample often used in public opinion polling. RDD relies on dialing telephone numbers according to a strategy that yields representative samples. RDD suffers from several potential biases. RDD will not select individuals without phones, although it can compensate for households with multiple telephone lines. Furthermore, many people refuse to respond to telephone surveys, especially since the advent of answering machines (*see* **Telephone Sampling**). Empirically, controls chosen by RDD seem to be of higher socioeconomic class than a truly random sample would be. This violation of the study-base principle may be alleviated by adjustment for income or socioeconomic status.

Requirements for individual controls vary. In *incidence-density sampling* [14, 19, 22], used most commonly in primary-base studies, controls must be disease free at the time of diagnosis of the case to which they are matched. As in the nested case–control study, this design allows estimation of an incidence rate-ratio (and **relative hazard**) and eliminates the need for the rare-disease assumption [14, 19]. For *cumulative-incidence sampling*, controls are selected from among those who survive the study period without developing disease. Cumulative-incidence sampling of controls allows estimation of the risk ratio (**relative risk**), which approximates the relative hazard only when the rate of disease is low.

Secondary-Base Studies.   Some diseases, including those not consistently detected in the general population, dictate an alternative to primary-base studies. For example, when case identification is incomplete, population controls may not be appropriate when completeness of case identification is differential by exposure and the selection bias cannot be corrected by adjustment for another variable. The most common secondary-base study is the *hospital-based case–control* study. Controls are patients seen at the same hospital as the cases, but for a different condition. This approach works well when two requirements are met. First, both cases and controls must be people who would have presented at the same hospital if they had *either* the case-defining illness or the control-defining condition. Secondly, the conditions used to select controls cannot be associated with the exposure. If these requirements are met, the distribution of the exposure in the controls reflects the distribution in the study base. The investigator seldom knows with certainty that both criteria are met, so compliance with the study-base criterion remains hard to verify convincingly.

A possible advantage of the hospital-based control group is more confidence that the equal accuracy criterion will be met. With equally serious illnesses, cases and controls ought to provide similarly complete and accurate reporting of past exposures. Thus, for the study of a specific birth defect, controls could be chosen from babies born with another birth defect of similar severity but known not to be related to the exposure of interest. Using controls with cancer at other sites for a study of a form of cancer may help with the equal-accuracy principle, but care must be taken so that cancer at the control site is not related to exposure.

Other Kinds of Control Groups.   While population and hospital controls are the most commonly used kinds of control groups, investigators have used other options [32]. Use of patients from the *same primary care provider* as the case helps to insure that a control who developed the disease of interest would have become a case in the study. Use of *friends* of the cases can lead to bias in studies of factors related to

sociability. Use of *relatives*, often siblings, as controls may reduce confounding by genetic factors. Each of these control groups requires a careful selection procedure to make sure that individuals are not being picked to be controls in a way that is related, directly or indirectly, to the factors under study.

Design Options.   **Matching** on well-established confounders is a common practice in case–control studies. In case–control studies, matching serves to increase the precision of the estimated effect of exposure by making the distribution of the confounder identical in the cases and controls. Usually, the efficiency advantage from matching is small, and may not compensate for the extra cost and complexity, the exclusion of cases for whom no match is found, and the reduced flexibility of the analysis [33]. Other justifications of matching include control for non-quantitative variables such as neighborhood and the ability to control for confounding without making assumptions about the effect of the confounder in the risk model [33].

Only strong confounders should be considered as matching variables. Two-phase designs, discussed below, are more appropriate if one wants to estimate the effect of a variable considered for matching. Demographic variables such as race and sex and temporal variables such as age and calendar year (or decade) of first employment are the most suitable matching variables. Matching is always inappropriate on a factor that is a consequence of exposure.

Two-Phase Designs.   These techniques [2, 36] (*see* **Case–Control Study, Two-Phase**) are a more flexible generalization of matching, also used to increase efficiency or to reduce the cost of exposure assessment. In two-phase designs, detailed information on exposures and confounders is not ascertained for everyone, but only for subsets of cases and controls, with the selection probability depending on case status and on the value of another variable that is available for everyone. Instead of requiring, as in matching, that the distribution of the variable be the same in the control as in the cases, essentially arbitrary distributions in each group are specified. These two-stage designs allow the estimation of both main effects and **interactions**. For example, in a study designed to investigate the joint effects of domestic radon exposure, requiring expensive measurements, and smoking, which is easier to ascertain, on the risk of lung cancer, taking all cases and a random sample of controls would lead to a study with a preponderance of smoking cases and nonsmoking controls; matching controls to cases on smoking status would lead to small numbers of control nonsmokers as well. The assessment of interaction is much more efficient in the two-phase design where nonsmoking cases and smoking controls are oversampled [35].

Sample Size.   There is an extensive literature on sample size determination for case–control studies [4, 24, 25]. As in the full cohort study, needed sample size is dependent on the variation in exposure in the study base. A key point is that increasing the ratio of controls to the harder-to-find cases increases the precision of the odds ratio estimate in an increasingly marginal way, especially for small effects. Ratios of controls to cases beyond four or five are usually not advisable because the successive gains in efficiency diminish. Indeed, the asymptotic relative efficiency for a study involving k controls per case is $k/(k + 1)$, which takes on values of 0.5, 0.67, 0.75, 0.8, and 0.83 for k from 1 through 5 [28].

Fieldwork

The best-designed study will not be convincing unless the fieldwork is sound. In the field, case–control studies face the usual challenges of observational research: identifying all members of the study population, achieving an adequate response rate, collecting accurate data, and measuring potential confounders.

Most case–control studies include a questionnaire, because seldom have all of the exposure variables of interest been recorded in documents easily available to the investigator. Sometimes the study subject, or his surrogate, completes the questionnaire ("self-administered"); alternatively, an interviewer can pose the questions. A questionnaire can be computerized or on paper; an interview can be in-person or by telephone. Depending on the hypotheses, investigators may also collect biologic specimens, samples of the study subject's present or past environment, and permission to contact agencies that have documented data about the exposures.

The case–control design poses some specific problems, as well. Since the cases have already developed the disease, it will not be possible to estimate the effects of exposure measures that are distorted by

the disease, including weight and body biochemistry, unless the investigator has access to stored measures that were collected before disease onset. If it is not clear whether a measure is likely to be valid once the disease is clinically manifest, the investigator may conduct a specific methodologic pilot study. Sometimes, it is possible to examine the effects specific for stage of disease, in the expectation that post-onset distortions will be more pronounced with more advanced disease. In a similar fashion, the investigator will consider whether therapy influences the level of the exposure variable. If so, then cases need to be studied before therapy begins, or well after any of its influence has waned.

Just as diagnosis and treatment of a serious disease can cause biological changes in exposure variables, they also can cause changes in a patient's recollection or willingness to report various exposures. The resulting **recall bias** does not always go in a particular direction; the specific exposure needs to be considered, preferably with data on reporting bias from ancillary sources. Some exposures lend themselves to internal validation by studying a higher-quality exposure variable on a subset of subjects or by collection of validation data from other sources, such as medical records (*see* **Validation Study**). In that circumstance, some or all of the subjects reporting an illness or hospitalization will be asked to give permission for review of records; ideally, some of the reports of no hospitalization ought to be selected for review, too, although this is seldom practical. To minimize recall bias, the investigator also attends to the exact phrasing of questions, trying to leave very little room for interpretation or rumination. Sometimes investigators attempt to blind the interviewer to the case–control status of subject, but often the status of the subject becomes apparent anyway.

With access to prospectively collected data stored in records, the investigator can avoid the problem of differential misclassification stemming from the fact of diagnosis. Even with stored records, however, one source of differential misclassification could be present: minor abnormalities noted because of greater medical surveillance of the exposed may not have been detected in the unexposed.

Analysis

The goal of the analysis of case–control studies is almost always to identify risk factors that are related to disease and to determine whether in fact the risk factors are causes of the disease (*see* **Causation**). As in other nonrandomized situations, the analysis must address the possibility of *confounding* and **effect-modification** by measured covariates.

The primary difficulty that is inherent to analysis of case–control studies is that the sampling is based on disease status while the parameters of interest relate to risk or rate of disease. Thus, it is not the difference in exposure frequency or means between cases and controls that is of direct interest, but estimates of the effect of determinants of disease on the rate of disease or on the probability of developing disease.

The analysis of case–control data can be exquisitely simple or tremendously complex. When the exposure and disease are each dichotomous and there are no other factors to consider, the analysis reduces to a two-by-two table of exposure by disease status. Originally, Cornfield [7] proposed that the *odds ratio*, or cross product ratio in the two-by-two table could be used as an estimate of the risk ratio (or relative risk) when the disease was rare. **Mantel & Haenszel** [16] developed an estimator and a test statistic that could be used when combining tables over several strata, thereby controlling for confounding. Exact conditional approaches, not relying on asymptotic theory, are also available for obtaining inference on the common odds ratio, adjusted for confounders by **stratification** [3, 13, 18].

While discriminant analysis seems a natural tool to distinguish cases and controls, **logistic regression**, in which the dependent variable is the logarithm of the odds of disease, has two distinct advantages. It allows for exposures, confounders and effect-modifiers that are discrete or continuous, regardless of distribution [9] and yields valid estimates of relative-odds parameters from case–control data. Prentice & Pyke [23] proved that prospective logistic modeling – that is, of disease as a function of exposure – estimated relative risk parameters correctly and with full efficiency. If the sampling fractions of cases and controls are known, as in some population-based case–control studies, the intercept estimate from the case–control analysis can be combined with the ratio of the sampling fractions to yield a valid estimate of absolute risk. Logistic regression is now the most commonly used approach to analyze case–control data. Carroll et al. [6] extended the Prentice–Pyke result to show that many variations of case–control designs could be analyzed by logistic regression and given a prospective interpretation. Extensions to the logistic framework allow the handling of more complex sampling schemes, such as two-phase designs, of nonlinear regression effects of covariates, and of alternative models of joint effects of two risk factors, such as **additive** rather than **multiplicative** effects.

Control for a small number of categorical confounders can be achieved by the Mantel–Haenszel estimator of the odds ratio and corresponding hypothesis test. These simple procedures have excellent statistical properties. Nonetheless, logistic modeling is used routinely, because of its greater flexibility, for instance, in handling continuous variables [3]. In most modern studies, there will be more than two levels of exposure or one or more confounders and effect-modifiers to consider.

The analysis of matched pairs with a single dichotomous exposure variable uses only discordant pairs. It takes the ratio of pairs with the case exposed to those with the control exposed as the odds ratio estimate. The corresponding test of the null hypothesis that the odds ratio is one is equivalent to the hypothesis that the number of pairs with exposed cases among the discordant ones is binomial with probability 0.5 (*see* **Matched Analysis**). While several extensions to more complex exposure variables and matching schemes were developed, the breakthrough in the analysis of matched data was the introduction by Breslow et al. [5] of **conditional logistic regression**, which allows general matching schemes, arbitrary exposures, continuous or discrete confounders (other than those used in the matching), and effect-modifiers.

An important variation of the analysis of case–control data allows for estimation of a hazard ratio rather than an odds ratio or risk ratio, as in nested case–control and case–cohort studies [21, 26, 27]. These designs are particularly useful when exposures vary with time, as does, for example, lifetime exposure to an environmental or occupational chemical. A conditional likelihood approach can be used here as well as where the matching is on time. In the contribution to the conditional likelihood at each event time, the exposure is accumulated only until the event time, exactly as if the analysis were prospective and no future data were available [21]. Furthermore, the same structure of the conditional likelihood as in the matched case–control study is used. As long as the controls are selected randomly from those at risk – that is, including future cases and independently of past use as a control or time of follow-up – the estimates of hazard ratio are valid, again reflecting the close relationship to the full cohort design. When the same controls are used for each case diagnosed during the control's follow-up, as in the case–cohort design, the estimates of the hazard ratio are also valid, but the variance estimate is more complex because the scores at each event time are not independent.

In most reports of case–control studies, no estimate of *absolute risk* or *absolute rate* is given. Methods are available for population-based case–control studies when the crude risk of disease is known [1, 7], and generally for nested case–control and case–cohort studies [17, 37]. Furthermore, risk or rate difference and other nonlogistic models can be fit [30]. Methods for estimating the attributable risk and its variance in a general setting are also available [8].

Summary

The case–control study remains the most popular approach in **analytic epidemiology** because of its relatively low cost and high speed. Ascertainment of disease, selection of controls and measurement of exposure present substantial difficulties in almost every case–control study, but a large body of epidemiologic theory and experience provides guidance to meet these challenges.

References

[1]   Benichou, J. & Wacholder, S. (1994). Epidemiologic methods: a comparison of the approaches to estimate exposure-specific incidence rates from population-based case–control data, *Statistics in Medicine* **13**, 651–661.

[2]   Breslow, N.E. & Cain, K.C. (1988). Logistic regression for two-stage case–control data, *Biometrika* **75**, 11–20.

[3]   Breslow, N.E. & Day, N.E. (1980). *Statistical Methods in Cancer Research*. Vol. I: *The Analysis of Case–Control Studies*. International Agency for Research on Cancer, Lyon.

[4]   Breslow, N.E. & Day, N.E. (1987). *Statistical Methods in Cancer Research*, Vol. II: *The Design and Analysis of Cohort Studies*. International Agency for Research on Cancer, Lyon.

[5]   Breslow, N.E., Day, N.E., Halvorsen, K.T., Prentice, R.I. & Sabai, C. (1978). Estimation of multiple relative risk functions in matched case–control studies, *American Journal of Epidemiology* **108**, 299–307.

[6]   Carroll, R.J., Wang, S. & Wang, C.Y. (1995). Prospective analysis of logistic case–control studies, *Journal of the American Statistical Association* **90**, 157–169.

[7]   Cornfield, J. (1951). A method of estimating comparative rates from clinical data. Applications to cancer of the lung, breast and cervix, *Journal of the National Cancer Institute* **11**, 1269–1275.

[8]   Coughlin, S.S., Benichou, J. & Weed, D.L. (1994). Attributable risk estimation in case–control studies, *Epidemiological Reviews* **16**, 51–64.

[9]   Cox, D.R. (1966). Some procedures connected with the logistic qualitative response curve, in *Research Papers in Statistics: Festschrift for Neyman J.*, F.N. David, ed. Wiley, New York, pp. 55–71.

[10] Doll, R. & Hill, A.B. (1950). Smoking and carcinoma of the lung: preliminary report, *British Medical Journal* **2**, 739–748.

[11] Feinstein, A.R. (1988). Scientific standards in epidemiologic studies of the menace of daily life, *Science* **242**, 1257–1263.

[12] Gail, M.H., Brinton, L.A., Byar, D.P., Corle, D.K., Green, S.B., Schairer, C. & Mulvihill, J.J. (1989). Projecting individualized probabilities of developing breast cancer for white females who are being examined annually, *Journal of the National Cancer Institute* **81**, 1879–1886.

[13] Gart, J.M. (1970). Point and interval estimation of the common odds ratio in the combination of 2×2 tables with fixed marginals, *Biometrika* **57**, 471–475.

[14] Greenland, S. & Thomas, D.C. (1982). On the need for the rare disease assumption in case–control studies, *American Journal of Epidemiology* **116**, 547–553.

[15] Lubin, J. & Gail, M.H. (1984). Biased selection of controls for case–control analyses of cohort studies, *Biometrics* **40**, 63–75.

[16] Mantel, N. & Haenszel, W. (1959). Statistical aspects of the analysis of data from retrospective studies of disease, *Journal of the National Cancer Institute* **22**, 719–748.

[17] McMahon, B. (1962). Prenatal X-ray exposure and childhood cancer, *Journal of the National Cancer Institute* **28**, 1173–1191.

[18] Mehta, C.R., Patel, N.R. & Gray, R. (1985). Computing an exact confidence interval for the common odds ratio in several 2×2 contingency tables, *Journal of the American Statistical Association* **80**, 969–973.

[19] Miettinen, O.S. (1976). Estimability and estimation in case–referent studies, *American Journal of Epidemiology* **103**, 226–235.

[20] Miettinen, O.S. (1985). The "case–control" study: valid selection of subjects, *Journal of Chronic Diseases* **38**, 543–548.

[21] Prentice, R.L. (1986). A case–cohort design for epidemiologic cohort studies and disease prevention trials, *Biometrika* **73**, 1–11.

[22] Prentice, R.L. & Breslow, N.E. (1978). Retrospective studies and failure time models, *Biometrika* **65**, 153–158.

[23] Prentice, R.L. & Pyke, R. (1979). Logistic disease incidence models and case–control studies, *Biometrika* **66**, 403–411.

[24] Schlesselman, J.J. (1982). *Case–Control Studies: Design, Conduct, Analysis*. Oxford University Press, New York.

[25] Self, S.G. & Mauritsen, R.H. (1988). Power/sample size calculations for generalized linear models, *Biometrics* **44**, 79–86.

[26] Sheehe, R.R. (1962). Dynamic risk analysis in retrospective matched pair studies of disease, *Biometrics* **18**, 323–341.

[27] Thomas, D.C. (1977). Addendum to a paper by Liddell, F.D.K., McDonald, J.C. & Thomas, D.C., *Journal of the Royal Statistical Society, Series A* **140**, 483–485.

[28] Ury, H.K. (1975). Efficiency of case–control studies with multiple controls per case: continuous or dichotomous data, *Biometrics* **31**, 643–649.

[29] Wacholder, S. (1995). Design issues in case–control studies, *Statistical Methods in Medical Research* **4**, 293–309.

[30] Wacholder, S. (1996). The case–control study as data missing by design: estimating risk differences, *Epidemiology* **7**, 144–150.

[31] Wacholder, S., McLaughlin, J.K., Silverman, D.T. & Mandel, J.S. (1992). Selection of controls in case–control studies, I. Principles, *American Journal of Epidemiology* **135**, 1019–1028.

[32] Wacholder, S., Silverman, D.T., McLaughlin, J.K. & Mandel, J.S. (1992). Selection of controls in case–control studies, II. Types of controls, *American Journal of Epidemiology* **135**, 1029–1041.

[33] Wacholder, S., Silverman, D.T., McLaughlin, J.K. & Mandel, J.S. (1992). Selection of controls in case–control studies, III. Design options, *American Journal of Epidemiology* **135**, 1042–1051.

[34] Waksberg, J. (1978). Sampling methods for random digit dialing, *Journal of the American Statistical Association* **73**, 40–46.

[35] Weinberg, C.R. & Sandler, D.P. (1991). Randomized recruitment in case–control studies, *American Journal of Epidemiology* **134**, 421–432.

[36] White, J.E. (1982). A two stage design for the study of the relationship between a rare exposure and a rare disease, *American Journal of Epidemiology* **115**, 119–128.

[37] Willett, W.C., Stampfer, M.J., Colditz, G.A., Rosner, B.A. & Speizer, F.E. (1992). Relation of meat, fat and fiber intake to the risk of colon cancer in a prospective study among women, *New England Journal of Medicine* **323**, 73–77.

SHOLOM WACHOLDER & PATRICIA HARTGE

Case–Control Study, Hospital-Based

A hospital-based case–control study is a **case–control study** in which cases with a given disease are selected from persons with that disease in a given hospital or group of hospitals, and **controls** are patients with other diseases from those hospitals. Hospital-based case–control studies are relatively convenient to conduct and offer some advantages, compared with **population-based case–control studies**. First, a higher proportion of persons invited to join a hospital-based case–control study may agree to participate, especially when biologic samples such as blood specimens are required. This reduces the chance for one type of **selection bias** known as **nonresponse** bias. Secondly, cases and controls with other diseases may provide a similar quality of information when asked about previous exposures, thus reducing the chance of **recall bias** compared with **population-based studies** in which most controls are healthy.

There are two serious sources of **bias** that may affect hospital-based case–control studies and that are not present in population-based case–control studies. First, the pattern of referral of cases to a hospital may differ from the pattern of referral for persons with control diseases, resulting in selection bias because the controls are not representative of the source population from which the cases arise. Secondly, the exposure under study may affect the risk of the control conditions, causing a distortion of the **relative risk**.

(*See also* **Bias in Case–Control Studies**; **Bias in Observational Studies**; **Bias, Overview**)

M.H. GAIL

Case–Control Study, Nested

The nested **case–control** design is a method of sampling from an assembled epidemiologic **cohort study** or a clinical trial that involves randomly sampling from eligible **controls** for each case. It is generally used when basic disease outcome and time on study information has been obtained for the cohort but it is too expensive to collect information on covariates of interest (e.g. exposure information) for all subjects in the cohort. This is especially advantageous when this information is "banked", either actively or passively, for the entire cohort, but is expensive to retrieve or process. For example, sera may be stored for all members of the cohort, but it may be expensive to analyze the sera for a particular substance. In the nested case–control design, such analyses would only be required for cases and selected controls. In such circumstances, a nested case–control study has the cost–efficiency associated with retrospective case–control studies but without the possibility of selection or information bias often associated with case–control studies (*see* **Bias in Case–Control Studies**). Even if covariate information is available for the full cohort, a nested case–control study is sometimes drawn to reduce the quality control costs or computational burden associated with fitting complex models to large cohort data sets.

The method appears to have been first elucidated in an appendix in an article on analysis of lung cancer risk in a cohort of asbestos miners [10]; it is now the most widely used method of sampling from cohorts. Nested case–control studies are closely related to population-based matched (*see* **Matching**) case–control studies (*see* **Case–Control Study, Population-Based**). The latter are often nested case–control studies where the underlying cohort is based on a geographic area, perhaps somewhat poorly defined. While both designs have adequate information for the estimation of rate ratios, the fact that "sampling fractions" from the cohort are known in nested case–control studies makes it also possible to estimate **absolute risk** reliably (see below). Thus, the study of nested case–control methodology has direct relevance for matched case–control studies, the most widely used study design for epidemiologic research. A comparison of this design with the case–cohort method is given in the article **Case–Cohort Study**.

The Design

Nested case–control sampling is closely related to the partial likelihood approach to the analysis of

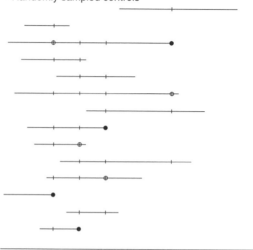

Figure 1 Cohort of 15 subjects. Each failure determines a risk set. A single control is sampled for each case to form a one-to-one matched nested case–control study

cohort data (*see* **Cox Regression Model**). Figure 1 illustrates the basic features of a small hypothetical cohort study of 15 subjects. Each subject enters the study at some *entry time*, is *at risk*, denoted by the horizontal line, over some time period, and exits the study at some *exit time*. A subject may contract or die from the disease of interest, and thus be a *failure* (represented by solid circle in Figure 1) or be censored, i.e. be alive at the end of the study, died never having had the disease of interest, or be lost to follow-up.

In this method, at each failure time a *risk set* is formed that includes the *case*; namely, the failure at that failure time, and all *controls*; namely, any other cohort members who are at risk at the failure time (these are denoted by a vertical tick mark in Figure 1). These risk sets are "case–control" sets as used in the partial likelihood approach to the analysis of cohort data.

A one-to-$m - 1$ case–control design consists of case–control sets with the case and $m - 1$ sampled controls, sampled without replacement from the controls in the risk set. Sampling is done independently across risk sets so subjects may serve as controls for multiple cases and cases may serve as controls for other cases that failed at a time when the case was at risk. So, for instance, for one-to-one nested case–control sampling ($m = 2$), each sampled risk set consists of two subjects, the case and one randomly sampled control, the pairs of solid and open circles in Figure 1. An important variant of this design is to sample within strata defined by levels of a *matching factor*. In this case, in addition to the failure time, the risk sets consist of subjects with the same matching factor level as the failure so that (sampled) case–control sets will be homogeneous in the matching factor. This corresponds to a **stratified proportional hazards** model. Restricting controls to be used only once or using "pure" controls, those that never become cases, will typically result in **biased** estimation [11] unless special analysis methods are used [15]. Other variants of these standard designs are discussed below.

Examples

Occupational Cohort Study of TCDD Exposure and soft-tissue sarcoma (STS) and non-Hodgkin's lymphoma (NHL). The International Agency for Research Against Cancer (IARC) maintains an international register of 21 183 workers exposed to phenoxy herbicides, chlorophenols, and dioxins [17]. In a cohort mortality study analysis, standardized mortality ratios (SMRs) (*see* **Standardization Methods**) of 1.96 and 1.29 were found for STS and NHL, respectively, comparing exposed with unexposed workers. These are somewhat smaller SMRs than observed in previous studies. To explore the effect of exposure to various agents more fully, a nested case–control study was undertaken in which, for each of the 11 STS and 32 NHL cases, five controls were sampled from those from the same country, of the same gender, and same year of birth as the case [6]. For each subject in the nested case–control study, investigators assessed the degree of exposure to 21 chemicals or mixtures. Increasing trends of risk of STS and NHL were observed for a number of phenoxy herbicides including 2,4D and TCDD. Based on the $(m-1)/m$ relative efficiency rule (see below), these nested case–control studies provide $5/6 = 83\%$ efficiency relative to an analysis of the entire cohort for testing associations between single exposures and disease.

Nested Case–Control Study of the Colorado Plateau Uranium Miners. The Colorado Plateau uranium miners cohort data were collected to study the effects of radon exposure and smoking on the rates of lung cancer. This study has been described in detail in earlier publications (see, for example, [5], [12] and [13]). The cohort consists of 3347 Caucasian male miners who worked underground at least one month in the uranium mines of the four-state Colorado Plateau area and were examined at least once by Public Health Service physicians between 1950 and 1960. These miners were traced for mortality outcomes through December 31, 1982, by which time 258 lung cancer deaths had occurred. Entry time into the cohort was the date of first examination or first underground work, whichever came later. Exit time was the date at death, December 31, 1982, if known alive at that time, or date last known to be alive if lost to follow-up. Subjects who died of lung cancer were taken to be the failures and all others were censored at their exit times. Miner radon exposure histories were estimated using job histories and mine radon levels. A smoking history was taken at the first examination and updated with each subsequent exam. Thus, for any age on study, it is possible to compute summary measures of radon and smoking exposures. Although radon and smoking information are available on all cohort members, a nested case–control study with 15 controls per case was used to reduce the required "data cleaning" and the computational burden required to fit complex models exploring the timing of exposures [18]. Each of the risk sets was formed by all those who were alive and had entered the study by the age of death of the case and had attained that age in the same five-year calendar period as the case's date of death (matching by calendar time). Models that explored the change in lung cancer mortality with **latency**, rate of exposure, and the relative timing of radon and smoking exposure were explored with this reduced data set. Absolute risk of lung cancer given radon and smoking histories were estimated from a nested case–control study in Langholz & Borgan [8].

Statistical Analysis

Inference about rates of disease from a nested case–control study are usually based on the semiparametric approach to the analysis of cohort data, including partial likelihood methods for **relative risk** parameters and nonparametric methods (based on the Nelson–Aalen estimator of **cumulative hazard**) for estimation of **absolute risk**. The underlying model is assumed to have a **multiplicative** form

$$\lambda(t; z(t)) = \lambda_0(t) r(z(t); \beta_0), \qquad (1)$$

where $r(z(t); \beta_0)$ is the relative risk (actually rate ratio) of disease for an individual with covariates $z(t)$ at time t and $r(0; \beta) = 1$, so $\lambda_0(t)$ is the rate of disease in subjects with $z = 0$.

Partial Likelihood Analysis of Relative Risk

The conditional probability that a subject is the case and the set of sampled controls is sampled given the case–control set is given by

$$\frac{\lambda_0 r_{\text{case}}(\beta_0) \pi}{\displaystyle\sum_{\text{case–control set}} \lambda_0 r_k(\beta_0) \pi},$$

where $\pi = \binom{n-1}{m-1}^{-1}$ is the probability of picking the particular set of $m - 1$ from the $n - 1$ risk set controls and the r_k are computed at the failure time. Multiplying such conditional probability terms with cancellation of λ_0 and π from numerator and denominator yields the partial likelihood

$$\prod_{\text{failure times}} \frac{r_{\text{case}}(\beta)}{\displaystyle\sum_{\text{case–control set}} r_k(\beta)}, \qquad (2)$$

from which the maximum partial likelihood estimators of β_0 can be calculated. This partial likelihood is formally the same as the conditional logistic likelihood for matched case–control data (*see* **Matched Analysis**). Standard conditional logistic regression software may be used to estimate the rate ratio (β_0) parameters (*see* **Software, Biostatistical**).

Absolute Risk Estimation

It is commonly believed that only relative risks are estimable from case–control studies. While estimation of relative risk has been the focus of most nested case–control studies, it is also possible to estimate the baseline **hazard rate** function and, in particular, absolute risk quantities that are functions of the hazard, if one has additional information linking the

sample to the full cohort. One approach adapts methods for unmatched case–control studies and links the case–control study to cohort rates using the overall incidence of disease in the cohort [1]. A second creates this link using the number at risk at each failure time [8]. Let $z^0(t)$ be a covariate history and $r^0 = r(z^0(t); \beta_0)$ be the relative risk associated with z^0 according to the model. An approximate measure of the pure risk of disease associated with that history between times s and t, which is valid for rare diseases, is the cumulative hazard,

$$\int_s^t \lambda_0(u) r(z^0(u); \beta_0) \, du. \qquad (3)$$

With n the number at risk and $\hat{r}_k = r(z_k, \hat{\beta})$, the relative risk for individual k predicted using $\hat{\beta}$, the estimator of (3), is the sum of contributions of the form

$$\hat{r}^0 \left/ \frac{n}{m} \sum_{\text{case–control set}} \hat{r}_k \right., \qquad (4)$$

over all failure times between s and t. Note that setting $m = n$ and $z^0(t) = 0$ yields the Breslow estimator of the baseline cumulative hazard for the full cohort. Langholz & Borgan [8] provide a relatively simple variance estimator which takes the estimation of β_0 into account [8]. They also give a Kaplan–Meier type estimator of risk, which is valid even if the disease is not rare and an Aalen–Johansen type estimator of crude (absolute) risk in the presence of competing causes of failure. Parallel methods have been described for absolute risk that take **competing risks** into account and that adapt methods for unmatched case–control studies [1].

Methods for modeling excess risk and estimation of absolute risk based on the Aalen additive regression model from nested case–control studies have also been developed [3].

Asymptotic Properties and Efficiency

Although formally the same as the conditional logistic likelihood for matched case–control studies, (2) is a "partial likelihood" in the same sense as the Cox partial likelihood for full cohort data [14]. In particular, the "matched sets" are not independent since subjects are available to serve as sampled controls for multiple risk sets. Using counting process and martingale methods, Goldstein & Langholz [4] proved that the partial likelihood for rate ratio parameters β_0 in the Cox model has the same basic properties as conventional likelihoods and they develop the asymptotic theory [4]. They also examined the asymptotic relative efficiency of nested case–control sampling relative to the full cohort. For instance, in a result analogous to the independent matched sets situation, when $\beta_0 = 0$, the asymptotic covariance matrix of the nested case–control estimator equals $m/(m-1)$ times the asymptotic covariance of the full cohort. Borgan et al. give further results including the joint asymptotic distribution of the estimated cumulative baseline hazard and estimated log rate ratio parameters in the Cox model [2].

Extensions

Nested case–control sampling is one example of sampling from the risk set. Other methods of sampling controls may be desirable depending on the goals of the study and the costs of collecting information. Methods for the analysis and asymptotic theory for a large class of risk set sampling designs when the sampling is "predictable" have been described [2, 9].

Counter-Matching

This method is appropriate when exposure or a correlate of exposure is available on the entire cohort. In 1:1 counter-matching, the exposure is dichotomized into high or low categories. For each case, a control is randomly sampled from controls in the risk set with opposite exposure status of the case. A better measure of exposure or **confounders** is collected for the counter-matched sample. In the analysis, the relative risk term from each subject (case or control) is weighted by the number of subjects of the same dichotomized exposure status in the risk set [2, 7, 9].

Nonrepresentative Sampling of Cases

This can be accommodated by including the case according to a Bernoulli "coin flip" where the probability of inclusion may depend on characteristics of the case. Thus, exposed cases could be included with higher probability than unexposed cases [7, 9].

Randomized Recruitment

In this design, inclusion of a control into the substudy is determined by a Bernoulli coin flip where the probability of inclusion would depend on characteristics of the control. This would be done for all (or a random sample) of controls in the risk set. Combined with the nonrepresentative sampling of cases described above, this is the "matched case–control" version of the design of Weinberg & Wacholder [19, Appendix].

Sampling the Risk Set with Replacement

This variant simply requires allowing the case to be included for available with-replacement sampling, i.e. the case is allowed to serve as its own control [16]. Then the partial likelihood and absolute risk estimators above are valid with each with-replacement sampled subject treated as a separate control (i.e. if a subject is picked multiple times, then their contribution in the sum is multiplied by the number of occurrences).

A number of other potentially useful designs, including quota sampling, sequential sampling of controls until a prespecified number of exposed subjects is reached, and varying the number of controls selected based on the exposure status of the case, have been described [2].

References

[1]   Benichou, J. & Gail, M.H. (1995). Methods of inference for estimates of absolute risk derived from population-based case–control studies, *Biometrics* **51**, 182–194.

[2]   Borgan, Ø., Goldstein, L. & Langholz, B. (1995). Methods for the analysis of sampled cohort data in the Cox proportional hazards model, *Annals of Statistics* **23**, 1749–1778.

[3]   Borgan, Ø. & Langholz, B. (1997). Estimation of excess risk from case–control data using Aalen's linear regression model, *Biometrics* **53**, 690–697.

[4]   Goldstein, L. & Langholz, B. (1992). Asymptotic theory for nested case–control sampling in the Cox regression model, *Annals of Statistics* **20**, 1903–1928.

[5]   Hornung, R.W. & Meinhardt, T.J. (1987). Quantitative risk assessment of lung cancer in U.S. uranium miners, *Health Physics* **52**, 417–430.

[6]   Kogevinas, M., Kauppinen, T., Winkelmann, R., Becher, H., Bertazzi, P.A., Bueno de Mesquita, H.B., Coggon, D., Green, L., Johnson, E., Littorin, M., Lynge, E.,

Marlow, D.A., Mathews, J.D., Neuberger, M., Benn, T., Pannett, B., Pearce, N. & Saracci, R. (1995). Soft tissue sarcoma and non-Hodgkin's lymphoma in workers exposed to phenoxy herbicides, chlorophenols, and dioxins: two nested case–control studies, *Epidemiology* **6**, 396–402.

[7]   Langholz, B. & Borgan, Ø. (1995). Counter-matching: a stratified nested case–control sampling method, *Biometrika* **82**, 69–79.

[8]   Langholz, B. & Borgan, Ø. (1997). Estimation of absolute risk from nested case–control data, *Biometrics* **53**, 767–774.

[9]   Langholz, B. & Goldstein, L. (1996). Risk set sampling in epidemiologic cohort studies, *Statistical Science* **11**, 35–53.

[10]   Liddell, F.D.K., McDonald, J.C. & Thomas, D.C. (1977). Methods of cohort analysis: appraisal by application to asbestos miners, *Journal of the Royal Statistical Society, Series A* **140**, 469–491.

[11]   Lubin, J.H. & Gail, M.H. (1984). Biased selection of controls for case–control analyses of cohort studies, *Biometrics* **40**, 63–75.

[12]   Lubin, J.H., Boice, J.D., Edling, C., Hornung, R.W., Howe, G., Kunz, E., Kusiak, R.A., Morrison, H.I., Radford, E.P., Samet, J.M., Tirmarche, M., Woodward, A., Xiang, Y.S. & Pierce, D.A. (1994). *Radon and Lung Cancer Risk: a Joint Analysis of 11 Underground Miners Studies*, NIH Publication 94-3644. US Department of Health and Human Services, Public Health Service, National Institutes of Health, Bethesda.

[13]   Lundin, F.D., Wagoner, J.K. & Archer, V.E. (1971). Radon daughter exposure and respiratory cancer, quantitative and temporal aspects, *Joint Monograph 1*. US Public Health Service, Washington.

[14]   Oakes, D. (1981). Survival times: aspects of partial likelihood (with discussion), *International Statistical Review* **49**, 235–264.

[15]   Prentice, R.L. (1986). On the design of synthetic case–control studies, *Biometrics* **42**, 301–310.

[16]   Robins, J.M., Gail, M.H. & Lubin, J.H. (1986). More on "Biased selection of controls for case–control analysis of cohort studies", *Biometrics* **42**, 293–299.

[17]   Saracci, R., Kogevinas, M., Bertazzi, P.A., Bueno de Mesquita, B.H., Coggon, D., Green, L.M., Kauppinen, T., L'Abbé, K.A., Littorin, M., Lynge, E., Mathews, J.D., Neuberger, M., Osman, J., Pearce, N. & Winkelmann, R. (1991). Cancer mortality in workers exposed to chlorophenoxy herbicides and chlorophenols, *Lancet* **338**, 1027–1032.

[18]   Thomas, D.C., Pogoda, J., Langholz, B. & Mack, W. (1994). Temporal modifiers of the radon-smoking interaction, *Health Physics* **66**, 257–262.

[19]   Weinberg, C.R. & Wacholder, S. (1990). The design and analysis of case–control studies with biased sampling, *Biometrics* **46**, 963–975.

BRYAN LANGHOLZ

Case–Control Study, Population-Based

A population-based **case–control study** is based on a well-defined source population from which all cases that arise in a given time period can be enumerated. **Controls** consist of random samples of persons without the disease of interest from the source population. Cases consist of all cases or a random sample of those cases. Because the total number of cases is known and the size of the source population can usually be estimated from census data or other sources, a population-based case–control study yields information not only on **relative risk**, but also, by combining information on relative risk with information on overall disease risk, on exposure-specific **absolute risk**.

Compared with **hospital-based case–control studies**, population-based case–control studies can, in principle, avoid **selection biases** that produce nonrepresentative samples of cases and controls. Moreover, there is no ambiguity about what constitutes an appropriate control. In practice, however, selection biases can arise if all cases are not identified or if persons selected for inclusion in the study refuse to participate. In addition, **recall bias** can distort the results of such a study if persons with disease provide a different quality of information on exposure from healthy controls selected from the general population.

(*See also* **Bias in Case–Control Studies**; **Bias in Observational Studies**; **Bias, Overview**)

M.H. GAIL

Case–Control Study, Prevalent

Incident cases represent the change from a non-diseased to a diseased state. For research purposes, a population at risk is defined as one whose members are, as of some arbitrary time point, disease-free. Over time, incident cases emerge from that population. In a study with incident cases, the underlying assumption is that either all of the cases produced by the population are available for study, or that the study includes what may be taken as a random sample of all of the cases [18]. In this way the experience of the cases and the population at risk can, in principle, be used to investigate the etiology of the disease, conditional on adjustment for potential **confounding** [16, 18, 24]. When, for efficiency, a **case–control study** is done, the measure of effect estimated by the exposure **odds ratio** will be either the **incidence density ratio**, the **cumulative incidence ratio**, or the disease odds ratio, depending upon the sampling scheme that was used to select the **controls** [17, 20, 23]. However, whatever the estimated parameter, the potential for etiologic inference remains, conditional on adjustment for potential confounding.

The situation is more complex when prevalent cases are included and the intent of the research remains etiologic. Prevalent cases have made the transition from a nondiseased to a diseased state. However, they also *survived* to the time the study sample was obtained [6, 16, 29]. All prevalent cases were once incident cases; but not all incident cases survive long enough to become prevalent cases.

When a study includes prevalent cases, the question arises as to whether the prevalent case series can reasonably be taken to represent a random sample of all incident cases with respect to the distribution of etiologically relevant factors (and potential confounders). For the answer to be "yes", incident cases that did not survive long enough to become prevalent cases must be assumed to have been etiologically similar to the incident cases that survived and became prevalent cases [3]. Survival would thus be unrelated to any etiologically important factor [16, 17, 24]. For this special situation, the prevalent case–control study is interchangeable with the incident case–control study with respect to the validity of the relative measure of effect, though it may differ with respect to power [2].

In the more likely situation, the prevalent case series cannot reasonably be taken to represent a random sample of all incident cases [2, 16, 29]. In particular, cases with short survival times will be under-represented; longer surviving cases will be over-represented; and most significantly, the duration of survival may well be related to etiologically relevant factors. Risk factors for the disease therefore will be simultaneously related to etiology *and* prognosis [6, 17, 29]. The exposure odds ratio will not directly estimate the incidence ratios that are the target for etiologic research. Table 1 illustrates

Table 1 Estimation of relative effects in incident and prevalent case–control studies

Frame A: Hypothetical data from an incident case–control study:

	Exposed	Unexposed	
Cases	50	50	
Controls	100	900	$OR = 9.0$

Frame B: Hypothetical data from a prevalent case–control study, where 50% of all cases do not survive long enough to be included in the study. Survival, however, is unrelated to exposure status:

	Exposed	Unexposed	
Cases	25	25	
Controls	100	900	$OR = 9.0$

Frame C: Hypothetical data from a prevalent case–control study, where 50% of exposed cases do not survive long enough to be included in the study. Survival is therefore related to exposure status:

	Exposed	Unexposed	
Cases	25	50	
Controls	100	900	$OR = 4.5$

Frame D: Hypothetical data from a prevalent case–control study, where 50% of unexposed cases do not survive long enough to be included in the study. Survival is therefore related to exposure status:

	Exposed	Unexposed	
Cases	50	25	
Controls	100	900	$OR = 18.0$

how estimates of relative effects from a case–control study with prevalent cases will or will not validly duplicate the estimate from a case–control study with incident cases.

Linking Prevalence- and Incidence-Based Studies

Freeman & Hutchison [7, 8] have demonstrated the interrelations between incidence and prevalence (*see* **Incidence–Prevalence Relationships**)–in particular, that prevalence, incidence, and duration of a condition or illness ... are interrelated in such a way that two of these quantities may be used to obtain the third. Data may be collected in the most expedient manner and the results expressed as both incidence and prevalence [7, p. 707].

At the core of these interrelationships is the assumption that the population is "steady" or "stationary" [1, 2, 7, 8, 16, 17, 21, 24]. For a population in a steady state, the immigration rate into the candidate pool equals the emigration rate from the candidate pool, so that the size of the candidate pool is constant over time. Similarly, the immigration rate into the prevalence pool equals the emigration rate from the prevalence pool, so that the size of the prevalence pool is constant over time. A corollary of these conditions is that the distribution of survival of incident cases remains constant. A practical consequence is that if the population is in a steady state, then estimates of disease incidence are not dependent upon the time period of the study. In a steady-state population, the prevalence odds (PO) equals the product of incidence density (ID) and the average duration ($\overline{D}$) of the illness or condition (see Appendix A). If this relation is calculated for the exposed and unexposed segments of the population (with a subscript 1 indicating exposure and a subscript zero indicating nonexposure), then the prevalence odds ratio (POR) is

$$POR = PO_1/PO_0 = [ID_1 \times \overline{D}_1]/[ID_0 \times \overline{D}_0]$$

$$= IDR \times \overline{D}_1/\overline{D}_0. \quad (1)$$

In a case–control study with prevalent cases, the POR estimates the incidence density ratio (IDR) if the population is in a steady state, and if the duration of disease among the exposed equals the duration of disease among the unexposed, that is, if survival is not related to an etiologically important factor (as in Table 1, Frame B).

Example 1: Nosocomial Infections

Freeman and his coauthors have used data from a "bed-to-bed" prevalence survey at a municipal hospital to illustrate the relations between prevalence and incidence [7, 8] and to study predictors of nosocomial infection [9–11]. They argue that it is reasonable to expect a hospital population to be in a steady state. Moreover, since admission, discharge, and occupancy

data are collected daily, the conditions underlying a steady state can be empirically checked.

Data from their report on risk factors for nosocomial infection [9] are reproduced in Table 2, Frame A. Suppose the data represent a complete **cross-sectional** survey, and, for illustrative purposes, that the relation between use of an endotracheal tube and nosocomial infection is unconfounded. We can compute the prevalence ratio (PR) and the POR. The $PR = [7/11]/[90/634] = 4.5$; the $POR = [7/4]/[90/544] = 10.6$. While both point estimates are large, the POR is not a good estimate of the PR because the overall prevalence is not low (15%) and the exposure rate in the noncases is less than half the exposure rate in the total population surveyed (0.7% and 1.7%, respectively).

Table 2, Frame B shows data from a potential case–control study drawn from this prevalence survey. Suppose, for example, that determination of the exposure status of the 645 subjects was expensive. For efficiency, the exposure status could be determined for all cases and for a 50% sample of controls (again assuming no confounding). Since the parameter of interest is the POR (because of its relation to the IDR), the controls are drawn from the noncases. The POR of 10.6 will be a valid estimate of the incidence density ratio *if*:

Table 2 Prevalence data on the relation between the need for an endotracheal tube and nosocomial infection

Frame A: Prevalence survey data:[a]

	Need for an endotracheal tube	
	Present	Absent
Nosocomial infection		
Present	7	90
Absent	4	544
$POR = 10.6$		

Frame B: Prevalent case–control data, with 50% sampling of controls:

	Need for an endotracheal tube	
	Present	Absent
Nosocomial infection		
present	7	90
absent	2	272
$POR = 10.6$		

[a]The data are from [9, Table 1, p 814].

1. the hospital population is in a steady state, i.e. if "the rate at which patients were admitted equaled the rate at which they were discharged, and the rate at which patients acquired active nosocomial infections and entered the prevalence pool equaled the rate at which they left the prevalence pool through recovery, death, or discharge ... [and] the rates at which new patients entered the hospital and new infections were acquired were ... constant ... [and the] distributions of durations of hospitalization and durations of infections were also ... constant" [11, p. 734]

and

2. the duration of nosocomial infection is equal for those who acquire an infection and have had an endotracheal tube and those who acquire an infection and have not had an endotracheal tube, i.e. that the exposure is not associated with the duration of the disease.

Freeman & McGowan [9, p. 815] report that the duration of nosocomial infection in the incident cases did not differ by the need for an endotracheal tube. The duration of infection was estimated from durations-to-date in the prevalent cases (the time from the onset of the infection to the time of the prevalence survey). Suppose, however, for illustrative purposes, that the durations of infection differed. The distribution of observed durations-to-date in the prevalent series can be converted into the distribution of durations of infection *from disease incidence* in the same steady-state population, as shown by Freeman & Hutchison [7]. In particular:

$$p_i(D) = [\overline{D}_i \times p_p(D)]/D, \tag{2}$$

where

$p_i(D)$ = the proportion from the incidence series (designated by i) with duration D;

$\overline{D}_i$ = the average duration of the disease or condition from a series of incident cases;

$p_p(D)$ = the proportion from the prevalence series (designated by p) with duration D; and

D = a specific duration of the disease or condition from onset to termination of the disease or condition, or to removal from observation.

Suppose infections associated with a poor underlying condition have a longer duration than infections associated with a less serious underlying condition, and that the need for an endotracheal tube is a marker for a poor underlying condition. Table 3 (Frame A) shows hypothetical data from a prevalent case–control study, along with information on the distribution of durations-to-date for the prevalent cases, by exposure categories.

From (2) we obtain the distribution of durations from disease incidence in exposed and unexposed cases (Table 3, Frame B) up to a constant multiplier

Table 3 Use of duration-to-date data to estimate duration of disease

Frame A: Hypothetical duration-to-date data:

	Need for an endotracheal tube	
	Present	Absent
Nosocomial infection		
present	7	90
absent	4	544
Duration		
10 days	5	27
5 days	2	63

Frame B: Calculation of distribution of duration of disease:

$$p_i(D) = [\overline{D}_i \times p_p(D)]/D$$

For exposed cases:
$$p_i(5) = [\overline{D}_i \times (2/7)]/5 = \overline{D}_i \times 0.057$$
$$p_i(10) = [\overline{D}_i \times (5/7)]/10 = \overline{D}_i \times 0.071$$

For unexposed cases:
$$p_i(5) = [\overline{D}_i \times (63/90)]/5 = \overline{D}_i \times 0.14$$
$$p_i(10) = [\overline{D}_i \times (27/90)]/10 = \overline{D}_i \times 0.03$$

Distribution of duration for incidence series:
exposed cases: 5 days for 45%; 10 days for 55%
unexposed cases: 5 days for 82%; 10 days for 18%

Average duration of disease for incidence series:
exposed cases: $\overline{D}_{i1} = 7.8$ days
unexposed cases: $\overline{D}_{i0} = 5.9$ days

Frame C: Calculation of *IDR*:
$$IDR = POR \times \overline{D}_0/\overline{D}_1$$
$$IDR = 10.6 \times 5.9/7.8 = 8.0$$

$\overline{D}_i$. For example, $p_i(5) = \overline{D}_i \times 0.057/[\overline{D}_i \times 0.057 + \overline{D}_i \times 0.071] = 0.45$ for exposed cases. Using these distributions, we calculate $\overline{D}_i = 7.8$ days for the group needing endotracheal tubes and 5.9 days for the group not needing endotracheal tubes (Table 3, Frame B).

A comparison of the observed distribution of durations-to-date from the prevalent series and the calculated distribution of the durations of disease in the incident series illustrates the length-biased sampling that can occur when prevalent rather than incident cases are studied [16, 25, 29]. In particular, cases of long duration represent 71% of the prevalent series of exposed cases, but would constitute only 55% of the incident series. For the unexposed group, the cases of long duration represent 30% of the prevalent series, but would constitute only 18% of the incident series.

By using (1) and solving for the IDR, the POR can be adjusted by the *inverse* average duration ratio to provide an estimate of the IDR. In particular:

$$IDR = POR \times \overline{D}_0/\overline{D}_1. \qquad (3)$$

For the example in Table 3, the POR of 10.6 can be adjusted by a factor of 0.76 to provide an estimate of the IDR of 8.0 (Table 3, Frame C).

Example 2: Neural Tube Defects

Length-biased sampling can be especially problematic in the study of risk factors for congenital malformations [12–15, 22, 28]. In principle, the goal would be to enroll women from the time of pregnancy and follow all of them through the termination of the pregnancy. All incident cases of malformations could be captured, and etiologic factors could be investigated. In practice, however, the situation is quite different. Women are often enrolled at the time of delivery of live or stillborn infants, so that only *prevalent cases* of malformations are available for study. Malformations at birth represent the *survivors* of early pregnancy, a time during which spontaneous and induced abortions occur, both of which are more likely in the presence of fetal malformations [13, 14, 22, 27, 31, 33]. If the duration of survival (early pregnancy loss versus survival to birth) is associated with an etiologically relevant factor, then the estimate of effect using only birth data will be biased because of either a toxic or a protective effect of the exposure on the fetus during the early prenatal period [13, 14, 22].

Consider the example of neural tube defects (NTDs), which include anencephaly, spina bifida,

craniorrhachischisis, and iniencephaly. Leaving aside the issue of early spontaneous abortions [34], over the last two decades prenatal screening for these malformations has increased, and as a result, induced abortions post-screening have also increased [30, 33]. Prevalent cases of NTDs at birth may thus be systematically different from incident cases with respect to any etiologic factor that is associated with obtaining prenatal screening and acting on the results of the screen. Velie & Shaw [32] demonstrate the magnitude of this bias by comparing the estimates of effect for a number of variables from a typical birth prevalence case–control study and from a case–control study that is more "incident-like" in that cases from induced abortions are included along with cases ascertained at birth. For illustrative purposes, we consider estimates of the effect of folic acid use on the occurrence of NTDs. Table 4 presents data adapted from Velie & Shaw [32].

Table 4   Prevalence and "incidence-type" data on the relation between folic acid and neural tube defects (NTDs)[a]

Frame A: Prevalent case–control data (cases from still and livebirths only):

	Folic acid use	
	Yes	No
Cases	151	164
Controls	374	149
POR = 0.37		

Frame B: "Incidence-type" case–control data (cases from electively aborted fetuses as well as still and livebirths):

	Folic acid use	
	Yes	No
Cases	319	207
Controls	374	149
POR = 0.61		

Frame C: The association of survival and exposure:

	Folic acid use	
	Yes	No
Survival to birth		
Yes	151	164
No	168	43
OR = 0.24		

[a]Data are adapted from [32, Tables 2 and 3, pp. 476–477].

Data from the prevalence case–control study show a strong protective effect of folic acid on the prevalence of NTDs, $POR = 0.37$. When the study is broadened to include early fetal deaths due to induced abortions following screening for NTDs that have been excluded from the birth prevalence study, the protective effect of folic acid remains, but it is considerably attenuated, $POR = 0.61$. The reason for this attenuation is that folic acid use is strongly and negatively associated with the odds of surviving early pregnancy and thereby being available for inclusion in the prevalence at birth study ($OR = 0.24$). Folic acid use may be associated with early prenatal care, which itself is associated with prenatal screening; and prenatal screening is associated with termination of affected fetuses.

The availability of data from "incident-like" and prevalence studies from the same population, in which the duration of survival is associated with a number of potential etiologic factors, allows for a demonstration of the way length-biased sampling can bias the estimate of effect. In particular:

1. From Eq. (1), $POR = IDR \times \overline{D}_1/\overline{D}_0$, the duration ratio can be estimated to be 0.61.
2. Alternatively, (4) below (from Freeman & Hutchison [8]) can be used to estimate the duration ratio:

$$\overline{D}_{i1}/\overline{D}_{i0} = [\pi_p(1)/\pi_i(1)]/[\pi_p(0)/\pi_i(0)], \quad (4)$$

where

$\overline{D}_{i1}$ = the average duration of the disease or condition from a series of incident cases from the exposed group;

$\overline{D}_{i0}$ = the average duration of the disease or condition from a series of incident cases from the unexposed group;

$\pi_p(1)$ = the proportion of exposed cases in a prevalence series;

$\pi_p(0)$ = the proportion of unexposed cases in a prevalence series;

$\pi_i(1)$ = the proportion of exposed cases in an incidence series; and

$\pi_i(0)$ = the proportion of unexposed cases in an incidence series.

Again, the duration ratio would be estimated to be 0.61. From this calculation, the POR of 0.37 can be adjusted by the inverse duration ratio of 1.65 to obtain an estimate of the IDR of 0.61.

For this last sequence of calculations, information about the exposure frequency of the prevalent cases might be obtained from data on hand. A series of potential exposure frequencies of the *un*observed incident cases could be postulated, based on the best available extra-study information. These frequencies could then be used to estimate a range of plausible duration ratios. These ratios could then be used to produce a band of plausible incidence density ratios. The main purpose of this exercise would be to show the sensitivity of the observed POR to length-biased sampling when the potential etiologic factor under investigation could plausibly be related to survival.

Separating Prevalence- and Incidence-Based Studies

We have illustrated some of the relations between estimates based on prevalence data and those based on incidence data when the steady-state assumption holds [7, 8]. Provided exposures are not strongly related to survival, the calculations suggest that qualitative conclusions from prevalence studies will often agree with those from incidence-based data. Experience confirms this expectation. Yet, in "strict logic, ... there is no reason why [incidence based and prevalence based studies] should yield even qualitatively similar results" [5, p. 524].

Neyman illustrates this point with hypothetical data which he describes as "somewhat implausible" [19, p. 404]. Using only prevalent cases to study the relation between smoking and lung cancer, it is possible that a positive association in the prevalent series could mask a protective effect in the population as a whole, if the majority of cases in nonsmokers were highly lethal and therefore did not survive long enough to be included in the prevalence study. However implausible the substance of this example, the point is that in such situations the duration of survival will be strongly associated with the exposure and thereby bias the POR as an estimate of the IDR. In principle, the bias may be so large as to reverse the direction of the effect.

The plausibility of "balancing" or "off-setting" effects of a potential risk factor among a segment of the population that does not survive long enough to be eligible for prevalence studies has been examined in detail in the study of risk factors for congenital malformations [13, 14, 22]. Evidence for potential teratogens typically comes from studies of livebirths, which involve prevalent cases. However, the object of these studies is to discover the potential teratogenic effects on *all* the products of conception, in principle, through incident cases. The results from studies of livebirths may not agree *even qualitatively* with results applicable to all conceptuses. For example, regarding the relation between maternal cigarette smoking and the occurrence of Down's syndrome, Hook & Regal [14] have shown that an apparent protective relative effect as low as 0.3 among livebirths could be consistent with a null effect among all conceptuses if smoking increased the risk of embryonic and fetal deaths by a factor of only 1.1. Regal & Hook [22] provide general formulas for estimating the magnitude of effect on embryonic and fetal deaths that could account for the observed effect in livebirths. Hook & Regal [13] also describe the following variant of the "Yule–Simpson" paradox (*see* **Simpson's Paradox**). The relative exposure effects can be protective among embryonic and fetal deaths and protective among livebirths, yet among all conceptuses the effect is null. Alternately, the exposure can increase the risk both among embryos and fetuses who died and among livebirths, yet among all conceptuses the exposure effect is null. (This situation is statistically similar to confounding, but it is substantively distinct since the "confounding" variable is duration of survival.) Appendix B contains an example of data embodying the "Yule–Simpson" paradox. Hook & Regal [14] develop the concept of a "boundary value", namely a value such that if the observed risk from a suspected teratogen derived from a prevalent series of livebirths exceeds this value, then the explanation of the finding is unlikely to be due solely to selection factors related to the exclusion of cases that did not survive long enough to be included in the prevalence study. The boundary value is a function of the following: the proportion of unexposed subjects that do not survive to be included in the prevalence study; the proportion of unexposed cases that do not survive to be included in the prevalence study; and the proportion of exposed subjects that do not survive to be included in the prevalence study. Where estimates of these quantities are available, a boundary value can be calculated. Tables of boundary values are given for a range of determinants.

Conducting and Interpreting Prevalence-Based Studies

Bias from the inclusion of prevalent cases is a concern when the goal of the study is to discover potential etiologic factors. In this case, if the exposure is related to the duration of survival, then a series of prevalent cases will not mirror the targeted series of incident cases. However, there are situations where etiologic research is not the goal [18]. At times one may be mainly interested in factors that influence disease *prevalence*. The question, for example, may not be, "What factors *cause* infection in neonatal intensive care units (NICUs)?" but rather, "What factors *predict* the number of NICU beds needed to treat the infections that occur?" Concern with length-biased sampling is central to the etiologic question, but irrelevant for estimating factors that influence prevalence. For determining required medical services, the prevalent series is the direct research target; it is not intended to duplicate the incidence series.

The assumption of steady-state conditions is important for both descriptive and etiologic research with prevalent cases. If a population is in a steady state, then the size of the prevalence pool is constant. In this case a prevalence-based study of service needs at time t will be applicable to $T > t$, provided the population remains in a steady state. For etiologic research, the steady-state assumption underlies the conversion formulas presented by Freeman & Hutchison [7, 8]. While the assumption of steady-state conditions may well be "unrealistic in a literal sense, it [may well] be approximately true in many applications" [2, p. 194]. For example, in a steady-state population, there should be "a stable pattern in terms of how disease gets diagnosed," [6, p. 1110], and treatment should be reasonably stable. Medical advances that change the way a disease is diagnosed or treated will perturb, at least temporarily, the steady state of the population. Studies done with prevalent cases during the early introduction of zidovudine (AZT) for the treatment of acquired immune deficiency syndrome (AIDS), or with livebirths following the introduction of prenatal screening, can be misleading. For more detailed arguments regarding the difficulties of studying the risk factors for AIDS in a setting of changing criteria for diagnosis and methods of treatment, see Brookmeyer & Gail [4]. Hook & Regal [12–14, 22] offer cautions concerning the effects of changing prenatal practices on the study of risk factors for congenital malformations.

When the assumption of a steady-state population is plausible, the formulae from Freeman & Hutchison [7, 8] can be used to convert information obtained from prevalence studies to estimates that would result from incidence studies from the same population. The formulas are applicable where exposure–outcome relations are either unconfounded or can be conveniently stratified on confounders. Begg & Gray [2] have developed multivariate methods and proposed quasi-likelihood estimates for bias correction that can be obtained using GLIM with a log link function and a gamma error distribution. (When the exposure is dichotomous, and there is no confounding, the correction factor proposed by Begg & Gray reduces to the inverse duration ratio as described by Freeman & Hutchison [7, 8].)

When a population is in a steady state (or stationary), the size of the candidate pool and the prevalence pool are constant, and the age distribution of the population is stable [1, 2, 7, 8, 16, 17, 21, 24]. The population, or segment of the population considered, is not growing. Alho [1] considered the basic relation examined by Freeman & Hutchison [7, 8] and Begg & Gray [2] in the more general situation where the size of the population is either increasing or decreasing, that is, a situation where the population is "stable" but is not "stationary" or in a "steady state". Under this situation, when, for example, incidence is increasing with age and duration of disease is declining with age, the standard relation of the prevalence odds as the product of incidence density and average duration of disease will be an overestimate. Instead, the prevalence odds will equal "a weighted average of the age specific products of incidence and (discounted) expected duration" [1, p. 587] (*see* **Incidence–Prevalence Relationships**).

Suppose that a population (or a segment of a population) can be assumed to approximate a steady state, such that the relations described by Freeman & Hutchison [7, 8] and Begg & Gray [2] hold. In this case inferences about incidence densities can be made from either incidence- or prevalence-based studies. Begg & Gray [2] have compared the relative efficiency of prevalence studies to incidence studies, where the determinants of efficiency included the proportion of cases in the sample, the exposure frequency among controls, the true relative effect, and the duration of disease ratio. There was substantial

variation in the relative efficiency of the prevalence-based study compared with the incidence-based study over a wide range of these determinant values. However, the authors conclude that

> for less extreme configurations [of the determinants of efficiency], the relative efficiency ranges from about 50% to 90%, so that an approximate rule of thumb is that on average, to achieve comparable precision, a prevalence study will require about three subjects for every two in an incidence study [2, p. 194].

While a prevalence-based study should be larger than the corresponding incidence-based study, it may be easier and less costly to enroll prevalent cases. However, the concerns about the precision of the study should always be subordinated to concerns about the validity of the study. Moreover, the validity of the study based on prevalent cases and aimed at etiologic investigation will depend on two factors: (i) the feasibility of obtaining accurate duration-to-date information on the duration from the onset of disease to the enrollment in the prevalence study, and (ii) the plausibility that the population (or population segment) approximates the steady-state requirements.

Conclusion

Examples from research on plausible teratogens highlight the importance of considering the possibility that prevalent studies can yield misleading estimates of exposure effects on incident disease. A comment from Sartwell & Merrell [26, p. 583] broadens this concern beyond studies that are traditionally described as "prevalence based":

> While the foregoing illustrations have dealt with limitations of prevalence and mortality rate, the interpretation of observed incidence rates also offers a challenge. What is actually obtained may more properly be termed a discovery rate, which may be quite different from the true incidence rate. Of the cases with onset in any time period, some will be discovered early, others late, perhaps at death, and still others will escape recognition entirely. Thus, the discovery rate of any period will include cases with onsets covering a long time span, and moreover will be influenced by the clinical level at which cases are recognized.

Sartwell & Merrell [26] remind us that even a typical incidence series may well contain a trace of prevalence. To the extent that any survival (or persistence) criterion is required to allow the diagnosis of a disease, estimates of exposure effect may be distorted, as in the prevalent case–control study.

Appendix A: Derivation of PO = ID × $\overline{D}$

Prevalence (P), incidence density (ID), and average duration ($\overline{D}$) are readily linked when the population is in a "steady state" [1, 2, 7, 8, 16, 17, 21, 24]. In a steady state the number of people entering the prevalence pool from the population at risk is equal to the number of people exiting the prevalence pool, through recovery or death.

At any time, the total population (N) can be divided into those individuals who have the disease (P) and those who are at risk for the disease ($N - P$). Entry into the prevalence pool is governed by the size of the population at risk ($N - P$), the rate of disease (ID), and the time period (δt) such that

$$\text{inflow} = ID \times \delta t \times (N - P).$$

Exit from the prevalence pool is governed by the size of the prevalence pool (P), the exit rate (ID_{exit}), and the time period (δt) such that

$$\text{outflow} = ID_{\text{exit}} \times \delta t \times P.$$

In a steady state, any rate is equal to the reciprocal of the average time to the event. Therefore, $ID_{\text{exit}} = 1/\overline{D}$, where $\overline{D}$ is the average duration of disease. In a steady state, inflow (to the prevalence pool) equals outflow (from the prevalence pool). Therefore

$$ID \times \delta t \times (N - P) = 1/\overline{D} \times \delta t \times P.$$

By algebraic manipulation:

$$ID \times \overline{D} = P/(N - P) = PO.$$

Appendix B: Hypothetical Data Embodying the "Yule–Simpson" Paradox

The data in this appendix are from [13, Table 2, p. 56].

Stratum 1: Embryonic and fetal deaths

	Exposed	Unexposed	Total
Down's syndrome	732	1251	1983
Unaffected	58 359	89 658	148 017
All	59 091	90 909	150 000

Relative risk of Down's syndrome = 0.9

Stratum 2: Livebirths

	Exposed	Unexposed	Total
Down's syndrome	213	637	850
Unaffected	274 029	575 121	848 150
All	274 242	575 758	850 000

Relative risk of Down's syndrome = 0.7

Total population: All (recognized conceptuses)

	Exposed	Unexposed	Total
Down's syndrome	945	1888	2833
Unaffected	332 388	663 834	997 167
All	333 333	666 667	1 000 000

Relative risk of Down's syndrome = 1.0

References

[1]   Alho, J.M. (1992). On prevalence, incidence and duration in general stable populations, *Biometrics* **48**, 587–592.

[2]   Begg, C.B. & Gray, R.J. (1987). Methodology for case–control studies with prevalent cases, *Biometrika* **74**, 191–195.

[3]   Borman, B. & Cryer, C. (1990). Fallacies of international and national comparisons of disease occurrence in the epidemiology of neural tube defects, *Teratology* **42**, 405–412.

[4]   Brookmeyer, R. & Gail, M.H. (1994). *AIDS Epidemiology: A Quantitative Approach*. Oxford University Press, New York.

[5]   Cornfield, J. & Haenszel, W. (1960). Some aspects of retrospective studies, *Journal of Chronic Diseases* **11**, 525–534.

[6]   Dunn, J.E. (1962). The use of incidence and prevalence in the study of disease development in a population, *American Journal of Public Health* **52**, 1107–1118.

[7]   Freeman, J. & Hutchison, G.B. (1980) Prevalence, incidence, and duration, *American Journal of Epidemiology* **112**, 707–723.

[8]   Freeman, J. & Hutchison, G.B. (1986). Duration of disease, duration indicators, and estimation of the risk ratio, *American Journal of Epidemiology* **124**, 134–149.

[9] Freeman, J. & McGowan, J.E., Jr (1978). Risk factors for nosocomial infection, *Journal of Infectious Diseases* **138**, 811–819.

[10] Freeman, J. & McGowan, J.E., Jr (1981). Day-specific incidence of nosocomial infection estimated from a prevalence survey, *American Journal of Epidemiology* **114**, 888–901.

[11] Freeman, J., Rosner, B.A. & McGowan, J.E. Jr (1979). Adverse effects of nosocomial infection, *Journal of Infectious Diseases* **140**, 732–740.

[12] Hook, E.B. (1982). Incidence and prevalence as measures of the frequency of birth defects, *American Journal of Epidemiology* **116**, 743–747.

[13] Hook, E.B. & Regal, R.R. (1991). Conceptus viability, malformation, and suspect mutagens or teratogens in humans: the Yule–Simpson paradox and implications for inferences of causality in studies of mutagenicity or teratogenicity limited to human livebirths, *Teratology* **43**, 53–59.

[14] Hook, E.B. & Regal, R.R. (1993). Representative and misrepresentative associations of birth defects in livebirths. Conditions under which relative risks greater than unity in livebirths necessarily imply relative risks greater than unity in all conceptuses, *American Journal of Epidemiology* **137**, 660–675.

[15] Khoury, M.J., Flanders, W.D., James, L.M. & Erickson, J.D. (1989). Human teratogens, prenatal mortality, and selection bias, *American Journal of Epidemiology* **130**, 361–370.

[16] Kleinbaum, D.G., Kupper, L.L. & Morgenstern, H. (1982). *Epidemiologic Research: Principles and Quantitative Methods*. Lifetime Learning Publications, Belmont.

[17] Miettinen, O.S. (1976). Estimability and estimation in case-referent studies, *American Journal of Epidemiology* **103**, 226–235.

[18] Miettinen, O.S. (1985). *Theoretical Epidemiology: Principles of Occurrence Research in Medicine*. Wiley, New York.

[19] Neyman, J. (1955). Statistics–servant of all sciences, *Science* **122**, 401–406.

[20] Pearce, N. (1993). What does the odds ratio estimate in a case–control study?, *International Journal of Epidemiology* **22**, 1189–1192.

[21] Preston, S.H. (1987). Relations among standard epidemiologic measures in a population, *American Journal of Epidemiology* **126**, 336–345.

[22] Regal, R.R. & Hook, E.B. (1992). Interrelationships of relative risks of birth defects in embryonic and fetal deaths, in livebirths, and in all conceptuses, *Epidemiology* **3**, 247–252.

[23] Rodrigues, L. & Kirkwood, B.R. (1990). Case–control designs in the study of common diseases: updates on the demise of the rare disease assumption and the choice of sampling scheme for controls, *International Journal of Epidemiology* **19**, 205–213.

[24] Rothman, K.J. (1986). *Modern Epidemiology*. Little, Brown, & Company, Boston.

[25] Rozencweig, M., Zelen, M., Von Hoff, D.D. & Muggia, F.M. (1978). Waiting for a bus: does it explain age-dependent differences in response to chemotherapy of early breast cancer?, *New England Journal of Medicine* **299**, 1363–1364.

[26] Sartwell, P.E. & Merrell, M. (1952). Influence of the dynamic character of chronic disease on the interpretation of morbidity rates, *American Journal of Public Health* **42**, 579–584.

[27] Seller, M.J. (1987). Unanswered questions on neural tube defects, *British Medical Journal* **294**, 1–2.

[28] Sever, L.E. (1983). Re: "Incidence and prevalence as measures of the frequency of birth defects", *American Journal of Epidemiology* **118**, 608–609.

[29] Simon, R. (1980). Length biased sampling in etiologic studies, *American Journal of Epidemiology* **111**, 444–452.

[30] Slattery, M.L. & Janerich, D.T. (1991). The epidemiology of neural tube defects: a review of dietary intake and related factors as etiologic agents, *American Journal of Epidemiology* **133**, 526–539.

[31] Stein, Z., Susser, M., Warburton, D., Wittes, J. & Kline, J. (1975) Spontaneous abortion as a screening device: the effect of fetal survival on the incidence of birth defects, *American Journal of Epidemiology* **102**, 275–290.

[32] Velie, E.M. & Shaw, G.M. (1996). Impact of prenatal diagnosis and elective termination on prevalence and risk estimates of neural tube defects in California, 1989–1991, *American Journal of Epidemiology* **144**, 473–479.

[33] Wald, N.J. (1984). Neural-tube defects and vitamins: the need for a randomized clinical trial, *British Journal of Obstetrics and Gynaecology* **91**, 516–523.

[34] Wilcox, A.J., Weinberg, C.R., O'Connor, J.F., Baird, D.D., Schlatterer, J.P., Canfield, R.E., Armstrong, E.G. & Nisula, B.C. (1988). Incidence of early loss of pregnancy, *New England Journal of Medicine* **319**, 189–194.

(*See also* **Bias in Case–Control Studies**; **Biased Sampling of Cohorts in Epidemiology**; **Cross-Sectional Study**; **Prevalence–Incidence Bias**)

JANET M. LANG

Case–Control Study, Sequential

Many **case–control studies** are based on previously identified cases and **controls**, together with their information on exposure and **confounders**. Some studies, however, require that data on newly **incident cases** and controls be collected and accumulated prospectively, not unlike the data collection for a controlled clinical trial. For example, when a new drug or exposure is introduced into a population, there may be no medical database or method to link records (*see* **Record Linkage**) to determine exposure and case status. When a concern exists about risk associated with these exposures and a case–control design is capable of addressing the issue, the conduct of a case–control study to evaluate and test the hypothesis requires the accumulation of new records and exposure information.

In these situations an investigator may wish to test the hypothesis repeatedly as the data accumulate in order to reduce the average sample size required by the study and obtain results sooner. Sequential case–control designs are proposed first, to take account more efficiently of the accumulating collection of exposure data on cases and controls and, thus, decide when sufficient data are in hand to address the question and, secondly, to preserve the integrity of the inferences drawn from case–control studies when these studies are repeatedly analyzed as data accumulate.

The statistical methods developed for monitoring randomized clinical studies can be applied to the analysis of accumulating data in matched or unmatched case–control designs, and to the repeated analyses of measures of association, such as the **odds ratio** or **relative risk**. In a clinical trial, ethical concerns usually drive the need to terminate a study early in order to minimize exposure of study subjects to harmful treatments. The ethical concerns are different for case–control studies, but there may be ethical motivations for trying to terminate a case–control early. For example, a case–control study may be used to identify or confirm an important risk that requires expeditious public health policy decisions.

Sequential methods can also be used to continue accumulating data until the odds ratio has been estimated with acceptable precision. In this article, we concentrate on hypotheses testing, though we discuss applications to sequential estimation.

Implementing the Sequential Approach

The following discussion is based upon O'Neill & Anello [13]. Assume that an investigator is interested

in studying whether or not there is an increased risk of an adverse outcome (cases) associated with exposure to a specified factor. Assume that there is a mechanism for uniformly identifying and collecting cases with the adverse outcome from a defined population and then, according to predetermined criteria, **matching** each case with respect to a matching variate to a control (person without the adverse outcome) at the time the case becomes available. Furthermore, assume that there is a mechanism for identifying in an unbiased manner the exposure to a risk factor for both case and matched controls. Thus, case and control matches become available over time, and at any point in time T a cumulative set of N_T cases and their matched controls is available. While it is not necessary that all cases be matched to the same number of controls, the example we provide assumes a constant matching ratio for ease of exposition. We will also assume that the relative risk is constant and independent of the matching variables and/or other covariables.

For one-to-one matching, the information is in the case–control pairs that are discordant with respect to the presence or absence of the risk factor. For multiple matching on **confounding** variables, the situation is somewhat more complex (e.g. [6]).

We illustrate two sequential designs with one-to-one matching. The first design monitors outcomes after each case–control pair is ascertained and uses the Wald [21] sequential probability ratio test (SPRT). The second design analyzes the data after successive groups of matched pairs have been accrued and is based on the theory of repeated significance testing for group sequential data. The group sequential approach can also be used for multiple-matched and unmatched case–control designs, as discussed in Pasternak & Shore [14, 15].

The Wald SPRT for a One-to-One Matched Design

For the ith case–control pair, let Y_{11} denote the exposure value (1 if exposed, 0 otherwise) assumed by the case and Y_{21} denote the value assumed by the control. For the ith case–control pair, let $P_{1i} = \mathrm{Pr}$(case is exposed to the factor under study) and $P_{2i} = \mathrm{Pr}$(control is exposed to the factor under study). The data from N matched case–control pairs may be summarized as in Table 1, where Z_{11} denotes the

Table 1 Summary of data from N matched case–control pairs

		Control (Y_2)		
		1	0	Total
Case (Y_1)	1	Z_{11}	Z_{10}	Z_1
	0	Z_{01}	Z_{00}	$N - Z_1$
	Total	Z_2	$N - Z_2$	N

number of pairs in which both case and control are exposed, Z_{10} the number of pairs where only the case is exposed, and so forth.

In an individually matched retrospective case–control study, the maximum likelihood estimate of relative risk ρ is based upon the pairs with discordant exposure and is given by $\rho = Z_{10}/Z_{01}$. Thus, the effective sample size for interval estimation of ρ is $Z_{10} + Z_{01} = n$. In testing whether this estimate of the relative risk differs significantly from one, attention is restricted to the discordant pairs. In the ith such pair, the probability that the case is exposed and the control is not exposed is

$$\pi_i = \frac{P_{1i}(1 - P_{2i})}{P_{1i}(1 - P_{2i}) + (1 - P_{1i})P_{2i}}. \tag{1}$$

The relative risk is $\rho = \pi/(1 - \pi)$ and is assumed constant for all pairs. The test of whether ρ differs significantly from one is equivalent to testing whether the conditionally binomial variate Z_{10}, based on n observations, has probability $\pi = \frac{1}{2}$ against an alternative that $\pi \neq \frac{1}{2}$.

To carry out the SPRT, it is essential that one specifies two simple hypotheses before the data are collected. That is, one specifies that the null hypothesis is $\rho_0 = 1$ and chooses a value of ρ for the alternative hypothesis H_1, call it ρ_1, which is of interest to detect. Furthermore, one must specify the type I and type II errors, α and β, respectively. Since we choose to examine the one-sided test in which the alternative of the form $\rho > 1$ is of interest, the SPRT tests the null hypothesis that $H_0 : \rho = 1$ vs. $H_1 : \rho = \rho_1$, which is equivalent to $H_0 : \pi = \frac{1}{2}$ vs. $H_1 : \pi_1 = \rho_1/(1 + \rho_1)$.

The SPRT is carried out as each case–control pair becomes available over time. The cumulative number of cases exposed to the factor, Z_{10}, among the subset of n exposure-discordant pairs is then compared with two parallel boundaries (see [13, Appendix A]). Crossing one boundary causes rejection of H_0 and crossing the other causes rejection of H_1.

The Group Sequential Design for a One-to-One Matched Design

Rather than analyze the data after each matched pair accrues, one can perform only K analyses after successive groups of M discordant pairs have accrued, giving rise to a maximum total sample size of $KM = N$ discordant pairs. Pasternak & Shore [16] described this group sequential approach for repeated tests of a hypothesis. The approach is based on the sequential use of the signed square root of the McNemar test statistic χ for accumulating discordant case–control pairs, namely

$$\chi_k^2 = \frac{(|Z_{10} - Z_{01}| - 1)^2}{Z_{10} + Z_{01}}. \tag{2}$$

While we emphasize this application, one could also use the estimate of the log odds ratio from the conditional logistic model (see **Logistic Regression, Conditional**) divided by its standard error.

Letting χ_k denote the signed square root of (2) after k groups, the decision rule for the kth ($1 \leq k \leq K$) group sequential test of $\rho = 1$ vs. $\rho \neq 1$ is

1. If $\chi_k > Z_\alpha$ reject the null hypothesis that $\rho = 1$ in favor of the alternative, $\rho \neq 1$; then no additional accumulation of data is required.

2.   (i) If $\chi_k < Z_\alpha$ and $k < K$, accumulate additional discordant pairs and then apply the $(k + 1)$th group sequential test.
  (ii) If $\chi_k < Z_\alpha$ and $k = K$, end the study and do not reject the null hypothesis that $\rho = 1$.

Note that Z_α is a constant in this "repeated testing design". To control the overall type I error at α, Z_α at each interim analysis will need to be adjusted. For example, for planned three-group sequential analyses controlled at $\alpha = 0.05$, $Z_\alpha = 2.289$, corresponding to a nominal $\alpha' = 0.022$ for each analysis (see Pocock [17, Table 2]). Other group sequential

Table 2 Average number of exposure discordant pairs for SPRT and fixed sample designs, for selected relative risk ρ : $\alpha = 0.05$, $\beta = 0.10$ (one-sided)[a]

	$\rho = 2$			$\rho = 3$		
Fixed plan	73			30		
SPRT	H_0	H_1	H_ρ^-	H_0	H_1	H_ρ^-
	34	42	56	14	18	23

[a]Extracted from O'Neill & Anello [13]

designs, referred to in the discussion section, allow for varying the boundary with k.

A Comparison of Sample Sizes for Fixed and Sequential Designs

One of the main benefits of a sequential design is that fewer observations are needed on average than for a fixed sample size plan to reject the null hypothesis when the alternative hypothesis is true, thereby being a more efficient design by offering the chance of yielding a conclusion before the final fixed sample size is needed. The difference in sample size needed for the fixed and sequential designs for the one-to-one individually matched design method was described by O'Neill & Anello [13] for the SPRT, and by Pasternak & Shore [16] for the group sequential designs using repeated significance-testing methods.

For the SPRT, formulas exist [13, Appendix A] to calculate the average number of exposure discordant pairs needed to arrive at a decision when the null and alternative hypotheses are assumed true and for a value of ρ; namely, $\bar{\rho}$, midway between ρ_0 and ρ_1. These sample sizes can be compared with those needed in a fixed sample design. Table 2, adapted from O'Neill & Anello [13], presents the average number of exposure discordant pairs required in a SPRT and fixed sampling design for selected protocol parameters. The SPRT offers a substantial advantage in average required sample size, although there is no upper limit on the sample size.

For the group sequential designs based upon repeated significance testing, one can calculate the maximum sample size N needed and the average sample size $\bar{N}$ needed for a prespecified number, K, of interim analyses of accruing case–control exposure discordant pairs. This calculation depends on the number of interim analyses, K, or independent groups of exposure discordant pairs, planned in advance, and on the per-test significance level α' and its corresponding standard normal deviate Z for use in normal group sequential testing ([16, Table 2]). Table 3, extracted from Pasternak & Shore [16], who provide further discussion of the calculations, presents a comparison of the number of discordant pairs needed for the group sequential design relative to a fixed sample plan for a two-sided hypothesis test. For example, for $\rho = 2$, the fixed sample plan ($K = 1$) requires

Table 3 Comparison of the number of discordant pairs needed for the group sequential design relative to a fixed sample plan for a two-sided hypothesis test: $\alpha = 0.05$, $\beta = 0.10$ (two-sided). $N =$ Maximum number ofs discordant pairs per group; $\bar{N} =$ Average number of discordant pairs per group[a]

Number of interim analyses (groups) K	$\rho = 2$		$\rho = 3$	
	N	$\bar{N}$	N	$\bar{N}$
1	91	91	38	38
2	100	71	42	30
3	105	66	45	28
4	108	64	44	27

[a]Extracted from Pasternak & Shore [16].

$N = 91$ pairs, compared with an average of only 64 pairs with $K = 4$. Note, however, with $K = 4$, the maximum trial size, 108, exceeds the fixed sample size, 91.

In Tables 2 and 3, the sample sizes presented for the average number of discordant pairs using the SPRT, the group sequential design, and the fixed sample design need to be adjusted to arrive at the expected total number of pairs required. To make the adjustment, one needs to divide the sample sizes in Tables 2 and 3 by the probability of obtaining a discordant pair, which is

$$Y = P_1(1 - P_2) + P_2(1 - P_1). \tag{3}$$

values for which are provided in [13, Table 3].

Discussion

To date, there are few examples of sequentially designed and analyzed case–control studies, though there are many examples of prospective collection of exposure information on cases and controls that could easily adapt the sequential strategy. Several variants of the group sequential approach can be used for monitoring case–control studies. Rather than using the same boundary (i.e. the same nominal Type 1 error) at each interim analysis as proposed by Armitage et al. [3] and Pocock [17], we can use different critical levels for each k. For example, O'Brien & Fleming [11] proposed a monotonically decreasing set of nominal α levels, and Lan & DeMets [10] introduced a flexible method for allocating the Type 1 error over the number of testing times used. Rather than applying group sequential statistic methods to simple statistics such as the McNemar statistic, one can also use score statistics derived from logistic models in sequential tests, as described by Whitehead [22].

Despite the attractiveness of the group sequential design for reducing required sample sizes when performing hypothesis testing in case–control studies, we are unaware of completed case–control studies that formally use this methodology.

Only in unusual circumstances will there be a pressing need to terminate an **observational study** early, unlike a clinical trial. It may be important to obtain a large number of cases and controls to pursue analyses of the effects of confounding. Issues of data quality and case ascertainment may play a role also. For example, it may be necessary to validate exposure assessments and histopathologic diagnoses of disease. Such quality control activities may be logistically difficult to accomplish during the conduct of the sequential acquisition of cases and controls. These factors may make it more attractive to design and conduct a large fixed sample size study rather than to attempt a sequential design. However, one should be aware that if one initiates a fixed sample design but terminates the study early on the basis of interim analyses, one risks increasing the chance of type I error.

More often, an epidemiologist may be interested in obtaining a precise estimate of a risk parameter rather than in rejecting a null hypothesis expeditiously. To the extent that precise and valid estimation of exposure effects is the dominant goal of the observational study, sequential strategies may play a greater role in the future by requiring that data continue to be accrued until precise estimates of exposure risks are obtained.

Generally, sample sizes to test a hypothesis will be inadequate to provide a confidence interval for the odds ratio whose width is sufficiently narrow for precise estimation [12]. Many authors have considered sequential estimation procedures in a univariate and multivariate context, which may be relevant for the medical and public health applications for which case–control studies have found utility [1, 2, 4, 5, 7–9, 18–20].

References

[1]   Anscombe, F.J. (1952). Large-sample theory of sequential estimation, *Proceedings of the Cambridge Philosophical Society* **48**, 600–607.

[2]   Anscombe, F.J. (1953). Sequential estimation, *Journal of the Royal Statistical Society, Series B* **15**, 1–21.

[3]   Armitage, P., MacPherson, C.K. & Rowe, B.C. (1969). Repeated significance tests on accumulating data, *Journal of the Royal Statistical Society, Series A* **132**, 235–244.

[4]   Cabilio, P. (1977). Sequential estimation in Bernoulli trials, *Annals of Statistics* **5**, 342–356.

[5]   Chow, Y.S. & Robbins, H. (1965). On the asymptotic theory of fixed-width sequential confidence intervals for the mean, *Annals of Mathematical Statistics* **36**, 457–462.

[6]   Connett, J., Ejigou, A., McHugh, R. & Breslow, N. (1982). The precision of the Mantel–Haenszel estimator in case–control studies with multiple matching, *American Journal of Epidemiology* **116**, 875–877.

[7]   Gleser, L.F. (1966). On the asymptotic theory of fixed size sequential confidence bounds for linear regression parameters, *Annals of Mathematical Statistics* **36**, 463–467. (See correction note: *Annals of Mathematical Statistics* **36** (1966) 1053–1055.)

[8]   Grambsch, P. (1983). Sequential sampling based on the observed Fisher information to guarantee the accuracy of the maximum likelihood estimator, *Annals of Statistics* **11**, 68–77.

[9]   Jennison, C. & Turnbull, B.W. (1993). Sequential equivalence testing and repeated confidence intervals, with applications to normal and binary responses, *Biometrics* **49**, 31–44.

[10]   Lan, K.K.G. & DeMets, D.L. (1983). Discrete sequential boundaries for clinical trials, *Biometrika* **70**, 659–662.

[11]   O'Brien, P.C. & Fleming, T.R. (1979). A multiple testing procedure for clinical trials, *Biometrics* **35**, 549–556.

[12]   O'Neill, R.T. (1983). Sample size for estimation of the odds ratio in unmatched case–control studies, *American Journal of Epidemiology* **120**, 145–153.

[13]   O'Neill, R.T. & Anello, C. (1978). Case–control studies: a sequential approach, *American Journal of Epidemiology* **108**, 415–424.

[14]   Pasternack, B.S. & Shore, R.E. (1980). Sample sizes for group sequential cohort and case–control study designs, *American Journal of Epidemiology* **113**, 778–784.

[15]   Pasternack, B.S. & Shore, R.E. (1980). Group sequential methods for cohort and case–control studies, *Journal of Chronic Diseases* **33**, 365–373.

[16]   Pasternack, B.S. & Shore, R.E. (1981). Sample sizes for individually matched case–control studies, *American Journal of Epidemiology* **115**, 778–784.

[17]   Pocock, S.J. (1977). Group sequential methods in the design and analysis of clinical trials, *Biometrika* **64**, 191–199.

[18]   Robbins, H. & Sigmund, D.O. (1974). Sequential estimation of *p* in Bernoulli trials, in *Studies in Probability and Statistics*, E.J. Williams, ed. University of Melbourne.

[19] Srivastava, M.S. (1967). On fixed width confidence bounds for regression parameters and mean vector, *Journal of the Royal Statistical Society, Series B* **29**, 132–140.

[20] Srivastava, M.S. (1971). On fixed width confidence bounds for regression parameters, *Annals of Mathematical Statistics* **42**, 1403–1411.

[21] Wald, A. (1947). *Sequential Analysis*. Wiley, New York.

[22] Whitehead, J. (1983). *The Design and Analysis of Sequential Clinical Trials*. Ellis Horwood, Chichester.

ROBERT T. O'NEILL

Case–Control Study, Two-Phase

Double sampling, also known as two-phase sampling, is a standard technique for **stratification** [19]. The investigator first draws a random sample from the population to measure the covariates needed for stratification. At phase two, random subsamples of varying size are drawn from within each stratum and the collection of data is completed for subjects selected at both phases. By using larger sampling ratios for the most informative strata, the efficiency of estimates of population parameters is enhanced.

The **case–control study** embodies a stratified sampling design where the strata depend on the outcome [4]. Case–control studies in epidemiology typically sample a large fraction of the **incident cases** of disease and a much smaller fraction of disease-free **controls** to evaluate the association between disease outcome and risk factors. This design is much more efficient than alternative **cohort** or **cross-sectional designs** for the study of a rare disease.

More complex double-sampling techniques offer the potential to enhance efficiency further and to reduce cost. White [33] proposed studying the association between a rare exposure and a rare disease by sampling at phase two on the basis of *both* disease and exposure status. She noted that the initial sample might itself be stratified by outcome, as in a case–control study, or not, as in a cohort or cross-sectional study. Another example of double sampling arises from secondary analysis, where the collection of data on a new covariate is limited to a subset of the original study group [8]. A third example is

the **validation study**. Here subsamples of cases and controls are drawn to make error-free measurements, so that parameter estimates may be adjusted for the attenuation caused by **measurement error** [9]. In all three examples, subjects not sampled for phase two have a portion of their data missing by design. There is a strong connection with the literature on **missing data** [17, 22].

This article reviews double sampling techniques for the study of binary outcomes, with particular emphasis on methods of fitting **logistic regression** models that appropriately utilize the data from both phases of sampling.

Stratified Sampling

Under the usual superpopulation model, the population from which subjects are sampled at phase one is regarded as infinite. Let S denote a random variable defined on this population whose values $S = j$ indicate the stratum and set $\pi_j = \Pr(S = j)$, $j = 1, \ldots, J$. Suppose for the moment that the object is to estimate the mean value, μ, of another random variable, U, and note that $\mu = \sum_j \pi_j \mu_j$, where $\mu_j = \mathrm{E}(U|S = j)$. Assuming that the π_j are known, appropriately stratified sampling yields a more informative estimate than does a simple random sample of like size [11].

Double Sampling for Stratification

Often the information needed for classification of population units into strata is not known in advance. Neyman [19] developed the theory of double sampling to handle this problem. At the first phase of sampling one draws a simple random sample of size N for stratum ascertainment and observes N_j, the number of sampled subjects, with $S = j$. At the second phase, subsamples of specified size n_j are drawn at random and without replacement from among the N_j in stratum j, for a total sample size of $n = \sum_j n_j$. Denote by U_{jk} the value of U for the kth subject in stratum j, $k = 1, \ldots, n_j$; by $f_j = n_j/N_j$ the known sampling fraction; and by $\overline{U}_j = n_j^{-1} \sum_k U_{jk}$ the stratum specific sample mean. With $\hat{\pi}_j = N_j/N$ and $\hat{\mu}_j = \overline{U}_j$, an obvious estimate of μ is

$$\hat{\mu} = \sum_{j=1}^{J} \hat{\pi}_j \hat{\mu}_j = N^{-1} \sum_{j=1}^{J} f_j^{-1} \sum_{k=1}^{n_j} U_{jk}. \quad (1)$$

The Horvitz–Thompson Estimator

When regarded as an estimator of the (unknown) finite population mean of the N values of U for subjects sampled at phase one, $\hat{\mu}$ weights each of the n phase two observations by the inverse of its selection probability. This is the defining property of the famous Horvitz–Thompson [13] estimator. The variance as given in standard texts [11] is

$$\text{var}(\hat{\mu}) = \frac{1}{N} \sum_{j=1}^{J} \pi_j (\mu_j - \mu)^2 + \sum_{j=1}^{J} \frac{\pi_j^2 \sigma_j^2}{n_j}$$
$$+ \frac{1}{N} \sum_{j=1}^{J} \frac{\pi_j (1 - \pi_j) \sigma_j^2}{n_j}, \qquad (2)$$

where $\sigma_j^2 = \text{var}(U|S = j)$. The first two terms dominate under an asymptotic scheme where each of the n_j increases proportionately with N. For fixed n, efficiency is enhanced by oversampling large strata or those with large σ_j^2 since this will reduce the value of the middle term in (2).

Weighted Likelihood and the Horvitz–Thompson Estimator

In case–control studies the parameters of interest are not the mean values of random variables but rather the regression coefficients in probability models for the association between a binary outcome variable Y and a vector $\mathbf{X}$ of explanatory variables. Suppose that

$$\Pr(Y = 1|\mathbf{X} = \mathbf{x}, S = j) = \Pr(Y = 1|\mathbf{X} = \mathbf{x}) = F(\mathbf{x}'\beta), \qquad (3)$$

where F denotes a known cumulative distribution function. Typical choices for F are the logistic distribution for logistic regression and the unit normal distribution for probit regression. The assumption of conditional independence between Y and S given $\mathbf{X}$ means simply that any dependence of the outcome probability on stratum is modeled in $\mathbf{X}$.

Under standard regularity conditions, likelihood theory tells us that β satisfies the expected score equation

$$\mu(\beta) = \text{E}[\mathbf{U}(\beta)] = \text{E} \left[\frac{\partial \log \Pr(Y|\mathbf{X}; \beta)}{\partial \beta} \right] = 0, \quad (4)$$

where $\mathbf{U}(\beta)$ is defined as the term in brackets. Even if (3) does not hold, the solution to (4) defines a

parameter of interest since it identifies that member of a set of hypothesized models that best describes the population association. If observations on $(Y_t, \mathbf{X}_t)$ were available for all N subjects sampled at phase one, then β would be estimated by solving the score equations $\mathbf{U}(\beta) = \sum_{t=1}^{N} \mathbf{U}_t(\beta) = 0$. In a two-phase study, the unknown $\mathbf{U}$ is estimated using (1). Thus, following Whittemore [34], we define the Horvitz–Thompson estimator, $\hat{\beta}$, as the solution to the Horvitz–Thompson estimating equations

$$\hat{\mathbf{U}}(\beta) = \sum_{j=1}^{J} f_j^{-1} \sum_{k=1}^{n_j} \mathbf{U}_{jk}(\beta) = 0, \qquad (5)$$

where $\mathbf{U}_{jk}(\beta)$ denotes the score for the kth subject sampled from stratum j. The consistency and asymptotic normality of $\hat{\beta}$ follow from Huber's [15] theory of M-estimation. The asymptotic variance is given by the "information sandwich"

$$\text{var}_A(\hat{\beta}) = \left[\frac{\partial \hat{\mathbf{U}}(\beta)}{\partial \beta} \right]^{-1}$$
$$\times \text{var}_A[\hat{\mathbf{U}}(\beta)] \left\{ \left[\frac{\partial \hat{\mathbf{U}}(\beta)}{\partial \beta} \right]' \right\}^{-1} \Bigg|_{\beta = \hat{\beta}}, \qquad (6)$$

where the middle expression is obtained by extending (2) to vector-valued random variables.

The Horvitz–Thompson estimator and its analog have a long history. In econometrics it is known as the weighted exogenous sampling maximum likelihood estimator [18]. A finite population version was studied by Binder [3] and Chambless & Boyle [10]. Others have referred to the weighted likelihood method alternatively as pseudo-maximum likelihood [28], design-based [24], pseudo-likelihood [12, 16], and mean score [21].

Two-Phase Case–Control Studies

The distinguishing feature of a case–control study is that the variables used for stratification and sample selection include the outcome (case–control) status. Were this not the case, and the sample was stratified using explanatory variables alone, standard methods of binary regression analysis could be used to estimate the regression coefficients in the model (3).

Such methods generally yield biased estimates, however, when applied to case–control data. Horvitz–Thompson estimation solves the **bias** problem.

Population-Based Case–Control Samples

Suppose the population from which the cases and controls are sampled has been completely enumerated and that disease status Y and stratum S are known for everyone. This (finite) population may itself then be regarded as the preliminary random sample in the two phase design. Since the sampling fractions are known for both cases and controls, no restrictions need be placed on F and both **absolute** and **relative risk** parameters may be estimated [2].

To apply the Horvitz–Thompson estimator to **population-based case–control studies**, we extend the notation to allow the phase one strata to depend on both Y and S. Thus, denote by N_{1j} the number of cases ($Y = 1$) and by N_{0j} the number of controls ($Y = 0$) with $S = j$ at phase one, and let n_{ij} denote the numbers in the corresponding subsample at phase two. The Horvitz–Thompson estimator is the solution to

$$\hat{\mathbf{U}}(\beta) = \sum_{i=0}^{1}\sum_{j=1}^{J} f_{ij}^{-1}\sum_{k=1}^{n_{ij}} \mathbf{U}_{ijk}(\beta) = 0, \qquad (7)$$

where now $f_{ij} = n_{ij}/N_{ij}$ and $\mathbf{U}_{ijk}(\beta)$ denotes the likelihood score for the kth subject in stratum (i, j).

Scott & Wild [25, 26] and Wild [36] studied the semiparametric efficient maximum likelihood estimator for this problem. For the special case of logistic regression, they provided a computational algorithm that involves repeated fitting of logistic models with offsets dependent on results obtained at the previous iteration.

Separate Preliminary Samples of Cases and Controls

More typically, a complete enumeration of the population at risk is not available, and one simply samples controls from the same communities or hospital service areas in which the cases arose. Then the appropriate model treats the phase one subjects as separate random samples of N_1 cases and N_0 controls. Since the case and control sampling fractions are not known, the only quantities that may be estimated consistently are **odds ratio** (**relative risk**) parameters in "multiplicative intercept" models [14]. Attention is confined here to the logistic model $F(x) = 1/(1 + e^{-x})$. Provided that the linear predictor $x'\beta$ includes a constant term β_0, the remaining βs represent log relative risks that are in principle estimable from the case–control sample. The logistic scores appearing in (7) are given by $\mathbf{U}_{ijk}(\beta) = \{Y_{ijk} - 1/[1 + \exp(-\mathbf{X}'_{ijk}\beta)]\}\mathbf{X}_{ijk}$.

Assume momentarily that the marginal outcome probabilities are known and set $\alpha = \log[\Pr(Y = 1)/\Pr(Y = 0)]$. If the constant term $\log(N_1/N_0) - \alpha$ is added to β_0, then the Horvitz–Thompson estimating equations (7) are unbiased for all parameters, including the intercept, and the corresponding estimator is consistent [6, 12]. The equations are easily solved using standard programs for logistic regression by treating the inverse sampling fractions f_{ij}^{-1} as prior weights (*see* **Software, Biostatistical**). The asymptotic variance is again given by (6), except that now the middle term is estimated by

$$\sum_{i=0}^{1}\sum_{j=1}^{J} f_{ij}^{-2}\left\{\sum_{k=1}^{n_{ij}} \mathbf{U}_{ijk}^{\otimes 2} - \frac{1 - f_{ij}}{n_{ij}}\left(\sum_{k=1}^{n_{ij}} \mathbf{U}_{ijk}\right)^{\otimes 2}\right\}$$

$$- \sum_{i=0}^{1}\frac{1}{N_i}\left(\sum_{j=1}^{J} f_{ij}^{-1}\sum_{k=1}^{n_{ij}} \mathbf{U}_{ijk}\right)^{\otimes 2},$$

where $\mathbf{u}^{\otimes 2}$ for any vector $\mathbf{u}$ denotes the matrix $\mathbf{uu}'$. The last expression involving the N_i, which only affects the variance of $\hat{\beta}_0$, reflects the extra information obtained by assuming α to be known and has no counterpart in (2). In practice, α is not known. Since its value only affects the free parameter β_0, however, this does not matter. One simply ignores $\hat{\beta}_0$ and its standard error.

Breslow & Holubkov [7] studied the maximum likelihood estimator of logistic regression coefficients for the two-phase design with separate sampling of cases and controls at phase one. They showed that it was identical to Scott & Wild's estimator, for which the phase one sampling was not outcome dependent. They also provided a faster iterative logistic regression computing algorithm and a simplified formula for the asymptotic variance. Although one can concoct exceptional data sets for which the maximum likelihood estimator is substantially more efficient than Horvitz–Thompson, in most practical settings the loss of information is slight. Many researchers prefer the Horvitz–Thompson approach because, at least for the **population-based study**, it provides a consistent estimator of a meaningful population parameter even if the model (3) does not hold.

Pseudo-Likelihood Estimators

A third method of estimation of logistic regression coefficients, which is typically of intermediate efficiency, was developed by Breslow & Cain [5] and by Schill et al. [23]. This is a pseudo-likelihood method in the sense that it uses unbiased estimating equations that arise from maximization of a product of conditional probabilities. For the Breslow–Cain version one fits the logistic regression model (3) to the phase two data, using as offsets in the linear predictor the terms $\log(n_{1j}N_{0j}) - \log(n_{0j}N_{1j})$ for observations in stratum j to adjust for the biased sampling. A matrix formula is available that corrects the usual asymptotic variance matrix to account for the additional information coming from the phase one data. The Schill version of the pseudo-likelihood estimator involves fitting a logistic regression model jointly to the phase one and phase two data and also requires offsets. Whenever the linear predictor contains a separate term for the main effect of each stratum, the two pseudo-likelihood estimators and the maximum likelihood estimator are identical.

Fixed vs. Random Phase Two Sample Sizes

So far we have assumed that the sample sizes, n_{ij}, at the second phase of sampling are fixed by the investigator after considering results of the phase one data collection. An alternative sampling strategy uses a random device to decide independently for each phase one subject, using selection probabilities p_{ij} that depend on (Y, S), whether to include the subject at phase two. This is known by econometricians as Manski–Lerman [18] sampling. In the context of case–control studies, Weinberg & Sandler [31] called it the randomized recruitment method and suggested it as an alternative to **frequency matching**. Others have referred to it as Bernoulli sampling. The associated sampling theory is simplified by the fact that the phase two observations are rendered statistically independent.

Both Horvitz–Thompson and pseudo-likelihood estimation procedures may be applied to data collected in randomized recruitment designs. Instead of dividing the log likelihood contributions by the observed sampling ratios, f_{ij}, one divides by the expected ones, p_{ij}. Use of the observed ratios is also justified; just condition on the n_{ij} and use the previous theory. Both empirical [32] and theoretical [22] studies show that use of the known selection probabilities results in less efficient estimates, however, so it is best to treat the phase two sample sizes as fixed even when they are not.

An Example

Cain & Breslow [8] gave an example of a two-phase study that illustrates basic concepts. Table 1 shows sample sizes at phases one and two for a study of the association of operative mortality and gender in patients undergoing coronary bypass surgery. Two different designs were used at phase two: a "case–control" design in which the subsamples of 100 cases (deceased) and 100 controls (alive) were drawn without consideration of the stratum variable gender; and a "balanced" design in which equal numbers ($n_{ij} = 50$) were drawn from within each of the four cells defined by both outcome and gender. More generally a balanced design involving n phase two subjects would set $n_{ij} = \min(n/2J, N_{ij})$. Since the "case–control" design involves sampling only with regard to outcome, fitting ordinary logistic regression models yields valid estimates of relative risk parameters [20]. Fitting of ordinary logistic regression models to data from the "balanced" design, however, results in biased estimates of the gender effect since the association between outcome and gender at

Table 1 Sample sizes for a study relating operative mortality to gender for patients undergoing coronary artery bypass surgery

	Male ($S = 1$)	Female ($S = 2$)
First phase sample (N_{ij})		
Alive ($Y = 0$)	6,666	1,228
Deceased ($Y = 1$)	144	58
Second phase sample: case–control (n_{ij})		
Alive	81	19
Deceased	67	33
Second phase sample: balanced (n_{ij})		
Alive	50	50
Deceased	50	50

Source: Cain & Breslow [8], reproduced by permission of the publisher.

Table 2 Logistic regression coefficients (and standard errors) for the data in Table 1

Model term	First phase sample	Second phase sample: case–control		Second phase sample: balanced	
		Unadjusted	Adjusted	Unadjusted	Adjusted
Constant	−3.271 (0.285)	−0.167 (0.615)	−3.812 (0.594)	0.990 (0.637)	−2.845 (0.606)
Female sex	0.634 (0.171)	0.650 (0.348)	0.690 (0.190)	−0.061 (0.301)	0.722 (0.189)
Diameter of arteries	−0.065 (0.016)	−0.030 (0.034)		−0.080 (0.033)	
Congestive heart failure (CHF) score	0.445 (0.072)	0.395 (0.160)		0.348 (0.165)	
Priority of surgery[a]					
Urgent	0.706 (0.181)	0.631 (0.365)		0.412 (0.350)	
Emergency	2.004 (0.232)	2.605 (1.072)		1.853 (0.800)	

Source: Cain & Breslow [8], reproduced by permission of the publisher.
[a]Relative to elective surgery.

phase two is completely distorted by the nonproportional sampling ratios.

Table 2 reports results of estimating logistic regression coefficients for gender and other covariates by two methods: ordinary logistic regression and "adjusted" logistic regression. Since gender is included in the model, simple adjustments may be applied directly to the results from ordinary logistic regression programs to calculate the maximum likelihood estimates and their standard errors [8]. Furthermore, adjusted and unadjusted results for the covariates other than gender are identical [5]. Note the severe distortion of the gender coefficient for the unadjusted analysis of the balanced data, and the substantial reduction in its standard error, when adjustment is made for the information available at phase one. Results of fitting the same model to the entire phase one data set, for which all the covariate values were in fact known, are shown for comparison.

Efficiency Gains from Stratification

The standard errors shown in Table 2 suggest there was little benefit with these data from use of the balanced design at phase two. In other situations one should expect the balanced design to yield more efficient estimates of coefficients that model stratum effects and their **interactions**, at the possible cost of some mild loss of efficiency for estimates of the other covariate effects. This conclusion is based on the asymptotic efficiencies shown in Table 3 for models with a binary stratum coefficient, β_1, and a binary covariate, β_2, with and without an interaction term, β_3. Part (a) of the table shows results for a study where all cases identified at phase one are also used at phase two. Here the principal efficiency gain is for

Table 3 Large-sample efficiencies of the balanced design relative to the case–control design
(a) Second phase sample contains all the cases but only a fraction of the controls from the first phase sample

e^{β_2}	θ^a	Relative efficiency		
		β_1	β_2	β_3
0.2	0.2	1.02	0.83	1.43
0.2	1.0	1.18	0.88	1.45
0.2	5.0	1.34	0.93	1.65
1.0	0.2	0.99	0.74	2.30
1.0	1.0	1.00	0.81	2.09
1.0	5.0	0.98	0.82	2.06
5.0	0.2	1.14	0.76	2.94
5.0	1.0	1.22	0.81	2.12
5.0	5.0	1.00	0.76	1.74

(b) Second phase sample contains a small fraction of both cases and controls from the first phase sample

e^{β_2}	θ^a	Relative efficiency		
		β_1	β_2	β_3
0.2	0.2	1.37	0.68	4.41
0.2	1.0	4.35	1.01	3.51
0.2	5.0	3.56	1.47	3.30
1.0	0.2	0.71	0.71	5.77
1.0	1.0	1.00	1.01	4.08
1.0	5.0	1.05	1.05	3.90
5.0	0.2	1.84	0.78	6.48
5.0	1.0	3.72	1.01	4.10
5.0	5.0	1.36	0.83	3.44

Source: Cain & Breslow [8], reproduced by permission of the publisher.
[a]θ = odds ratio measure of association between S and X among controls.

the interaction effect. When subsamples of both cases and controls are taken at phase two, as shown in part (b), stratum and interaction effects are both estimated more efficiently using the balanced design.

While the balanced design seems reasonable on general grounds and has good efficiency properties over a large region of the parameter space, other designs offer greater efficiency in particular circumstances. For the measurement error problem with Horvitz–Thompson estimation, Reilly & Pepe [21] derived expressions for the optimal sampling fractions, f_{ij}, needed for estimation of a particular regression coefficient. They presented numerical results for a logistic regression model with a single explanatory variable, X, assumed to have a standard normal distribution. Stratification was based on a binary, S, indicating whether or not X, when measured with normally distributed error, is positive. Although intended for cohort sampling at phase one, their results apply also to the two-phase case–control study provided that the intercept parameter, β_0, is interpreted as applying to the case–control sample rather than the source population.

Table 4 shows the optimal sampling fractions for a study involving $N = 500$ phase one subjects, 25% of whom are to be selected for the validation sample at phase two. Note that the balanced design here is optimal only when $\beta_0 = \beta_1 = 0$. As with all design problems, the optimal sampling fractions depend on the values of unknown parameters, so that prior information or a good guess is needed to achieve

near optimality. Tosteson & Ware [29] considered a similar problem in which the outcome, Y, is also **misclassified** at the first phase of sampling.

Other Complex Sampling Designs

Whittemore [34] studied Horvitz–Thompson estimation for designs with three or more sampling phases based on nested partitions of the sample space into increasingly fine strata. Noting that the selection probabilities for observations with complete covariate data were given by products of the inverse sampling fractions at each phase, she derived an explicit expression for the variance of the scores used in the information sandwich formula (6). Results were given for both fixed sample size and random recruitment at the second and each succeeding phase.

Whittemore & Halpern [35] gave an example of a three-phase study of the association between prostatic cancer and lifestyle factors. The first phase involved a case–control sample of men with and without a history of prostate cancer. Each was asked if he had a brother with the disease, and subsamples were drawn at phase two according to whether or not there was a positive reply. A complete family history was taken for those so selected. In a third phase of sampling all the subjects whose families had three or more cases of prostate cancer were asked to provide blood or tissue specimens for deoxyribonucleic acid (DNA) analysis. Data of interest for statistical modeling included the complete family histories and the DNA results. Variance formulas were used to determine optimal sampling fractions at phases two and three for estimation of parameters in genetic models. Stratification of the phase two sample, using the reply to the simple question posed at phase one, remarkably improved efficiency.

Benichou et al. [1] provided another example of three-phase sampling involving women participating in a large-scale breast cancer demonstration project. Data on age, treatment center, and date of entry into the study were available initially for 280 000 women. The second phase involved selection of approximately 3000 breast cancer cases and 3000 controls with data on family history and clinical and reproductive risk factors. At the third phase, subsamples were selected on the basis of the availability of mammographic information. This example is best characterized as a problem with a complex pattern of

Table 4 Optimal sampling fractions f_{ij}

		$\sigma = 0.25^a$				
(β_0, β_1):	(0,0)	(0,1)	(0,2)	(1,0)	(1,1)	(2,2)
f_{01}	0.25	0.46	0.12	0.28	0.11	0.21
f_{02}	0.25	0.47	0.52	0.61	0.75	0.80
f_{11}	0.25	0.17	0.54	0.43	0.72	0.56
f_{12}	0.25	0.17	0.12	0.04	0.11	0.06
		$\sigma = 1.00^a$				
(β_0, β_1):	(0,0)	(0,1)	(0,2)	(1,0)	(1,1)	(2,2)
f_{01}	0.25	0.46	0.17	0.30	0.16	0.23
f_{02}	0.25	0.46	0.37	0.52	0.44	0.56
f_{11}	0.25	0.17	0.38	0.31	0.42	0.35
f_{12}	0.25	0.17	0.18	0.11	0.18	0.13

Source: Reilly & Pepe [21], reproduced by permission of the publisher.

[a]σ = standard deviation of measurement error distribution.

missing data, because at phases two and three only those cases and controls with complete data on the relevant covariates were retained. The authors developed their own pseudo-likelihood analysis, using the parametric bootstrap for calculation of standard errors.

The essential feature of the multiphase sampling design [34] that makes it amenable to simple Horvitz–Thompson estimation is the fact that the resulting data are subject to a *monotone* pattern of *missingness* [17]. The covariates may be ordered so that the groups of subjects missing each one of them are nested within each other. For other complex sampling designs the data analysis is inherently more difficult and may require additional parametric assumptions. Wacholder et al. [30], for example, proposed the *partial questionnaire* design for case–control studies as a means of reducing the length of the questionnaire administered to most subjects. Different subgroups of subjects are given distinct questionnaires that are missing different blocks of questions, so that the missingness pattern is *nonmonotone*. They developed a pseudo-likelihood estimation procedure that requires explicit estimation of the joint covariate distribution in the sample. Consequently, the technique is currently restricted to studies with a small number of discrete covariates.

Conclusions

Relatively few examples of two- and three-phase sampling designs for case–control studies have appeared to date in the epidemiologic literature. This is unfortunate, because the stratified designs are easy to implement and can result in substantial savings. Procedures for Horvitz–Thompson estimation of logistic regression coefficients have been implemented in software designed specially for complex sample surveys [27]. Development of macros for Horvitz–Thompson, pseudo-likelihood, and maximum likelihood estimation of logistic regression parameters for data from two-phase studies, using the flexibility provided by many of the more popular general purpose computing packages, would help to stimulate interest in and use of these valuable statistical methods. Further work is required to develop efficient estimation methods for other complex sampling designs that may be equally valuable in practice.

Acknowledgment

This work was supported in part by a US Public Health Services Grant CA 40644.

References

[1] Benichou, J., Byrne, C. & Gail, M. (1997). An approach to estimating exposure-specific rates of breast cancer from a two-stage case–control study within a cohort, *Statistics in Medicine* **16**, 133–151.

[2] Benichou, J. & Wacholder, S. (1994). Epidemiologic methods: a comparison of three approaches to estimate exposure-specific incidence rates from population-based case–control data, *Statistics in Medicine* **13**, 651–661.

[3] Binder, D.A. (1983). On the variances of asymptotically normal estimators from complex surveys, *International Statistical Review* **51**, 279–292.

[4] Breslow, N.E. (1996). Statistics in epidemiology: the case–control study, *Journal of the American Statistical Association* **91**, 14–28.

[5] Breslow, N.E. & Cain, K.C. (1988). Logistic regression for two-stage case–control data, *Biometrika* **75**, 11–20.

[6] Breslow, N.E. & Holubkov, R. (1997). Weighted likelihood, pseudo-likelihood and maximum likelihood methods for logistic regression analysis of two-stage data, *Statistics in Medicine* **16**, 103–116.

[7] Breslow, N.E. & Holubkov, R. (1997). Maximum likelihood estimation of logistic regression parameters under two-phase, outcome-dependent sampling, *Journal of the Royal Statistical Society, Series B* **59**, 447–461.

[8] Cain, K.C. & Breslow, N.E. (1988). Logistic regression analysis and efficient design for two-stage studies, *American Journal of Epidemiology* **128**, 1198–1206.

[9] Carroll, R.J., Ruppert, D. & Stefanski, L.A. (1995). *Measurement Error in Nonlinear Models*. Chapman & Hall, New York.

[10] Chambless, L.E. & Boyle, K.E. (1985). Maximum likelihood methods for complex sample data: logistic regression and discrete proportional hazards models, *Communications in Statistics – Theory and Methods* **14**, 1377–1392.

[11] Cochran, W.G. (1963). *Sampling Techniques*, 2nd Ed. Wiley, New York.

[12] Flanders, W.D. & Greenland, S. (1991). Analytic methods for two-stage case–control studies and other stratified designs, *Statistics in Medicine* **10**, 739–747.

[13] Horvitz, D.G. & Thompson, D.J. (1951). A generalization of sampling without replacement from a finite universe, *Journal of the American Statistical Association* **47**, 663–685.

[14] Hsieh, D.A., Manski, C.F. & McFadden, D. (1985). Estimation of response probabilities from augmented retrospective observations, *Journal of the American Statistical Association* **80**, 651–662.

[15] Huber, P.J. (1967). The behavior of maximum likelihood estimates under nonstandard conditions,

in *Proceedings of the Fifth Berkeley Symposium on Mathematical Statistics and Probability*, J. Neyman, ed. University of California Press, Berkeley, pp. 221–233.

[16] Kalbfleisch, J.D. & Lawless, J.F. (1988). Likelihood analysis of multi-state models for disease incidence and mortality, *Statistics in Medicine* **7**, 149–160.

[17] Little, R.J.A. & Rubin, D.B. (1987) *Statistical Analysis with Missing Data*. Wiley, New York.

[18] Manski, C.F. & Lerman, S.R. (1977). The estimation of choice probabilities from choice based samples, *Econometrica* **45**, 1977–1988.

[19] Neyman, J. (1938). Contribution to the theory of sampling human populations, *Journal of the American Statistical Association* **33**, 101–116.

[20] Prentice, R.L. & Pyke, R. (1979). Logistic disease incidence models and case–control studies, *Biometrika* **66**, 403–411.

[21] Reilly, M. & Pepe, M.S. (1995). A mean score method for missing and auxiliary covariate data in regression models, *Biometrika* **82**, 299–314.

[22] Robins, J.M., Rotnitzky, A. & Zhao, L.P. (1994). Estimation of regression coefficients when some regressors are not always observed, *Journal of the American Statistical Association* **89**, 846–866.

[23] Schill, W., Jöckel K.-H., Drescher, K. & Timm, J. (1993). Logistic analysis in case–control studies under validation sampling, *Biometrika* **80**, 339–352.

[24] Scott, A.J. & Wild, C.J. (1985). Selection based on the response variable in logistic regression, in *Analysis of Complex Surveys*, C.J. Skinner, D. Holt & T.M.F. Smith, eds. Wiley, New York, pp. 191–205.

[25] Scott, A.J. & Wild, C.J. (1991). Fitting logistic regression models in stratified case–control studies, *Biometrics* **47**, 497–510.

[26] Scott, A.J. & Wild, C.J. (1997). Fitting regression models to case–control data by maximum likelihood, *Biometrika* **84**, 57–71.

[27] Shah, B.V., Folsom, R.E., LaVange, L.M., Wheeless, S.C., Boyle, K.E. & Williams, R.L. (1993). *Statistical Methods and Mathematical Algorithms Used in SUDAAN*. Research Triangle Institute, Research Triangle Park, North Carolina.

[28] Skinner, C.J. (1985). Domain means, regression and multivariate analysis, in *Analysis of Complex Surveys*, C.J. Skinner, D. Holt, & T.M.F. Smith, eds. Wiley, New York, pp. 59–87.

[29] Tosteson, T.D. & Ware, J.H. (1990). Designing a logistic regression study using surrogate measures for exposure and outcome, *Biometrika* **77**, 11–21.

[30] Wacholder, S., Carroll, R.J., Pee, D. & Gail, M. (1994). The partial questionnaire design for case–control studies, *Statistics in Medicine* **13**, 623–634.

[31] Weinberg, C.R. & Sandler, D.P. (1991). Randomized recruitment in case–control studies, *American Journal of Epidemiology* **134**, 421–432.

[32] Weinberg, C.R. & Wacholder, S. (1990). The design and analysis of case–control studies with biased sampling, *Biometrics* **46**, 963–975.

[33] White, J.E. (1982). A two stage design for the study of the relationship between a rare exposure and a rare disease, *American Journal of Epidemiology* **115**, 119–128.

[34] Whittemore, A.S. (1997). Multistage sampling designs and estimating equations. *Journal of the Royal Statistical Society, Series B* **59**, 589–602.

[35] Whittemore, A. & Halpern, J. (1997). Multistage sampling in genetic epidemiology, *Statistics in Medicine* **16**, 153–167.

[36] Wild, C.J. (1991). Fitting prospective regression models to case–control data, *Biometrika* **78**, 705–717.

N.E. BRESLOW

Case–Control Surveillance *see* Pharmacoepidemiology, Study Designs

Case-Crossover Design *see* Pharmacoepidemiology, Overview

Case-Dependent Disease Process *see* Geographical Analysis

Case-Independent Disease Process *see* Geographical Analysis

Case–Referent Study *see* Case–Control Study

Case–Time-Control Design *see* Pharmacoepidemiology, Overview

Catalytic Models *see* Communicable Diseases

Category Matching *see* Frequency Matching

Causality, Hill's Criteria *see* Hill's Criteria for Causality

Causation

The concepts of cause and effect are central to most areas of scientific research, so it is not surprising that the literature on them could fill a small library. What may be surprising, given their importance, is that consensus about basic definitions and methods for causal inference is (at best) limited, despite some three centuries of debate. A brief review cannot do justice to the history and details of this debate, nor to all the schools of thought on causation. This article will, therefore, focus on a few major themes that have affected modern biostatistical practice. Of necessity, some aspects of the discussion are simplified relative to the literature, and the references should be consulted for more thorough descriptions. Entries on related topics are given in the final section.

Counterfactual Causation

At least as far back as the early eighteenth century, philosophers noted serious deficiencies in ordinary definitions of causation (e.g. see Hume [8]). For example, *Webster's New Twentieth Century Dictionary* [12] offers "that which produces an effect or result" as a definition of "cause". The circularity of this definition becomes apparent when one discovers "to cause" among the definitions of "produces". In early scientific treatises, an event (or set of events)

A was said to cause a later event B if there was "constant conjunction" or "regularity" of the events, in that A (the cause) was inevitably followed by B ("the effect"). Mill [13] pointed out that such "constant conjunction" could always be the effect of a third event C preceding A and B; in other words, the regularity of B following A might only be due to **confounding**. Informal definitions of "effect" suffer from the same problems, because "effect" as a verb is merely a synonym for "cause", while "effect" as a noun is defined as a "result", which is, in turn, defined as an "effect" in causal contexts.

Hume [7], however, offered in passing another view of causation that pointed a way out of circularity or confounding in the definition (even if confounding might be inevitable in the observation). In the present terminology, Hume proposed that A caused B if failure of A to occur would have been sufficient for failure of B to occur (see Lewis [10]). That is, by focusing on specific instances of causation, we could say that a specific event A caused a specific event B if occurrence of A was necessary for B under the observed background circumstances. Essentially, the same concept of causation can be found in [3] and [13] (both quoted in [22]).

Of course, the preceding definition falls short of the formalism necessary for rigorous logical analysis. Such analysis first appeared in the statistics literature in [14]. The basic idea is as follows: Suppose N units indexed by $i = 1, \ldots, N$ are to be observed in an experiment that will assign each unit to one of K treatments $x_1, \ldots, x_K$. For each unit, the outcome of interest is the value of a response variable Y_i. It is assumed that Y_i will equal y_{ik} if unit i is assigned treatment x_k. Suppose that one treatment level, say x_1, is designated the reference treatment against which other treatments are to be evaluated (typically, x_1 is "no treatment", placebo, or standard treatment). We may then define the causal *effect* of $x_k (k > 1)$ on Y_i relative to x_1 (the reference) to be $y_{ik} - y_{i1}$. Alternatively, if the response is restricted to positive values (such as blood pressure), we may define causal effect as y_{ik}/y_{i1} or $\log y_{ik} - \log y_{i1}$.

This definition of effect leads naturally to a precise usage for the word "cause". Prior to treatment, we say y_k would cause a change of $y_{ik} - y_{i1}$ in Y_i; if $y_{ik} - y_{i1} = 0$, we say x_k would cause no change in Y_i. After the experiment, if unit i had received treatment k, then we say that x_k caused a change of

$y_{ik} - y_{i1}$ in Y_i; otherwise, we say that x_k would have caused a change of $y_{ik} - y_{i1}$ in Y_i.

There are four crucial restrictions that the preceding formalism places on the notion of effect (and, hence, cause). First, effects are defined only within comparisons of treatment levels. To say that "drinking two glasses of wine a day lengthened Smith's life by four years" is meaningless by itself. A reference level must be at least implicit to make sense of the statement. Smith might have lived even longer had she consumed one rather than two glasses per day. As given, the statement could refer to no wine or four glasses per day or any other possibility.

Secondly, more subtly and profoundly, the formalism assumes that y_{ik}, the response of unit i under treatment k, remains well defined even if unit i is *not* given treatment k. In the philosophy literature, this assumption and the problems attendant with it are recognized as problems of *counterfactual* analysis [10, 11, 24] (see also the discussion of Holland [6]). The statement "if x_k had been administered, then the response Y_i of unit i would have been y_{ik}" is called a *counterfactual conditional*: it asserts that Y_i would equal y_{ik} if, *contrary to fact*, x_k had been administered to unit i. Consider again Smith's drinking. Suppose she would contract cancer at age 70 if she drank two glasses of wine a day, but would instead die of a stroke at age 68 if she drank no wine. If Y_i is her time to cancer and she drank two glasses per day, how could we define her counterfactual time to cancer given no wine? Without this definition, the effect of two glasses of wine vs. none would be undefined.

The preceding problem is common in **survival analysis** when **competing risks** are present. The problem is not solved by attempting to condition on "absence of competing risks": such hypothetical absence is itself not a well-defined counterfactual state, even though standard probability calculations (as used in product-limit estimates) make it appear otherwise (see Kalbfleisch & Prentice [9, p. 166], and Prentice & Kalbfleisch [18], for further discussion). Rather, the definition of the response must be amended to include the competing risks if the counterfactual definition is to be applied. For example, Y_i could become the pair comprising time of cancer or competing risk and an indicator marking the event at that time.

Thirdly, the effects captured by the counterfactual definition are *net effects*, in that they include all indirect effects and **interactions** not specifically excluded by the treatment definition. For example, Smith's consumption of two glasses of wine per day rather than none may have given her four extra years of life solely because one night at a formal dinner it made her feel unsteady and she had a friend drive her home; had she not drunk, she would have driven herself and been hit and killed by a drunk driver. This sort of indirect effect is not one we would wish to capture when studying biological effects of wine use. It is, nonetheless, included in our measure of effect (as well as any estimate) unless we amend our treatment definition to include holding constant all "risky" activities that take place during Smith's life. Such amendment is sometimes (simplistically) subsumed under the clause of "all other things being equal (apart from treatment)", but can be a serious source of ambiguity when the intervention that enforces the amendment is not well defined.

A fourth restriction, which may be considered an aspect of the third, is that the formalism assumes that treatments not applied to a unit could have been applied. Suppose Smith would not, and could not, stop daily wine consumption unless forced physically to do so. The effect of her actual two-glass-a-day consumption vs. the counterfactual "no wine" would now be undefined without amending the treatment definition to include forcing Smith to drink no wine, e.g. by forcibly injecting Smith with antabuse each day of her life. Such amendment would be of little interest, not just because of its wild impracticality, but because of the side effects it would introduce.

The preceding restriction is sometimes accounted for by requiring that the counterfactual definition of "effect" applies only to "treatment variables". The latter are defined informally as variables subject to manipulation of their levels; an additional restriction is made that each possible level (treatment) for the treatment variable has nonzero probability of occurrence (e.g. see Holland [6]). One may sense here an echo of the circularity in ordinary definitions of cause, for this notion of manipulation embodies having an effect on treatment levels. Nonetheless, it has been argued that one strength of the counterfactual approach is its explication of the ambiguities inherent in defining cause and effect [10, 22].

One model of causation that has enjoyed some popularity in epidemiology is the sufficient-component cause (SCC) model introduced by Rothman [20]. This model presents causal mechanisms via schematic "pie charts" composed of slices representing necessary causal components of mechanisms. It can be shown that this model can be mapped into the general counterfactual framework, although it involves certain nonidentifiable elaborations [4].

Probabilistic Causation

A number of authors have attempted to formalize causation through axioms governing the evolution of probabilities over time (e.g. see Suppes [25] and Eells [2]). Such systems have attracted little attention in biostatistics. Other approaches include probabilistic extensions of the counterfactual approach. One is based on the distribution of fixed potential responses; that is, the joint distribution $F(y_1, \ldots, y_K)$ of $y_{i1}, \ldots, y_{iK}$ in a population of units. We may also consider conditional distributions in subpopulations defined by covariates such as age, sex, and received treatment. Population effects can be defined as averages of individual effects over populations; statistical procedures for inferences about these effects follow from assumptions about sampling and treatment assignment mechanisms. The basic ideas were present in Fisher [3] and Neyman [14], and elaborated more generally in Rubin [21–23].

Another extension considers potential responses that are distributional parameters specific to units. For example, we could consider the probability that a given atom emits a photon in the second following absorption of a photon ("treatment 2") minus the probability of emission in the same second if no photon had been absorbed ("treatment 1"). This probability difference is the effect of photon absorption on the atom relative to no absorption. In quantum mechanics, this difference (effect) is well defined *whether or not a photon is actually emitted*. In fact, under the standard quantum model, the emission indicator ($Y_i = 1$ if the atom emits a photon in the second, 0 if not) is *not* well defined under counterfactual alternatives to the actual history of the atom. Fortunately, the latter ambiguity appears to have no practical implications for the gross phenomena studied in biostatistics. It

does, however, illustrate the possibility of considering probabilities and expectations (rather than events) as responses in the counterfactual definition, even for macrophenomena.

Causal Inference

Of causal inference there may be even more written and less agreed than for the basic definitions of cause and effect. A discussion of this literature is beyond the scope of the present article. Issues of **bias**, validity, and generalizability in causal inference are discussed elsewhere (*see* **Bias in Case–Control Studies**; **Bias in Observational Studies**; **Confounding**; **Validity and Generalizability in Epidemiologic Studies**). A discussion of criteria for causal inference [5] may be found in **Hill's Criteria for Causality**; most of these criteria are informal, and the article notes many objections to their use.

Formalisms for causal inference in biostatistics have thus far been restricted to counterfactual-based procedures, as in [1, 14, 21, 23], and to methods based on path diagrams or directed graphs. Starting with Wright [26], path diagrams (more recently called causal diagrams) have been used to display assumptions about the absence of particular effects and to provide a basis for algorithms useful in determining whether effects are identifiable from a given observational process (e.g. Robins [19], Pearl [16], and Pearl & Robins [17]). Most of these approaches take the notion of cause as a primitive; a few define effects in a manner formally equivalent to the counterfactual definition extended to probabilistic domains [15]. The counterfactual approaches emphasize the importance of randomization in assuring identifiability of causal effects [19, 23].

References

[1]   Angrist, J.D., Imbens, G.W. & Rubin, D.B. (1996). Identification of causal effects using instrumental variables (with discussion), *Journal of the American Statistical Association* **91**, 444–472.

[2]   Eells, E. (1991). *Probabilistic Causality*. Cambridge University Press, New York.

[3]   Fisher, R.A. (1918). The causes of human variability, *Eugenics Review* **10**, 213–220.

[4]   Greenland, S. & Poole, C. (1988). Invariants and noninvariants in the concept of interdependent effects,

Scandinavian Journal of Work Environment and Health **14**, 125–129.

[5] Hill, A.B. (1965). The environment and disease: association or causation?, *Proceedings of the Royal Society of Medicine* **58**, 295–300.

[6] Holland, P.W. (1986). Statistics and causal inference (with discussion), *Journal of the American Statistical Association* **81**, 945–970.

[7] Hume, D. (1739; reprinted 1888). *A Treatise of Human Nature*. Oxford University Press, Oxford.

[8] Hume, D. (1748; reprinted 1988). *An Enquiry Concerning Human Understanding*. Open Court Press, LaSalle.

[9] Kalbfleish, J.D. & Prentice, R.L. (1980). *The Statistical Analysis of Failure-Time Data*. Wiley, New York.

[10] Lewis, D. (1973). Causation, *Journal of Philosophy* **70**, 596–567.

[11] Lewis, D. (1973). *Counterfactuals*. Blackwell, Oxford.

[12] McKechnie, J.L., ed. (1979). *Webster's New Twentieth Century Dictionary*. Simon & Schuster, New York.

[13] Mill, J.S. (1862). *A System of Logic, Ratiocinative and Inductive*, 5th Ed. Parker, Son & Bowin, London.

[14] Neyman, J. (1923). Sur les applications de la théorie des probabilités aux experiences agricoles: essai des principes. English translation by Dabrowska, D. & Speed, T. (1990), *Statistical Science* **5**, 463–472.

[15] Pearl, J. (1993). Comment: graphical models, causality, and intervention, *Statistical Science* **8**, 266–269.

[16] Pearl, J. (1995). Causal diagrams for empirical research, *Biometrika* **82**, 669–710.

[17] Pearl, J. & Robins, J.M. (1995). Probabilistic evaluation of sequential plans from causal models with hidden variables, in *Uncertainty in Artificial Intelligence*, R.L. Mantaras & D. Poole, eds. Morgan Kaufman, San Francisco, pp. 444–453.

[18] Prentice, R.L. & Kalbfleisch, J.D. (1988). Author's reply, *Biometrics* **44**, 1205.

[19] Robins, J.M. (1987). A graphical approach to the identification and estimation of causal parameters in mortality studies with sustained exposure periods, *Journal of Chronic Diseases* **40**, Supplement 2, 139S–161S.

[20] Rothman, K.J. (1976). Causes, *American Journal of Epidemiology* **104**, 587–592.

[21] Rubin, D.B. (1974). Estimating causal effects of treatments in randomized and nonrandomized studies, *Journal of Educational Psychology* **66**, 688–701.

[22] Rubin, D.B. (1990). Comment: Neyman (1923) and causal inference in experiments and observational studies, *Statistical Science* **5**, 472–480.

[23] Rubin, D.B. (1991). Practical implications of modes of statistical inference for causal effects and the critical role of the assignment mechanism, *Biometrics* **47**, 1213–1234.

[24] Stalnaker, R.C. (1968). A theory of conditionals, in *Studies in Logical Theory*, N. Rescher, ed. Blackwell, Oxford.

[25] Suppes, P. (1970). *A Probabilistic Theory of Causality*. North-Holland, Amsterdam.

[26] Wright, S. (1921). Correlation and causation, *Journal of Agricultural Research* **20**, 557–585.

SANDER GREENLAND

Cause of Death, Automatic Coding

Accurate selection and coding of the underlying cause of death based on death certificates using the **International Classification of Diseases (ICD)** is a labor-intensive task requiring special training and knowledge. Persons without a medical background must learn basic anatomy and physiology as a prerequisite to cause of death coding training, but even trained nurses and physicians must learn the detailed procedures and rules embodied in the ICD. **Vital statistics** offices have had a continuing burden to maintain a well-trained and experienced mortality coding staff. However, it was not until there was a heightened interest in coding not only the underlying cause of death but the other causes on the death certificate as well, that efforts to utilize computer technology to code death certificates began in earnest (*see* **Cause of Death, Underlying and Multiple**). The dual coding burden of the different procedures required to produce the two kinds of mortality data was prohibitive for most, if not all, countries interested in producing enhanced mortality statistics.

There were several independent approaches to automation of the international selection and modification rules, most notably in England and Wales and in the United States (US). Responsible government authorities in these two countries kept in close touch with each other's progress, but resource constraints in the former left the US National Center for Health Statistics as the single remaining major investor in research and development of an automated mortality coding system.

Originally designed for a large mainframe computer, the US system consisted of two subsystems, Medical Information, Classification, and Retrieval (MICAR) and Automated Classification of Medical Entities (ACME). MICAR required an ICD code or a standardized diagnostic abbreviation to be assigned by a coder to each condition reported, along with a location code indicating where the condition was written in relation to the other conditions entered on the death certificate (*see* **Death Certification**). This information was entered into the computer. The MICAR software searched its internal dictionary until the condition was found and then it assigned a dictionary reference number to each such term. The reference numbers and their death certificate location codes (i.e. MICAR output) formed the input to the ACME module which then, through a series of logical decision tables, applied the international selection and modification rules to arrive at the underlying cause of death. The MICAR output data could then also be used to produce multiple cause of death tabulations by applying additional computer procedures designed for that purpose.

The original versions of both MICAR and ACME have undergone many iterations since their early development in the late 1960s. The current versions are designed to run on a personal computer and are based on the latest revision of the ICD. The MICAR module, now known as SuperMICAR, accepts English language diagnostic text as well as standard disease abbreviations as input while earlier versions required a coder to assign code numbers to each diagnostic term. This allows the data to be entered by persons who can operate a keyboard but who have no need for familiarity with the ICD.

The main features of the MICAR/ACME approach are as follows:

1. The coding of death certificates can be done by coders with less training and knowledge than is required of underlying cause of death coders, although the total number of individual codes to be assigned is greater.
2. The ACME decision tables residing in the computer are logical reflections of the steps an underlying cause of death coder is trained to follow in the application of the international selection and modification rules and therefore result in underlying cause codes with a very high degree of agreement with those resulting from the work of highly experienced human coders.
3. The same original coding of death certificates can be used to produce both underlying cause of death statistics and multiple cause of death statistics.
4. There is a higher degree of consistency in the results, since variation due to differences in interpretation of the rules by coders is eliminated.

5. Changes in the ICD, its rules, or their interpretation can be implemented at any time by modifying the appropriate decision table(s) and reprocessing the records that have been processed prior to the change.

A number of countries plan to implement this automated system when they begin using the Tenth Revision of the ICD. Because of this widespread interest, there will be increased international involvement with the content and possible future modification of the decision tables and in the way multiple cause of death data are manipulated and presented. Countries planning to use this automated system have participated in planning meetings with the system designers and, in the case of the UK, have assisted in some of the research for the latest version. In addition, a few other automated systems in languages other than English have been developed using, in part, the ACME decision table logic. This broader involvement of many countries in the same or highly similar automated programs is expected to contribute to greater uniformity and comparability of international mortality data.

ROBERT A. ISRAEL

Cause of Death, Underlying and Multiple

The underlying cause of death is defined by the World Health Organization (WHO) as "(a) the disease or injury which initiated the train of morbid events leading directly to death, or (b) the circumstances of the accident or violence which produced the fatal injury" [5]. This definition recognizes the importance of the public health principle of prevention. By having information on the sequence of conditions leading to death, from the initial disease or condition, through diseases arising as consequences of the initial disease, on to the final or terminal condition, it is believed that interventions can be found to break the train of events and reduce mortality from selected causes of death.

The concept of attributing to each death a single cause for statistical tabulation and analytic purposes is rooted in the early development of disease classifications. From the outset and through the first part of the twentieth century, disease classifications were focused primarily on the causes of mortality, and it was the principal cause of death – not symptoms, other concurrent conditions, nor modes of dying – that was of primary interest. At the First International Revision Conference for the **International Classification of Diseases (ICD)**, convened in 1900, Bertillon proposed a set of rules for selecting the single cause of death to be used for statistical purposes when more than one condition was reported [4]. In subsequent years, however, there was little uniformity in practice among countries for the selection of a single cause of death and it was not until 1938, at the Fifth Decennial Revision Conference, that formal recognition at the international level was given to the statistical problem of selecting a single cause of death where more than one cause was given on the death certificate (joint causes of death). This question had been under study in the United States (US), and the Conference requested the US government to continue its investigations in this regard. Accordingly, the US government established the US Committee on Joint Causes of Death, comprised of members from the US, Canada, the United Kingdom (UK), and representatives in an advisory capacity from the Interim Commission of the WHO [2]. In recognition of the work of this committee and the recommendations of the WHO Expert Committee for the Preparation of the Sixth Revision of the International Lists of Diseases and Causes of Death, the Sixth Decennial Revision Conference, at its meeting in 1948, not only adopted the Sixth Revision of the International Lists but also an International Form of Medical Certificate of Cause of Death, a formal definition of underlying cause of death, and a standardized set of selection rules for arriving at an underlying cause of death when more than one condition is reported (*see* **Death Certification**). The recommendations of the Conference were accepted by the World Health Assembly in 1948 and incorporated into Regulations No. 1 under Article 21(b) of the WHO Constitution. The regulations serve as guidelines to Member States for the compilation of morbidity and mortality statistics in accordance with the ICD [3]. This acceptance of a standard form for certifying causes of death, the definition of the underlying cause, and the rules for selecting it from more than one reported cause was a major step in the quest for international comparability of mortality data.

While the underlying cause of death continues to form the basis for mortality data for countries with medically certified deaths, some have observed that there is a loss of potentially useful information when several diseases or conditions are reported on a death certificate but only one is used for statistical reporting and analysis. With the decline in importance, especially in developed countries, of infectious diseases and a concomitant rise in **life expectancy**, the number of death certificates listing several conditions, particularly chronic illnesses, has risen noticeably. In those cases in which more than one disease is reported, all of the diagnostic entries on the death certificate are known collectively as "multiple causes of death". From the group of multiple causes on a death certificate, an underlying cause is chosen in accordance with the standard definition and procedures, but unless additional steps are taken, the remainder of the entries on the medical certification of cause of death contribute nothing to the statistical collection of mortality data. Recognizing this, several countries, particularly England and Wales, France, Sweden, and the US, began experimenting in the 1960s and subsequent years with ways to capture the additional information and analyze and present the findings [1]. At the international level, the WHO convened several meetings of interested countries, the first in London in 1969, to review multiple cause of death coding procedures and to compare findings. At those international meetings it was generally agreed that there was not enough similarity of approach, nor a clearly superior methodology, to recommend a single international procedure. However, the growing number of interested countries were encouraged to continue to develop and use their own methodologies and to continue to keep each other informed of results. Furthermore, it was emphasized that some form of multiple cause of death analysis and data presentation was an important adjunct to the traditional underlying cause approach. Late in the 1990s, with a growing number of countries beginning to rely on a common automated computer coding scheme (*see* **Cause of Death, Automatic Coding**), there appeared to be more likelihood that several countries would mutually agree to a uniform procedure for multiple cause of death coding and analysis. This, when realized, would form an important step toward international comparability of multiple cause data to enhance the traditional underlying cause of death statistics.

References

[1]   Israel, R.A., Rosenberg, H.M. & Curtin, L.R. (1986). Analytic potential for multiple cause-of-death data, *American Journal of Epidemiology* **124**, 161–179.

[2]   United States Bureau of the Census (1939). *Manual of the International List of Causes of Death (Fifth Revision) and Joint Causes of Death (Fourth Revision)*. US Government Printing Office, Washington.

[3]   World Health Organization (1967). *WHO Nomenclature Regulations*. World Health Organization, Geneva.

[4]   World Health Organization (1977). *Manual of the International Statistical Classification of Diseases, Injuries and Causes of Death*, Vol. 1. World Health Organization, Geneva.

[5]   World Health Organization (1992). *International Statistical Classification of Diseases and related health problems: 10th revision*, Vol. 2. World Health Organization, Geneva, p. 30.

ROBERT A. ISRAEL

Chloropleth Mapping *see* Mapping Disease Patterns

Classical Error Model *see* Measurement Error in Epidemiologic Studies

Clinical Economics *see* Clinical Epidemiology, Overview

Clinical Epidemiology, Overview

Clinical epidemiology involves the application of methods derived from epidemiology and other fields to the study of clinical phenomena, particularly diagnosis, treatment decisions, and outcomes. Clinical epidemiology has been characterized, somewhat immodestly but fairly accurately, as the basic science of clinical medicine. Clinical epidemiology is not a clearly delimited field. In its concern with the accuracy of diagnosis, the elements of treatment decisions, and the measurement of outcomes, clinical epidemiology overlaps substantially with clinical medicine. In its focus on physician and patient choices and the interactions between patients and physicians in clinical processes, it overlaps substantially with health services research. In its use of various quantitative methodologies to address questions of clinical relevance, clinical epidemiology overlaps substantially with epidemiology, economics, and other disciplines.

To facilitate an understanding of this broad field, it is helpful, if somewhat arbitrary, to consider clinical epidemiology in terms of its major areas. These include clinical measurement, diagnosis and screening, clinical decision making, measurement of treatment effects, clinical economics, and clinical study design.

Clinical Measurement

Clinical measurement, or clinimetrics, as it is sometimes called, is the foundation for all of clinical epidemiology. Sound measurements are the raw material for the various methodologies of the clinical epidemiologist. If this raw material is flawed, then it is very likely that the results and conclusions derived from it will also be flawed.

Clinical measurement involves some issues that are common to all forms of measurement and others that are almost uniquely applicable to measurement as a clinical process. The common issues for any measure include its reliability, validity, responsiveness, and generalizability. A measure is reliable if it provides consistent results when used to measure an unchanged phenomenon at different times or in different settings. A measure is valid if it truly measures the construct it is assumed to measure. A measure is responsive if it is sensitive to clinically meaningful change. A measure is generalizable if it can be usefully applied to subjects who differ by age, gender, race, diagnosis, or some other major characteristic (*see* **Validity and Generalizability in Epidemiologic Studies**).

Other issues in clinimetrics arise from the fact that clinical measurement typically involves an examiner, an examinee, and an examination technique, all of which are subject to **measurement error**. The clinical examiner may be inadequately trained or may be prone to **biased** measurement. The clinical examinee is subject to physiological variation and is prone to reporting bias. The examination methodology may be affected by a variety of factors, including calibration errors and changes in technique. The effects of the sources of measurement error can be cumulative, making clinical measurement a particularly challenging proposition.

Diagnosis and Screening

Diagnosis is a critical step in the clinical process, and the analysis of the diagnostic process is a major focus for clinical epidemiology. Diagnosis refers to the categorization of individuals who have come to a clinician with symptoms. **Screening** refers to the categorization of asymptomatic individuals in a clinical setting or in the general population.

The analysis of diagnosis in clinical epidemiology focuses on the performance of **diagnostic tests**. The key properties of a diagnostic test are its **sensitivity** and **specificity**. Sensitivity refers to the frequency with which a test is positive when it is applied to a group of individuals known to have a particular disease. Specificity refers to the frequency with which a test is negative when it is applied to a group of individuals known to be without a particular disease.

In the clinical setting, the sensitivity and specificity of a test, combined with the estimated **prevalence** of the expected diagnosis (sometimes referred to as the pretest probability of disease) determine the **predictive value** of a test. A positive predictive value estimates the probability that an individual with a positive diagnostic test result will actually have a particular disease. A negative predictive value estimates the probability that an individual with a negative test will actually be free of disease. Since pretest probability is substantially lower for screening than it is for diagnosis, the predictive value of diagnostic tests may be substantially lower when they are used for screening.

Diagnosis in medicine is seldom based on the positive or negative result of a single test. In most diagnostic situations several diagnostic tests are available, with each providing a range of results rather than a simple positive or negative. Methods have been adopted to compare the diagnostic efficiency of different clinical tests across their range (receiver operating characteristic (ROC) curves) and to determine the probability of a diagnosis given the level of a diagnostic test result (likelihood ratios).

In many diagnostic or screening situations several tests are used in combination. In circumstances in which a diagnosis should not be missed, such as a highly treatable infectious disease, one or more diagnostic tests may be applied in parallel with any positive result leading to a diagnosis. This approach enhances the sensitivity of a diagnostic or screening strategy. In other settings, serial testing, in which a second test is done only if a first one is positive, minimizes the use of costly or dangerous second-stage tests. Serial testing lowers the sensitivity of the diagnostic or screening strategy, but it maximizes specificity and minimizes false positive rates.

Clinical epidemiologists also concern themselves with issues of intra- and interobserver agreement. In the realm of diagnosis, intraobserver agreement estimates the extent to which a clinician reproducibly categorizes subjects into diagnostic categories. Interobserver agreement estimates the extent to which two or more clinicians agree on the dia1gnostic categorization of subjects. Since agreement in either situation may occur by chance, **kappa** and other statistics are used as measures of agreement that adjust for chance. Clinical epidemiologists have repeatedly demonstrated that the adjusted diagnostic agreement between two trained clinicians may be surprisingly low.

Clinical Decision Making

The key methodology for the study of clinical decision making is formal **decision analysis**. Decision analysis involves the construction of detailed trees in which each decision point in a clinical treatment cascade is specified, probabilities are assigned to an exhaustive group of potential outcomes, and values are assigned to each outcome. To guide clinical practice, formal decision analysis can be quite helpful in clearly specifying the issues and potential outcomes in a given clinical decision. At the level of clinical epidemiology, formal decision analysis forms the basis for explicit cost and benefit estimates that serve to inform the choice between treatment alternatives.

Measurement of Treatment Effects

A central topic in clinical epidemiology is the estimation of benefits and side-effect rates that result from clinical therapies. The estimation of benefits involves the specification and measurement of the major components of treatment outcome. Until recently, treatment outcome was usually estimated in terms of reduced mortality or improvements in the physiological manifestations of a particular disease, such as blood pressure reduction in hypertension treatment and blood sugar control in diabetes treatment.

In recent years, clinical epidemiologists, in concert with health services researchers, have expanded the measurement of treatment benefits to include the four major components of health status: physical function, psychological function, social function, and symptoms. These elements of health status are measured using a variety of methods, with an emphasis on recently developed questionnaire approaches. These questionnaires have proven to be as reliable, valid, responsive, and generalizable as more traditional clinical measures of benefit. In addition, these newer measures have more relevance for patients because they assess treatment benefits, such as functional capacity and symptom reduction, that are of particular concern to patients.

Treatment benefits may be measured using general methods that apply across diagnostic categories. The SF-36 health status questionnaire is the most widely used example of this approach. Other questionnaires are designed to measure the major elements of health status in particular categories of disease, such as arthritis or respiratory disease-specific measures.

Treatment benefits may also be estimated in terms of patient utilities. In this approach, such methods as time tradeoff and standard gamble are used to estimate patient-specific preferences for potential benefits. Although utility estimation may be methodologically difficult, it is conceptually appealing, and it provides a basis for comparing treatment benefits across different disease categories and patient groups.

There is no such thing as a treatment without costs. So in their efforts to develop an accurate and balanced assessment of medical treatments, clinical epidemiologists must measure the rate of adverse events and their severity as well as benefits. Drug toxicities, or adverse effects, may result from an overshoot in the intended effect (e.g. low blood sugar caused by a diabetes treatment), from undesirable but related physiological effects (e.g. stomach ulcers from arthritis drugs), and from apparently idiosyncratic effects (e.g. headache or skin rash from various drugs).

The study of the frequency and severity of adverse events falls into the realm of pharmacoepidemiology. For common treatment side-effects, follow-up of patients on medication or even data from clinical trials can be utilized to characterize the frequency and severity of side-effects. The rate of common side-effects can be characterized with the highest level of validity because these rates are often derived from close observations by practitioners who are actively monitoring clinical subjects for drug side-effects. For rarer adverse events, computerized clinical databases or claims databases are increasingly being used, for they are the best source of information on large numbers of people under treatment. Both approaches typically utilize the prescription as their measure of treatment exposure. Any side-effect of treatment that occurs outside the medical record or claims file may be difficult to capture and count. There is also an inherent problem in large-scale **observational studies** of drug use in that certain drugs may be given only to persons at high risk of certain side-effects, so that an association with those side-effects is to be expected. This **confounding** by indication has made it nearly impossible to perform pharmacoepidemiologic studies of drugs that are supposed to protect against other drug side-effects. Notwithstanding these difficulties, large-scale, computer-based pharmacoepidemiology studies offer promise in terms of identifying and quantifying the serious adverse effects of drugs.

Clinical Economics

Dollars are the other major cost of treatment, so clinical epidemiology must concern itself with the estimation of dollar costs. The first issue in doing any clinical cost study is to define the perspective from which costs are estimated. For example, a vaccination program will have different costs depending on whether costs are analyzed from the perspective of the State Health Department, the clinic providing the vaccinations, or the family whose child is vaccinated.

There are three major types of clinical cost study. The first is a descriptive study in which the costs of a treatment are measured in terms of direct medical costs (e.g. the cost of a clinic visit and the prescription), direct nonmedical costs (e.g. the cost of losing time from work to receive treatment), and indirect costs (e.g. the cost of reduced productivity caused by disease-related disability or death). Cost estimates may then be used in a cost-effectiveness study in which the costs of treatment are compared to benefits measured in terms of clinical or health status improvements. The third type of cost study is a cost–benefit study in which both the costs and benefits of treatment are measured in dollar terms. Although it is the most difficult form of cost study to carry out, the cost–benefit study has the advantage of allowing comparisons of very different treatments, such as a vaccination program for children vs. a hip replacement program for the elderly, because the benefits of each approach are measured using a single metric: dollars.

Clinical Study Design

The distinguishing characteristic of clinical studies is that they begin with subjects who have a particular diagnosis. Clinical study designs include natural history studies, randomized clinical trials, and N of 1 studies. The natural history study focuses on analyzing prognosis in subjects who have a particular disease. Using the natural history design, one can evaluate the effects of treatments including important and common adverse events. One can also identify persons at high risk of experiencing a poor disease course who might be appropriate subjects for more aggressive treatment and other subjects who experience a benign disease outcome in whom aggressive treatment may not be indicated. In addition, data on prognosis can be utilized to develop "predictive models" identifying which patients might benefit from extensive, costly clinical evaluation. Thus natural history studies of people with a particular disease provide valuable diagnostic and therapeutic information that can guide clinical decisions.

Clinical epidemiologists have identified several critical methodologic concerns in performing a natural history study. These concerns are similar to those of epidemiologic **cohort studies**, the main differences being that in natural history studies subjects already have disease. The **controls** in a natural history study are internal controls, and comparisons are made between different subsets of people with disease. Natural history studies are most accurate in so-called inception cohorts, in which patients are

entered into the study just after diagnosis. If patients are entered long after diagnosis, patients who die or go into remission soon after diagnosis may be missed, thus biasing the study. Right censoring, or loss to follow-up of patients enrolled in the natural history study, must be avoided to give an accurate picture of the prognosis of disease. If dropouts tend to have poor prognosis, then the study would arrive at an inaccurately optimistic prediction of disease prognosis.

Prognostic information can be used to build prediction rules that will estimate patient prognosis based on the presence or absence of key clinical characteristics. To develop prediction rules, investigators generally study two different groups of subjects with disease. Using the first group, they develop the rule identifying those factors which affect prognosis. Using the second group, they test this prediction rule, attempting to confirm that the factors identified in the first sample generalize to the second. Such repeatability of a prediction role in two independent samples augurs well for the general applicability of this rule to yet other patient samples.

Summary

Clinical epidemiology is a heterogeneous and dynamic field in which methodologies drawn from epidemiology, economics, and psychometrics are applied to issues related to clinical measurement and clinical decision making. This applied science will undoubtedly continue to grow and become even more important as clinical scientists apply additional methodologies to the analysis of clinical problems.

Several general references on clinical epidemiology are listed in the Bibliography.

Bibliography

Fletcher, R.H., Fletcher, S.W. & Wagner, E.H. (1996). *Clinical Epidemiology: The Essentials*, 3rd Ed. Williams & Wilkins, Baltimore.

Murphy, E.A. (1976). *The Logic of Medicine*. Johns Hopkins University Press, Baltimore.

Sackett, D.L., Haynes, R.B., Guyatt, G.H. & Tugwell, P. (1991). *Clinical Epidemiology: A Basic Science for Clinical Medicine*, 2nd Ed. Little, Brown, & Company, Boston.

Spilker, B. (1996). *Quality of Life and Pharmacoeconomics in Clinical Trials*, 2nd Ed. Lippincott-Raven, Philadelphia.

Weiss, N.S. (1996). *Clinical Epidemiology: The Study of the Outcomes of Illness*, 2nd Ed. Oxford University Press, New York.

ROBERT F. MEENAN & DAVID T. FELSON

Clinical Latency Period *see* Incubation Period of Infectious Diseases

Clinimetrics *see* Clinical Epidemiology, Overview

Clustering

Clustering can be defined as the "irregular" grouping of events from a stochastic process in either space or time or simultaneously in both space and time. More generally, it can be studied in any metric space that possesses a uniform or baseline "nonclustered" probability measure for the location of events (point process) under the null hypothesis of no clustering.

A major issue in this area, which is particularly acute in the medical context, is the differentiation between clustering as a general phenomenon, and the usually *post hoc* attempt to establish "significance" or "likelihood" of a real causal agent for a previously observed "cluster". The former question is amenable to reasonably standard statistical analysis. Usually, data are available from a large area or time period and a null hypothesis of "no clustering" can be formed. The description of a realistic alternative "clustered" hypothesis or family of hypotheses is usually more difficult, but a number of model cluster processes exist, and various *ad hoc* tests have been developed that will consistently detect a wide range of departures from the nonclustered null hypothesis. In many cases, these *ad hoc* tests have much to offer, since most clustering models are too inflexible to encompass the full range of possibilities seen in practice, and likelihood ratio tests based on them are usually complicated and may not have good power against other alternatives.

Unfortunately, it is far more common to encounter the latter situation, where some measure of "reality" is demanded for a "cluster" that has been identified before any statistical analysis has taken place. In this case, the temporal and/or spatial aspects of the cluster have been well circumscribed in advance and formal hypothesis testing is not valid. The problem is aptly illustrated by the Texas sharpshooter who fires his shots first and then positions the target to best advantage *afterwards*. Attempts to allow for this by adjusting for multiple potential comparisons are not very helpful, because the adjustment factor depends on the domain used for this, and by taking a large enough spatial or temporal domain, any cluster can be reduced to nonsignificance. In the end, the "reality" of any cluster ultimately depends on finding a cause and establishing that it also causes the disease in question in other circumstances. However, this is a costly and time-consuming process, and the "art of statistics" has an important role to play in helping to focus attention on "clusters" that still appear "highly unusual" after a range of statistical tests have been employed.

Such investigations usually start with readily available information, and clusters that are still interesting are then subjected to more stringent tests that may require the gathering of more data. A guideline for approaching this has been developed by the Centers for Disease Control, Atlanta, Georgia, USA [7, 49]. They propose a four-stage process of increasing complexity and cost, in which the investigation can be terminated after any stage if alternative explanations can be found or the evidence for clustering is no longer very compelling. In outline form, the stages are as follows:

Stage 1: Initial contact.   The purpose at this stage is to collect information from the person(s) or group(s) first reporting a perceived cluster (hereafter referred to as the caller). The caller must be referred quickly to the responsible health agency unit, and the problem should never be dismissed summarily. The majority of potential cluster reports can be brought to successful closure at the time of initial contact, and the first encounter is often one of the best opportunities for communication with the caller about the nature of clusters.

Stage 2: Assessment.   Once the decision has been made at Stage 1 to proceed further with an assessment, it is important to separate two concurrent issues: whether an excess number of cases has actually occurred, and whether the excess can be tied etiologically to some exposure. The first usually has precedence, and may or may not lead to the second. This stage initiates a mechanism for evaluating whether an excess has occurred. Three separate elements are identified:

1. a preliminary evaluation (Stage 2(a)) to assess quickly from the available data whether an excess may have occurred;
2. confirmation of cases (Stage 2(b)) to assure that there is a biological basis for further work; and
3. an occurrence investigation (Stage 2(c)) whose purpose is a more detailed description of the cluster through case-finding, interaction with the community, and **descriptive epidemiology**.

If an excess is confirmed, and the epidemiologic and biologic plausibility is compelling, proceed to Stage 3.

Stage 3: Major feasibility study. The major feasibility study examines the potential for relating the cluster to some exposure. It should consider all the options for geographic and temporal analysis, including the use of cases that are from a different geographic locale or time period and not part of the original cluster. In some instances the feasibility study itself may provide answers to the question under study.

If the feasibility study suggests that there is merit in pursuing an etiologic investigation, then the health agency should proceed to Stage 4. This may entail extensive resource commitment, however, and the decision to conduct a study will be tied to the process of resource allocation.

State 4: Etiologic investigation. Perform an etiologic investigation of a potential disease–exposure relationship. Using the major feasibility study as a guide, a specific protocol for the study should be developed and the study implemented.

Reporting of results. At whatever stage an investigation terminates, administrative closure is critical. Health authorities must remain aware that even internal reports are, in many circumstances, public documents, and can become part of legal proceedings. Even a brief memorandum to the record or a handwritten note summarizing a telephone call are subject to use in court and should be handled accordingly.

Issues of *Statistics in Medicine* (April–May 1996, Vol. 15) and the *American Journal of Epidemiology* (July 1990, Vol. 132) have been devoted exclusively to theoretical and practical issues related to clustering. These publications and the book edited by Elliot et al. [16] provide fuller details of points raised below.

Statistical Tests for Clustering

Tests for clustering, either spatially or temporally, fall into four main classes:

1. Methods based on cell occupancy counts for a partition of the region of interest.
2. Methods based on overlapping cells or adjacencies of cells with "high counts".
3. Distance methods.
4. Space–time clustering methods.

Methods can also be distinguished by the form of the null hypothesis. In nonmedical settings, often a uniform process is appropriate in which events occur according to a homogeneous Poisson process on the time axis (for temporal clustering) or the plane (for spatial clustering). For medical applications often some degree of inhomogeneity is appropriate for the nonclustered process. For time series, seasonal effects may need to be accounted for, and in studying spatial clustering, the nonuniform nature of the population density needs to be considered. In these circumstances, some form of **control** series is needed to allow for variations not related to short-range clustering.

Cell Occupancy Methods

These methods are equally appropriate to both temporal and spatial clustering as they take no account of the geometric structure of the region once it has been partitioned into nonoverlapping cells.

Dispersion Test. The simplest test for clustering is a heterogeneity or dispersion test [10]. When there are n cells, this is a simple chi-square test for an $n \times 1$ table. If E_i denotes the expected number of events in cell i, and N_i is the observed number, then the test is given by

$$T_D = \sum_{i=1}^{n} \frac{(N_i - E_i)^2}{E_i}.$$

When all the E_i are large (≥ 5), the test has an approximately χ^2 distribution on n degrees of freedom. However, this is usually not the case. Nevertheless, T tends to a normal distribution as $n \to \infty$, in general. The mean and variance depend on whether one conditions on the total number of events $N = \sum N_i$. Usually, this is the case so that the N_i have a multinomial distribution with cell probabilities $p_i = E_i/E$, where $E = \sum E_i$, and total number of observations N. In that case [24, 38],

$$E(T_D) = n - 1,$$

$$\text{var}(T_D) = 2(n-1) + \sum E_i^{-1} - \frac{1}{N}(n^2 - 2n + 2),$$

and $[T_D - E(T_D)]/\text{var}^{1/2}(T_D)$ is approximately a standard normal deviate.

Pothoff & Whittinghill's Test.   Pothoff & Whittinghill [46, 47] considered a cell occupancy model in which the cell counts were Poisson with mean E_i under the null hypothesis. Under the alternative, the E_i were assumed to be multiplied by independent gamma-distributed variables with mean one, so that the observed counts had a negative binomial distribution (i.e. a compound Poisson-gamma distribution). They computed the score test as the variance of the gamma distribution tended to zero while keeping the means fixed, and arrived at a test of the form:

$$T_{PW} = \sum_{i=1}^{n} \frac{N_i(N_i - 1)}{E_i}.$$

Again, the N_i are multinomial and if $\max_i p_i \to 0$ as $n \to \infty$,

$$E(T_{PW}) = N - 1,$$

$$\text{var}(T_{PW}) \cong 2(N-1)^2/N,$$

and

$$[T_{PW} - E(T_{PW})]/\text{var}^{1/2}(T_{PW}) \to \mathcal{N}(0, 1).$$

Note that cells contribute nothing to T_{PW} unless there are at least two events in the cell. Also, when all the E_i are the same, this test is equivalent to the dispersion test given above. In general, T_{PW} gives less weight to cells with larger expected values than does T_D.

Dispersion Tests with Controls.   In some circumstances, it is appropriate to consider whether the variability in a time series of events is greater than that in a control series. The control series may account for seasonal disease patterns or changing referral patterns and is used as a surrogate for the cell probabilities p_i defined above. An approach based on a chi-square test for independence in a $2 \times n$ table has been proposed by Fleiss & Cuzick [18] in which the case and control series comprise the two rows. The asymptotic distribution is *not* χ^2 on (n − 1) degrees of freedom (df) unless all cell counts are large, but as $n \to \infty$ the test does tend to be a normal with mean $(n - 1)$ and variance [25, 38]

$$\text{var}(T_D) \cong 2(n - 1 - N^*) + (p^* - 2)\left(N^* - \frac{n^2}{N}\right)$$

$$+ 2\left(\frac{n}{N}\right)(1 - p^*)$$

$$- \left(\frac{n}{N}\right)^2 (5 - p^*) + O\left(\frac{1}{n}\right),$$

where

$$p^* = \overline{p}^{-1} + (1 - \overline{p})^{-1},$$

$$N^* = \sum_{i=1}^{n} N_i^{-1},$$

$\overline{p}$ is the proportion of all events that are in the case series, and N_i is the total number of events in period i for cases and controls combined.

Tests Based on the Maximum Cell Count.   When looking for a single cluster, tests based on the maximum cell count are an obvious choice. When done in a *post hoc* fashion, i.e. when the cluster has already been identified, the significance is completely dependent on the number of cells included in the sample. A more attractive option is to examine the maximum cell count in a number of short subsets of the data. This approach has an intuitive appeal, and will detect multiple clusters. A weakness is that the cells are chosen in advance and clusters that are split over two cells will not be fully scored. Also, the method assumes equal expected numbers in the different cells. The method was first proposed by Ederer et al. [15]. For their test, the cells are first partitioned into a number of nonoverlapping time series. For example, if the data consisted of quarterly event rates over a 20-year period in a number of localities, the individual time series might be chosen to be the event rates over a five-year period for each locality. These individual series are then self-normalized by conditioning on the total number of events in that subseries. Thus, if N_{ij} denotes the number of events in cell i of series j, $i = 1, \ldots, I$, $j = 1, \ldots, J$, one computes $M_j = \max_{1 \le i \le I} N_{ij}$ conditional on $N_j = \sum_{i=1}^{I} N_{ij}$.

The overall test statistic is then

$$T_{\text{EMM}} = \sum_{j=1}^{J} M_j,$$

and is normalized by the conditional means:

$$\mathrm{E}(T_{\text{EMM}}) = \sum \mathrm{E}(M_j | N_j),$$

and conditional variances

$$\mathrm{var}(T_{\text{EMM}}) = \sum \mathrm{var}(M_j | N_j)$$

to form an approximately standard normal deviate in the usual way.

Thus, this test only looks for evidence of clustering within the subseries and by appropriate choice of the space and time groups can be viewed as a space–time clustering method as well. However, by including only one geographic entity and allowing the subseries to be rather long, it takes on more the character of a purely temporal statistic. An underlying assumption is that all cells in the same subseries have the same expected event rate under the null hypothesis. Thus, some adjustment for seasonal variation can be made by creating subseries based on the same months in successive years, and temporal trends can be accounted for by using short time periods, but it is not possible to adjust for both simultaneously.

Ederer et al. rely on the asymptotic normality of their test and thus it is only necessary to compute $\mathrm{E}(M_i | N_i)$ and $\mathrm{var}(M_i | N_i)$, for which Mantel et al. [35] have given tables for small values of N_i and I. Grimson [22] has obtained the exact distribution of the maximum, based on factorial moments and the inclusion–exclusion formula. Specifically, he shows that when $N_i = r$ and $I = c$:

$$\Pr(M_i \ge m) = i^r \sum_{k=1}^{r} (-1)^{k+1} \binom{c}{k}$$

$$\times \sum_{j_1, \ldots, j_k = m}^{r} (c - k)^{r - j_1 - \cdots - j_k} \binom{r}{j_1, \ldots, j_k}.$$

Levin [31] has given a large sample approximation based on Edgeworth expansions.

Overlapping or Adjacent Cells Methods

One of the problems with cell occupancy methods is that clusters may span more than one cell. To be valid, the partitioning of space for these methods must be independent of the location of events so that it is likely that any clusters will not match up with the partitioning. Attempts to address this problem have led to tests based on overlapping or neighboring cells.

Scan Tests.   For temporal clustering, where events are distributed on a line and cells are often based on equal length intervals (e.g. months), an obvious solution exists. Instead of looking only at the number of events in prespecified intervals (e.g. six months), it is also possible to look at overlapping intervals (e.g. six-monthly intervals beginning every quarter). The most thorough method is to look at all intervals of a fixed size (e.g. six-monthly intervals beginning every day), and consider the maximum number of events in any such interval. However, the fact that overlapping intervals are now being considered greatly complicates the problem of determining the distribution of the scan test. To simplify matters, one usually assumes that the time axis is broken into sufficiently small intervals (e.g. one day) so that one can safely assume that the scan is continuous. Under the null hypothesis, the problem is then transformed into determining the distribution of $n(t, N)$, the maximum number of events in an interval of length t when N events are uniformly distributed on the unit interval. Computations for this probability go back at least as far as the 1940s [2, 33], but Naus [39, 41, 42] was the first to develop this as a test for temporal clustering. Exact calculations require detailed combinational expressions and are very computationally time-consuming in the important case when t is small. Various approximations have been proposed [3, 13, 19, 21, 30, 42, 51] (*see* **Scan Statistics for Disease Surveillance**).

The primary quantity of interest is $p(n, t, N) = \Pr(n(t, N) \ge n)$, and approximations are given in terms of the binomial probabilities $b(j, n, p) = \binom{n}{j} p^j (1 - p)^{n-j}$. Wallenstein & Neff [51] give the simple approximation:

$$p(n, t, N) \cong (n/t - N + 1)b(n, N, t)$$

$$+ 2 \sum_{j=n+1}^{N} b(j, N, t),$$

which is accurate when $p(n, t, N)$ is small and, in fact, exact when $n > N/2$ and $t < \frac{1}{2}$. Berman & Eagleson [3] give an upper bound of similar complexity based on a second-order inclusion–exclusion (Bonferroni) approximation:

$$P(n, t, N) \leq (N - n + 1) \sum_{j=n-1}^{N} b(j, N, t)$$

$$- \sum_{j=n-1}^{N} (-1)^{j+n-1} b(j, N, t),$$

which is also a good approximation in some cases. Glaz [20, 21] has developed more complicated expressions on the basis of higher-order Bonferroni inequalities and a product-type inequality, all of which have greater accuracy. Two series of expressions are given that increase in complexity (and hopefully accuracy) as L increases.

The first is an upper bound: for $1 \leq L \leq n \leq N/2$:

$$P(n, t, N) \leq \sum_{j=1}^{L-1} Q_j^* + (N - n + 2 - L)Q_L^*,$$

where

$$Q_1^* = \sum_{J=n-1}^{N} b(j, N, t),$$

$$Q_2^* = Q_1^* - \sum_{j=n-1}^{N} (-1)^{j+n-1} b(j, N, t),$$

and for $j \geq 3$

$$Q_j^* = b(n - 1, N, t) - b(n, N, t)$$

$$+ \sum_{k=j}^{N-n+1} (-1)^k \prod_{i=1}^{j-2} [1 - k(k - 1)/i(i + 1)]$$

$$\times b(n + k - 1, N, t).$$

A more accurate approximation is given by

$$P(n, t, N)$$

$$\cong 1 - \left(1 - \sum_{j=1}^{L} Q_j^*\right)$$

$$\times \left[\left(1 - \sum_{j=1}^{L} Q_j^*\right) \bigg/ \left(1 - \sum_{j=1}^{L-1} Q_j^*\right)\right]^{N-n+1-L},$$

which is said to be most accurate when $L = n$. Neff & Naus [43] have tabulated $P(n, t, N)$ for $t < \frac{1}{2}$, $3 \leq n < N \leq 25$.

Approximations for $P(n, t, N)$ under various clustering alternatives are described in Wallenstein et al. [52], which are important for power calculations.

Glaz [21] gives references for approximations of the moments of $n(t, N)$ and various related quantities. He also discusses scan statistics based on the use of a range of different window widths, t_i. Nagarwalla [37] also discusses a scan test with variable window width. Simulation is required to approximate its null distribution.

Extensions of the scan statistic to the plane or higher dimensions have not been very fully developed. There are problems in the choice of metric (e.g. circles or squares) and the structure of overlapping cells is much more complicated in the plane. Naus [40] has some theoretical results for the plane, and Openshaw et al. [44] give an example of an application that uses circles of different radii. This approach is very descriptive, however.

Runs Test.   The runs test is a well-established method for evaluating clustering in sequences of binary data. For temporal data, such sequences can be created by looking at intervals of fixed length and recording whether one or more events occur in each interval, or, when events are more common, intervals in which an excessive number of events have occurred. The elements of the sequence are then treated as independent Bernoulli trials with fixed success probabilities. As the success probability is usually unknown, one usually is interested in the probability of a run of length at least m in n trials in which there are known to be s successes overall. Denoting this as $P_R(m, s, n)$, the exact distribution is (cf. [5, p. 257])

$$P_R(m, s, n) = \sum_{i=1}^{[s/m]} (-1)^{i+1}$$

$$\times \binom{n-s+1}{i} \binom{n-im}{n-s} \Big/ \binom{n}{s}.$$

Burr & Cane [6] have developed and surveyed various approximations and Naus [42], on the basis of ideas used for the scan test, suggested

$$P_R(m, s, n) \cong 1 - Q_2^{**}(Q_3^{**}/Q_2^{**})^{(n/m)-2},$$

where

$$Q_2^{**} = \left[m\binom{n-m-1}{s-m} + \binom{n-m}{s-m}\right] \Big/ \binom{n}{s},$$

$$Q_3^{**} = \left[2m\binom{n-m-1}{s-m} + \binom{n-m}{s-m}\right.$$

$$- \binom{m}{2}\binom{n-2m-2}{s-2m}$$

$$\left. -m\binom{n-2m-1}{s-2m}\right] \Big/ \binom{n}{s}.$$

A simple, but less accurate, approximation is given by Feller [17]:

$$P_R(m, s, n) \cong 1 - \exp(-nqp^m),$$

where $p = 1 - q = s/n$. Tests have also been based on the number of runs greater than a certain size or the total number of runs (change from zero to one or vice versa) in a series [27].

Join–Count Statistics. This approach was first developed by Moran [36], and the test is sometimes called the Geary–Moran statistic. It has been developed for two-dimensional maps, but the ideas are quite general and suitable for other dimensions as well. It can be seen as a hybrid between a cell occupancy method and a distance method. The basic approach is as follows: one starts with a map in which a partition into cells is given. Cells with "large" numbers of events are determined by some scheme chosen separately by the investigator. Common approaches are to choose cells in which the observed number of events exceeds the expected number by a given percentage (standardized incidence ratio) (*see* **Standardization Methods**) or is significantly different at

a predetermined level (say 5%). The number of pairs of "such" extreme cells that are adjacent, i.e. that share a common boundary (denoted T_{JC}), is then determined and compared against expected numbers. The problem can be reduced to the analysis of a graph in which the cells are vertices and adjacent cells are connected by edges. The null hypothesis is that the "extreme cells" are chosen at random (permutational distribution). Under this hypothesis, the expected number of adjacent cells is

$$E(T_{JC}) = Np_1,$$

where N is the total number of joins (adjacent cells) and for $j = 0, 1, 2, \ldots,$

$$p_j = \prod_{i=0}^{j} \frac{n_0 - l}{n - l},$$

$n =$ number of points, and $n_0 =$ number of "extreme" points, and the variance is

$$\text{var}(T_{JC}) = N(p_1^2 - p_3) - N^2(p_1^2 - p_3)$$

$$+ p_2 \sum_{i=1}^{n} M_i(M_i - 1) - p_3 \sum_{j=1}^{n} K_j,$$

where M_i is the number of joins emanating from point i, and K_j is the number of points to which the points at the ends of join j are both joined.

Asymptotic normality of $[T_{JD} - E(T_{JC})]/\text{var}^{1/2}$ (T_{JC}) can be established. Besag [4] has noted that even in the absence of clustering, the null hypothesis may not hold when extreme cells are determined by observed to expected ratios. When the populations in different cells are not the same, and low population cells are next to each other (e.g. rural areas), those cells are more likely to be extreme because of greater random fluctuations, and artefactual aggregation could arise. Contrariwise, if there is general, but unaccounted for, extra Poisson variation, and significance levels based on the Poisson distribution are used to determine extreme cells, then cells with large underlying populations could be over-represented. In these circumstances, more complicated expressions for the mean and variance of T_{JC} are needed, or simulation must be used to assess the significance level.

Distance Methods

Nearest Neighbor Tests for Uniform Populations.
Under the assumption of a uniform (or homogeneous
Poisson) distribution, tests for clustering have been
based on the distance to the kth nearest neighbor of
any particular case [9, 32]. If d_k denotes the distance
to the kth nearest point from any arbitary point in
the plane, then when the number of points is large
(so edge effects can be discounted), d_k has a gamma
(μ, k) distribution:

$$P(d_k > t) = \sum_{j=0}^{k-1} \mu^j e^{-\mu}/j!,$$

where $\mu = 2\pi\lambda d_k^2$ and λ is the event rate of the
underlying Poisson process. Tests have been based
on the mean of d_k, often with $k = 1$, i.e. the average
distance from an arbitrary point to its nearest neighbor. Other approaches based on more complicated
sampling plans are surveyed in [48, Chapter 7].

Covariance Function.   An alternative approach is
to use the k function associated with homogeneous
point processes [13]. Specifically, for a homogeneous
point process with event rate λ per unit area, define
$k(t) = \lambda^{-1}E$ (number of events within distance t of
an arbitrary event). For a Poisson process with unit
intensity, $k(t) = \frac{1}{2}\pi t^2$. Empirical estimates $\hat{k}$ can be
formed in an obvious way and compared with $k(t)$ to
see if more or fewer events are occurring near to an
arbitrary event.

**Nearest Neighbor Tests for Nonuniform Popula-
tions.**   Work with homogeneous populations arose
from questions in ecology and geography and is generally not applicable to questions of disease association in populations because of the nonhomogeneous
distribution of the population. In this case, some estimate of the local population density is also required.
Cuzick & Edwards [11, 12] have developed a variety
of tests in this setting. When the population density is
known precisely, this test consists of creating circles
of different radius but constant expected number of
events around each case and counting the number of
observed events in all such circles. If the expected
number is taken to be λ and O_i is the observed number of events in the circle around event i, then this

takes the form

$$T_{1s} = \sum_i (O_i - \lambda),$$

with

$$E(T_{1S}) = 0,$$
$$\text{var}(T_{1S}) = n\lambda + 2n^{-1}N_S + n^{-1}N_t - n\lambda^2,$$

where n is the number of points, N_S is the number
of pairs of points in each other's neighborhood, and
$N_t = \sum M_i(M_i - 1)$, where M_i is the number of
points for which point i falls in its neighborhood. In
many circumstances, precise information about the
geographic location of the population is unavailable
and information about this must be replaced by a
control series selected in an appropriate way. Cuzick
& Edwards [11] developed a test on the basis of the
number of cases in the k nearest neighbors ($k - NN$)
to each case; see also Schilling [50] and Henze
[26]. Specifically, cases and controls are labeled from
$1, \ldots, N$ and

$$T_k = \sum_{i=1}^{N} \sum_{j=1}^{N} a_{ij} \delta_i \delta_j,$$

where δ_i is the indicator for the ith event to be a case
and a_{ij} is the indicator for event j to be among the
$k - NN$s of event i. This test can also be viewed as
formally similar to a join–count test, except that the
a_{ij} is not in general symmetric (although it is easily
converted by replacing a_{ij} with $\frac{1}{2}(a_{ij} + a_{ji})$). The
permutational distribution of T_k can be computed as
before (assuming cases are selected at random from
the set of cases and controls) and yields

$$E(T_k) = p_1 kn,$$

where p_1 is as in the section on join–count statistics,
where n_o denotes the number of cases and n the total
number of points, and

$$\text{var}(T_k) = (kn + N_s)p_1(1 - p_1)$$
$$+ [(3k^2 - k)n + N_t - 2N_s](p_2 - p_1)^2$$
$$- [k^2(n^2 - 3n) + N_s - N_t](p_1^2 - p_3),$$

where N_s is the number of pairs of points for which
the $k - NN$ relation is symmetric, i.e. pairs that are
$k - NN$s of each other and $N_t = \sum_{i=1}^{n} M_i(M_i - 1)$,

and where M_i is the number of points for which point i is a $k - NN$.

Diggle [14] has suggested an alternative based on comparing the k function of the cases with that of the controls. His approach essentially uses circles of the same geographic size, whereas the Cuzick–Edwards approach uses circles of approximately equal population. The choice of approach depends on the type of alternative envisaged. Cuzick & Edwards [11] have also considered tests based on the number of cases encountered before k controls. When $k = 1$, this is similar to the runs test sometimes used to look for clustering in one dimension.

Space–Time Clustering Methods

When events are thought to be closely related to exposures both in time and distance, such as in epidemics of disease associated with contagious infectious agents, then tests based on space–time clustering are most appropriate. Such tests are self-normalizing in the sense that any overall nonhomogeneity in the time course of the events or their spatial distribution is automatically accounted for. This has great advantages in terms of automatically cancelling out seasonal effects of nonhomogeneous population distributions, but, of course, limits the ability of the test to detect alternatives that vary both in time and space. Thus, a point source of events or a change that affected the entire geographic region under consideration would not be detected. Thus, these tests are appropriate for infectious diseases with short incubation times, but Chen et al. [8] have shown they have low power for the type of clustering expected in adult cancer or other chronic diseases where the **latent period** between exposure and disease is long.

The simplest space–time tests partition space and time separately and then perform a chi-square test for independence on the associated two-way contingency table in which spatial cells are rows and temporal cells are columns. However, more interest has been generated by the work of Knox [28, 29], in which distances and times are computed between all pairs of points and tests are developed to determine whether events that are close spatially are also close in time. By partitioning distances and time intervals, these data can be summarized in a two-way table, but the induced correlations arising from considering pairs of points means that the chi-square distribution is invalid

for assessing independence. Knox only considered a two by two table formally by dichotomizing time and spatial pairs as close or distant in each variable. One problem with Knox's approach is the arbitrary dichotomy on the close and distant pairs. Related tests have been proposed by Pinkel & Nefzger [45], Barton & David [1] and Mantel [34]. Mantel [34] considered a more general approach giving weights to distances that decrease as the distance increases. Knox's tests is then a special case in which the weight changes from one to zero, once the cut-off is exceeded. Mantel's test can be written in the very general form:

$$T_{\mathrm{M}} = \sum_{i \neq j} \sum X_{ij} Y_{ij},$$

where $X_{ij} = a(i, j)$ is a score for the pair of spatial variables and $Y_{ij} = b(i, j)$ is a score for the pair of temporal variables. Under the assumption that the spatial variables are unrelated to the temporal variables, the permutational distribution of T_{M} can be simulated or approximated. For large samples, the permutational mean and variance can be computed and asymptotic normality assumed, although conditions for this are not clearly known [23]. Even the computation of the permutational variance can be quite involved [34].

References

[1]   Barton, D.E. & David, F.N. (1966). The random intersection of two graphs, in *Research Papers in Statistics*, F.N. David, ed. Wiley, New York, pp. 455–459.

[2]   Berg, W. (1945). Aggregates in one- and two-dimensional random distributions, *London, Edinburgh, and Dublin Philosophical Magazine and Journal of Science* **36**, 319–336.

[3]   Berman, M. & Eagleson, G.K. (1985). A useful upper bound for the tail probabilities of the scan statistic when the sample size is large, *Journal of the American Statistical Association* **80**, 886–889.

[4]   Besag, J. (1990). Discussion of the paper by Cuzick and Edwards, *Journal of the Royal Statistical Society, Series B* **52**, 96–104.

[5]   Bradley, J.V. (1968). *Distribution-Free Statistical Tests*. Prentice-Hall, Englewood Cliffs.

[6]   Burr, E.J. & Cane, G. (1961). Longest run of consecutive observations having a specified attribute, *Biometrika*, **48**, 461–465.

[7]   CDC (1990). Guidelines for investigating clusters of health events, *Morbidity and Mortality Weekly Report* **39**, (RR-11), 1–23.

[8]   Chen, R., Mantel, N. & Klingberg, M.A. (1984). A study of three techniques for time–space clustering in Hodgkin's disease, *Statistics in Medicine* **3**, 173–184.

[9]   Clark, P.J. & Evans, F.C. (1955). On some aspects of spatial pattern in biological populations, *Science* **121**, 397–398.

[10] Cox, D.R. & Lewis, P.A.W. (1966). *The Statistical Analysis of Series of Events*. Methuen, London.

[11] Cuzick, J. & Edwards, R. (1990). Spatial clustering for inhomogeneous populations, *Journal of the Royal Statistical Society, Series B* **52**, 73–104.

[12] Cuzick, J. & Edwards, R. (1996). Clustering methods based on k nearest neighbour distributions, in *Methods for Investigating Localized Clustering of Disease*, F.E. Alexander & P. Boyle, eds. IARC Scientific Publication No. 135, Lyon.

[13] Diggle, P.J. (1983). *Statistical Analysis of Spatial Point Patterns*. Academic Press, London.

[14] Diggle, (1990). A point process modelling approach to raised incidence of a rare phenomenon in the vicinity of a pre-specified point, *Journal of the Royal Statistical Society, Series A* **153**, 349–362.

[15] Ederer, F., Myers, M.H. & Mantel, N. (1964). A statistical problem in space and time: do leukemia cases come in clusters?, *Biometrics* **20**, 626–638.

[16] Elliott, P., Cuzick, J., English, D. & Stern, R. (1992). *Geographical and Environmental Epidemiology Methods for Small-Area Studies*. Oxford University Press, Oxford.

[17] Feller, W. (1957). *An Introduction to Probability Theory and its Application*, Vol. 1, 2nd Ed. Wiley, New York.

[18] Fleiss, J.L. & Cuzick, J. (1979). The reliability of dichotomous judgments: unequal numbers of judges per subject, *Applied Psychological Measurement* **3**, 537–542.

[19] Gates, D.J. & Westcott, M. (1984). On the distributions of scan statistics, *Journal of the American Statistical Association* **79**, 423–429.

[20] Glaz, J. (1992). Approximations for tail probabilities and moments of the scan statistic, *Computational Statistics and Data Analysis* **14**, 213–227.

[21] Glaz, J. (1993). Approximations for the tail probabilities and moments of the scan statistic, *Statistics in Medicine* **12**, 1845–1852.

[22] Grimson, R. (1993). Disease cluster, exact distributions of maxima, and P-values, *Statistics in Medicine* **12**, 1773–1794.

[23] Guttorp, P. & Lockhart, R.A. (1988). On the asymptotic distribution of quadratic forms in uniform order statistics, *Annals of Statistics* **16**, 433–449.

[24] Haldane, J.B.S. (1937). The exact value of the moments of the distribution of χ^2, used as a test of goodness of fit, when expectations are small, *Biometrika* **29**, 133–143.

[25] Haldane, J.B.S. (1940). The mean and variance of χ^2, when used as a test of homogeneity, when expectations are small, *Biometrika* **31**, 346–355.

[26] Henze, N. (1988). A multivariate two-sample test based on the number of nearest neighbour type coincidence, *Annals of Statistics* **16**, 772–783.

[27] Johnson, N.L. & Kotz, S. (1969). *Discrete Distributions*. Wiley, New York.

[28] Knox, E.G. (1964). The detection of space–time interactions, *Applied Statistics* **13**, 25–29.

[29] Knox, E.G. (1964). Epidemiology of childhood leukaemia in Northumberland and Durham, *British Journal of Preventive and Social Medicine* **18**, 17–24.

[30] Krauth, J. (1988). An improved upper bound for the tail probability of the scan statistic for testing non-random clustering, in *Classification and Related Methods of Data Analysis*, Proceeding of the First Conference of the International Federation of Classification Society. Technical University of Aachen, Germany, pp. 237–244.

[31] Levin, B. (1981). A representation for multinomial cumulative distribution functions, *Annals of Statistics* **9**, 1123–1126.

[32] Lewis, M.S. (1980). Spatial clustering in childhood leukaemia, *Journal of Chronic Diseases* **33**, 703–712.

[33] Mack, C. (1948). An exact formula for $Q_k(n)$, the probable number of k-aggregates in a random distribution of n points, *The London, Edinburgh, and Dublin Philosophical Magazine and Journal of Science* **39**, 778–790.

[34] Mantel, N. (1967). The detection of disease clustering and a generalized regression approach, *Cancer Research* **27**, 209–220.

[35] Mantel, M., Kryscio, R.J. & Myers, M.H., (1976). Tables and formulas for extended use of the Ederer–Myers–Mantel disease clustering procedure, *American Journal of Epidemiology* **104**, 576–584.

[36] Moran, P.A.P. (1948). The interpretation of statistical maps, *Journal of the Royal Statistical Society, Series B* **10**, 243–251.

[37] Nagarwalla, N. (1996). A scan statistic with a variable window, *Statistics in Medicine* **15**, 845–850.

[38] Nass, C.A.G. (1959). The χ^2 test for small expectations in contingency tables, with special reference to accidents and absenteeism, *Biometrika* **46**, 365–385.

[39] Naus, J.I. (1965). The distribution of the size of the maximum cluster of points on a line, *Journal of the American Statistical Association* **60**, 532–538.

[40] Naus, J.I. (1965). Clustering of random points in two dimensions, *Biometrika* **52**, 263–267.

[41] Naus, J.I. (1966). Some probabilities, expectations and variances for the size of the largest clusters and smallest intervals, *Journal of the American Statistical Association* **61**, 1191–1199.

[42] Naus, J.I. (1982). Approximations for distributions of scan statistics, *Journal of the American Statistical Association* **77**, 177–183.

[43] Neff, N.D. & Naus, J.I. (1980). The distribution of the size of the maximum cluster of points on a line, in *IMS Series of Selected Tables in Mathematical Statistics*, Vol. 6 American Mathematical Society, Providence.

[44] Openshaw, S., Craft, A.W., Charlton, M. & Birch, J.M. (1988). Investigation of leukaemia clusters by use of a geographical analysis machine, *Lancet* **i**, 272–273.

[45] Pinkel, D. & Nefzger, D. (1959). Some epidemiological features of childhood leukemia in the Buffalo, N.Y. area, *Cancer* **12**, 351–358.

[46] Potthoff, R.F. & Whittinghill, M. (1966). Testing for homogeneity. I. The binomial and multinomial distributions, *Biometrika* **53**, 167–182.

[47] Potthoff, R.F. & Whittinghill, M. (1966). Testing for homogeneity. II. The Poisson distribution, *Biometrika* **53**, 183–190.

[48] Ripley, B.D. (1981). *Spatial Statistics*. Wiley, New York.

[49] Rothenberg, R.B. & Thacker, S.B. (1992). Guidelines for the investigation of clusters of adverse health events, in *Geographical and Environmental Epidemiology. Methods for Small-Area Studies*, P. Elliott, J. Cuzick, D. English & R. Stern, eds. Oxford University Press, Oxford, 264–277.

[50] Schilling, M.F. (1986). Multivariate two-sample tests based on nearest neighbors, *Journal of the American Statistical Association* **81**, 799–806.

[51] Wallenstein, S. & Neff, N. (1987). An approximation for the distribution of the scan statistic, *Statistics in Medicine* **6**, 197–207.

[52] Wallenstein, S., Naus, J. & Glaz, J. (1993). Power of the scan statistic for detection of clustering, *Statistics in Medicine* **12**, 1829–1843.

JACK CUZICK

Cochran's Q Statistic *see* Agreement, Measurement of

Cohort Study

Cohort studies constitute a central epidemiologic approach to the study of relationships between personal characteristics or exposures and the occurrence of health-related events, and hence to the identification of disease prevention hypotheses and strategies.

Consider a conceptually infinite population of individuals moving forward in time. A cohort study involves sampling a subset of such individuals, and observing the occurrence of events of interest, generically referred to as disease events, over some follow-up period. Such a study may be conducted to estimate the rates of occurrence of the diseases to be ascertained, but most often estimation of relationships between such rates and individual characteristics or exposures is the more fundamental study goal. If cohort study identification precedes the follow-up period, then the study is termed prospective, while a retrospective or historical cohort study involves cohort identification after a conceptual follow-up period (*see* **Cohort Study, Historical**). The subsequent presentation assumes a prospective design.

Other research strategies for studying exposure–disease associations, and for identifying disease prevention strategies, include **case-control studies** and randomized controlled disease prevention trials. Compared with case-control studies, cohort studies have the advantages that a wide range of health events can be studied in relation to exposures or characteristics of interest, and that prospectively ascertained exposure data are often of better quality than the retrospectively obtained data that characterize case-control studies. However, a cohort study of a particular association would typically require much greater cost and longer duration than would a corresponding case-control study, particularly if the study disease is rare. Compared with randomized controlled trials, cohort studies have the advantage of allowing the study of a broad range of exposures or characteristics in relation to health outcomes of interest, and typically of much simplified study logistics and reduced cost. Randomized intervention trials can also examine a broad range of exposures and disease associations in an observational manner, but the randomized assessments are necessarily restricted to examining the health consequences of a small number of treatments or interventions. However, disease prevention trials have the major advantage that these comparisons are not confounded (*see* **Confounding**) by pre-randomization disease risk factors, whether or not these are even recognized. The choice among these and other research strategies may depend on the distribution of the exposures in the study population and especially on the ability to measure such exposures reliably, on the knowledge and measurement of confounding factors, on the reliability of outcome ascertainment, and on study costs in relation to the public health potential of study results. These issues will be returned to in the final section of this article.

There are many examples of associations that have been identified or confirmed using cohort study techniques, including that between cigarette smoking and lung cancer; between blood pressure, blood cholesterol, cigarette smoking, and coronary heart disease; between current use of the original combined oral contraceptives and the risk of various vascular diseases; and between atomic bomb radiation exposure and the risk of leukemia or of various solid tumors, to name a few. In recent years there have also been many examples of the use of cohort study designs to examine the association between exposures that are difficult to measure, or that may have limited within-cohort exposure variability, and the occurrence of disease. Such examples may involve, for example, physical activity, dietary, environmental, or occupational exposures. In these settings cohort studies seem often to yield weak or equivocal results, and multiple cohort studies of the same general association may yield contradictory results. It is important to be able to anticipate the reliability and power of cohort studies, to be aware of strategies for enhancing study power and reliability, and to consider carefully optimal research strategies for assessing specific exposure–disease hypotheses.

This article relies substantially on a recent review of cohort study design issues by the author [66]. The reader is also referred to a number of books and review articles focusing on cohort study methodology, including Kleinbaum et al. [41], Miettinen [52], Kelsey et al. [40], Rothman [80], Breslow & Day [7], Kahn & Sempos [38], Checkoway et al. [16], Willett [101], and Morganstern & Thomas [57].

Basic Cohort Study Elements

Exposure Histories and Disease Rates

A general regression notation can be used to represent the exposures (and characteristics) to be ascertained in a cohort study. Let $z_1(u)^{\mathrm{T}} = [z_{11}(u), z_{12}(u), \ldots]$ denote a set of numerically coded variables that describe an individual's characteristics at "time" u, where, to be specific, u can be defined as time from selection into the cohort, and "T" denotes vector transpose. Let $Z_1(t) = [z_1(u), u < t]$ denote the history of such characteristics at times less than t. Note that the "baseline" exposure data, $Z_1(0)$, may include information that pertains to time periods prior to selection into the cohort. Denote by $\lambda[t; Z_1(t)]$ the

population **incidence rate** at time t for a disease of interest, as a function of an individual's preceding "covariate" history. A typical cohort study goal is the elucidation of the relationship between aspects of $Z_1(t)$ and the corresponding disease rate $\lambda[t; Z_1(t)]$. As mentioned above, a single cohort study may be used to examine many such covariate–disease associations.

The interpretation of the relationship between $\lambda[t; Z_1(t)]$ and $Z_1(t)$ may well depend on other factors. Let $Z_2(t)$ denote the history up to time t of a set of additional characteristics. If the variates $Z_1(t)$ and $Z_2(t)$ are related among population members at risk for disease at time t, and if the disease rate $\lambda[t; Z_1(t), Z_2(t)]$ depends on $Z_2(t)$, then an observed relationship between $\lambda[t; Z_1(t)]$ and $Z_1(t)$ may be attributable, in whole or in part, to $Z_2(t)$. Hence, toward an interpretation of causality (*see* **Causation**) one can focus instead on the relationship between $Z_1(t)$ and the disease rate function $\lambda[t; Z_1(t), Z_2(t)]$, thereby controlling for the "confounding" influences of Z_2. In principle, a cohort study needs to control for all pertinent confounding factors in order to interpret a relationship between Z_1 and disease risk as causal. It follows that a good deal must be known about the disease process and disease risk factors before an argument of causality can be made reliably. This feature places a special emphasis on the replication of results in various populations, with the idea that unrecognized or unmeasured confounding factors may differ among populations. As noted above, the principal advantage of a randomized disease prevention trial, as compared with a purely observational study, is that the randomization indicator variable $Z_1 = Z_1(0)$, where here $t = 0$ denotes the time of randomization, is unrelated to the histories $Z_2(0)$ of all confounding factors, whether or not such are recognized or measured. See, for example, Rubin [82], Robins [74, 76], and Greenland [27], for a fuller discussion of causal inference criteria and strategies.

The choice as to which factors to include in $Z_2(t)$, for values of t in the cohort follow-up period, can be far from straightforward. For example, factors on a causal pathway between $Z_1(t)$ and disease risk may give rise to "overadjustment" if included in $Z_2(t)$, since one of the mechanisms whereby the history $Z_1(t)$ alters disease risk has been conditioned upon. However, omission of such factors may leave a confounded association, since the relationship between Z_2 and disease risk may not be wholly attributable to the effects of Z_1 on Z_2. See Robins [76] for a detailed discussion of the assumptions and procedures needed to argue causality in such circumstances.

Cohort Selection and Follow-Up

Upon identifying the study diseases of interest and the "covariate" histories $Z(t) = [Z_1(t), Z_2(t)]$ to be ascertained and studied in relation to disease risk, one can turn to the estimation of $\lambda[t; Z(t)]$ based on a cohort of individuals selected from the study population. The basic cohort selection and follow-up requirement for valid estimation of $\lambda[t; Z(t)]$ is that at any $[t, Z(t)]$ a sample that is representative of the population in terms of disease rate be available and under active follow-up for disease occurrence. Hence, conceptually, cohort selection and censoring rates (e.g. loss to follow-up rates) could depend arbitrarily on $[t, Z(t)]$, but selection and follow-up procedures cannot be affected in any manner by knowledge about, or perception of, disease risk at specified $[t, Z(t)]$.

Cohort selection rates typically depend on a variety of pre-enrollment characteristics. Potential study subjects may be excluded if they fail to meet certain conditions, perhaps related to prior health events or to their likelihood of completing all study requirements. Similarly, potential study subjects may choose not to participate in a cohort study for a myriad reasons that may be impossible to quantify. How do such selection factors affect the validity or interpretation of estimates of $\lambda[t; Z(t)]$?

In the presence of selection factors the estimation of $\lambda[t; Z(t)]$ applies not to the original conceptual population, but to a reduced population satisfying cohort exclusionary and "willingness" criteria. The magnitude of disease rates may well differ between these two populations, particularly if certain health criteria must be met for inclusion, or if study subjects tend to be more or less healthy than the broader population from which they arise. The magnitude of associations between $\lambda[t; Z(t)]$ and elements of $Z(t)$ may be affected by cohort selection, thereby limiting the ability to "generalize" the estimated association to the larger population. In general, issues of bias and **effect modification** can be addressed satisfactorily only if the selection factors are accurately measured and properly incorporated into the disease rate model. The ability to generalize to the larger population additionally requires knowledge about, or estimates of, cohort selection rates as a function of selection factor values (*see* **Validity and Generalizability in Epidemiologic Studies**).

As noted previously, censoring rates at a typical follow-up time t may depend on aspects of $Z(t)$ without biasing the estimation of $\lambda[t; Z(t)]$. Note, however, that elements of $Z(t)$ that relate to censoring then typically need to be included in the disease rate model and analysis in order to avoid bias. For this reason, as well as reasons of overall study power, it is important to strive to minimize losses to follow-up in cohort study conduct. Certainly, a dependence of selection or censoring rates on characteristics that may be affected by the exposures of interest can much complicate the interpretation of corresponding estimated relationships with disease risk.

The reader is referred to Miettinen [52] and the texts previously listed, as well as to Greenland [24], Miettinen [53, 54], and Poole [63], for discussion of the definition of the study population, and of the "study base" subset thereof from which a cohort is selected, and to these same sources and Greenland [25], Kalbfleisch & Prentice [39, Chapter 5], and Robins [75] for further discussion of cohort study follow-up bias (*see* **Bias in Cohort Studies**).

Covariate History Ascertainment

In general, valid estimation of $\lambda[t; Z(t)]$ within the subpopulation defined by the selection and follow-up procedures requires the accurate and timely ascertainment of the histories $Z(t)$ during the cohort study follow-up period. As before, let $t = 0$ denote the time of enrollment into the cohort. Then one seeks accurate ascertainment of $Z(t)$ for values of $t \geq 0$ in the follow-up period for each cohort member. Characteristics or exposures prior to cohort enrollment ($t < 0$) may be of considerable interest, but there may be a limited ability to obtain such information retrospectively. Hence, it may sometimes be necessary to restrict the covariate history $Z(0)$ to time-independent factors, or to the current or recent values of time-varying factors. Reliable measurement tools may not be available, even for current values of exposures of interest, or for corresponding confounding factor histories. Similarly, during cohort follow-up ($t > 0$) reliable means of updating covariate histories may or may not be available, and such updates would typically be practicable only at a few selected time points. Also, some of the measurements of interest to be included in $Z(t)$ may be too expensive to obtain on all cohort members. For example, such measurements may involve biochemical or molecular analysis of blood components, or hand extraction of occupational exposure histories from employer records. Hence, a covariate subsampling plan may be an important element of a cohort study concept and design.

Disease Event Ascertainment

A cohort study will often involve a system for regularly updating disease event information. This may involve asking study subjects to self-report a given set of diagnoses, or to self-report all hospitalizations. Hospital discharge summaries may then be examined for diagnoses of interest with confirmation by other medical and laboratory records. Sometimes disease events of interest will be actively ascertained by taking periodic measurements on all cohort members. For example, electrocardiographic tracings toward coronary heart disease diagnosis or screening breast mammograms toward breast cancer diagnosis may be a part of a basic study protocol. Diagnoses that require considerable judgment may be examined by a committee of experts toward enhancing the standardization and accuracy of disease event diagnoses. In spite of the application of the best practical outcome ascertainment procedures, there will usually be some misclassification (*see* **Misclassification Error**) of whether or not certain disease events have occurred with resulting bias in the estimation of $\lambda[t; Z(t)]$. A dependence of ascertainment rates on factors other than those included in $Z(t)$ may be able to be accommodated by including such factors as control variables in $Z_2(t)$.

Unbiased ascertainment of the timing of disease events relative to $Z(t)$ is also important for valid inference. For example, if disease screening activities vary with aspects of $Z(t)$, leading to earlier reporting at some covariate values than at others, then biased associations will typically arise. Similarly, differential lags in the reporting of disease events may cause bias unless specifically accommodated in data analysis.

Data Analysis

Suppose now that covariate disease associations of interest have been identified, and that procedures for selecting a cohort and for accurately ascertaining pertinent covariate histories and disease event times have

been established. What then can be said about the ability to detect an association between a particular characteristic or exposure and a corresponding disease risk? Typically, a test of association would be formulated in the context of a descriptive statistical model, though in some settings a mechanistic or biologically based model may be available (e.g. Armitage & Doll [2], Whittemore & Keller [99], and Moolgavkar & Knudson [56] (*see* **Multistage Carcinogenesis Models**).

A very useful and flexible descriptive modeling approach formulates the association in terms of relative risk. Specifically, one supposes [18] that

$$\lambda\{t; Z(t)\} = \lambda_0(t)\exp\{z(t)^T\beta\}, \qquad (1)$$

where $z(t)^T = \{z_1(t), \ldots, z_p(t)\}$ is a modeled regression vector formed from $Z(t)$, $\beta^T = (\beta_1, \ldots, \beta_p)$ is a corresponding relative risk parameter to be estimated, and $\lambda_0(\cdot)$ is an unrestricted baseline disease rate (**hazard**) function corresponding to a modeled regression vector $z(t) \equiv 0$. A test of the null hypothesis of no association between, say, $z_1(t)$ and disease risk then corresponds to $\beta_1 = 0$. Estimation and testing can be conducted by applying standard likelihood procedures to the partial likelihood function

$$L(\beta) = \prod_{i=1}^{k}\left\{\exp[z_i(t_i)^T\beta] \Big/ \sum_{l\in R(t_i)}\exp[z_l(t_i)^T\beta]\right\}, \qquad (2)$$

where $t_1, \ldots, t_k$ denotes the disease incidence times in the cohort, $z_i(t_i)$ is the modeled covariate at time t_i for the cohort member diagnosed at t_i, and $R(t_i)$ denotes the set of cohort members being followed for disease occurrence at time t_i. Consideration of the distribution of the score statistics $U_1(0) = \partial \log L(\hat{\beta}_0)/\partial\hat{\beta}_0^T$, where $\hat{\beta}_0$ maximizes $L(\beta)$ subject to $\beta_1 = 0$, makes it clear that the power of the test for $\beta_1 = 0$ depends primarily on the magnitude, β_1, of the regression coefficient, the expected number of disease events, k, during cohort follow-up, and the "spread" of the primary regression variable distribution $[z_{1l}(t); l \in R(t)]$ across the cohort follow-up times. The power will also depend somewhat on the distributions of the other (control) variables included in $z(t)$ and on the sampling variation in $\hat{\beta}_0$. A useful generalization of (1) allows the baseline disease rate function $\lambda_0(\cdot)$ to differ arbitrarily among strata that may be time dependent, typically defined by categorizing the histories $Z_2(t)$. Estimation and testing can then be based on a likelihood function that is simply the product of terms (2) over strata.

Conditions for the avoidance of confounding and other biases in the estimation, of a **relative risk** parameter β_1 are naturally less restrictive than are those for accurate estimation of the entire disease rate process $\lambda[t; Z(t)]$. For example, selection, follow-up, and disease ascertainment rates can depend on factors not included in $Z(t)$ provided such factors are unrelated to $Z_1(t)$, conditional on $[t, Z_2(t)]$, without implying bias in the estimation of β_1, assuming that a relative risk model of the form (1) holds conditional on such factors. There is a considerable epidemiologic literature exploring such issues. In addition to the texts previously cited see, for example, Miettinen & Cook [55], Boivin & Wacholder [5], and Greenland & Robins [29]. Though the use of relative risk, and of closely associated **odds ratios** is ubiquitous in epidemiology, other measures of association, including disease rate difference measures, also have utility and their own criteria for valid estimation. See, for example, the texts previously cited and Greenland [25]. The evolution of the covariate histories $Z(t)$, over time, may also be of substantive interest. For example, the extent to which disease risk factors track over time may have clinical implications, or the extent to which an intermediate outcome in $Z_2(t)$ can explain an exposure disease association may provide insights into disease mechanisms. Joint analyses of an exposure in relation to two or more disease processes may also be of considerable practical interest.

Subsequent sections expand upon these basic cohort study features.

Study Design

Cohort Study Power

A number of authors have provided a methodology for cohort study sample size and power determination (e.g. Gail, [22], Casagrande et al. [15], Fleiss et al. [20], Whittemore [97], Brown & Green [11], Greenland [23], and Self et al [85]. Breslow & Day [7, Chapter 7] provide a detailed account of this topic, including consideration of the impact of varying the exposure distribution, of confounding factor control, of **matching**, and of nested case-control sampling (*see* **Case–Control Study, Nested**), on study power. See also Whittemore & McMillan [100].

As suggested above, a comprehensive approach to the issue of study power for a particular association would require a range of design assumptions, including assumptions about the exposure distribution and its variation across time, about the magnitude of the regression parameter β_1, and concerning the baseline disease incidence rates. Though such a comprehensive approach may be useful, and flexible power calculation procedures permitting the use of complex assumptions are available (e.g. Self et al. [85]), power calculations for the simple odds ratio special case can provide valuable guidance concerning cohort study power and related design choices. Suppose that a baseline characteristic or exposure of interest is dichotomized into an "exposed" group ($Z_1 = 1$) comprised of the fraction, γ, of the population having a high value of an exposure, and an "unexposed" group ($Z_1 = 0$) comprised of the fraction, $1 - \gamma$, of the population having a comparatively low value. Let p_1 denote the probability that an exposed subject experiences a study disease of interest during a prescribed cohort follow-up period and let p_2 be the corresponding probability for an unexposed subject. Note that p_1 and p_2 can be thought of as average probabilities over the respective distributions of cohort follow-up times and over the exposure distributions within the exposed and unexposed categories. A simple sample size formula, based on the well-known approximate normality of logarithm of the simple odds ratio estimator, indicates that the cohort sample size must be at least

$$n = [p_2(1 - p_2)]^{-1}(\log \lambda)^{-2}Q, \qquad (3)$$

where $\lambda = p_1(1 - p_2)[p_2(1 - p_1)]^{-1}$ is the exposed vs. unexposed odds ratio, and $Q = [\gamma(1 - \gamma)]^{-1}\{W_{\alpha/2} - W_{1-\eta}[\gamma + \lambda^{-1}(1 - p_2 + \lambda p_2)^2(1 - \gamma)]^{1/2}\}^2$, to ensure that a two-sided α-level test (e.g. $\alpha = 0.05$) of the null hypothesis of no exposure effect ($\lambda = 1$) will be rejected with probability (power) η, where $W_{\alpha/2}$ and $W_{1-\eta}$ denote the upper $\alpha/2$ and $1 - \eta$ percentiles of the standard normal distribution, respectively.

Note that Q in Eq. (3) is a rather slowly varying function of λ and p_2 at specified α and η, so that the sample size necessary to achieve a specified power is approximately inversely proportional to $p_2(1 - p_2)$, where p_2 is again the unexposed disease probability, and inversely proportional to $(\log \lambda)^2$, the square of the exposed vs. unexposed log-odds ratio. Hence there is considerable sample size sensitivity to the magnitude of the odds ratio, with an odds ratio of 1.5 requiring about three times the cohort size of an odds ratio of 2.0, and an odds ratio of 1.25 requiring about ten times the sample size of that for an odds ratio of 2.0. The magnitude of the basic disease incidence rates (i.e. p_2) are also of considerable importance in the choice of a cohort size and average follow-up duration. Prentice [66] displayed selected power, η, calculations, developed in planning the cohort study component of the Women's Health Initiative [79, 103] which is currently enrolling 100 000 post-menopausal American women in the age range 50–79, based on (3) for selected cohort sizes, n, odds ratios, λ, and exposure fractions, γ. The power calculations are shown as a function of unexposed average incidence rates and average cohort follow-up duration, the product of which is the unexposed incidence rate p_2.

Measurement error in the modeled regression variable in (1) can involve a substantial loss of power and, except in idealized situations, can invalidate the null hypothesis test. The impact of covariate measurement error on the study design, conduct, and interpretation is one of the least developed, and potentially most important, aspects of cohort study methodology. For example, consider a binary exposure variable subject to misclassification. Suppose also that the misclassification rates do not vary within the exposed and unexposed groups, according to quantitative exposure levels or other study subject characteristics, and that all necessary confounding variables are included in the analysis and are measured without error. Under this circumstance, misclassification in the binary exposure variable effectively reduces the odds ratio λ in the sample size–power relationship (3). To cite a specific example, suppose that $Z_1 = 1$ denotes values above the median for a specific exposure while $Z_1 = 0$ denotes values below the median, so that $\gamma = 0.5$, $\lambda = 2.0$, and $p_2 = 0.02$. Suppose that rather than Z_1 one can only measure a variable X_1 which, when dichotomized at its median, gives $p(X_1 = 1|Z_1 = 1) = p(X_1 = 0|Z_1 = 0) = 1 - \Delta$ and $p(X_1 = 1|Z_1 = 0) = p(X_1 = 0|Z_1 = 0) = \Delta$. Suppose that this common misclassification probability takes the value $\Delta = 0.2$. The odds ratio based on the measured dichotomous variate X can then be calculated to be 1.50, so that a 20% exposure misclassification leads in these circumstances to a substantially attenuated odds ratio and requires an increase in cohort sample size by a factor of

about 3 to preserve power for the null hypothesis test. See, for example, Walter & Irwig [93] and Holford & Stack [33] for additional discussion of exposure measurement error effects on study design and power. In general, the effects of covariate measurement error may be much more profound than simply relative risk attenuation and loss of power, as will be discussed further below (*see* **Misclassification Error**; **Measurement Error in Epidemiologic Studies**).

Study Population

Typically a cohort study will be conceived with a set of motivating hypotheses in mind. The study population may then be selected as one in which such hypotheses and related associations may be able to be efficiently and reliably tested. For example, a range of studies of the health risks following from human exposure to ionizing radiation have been carried out in cohorts of atomic bomb exposed populations in Hiroshima and Nagasaki. A principal "Life Span Study" cohort consists of over 100 000 persons with residence in either city as of 1 October 1950 [4]. Decisions needed to be made concerning the inclusion of such residents who were some distance from the epicenter at the time of bombing or who were "not-in-city" at the time of bombing. The latter group has been variably included in reports from this study. The generalizability of the Life Span Study results is somewhat impacted by selection factors related to survival of the acute exposure and factors related to continuing residence in either of the two cities during the time period 1945–1950, but otherwise appears to be representative of a hypothetical population "like that of Hiroshima and Nagasaki residents" at the time of radiation exposure.

There are several ongoing cohort studies that are motivated in part by hypotheses related to diet and cancer. Recent examples include studies of US nurses (e.g. Willett et al. [102]), studies of women participating in a randomized trial of breast screening to prevent breast cancer mortality (e.g. Howe et al. [34]), studies of Iowa women (e.g. Kushi et al. [43]), and studies of men of Japanese heritage living in Hawaii (e.g. Stemmerman et al. [89]). Such studies appear to be limited (e.g. Prentice et al. [69]) by modest within-population variability in nutrient exposures of interest, substantial exposure measurement error in dietary assessment, and many highly correlated dietary exposure variables. These factors may combine to cast doubt on study reliability. Recent diet and cancer cohort study developments attempt to address such concerns by studying populations having a broader than usual range in dietary habits, by enhancing dietary assessment methodology, and by employing multiple dietary assessment tools in subsets of the cohort. Specifically, recently initiated diet and cancer cohort studies include a study among members of the American Association of Retired Persons with an overrepresentation of persons having estimated fat intake within certain extreme percentiles of the overall fat intake distribution; a multiethnic cohort study taking place in Los Angeles and Hawaii; and a multipopulation cohort study in Europe entitled the European Prospective Investigation into Cancer and Nutrition (EPIC) (e.g. Riboli [73]).

Much valuable information on cardiovascular disease risk factors has arisen in the context of randomized prevention trials, including, for example, cohort studies of persons enrolled in the Multiple Risk Factor Intervention Trial (MRFIT) [58], the Lipid Research Clinic Primary Prevention Trial [49], and the Hypertension Detection and Follow-up Program Trial [35]. Persons screened for possible enrollment in such trials include another potential source of cohort study enrollees. For example, the approximately 300 000 men screened for possible enrollment in MRFIT, a trial involving about 12 000 randomized men, yielded precise information on the relationship between blood cholesterol and mortality from various diseases (e.g. Jacobs et al. [37]).

In each of the cohort studies mentioned above consideration of inclusion and exclusion criteria is required in interpreting study results, particularly concerning the degree of generalizability of results to a broader source population.

Sample Size and Study Duration

One approach to establishing the size of the cohort is to list motivating hypotheses along with corresponding design assumptions, and to select a cohort size that will yield acceptable power (e.g. >80%) for all, or most, key hypotheses within a practical follow-up period. In fact, cohort studies are often initiated with the hope that active follow-up will continue for some decades, but for scientific and logistic reasons study planning exercises may need to be based on an average follow-up period of, say, 5–10 years. These

reasons include funding cycle logistics, the desire of investigators to produce new information in a practicable time period, and a possible reduced relevance of baseline covariate data to disease risk determination beyond a few years of follow-up. Exercises to determine a cohort size should make provisions for the power-influencing factors mentioned previously, particularly exposure measurement error influences.

A more empirical approach to cohort size determination can be based on the consideration of previous cohort study sizes and of the corresponding range of associations tested. Specifically, cohort studies that have yielded much useful information on cardiovascular disease risk factors have often been in the range of 5000 to 20 000 persons, including, for example, the Framingham Study, observational studies within the MRFIT study and other coronary heart disease prevention trials, the Adult Health Study of atomic bomb survivors, and the Cardiovascular Health Study. Cohort sizes in the vicinity of 5000 may be adequate for cardiovascular disease studies among older persons, as in the Cardiovascular Health Study [21] that is restricted to persons of age 65 or older, whereas considerably larger cohort sizes may be indicated for studies among younger persons, as in the Royal College of General Practitioners' study of the health effects of oral contraceptive use [81] that enrolled 46 000 younger women.

Most cohort studies of diet and cancer to date have involved sample sizes in the vicinity of 50 000–100 000, including, for example, the Nurses Health Study, the Canadian National Breast Screening study, and the Iowa Women's study. Consideration of range of nutrient intake and likely magnitude of random measurement error in dietary assessment, however, suggests that some pertinent odds ratios following measurement error influences can be hypothesized to be in the range 1.1–1.2 (e.g. Prentice et al. [69], Prentice & Sheppard [70], Prentice [67]). These types of considerations support the recently initiated cohort studies involving larger sample sizes (e.g. 100 000–400 000) in populations having an unusual degree of diversity of dietary habits.

Study Conduct and Analysis

Protocol and Procedures

A cohort study requires a clear, concise protocol that describes study objectives, design choices, performance goals and monitoring and analysis procedures. A detailed manual of procedures, which describes how the goals will be achieved, is necessary to ensure that the protocol is applied in a standardized fashion. Carefully developed data collection and management tools and procedures, with as much automation as practicable, can also enhance study quality. Centralized training of key personnel may be required to ensure that the protocol is understood, and to enhance study subject recruitment and comparability of outcome ascertainment as a function of exposures and confounding factors.

Analysis and reporting procedures should acknowledge the large number of exposure–disease associations that may be examined in a given cohort study, as well as the multiple time points at which hypotheses concerning each such exposure may be tested. In fact, even though such multiple testing considerations are routinely acknowledged in randomized clinical trials, their inclusion in cohort study reporting seems to be uncommon.

Covariate Data Ascertainment and Reliability

The above framework assumes that pertinent covariate histories $Z(t)$ are available for all cohort members at all times t during the cohort follow-up period. Conceptually, the availability of such data would require baseline covariate data collection to ascertain all pertinent exposures and characteristics prior to enrollment in the cohort study followed by the continuous updating of evolving covariates of interest during cohort follow-up. In practice, however, there may be a limited ability to ascertain retrospectively such covariate information at baseline, unless relevant specimens and materials had fortuitously been collected and stored for other reasons. Furthermore, there will be a limit to the frequency and extent of covariate data updating that can be carried out during covariate follow-up. Such evolving covariate data may be a key to adequate confounding control [76], and may be fundamental to such issues as the estimation of time lags between exposure and disease risk, and estimation of the relationship between covariate change and disease risk more generally.

The fact that the desired covariates may be poorly measured, or completely missing, can be a substantial impediment to the analysis and interpretation of study results. The effects of mismeasured or missing exposure or confounding factor data on relative risk parameter estimation may be much more profound than simple attenuation. In fact, if the measurement error variances are at all large (e.g. more than 10%–20%) relative to the variance of the true regression variables, then it will often be important to undertake additional data collection in the form of validation or calibration substudies, toward accommodating such measurement errors in data analysis. These substudies can also aid in the accommodation of missing covariate data, as it is otherwise necessary to make a missing at random assumption; that is, to assume that missingness rates are independent of the true covariate value, given the accumulated data at earlier time points (*see* **Missing Data in Epidemiologic Studies**).

Validation and Calibration Substudies

In some circumstances it may be possible to design a cohort study to include a validation subsample in which covariate measurements that are essentially without measurement error are taken in a random subset of the cohort. Such measurements may be too expensive or too demanding on study subjects to be practicable for more than a small subset of the cohort. See Greenland [26], Marshall [50], and Spiegelman & Gray [88] for discussion of the role and design of validation substudies (*see* **Validation Study**).

Consistent estimation of the relative risk parameter β is possible by making use of a validation substudy (e.g. Pepe & Fleming [59], Carroll & Wand [14], Lee & Sepanski [46]), though the loss of efficiency arising from substantial measurement errors presumably may be large. The validation sample permits nonparametric estimation of the expectation of $\exp[z(t)^T\beta]$ given the measured covariate and study subject "at risk" status at t, obviating the need for specific measurement error assumptions, and giving rise to estimated likelihood or estimated score procedures for the estimation of β. An alternate data analysis strategy, in the presence of a validation subsample, simply replaces the mismeasured covariate by its estimated conditional expectation, given the accumulated data on the study subject at preceding times. This so-called regression calibration approach is quite convenient, and it performs well in a variety of circumstances even though typically technically inconsistent under (1) and other nonlinear models (e.g. Prentice [64], Rosner et al. [77, 78], Carroll et al. [12], and Wang et al. [94]). If a validation study is possible for some or all important covariates, then the inclusion of a validation sample of appropriate size may be a critically important aspect of cohort study design and conduct.

The regression calibration procedure just mentioned extends fairly readily even if the subsample measure is not the true covariate value but is contaminated by measurement error that is independent of both the routinely available measurement and the true covariate values. See, for example, Greenland & Kleinbaum [28], Kupper [42], Whittemore [98], Rosner et al. [78, 79], Pierce et al. [61], Carroll et al. [13], Armstrong [3], Clayton [17], Thomas et al. [90], and Sepanski et al. [86] for various approaches to cohort data analyses in the presence of calibration subsamples.

Unfortunately, the situation changes dramatically if the subsample measurement error does not satisfy such independence properties. For example, Prentice [67] considers a measurement model for two self-report measures of dietary fat in an attempt to interpret a combined cohort study analysis of dietary fat in relation to breast cancer. One self-report measure, based on food frequency assessment, was available in all cohort study members, while a more detailed measure, based on multiple days of food recording, was available on a small subset of the cohorts in question. By using food frequency and food record data from the Women's Health Trial feasibility study [36] and allowing the dietary fat measurement errors for the two instruments to be correlated and to depend on an individual's body mass index, Prentice [67] showed that even the strong relative risk relationship between fat and postmenopausal breast cancer suggested by international correlation studies (e.g. Prentice & Sheppard [70] could be projected to be essentially undetectable in a cohort study using a food frequency instrument, regardless of its size. Specifically, relative risks of 1, 1.5, 2.0, 2.7, and 4.0 across fat intake quintiles if measurement errors were absent are reduced to projected values of 1, 1.0, 1.0, 1.1, and 1.1 upon allowing for both random and systematic aspects of dietary fat measurement error. This illustration suggests that covariate measurement errors may be at the root of many controversial associations in epidemiology, and motivates the importance of objective measures of exposure. Biomarker exposure measures may be quite valuable in such contexts even if such measures include considerable noise. For example,

in the dietary area, total energy expenditure can be objectively measured over short periods of time using doubly labelled water techniques while protein expenditure can be measured by urinary nitrogen (e.g. Lichtman et al. [47], Heitmann & Lessner [32], Martin et al. [51], Sawaya et al. [84]). Plummer & Clayton [62] use urinary nitrogen data to demonstrate correlated measurement errors among dietary protein self-report measures.

Additional Sampling Strategies

It will often be efficient when conducting a cohort study to assemble the raw materials for covariate history assembly on the entire cohort, but to restrict the processing and analysis of such materials to appropriate subsamples. For example, a random sample, or stratified random sample, of the cohort may be selected, along with all persons experiencing disease events of interest, for covariate data processing. Such a case–cohort approach allows relative risk estimation (e.g. Prentice [65]) based on (2) with $R(t_i)$ consisting of the person developing a disease at t_i (the case) along with all "at risk" members of the selected sample (the subcohort), though (2) no longer has a likelihood function interpretation and specialized variance estimators are required (*see* **Case–Cohort Study**). Alternatively, a case of a specific disease at time t_i may be matched to one or more controls randomly selected from the risk set at t_i, with ordinary likelihood methods applied to (2) except that $R(t_i)$ is replaced by the case and time-matched controls (e.g. Liddell et al. [48], Prentice & Breslow [68]) (*see* **Case–Control Study, Nested**). Recently Samuelson [83] has proposed an alternate analysis of such nested case-control samples that appears to yield meaningful efficiency improvements relative to the standard procedure just described.

The nested case-control sampling approach allows cases and controls to be matched on various study subject characteristics, including time from enrollment into the cohort, as may be important if some covariate measurements (e.g. blood concentrations of selected nutrients) degrade with storage time. Such issues may be accommodated under case–cohort sampling by stratifying the subcohort selection on cohort enrollment data and by analyzing all case and subcohort specimens and materials at a common point in time. In fact, it may be useful to delay subcohort selection to the time of data analysis in order to match subcohort sizes in each stratum to the corresponding numbers of disease events. See Langholz & Thomas [44, 45] and Wacholder [91] for further discussion and comparison of nested case-control and case–cohort sampling.

A related topic includes a two-stage process in establishing a cohort. A first stage would involve collecting information on the exposures of primary interest, or perhaps collecting fairly crude estimates of such exposures. The second stage would then involve selecting a subset of the stage 1 study subjects that give a desirable exposure distribution for more detailed data collection. The diet and cancer cohort study among members of the American Association of Retired Persons provides an example in which subjects are oversampled for the second stage if their food frequency estimated fat intakes are in certain extreme percentiles. A two-stage sampling approach is also natural for the study of rare exposures. A considerable literature exists on the design and analysis of two-stage sampling schemes, mostly in the context of case-control studies (e.g. White [96], Walker [92], Breslow & Cain [8], Breslow & Zhao [9], Flanders & Greenland [19] (*see* **Case–Control Study, Two-Phase**).

Additional Data Analysis Topics

The above discussion assumes that the basic time variable is time from selection into the cohort. This choice is attractive in that relative risk estimation [i.e. each factor in (2)] is then based on comparisons among individuals at the same length of time since cohort entry. Other important time variables, such as study subject age and chronologic time, can be accommodated by regression modeling, or stratification with (2) replaced by a product of like terms over strata. Alternatively, if cohort eligibility criteria or recruitment strategies changed markedly over time, or if covariate data or outcome data ascertainment procedures changed markedly over time, one may prefer to define t to be chronologic time so that relative risk estimates are based on comparisons of measurement taken under common procedures, with age and time since study enrollment controlled by stratification or modeling. In this case a study subject begins contributing to (2) at the time (date) of study enrollment.

If the study is conducted to estimate disease rates, or cumulative disease rates and **absolute risks**, then it may be natural for interpretation to define t to be age,

or time from some significant event (e.g. infection with human immunodeficiency virus). Depending on the means of study subject identification such significant event data may only be known to be earlier than a specified time, giving rise to interval censored event time data and a range of interesting statistical estimation issues (e.g. Brookmeyer & Gail [10, Chapter 5]) (*see* **Biased Sampling of Cohorts in Epidemiology**).

The fact that multiple outcomes are typically ascertained in a cohort study allows for the possibility of relating an exposure jointly to two or more event rates and, of course, there may be multiple events of a given type during the cohort study follow-up of an individual. The literature includes generalization of (1) to repeat failure times on an individual study subject (e.g. Prentice et al. [72], Andersen et al. [1]), while for single occurrences of multiple types of events one can consider the use of (2) for each failure type in conjunction with a modified variance estimation procedure for the joint estimation of relative risks for several diseases (e.g. Wei et al. [95]). This latter procedure will have acceptable efficiency under most situations of practical interest.

The above presentation assumes that failure times among distinct cohort study members are independent. This assumption may be violated if study subjects share environmental or genetic factors. In fact, in **genetic epidemiology** one may use the relationships among the failure time data of family members in a pedigree cohort study in an attempt to identify the existence (aggregation analysis), inheritance pattern (segregation analysis) and physical location (linkage analysis) of genes that play a role in determining disease risk. Such studies or, more practically, case-control subsamples of population-based family studies, may also be used to study gene–environment interaction.

Cohort Study Role

Cohort studies properly play a central role in epidemiologic research. Disease associations that are relatively strong can often be reliably studied using cohort study techniques, especially if there is sufficient knowledge of disease risk factors and exposure correlates to permit comprehensive efforts to control confounding. Relative risk analyses are unlikely to be misleading under these circumstances since residual **confounding** will tend to be small compared with the relative risk trend under study. If the exposures and other covariates of interest can be reliably ascertained retrospectively, then a case-control design may introduce considerable economies relative to a cohort study; in fact, the case-control design is very commonly employed, particularly if the study diseases are rare and good disease registries are available for case ascertainment.

If the relative risk trends to be studied are more modest, then the reliability of the cohort study may be less clear, as uncontrolled confounding, or other biases, may have a salient impact on the estimated associations. If, in addition, the exposures of interest or strong confounding factors or disease outcomes involve measurement errors that are substantial, but of unknown properties, then the cohort study reliability may be poor.

In these circumstances one can turn to an experimental approach, as has been done to study the role of diet in disease in various studies of micronutrient supplementation, and of a low fat eating pattern. Such clinical trials permit a valid test of the intervention applied in relation to a range of diseases without concern about "baseline" confounding, and without the need for precise dietary assessment. Dietary assessment, in such contexts, enters in a secondary fashion to document that a sufficiently powerful hypothesis test has been conducted, and in attempts to isolate intervention activities responsible for any observed disease risk difference. However, primary disease prevention clinical trials are logistically difficult and expensive, so that only a few can be conducted at any time point, preferably those that are motivated by hypotheses having great public health potential.

The recent movement mentioned above, toward multipopulation cohort studies (e.g. the EPIC study) to enhance exposure heterogeneity seems attractive in the type of circumstances alluded to above. Such a multipopulation cohort can be expected to involve a broadened exposure range, perhaps in a manner that does not increase covariate measurement errors, thereby enhancing both reliability and power. The relative risk information in such a multipopulation study can be partitioned into between-population and within-population components under standard random effects modeling assumptions (e.g. Sheppard & Prentice [87]). In fact, it may often happen that much of the retrievable information arises from between-population sources. Also, between-population, but not within-population, relative risk estimates tend to be

highly robust to independent mean zero measurement errors in covariates, essentially because such estimates are based on covariate function averages over large numbers of study subjects that are little affected by such errors. Furthermore, the between-population relative risk information may be able to be extracted efficiently by relating covariate history data on modest numbers of persons in each population (e.g. 100–200) to corresponding population disease rates, as may be available from disease registers in each population [71]. These points suggest that studies of relatively modest relative risk trends associated with exposures that are measured with considerable noise may sometimes be efficiently studied using an aggregate data (ecologic) approach that involves covariate surveys in disease populations covered by good quality disease registers. Note, however, that confounding control across heterogeneous populations may pose particular challenges, and that careful data analysis will be required to avoid aggregation and other biases in such a study. See Piantadosi et al. [60], Greenland & Morganstern [30], Brenner et al. [6], and Greenland & Robins [31] for further discussion of these bias issues (*see* **Ecologic Study**; **Ecologic Fallacy**).

Statistical thinking and methodology have come to play an important role in the design, conduct, and analysis of cohort studies. Cox regression and closely related logistic regression methods play a central role in data analysis and reporting, and in related study planning efforts. Cohort sampling techniques are widely used and have enhanced cohort study efficiency. A topic of continuing importance relates to the methodology for measurement error assessment, and to analytic methods to reduce the sensitivity of results to measurement error influences.

Acknowledgment

This work was supported by grant CA-53996 from the National Institutes of Health.

References

[1]   Andersen, P.K., Borgan, D., Gill, R.D. & Keiding, N. (1961). *Statistical Models Based on Counting Processes.* Springer-Verlag, New York.

[2]   Armitage, P. & Doll, R. (1961). Stochastic models for carcinogenesis, in *Proceedings of the Fourth Berkeley Symposium on Mathematical Statistics and*

Probability, vol. IV University of California Press, Berkeley, pp. 19–38.

[3]   Armstrong, B.G. (1991). The effect of measurement error on relative risk regressions, *American Journal of Epidemiology* **132**, 1176–1184.

[4]   Beebe, G.W. & Usagawa, M. (1968). The major ABCC samples, *Atomic Bomb Casualty Commission Technical Report* 12–68.

[5]   Boivin, J.F. & Wacholder, S. (1985). Conditions for confounding of the risk ratio and the odds ratio, *American Journal of Epidemiology* **121**, 152–158.

[6]   Brenner, H., Savitz, D.A., Jöckel, K.H. & Greenland, S. (1992). The effects of non-differential exposure misclassification in ecological studies, *American Journal of Epidemiology* **135**, 85–95.

[7]   Breslow, N.E. & Day, N.E. (1987). *Statistical Methods in Cancer Research*, Vol. 2: *The Design and Analysis of Cohort Studies*. IARC Scientific Publications No. 82, International Agency for Research on Cancer, Lyon, France.

[8]   Breslow, N.E. & Cain, K.C. (1988). Logistic regression for two-stage case-control data, *Biometrika* **74**, 11–20.

[9]   Breslow, N.E. & Zhao, L.P. (1988). Logistic regression for stratified case-control studies, *Biometrics* **44**, 891–899.

[10]   Brookmeyer, R. & Gail, M.H. (1994). *AIDS Epidemiology: A Quantitative Approach*. Oxford University Press, New York.

[11]   Brown, C.C. & Green, S.B. (1982). Additional power computations for designing comparative Poisson trials, *American Journal of Epidemiology* **115**, 752–758.

[12]   Carroll, R.J., Ruppert, D. & Stefanski, L.A. (1995). *Measurement Error in Nonlinear Models*. Chapman & Hall, New York.

[13]   Carroll, R.J. & Stefanski, L.A. (1990). Approximate quasi-likelihood estimation in models with surrogate predictors, *Journal of the American Statistical Association* **85**, 652–663.

[14]   Carroll, R.J. & Wand, M.P. (1991). Semiparametric estimation in logistic measurement error models, *Journal of the Royal Statistical Society, Series B* **53**, 573–585.

[15]   Casagrande, J.T., Pike, M.C. & Smith, P.G. (1978). An improved approximate formula for calculating sample sizes for comparing two binomial distributions, *Biometrics* **34**, 483–486.

[16]   Checkoway, H., Pearce, N. & Crawford-Brown, D.J. (1989). *Research Methods in Occupational Epidemiology*. Oxford University Press, New York.

[17]   Clayton, D.G. (1992). Models for the analysis of cohort and case-control studies with inaccurately measured exposures, in *Statistical Models for Longitudinal Studies of Health*, J.H. Dwyer, P. Lippert, M. Feinleib & H. Hoffmeister, eds. Oxford University Press, Oxford, pp. 301–331.

[18]   Cox, D.R. (1972). Regression models and life tables (with discussion), *Journal of the Royal Statistical Society, Series B* **34**, 187–220.

[19]   Flanders, W.D. & Greenland, S. (1991). Analytic methods for two-stage case-control studies and other stratified designs, *Statistics in Medicine* **10**, 739–747.

[20]   Fleiss, J.L., Tytun, A. & Ury, U.K. (1980). A simple approximation for calculating sample sizes for comparing independent proportions, *Biometrics* **36**, 343–346.

[21]   Fried, L.P., Borhani, N., Enright, P., Furberg, C., Gardin, J.M., Kronmal, R.A., Kuller, L.H., Manolio, T., Mittlemark, M.B., Newman, A., O'Leary, D.H., Psaty, B., Rautaharju, P., Tracy, R.P., Weiler, P.G. for the Cardiovascular Health Study Research Group (CHS) (1991). The cardiovascular health study: design and rationale, *Annals of Epidemiology* **1**, 263–276.

[22]   Gail, M. (1974). Power computations for designing comparative Poisson trials, *Biometrics* **30**, 231–237.

[23]   Greenland, S. (1985). Power, sample size and smallest detectable effect determination for multivariate studies, *Statistics in Medicine* **4**, 117–127.

[24]   Greenland, S. (1986). Cohorts versus dynamic populations: A dissenting view, *Journal of Chronic Diseases* **39**, 565–566.

[25]   Greenland, S. (1987). Interpretation and choice of effect measures in epidemiologic analyses, *American Journal of Epidemiology* **125**, 761–768.

[26]   Greenland, S. (1988). Statistical uncertainty due to misclassification: implications for validation substudies, *Journal of Clinical Epidemiology* **41**, 1167–1174.

[27]   Greenland, S. (1990). Randomization, statistics and causal inference, *Epidemiology* **1**, 421–429.

[28]   Greenland, S. & Kleinbaum, D.G. (1983). Correcting for misclassification in two-way tables and matched-pair studies, *International Journal of Epidemiology* **12**, 93–97.

[29]   Greenland, S. & Robins, J.M. (1986). Identifiability, exchangeability, and epidemiological confounding, *International Journal of Epidemiology* **15**, 412–418.

[30]   Greenland, S. & Morganstern, H. (1989). Ecological bias, confounding and effect modification, *International Journal of Epidemiology* **18**, 269–274.

[31]   Greenland, S. & Robins, J. (1994). Invited commentary: Ecologic studies. Biases, misconceptions and counterexamples, *American Journal of Epidemiology* **139**, 747–760.

[32]   Heitman, B.L. & Lessner, L. (1995). Dietary underreporting by obese individuals – is it specific or nonspecific? *British Medical Journal* **311**, 986–989.

[33]   Holford, T.R. & Stack, C. (1995). Study design for epidemiologic studies with measurement error, *Statistical Methods in Medical Research* **4**, 339–358.

[34]   Howe, G.R., Friedenreich, C.M., Jain, M. & Miller, A.B. (1991). A cohort study of fat intake and risk of breast cancer, *Journal of the National Cancer Institute* **83**, 336–340.

[35]   Hypertension Detection and Follow-up Program Cooperative Group (1979). Five year findings of the Hypertension Detection and Follow-up Program I. Reductions

in mortality of persons with high blood pressure, including mild hypertension, *Journal of the American Medical Association* **242**, 2562–2571.

[36] Insull, W., Henderson, M.M., Prentice, R.L., Thompson, D.J., Clifford, C., Goldman, S., Gorbach, S., Moskowitz, M., Thompson, R. & Woods, M. (1990). Results of a feasibility study of a low fat diet, *Archives of Internal Medicine* **150**, 421–427.

[37] Jacobs, D., Blackburn, H., Higgins, M., Reed, D., Iso, H., McMillan, G., Neaton, J., Nelson, J., Potter, J., Rifkind, B., Rossouw, J., Shekelle, R., Yusuf, S., for Participants in the Conference on Low Cholesterol: Mortality Associations (1992). Report of the conference on low blood cholesterol: Mortality associations, *Circulation* **86**, 1046–1060.

[38] Kahn, H.A. & Sempos CT (1989). *Statistical Methods in Epidemiology*. Oxford University Press, New York.

[39] Kalbfleisch, J.D. & Prentice, R.L. (1980). *The Statistical Analysis of Failure Time Data*. Wiley, New York.

[40] Kelsey, J.L., Thompson, W.D. & Evans, A.S. (1986). *Methods in Observational Epidemiology*. Oxford University Press, New York.

[41] Kleinbaum, D.G., Kupper, L.L. & Morganstern, H. (1982). *Epidemiologic Research: Principles and Quantitative Methods*. Lifetime Learning Publications, Belmont.

[42] Kupper, L.L. (1984). Effects of the use of unreliable surrogate variables on the validity of epidemiologic research studies, *American Journal of Epidemiology* **120**, 643–648.

[43] Kushi, L.H., Sellers, T.A., Potter, J.D., Nelson, C.L., Munger, R.G., Kaye, S.A. and Folson, A.R. (1992). Dietary fat and postmenopausal breast cancer, *Journal of the National Cancer Institute* **84**, 1092–1099.

[44] Langholz, B. & Thomas, D.C. (1990). Nested case-control and case–cohort methods for sampling from a cohort: a critical comparison, *American Journal of Epidemiology* **31**, 169–176.

[45] Langholz, B. & Thomas, D.C. (1991). Efficiency of cohort sampling designs: some surprising results, *Biometrics* **47**, 1553–1571.

[46] Lee, L.F. & Sepanski, J.H. (1995). Estimation in linear and nonlinear errors in variables models using validation data, *Journal of American Statistical Association* **90**, 130–140.

[47] Lichtman, S.W., Pisarka, K., Berman, E.R., Pestone, M., Dowling, H., Offenbacker, E., Weisel, H., Heshka, S., Matthews, D.E. & Heymsfield, S.B. (1992). Discrepancy between self-reported and actual calorie intake and exercise in obese subjects, *New England Journal of Medicine* **327**, 1893–1898.

[48] Liddell, F.D.K., McDonald, J.C. & Thomas, D.C. (1977). Methods for cohort analysis: appraisal by application to asbestos mining, *Journal of the Royal Statistical Society, Series A* **140**, 469–490.

[49] Lipid Research Clinic Program: The Lipid Research Clinic Coronary Primary Prevention Trial Results I (1984). Reduction in incidence of coronary heart disease, *Journal of the American Medical Association* **251**, 351–364.

[50] Marshall, R.J. (1990). Validation study methods for estimating exposure proportions and odds ratios with misclassified data, *Journal of Clinical Epidemiology* **43**, 941–947.

[51] Martin, L.J., Su, W., Jones, P.J., Lockwood, G.A., Tritchler, D.L. & Boyd, N.F. (1996). Comparison of energy intakes determined by food records and doubly labeled water in women participating in a dietary intervention trial, *American Journal of Clinical Nutrition* **63**, 483–490.

[52] Miettinen, O.S. (1985). *Theoretical Epidemiology: Principles of Occurrence Research in Medicine*. Wiley, New York.

[53] Miettinen, O.S. (1986). Response, *Journal of Chronic Diseases* **39**, 567.

[54] Miettinen, O.S. (1990). The concept of secondary base, *Journal of Clinical Epidemiology* **43**, 1017–1020.

[55] Miettinen, O.S. & Cook, E.F. (1981). Confounding: essence and detection, *American Journal of Epidemiology* **114**, 593–603.

[56] Moolgavkar, S.H. & Knudson, A. (1981). Mutation and cancer: a model for human carcinogenesis, *Journal of the National Cancer Institute* **66**, 1037–1052.

[57] Morganstern, H. & Thomas, D. (1993). Principles of study design in environmental epidemiology, *Environmental Health Perspectives* **101**, 23–38.

[58] Multiple Risk Factor Intervention Trial (MRFIT) Research Group (1982). Multiple risk factor intervention trial: risk factor changes and mortality results, *Journal of the American Medical Association* **248**, 1465–1477.

[59] Pepe, M. & Fleming, T.R. (1991). A nonparametric method for dealing with mis-measured covariate data, *Journal of the American Statistical Association* **86**, 108–113.

[60] Piantadosi, S., Byar, D.P. & Green, S.B. (1988). The ecological fallacy, *American Journal of Epidemiology* **127**, 893–904.

[61] Pierce, D.A., Stram, D. & Vaeth, M. (1990). Allowing for random errors in radiation dose estimates for the atomic bomb survivors, *Radiation Research* **126**, 36–42.

[62] Plummer, M. & Clayton, D. (1993). Measurement error in dietary assessment: an assessment using covariance structured models. Part II, *Statistics in Medicine* **12**, 937–948.

[63] Poole, C. (1990). Would vs. should in the definition of secondary study base, *Journal of Clinical Epidemiology* **43**, 1016–1017.

[64] Prentice, R.L. (1982). Covariate measurement errors and parameter estimation in Cox's failure time regression model, *Biometrika* **69**, 331–342.

[65] Prentice, R.L. (1986). A case–cohort design for epidemiologic cohort studies and disease prevention trials, *Biometrika* **73**, 1–11.

[66] Prentice, R.L. (1995). Design issues in cohort studies, *Statistical Methods in Medical Research* **4**, 273–292.

[67] Prentice, R.L. (1996). Measurement error and results from analytic epidemiology: Dietary fat and breast cancer, *Journal of the National Cancer Institute* **88**, 1738–1747.

[68] Prentice, R.L. & Breslow, N.E. (1978). Retrospective studies and failure time models, *Biometrika* **65**, 153–158.

[69] Prentice, R.L., Pepe, M. & Self, S.G. (1989). Dietary fat and breast cancer: a quantitative assessment of the epidemiologic literature and a discussion of methodologic issues, *Cancer Research* **49**, 3147–3156.

[70] Prentice, R.L. & Sheppard, L. (1990). Dietary fat and cancer: consistency of the epidemiologic data and disease prevention that may follow from a practical reduction in fat consumption, *Cancer Causes and Control* **1**, 87–97.

[71] Prentice, R.L. & Sheppard, L. (1995). Aggregate data studies of disease risk factors, *Biometrika* **82**, 113–125.

[72] Prentice, R.L., Williams, B.J. & Peterson, A.V. (1981). On the regression analysis of multivariate failure time data, *Biometrika* **68**, 373–379.

[73] Riboli, E. (1992). Nutrition and cancer: background and rationale of the European Prospective Investigation into cancer and nutrition (EPIC), *Annals of Oncology* **3**, 783–791.

[74] Robins, J. (1987). A graphical approach to the identification and estimation of causal parameters in mortality studies with sustained exposure periods, *Journal of Chronic Diseases, Suppl.* **2**, 139–161.

[75] Robins, J. (1989). The control of confounding by intermediate variables, *Statistics in Medicine* **8**, 679–701.

[76] Robins, J. (1997). Causal inference from complex longitudinal data, in *Latent Variable Modeling and Application to Causality, Springer Lecture Notes in Statistics*, Vol. 120, M. Berkane, ed. Springer-Verlag, New York, pp. 69–117.

[77] Rosner, B., Spiegelman, D. & Willett, W.C. (1990). Correction of logistic regression relative risk estimates and confidence intervals for measurement error: the case of multiple covariates measured with error, *American Journal of Epidemiology* **132**, 734–745.

[78] Rosner, B., Willett, W.C. & Spiegelman, D. (1989). Correction of logistic regression relative risk estimates and confidence intervals for systematic within-person measurement error, *Statistics in Medicine* **8**, 1051–1070.

[79] Rossouw, J., Finnegan, L.P., Harlan, W.R., Pinn, V.W., Clifford, C. & McGowan, J.A. (1995). The evolution of the Women's Health Initiative: perspectives from the NIH, *Journal of the American Medical Association* **50**, 50–55.

[80] Rothman, K.J. (1986). *Modern Epidemiology*. Little, Brown & Co., Boston, MA.

[81] Royal College of General Practitioners (RCGP) Oral Contraception Study (1974). *Oral Contraceptives and Health: An Interim Report*. Pitman, London.

[82] Rubin, D.B. (1978). Bayesian inference for causal effects: the role of randomization, *Annals of Statistics* **6**, 34–58.

[83] Samuelson, S.D. (1996). A Pseudo-Likelihood Approach to Analysis of Nested Case-Control Studies. *Technical Report No. 2*. Institute of Mathematics, University of Oslo.

[84] Sawaya, A.L., Tucker, K., Tsay, R., Willett, W., Saltzman, E., Dallal, G.E. & Roberts, S.B. (1996). Evaluation of four methods for determining energy intake in young and older women: comparison with doubly labeled water measurements of total energy expenditure, *American Journal of Clinical Nutrition* **63**, 491–499.

[85] Self, S.G., Mauritsen, R.H. & Ohara, J. (1992). Power calculations for likelihood ratio tests in generalized linear models, *Biometrics* **48**, 31–39.

[86] Sepanski, J.H., Knickerbocker, R. & Carrol, R.J. (1994). A semiparametric correction for attenuation, *Journal of the American Statistical Association* **89**, 1366–1373.

[87] Sheppard, L. & Prentice, R.L. (1995). On the reliability and precision of within and between population estimates of relative risk parameters, *Biometrics* **51**, 853–863.

[88] Spiegelman, D. & Gray, R. (1991). Cost efficient study designs for binary response data with Gaussian covariate measurement error, *Biometrics* **47**, 851–870.

[89] Stemmerman, G.N., Nomura, A.M.Y. & Heilbrun, L.K. (1984). Dietary fat and risk of colorectal cancer, *Cancer Research* **44**, 4633–4637.

[90] Thomas, D., Stram, D. & Dwyer, J. (1993). Exposure measurement error: influence on exposure–disease relationships and methods of correction, *Annual Review of Public Health* **14**, 69–93.

[91] Wacholder, S. (1991). Practical considerations in choosing between the case–cohort and nested case-control designs, *Epidemiology* **2**, 155–158.

[92] Walker, A.M. (1982). Anamorphic analysis: sampling and estimation for covariate effects when both exposure and disease are known, *Biometrics* **38**, 1025–1032.

[93] Walter, S.D. & Irwig, L.M. (1988). Estimation of test error rates, disease prevalence and relative risk from misclassified data: a review, *Journal of Clinical Epidemiology* **41**, 923–927.

[94] Wang, C.Y., Hsu, L., Feng, Z.D. & Prentice, R.L. (1997). Regression calibration in failure time regression with surrogate variables, *Biometrics*, 131–.

[95] Wei, L.J., Lin, D.Y. & Weissfeld, L. (1989). Regression analysis of multivariate incomplete failure time data by modeling marginal distributions, *Journal of the American Statistical Association* **84**, 1065–1073.

[96] White, J.E. (1982). A two-stage design for the study of the relationship between a rare exposure and a rare disease, *American Journal of Epidemiology* **115**, 119–128.

[97] Whittemore, A.S. (1981). Sample size for logistic regression with small response probabilities, *Journal of the American Statistical Association* **76**, 27–32.

[98] Whittemore, A.S. (1989). Errors-in-variables regression using Stein estimates, *American Statistician* **43**, 226–228.

[99] Whittemore, A.S. & Keller, J.B. (1978). Quantitative theories of carcinogenesis, *SIAM Review* **20**, 1–30.

[100] Whittemore, A.S. & McMillan, A. (1982). Analyzing occupational cohort data: application to US uranium miners, in *Environmental Epidemiology: Risk Assessment*, R.L. Prentice & A.S. Whittemore, eds. SIAM, Philadelphia, pp. 65–81.

[101] Willett, W.C. (1989). *Nutritional Epidemiology*. Oxford University Press, New York.

[102] Willett, W.C., Hunter, D.J., Stampfer, M.J., Colditz, G., Manson, J.E., Spiegelman, D., Rosner, B., Hennekens, C.H. & Speizer, F.E. (1992). Dietary fat and fiber in relation to risk of breast cancer, *Journal of the American Medical Association* **268**, 2037–2044.

[103] Women's Health Initiative Study Group (1997). Design of the Women's Health Initiative Clinical Trial and Observational Study, *Controlled Clinical Trials*, in press.

ROSS L. PRENTICE

Cohort Study, Historical

In **cohort study** design, participants are enrolled, often with selection based on one or more exposures of interest, and observed over time for disease incidence or mortality. Cohort studies are further classified by the timing of the enrollment and follow-up in relation to actual calendar time. Cohort studies involving identification of participants and follow-up into the future are termed "prospective cohort studies", while those involving follow-up and events in the past are referred to as "historical cohort studies". Other designations used for historical cohort design include "retrospective cohort study" and "nonconcurrent cohort study". A study may be initiated as an historical cohort study, but subsequently follow-up could be maintained into the future. The study of bladder cancer in British chemical industry workers, conducted by Case et al. [1], represents one of the first comprehensive applications of historical cohort design. Beginning the study in the 1950s, Case et al. traced a group of chemical industry workers employed subsequent to 1920 and showed a clear excess of deaths from bladder cancer, which was attributed to exposures to anilines. The researchers compared the data with expected mortality, on the basis of the experience of males in the general population, over the same time interval. Frost [3] and others had previously applied a similar method in studying infectious diseases.

Historical cohort design can be applied if records are available for the retrospective identification of study participants, the classification of the exposure(s) of interest, and the follow-up of the participants for the relevant outcomes. For example, historical cohort design has been widely applied in investigating the effects of specific occupations and industries (*see* **Occupational Epidemiology**), because of the availability of records appropriate to these purposes. Employment records can be used to identify cohort members and, in some instances, to estimate exposures; follow-up for mortality can be accomplished using pension records and national death registries. In the absence of an internal reference population, comparison has been made in many studies to mortality in the general population. For example, Samet et al. [6] conducted an historical cohort study of lung cancer mortality in underground uranium miners who had worked in the state of New Mexico, USA, using industry and health clinic records to define the cohort. The investigation began in 1978; the records were used to identify men who had worked for at least 12 months in an underground uranium mine in New Mexico by December 31, 1976. Follow-up for mortality was accomplished by using listings of deaths in the state and by matching the study roster against two national databases, the files of the Social Security Administration and the National Death Index. The initial report of study findings involved follow-up through 1985; follow-up has continued.

A variety of approaches may be used to estimate exposures in historical cohort studies of occupational groups, depending on the nature of the exposure(s) and the extent and quality of data available on exposures [2]. The occupation or industry may serve as a surrogate for associated exposures, and job information may be used in a job–exposure matrix to link occupation and industry pairs to specific exposures. General systems have been created for this purpose and the same approach has been tailored to specific occupational groups. If data are available on concentrations of workplace contaminants, it may be possible to calculate estimates of exposure for specific study participants by combining the concentration data with the time spent in jobs involving the exposure. For example, in the study of New Mexico uranium miners, information on concentrations of radon progeny in specific mines was used in combination with data on time spent in the mines to estimate exposures to radon progeny [6].

Historical cohort design has the advantage of rapidity of execution. While the task of conducting an historical cohort study may be formidable, the investigator does not need to wait for follow-up time to accumulate, as in a prospective cohort study. Costs tend to be modest as a result, and many historical cohort studies can be completed in only a few years, depending on the status and complexity of the involved databases.

Historical cohort studies, similar to prospective cohort studies, are subject to limitation by information bias, selection bias (*see* **Selection Bias**; **Bias in Cohort Studies**) and confounding (*see* **Bias in Observational Studies**). The limitations of the design primarily reflect the availability of the relevant historical data to ascertain the cohort participants and to estimate exposures of interest and potential confounding and modifying factors. Information bias is a particular concern. There is a strong potential for exposure misclassification (*see* **Misclassification Error**) and for bias from uncontrolled confounding. Because databases used to estimate exposures and covariates may be most complete in the more recent years, there is a potential for complex time-dependent exposure misclassification. The design may be further compromised by losses to follow-up and misclassification of the health outcome(s), because of reliance on historical records and death certificate assignment of cause of death. Historical cohort studies of workers involving mortality as the outcome measure are subject to a bias that has been widely termed "the healthy worker effect" [4]. Employed persons tend to be healthier than unemployed persons and consequently fewer deaths than expected are typically observed. The healthy worker effect has been characterized as a form of selection bias [2], although it can also be viewed as a reflection of confounding from uncontrolled differences between employed and unemployed persons. Selection bias could also be introduced in defining a cohort on the basis of incomplete records; for example, the findings of an historical cohort study could be affected by selection bias if records used to define the cohort were more complete in the most recent years of exposure

and exposures had declined over the period of eligibility. Furthermore, investigating disease incidence may not be possible using historical cohort design, unless special mechanisms have been put in place to track outcomes of interest, or unless it is possible to match records against an incidence registry for the disease(s) of interest, e.g. a cancer registry.

Historical cohort design may be strengthened by the addition of complementary, nested studies that involve additional collection of data on exposures, confounders, or modifiers from samples of the cohort members. Using case-based sampling methods (*see* **Case–Control Study, Nested**; **Case–Cohort Study**), more detailed data may be obtained for participants who have developed the outcome of interest and for an appropriate sample of controls. For example, in the study of New Mexico uranium miners, the effect of silicosis (a chronic respiratory disease arising from silica dust exposure) on lung cancer risk was assessed using a nested case-control design [5]. Chest radiographs were interpreted for lung cancer cases ($N = 65$) and for controls ($N = 216$) sampled from a total cohort of 3400 miners.

Historical cohort design has proven to be useful for studying the effects of occupational and other exposures. We may see increasing application of this design as implementation of disease registries expands and large administrative databases developed by health care organizations are used for research on health care outcomes and effectiveness.

References

[1]   Case, R.A.M., Hosker, M.E., McDonald, D.B. & Pearson, J.T. (1954). Tumors of the urinary bladder in workmen engaged in the manufacture and use of certain dyestuff intermediates in the British chemical industry, *British Journal of Industrial Medicine* **11**, 75–104.

[2]   Checkoway, H., Pearce, N.E. & Crawford, D.J. (1989). *Research Methods in Occupational Epidemiology*. Oxford University Press, New York.

[3]   Frost, W.H. (1933). Risk of persons in familial contact with pulmonary tuberculosis, *American Journal of Public Health* **23**, 426–432.

[4]   McMichael, A.J. (1976). Standardized mortality ratios and the "healthy worker effect": scratching below the surface, *Journal of Occupational Medicine* **18**, 165–168.

[5]   Samet, J.M., Pathak, D.R., Morgan, M.V., Coultas, D.B. & Hunt, W.C. (1994). Silicosis and lung cancer risk in underground uranium miners, *Health Physics* **66**, 450–453.

[6]   Samet, J.M., Pathak, D.R., Morgan, M.V., Key, C.R. & Valdivia, A.A. (1991). Lung cancer mortality and exposure to radon decay products in a cohort of New Mexico underground uranium miners, *Health Physics* **61**, 745–752.

JONATHAN M. SAMET

Collapsibility

Consider the $I \times J \times K$ contingency table representing the joint distribution of three discrete variables, X, Y, and Z, the $I \times J$ marginal table representing the joint distribution of X and Y, and the set of conditional $I \times J$ subtables (strata) representing the joint distributions of X and Y within levels of Z. A measure of association of X and Y is said to be *strictly collapsible* across Z if it is constant across the conditional subtables *and* this constant value equals the value obtained from the marginal table. Noncollapsibility (violation of collapsibility) is sometimes referred to as **Simpson's paradox** after a celebrated article by Simpson [10], but the same phenomenon had been discussed by earlier authors, including Yule [13]; see also Cohen & Nagel [3]. The term *collapsibility*, however, seems to have arisen later in the work of Bishop and colleagues; see Bishop et al. [1].

Table 1 provides some simple examples. The difference of probabilities that $Y = 1$ (the risk difference) is strictly collapsible. Nonetheless, the ratio of probabilities that $Y = 1$ (the risk ratio) is not collapsible because the risk ratio (*see* **Relative Risk**) varies across the Z strata, and the **odds ratio** is not collapsible because its marginal value does not equal the constant conditional (stratum-specific) value. Thus,

collapsibility depends on the chosen measure of association.

Now suppose that a measure is not constant across the strata, but that a particular summary of the conditional measures does equal the marginal measure. This summary is then said to be *collapsible* across Z. As an example, in Table 1 the risk ratio standardized to the marginal distribution of Z is

$$\frac{\begin{aligned}&\Pr(Z=1)\Pr(Y=1|X=1,Z=1)\\&+\Pr(Z=0)\Pr(Y=1|X=1,Z=0)\end{aligned}}{\begin{aligned}&\Pr(Z=1)\Pr(Y=1|X=0,Z=1)\\&+\Pr(Z=0)\Pr(Y=1|X=0,Z=0)\end{aligned}}$$
$$=\frac{0.50(0.80)+0.50(0.40)}{0.50(0.60)+0.50(0.20)}=1.50,$$

equal to marginal (crude) risk ratio. Thus, this measure is collapsible in Table 1. Various tests of collapsibility and strict collapsibility have been developed [4, 7, 12].

The definition of collapsibility also extends to regression contexts. Consider a generalized linear model for the regression of Y on three regressor vectors $\mathbf{W}$, $\mathbf{X}$, and $\mathbf{Z}$:

$$g[E(Y|\mathbf{W}=\mathbf{w}, \mathbf{X}=\mathbf{x}, \mathbf{Z}=\mathbf{z})]$$
$$= \alpha + \mathbf{w}\beta + \mathbf{x}\gamma + \mathbf{z}\delta.$$

The regression is said to be *collapsible* for β over $\mathbf{Z}$ if $\beta = \beta^*$ in the regression omitting $\mathbf{Z}$ [2],

$$g[E(Y|\mathbf{W}=\mathbf{w}, \mathbf{X}=\mathbf{x})] = \alpha^* + \mathbf{w}\beta^* + \mathbf{x}\gamma^*.$$

Thus, if the regression is collapsible for β over $\mathbf{Z}$ and β is the parameter of interest, then $\mathbf{Z}$ need not be measured to estimate β. If $\mathbf{Z}$ is measured, however, tests of $\beta = \beta^*$ can be constructed [2, 8].

The preceding definition generalizes the original contingency-table definition to arbitrary variables.

Table 1 Examples of collapsibility and noncollapsibility in a three-way distribution

	$Z=1$		$Z=0$		Marginal	
	$X=1$	$X=0$	$X=1$	$X=0$	$X=1$	$X=0$
$Y=1$	0.20	0.15	0.10	0.05	0.30	0.20
$Y=0$	0.05	0.10	0.15	0.20	0.20	0.30
Risks[a]	0.80	0.60	0.40	0.20	0.60	0.40
Risk differences	0.20		0.20		0.20	
Risk ratios	1.33		2.00		1.50	
Odds ratios	2.67		2.67		2.25	

[a]Probabilities of $Y = 1$.

However, there is a technical problem with the regression definition: if the first (full) model is correct, then it is unlikely that the second (reduced) regression will follow the given form. If, for example, Y is Bernoulli and g is the logit link function, so that the full regression is first-order **logistic**, the reduced regression will not follow a first-order logistic model except in special cases. One way around this dilemma (and the fact that neither of the models is likely to be exactly correct) is to define the model parameters as the asymptotic means of the maximum likelihood estimators. These means are well defined and interpretable even if the models are not correct [11].

It may be obvious that, if the full model is correct, $\delta = 0$ implies collapsibility for β and γ over $\mathbf{Z}$. Suppose, however, that neither β nor δ is zero. In that case, independence of the regressors does not ensure collapsibility for β over $\mathbf{Z}$ except when g is the identity or log link [5, 6]; conversely, collapsibility can occur even if the regressors are dependent [12]. Thus, it is not correct to equate collapsibility over $\mathbf{Z}$ with simple independence conditions.

Consider a situation in which the full regression is intended to represent the causal effects of the regressors on Y. One point, overlooked in much of the literature, is that noncollapsibility over $\mathbf{Z}$ (that is, $\beta \neq \beta^*$) does not correspond to **confounding** of effects unless g is the identity or log link. That is, it is possible for β to represent unbiasedly the effect of manipulating $\mathbf{W}$ within levels of $\mathbf{X}$ and $\mathbf{Z}$, and, at the same time, for β^* to represent unbiasedly the effect of manipulating $\mathbf{W}$ within levels of $\mathbf{X}$, even though $\beta^* \neq \beta$. Such a divergence is easily shown for logistic models, and points out that noncollapsibility does not always signal a **bias**. In the literature on random effects logistic models, the divergence corresponds to the distinction between cluster-specific and population-averaged effects [9]. The cluster-specific model corresponds to the full model in which $\mathbf{Z}$ is an unobserved cluster-specific random variable independent of $\mathbf{W}$ and $\mathbf{X}$, with mean zero and unit variance; δ^2 is then the vector of random-effects variances. For further discussion and an example in which confounding and noncollapsibility diverge, (*see* **Confounding**).

References

[1]   Bishop, Y.M.M., Feinberg, S.E. & Holland, P.W. (1975). *Discrete Multivariate Analysis: Theory and Practice*. MIT Press, Cambridge, Mass.

[2]   Clogg, C.C., Petkova, E. & Shihadeh, E.S. (1992). Statistical methods for analyzing collapsibility in regression models, *Journal of Educational Statistics* **17**, 51–74.

[3]   Cohen, M.R. & Nagel, E. (1934). *An Introduction to Logic and the Scientific Method*. Harcourt, Brace & Company, New York.

[4]   Ducharme, G.R. & LePage, Y. (1986). Testing collapsibility in contingency tables, *Journal of the Royal Statistical Society, Series B* **48**, 197–205.

[5]   Gail, M.H. (1986). Adjusting for covariates that have the same distribution in exposed and unexposed cohorts, in *Modern Statistical Methods in Chronic Disease Epidemiology*, S.H. Moolgavkar & R.L. Prentice, eds. Wiley, New York.

[6]   Gail, M.H., Wieand, S. & Piantadosi, S. (1984). Biased estimates of treatment effect in randomized experiments with nonlinear regressions and omitted covariates, *Biometrika* **71**, 431–444.

[7]   Greenland, S. & Mickey, R.M. (1988). Closed-form and dually consistent methods for inference on collapsibility in $2 \times 2 \times K$ and $2 \times J \times K$ tables, *Applied Statistics* **37**, 335–343.

[8]   Hausman, J. (1978). Specification tests in econometrics, *Econometrica* **46**, 1251–1271.

[9]   Neuhas, J.M., Kalbfleisch, J.D. & Hauck, W.W. (1991). A comparison of cluster-specific and population-averaged approaches for analyzing correlated binary data, *International Statistical Review* **59**, 25–35.

[10]   Simpson, F.H. (1951). The interpretation of interaction in contingency tables, *Journal of the Royal Statistical Society, Series B* **13**, 238–241.

[11]   White, H.A. (1994). *Estimation, Inference, and Specification Analysis*. Cambridge University Press, New York.

[12]   Whittemore, A.S. (1978). Collapsing of multidimensional contingency tables, *Journal of the Royal Statistical Society, Series B* **40**, 328–340.

[13]   Yule, G.U. (1903). Notes on the theory of association of attributes in statistics, *Biometrika* **2**, 121–134.

Sander Greenland

Communicable Diseases

The epidemiology of communicable diseases typically involves an interplay between the natural history of infective organisms, evolving largely within infected individuals, and their transmission dynamics, governed by direct or indirect contacts between individuals. While most fields of epidemiology comprise a social dimension, for infectious diseases this element enters at the level of mechanism, and is therefore central to our understanding of these diseases. The application of statistics to infectious diseases thus requires both a biological and a sociological perspective. This dialectic is strikingly illustrated by the epidemiology of the human immunodeficiency virus (HIV), the study of which motivated a large-scale investigation of sexual attitudes and lifestyles [59].

The Scope of Statistics in Infectious Disease Epidemiology

In spite of the distinct characteristics of infectious disease epidemiology, many of the statistical methods most commonly used are entirely standard. Thus, for instance, **observational studies** based on **surveillance** data, and epidemiological investigations using **case–control** or **cohort** designs, employ broadly the same statistical methodology whether the disease involved is measles or cancer. Nevertheless, statistical science has made distinct contributions to many areas of infectious disease epidemiology. The most prominent include catalytic and transmission models (*see* **Infectious Disease Models**), the study of the natural history of infectious disease, the detection of infectiousness, and the statistics of vaccination. These are the major topics around which this article is organized. In addition, statistics has played a key role in promoting our understanding of specific infectious diseases, as witnessed by the large statistical literature on the acquired immune deficiency syndrome (AIDS) [17]. Historically, many statistical techniques which are today widely employed were originally developed in the context of infectious disease epidemiology. Thus John Snow's famous study [92] of cholera and his investigation of an outbreak of cases around the Broad Street pump is an early demonstration of space–time clustering. A more recent example is provided by Bradford Hill's pioneering influence on field trials of pertussis vaccines [73], of streptomycin against pulmonary tuberculosis [71], and antihistamines against the common cold [72], which did much to establish the randomized controlled trial as a basic tool in medical research. More broadly, many of the principles governing the transmission of infectious diseases are of a more general nature, as originally alluded to by Ross in his "theory of happenings" [85], and similar models have been applied to such diverse topics as the spread of drug addiction and of scientific ideas [24].

Historical Background

The application of formal mathematical methods to infectious diseases dates back to Daniel Bernoulli's 1760 publication [15] of a mathematical model to evaluate the impact of smallpox on **life expectancy**. Later, William Farr [28] sought to describe the course of epidemics by fitting curves to smallpox data, and used this technique to predict the course of an epidemic of rinderpest among cattle [29]. Brownlee [18] also pursued this approach, fitting Pearson distribution curves to outbreak data on numerous diseases in support of his theory, later disproved, that pathogens decline in infectiousness during the course of an epidemic [40] (*see* **Epidemic Models, Deterministic**).

This early phase of largely empirical investigations was followed by the more analytical work of Hamer [55] and Ross [85], who sought to understand the mechanisms governing disease transmission. Hamer first formulated what was later to be known as the mass action principle, according to which the number of cases in generation $t + 1$ is proportional to the numbers of susceptibles and infectives in generation t. Ross developed transmission models for malaria, and formulated the first threshold theorem, on the critical density of mosquitoes required for malaria to remain endemic [39]. The ideas of Hamer and Ross were later elaborated by Kermack & McKendrick [62]. Chain binomial models of disease spread may be traced back to En'ko [27], who, as argued by Dietz [23], anticipated the Reed–Frost model (1928) (published as Frost [46]). The fully stochastic treatment of the chain binomial model is primarily due to Greenwood [48].

The pioneering approach of Bernoulli was extended by Muench [76, 77], who investigated the age distribution of susceptibles in a population using survival analytic methods (*see* **Survival Analysis, Overview**). Drawing upon an analogy from chemistry, Muench described his models as catalytic. Dietz [22] clarified the connections between transmission models and catalytic models, and demonstrated how key transmission parameters can be estimated from epidemiological data.

Catalytic Models

The great variety in the ecology and natural history of different infections generally requires different models for different diseases. However, some of the key features of all infectious disease models are captured by the simple case of person-to-person transmission of an infection conferring permanent immunity to those infected. The emphasis here is on endemic diseases that have reached a state of dynamic equilibrium.

The Basic Relationships

Let the random variable X denote the age at which individuals acquire infection. Let $S(x)$ denote the survivor function (*see* **Survival Analysis, Overview**):

$$S(x) = \Pr\{X > x\}$$

and $\lambda(x)$ the age-specific **hazard rate** of infection. In the context of infectious disease epidemiology, this is often called the force of infection, and depends on a variety of factors, including the rate at which individuals come into contact with one another, and the ease with which the organism is transmitted, given a suitable contact.

Assume, for simplicity, that all individuals in the population die at a fixed age, L, the life expectancy, and that the disease concerned is not fatal. In addition, we allow for the possibility that individuals are protected by maternally acquired immunity from birth to some age, M. These assumptions are broadly applicable to common childhood diseases such as measles, mumps, rubella, and whooping cough in developed countries. For these diseases, $\lambda(x)$ is typically a non-negative unimodal function, formally set to zero for $x \leq M$, and

$$S(x) = \exp\left(-\int_0^x \lambda(u)\mathrm{d}u\right).$$

The survivor function equals 1 for $x \leq M$, and hence differs from the probability that an individual of age x is susceptible, which is 0 for $x \leq M$ and $S(x)$ for $x > M$. Let A denote the expectation of X, or average age at infection. The average force of infection acting on susceptibles, $\bar{\lambda}$, is related to A by

$$\bar{\lambda} = \frac{\int_M^L \lambda(x)S(x)\mathrm{d}x}{\int_M^L S(x)\mathrm{d}x} = \frac{1 - S(L)}{A - M}.$$

For endemic infections, the proportion of the population escaping infection is negligible, and hence $S(L)$

is effectively zero. Thus,

$$\bar{\lambda} \doteq \frac{1}{(A - M)}.$$

It follows that if the average force of infection is reduced, for instance by vaccination, then the average age at infection will rise. Assuming a uniform age distribution, the proportion of the population remaining susceptible is

$$\pi = \int_M^L \frac{S(x)}{L - M}\mathrm{d}x = \frac{A - M}{L - M}. \tag{1}$$

Since the duration of protection by maternal antibodies is usually much less than A, the following approximations hold:

$$\pi \doteq \frac{A}{L} \doteq \frac{1}{\bar{\lambda}L}.$$

So far, the methods described are essentially those of survival analysis, and apply to any event occurring with hazard $\lambda(x)$. We now make the connection with infectious diseases.

An important summary measure of the infectiousness of a disease in a given population is the basic reproduction number, R_0. This is the mean number of secondary cases generated by a single infective in a totally susceptible population. It is a parameter of fundamental importance in infectious disease epidemiology. The higher the value of R_0, the more infectious the disease. However, if the basic reproduction number is equal to or below 1, transmission of the infection cannot be sustained and will eventually die out with probability 1.

R_0 depends on the effective contact rate, β. The term "contact" is taken to mean one of such a nature as to enable transmission of infection to occur. This of course depends on the mode of transmission of each organism. The effective contact rate, β, is defined as follows. Let η denote the rate at which contacts occur in the population, that is, the average number of contacts that an individual makes per unit time, and let θ denote the conditional probability of infection, given a contact between an infective and a susceptible. Then the effective contact rate is

$$\beta = \eta\theta.$$

It follows from this definition that

$$R_0 = \beta D,$$

where D is the mean duration of the infectious period.

In general, the contact rate, η, and hence β and R_0, vary with age. For simplicity, we assume that the population mixes in a homogeneous fashion, so that η is independent of age. Then β, R_0, and the force of infection are also independent of age. For long-established endemic diseases in dynamic equilibrium, the proportion susceptible fluctuates around the constant value π given by (1). Thus the average number of secondary cases produced by one infective is πR_0. But since the disease is in equilibrium, this must on average equal 1, since otherwise the proportion susceptible will not remain constant. It follows that

$$\pi R_0 = 1,$$

and hence

$$R_0 = \frac{1}{\pi} \doteq \frac{L}{A} \doteq \lambda L,$$

$$\beta = \frac{1}{\pi D} \doteq \frac{L}{AD} \doteq \frac{\lambda L}{D}. \tag{2}$$

Thus, in a homogeneously mixing population, the basic reproduction number and the effective contact rate may be estimated from the average age at infection, the life expectancy, and the duration of the infectious period.

These fundamental relationships also have important consequences for the control of infectious diseases. If the proportion of susceptible individuals in the population is reduced by vaccination below the equilibrium level π, then the number of secondary cases produced by each infective will be reduced below 1. Thus the infection will no longer be self-sustaining, and will eventually die out. Assuming that vaccination confers complete protection, and letting V denote the minimum proportion that must be vaccinated for eradication of the infection, we therefore have

$$V = 1 - \pi \doteq 1 - \frac{A}{L} \doteq 1 - (\lambda L)^{-1}.$$

In particular, note that it is not necessary to vaccinate the entire population to eradicate infection. This is the phenomenon of herd immunity: the effect of vaccination is not simply to protect vaccinated individuals, but also to impart indirect protection to unvaccinated susceptibles by impeding the circulation of the infection in the population.

This discussion shows how key epidemiologic parameters, such as the basic reproduction number and the proportion to vaccinate for eradication of infection, may be estimated from observable quantities such as the hazard of infection. Clearly, the assumption of homogeneous mixing is untenable for many populations. More complex versions of the results described above may be derived for age-dependent mixing patterns [3]. Similarly, the concepts introduced above in the case of person-to-person transmission have direct counterparts for other types of infection. For instance, in the case of helminth infections, the force of infection is the rate at which uninfected individuals acquire parasites, and R_0 is the average number of offspring produced throughout the reproductive life span of a mature parasite that themselves survive to maturity, in the absence of density-dependent constraints on population growth [3].

Estimation of the Force of Infection

As shown above, knowledge of the age-specific force of infection, or infection hazard $\lambda(x)$, is central to control strategies for infectious diseases. In the case of endemic infections conferring long-lasting immunity, with no differential mortality, in unvaccinated populations, it is most readily estimated from serological surveys, in which a **cross-sectional** sample of the population is tested for the presence or absence of relevant antibodies. Suppose that n_x individuals of age x are tested, with $x > M$, the duration of protection from maternal antibodies. The number r_x who display no evidence of past infection may be regarded as binomial $[n_x, S(x)]$, where $S(x)$ is the survivor function. Given a parametric form for the hazard function, the likelihood is proportional to

$$\prod_{x=1}^{L} S(x; \beta)^{r_x} [1 - S(x; \beta)]^{n_x - r_x}, \tag{3}$$

where

$$S(x; \beta) = \exp\left(-\int_0^x \lambda(u; \beta) du\right).$$

Individuals below age M are excluded from this analysis because they may be protected by maternally acquired antibodies. The decline of maternal protection after birth is of course of interest in its own right, and may be modeled provided sufficient data are available on infants. Note also that in the presence of vaccination, the hazard function can no longer be interpreted as the hazard of infection, but is the combined effect of natural infection and immunization.

For diseases with short **incubation periods**, the force of infection may also be estimated from case reports or routine notification data, provided it is reasonable to assume that these are not subject to age-specific bias in diagnosis or reporting. It is also necessary to assume that the age distribution of the population from which the cases are drawn is uniform, at least up to some age x_k above which few infections occur. Let $\mathbf{n} = (n_1, \ldots, n_k)$ denote the numbers of cases in the different age groups, where the subscript i indexes the age range $[x_{i-1}, x_i), i = 1, \ldots, k$. Thus $\mathbf{n}$ is multinomial and the likelihood is proportional to

$$\prod_{i=1}^{k} \left[\frac{S(x_{i-1}; \beta) - S(x_i; \beta)}{1 - S(x_k; \beta)} \right]^{n_i}.$$

Parametric models for the force of infection are discussed by Griffiths [51], Grenfell & Anderson [50], and Farrington [30]. Keiding [61] discusses nonparametric estimation, with an application to hepatitis A data. Alternately, the hazard may be assumed piecewise constant, taking the value λ_j in age group $[x_{j-1}, x_j), j = 1 \ldots k$. This enables regression models to be fitted using standard modeling software. Given fixed covariates $\mathbf{z}$ and letting $t_j(x)$ denote the time spent by an individual of age x in the jth interval, we have

$$\ln[S(x; \beta, \lambda)] = \beta^{\mathrm{T}} z + \sum_{j=1}^{k} \lambda_j t_j(x),$$

and hence the likelihood (3) may be maximized by generalized linear modeling with logarithmic link function.

The methods described above apply to infections having reached a dynamic equilibrium, in which the age-specific incidence fluctuates around a constant value according to stable epidemic cycles. For emerging infections, such as HIV, the age-specific incidence will initially increase over time. For others, such as hepatitis A, it may decline as contact rates change. The methods described above may be extended to model secular changes in the hazard of infection, using data from sequential seroprevalence surveys in the same population. In this context the

hazard $\lambda(x, t)$ depends on both age and time, and the survivor function is

$$S(x, t) = \exp\left(-\int_0^x \lambda(u, t - x + u) du \right).$$

Ades & Nokes [2] discuss an application to the incidence of toxoplasma infection. In some circumstances data may be available on repeat tests for the same individuals. One example is repeat tests for HIV on attenders at genito-urinary medicine clinics. This sampling scheme gives rise to interval-censored data, in which the time of infection is bracketed between the times of the last negative and the first positive tests. Denoting these, respectively, by U and V, where U may be zero (denoting a left-censored observation) and V may be infinite (denoting a right-censored observation), the likelihood is

$$\prod_{i=1}^{n} [S(U_i) - S(V_i)].$$

The estimation method based on case reports can similarly be extended to incorporate secular changes in incidence, provided the incubation period of the disease is short. For diseases with long incubation periods, for example AIDS and the chronic sequelae of hepatitis C infection, symptoms may appear many years after infection, and hence case reports alone provide little information on the date or age of infection. Data on case reports must be combined with information about the incubation period to estimate the incidence function. This is the **back calculation** approach, developed by Brookmeyer & Gail [16] to model the incidence of HIV infection.

For simplicity we ignore age effects. Let $\mu(t)$ denote the rate at which case reports arise, and $F(t)$ denote the distribution function for the incubation period. These are related to the force of infection by the convolution equation

$$\mu(t) = \int_{-\infty}^{t} \lambda(s) S(s) F(t - s) ds.$$

The product $\lambda(s) S(s)$ is sometimes combined into a single term, $\alpha(s)$, denoting the incidence of infection in the population. For uncommon or emerging infections, virtually the entire population is susceptible, hence $\alpha(s)$ and $\lambda(s)$ are practically identical.

Many methods have been proposed to estimate $\lambda(t)$ from this basic equation, given observed case reports and knowledge of the incubation period distribution. A comprehensive account is given in Brookmeyer & Gail [17]. For instance, given a parametric form $\alpha(s; \beta)$ for the incidence curve and assuming that infections arise in a Poisson process, then the number of cases, Y_i, arising in time period $[t_{i-1}, t_i)$ is also Poisson with mean

$$\mu_i = \int_{t_{i-1}}^{t_i} \alpha(s; \beta)[F(t_i - s) - F(t_{i-1} - s)]ds,$$

and hence the parameters β may be estimated by maximizing the Poisson log likelihood:

$$\sum_{i=1}^{n} [n_i \ln(\mu_i) - \mu_i - \ln(n_i!)].$$

Transmission Models

Catalytic models describe the age distribution of susceptibles for an endemic infection in dynamic equilibrium. However, they only capture the steady-state characteristics of the infection process, averaged over a long period of time. In particular, they fail to account for epidemic cycles. These constitute one of the most striking features of endemic infectious diseases with short incubation periods, at least those conferring life-long immunity and not involving a carrier state. In addition, catalytic models cannot be used for infections that have not reached a dynamic equilibrium, such as emerging diseases. By contrast, transmission models, whether deterministic or stochastic, attempt to incorporate the mechanism by which infection is spread in a population.

Dynamic Models for Large Populations

As seen above, the mechanism of disease spread is governed by the effective contact rate, β. This may be expressed more generally as a function $\beta(u, v)$ representing the number of effective contacts per unit time between an individual of age v and individuals of age u. The relationship between the contact rate and the force of infection at age x and at time t depends on the number of infectives in the population at time t. An intuitively appealing, though by no means unique, functional relationship is

$$\lambda(x, t) = \int_0^\tau \beta(u, x)Y(u, t)du,$$

where $Y(x, t)$ is the proportion of infectives of age x in the population at time t.

The basic ideas behind dynamic models may be illustrated using the simple example of a homogeneously mixing population, that is, one in which the contact rate is a constant β. It follows that the force of infection is also independent of age.

The population, of constant size, is divided into proportions $X(t)$ susceptible, $Y(t)$ infective, and $Z(t)$ recovered, who are immune from further infection. Individuals are born into the susceptible class with constant rate μ, and die at the same rate. There is no disease-associated mortality. The model is driven by the mass action principle, according to which the number of new infectives in a small time interval $[t, t + \delta t)$ is proportional to the number of infectives and to the number of susceptibles at time t. The dynamics of this three-stage model, often called a SIR (for susceptible–infectious–recovered) model, may be represented by the following system of differential equations:

$$\dot{X}(t) = -\beta X(t)Y(t) + \mu - \mu X(t),$$
$$\dot{Y}(t) = \beta X(t)Y(t) - \gamma Y(t) - \mu Y(t),$$
(4)

in which the dots represent derivatives with respect to t and γ is the reciprocal of the duration of the infectious period, D. Setting the derivatives to zero and solving for $X(t)$ gives the nontrivial equilibrium proportion susceptible:

$$\pi = \frac{\gamma + \mu}{\beta} \doteq \frac{1}{\beta D},$$

where the approximation is valid provided the duration of infectiousness is much smaller than life expectancy. Note that expression (2) is retrieved only approximately, owing to the different assumptions about the death rate.

Using standard methods for the analysis of small departures from equilibrium, it can be shown that these result in oscillations in the numbers of infectives. When the duration of the infectious period is small compared with the average age at infection, these have period

$$T = 2\pi(AD)^{1/2}.$$
(5)

This simple model thus exhibits the well-known phenomenon of epidemic cycles, typical of endemic immunizing infections with short infectious periods and no carrier state.

The second equation in (4) also illustrates the fact that the number of cases only grows if $\beta X(t) - \gamma - \mu > 0$, and hence in an initially susceptible population an epidemic can only occur if

$$R_0 = \frac{\beta}{\gamma + \mu} > 1.$$

Clearly, more sophisticated models can be developed to incorporate a latent period, protection by maternal antibodies, age-dependence, etc. In particular, if an infection has latent period E, D in expression (5) should be replaced by $D + E$. Anderson et al. [4] apply spectral analysis to the time series of some common childhood infections and show that the epidemic periods broadly correspond to those predicted by the model.

The transmission of infection in a population clearly involves a stochastic component, which is not captured by deterministic models. In small populations, stochastic effects become dominant, and deterministic models are of little use. In particular, they cannot readily account for the phenomenon of extinction, in which the transmission of infection is interrupted.

The stochastic version of (4) may be developed in terms of transition probabilities. Thus, letting $X'(t)$ and $Y'(t)$ denote, respectively, the number (rather than the proportions) of susceptibles and infectives at time t in a population of fixed size N, the corresponding transition probabilities in a short interval $(t, t + \delta t)$ are

$$\Pr[X'(t + \delta t) = X'(t) - 1; Y'(t + \delta t) = Y'(t) + 1]$$
$$= N^{-1}\beta X'(t)Y'(t)\delta t,$$

$$\Pr[X'(t + \delta t) = X'(t); Y'(t + \delta t) = Y'(t) - 1]$$
$$= (\gamma + \mu)Y'(t)\delta t,$$

$$\Pr[X'(t + \delta t) = X'(t) + 1; Y'(t + \delta t) = Y'(t)]$$
$$= N\mu\delta t,$$

$$\Pr[X'(t + \delta t) = X'(t) - 1; Y'(t + \delta t) = Y'(t)]$$
$$= \mu X'(t)\delta t.$$

Unfortunately the solution of such systems is far from straightforward. There is a substantial literature on the properties of general stochastic models, much of it of a highly mathematical nature [5–8, 94]. In practice, in large populations analytic solutions for the stochastic model become unmanageable. Using

Monte Carlo methods, Bartlett [7, 8] showed that a minimum population size is required for an infection to remain endemic.

The main purpose of the deterministic and stochastic dynamic models discussed above is to exhibit the qualitative aspects of the spread of infectious disease. One important application is in predicting the impact of vaccination strategies. The stochastic model may also, in principle, be used for parameter estimation. However, epidemics are rarely observed completely, and in consequence maximum likelihood methods are usually impracticable. Alternative methods include estimation via martingales [13, 14] and Markov Chain Monte Carlo [79]. Alternatively, simplified stochastic models may be used.

Branching Processes

In some cases it is possible to ignore the depletion of susceptibles, for instance during the initial stages of an epidemic. In these circumstances the spread of infection may be modeled by means of a branching process in discrete time [12, 13]. This approach is useful when the emphasis is on parameter estimation, rather than prediction. In such a model the epidemic begins with the introduction of an initial number of infectives, Y_0, at generation 0. These infect Y_1 individuals, who comprise the next generation of cases. In turn, these infect Y_2 individuals in the next generation of cases, and so on. Suppose that the number of infections directly caused by one individual is a random variable Z with probability distribution $g(z)$, the offspring distribution, and that the numbers of infections caused by two cases from the same generation are independent. Thus, for each i, $Y_i = Z_1 + \cdots + Z_{Y_{i-1}}$, where the Z_j are independent variables with density $g(z)$.

Let μ and σ^2 denote the mean and variance, respectively, of the offspring distribution. Thus μ is the expected number of infections caused by one case, and plays the same role as R_0 above. General results on branching processes show that if $\mu \leq 1$, then the process will become extinct with probability one [56]. Inference for branching processes is usually conditional on extinction or nonextinction.

For endemic diseases we proceed conditionally on nonextinction. Generation sizes $Y_0, \ldots, Y_k$ are observed for some value of k. In practice k is usually small, because generations soon become indistinguishable. Also the stock of susceptibles may be depleted, thus rendering the branching process model invalid. Harris [56] proposed the following nonparametric maximum likelihood estimator for μ:

$$\hat{\mu} = \frac{\sum_{i=1}^{k} Y_i}{\sum_{i=1}^{k} Y_{i-1}}.$$

The properties of this estimator are discussed by Keiding [60]. Heyde [57] and Dion [25] discuss nonparametric interval estimation. Alternatively, a parametric assumption may be made about the offspring distribution $g(z)$. Becker [12] suggests the alternative estimator:

$$\hat{\mu} = \begin{cases} (y_k/y_0)^{1/k}, & \text{if } I_k > 0, \\ 1, & \text{if } y_k = 0. \end{cases}$$

For outbreaks of diseases for which $\mu \leq 1$, it can be shown that if the offspring distribution has a power series distribution, then the total size of the outbreak also has a power series distribution [10], and the total outbreak size is a sufficient statistic for μ. The maximum likelihood estimate of μ is

$$\hat{\mu} = 1 - \frac{Y_0}{Y_+},$$

where Y_+ is the outbreak size. In particular for Poisson offspring distributions, the total number of cases follows the Borel–Tanner distribution and the asymptotic variance of the maximum likelihood estimator of μ is $\mu(1 - \mu)/Y_+$.

Heyde [58] discusses a Bayesian approach which allows the cases $\mu > 1$ and $\mu \leq 1$ to be treated without distinction. Becker [10, 11, 13] discusses several applications of branching processes to smallpox epidemics.

Chain Binomial Models and Extensions

The branching process offers a simple framework in which to investigate the early stages of epidemics, and outbreaks of nonendemic infections. However, its applicability is limited to situations in which it is reasonable to assume an unlimited pool of susceptibles. In particular, branching processes are unsuitable for the analysis of disease spread within households and small communities. In this context,

a more appropriate framework is provided by chain binomial models.

Consider a household with n individuals. At generation k there are X_k susceptibles exposed to Y_k infectives. The distribution of the number of cases in the next generation, Y_{k+1}, conditional on X_k and Y_k, is binomial:

$$\Pr(Y_{k+1} = z | X_k = x, Y_k = y)$$
$$= \frac{x!}{z!(x-z)!} p_k^z (1 - p_k)^{x-z},$$

where p_k is the probability that a susceptible of generation k will acquire infection from one of the y_k infectives. To parameterize p_k, some assumptions are required. A common assumption due to Reed & Frost (1928), published as [46], is that contacts with infectives occur independently, so that

$$p_k = 1 - (1 - \pi)^{y_k},$$

where π is the probability of an effective contact between two individuals. In continuous time, the mass action principle as incorporated in (4) coincides with the Reed–Frost model, in which π is replaced by $\beta \cdot \delta t$, where β is the contact rate. An alternate assumption, due to Greenwood [48], is

$$p_k = \begin{cases} \pi, & \text{if } y_k \geq 1, \\ 0, & \text{otherwise.} \end{cases}$$

The Greenwood model may be valid for diseases such as measles, in which infectious material is spread by aerosol. In these circumstances the number of infectives present will have little bearing on the number of susceptibles infected.

In some cases, data may be available on the actual chains of infection within the household, thus enabling the full likelihood to be written down. Thus, for one household with x_0 initial susceptibles the likelihood is

$$L = \prod_{i=1}^{m} \Pr(y_i | x_0, y_0, \dots, y_{i-1}),$$

where m is the total number of generations of cases in the household. For instance, in a household of size three, with one initial infective and two initial susceptibles, the possible chains of infection are $\{1\}$, $\{1, 1\}$, $\{1, 1, 1\}$, $\{1, 2\}$. The corresponding probabilities are, respectively, $(1 - \pi)^2$, $2\pi(1 - \pi)^2$, $2\pi^2(1 - \pi)$, π^2. In this case the probabilities are the same under the

Reed–Frost and Greenwood assumptions, although this is not generally the case. Bailey [5] contains tables of probabilities for households of up to five.

The parameter π may be estimated by directly maximizing the likelihood L. Alternately it may be maximized using generalized linear modeling techniques, since y_{k+1} is conditionally binomial(x_k, p_k). This enables household characteristics to be modeled in a straightforward manner. In the case of the Reed–Frost model, the appropriate link function is the complementary log–log, used with the offset $\ln(y_k)$. Thus, if

$$\ln[-\ln(1-\pi)] = \alpha + \beta^{\mathrm{T}} x$$

for covariates x, then

$$\ln[-\ln(1-p_k)] = \ln(y_k) + \alpha + \beta^{\mathrm{T}} x. \qquad (6)$$

The Reed–Frost assumption may also be tested formally, since omission of the offset term $\ln(y_k)$ in (6) corresponds to the Greenwood assumption.

In practice it is exceedingly rare to have such detailed data. In some situations, however, data may be available on the size of outbreaks in households. Assuming that information is also available on the numbers of introductory cases and initial susceptibles, the likelihood of an outbreak of any given size may be obtained by summing the probabilities of all chains with that number of cases. Thus, for instance, in a household of size three with one initial infective and two initial susceptibles, the probability of an outbreak of total size three is $2\pi^2(1-\pi) + \pi^2 = \pi^2(3-2\pi)$.

Bailey [5] discusses some of the problems involved in collecting data on household outbreaks. Bailey [5] and Becker [13] describe model checking for the chain binomial model, and extensions to random infectiousness, in which the parameter π may vary between households, for instance according to a beta distribution. Becker [13] gives a detailed application of chain binomial methods to the common cold.

The chain binomial models so far considered only seek to model the course of disease within households, and ignore the transmission of infection between households. This latter problem has been discussed by Longini et al. [67] and Longini & Koopman [66]. Suppose that an outbreak in a defined community of households is observed. Infections may be acquired within the household, or from the community, that is, from an individual from a different

household. Let π_c and π_h denote, respectively, the probabilities that a susceptible is infected from the community and from the household during the outbreak. Let p_{is} denote the probability that i of the s initial susceptibles within a given household are infected during the outbreak. Expressions for the p_{is} in terms of π_c and π_h are obtained recursively using the formula

$$p_{is} = \frac{s!}{i!(s-i)!} p_{ii} (1-\pi_c)^{s-i} (1-\pi_h)^{i(s-i)}.$$

Given a random sample of households from the community, the likelihood is the product of the p_{is} over the households in the sample and may be maximized to estimate the probabilities π_c and π_h. Becker [13], Longini & Koopman [66], and Longini et al. [67] give several applications of this method to data on various respiratory diseases.

The Natural History of Infectious Diseases

An important area of application of infectious disease statistics is in estimating key parameters describing the natural history of infection. This section describes methods for estimating the incubation, latent, and infectious periods, and the risk and severity of clinical disease following infection.

Estimation of the Incubation Period

The **incubation period** is defined as the interval between acquisition of infection and the appearance of symptoms. A related concept is that of generation time, also called the *serial interval*, which is the time between acquisition and transmission of infection. For many infections, such as measles, mumps, or chickenpox, the two are almost identical. Knowledge of the incubation period and generation time are important for several reasons. First, it enables cases in an epidemic to be classified into generations, thus allowing more detailed investigation of the spread of disease. Secondly, in the investigation of point source outbreaks, for instance involving food contaminated with Salmonella, knowledge of the incubation period is essential to define the time period over which food histories and other risk factor information should be collected. Thirdly, for evolving diseases with long incubation periods, the true incidence of infection can only be determined if the incubation period is known.

For diseases with short incubation periods, the incubation period distribution may be estimated directly using information on the time of exposure. In this way Sartwell [86] found that the incubation periods of many common diseases follow lognormal distributions. However, for diseases with long incubation periods, account must be taken of right-truncation: infected individuals who have not yet developed symptoms are not observed. If the incidence of infection varies over time, then ignoring the truncation of the data would produce biased estimates.

Several methods have been proposed for estimating the incubation period in this context. One simple method applicable to grouped data is by linear modeling. Let r_{ij} denote the number of observed cases infected in time period i with incubation period j, where $i = 1, \ldots, k$ and $j = 0, \ldots, k-1$ range over discrete time intervals with $i + j \leq k$, where k denotes the most recent time interval on which data are available. The incubation period distribution is estimated conditionally on the maximum observed interval, $k - 1$. Taking r_{ij} as Poisson with mean μ_{ij}, define the loglinear model

$$\log(\mu_{ij}) = h(i) + g(j)$$

for some parametric or nonparametric incidence function $\exp[h(i)]$ and incubation period distribution $\exp[g(j)]$ satisfying $\sum \exp[g(j)] = 1$. This method is described in Zeger et al. [102] and provides a simple way of jointly estimating the incidence function and the (conditional) incubation period distribution.

When data on individuals are available, an alternate method is as follows. Suppose that onsets are observed up to time t_0, resulting in n observations (t_i, s_i), where t_i is the date of onset of symptoms and s_i is the interval between infection and onset of symptoms, that is, the observed incubation period. Letting $\alpha(t)$ denote the incidence of infection at time t and $f(s)$ the density function of the incubation period, the log likelihood may be written

$$\sum_{i=1}^{n} \ln[\alpha(t_i)] + \sum_{i=1}^{n} \ln[f(s_i)] - \int_{-\infty}^{t_0} \alpha(u) F(t_0 - u) \, du,$$

$$(7)$$

where $F(s)$ is the distribution function of the incubation period. Suitable parameterizations of $\alpha(t)$ and $f(s)$ may be inserted into (7) and estimates obtained

by maximum likelihood. A slightly more general version of this approach was used by Medley et al. [74] to estimate the incubation period of AIDS.

A nonparametric approach has been suggested by Lagakos et al. [65]. In this approach the analysis is undertaken in "reverse time". Right-truncated observations in forward time become left-truncated in reverse time, and can be handled using nonparametric methods developed for left-truncated data. Suppose that n observations (t_i, s_i) are made over the time interval $[0, t_0]$, where t_i and s_i denote the same quantities as above. The distribution of the incubation period is estimated conditionally on the maximum observable interval, t_0. Thus, the distribution estimated is

$$F^*(s|t_0) = F(s)/F(t_0), \quad s \leq t_0.$$

Let $v_1, \ldots, v_k$ denote the distinct values of the s_i and define

$$n_j = \sum_{i=1}^{n} 1(s_i = v_j),$$

$$N_j = \sum_{i=1}^{n} 1(s_i \leq v_j \leq t_0 - t_i),$$

where $1(\cdot)$ is the indicator function. Then in reverse time measured from t_0 to 0, n_j is the number of events occurring at reverse time $t_0 - s_j$, and N_j is the number at risk. The nonparametric maximum likelihood estimate of $F^*(s|t_0)$ is then

$$\hat{F}^*(s) = \prod_{v_j \geq s} \left(1 - \frac{n_j}{N_j}\right)$$

for $0 \leq s \leq v_k$, and 1 for $v_k < s \leq t_0$.

All three methods may be used in other contexts, such as estimating the distribution of delays between the onset of disease and reporting or ascertainment.

Estimation of the Latent and Infectious Periods

For some diseases it is possible to identify the end of the infectious period. Thus, for instance, for measles infectiousness is minimal 2 days after the appearance of the rash. For such diseases it is possible to estimate the latency and incubation period from home contact studies, provided the chains of infection within the household are known. The method is described for households of two susceptibles.

For simplicity, assume that the infectious period is of fixed length, μ, and let Z denote the latency period, with probability density function (pdf) $g(z)$. For each case the end of the infectious period is observed, and occurs at time Y. The beginning of the infectious period for each individual is thus $Y - \mu$. Assume also that infectiousness is constant over the infectious period, so that infectious contacts occur in a Poisson process with constant rate β.

The contribution to the likelihood from a household with two co-primary cases infected at the same time with $Y_1 = y_1, Y_2 = y_2$, and $y_1 < y_2$, is

$$\int_0^\infty g(z)g(z + y_2 - y_1)\mathrm{d}z.$$

In the same notation, the contribution to the likelihood of a household in which the primary case infects the remaining susceptible is

$$\beta \int_0^\mu g(y_2 - y_1 - z)\exp(-\beta z)\mathrm{d}z,$$

while the contribution of a household with a single case with $Y_1 = y_1$ is

$$\exp(-\beta\mu).$$

Letting n_1, n_{11}, and n_2 denote the numbers of households of size two with chains $\{1\}$, $\{1, 1\}$, and $\{2\}$, respectively, the log likelihood is then

$$-n_1\beta\mu + n_{11}\log(\beta)$$
$$+ n_{11}\log\left[\int_0^\mu g(y_2 - y_1 - z)\exp(-\beta z)\mathrm{d}z\right]$$
$$+ n_2\log\left[\int_0^\infty g(z)g(z + y_2 - y_1)\mathrm{d}z\right].$$

Specification of a suitable parametric form $g(\cdot|\gamma)$ then enables the log likelihood to be maximized with respect to β, μ, and γ. This approach can be extended to households with more than two susceptibles. The assumption of a constant infective period can also be relaxed. These and other extensions are discussed in Bailey [5] and Becker [13]. Becker [13] gives a detailed application of this method to measles data.

Severity and Complications of Infectious Diseases

Infection and disease are not synonymous. Some infections are asymptomatic, and most produce a range of symptoms which can vary in severity. The clinical severity of disease may be directly quantified using clinical information. One important such measure is the **case fatality** rate, which is the proportion dying as a result of infection. Alternately, severity may be measured by proxy variables, such as the proportion of cases admitted to hospital, or socioeconomic variables, such as days off work. In most cases disease severity is age-dependent: for instance, for mumps and hepatitis A, severity of disease increases with age. Since the introduction of vaccination increases the average age at infection, vaccination programs can perversely produce an increase in the morbidity attributable to infection [3, 64].

The statistical methods commonly used to investigate risk factors for clinical disease typically involve **survival analysis** and regression. One perhaps distinctive application is to the estimation of the mortality attributable to influenza. For example, Serfling [87] applied regression techniques to model the seasonal and secular trends in mortality in selected cities in the US. In influenza epidemic years, large positive residuals are observed, from which an estimate of the **excess mortality** attributable to influenza may be derived.

Some infections, which are otherwise relatively benign, can have devastating consequences on the unborn child. For instance, rubella, toxoplasma, and cytomegalovirus infection in pregnancy can result in congenital abnormalities. The estimation of the number of infections in pregnancy is therefore of critical importance in assessing the value of screening and other prevention policies. Letting $\lambda(x)$ denote the force of infection at age x, $\eta(x)$ the number of births to women of age x, and τ the duration of pregnancy, the expected number of women infected in pregnancy is

$$\int_0^\infty \eta(z) \int_{z-\tau}^z \left[\lambda(x)\exp\left(-\int_0^x \lambda(u)\mathrm{d}u\right)\mathrm{d}x\right]\mathrm{d}z.$$

The force of infection may be estimated using the methods described above, while information on $\eta(z)$ may be derived from **vital statistics**. This and other methods are discussed by Ades [1].

Some complications have long induction periods. When the incidence of the originating infections varies over time, the estimation of the risk of complications following infection must take account of truncation effects. Similarly, transient effects due to changing incidence of infection may distort the induction period distribution. To see this let $\alpha(t)$ denote the incidence of originating infections, and $f(s)$ denote the pdf of the induction period distribution. Then the observed induction period distribution at time t is

$$f_t^*(s) = \frac{\alpha(t-s)f(s)}{\int_0^\infty \alpha(t-u)f(u)\mathrm{d}u}.$$

Thus, if the incidence is declining over time, the observed distribution of induction times is biased towards longer intervals. These effects are analyzed by Cox & Medley [21] in the context of AIDS. Farrington [31] discusses an application to subacute sclerosing panencephalitis (SSPE) after infection by wild measles virus.

Clustering of Infectious Diseases

One of the distinguishing features of many infectious diseases is their tendency to arise in clusters in space and time (*see* **Clustering**). While *cluster analysis* is a preoccupation common to most areas of epidemiology, in the case of infectious diseases it stems directly from the transmissibility of disease, rather than the influence of shared risk factors. The clearest example of this is the epidemicity of endemic infections, discussed above. This section describes two further areas in which statistical methods have been developed specifically for detecting clusters of infectious diseases.

Detection of an Infectious Etiology

For some diseases, such as leukemia, Hodgkin's disease, and multiple sclerosis, an infectious etiology has been suggested, but still remains unproven. Much effort has been devoted to detecting clustering of cases which might support such a hypothesis. From a statistical point of view, this requires the formulation of a suitable null hypothesis reflecting the distribution of cases expected if there was no infectious agent involved, and testing for departures from this hypothesis in a direction suggestive of infection.

There is a large literature on clustering of health events, much of which can be applied to the detection of infectiousness; see, for instance, Mantel [68]. This discussion is limited to some of the methods developed specifically for this purpose.

An early procedure was described by Mathen & Chakraborty [69], who considered the distribution of disease within a community of households. Regarding the total number of cases as fixed, they used as test statistic the total number of households containing at least one case. This idea was developed further by Walter [99] to take account of the actual numbers of cases within each household. Consider a population of n individuals in s households. The ith household comprises n_i individuals, of whom r_i become infected. Conditioning on the total $r = \sum r_i$ cases, the null distribution of r_i is hypergeometric. This corresponds to a null hypothesis of no clustering within households. The test statistic, T, is the number of distinct pairs of individuals, both of whom are infected, and both of whom are from the same household:

$$T = \frac{1}{2}\sum_{i=1}^{s} r_i(r_i - 1).$$

Walter [99] gives exact expressions for the null expectation and variance of T. Asymptotically, as $n \to \infty$ and $r/n \to p$, the proportion of the population infected, the null mean and variance of T tend to

$$\mathrm{E}(T) \to np^2(v_2 - 1)/2,$$

$$\mathrm{var}(T) \to np^2(1-p)[2pv_3 + (v_2 - 1)(1-p) - 2pv_2^2]/2.$$

where $v_2 = s\mathrm{E}(m_i^2)/n$ and $v_3 = s\mathrm{E}(m_i^3)/n$. The method may also be extended to the situation where only data on households with one or more infected individuals are collected. Various modifications have been proposed to this test statistic, by Smith & Pike [90] and Fraser [45].

Methods based on the distribution of cases within households are likely to lack power when applied to rare diseases. In addition, they do not use information on the times at which cases arise. These shortcomings are addressed by methods to detect space–time interactions. Many methods for detecting space–time clustering have been developed, the first being that of Knox [63]. Suppose that n cases of disease are identified, together with their locations and times of onset. Knox's test statistic is the number of distinct pairs of cases which lived within a distance d and had onsets within a time period t of each other, for fixed values of d and t. Barton & David [9] expressed Knox's statistic in graph-theoretic terms, proximity in space and time being represented by adjacency matrices, and derived the null expectation and variance of Knox's statistic.

Several enhancements of Knox's statistic have been proposed. In its original form it is applicable only to infections with short latent periods. To extend it to diseases with long latent periods, Pike & Smith [82] included information on the infectious and susceptible periods of each case. Evidence of contagion is given by any case being in the "right" place at the "right" time to have caught the disease from some other case. The test statistic measures the total effective contact between distinct pairs of cases, larger values providing evidence of infectiousness.

Pike & Smith [83] extend this approach further by including a control group, and apply the method to Hodgkin's disease. Given n cases of disease, let y_{ij} denote the presence ($y_{ij} = 1$) or absence ($y_{ij} = 0$) of an effective contact from case i to case j, that is, which may have resulted in case i transmitting the disease to case j, for $i, j = 1, \ldots, n$ and $i \neq j$. The test statistic is defined as the total contact between the n cases:

$$T = \sum_i \sum_{j \neq i} y_{ij}.$$

For each case a matched control is selected. The null distribution of T is obtained by calculating the total contact for each of the 2^n random selections of one individual from each of the n case–control pairs. This is most readily derived by Monte Carlo simulation. Pike & Smith [83] derive the exact null values of $E(T)$ and var(T), and propose a variety of related test statistics for the total numbers of linked patients.

The Detection of Outbreaks

A characteristic shared by many infectious diseases, at least those with short incubation periods, is the rapidity with which they evolve. It follows that if effective control measures are to be introduced, then outbreaks of infectious diseases must be detected in a timely fashion. In this context the emphasis is on the prospective detection of temporal clustering of disease, that is, as data accumulates, rather than the more usual retrospective identification of temporal clusters for epidemiologic analysis. Prospective outbreak detection is therefore necessarily based on incomplete data which are usually subject to delays in reporting, and is further complicated by fluctuations

in the historical data series due to seasonal cycles, secular trends, and past outbreaks (*see* **Surveillance of Diseases**).

Several statistical approaches to prospective outbreak detection have been suggested. Cumulative sum statistics have been used to detect the onset of influenza epidemics [97]. Time series methods have been suggested for the detection of outbreaks of Salmonella [101]. Nobre & Stroup [78] describe a different approach using exponential smoothing of the time series to identify the points at which the first derivative of the series departs significantly from zero.

The methods described above involve organism-specific modeling and hence are best suited to monitoring small numbers of data series. For the purposes of routine monitoring of large databases of infectious disease reports, however, robust methods are required applicable to a wide variety of organisms. Stroup et al. [96] describe a simple method for routinely detecting aberrations in reports of notifiable diseases in the US. Their method is to compare the current month's reports with the average of those received in comparable baseline periods over previous years. The current month's report is declared aberrant if it lies outside the limits $\hat{\mu} \pm 2\hat{\sigma}$, where $\hat{\mu}$ and $\hat{\sigma}$ are the estimated mean and standard deviation, respectively, of the baseline values.

This approach corrects for seasonal variation, though not for past outbreaks. Also, the method is applicable only for organisms with substantial monthly counts. An algorithm based on **Poisson regression** modeling, applicable to rare as well as frequent organisms, and incorporating an adjustment for past outbreaks, has been described by Farrington et al. [37]. A two-thirds power transformation is applied to preserve a roughly constant false positive probability for different organism frequencies.

Vaccination

One of the distinguishing features of infectious disease epidemiology is the ability to prevent disease by vaccination. Vaccination programs are generally acknowledged as among the most effective and cheapest public health measures available. It follows that the statistical issues raised by vaccination are central to the statistics of communicable diseases.

Vaccine Trials

The clinical trial is the method of choice for the evaluation of vaccines. Since the 1940s, when the method was first applied systematically to the evaluation of vaccines, a vast body of experience and methodology has developed. This section briefly reviews some of those aspects specific to vaccine trials. More detailed discussions may be found in Smith & Morrow [89] and Farrington & Miller [36].

Vaccine trials broadly fit within the Phase I, Phase II, and Phase III sequence of trial methodology. Most Phase I and II trials may be regarded as preliminary investigations, laying the groundwork for Phase III protective efficacy trials. However, in some cases Phase II trials take on a different purpose in that they are used to underpin major decisions about vaccination policy. This is the case, for instance, when a vaccine has already undergone a successful evaluation in a Phase III trial, possibly in another country. Additional data are required to support the introduction of the vaccine in a different population, possibly under a different immunization schedule from that used in the Phase III trial. Such Phase II trials may thus be described as confirmatory rather than exploratory.

The primary purpose of a Phase III trial is to assess the protective efficacy of the vaccine in the **target population**. Phase III trials may be large, especially when the disease concerned is rare. The 1954 field trial of Salk vaccine for polio involved 1.8 million children in the US, over 400 000 of whom were randomly assigned to vaccine or placebo and a much larger number enrolled in an open study [44]. Trials on such a gigantic scale are rare, but many nevertheless require sample sizes running into thousands. Vaccine efficacy trials are thus considerable logistic undertakings, and require clear procedures for handling vaccines, including their labeling, storage and transport, and monitoring their condition, for instance using temperature-sensitive devices.

The first stage in designing an efficacy trial is to define the outcome of primary interest. Many vaccines, such as those against pertussis [42] or rotavirus [98], alter the clinical course of the disease. Thus, a vaccine that is effective in preventing clinical disease may have a considerably lower efficacy against milder or asymptomatic infection. Clarity about the purpose of the trial and the intended use of the vaccine is, therefore, essential from the start if confusion resulting from contradictory interpretations of the trial results is to be avoided. In the special circumstances of measles vaccines in developing countries, it has been argued that it is more appropriate to use total mortality from any cause as the primary outcome, rather than measles morbidity, since the effect of vaccination may have nonspecific immunological consequences [53].

These considerations will guide the choice of primary case definitions, which should be chosen with due regard to potential **biases**. Clinical case definitions may lack **specificity**, unless corroborated by laboratory evidence, and hence will bias efficacy towards zero (*see* **Bias Toward the Null**), since the vaccine cannot be expected to protect against infections other than that for which it was developed. However, the use of laboratory methods for confirmation should be validated, since the **sensitivity** of the method may vary between vaccinated and unvaccinated cases. For example, there is some evidence that bacterial isolation rates of *B. pertussis* are lower in vaccinated than unvaccinated cases [95] which would result in an artificially high estimate of vaccine efficacy. As in other studies of vaccine efficacy, special care must be taken to ensure that individuals allocated to the different vaccine groups have the same probability of exposure to infection, for instance by using block randomization within suitably defined units of space and time.

Estimation of Vaccine Efficacy

Vaccine efficacy is defined as the percentage reduction in the attack rate attributable to the vaccine. This may be written:

$$VE = \left(\frac{p_\mathrm{u} - p_v}{p_\mathrm{u}} \right) \times 100, \qquad (8)$$

where p_u and p_v denote, respectively, the risk of infection in unvaccinated and vaccinated individuals over a specified observation period $[0, t]$ (*see* **Attributable Risk**). For notational simplicity, we omit the percentage multiplier and write

$$VE = 1 - \rho,$$

where ρ is the **relative risk** of infection, p_v/p_u. Alternately, one can define vaccine efficacy in terms of the **relative hazard** of infection:

$$VE = 1 - \frac{\lambda_v}{\lambda_u}, \tag{9}$$

where

$$p_u = 1 - \exp(-\lambda_u t), \qquad p_v = 1 - \exp(-\lambda_v t).$$

The two measures do not differ appreciably when $\lambda_u t$ is small.

These measures are used both to quantify vaccine efficacy in clinical trials and to evaluate vaccine effectiveness in the field. The term "effectiveness", rather than "efficacy", is often used to underline the distinction between estimates obtained in controlled experiments and those achieved under field conditions. The latter may be influenced by vaccine storage, variability of vaccination schedules, herd immunity, and other factors not directly attributable to the vaccine's direct biological effect. Henceforth, for reasons of economy, we use the term "efficacy" to cover both biological efficacy and field effectiveness.

Vaccine efficacy may be estimated directly in a **cohort study** involving vaccinated and unvaccinated individuals. This was the original approach of Greenwood & Yule [49]. Let n_v and n_u denote, respectively, the numbers of vaccinated and unvaccinated individuals. Suppose that r_v vaccinated and r_u unvaccinated cases arise during a specified observation period. The vaccine efficacy may then be estimated as

$$\widehat{VE} = 1 - \frac{r_v/n_v}{r_u/n_u}.$$

Confidence limits may be derived from those for the estimated relative risk $\hat{\rho} = (r_u/n_u)/(r_v/n_v)$.

Covariate effects may be estimated by modeling the number of cases as binomial, using a generalized linear model with logarithmic link. Thus, for instance, if each group is stratified according to covariates $\mathbf{x}_i, i = 1, \ldots, k$, then the main effects model for vaccine and covariate effects has the structure:

$$\ln(p_{ui}) = \alpha + \beta^{\mathrm{T}} X_i,$$

$$\ln(p_{vi}) = \alpha - \gamma + \beta^{\mathrm{T}} X_i,$$

and the corrected estimate of vaccine efficacy, allowing for covariate effects, is $\widehat{VE} = 1 - \mathrm{e}^{-\hat{\gamma}}$. The effect of the covariates on vaccine efficacy may also be investigated by fitting the relevant **interaction** terms.

A second method for estimating vaccine efficacy is by means of a **case–control study** [88]. A sample of cases is identified along with suitable controls, typically from the same age group and locality. Vaccination histories are obtained for both cases and controls. The **odds ratio** of vaccination in cases and controls is equal to the odds ratio of disease in vaccinated and unvaccinated children. Provided attack rates are low, this approximates the relative risk, so that

$$VE \doteq 1 - \frac{p_v/(1 - p_v)}{p_u/(1 - p_u)}.$$

The analysis uses standard case control methodology, regression models being fitted with conditional or unconditional **logistic regression** techniques.

A third method for estimating vaccine efficacy, called the *screening method*, is commonly used for routine monitoring purposes, or in circumstances in which only data on cases are available. Suppose that all or a random sample of cases of disease arising over a given period in a defined population are available. Let θ denote the proportion of cases vaccinated, and suppose that the proportion of the population vaccinated, π, is known. The vaccine efficacy is then

$$VE = 1 - \left(\frac{\theta}{1 - \theta}\right)\left(\frac{1 - \pi}{\pi}\right). \tag{10}$$

In the screening method, the vaccination coverage, π, is fixed, while θ is estimated.

Stratified analyses (*see* **Stratification**) using the screening method are possible provided suitably stratified vaccine coverage statistics are available. Suppose that cases are observed and classified into m strata, with n_i cases in stratum $i, i = 1, \ldots, m$. Suppose that of the n_i cases in stratum i, r_i, are vaccinated. For each stratum $i = 1, \ldots, m$, let θ_i denote the probability that a case is vaccinated, π_i the population vaccine coverage, and ρ_i the relative risk of disease. Suppose also that k covariates on each stratum are also available, the value of the jth covariate in the ith stratum being denoted by $x_{ij}, j = 1, \ldots, k$. Then, given a linear model for the relative risk,

$$\ln(\rho_i) = \alpha + \sum_{j=1}^{k} \beta_j X_{ij},$$

(10) may be re-expressed for each stratum as

$$\text{logit}(\theta_i) = \text{logit}(\pi_i) + \alpha + \sum_{j=1}^{k} \beta_j X_{ij}. \quad (11)$$

Assuming that cases of disease arise in a Poisson process, r_i is binomial (n_i, θ_i). Thus, the model specified by (11) may be fitted as a generalized linear model with binomial error and logistic link, with offsets $\text{logit}(\pi_i)$. Clearly, this method depends for its validity on the availability of accurate data on vaccine coverage. Given such data, the method allows vaccine efficacies to be calculated very simply from case reports or notifications. Applications of the method to measles and pertussis vaccine efficacy are given in [34].

Alternatively, if the population vaccine coverage is not known, then it may be estimated from a sample. This approach leads to **case–cohort** designs [75].

In all the methods described above, care must be taken to adjust for potential **confounders**. For instance, both vaccine coverage and incidence of infection may vary with age and location, which may therefore confound vaccine efficacy. In field investigations it is essential to document vaccination histories, and to ascertain cases independently of vaccination status. These and other methodological issues are discussed in detail in Clarkson & Fine [19], Fine & Clarkson [42], and Orenstein et al. [80].

In estimating vaccine efficacy it is also important to ensure that vaccinated and unvaccinated individuals have the same probability of exposure. In an attempt to control for exposure, vaccine efficacy is sometimes estimated from attack rates in household contacts of infected cases. Some of the methodological issues surrounding such studies are discussed in Fine et al. [43]. Concern about this issue has led to a further measure of vaccine efficacy being proposed, which controls for exposure:

$$VE = 1 - \frac{\theta_v}{\theta_u}, \quad (12)$$

where θ_u and θ_v are, respectively, the transmission probabilities of infection to unvaccinated and vaccinated individuals given contact with a single infective [52].

The various definitions of efficacy given above all represent direct efficacy, that is, they measure the individual benefit gained from vaccination, in a vaccinated population. In addition, the vaccine may confer an indirect benefit through herd immunity, by reducing the circulation of the infection, and hence indirectly protecting unvaccinated individuals. Direct and indirect measures of vaccine efficacy are discussed in [54].

Vaccine Models

Two contrasting models of vaccine mechanisms have been suggested [91]. In the first, the so-called "all-or-nothing" model, the vaccine imparts total, long-lasting protection to a proportion of vaccinees, and gives no protection to the remainder. The proportion protected may be estimated unbiasedly as one minus the relative risk of disease, that is, using (8) above. It has been suggested that this model of vaccine protection may apply to live viral vaccines such as measles vaccine. In the second model, sometimes called the "leaky" vaccine model, vaccination does not impart complete protection on any individual, but reduces the hazard of infection by a constant factor. This relative hazard corresponds to $1 - VE$, where the vaccine efficacy is estimated using (9) above. This mechanism might be appropriate for bacterial vaccines, such as whole cell pertussis vaccine. In a randomly mixing population, the vaccine efficacy measure, (12), based on transmission probabilities, has been shown to equal that based on attack rates, (8), for all-or-nothing vaccines, and (9) for leaky vaccines [52].

In practice it is extremely difficult to distinguish between the two vaccine mechanisms, since changes in one or other measure of vaccine efficacy over time can be attributed either to the vaccine mechanism or to waning vaccine efficacy. This confounding of vaccine mechanism and changes in efficacy over time poses particular problems for the evaluation of age-specific efficacy of the vaccine, since a decline in age-specific efficacy may be attributed to the vaccine mechanism, to bias in identifying susceptible individuals, or to waning efficacy of the vaccine. The problem of estimating and interpreting age-specific vaccine efficacy measures is discussed in [33].

Vaccine Safety Evaluation

Vaccine safety is clearly a critical issue, often generating considerable public interest, particularly in the case of vaccines administered to children on a large scale for preventive purposes. Clinical trials are usually too small to demonstrate the safety of vaccines with respect to rare, but potentially serious, adverse events. Instead, vaccine safety is monitored by surveillance and epidemiologic investigations after the vaccine is in widespread use. Such studies present considerable statistical challenges. For instance, for vaccines administered as part of a routine immunization program, unvaccinated individuals are a selected group which cannot be assumed representative of the population as a whole, and hence should not be included in the control group. Instead, for acute adverse reactions, such as febrile convulsions following measles or pertussis vaccine, or aseptic meningitis following mumps vaccine, the focus is to detect a clustering of events in the period following vaccination. This is achieved by estimating the relative rate at which events occur in a specified period following vaccination, compared with the background rate in control time periods, correcting for age effects which may confound the relationship between vaccination and adverse events. Commonly used methods include cohort and case–control studies. In the cohort approach, the analysis is conditional on vaccination times, the time of observation for each individual being divided into "at risk" and "control" periods. In the case–control approach, cases are matched to controls by date of birth and other relevant variables. The date of the reaction in the case is taken as the index date, and exposure in both case and control is defined as vaccination in a specified period prior to the index date. The methodologic issues associated with such studies are discussed in Ray et al. [84] and Fine & Chen [41].

A third method specifically designed for the analysis of acute, transient vaccine reactions combines the economy of the case–control method and the power of the cohort method. This is the case–series method [35]. The method is derived from a cohort model, by conditioning on the total number of events experienced by each individual. Individuals who do not experience any reactions thus make no contribution to the likelihood, and hence only data on cases are required. Thus, suppose that n cases are observed over a defined observation period. For the ith individual, let e_{ijk} denote the time spent in age group j and risk group k. The risk groups are defined in relation to vaccination: for instance, for febrile convulsions after pertussis vaccine, one might use the intervals 0–3 days, 4–7 days, 8–14 days after vaccination as distinct risk groups, all other times being included in the reference control group. The number of adverse events experienced by individual i in age group j and risk group k, r_{ijk}, is assumed Poisson with mean μ_{ijk}. A simple cohort model may be written

$$\ln(\mu_{ijk}) = \ln(e_{ijk}) + \alpha^{\mathrm{T}} x_i + \beta_j + \gamma_k,$$

where x_i are fixed covariates. Conditioning on the total number of events observed for individual i results in the product multinomial likelihood:

$$L = \prod_i \prod_{j,k} \left(\frac{e_{ijk} \exp(\beta_j + \gamma_k)}{\sum_{r,s} e_{irs} \exp(\beta_r + \gamma_s)} \right)^{r_{ijk}},$$

to which individuals with $r_{i..} = 0$ contribute 1, and hence may be ignored. This greatly simplifies the study of adverse events, since only a sample of individuals experiencing an event over a given period is required. This model assumes that events are potentially recurrent. However, for rare nonrecurrent events, such as sudden infant death syndrome (SIDS) or encephalopathy, the method can be applied with little bias. Note that with this approach the effect of fixed covariates on the incidence of adverse events cannot be estimated. However, their effect on the relative incidence of adverse events after vaccine can be estimated by including suitable interaction terms in the model. This method has been shown to be as powerful as the cohort method when vaccine coverage is high [38].

Other Methods

The collection of infectious disease data frequently relies on complex laboratory techniques, such as serological and other assays, electron microscopy, electrophoresis, typing, and other identification methods. Many of these involve statistical techniques, such as statistical taxonomy. A thorough discussion of laboratory methods is beyond the scope of this article. However, the laboratory methods used often also have a direct bearing on the analysis and interpretation of epidemiologic data. This section aims to illustrate this point using two examples.

Prevalence Estimation by Group Testing

In some situations it is necessary, for instance for reasons of economy, to pool samples of material for analysis, and test the combined pool rather than the individual samples. The statistical properties of this approach were originally investigated by Dorfman [26] to reduce the number of tests required to identify cases of syphilis. Today, group testing is often used to test for HIV in large population surveys [17]. In some cases it is possible, and indeed, for diagnostic tests, necessary, to retest the individual components of a positive pool. However, the approach may also be used directly to estimate population prevalence [93]. In this setting the retesting of individual samples is not necessary, and in some cases not possible, as for instance in the study of vertical transmission of yellow fever virus by mosquitoes discussed by Walter et al. [100].

Suppose that n pools have been formed, the ith pool including m_i samples from individuals with a common covariate vector $\mathbf{x}_i$, $i = 1, \ldots, n$. Let $r_i = 1$ if the ith pool is positive, 0 if it is negative. Let π_i be the probability that the ith pool tests positive, and θ_i be the probability that an individual in the ith pool is positive. Thus θ_i is the prevalence in the subpopulation with characteristics $\mathbf{x}_i$. Provided that the individuals within each pool are independent, the pool and population prevalences are related by

$$\pi_i = 1 - (1 - \theta_i)^{m_i}.$$

Thus, if the population prevalences satisfy the linear model

$$\log(-\log(1 - \theta_i)) = \beta^T x_i,$$

with regression parameters β, then the pool prevalences satisfy

$$\log(\pi_i) = \log(m_i) + \beta^T x_i.$$

Thus, the population prevalences and the regression parameters may be estimated by fitting a generalized model with dependent variable r_i, binomial error, complementary log–log link function, and fixed offset $\log(m_i)$. This method is further discussed in [32], with an application to estimating the prevalence of Salmonella contamination in eggs.

The concept of group testing may also be applied to estimating the most probable number (MPN) of coliform organisms in water samples, using the multiple fermentation tube method of McCrady [70]. A sample of water from a given source is taken and subdivided, with or without dilution, into subvolumes. These are then incubated in separate tubes, which are examined for evidence of growth, indicating that at least one organism was present in the subvolume. Let n_i denote the number of tubes containing a volume v_i of the original water sample, and r_i the number of positive tubes among these n_i. If coliforms are homogeneously distributed with density λ per unit volume, then r_i is binomial (n_i, π_i), where

$$\log(-\log(1 - \pi_i)) = \log(v_i) + \log(\lambda).$$

Hence the density, λ, and the MPN, λV, where V denotes the original volume of water, may be estimated using a binomial model with a complementary log–log link function and offset $\log(v_i)$.

Mixture Models for Quantitative Assay Data

Laboratory assays are widely used for diagnostic purposes on samples from individual patients. They may also be used in serological surveys to determine immunity levels in a population, and hence to monitor or design vaccination programs. Many commonly used assays, such as enzyme-linked immunosorbent assays (ELISAs), give quantitative results. When used for diagnostic purposes, it is necessary to define one or more cutoff values to classify the test results as negative, positive, or equivocal. These cutoff values also determine the diagnostic sensitivity and specificity of the assay. In serological surveys, on the other hand, the aim is not to classify individual test results, but to estimate the age-specific prevalence in the population.

The determination of cutoff values is problematic when there is no objective criterion by which to classify samples as "true" positives or negatives. For common infections, however, this may be achieved by fitting mixture models to data obtained from population-based serological surveys. Furthermore, when used for determining population prevalence, cutoff values are not required using these methods.

Each age group i is assumed to be a mixture of positives (immunes) and negatives (nonimmunes) in the proportions π_i and $1 - \pi_i$, respectively, where π_i is the proportion positive, which may be constrained to increase with age. Assay results in age group i are distributed with density:

$$f(x|\pi_i, \alpha_i, \beta_i) = (1 - \pi_i)g(x|\alpha_i) + \pi_i h(x|\beta_i),$$

where $g(x|\alpha_i)$ and $h(x|\beta_i)$ are the densities of assay results from negative and positive individuals, respectively. For instance, for an ELISA, the random variable X may be taken to be the logarithm of the optical density reading, and $g(\cdot)$ and $h(\cdot)$ may be normal with age-dependent means and constant variance. Let $x_0 = -\infty < x_1 < \ldots < x_k = \infty$ subdivide the range of X and suppose that there are n_{ij} values from age group i in interval $[x_{j-1}, x_j)$. The parameters π_i, α_i, and β_i may be estimated by maximizing the product multinomial log likelihood:

$$\sum_i \sum_j n_{ij} \log \left(\int_{x_{j-1}}^{x_j} f(x|\pi_i, \alpha_i, \beta_i) \mathrm{d}x \right).$$

Note that the parameters π_i are estimated without the need to specify cutoff values. Appropriate cutoff values may be derived by examining the receiver operating characteristic (ROC) curve using the estimated specificities and sensitivities corresponding to different cutoff values c:

$$\mathrm{spec}_i(c) = \int_{-\infty}^{c} g(x|\hat{\alpha}_i) \mathrm{d}x,$$

$$\mathrm{sens}_i(c) = \int_{c}^{\infty} h(x|\hat{\beta}_i) \mathrm{d}x.$$

The mixture modeling approach to the determination of cutoff values is discussed in [80] and applied to estimating prevalences in serological surveys by Gay [47], both in relation to parvovirus B19 infection.

Future Challenges

The substantial statistical literature on applications to AIDS and HIV demonstrates the vitality of infectious disease statistics. To this date, smallpox remains the only infectious disease which has been eradicated. The continued toll of infectious disease throughout the world, and the emergence of resistant forms of diseases like tuberculosis, unfortunately guarantees the continued relevance of infectious disease statistics.

It is perhaps surprising that our understanding of the mechanism of transmission of infectious diseases has not changed fundamentally since the work of the pioneers at the start of the twentieth century. Further work is required on understanding the epidemicity and seasonality of infectious diseases and it is likely that computer-intensive statistical methods will play

an increasingly important role in this area. Work is also needed on the geographic spread of infectious diseases. Though much mathematical modeling and some statistical work has been done in this area (see, for instance, Cliff & Haggett [20]), little data have so far been available. The development of combination vaccines will also bring new challenges, requiring the assessment of new vaccines against old in equivalence trials with multiple comparisons and surrogate endpoints. The potential risks of vaccines are likely to come under ever closer scrutiny, raising the difficult statistical issue of evaluating vaccine safety with respect to adverse events with long induction periods, in highly vaccinated populations.

References

[1] Ades, A.E. (1992). Methods for estimating the incidence of primary infection in pregnancy: a reappraisal of toxoplasmosis and cytomegalovirus data, *Epidemiology and Infection* **108**, 367–375.

[2] Ades, A.E. & Nokes, D.J. (1993). Modelling age- and time-specific incidence from seroprevalence: toxoplasmosis, *American Journal of Epidemiology* **137**, 1022–1034.

[3] Anderson, R.M. & May, R.M. (1991). *Infectious Diseases of Humans: Dynamics and Control*. Oxford University Press, Oxford.

[4] Anderson, R.M., Grenfell, B.T. & May, R.M. (1984). Oscillatory fluctuations in the incidence of infectious disease and the impact of vaccination: time series analysis, *Journal of Hygiene, Cambridge* **93**, 587–608.

[5] Bailey, N.T.J. (1975). *The Mathematical Theory of Infectious Diseases and its Applications*, 2nd Ed. Griffin, London.

[6] Bartlett, M.S. (1956). Deterministic and stochastic models for recurrent epidemics, in *Proceedings of the Third Berkeley Symposium on Mathematical Statistics and Probability*, Vol. 4. University of California Press, Berkeley, pp. 81–109.

[7] Bartlett, M.S. (1957). Measles periodicity and community size, *Journal of the Royal Statistical Society, Series A* **120**, 48–70.

[8] Bartlett, M.S. (1960). The critical community size for measles in the United States, *Journal of the Royal Statistical Society, Series A* **123**, 37–44.

[9] Barton, D.E. & David, F.N. (1966). The random intersection of two graphs, in *Research Papers in Statistics: Festschrift for J. Neyman*, F.N. David, ed. Wiley, New York, pp. 445–459.

[10] Becker, N. (1974). On parametric estimation for mortal branching processes, *Biometrika* **61**, 393–399.

[11] Becker, N. (1976). Estimation for an epidemic model, *Biometrics* **32**, 769–777.

[12] Becker, N. (1977). Estimation for discrete time branching processes with applications to epidemics, *Biometrics* **33**, 515–522.

[13] Becker, N.J. (1989). *Analysis of Infectious Disease Data*. Chapman & Hall, London.

[14] Becker, N.G. & Hasofer, A.M. (1997). Estimation in epidemics with incomplete observations, *Journal of the Royal Statistical Society, Series B* **59**, 415–429.

[15] Bernoulli, D. (1760). Essai d'une nouvelle analyse de la mortalité causée par la petite vérole et des avantages de l'inoculation pour la prévenir, *Mémoires de Mathematiques et de Physique*, pp. 1–45. In *Histoire de l'Académie Royale des Sciences, Paris* (1760).

[16] Brookmeyer, R. & Gail, M.H. (1988). A method for obtaining short-term projections and lower bounds on the size of the AIDS epidemic, *Journal of the American Statistical Association* **83**, 301–308.

[17] Brookmeyer, R. & Gail, M.H. (1994). *AIDS Epidemiology: A Quantitative Approach*. Oxford University Press, Oxford.

[18] Brownlee, J. (1907). Statistical studies in immunity: the theory of an epidemic, *Proceedings of the Royal Society of Edinburgh* **26**, 484–521.

[19] Clarkson, J.A. & Fine, P.E.M. (1987). An assessment of methods for routine local monitoring of vaccine efficacy, with particular reference to measles and pertussis, *Epidemiology and Infection* **99**, 485–499.

[20] Cliff, A.D. & Haggett, P. (1982). Methods for the measurement of epidemic velocity from time series data, *International Journal of Epidemiology* **11**, 82–89.

[21] Cox, D.R. & Medley, G.F. (1989). A process of events with notification delay and the forecasting of AIDS, *Philosophical Transaction of the Royal Society of London, Series B* **925**, 135–145.

[22] Dietz, K. (1975). Transmission and control of arbovirus diseases, in *Epidemiology*, D. Ludwig & K.L. Cooke, eds. SIAM, Philadelphia.

[23] Dietz, K. (1988). The first epidemic model: a historical note on P.D. En'ko, *Australian Journal of Statistics* **30A**, 56–65.

[24] Dietz, K. & Schenzle, D. (1985). Mathematical models for infectious disease statistics, in *A Celebration of Statistics*, A.C. Atkinson & S.E. Fienberg, eds. Springer-Verlag, New York.

[25] Dion, J.P. (1975). Estimation of the variance of a branching process, *Annals of Statistics* **3**, 1184–1187.

[26] Dorfman, R. (1943). The detection of defective members of large populations, *Annals of Mathematical Statistics* **14**, 436–440.

[27] En'ko, P.D. (1889). The epidemic course of some infectious diseases, *Vrach, St Petersburg* **10**, 1008–1010; 1039–1042; 1061–1063 (in Russian).

[28] Farr, W. (1840). *Progress of Epidemics. Second Report of the Registrar General of England and Wales*. HMSO, London, pp. 91–98.

[29] Farr, W. (1866). On the cattle plague, *Letter to the Editor of the Daily News*, February 19, London.

[30] Farrington, C.P. (1990). Modelling forces of infection for measles, mumps and rubella, *Statistics in Medicine* **9**, 953–967.

[31] Farrington, C.P. (1991). Subacute sclerosing panencephalitis in England and Wales: transient effects and risk estimates, *Statistics in Medicine* **10**, 1733–1744.

[32] Farrington, C.P. (1992). Estimating prevalence by group testing using generalized linear models, *Statistics in Medicine* **11**, 1591–1597.

[33] Farrington, C.P. (1992). The measurement and interpretation of age-specific vaccine efficacy, *International Journal of Epidemiology* **21**, 1014–1020.

[34] Farrington, C.P. (1993). Estimation of vaccine efficacy using the screening method, *International Journal of Epidemiology* **22**, 742–746.

[35] Farrington, C.P. (1995). Relative incidence estimation from case series for vaccine safety evaluation, *Biometrics* **51**, 228–235.

[36] Farrington, P. & Miller, E. (1996). Clinical trials, in *Methods in Molecular Medicine: Vaccine Protocols*, A. Robinson, G. Farrar & C. Wiblin, eds. Humana Press, Totowa.

[37] Farrington, C.P., Andrews, N.J., Beale, A.D. & Catchpole, M.A. (1996). A statistical algorithm for the early detection of outbreaks of infectious disease, *Journal of the Royal Statistical Society, Series A* **159**, 547–563.

[38] Farrington, C.P., Nash, J. & Miller, E. (1996). Case series analysis of adverse reactions to vaccine: a comparative evaluation, *American Journal of Epidemiology* **143**, 1165–1173.

[39] Fine, P.E.M. (1975). Ross's *a priori* pathometry: a perspective, *Proceedings of the Royal Society of Medicine* **68**, 547–551.

[40] Fine, P.E.M. (1979). John Brownlee and the measurement of infectiousness: an historical study in epidemic theory, *Journal of the Royal Statistical Society, Series A* **142**, 347–362.

[41] Fine, P.E. & Chen, R.T. (1992). Confounding in studies of adverse reactions to vaccines, *American Journal of Epidemiology* **136**, 121–135.

[42] Fine, P.E.M. & Clarkson, J.A. (1987). Reflections of the efficacy of pertussis vaccines, *Reviews of Infectious Diseases* **9**, 866–883.

[43] Fine, P.E.M., Clarkson, J.A. & Miller, E. (1988). The efficacy of pertussis vaccines under conditions of household exposure, *International Journal of Epidemiology* **17**, 635–642.

[44] Francis, T., Korns, R.F., Voight, T., Boisen, M., Hemphill, F.M., Napier, J.A. & Tochinsky, E. (1955). An evaluation of the 1954 poliomyelitis vaccine trials, *American Journal of Public Health, Part 2* **45**, 1–63.

[45] Fraser, D.W. (1983). Clustering of disease in population units: an exact test and its asymptotic version, *American Journal of Epidemiology* **118**, 732–739.

[46] Frost, W.H. (1976). Some conceptions of epidemics in general, *American Journal of Epidemiology* **103**, 141–151.

[47] Gay, N.J. (1996). Analysis of serological surveys using mixture models: application to a survey of parvovirus B19, *Statistics in Medicine* **15**, 1567–1573.

[48] Greenwood, M. (1931). On the statistical measure of infectiousness, *Journal of Hygiene, Cambridge* **31**, 336–351.

[49] Greenwood, M. & Yule, U.G. (1915). The statistics of anti-typhoid and anti-cholera inoculations, and the interpretation of such statistics in general, *Proceedings of the Royal Society of Medicine* **8**(2), 113–194.

[50] Grenfell, B.T. & Anderson, R.M. (1985). The estimation of age-related rates of infection from case notifications and serological data, *Journal of Hygiene, Cambridge* **95**, 419–436.

[51] Griffiths, D.A. (1974). A catalytic model of infection for measles, *Applied Statistics* **23**, 330–339.

[52] Haber, M., Longini, I.M. & Halloran, M.E. (1991). Measures of the effects of vaccination in a randomly mixing population, *International Journal of Epidemiology* **20**, 300–310.

[53] Hall, A.J. & Aaby, P. (1990). Tropical trials and tribulations, *International Journal of Epidemiology* **19**, 777–781.

[54] Halloran, M.E., Haber, M., Longini, I.M. & Struchiner, C.J. (1991). Direct and indirect effects in vaccine efficacy and effectiveness, *American Journal of Epidemiology* **133**, 323–331.

[55] Hamer, W.H. (1906). Epidemic disease in England: the evidence of variability and persistency of type, *Lancet* **ii**, 733–739.

[56] Harris, T.E. (1948). Branching processes, *Annals of Mathematical Statistics* **19**, 474–494.

[57] Heyde, C.C. (1974). On estimating the variance of the offspring distribution in a simple branching process, *Advances in Applied Probability* **6**, 421–433

[58] Heyde, C.C. (1979). On assessing the potential severity of an outbreak of a rare infectious disease: a Bayesian approach, *Australian Journal of Statistics* **21**, 282–292.

[59] Johnson, A.M., Wadsworth, J., Wellings, K. & Field J. (1994). *Sexual Attitudes and Lifestyles*. Blackwell, Oxford.

[60] Keiding, N. (1975). Estimation theory for branching processes, *Bulletin of the International Statistical Institute* **46**(4), 12–19.

[61] Keiding, N. (1991). Age-specific incidence and prevalence: a statistical perspective, *Journal of the Royal Statistical Society, Series A* **154**, 371–412.

[62] Kermack, W.O. & McKendrick, A.G. (1927). A contribution to the mathematical theory of epidemics, *Proceedings of the Royal Society, Series A* **115**, 700–721.

[63] Knox, E.G. (1964). The detection of space–time interactions, *Applied Statistics* **13**, 25–29.

[64] Knox, E.G. (1980). Strategy for rubella vaccination, *International Journal of Epidemiology* **9**, 13–23

[65] Lagakos, S.W., Barraj, L.M. & De Gruttola, V. (1988). Nonparametric analysis of truncated survival data, with application to AIDS, *Biometrika* **75**, 515–523.

[66] Longini, I.M. & Koopman, J.S. (1982). Household and community transmission parameters from final distributions of infections in households, *Biometrics* **38**, 115–126.

[67] Longini, I.M., Koopman, J.S., Monto, A.S. & Fox, J.P. (1982). Estimating household and community transmission parameters for influenza, *American Journal of Epidemiology* **115**, 736–751.

[68] Mantel, N. (1967). The detection of disease clustering and a generalized regression approach, *Cancer Research* **27**, 209–220.

[69] Mathen, K.K. & Chakraborty, P.N. (1950). A statistical study on multiple cases of disease in households, *Sankhyā* **10**, 387–392

[70] McCrady, M.H. (1918). Tables for rapid interpretation of fermentation-tube results, *Public Health Journal, Toronto* **9**, 201–220.

[71] Medical Research Council (1948). Streptomycin treatment of pulmonary tuberculosis, *British Medical Journal* **ii**, 769–782.

[72] Medical Research Council (1950). Clinical trials of antihistaminic drugs in the prevention and treatment of the common cold, *British Medical Journal* **ii**, 425–429.

[73] Medical Research Council (1951). The prevention of whooping cough by vaccination, *British Medical Journal* **i**, 1463–1471.

[74] Medley, G.F., Billard, L., Cox, D.R. & Anderson, R.M. (1988). The distribution of the incubation period for the acquired immunodeficiency syndrome (AIDS), *Proceedings of the Royal Society, Series B* **233**, 367–377.

[75] Moulton, L.H., Wolff, M.C., Brenneman, G. & Santosham, M. (1994). Case–cohort analysis of case-coverage studies of vaccine effectiveness, *American Journal of Epidemiology* **142**, 1000–1006.

[76] Muench, H. (1934). Derivation of rates from summation data by the catalytic curve, *Journal of the American Statistical Association* **29**, 25–38.

[77] Muench, H. (1959). *Catalytic Models in Epidemiology*. Harvard University Press, Cambridge, Mass.

[78] Nobre, F.F. & Stroup, D.F. (1994). A monitoring system to detect changes in public health surveillance data, *International Journal of Epidemiology* **23**, 408–418.

[79] O'Neill, P.D. & Roberts, G.O. (1999). Bayesian inference for partially obscured stochastic epidemics, *Journal of the Royal Statistical Society, Series A* **162**, 121–129.

[80] Orenstein, W.A., Bernier, R.H. & Hinman, A.R. (1988). Assessing vaccine efficacy in the field, *Epidemiologic Reviews* **10**, 212–241.

[81] Parker, R.A., Erdman, D.D. & Anderson, L.J. (1990). Use of mixture models in determining laboratory criterion for identification of seropositive individuals: application to parvovirus B19 serology, *Journal of Virological Methods* **27**, 135–144.

[82] Pike, M.C. & Smith, P.G. (1968). Disease clustering: a generalization of Knox's approach to the detection of space–time interactions, *Biometrics* **24**, 541–556.

[83] Pike, M.C. & Smith, P.G. (1974). A case–control approach to examine diseases for evidence of contagion, including diseases with long latent periods, *Biometrics* **30**, 263–279.

[84] Ray, W.A. & Griffin, M.R. (1989). Use of Medicaid data for pharmacoepidemiology, *American Journal of Epidemiology* **129**, 837–849.

[85] Ross, R. (1911). *The Prevention of Malaria*, 2nd Ed. John Murray, London.

[86] Sartwell, P.E. (1950). The distribution of incubation periods of infectious disease, *American Journal of Hygiene* **51**, 310–318.

[87] Serfling, R.E. (1963). Methods for current statistical analysis of excess pneumonia-influenza deaths, *Public Health Reports* **78**, 494–506.

[88] Smith, P.G. (1982). Retrospective assessment of the effectiveness of BCG vaccination against tuberculosis using the case–control method, *Tubercle* **63**, 23–35

[89] Smith, P.G. & Morrow, R.H. eds (1991). *Methods for Field Trials of Interventions Against Tropical Diseases: A Toolbox*. Oxford University Press, Oxford.

[90] Smith, P.G. & Pike, M.C. (1976). Generalization of two tests for the detection of household aggregation of disease, *Biometrics* **32**, 817–828.

[91] Smith, P.G., Rodrigues, L.C. & Fine, P.E.M. (1984). Assessment of the protective efficacy of vaccines against common diseases using case–control and cohort studies, *International Journal of Epidemiology* **13**, 87–93.

[92] Snow, J. (1855). *The Mode of Communication of Cholera*, 2nd Ed. Churchill, London.

[93] Sobel, M. & Elashoff, R.M. (1975). Group testing with a new goal, estimation, *Biometrika* **62**, 181–193.

[94] Stirzaker, D.R. (1975). A perturbation method for the stochastic recurrent epidemic, *Journal of the Institute for Mathematics and its Applications* **15**, 135–160.

[95] Storsaeter, J., Hallander, H., Farrington, C.P., Olin, P., Mollby, R. & Miller E. (1990). Secondary analyses of the efficacy of two acellular pertussis vaccines evaluated in a Swedish phase III trial, *Vaccine* **8**, 457–461.

[96] Stroup, D.F., Williamson, G.D. & Herndon, J.L. (1989). Detection of aberrations in the occurrence of notifiable diseases surveillance data, *Statistics in Medicine* **8**, 323–329.

[97] Tillett, H.E. & Spencer, I.-L. (1982). Influenza surveillance in England and Wales using routine statistics, *Journal of Hygiene, Cambridge* **88**, 83–94.

[98] Vesikari, T. (1993). Clinical trials of live oral rotavirus vaccines: the Finnish experience, *Vaccine* **11**, 255–261.

[99] Walter, S.D. (1974). On the detection of household aggregation of disease, *Biometrics* **30**, 525–538.

[100] Walter, S.D., Hildreth, S.W. & Beaty, B.J. (1980). Estimation of infection rates in populations of organisms using pools of variable size, *American Journal of Epidemiology* **112**, 124–128.

[101] Watier, L., Richardson, S. & Hubert, B. (1991). A time series construction of an alert threshold with application to *S. bovismorbificans* in France, *Statistics in Medicine* **10**, 1493–1509.

[102] Zeger, S.L., See, L.-C. & Diggle, P.J. (1989). Statistical methods for monitoring the AIDS epidemic, *Statistics in Medicine* **8**, 3–21.

C.P. FARRINGTON

Comparable-Accuracy Principle in Control Selection *see* Case–Control Study

Comparative Mortality Figure (CMF) *see* Standardization Methods

Competing Risks

"Competing risks" refers to the study of mortality patterns in a population of individuals, all subject to the same $k \geq 2$ competing risks or **causes of death**. Specifically, the objective is to isolate the effect of a given risk, or a subset of risks, acting on a population. The use of competing risks dates back to 1760 and evolved out of a controversy over smallpox inoculation.

According to Karn [22] and Todhunter [30], smallpox inoculation in the 1700s was administered by applying leeches to the body, a practice that could lead to acute illness and death. Physicians argued whether the benefits of inoculation outweighed the initial risk of death. Daniel Bernoulli [9], in a 1760 memoir entitled "Essai d'une nouvelle analyse de la mortalité causée par le petite vérole; et des advantages de l'inoculation pour le prévenir", tried to estimate the expected increase in lifespan (*see* **Life Expectancy**) if smallpox were eliminated. This calculation could then be used to weigh the pros and cons of smallpox inoculation.

Similarly, in the modern treatment of competing risks we are interested in isolating the effect of individual risks. For example, suppose we wish to assess a new treatment for heart disease. In a long-term study of this treatment on a sample of individuals, some will die of causes other than heart disease. The appropriate analysis of this problem must account for the competing effects of death from other causes.

Various methods have been proposed to study the problem of competing risks. For example, Makeham [24] formulated the law of composition of decremental forces and applied it to competing risks theory. A multiple decrement model is a time-continuous Markov model with one transient state and k absorbing states. An excellent account of the use of multiple decrement theory to explain competing risks may be found in Chiang [12].

Another approach to modeling competing risks is through the use of latent failure times. This method was first advocated by Sampford [28] who proposed an "accidental death model". In this approach each individual has latent failure times T_1 and T_2, where T_1 corresponds to time of natural death and T_2 to time to accidental death. Sampford assumed that T_1 and T_2 are independent and normally distributed and death occurred at time X equal to the minimum of T_1 and T_2. Berkson & Elveback [8] considered a similar model to study the effect of smoking on lung cancer assuming that the latent failure times were independent exponentially distributed random variables. Moeschberger & David [25] generalized these ideas to k causes of death with general survival distributions. Excellent reviews of the theory of competing risks are given by Gail [18, 19], David & Moeschberger [15], and Birnbaum [10].

In this article, latent failure times are used to describe competing risks models. We assume that all individuals in a population are subject to k competing causes of death, $D_1, \ldots, D_k$. For each possible cause of death, D_i, there corresponds a latent failure time, T_i, a positive random variable representing the age at death in the hypothetical situation in which D_i is the only possible cause of death. The joint distribution of the latent failure times is given by the multivariate survival distribution

$$H^C(t_1, \ldots, t_k) = P(T_1 > t_1, \ldots, T_k > t_k), \quad (1)$$

defined for all nonnegative values $t_1, \ldots, t_k$. We use a superscript C to highlight that this is the joint distribution of the complete set of risks acting on the population. The latent failure times are mostly unobservable and serve only as a theoretical construct. In contrast, the observable random variables for each member of a population of individuals are the actual times to death, denoted by the positive random variable X, and the cause of death, Δ, which may take one of the integer values $1, \ldots, k$. The observed time of death, X, is taken to be the minimum of $T_1, \ldots, T_k$, and Δ indexes this cause of death, i.e. $\Delta = i$ if $X = T_i$. For simplicity we assume the joint distribution is absolutely continuous so that Δ is uniquely defined.

The study of competing risks considers the interrelationship of three types of probabilities of death from specific causes. These are:

1. *The crude probability*: the probability of death from a specific cause in the presence of all other risks acting on the population. This is also referred to as **absolute risk**. An example of a crude probability is the answer to the question: What is the chance that a woman will die of breast cancer between ages 40 and 60?

2. *The net probability*: the probability of death if a specific risk is the only risk acting on a population, or conversely, the probability of death if a specific cause is eliminated from the population. For example, what is the chance of surviving to age 60 if cancer were the only cause of death?

3. *The partial crude probability*: the probability of death from a specific cause when some risks are eliminated from the population. For example, what is the chance that a woman would die from breast cancer between ages 40 and 60 if smallpox were eliminated?

In the next section we define notation and give some fundamental relationships between the three different types of probabilities. Then we consider the issue of identifiability of these probabilities and discuss some philosophical issues regarding the study of competing risks in light of nonidentifiability. Finally, we address statistical issues of estimation and hypotheses testing based on a sample of observable data.

Notation and Relationships

Crude Probability

Crude probability is a way of describing the probability distribution for a specific cause of death in the presence of all causes. Crude probability refers to quantities derived from the probability distribution of the observable random variables, X and Δ, where X is time to death, and $\Delta = 1, \ldots, k$ is cause of death. Two approaches have been used to describe the distribution of X and Δ. The first is through subdistribution functions:

$$F_i^C(x) = \Pr(X \le x, \Delta = i), \quad i = 1, \ldots, k.$$

The function $F_i^C(x)$ denotes the proportion of all individuals who are observed to die from cause D_i at or before time x in the presence of all causes of death. We use the superscript C to denote all causes of death, i.e. $C = \{1, \ldots, k\}$. For example, if D_1 represents death from breast cancer, then the chance that a woman dies from breast cancer between ages 40 and 60 would be equal to $[F_1^C(60) - F_1^C(40)]$. Note that $F_i^C(\infty)$ is the proportion of individuals who will be observed to die from cause D_i, and $\sum_{i=1}^k F_i^C(x) = F^C(x)$ defines the distribution function for death from any cause, i.e. $F^C(x) = \Pr(X \le x)$. We denote the overall survival distribution as $S^C(x) = 1 - F^C(x)$.

Another way to define the distribution of X and Δ is through the use of k cause specific **hazard rate** functions given by

$$\lambda_i^C(x) = \lim_{h \to 0} \left[\frac{\Pr(x \le X < x + h, \Delta = i | X \ge x)}{h} \right],$$
$$i = 1 \ldots, k.$$

The ith cause-specific hazard is the rate of death at time x from cause i among individuals who are still alive at time x. Calculus yields the following relationships:

$$\lambda_i^C(x) = \frac{dF_i^C(x)}{dx} \Big/ S^C(x),$$

$$\lambda^C(x) = \sum_{i=1}^k \lambda_i^C(x) = \frac{dF^C(x)}{dx} \Big/ S^C(x), \quad (2)$$

$$S^C(x) = \exp[-\Lambda^C(x)]; \quad \Lambda^C(x) = \int_0^x \lambda^C(u)du,$$

$$F_i^C(x) = \int_0^x \exp[-\Lambda^C(u)]\lambda_i^C(u)du.$$

Note that $\Lambda^C(x)$ is defined as the **cumulative hazard** function of death from any cause and is the sum of the individual cause-specific integrated hazards. The relationship given in (2) illustrates that there is a one-to-one relationship between subdistribution functions and cause-specific hazard functions.

The crude probability distributions may be derived from the joint distribution of the latent failure times as follows. Because $X = \min(T_1, \ldots, T_k)$, it follows that $S^C(x) = H^C(x, \ldots, x)$; hence, it is straightforward to show that

$$\frac{dF_i^C(x)}{dx} = - \frac{\partial H^C(t_1, \ldots, t_k)}{\partial t_i} \Big|_{t_1 = \cdots = t_k = x}.$$

Using (2), the cause-specific hazard function is given by

$$\lambda_i^C(x) = \frac{- \dfrac{\partial H^C(t_1, \ldots, t_k)}{\partial t_i} \Big|_{t_1 = \cdots = t_k = x}}{H^C(x, \ldots, x)}. \quad (3)$$

This relationship was derived by Gail [18] and Tsiatis [31].

Cause-specific hazard functions and cause-specific subdistribution functions may also be defined for a subset of risks. We use italicized capital letters to index a subset of the risks $1, \ldots, k$; for example, J may be used to denote such a subset of risks. The complement of J is equal to $C - J$ and is denoted by $\bar{J}$. The subdistribution function for failing from any of the causes in J is given by

$$F_J^C(x) = \Pr(X \le x, \Delta \in J) = \sum_{i \in J} F_i^C(x),$$

and the cause-specific hazard of failing from any of the causes in J is

$$\lambda_J^C(x) = \lim_{h \to 0} \left[\frac{\Pr(x \le X < x + h, \Delta \in J | X \ge x)}{h} \right]$$
$$= \sum_{i \in J} \lambda_i^C(x).$$

The Net Probability

The net probability is the probability distribution of time to death if only one cause of death acted on a population. If we are interested in the net probability distribution from cause D_i, then this would be the marginal probability distribution of the latent failure time, T_i, given by

$$S_i^i(x) = \Pr(T_i > x) = H^C(t_1, \ldots, t_k)|t_i = x,$$
$$t_j = 0, j \ne i.$$

We use superscript i to highlight the fact that we consider only the case where D_i is acting on a population. For example, if D_1 denotes death from cancer, then the chance of surviving to age 60 if cancer were the only cause of death would be given by S_1^1 (60).

The net distribution may be defined through the net or marginal hazard function for T_i, that is,

$$\lambda_i^i(x) = \lim_{h \to 0} \left[\frac{\Pr(x \le T_i < x + h | T_i \ge x)}{h} \right].$$

The net hazard function and net survival distribution are related to each other as follows:

$$\lambda_i^i(x) = -\frac{dS_i^i(x)}{dx} \Big/ S_i^i(x),$$

$$S_i^i(x) = \exp[-\Lambda_i^i(x)],$$

(4)

where $\Lambda_i^i(x) = \int_0^x \lambda_i^i(u) du$.

One of the key results in competing risks theory is for the case where the latent failure times are assumed to be statistically independent, i.e.

$$H^C(t_1, \dots, t_k) = \prod_{i=1}^{k} S_i^i(t_i).$$

From (1) it is a simple exercise to show that the ith cause-specific hazard function, $\lambda_i^C(x)$, is equal to the ith net-specific hazard function, $\lambda_i^i(x)$. This important fact allows one to use the crude probability distribution of the observables to obtain net probabilities. Specifically, formulas (1) and (2) may be used to show that the net survival distribution is related to the crude subdistribution functions by

$$H_i^i(x) = \exp \left[-\int_0^x \frac{dF_i^C(u)}{S^C(u)} \right].$$

(5)

Because $F_i^C(u)$ and $S^C(u)$ may be estimated from a sample of observable data, (5) suggests obvious methods for estimating net survival probabilities when the latent failure times are assumed independent, which are described in detail later. Although the crude cause-specific hazard is equal to the net-specific hazard when the latent failure times are independent, the converse is not true. Examples where nonindependent latent failure times have cause-specific hazards equal to the net-specific hazards, although mathematically possible, are generally artificial constructs and not important from an applied perspective.

For many applications it may not be reasonable to assume that the latent failure times are independent. In such cases the relationship between net and crude probabilities becomes more complicated. Without additional assumptions, there is a problem of nonidentifiability discussed in greater detail later.

Partial Crude Probability

We now show how to characterize the distribution of probability of death from a subset of causes acting on a population in the hypothetical situation where all other causes of death are eliminated. Similar to crude probabilities, partial crude probabilities may be expressed through partial crude subdistribution functions or partial crude cause-specific hazard functions. Define X^J and Δ^J respectively as the time of death and cause of death in the hypothetical case where individuals are only subject to the causes of death in J, i.e. the causes $\bar{J}$ are eliminated. In terms of latent failure times, $X^J = \min(T_i, i \in J)$ and $\Delta^J = i$, if $X^J = T_i, i \in J$. The partial crude subdistribution function is given by

$$F_i^J(x) = \Pr(X^J \le x, \Delta^J = i), \quad i \in J,$$

and the partial crude cause-specific hazard is given by

$$\lambda_i^J(x)$$
$$= \lim_{h \to 0} \left(\frac{\Pr(x \le X^J < x + h, \Delta^J = i | X^J \ge x)}{h} \right),$$
$$i \in J.$$

These definitions may be extended in a natural way to subsets K of J, i.e.

$$F_K^J(x) = \sum_{i \in K} F_i^J(x)$$

and

$$\lambda_K^J(x) = \sum_{i \in K} \lambda_i^J(x).$$

If $J = C$, then partial crude probabilities are the same as crude probabilities, and if $J = i$, so that there is only one cause of death, then partial crude probability is the same as net probability.

Using the same logic as for crude probabilities, we can derive the partial crude cause-specific hazard function from the joint distribution of the latent failure times in a manner similar to that for (3). The partial crude cause-specific hazard is given by

$$\lambda_i^J(x) = \frac{-\dfrac{\partial H^C(t_1,\ldots,t_k)}{\partial t_i}\bigg|_{t_j=x,\,j\in J;\,t_j=0,\,j\in\bar{J}}}{H^C(t_1,\ldots,t_k)|_{t_j=x,\,j\in J;\,t_j=0,\,j\in\bar{J}}},\quad(6)$$

and the partial crude subdistribution function may be expressed as

$$F_i^J(x) = \int_0^x \exp[-\Lambda_J^J(u)]\lambda_i^J(u)\,\mathrm{d}u,\quad i\in J,\quad(7)$$

where $\Lambda_J^J(u)=\int_0^u\lambda_J^J(v)\,\mathrm{d}v$.

Of particular interest is the case when the latent failure times in the set J are independent of the latent failure times in $\bar{J}$. Comparing (6) with (3) we see that the ith partial crude cause-specific hazard function, $\lambda_i^J(x)$, is equal to the overall crude cause-specific hazard function, $\lambda_i^C(x)$, $i\in J$. This allows us to express the unobservable partial crude probabilities in terms of the observable crude probabilities. So, for example, the partial crude subdistribution function may be expressed in terms of the observable crude subdistribution functions as follows:

$$F_i^J(x) = \int_0^x \exp[-\Lambda_J^C(u)]\lambda_i^C(u)\,\mathrm{d}u,\quad i\in J,\quad(8)$$

where

$$\lambda_i^C(u) = \frac{\mathrm{d}F_i^C(u)}{\mathrm{d}u}\bigg/S^C(u).$$

The above relationships hold whenever the latent failure times in J and $\bar{J}$ are independent. It is not necessary that the failure times within J or $\bar{J}$ be independent.

Issues Regarding the Use and Interpretation of Competing Risks

A major aim in many competing risks studies is the estimation of net survival probabilities. The ability to isolate the effect of one risk acting on a population is intuitively attractive, especially if the focus of a study is to evaluate the effect of an intervention that is targeted at reducing mortality from that specific cause. Of course, net survival probabilities are hypothetical quantities and not directly observable in a population; therefore they must be computed from the available information on the distribution of observables, or

what we refer to as *crude probabilities*. Previously, we derived the net survival distribution for a specific risk D_i as a function of the observable crude probabilities under the assumption that the different latent failure times were independent of each other. The independence assumption is critical, because in this case the crude cause-specific hazard function is equal to the net hazard function, which leads to the important relationship given by (5).

In some situations such an assumption of independence may be reasonable. For example, when studying cause of death from a specific disease, it may be reasonable to assume that death from accidental causes is independent of those causes associated with the disease. Of course, there are other scenarios for which the independence assumption is not plausible. It is therefore important to consider the relationship of net probabilities to crude probabilities in the case where the latent failure times are not independent.

As we showed in (3), given any joint distribution of latent failure times, there exists a corresponding set of crude cause-specific hazard functions, or equivalently a set of crude cause-specific subdistribution functions. Unfortunately, the converse is not true, as there exist many joint distributions, $H^C(t_1,\ldots,t_k)$, that would result in the same set of crude subdistribution functions, $F_i^C(x)$, $i=1,\ldots k$. These different joint distributions of latent failure times, each resulting in the same set of subdistribution functions, would lead to different net survival probabilities. Consequently we cannot identify net survival probabilities from corresponding crude probabilities. Because crude survival distributions define the observable random variables, we cannot estimate the net survival probabilities from observable data without making additional assumptions that cannot be verified from the observable data. Independence of the latent failure times is one assumption that would resolve the problem of identifiability and permit estimation of net probabilities; however, this assumption can never be verified. This problem of nonidentifiability was pointed out by Cox [13] and Tsiatis [31].

To get a sense of the extent of the nonidentifiability problem, Peterson [26] computed sharp bounds for net survival probabilities as a function of crude subdistribution functions. Specifically, he showed that

$$S^C(x) \le S_i^i(x) \le 1 - F_i^C(x).$$

Heuristically, these inequalities may be explained as follows. First, consider the hypothetical case that the causes of death are so highly correlated that an individual dying at time x from any cause other than D_i would have died from cause D_i immediately thereafter. For such a scenario the net survival probability at time x, $S_i^i(x)$, would be equal to the probability of surviving until time x from any cause, $S^C(x) = \Pr(X > x)$. At the other extreme, consider the hypothetical case where an individual who would die from any cause other than D_i would never die from cause D_i. Here, $\Pr(T_i \leq x) = 1 - S_i^i(x)$ would be equal to $F_i^C(x) = \Pr(X \leq x, \Delta = i)$. The upper and lower bounds for net survival probabilities may be quite substantial, as shown by Tsiatis [32].

This creates a philosophical dilemma in competing risks theory. Knowledge of the distribution of observable causes of death does not suffice to determine net survival probabilities. Only if additional assumptions are made on the joint distribution of the latent failure times are we able to identify uniquely the net survival probabilities. Two points of view have been taken in the literature. One is to restrict attention to certain dependency structures on the latent failure times that allow for identification or, at least, restrict to a class of joint distributions where the bounds for the net survival probability are much tighter than the Peterson bounds. This has been the focus of research by Slud & Rubinstein [29], Klein & Moeschberger [23], and Zheng & Klein [33].

Another perspective is as follows. Because nonidentifiability problems can only be handled by making additional assumptions that cannot be verified from the data, perhaps we should only consider making inference on the distribution of the observable random variables. That is, the focus should be on estimating cause-specific hazard and subdistribution functions and the comparison of such quantities under a variety of conditions that have practical importance. For example, comparisons may be made among different treatments or varying environmental conditions. This pragmatic point of view suggests that there is no reason to consider hypothetical quantities, such as net survival probabilities, because in fact we will never be in a position to evaluate one cause of death acting in isolation on a population. This point of view was eloquently presented by Prentice et al. [27].

This idea may be modified slightly in the case where a subset of the causes of death that are not of primary interest, denoted by $\bar{J}$, are thought a priori to be independent of the other causes of death, J, that are of interest. For example, certain accidental causes of death may fall into this category when studying treatment of disease. For these problems, inference using partial crude probabilities may be appropriate. We showed before how partial crude probabilities can be defined in terms of the distribution of the observable crude probabilities when causes J are independent of $\bar{J}$.

The Statistical Analysis of Competing Risk Data

Often, the data available for the analysis of competing risks are incomplete or right censored. This may be due to the termination of the study before all individuals fail, or to individuals who drop out of the study and subsequently are lost to follow-up. To accommodate this situation we extend the definition of competing risks to include censoring, i.e. we include an additional random variable, T_0, that denotes the latent time to censoring. With this extended definition of competing risks, the observable data are defined by X^* and Δ^*, where $X^* = \min(T_0, \ldots, T_k)$ and $\Delta^* = i$ if $X^* = T_i$, $i = 0, \ldots, k$. We note that $\Delta^* = 0$ means that the failure time was censored at time X^*.

In a typical competing risks study we observe a sample of data (X_j^*, Δ_j^*, Z_j), $j = 1, \ldots, n$, where for the jth individual, X_j^* denotes the time to failure or censoring, Δ_j^* corresponds to cause of death or censoring, and Z_j corresponds to covariate(s) which we may use for modeling the distribution of competing risks. Using this extended notation, the observable data include censoring as a competing risk. We use an asterisk to denote the competing risks model that includes censoring. Therefore, the complete set of observable risks will be denoted by $C^* = 0, \ldots, k$, in contrast to the risks of interest, $C = 1, \ldots, k$, or perhaps some subset, J. In the previous section we denoted the complement of the subset J by $\bar{J} = C - J$; in the extended definition of competing risks we denote the complement of J by $\bar{J}^* = C^* - J$. In what follows it will be assumed that censoring, or risk 0, is independent of the other risks C. Without this assumption, nonidentifiability problems would not allow for estimation of the competing risk probabilities of interest regarding causes C.

One Sample Problems

Here we consider the problem of estimating relevant competing risk probabilities from a single sample of data (X_j^*, Δ_j^*), $j = 1, \ldots, n$.

Estimating Cause-Specific Hazard Functions

We showed before that the partial crude cause-specific hazard function is equal to the observable crude cause-specific hazard function whenever the risks in J are independent of the risks in $\bar{J}^*$, i.e.

$$\lambda_i^J(x) = \lambda_i^{C^*}(x). \tag{9}$$

Because censoring, or risk 0, is always assumed independent of the other risks, (9) will follow as long as the risks in J are independent of $\bar{J}$. It is important to note that the crude cause-specific hazard functions discussed in the previous section, $\lambda_i^C(x)$, are actually partial crude cause-specific hazard functions when we include censoring as a competing risk. However, because of (9) applied to $J = C$, $\lambda_i^C(x)$ is equal to the observable $\lambda_i^{C^*}(x)$. In the case when cause of death D_i is independent of the other risks, the net-specific hazard function, $\lambda_i^i(x)$, is equal to $\lambda_i^{C^*}(x)$.

For certain independence assumptions, the cause-specific hazard functions are related to the observable crude cause-specific hazard functions, which by (2) is equal to

$$\lambda_i^{C^*}(x) = \frac{dF_i^{C^*}(x)}{dx} \bigg/ S^{C^*}(x),$$

where

$$F_i^{C^*}(x) = \Pr(X^* \leq x, \Delta^* = i)$$

and

$$S^{C^*}(x) = \Pr(X^* > x).$$

The natural estimate for the crude subdistribution function is the empirical subdistribution function, i.e.

$$\hat{F}_i^{C^*}(x) = n^{-1} \sum_{j=1}^{n} I(X_j^* \leq x, \Delta_j^* = i),$$

where $I(\cdot)$ denotes the indicator function. This estimate puts mass $1/n$ at each observed event time from cause i. Similarly,

$$\hat{S}^{C^*}(x) = n^{-1} \sum_{j=1}^{n} I(X_j^* > x)$$

puts mass $1/n$ at each event time.

Because crude cause-specific hazards are functions of the crude subdistribution probabilities, the obvious estimates are obtained by substituting the corresponding functions of the empirical subdistribution probabilities. For example, the estimate of the cumulative cause-specific hazard function is

$$\hat{\Lambda}_i^{C^*}(x) = \int_0^x \frac{d\hat{F}_i^{C^*}(u)}{\hat{S}^{C^*}(u)} = \sum_{j=1}^{n} \frac{I(X_j^* \leq x, \Delta_j^* = i)}{Y(X_j^*)},$$

where $Y(u) = \sum_{j=1}^{n} I(X_j^* > u)$ denotes the number of individuals in the sample who are at risk at time u, i.e. neither died nor were censored. This estimator is the so-called Nelson–Aalen estimator; see Aalen [1]. Aalen [2, 3] derived the theoretical large-sample properties, including consistency and asymptotic normality, using the theory of counting processes.

This estimator of the ith crude cause-specific cumulative hazard is the appropriate estimator for the partial crude cause-specific cumulative hazard whenever the causes in J are independent of the causes in $\bar{J}^*$, i.e.

$$\hat{\Lambda}_i^{J^*}(x) = \hat{\Lambda}_i^{C^*}(x), \quad i \in J.$$

In the special case where cause i is assumed independent of all other causes, the ith net-specific cumulative hazard function, $\Lambda_i^i(x)$, is estimated by $\hat{\Lambda}_i^{C^*}(x)$. The ith net survival distribution, $S_i^i(x)$, is equal to $\exp[-\Lambda_i^i(x)]$. Therefore, a natural estimator is the exponentiated negative of the Nelson–Aalen estimator. This estimator is

$$\hat{S}_i^i(x) = \exp - \left[\sum_{j=1}^{n} \frac{I(X_j^* \leq x, \Delta_j^* = i)}{Y(X_j^*)} \right].$$

Noting that this is equal to

$$\prod_{j=1}^{n} \exp \left[\frac{-I(X_j^* \leq x, \Delta_j^* = i)}{Y(X_j^*)} \right]$$

and that

$$\exp[-1/Y(u)] \approx [1 - 1/Y(u)],$$

yields the approximation

$$\hat{S}_i^i(x) \approx \prod_{j=1}^{n} [1 - 1/Y(X_j^*)]^{I(X_j^* \leq x, \Delta_j^* = i)}.$$

This is the well known Kaplan–Meier [21], or product-limit, estimator. The asymptotic equivalence of the exponentiated Nelson–Aalen estimator and the Kaplan–Meier estimator, and the large-sample properties of these estimators, are given by Breslow & Crowley [11].

It is important to note that the Kaplan–Meier estimator, by construction, is a consistent estimator of the exponentiated cumulative crude cause-specific hazard function. That this corresponds to an estimator of the net survival distribution follows only when the net hazard function is equal to the crude cause-specific hazard, i.e. when cause i is independent of all the other causes, including censoring. Without this assumption, the Kaplan–Meier estimator of the ith net-specific survival distribution does not estimate any interesting or relevant probability.

If we consider death from any cause, i.e. $\Delta \in C$, then the estimate of the corresponding survival distribution, $S^C(x)$, from a sample of potentially censored data (X_j^*, Δ_j^*), $j = 1, \ldots, n$, follows from applying the same logic:

$$\hat{S}^C(x) = \prod_{j=1}^{n} [1 - 1/Y(X_j^*)]^{I(X_j^* \leq x, \Delta_j^* \in C)}.$$

This estimator for the survival distribution from any cause of death in the presence of censoring is the Kaplan–Meier estimator as originally presented in the seminal paper [21] in 1958. Failure is considered a death from any cause, and an incomplete observation is a censored observation. The estimator of the ith net survival function given above is also referred to as a Kaplan–Meier estimator, since it may be derived via the same formula, letting failure be death from cause i and an incomplete observation be death from any cause other than i or censoring.

Estimating Subdistribution Functions

We may use the above results to derive nonparametric estimators for crude and partial crude subdistribution functions. Using (2), the ith crude subdistribution function may be expressed as

$$F_i^C(x) = \int_0^x S^C(u) \lambda_i^C(u) \mathrm{d}u.$$

Because censoring is independent of the other causes of death, $\lambda_i^C(u) = \lambda_i^{C*}(u)$. Therefore a natural estimator for the ith subdistribution function is

given by

$$\hat{F}_i^C(x) = \int_0^x \hat{S}^C(u) \frac{\mathrm{d}\hat{F}_i^{C*}(u)}{\hat{S}^{C*}(u)},$$

where $\hat{S}^C(u)$ is the Kaplan–Meier estimator for the survival distribution of time to death from any cause.

The large-sample statistical properties of this estimator may be derived using the theory of counting processes. Details may be found in Aalen [2, 3], Fleming [16, 17], Benichou & Gail [6], and Andersen et al. [5] when using **cohort** data, and in Benichou & Gail [7] when using **population-based case–control data**.

The Relationship of Competing Risks to Covariates

Often, we are interested in studying the relationship of time to death from one or many causes to other covariates. For example, we may be interested in the effect of different treatments on reducing the risk of death from specific causes, or we may wish to model the relationship of competing risk probabilities to other prognostic factors. These problems are generally posed in terms of hypothesis testing or estimation of regression parameters. There is a wide literature on inferential techniques for hypothesis testing and regression modeling for survival problems with censored data. Because of the close relationship between censoring and competing risks, many of the methods developed for analyzing censored survival data may also be applied to competing risks data (*see* **Survival Analysis, Overview**).

Hypothesis Testing

The most widely used methods for testing the null hypothesis of no treatment effect among K treatments with censored survival data are the logrank or weighted logrank tests. These tests were designed to test the equality of the hazard functions for death among K treatments when the censoring time is independent of time to death within each treatment group. If we study these tests carefully, then we realize that they actually compare the observable cause-specific hazard functions among the different treatment groups. Therefore, we can immediately apply these methods for testing equality of cause-specific hazard functions among different treatments. To be more precise, we denote by $\lambda_{il}^{C^*}(x)$, $l = 1, \ldots, K$, the ith cause-specific hazard function within treatment group l. The weighted logrank tests may then be used to test the null hypothesis that

$$\lambda_{i1}^{C^*}(x) = \cdots = \lambda_{iK}^{C^*}(x), \quad x > 0.$$

The theoretical development for these tests is given by Andersen et al. [4]. This is carried out by letting failure correspond to death from cause i and an incomplete observation to correspond to death from any cause other than i or censoring ($\Delta^* = 0$).

We reiterate the interpretation of this null hypothesis and the results of the logrank test. If we are willing to assume that time to death from cause i is independent of the times to death from other causes as well as time to censoring, within each treatment group $l = 1, \ldots, K$, then the cause-specific hazard function, $\lambda_{il}^{C^*}(x)$, is equal to the net-specific, or marginal, hazard function, $\lambda_{il}^{i}(x)$. Equality of net-specific hazard functions implies equality of net-specific survival probabilities. Therefore, with the assumption of independence, the logrank test is a test of the null hypothesis that the K net-specific survival distributions are equal. This is often the hypothesis of interest.

To illustrate, consider a clinical trial of several treatments to reduce breast cancer mortality. Because breast cancer clinical trials generally occur over many years, some patients may die from causes other than breast cancer. Because the treatments were targeted to reduce breast cancer mortality, the investigators are not interested in the effect that treatment may have on other causes of death; rather, they are mainly interested in the effect of the treatments on breast cancer mortality in the absence of causes of death other than breast cancer. This is the classic competing risks problem of comparing net survival distributions. When the logrank test is used, patients not dying from breast cancer are treated as censored observations. As previously discussed, this is an appropriate test for the equality of net survival probabilities when the time to death from other causes is independent of time to death from breast cancer within each treatment group. This assumption may not be true, and in fact cannot be verified with the data because of nonidentifiability problems alluded to above. If this independence assumption is not true, then it is not clear what we are testing when we use the logrank test.

One way around this philosophical dilemma is to consider only tests of observable population parameters. An important observable population parameter is the crude cause-specific hazard function, $\lambda_i^C(x)$. We again emphasize that the population cause-specific hazard function, $\lambda_i^C(x)$, is observable only if there is no additional censoring introduced. With the introduction of censoring, the observable parameter is $\lambda_i^{C^*}(x)$. However, by assumption, the censoring ($\Delta^* = 0$) is independent of the other causes of death, in which case $\lambda_i^C(x) = \lambda_i^{C^*}(x)$.

As we pointed out, the logrank test tests the equality of the cause-specific hazard functions, $\lambda_{il}^{C^*}(x)$, and, with independent censoring, the equality of $\lambda_{il}^C(x)$. Therefore, the logrank test would be a valid test of the equality of the breast cancer specific hazard functions among the K treatments. Although this cause-specific hazard function may not be directly related to net-specific breast cancer mortality, if independence does not hold, then it still may be an important comparison. This point of view is given by Prentice et al. [27].

Another observable quantity is the subdistribution function $F_{il}^C(x)$ for cause i within treatment group l. Very little work has been done on deriving tests for the equality of these K-sample subdistribution functions. One exception is a class of tests derived by Gray [20] to test the null hypothesis that

$$F_{i1}^C(x) = \cdots = F_{iK}^C(x).$$

Regression Modeling

The most popular framework for modeling the association of censored survival data to prognostic variables is with the **proportional hazards** model of Cox [14] (*see* **Cox Regression Model**). In this model the hazard for death is related to a vector of covariates by

$$\lambda(t|\mathbf{z}) = \lambda_0(t) \exp(\beta^T \mathbf{z}),$$

where $\mathbf{z}$ represents a vector of covariates, and $\lambda(t|\mathbf{z})$ is the hazard rate of death at time t given covariates $\mathbf{z}$. In this model, censoring is assumed to be independent of the failure time, conditional on the covariates. A careful study of the inferential procedure for estimating parameters in the Cox model reveals that this is actually the observable cause-specific hazard of death in the presence of censoring. That this corresponds to the actual net hazard function of death holds only when we add the assumption of independence of censoring time and failure time.

Consequently, this model may also be applied to competing risks data; that is, we may use the same inferential procedures to estimate the parameter β when considering the model

$$\lambda_i^{C^*}(t|\mathbf{z}) = \lambda_{i0}^{C^*}(t)\exp(\beta^{\mathrm{T}}\mathbf{z}).$$

To apply software for the Cox model, we must define a failure as death from cause i, and an incomplete observation as either death from a cause other than i or censoring. The interpretation of this model and the parameters is the same as discussed above. That is, if we are willing to assume that time to death from cause i is independent of the times to death from other causes and time to censoring, then the observable cause-specific hazard, $\lambda_i^{C^*}(t|\mathbf{z})$, is equal to the net-specific hazard, $\lambda_i^i(t|\mathbf{z})$.

Even if we are unwilling to make this nonidentifiable assumption, the relationship of the observable cause-specific hazard to covariates may be of interest. By assumption, censoring is independent of all other causes of death. This implies that $\lambda_i^C(t|\mathbf{z}) = \lambda_i^{C^*}(t|\mathbf{z})$. Therefore, the results of the Cox regression analysis may be used to estimate the parameters in the model of the cause-specific hazard function, given by

$$\lambda_i^C(t|\mathbf{z}) = \lambda_{i0}^C(t)\exp(\beta^{\mathrm{T}}\mathbf{z}).$$

Using cause-specific hazards thus allows useful interpretation of relevant observable quantities without an additional assumption of independence of the different causes of death.

References

[1] Aalen, O. (1976). Nonparametric inference in connection with multiple decrement models, *Scandinavian Journal of Statistics* **3**, 15–27.

[2] Aalen, O. (1978). Nonparametric estimation of partial transition probabilities in multiple decrement models, *Annals of Statistics* **6**, 534–545.

[3] Aalen, O. (1978). Nonparametric inference for a family of counting processes, *Annals of Statistics* **6**, 701–726.

[4] Andersen, P.K., Borgan, O., Gill, R.D. & Kieding, N. (1982). Linear nonparametric tests for comparison of counting processes, with applications to censored survival data, *International Statistical Review* **50**, 219–258.

[5] Andersen, P.K., Borgan, O., Gill, R.D. & Kieding, N. (1992). *Statistical Models Based on Counting Processes*. Springer-Verlag, New York, pp. 299–301.

[6] Benichou, J. & Gail, M.H. (1990). Estimates of absolute risk in cohort studies, *Biometrics* **46**, 813–826.

[7] Benichou, J. & Gail, M.H. (1995). Methods of interferences for estimates of absolute risk derived from population-based case–control studies, *Biometrics* **51**, 182–194.

[8] Berkson, J. & Elveback, L. (1960). Competing exponential risks with particular reference to the study of smoking and lung cancer, *Journal of the American Statistical Association* **55**, 415–428.

[9] Bernoulli, D. (1760). Essai d'une nouvelle analyse de la mortalité causée par la petite vérole, et des avantages de l'inoculation pour le prévenir. *Historie avec les Mémoires, Académie Royal des Sciences*. Paris, pp. 1–45.

[10] Birnbaum, Z.W. (1979). *On the Mathematics of Competing Risks*. US Department of Health, Education and Welfare, Washington.

[11] Breslow, N. & Crowley, J. (1974). A large sample study of the life table and product limit estimates under random censorship, *Annals of Statistics* **2**, 437–453.

[12] Chiang, C.L. (1968). *Introduction to Stochastic Processes in Biostatistics*. Wiley, New York, Chapter 11.

[13] Cox, D.R. (1959). The analysis of exponentially distributed life-times with two types of failure, *Journal of the Royal Statistical Society, Series B* **21**, 411–421.

[14] Cox, D.R. (1972). Regression models and life tables, *Journal of the Royal Statistical Society, Series B* **34**, 187–220.

[15] David, H.A. & Moeschberger, M.L. (1978). *The Theory of Competing Risks*, Griffin's Statistical Monograph No. 39. Macmillan, New York.

[16] Fleming, T.R. (1978). Nonparametric estimation for nonhomogeneous Markov processes in the problem of competing risks, *Annals of Statistics* **6**, 1057–1070.

[17] Fleming, T.R. (1978). Asymptotic distribution results in competing risks estimation, *Annals of Statistics* **6**, 1071–1079.

[18] Gail, M. (1975). A review and critique of some models used in competing risk analysis, *Biometrics* **31**, 209–222.

[19] Gail, M. (1982). Competing risks, in *Encyclopedia of Statistical Sciences*, Vol. 2, S. Kotz & N.L. Johnson, eds. Wiley, New York, pp. 75–81.

[20] Gray, R.J. (1988). A class of k-sample tests for comparing the cumulative incidence of a competing risk, *Annals of Statistics* **16**, 1141–1154.

[21] Kaplan, E.L. & Meier, P. (1958). Non-parametric estimation from incomplete observations, *Journal of the American Statistical Association* **53**, 457–481.

[22] Karn, M.N. (1931). An inquiry into various death rates and the comparative influence of certain diseases on the duration of life, *Annals of Eugenics* **4**, 279–326.

[23] Klein, J.P. & Moeschberger, M.L. (1988). Bounds on net survival probabilities for dependent competing risks, *Biometrics* **44**, 529–538.

[24] Makeham, W.M. (1874). On the law of mortality, *Journal of the Institute of Actuaries* **18**, 317–322.

[25] Moeschberger, M.L. & David, H.A. (1971). Life tests under competing causes of failure and the theory of competing risks, *Biometrics* **27**, 909–933.

[26] Peterson, A.V. (1976). Bounds for a joint distribution function with fixed subdistribution functions: applications to competing risks, *Proceedings of the National Academy of Sciences* **73**, 11–13.

[27] Prentice, R.L., Kalbfleisch, J.D., Peterson, A.V., Flournoy, N., Farewell, V.T. & Breslow, N.E. (1978). The analysis of failure time data in the presence of competing risks, *Biometrics* **34**, 541–554.

[28] Sampford, M.R. (1952). The estimation of response time distributions. II. Multistimulus distributions, *Biometrics* **8**, 307–353.

[29] Slud, E.V. & Rubinstein, L.V. (1983). Dependent competing risks and summary survival curves, *Biometrika* **70**, 643–650.

[30] Todhunter, J. (1949). *A History of the Mathematical Theory of Probability*. Chelsea, New York.

[31] Tsiatis, A.A. (1975). A nonidentifiability aspect of the problem of competing risks, *Proceedings of the National Academy of Sciences* **72**, 20–22.

[32] Tsiatis, A.A. (1978). An example of nonidentifiability in competing risks, *Scandinavian Actuarial Journal* **1978**, 235–239.

[33] Zheng, M. & Klein, J.P. (1994). A self-consistent estimator of marginal survival functions based on dependent competing risk data and the assumed copula, *Communications in Statistics – Theory and Methods* **23**, 2299–2311.

A.A. Tsiatis

Complete Case Analysis for Missing Data *see* Missing Data in Epidemiologic Studies

Concordance Correlation *see* Agreement, Measurement of

Confidentiality in Epidemiology

Respecting confidentiality is an important prerequisite in clinical and epidemiologic research. The term *confidentiality* is closely related to informational "privacy" and states the principle of the individual wish and right to decide about the disclosure of personal health data [1, 8]. Based on the Declarations of Helsinki (1964 and 1975) from the World Medical Association, it is a basic right of the patient to be assured that all his medical and personal data are confidential. The health professional who has obtained such data has a primary obligation to respect the confidentiality of the data and to safeguard them against any disclosure. Only in the case of a few well-defined exceptions is disclosure allowed, e.g. prevention of serious risk to public health, order by a court of law in a crime case, and, under certain safeguards, health research (including epidemiologic inquiry) [1, 10] (*see* **Epidemiology as Legal Evidence**).

According to Thompson, the concept of confidentiality refers to three principal values, namely "privacy", "confidence", and "secrecy" [8]. Privacy – and in epidemiology we mean in most cases "informational" privacy – deals with the right of individuals to control their own lives, while confidence is an essential requirement of the doctor–patient relationship. Abuse of the trust of confidence the patient places in his doctor would make the practice of medicine impossible. "Secrecy" can be seen as a complementary factor to individual privacy, but from the perspective of the professional dealing with the question of what the patient is allowed to know about his own records.

Ethical principles may affect research and the way we deal with confidentiality in many ways [2, 10, 11]. First, there is the question of the decision to do or not to do a study. Then the legal framework, including guidelines on how to conduct a study, is important. There is a considerable range of types of legislation to protect individual confidentiality in time and among countries. This perspective deals also with the data management and disclosure approaches in balancing the interests of science while respecting confidentiality rules and guidelines [6].

Ethical Principles

Respect for confidentiality of persons involved in clinical and epidemiologic research has its origins in the fulfillment of relevant ethical principles. In general, four ethical principles can be distinguished [2, 6].

1. *Beneficence*. People in general, and the same is true for epidemiologists, have a moral obligation to do "right", i.e. to benefit individuals and society. The results of a research project should add to the existing knowledge base of medicine in order to make patients better, to prevent health hazards, or to decrease mortality.
2. *Nonmaleficence*. This principle reflects a moral obligation not to do harm to the persons involved in a scientific study. Harm can, under certain circumstances, be justified when the population benefits outweigh the individual harm: e.g. a Phase I trial in oncology almost never benefits the patients in the study, but may benefit other patients in the future.
3. *Autonomy*. The principle of autonomy states the moral obligation to respect the right to self-determination. Autonomy is the key principle for respecting confidentiality [1]. The demand for informed consent given by the persons involved in a study reflects the fulfillment of the principle of autonomy.
4. *Justice*. Justice can be considered as the principle of a fair distribution of burdens and benefits between individuals, and between groups in society. This principle may mean equal access to study participation and subsequent benefit (e.g. in acquired immune deficiency syndrome (AIDS) trials), as well as equal exposure when certain outcomes are still uncertain (e.g. postmarketing studies with new drugs).

A useful approach in applying such principles is the assessment of each ethical principle in the context (or scope) of a specific study. Nilstun & Westrin have proposed to apply these principles from the perspective of each of the parties involved and then to assess the ethical "benefits" and "costs" in the event the study is or is not conducted [6]. This process can be illustrated by an example, in deciding whether to do or not a **pharmacoepidemiologic** study on the risk of hip fracture in patients using benzodiazepines [3]. In this example we may identify two relevant parties, i.e. the persons included in the study and society at large. In Table 1 a possible outcome of an analysis of the most relevant "benefits" and "costs" is listed concerning the two dimensions of ethical principles and parties involved in the event that the study is conducted. "Benefits" and "costs" are essentially exchanged if the study is not conducted.

Table 1 The most important possible "benefits" and "costs" when the study is done [3]

	Bene-ficence	Nonmale-ficence	Auto-nomy	Justice
Persons in the study			Costs	
Society at large	Benefit			Benefit

If the study is done, there are possible "benefits" for society at large because the study strengthened a hypothesis based on earlier findings and its results can guide prescribers in rationing the use of these drugs. There could be potential costs with respect for autonomy by violating the privacy of the patients in the study. Data on prescription drug use had to be linked to cases of hospitalizations for hip fracture without knowing the patient's identity. All this was done with existing data and applying a probabilistic approach in relating different datafiles to the same individual using dates of birth, gender, and physician practice [3]. For society at large, potential "benefits" to the principle of justice can be stated. Justice means a fair contribution to the gain of relevant medical knowledge, obviously within the boundaries of economics and other structural conditions. By "participating" in such a study the population involved took its share in the solidarity of bringing together relevant pieces of clinical and epidemiologic insight.

Legal Framework and Guidelines

There is great international variety in legislation and practice guidelines on protecting violation of confidentiality. Several international professional organizations have developed ethical guidelines and recommendations for epidemiologic studies, including those produced by the World Health Organization (WHO), the Industrial Epidemiology Forum (IEF), the International Epidemiological Association (IEA), and the Council of International Organizations of Medical Sciences (CIOMS), and the guidelines of the International Society for Pharmacoepidemiology (ISPE).

Recently, the greatest attention has been paid to the directives of the European Union [4]. There has been ample expression of public and professional concern against these directives, principally because "privacy" is deemed to be violated even in epidemiologic studies where confidentiality is assured, unless the particular purpose is approved by all individuals [5, 7, 9]. The intent of the European directives is to protect individuals from improper administrative use of personal data, including medical data, although no specific details in this direction were given. The definition of "personal data" is crucial here, because it relates to the question of how much effort is needed to identify an individual person within the format of the data. Apart from many other criteria for and conditions about data confidentiality, "express and written informed consent" and "personal data" are the two basic features of European directives that are most critical.

Record linkage is a key methodology in epidemiology and various techniques (e.g. Probabilistic matching and encryption techniques) have been developed to cope with the confidentiality issue [3, 5]. Some privacy advocates, however, continue to argue that written informed consent from all patients would be required to do such linkage studies, even if all the data are processed in a fully anonymous fashion. The creation of unbiased personal histories (including both data on various exposure and outcomes) is a crucial requirement in epidemiology. Record linkage, as was done in the case study on hip fractures, would be virtually impossible if a requirement of full written informed consent were imposed.

Discussion

Protecting confidentiality in the context of scientific inquiry is one of today's paradoxes. The paradox confuses us because it requires us to live simultaneously with opposites. The paradox here is the growing ability and need to apply advanced data systems to investigate health hazards related to various exposures, and on the other hand the increase of legal control over data collection and procedures to use these data for epidemiologic research. Major progress is being made in automated databases and information technology to establish effective strategies in the use of data for epidemiologic research. Linking existing data can be an effective and efficient way to study various exposures and population outcomes. However, society is increasingly concerned about violating the privacy of individuals. Ethical controversies on confidentiality may affect and obstruct epidemiologic research in a significant way [4, 9]. On the other hand, ethical principles may be important to support the conduct

of research and to guide decision making in this respect.

Westrin & Nilstun have compared the aims and tasks of both epidemiologists and journalists in terms of their responsibility towards the protection of confidentiality [11]. Society seems willing to accept that, in the interests of wider public good, journalism may sometimes invade individuals' privacy and do them harm, but it is not prepared to offer epidemiology an equal measure of tolerance. Confusion still surrounds the question of whether confidentiality can be fundamentally violated by data drawn from personal records. Ethical conflicts between moral principles and methodologic standards affecting epidemiologic research will remain. The future lies in thoughtful weighing of the various "costs" and "benefits" in such conflicts.

References

[1]   Beauchamp, T.L. & Childres, J.F. (1989). *Principles of Biomedical Ethics*, 3rd Ed. Oxford University Press, New York.

[2]   Gillon, R. (1994). Medical ethics: four principles plus attention to scope, *British Medical Journal* **309**, 184–188.

[3]   Herings, R.M.C., Stricker, B.H.Ch., Boer, de A., Bakker, A. & Sturmans, F. (1995). Benzodiazepines and the risk of falling leading to femur fractures: dosage more important than elimination half-life, *Archives of Internal Medicine* **155**, 1801–1807.

[4]   Knox, E.G. (1992). Confidential medical records and epidemiological research, *British Medical Journal* **304**, 727–728.

[5]   Newcombe, H.B. (1995). When "privacy" threatens public health, *Canadian Journal of Public Health*, **86**, 188–192.

[6]   Nilstun, T. & Westrin, C.G. (1994). Analyzing ethics, *Health Care Analysis*, **2**, 43–46.

[7]   Olsen, J., Breart, G., Feskens, E., Grabauskas, V., Noah, N., Olsen, J., Porta, M. & Saracci, R. The International Epidemiological Association–IEA European Epidemiological Group (1995). Directive of the European Parliament and of the council on the protection of individuals with regard to the processing of personal data and on the free movement of such data, *International Journal of Epidemiology* **24**, 462–463.

[8]   Thompson, I.E. (1979). The nature of confidentiality, *Journal of Medical Ethics*, **5**, 5.

[9]   Vandenbroucke, J.P. (1992). Privacy, confidentiality and epidemiology: the Dutch ordeal, *International Journal of Epidemiology* **21**, 825–826.

[10] Weed, D.L. (1994). Science, ethics guidelines, and advocacy in epidemiology, *Annals of Epidemiology* **4**, 166–171.

[11]   Westrin, C.G. & Nilstun, T. (1994). The ethics of data utilisation: a comparison between epidemiology and journalism, *British Medical Journal* **308**, 522–523.

HUBERT G. LEUFKENS

Confounder

As used in epidemiology, a confounder is a factor that is associated with the risk of disease in subjects unexposed to the exposure of interest, that is not affected by exposure or disease, and that is associated with exposure in the source population from which cases arise. For example, the risk of cancer increases with age. To study an exposure that is associated with age, such as cumulative coffee consumption, as a risk factor for cancer, one needs to control for the **confounding** effects of age. Because the confounder is associated both with disease risk and with exposure status, failure to account for the confounder either by appropriate choice of study design, such as a restricted design or a stratified design (*see* **Stratification**), or by analytical adjustments (*see* **Standardization Methods**) can lead to misleading estimates of the relationship between the exposure of interest and the risk of disease (*see* **Confounding**; **Matched Analysis**; **Matching**). However, applying such adjustment methods to a factor that is affected by exposure or disease, such as an intermediate effect of exposure on the pathway leading from exposure to disease (*see* **Causation**) can misleadingly reduce estimates of the strength of association between exposure and disease (*see* **Odds Ratio**; **Relative Risk**).

Confounding can be described more fundamentally as a distortion in estimates of **exposure effect** that results when responses from an unexposed **control** population are used to estimate the hypothetical responses that would have been observed in the exposed population had that population been unexposed. In this context, confounders are factors that account for differences between observed control responses and the hypothetical responses in the exposed group that would have been observed had that group been unexposed. A disadvantage of this formulation is that one cannot verify directly that confounding is present, because one does not observe the hypothetical responses of the exposed population had it been unexposed. The criteria for confounding in the previous paragraph, although less fundamental than the definition just given, are at least useful indicators of confounding, although they can be misleading in some situations [1, 2].

References

[1]   Greenland, S. & Robin, J.M. (1986). Identifiability, exchangeability, and epidemiological confounding, *International Journal of Epidemiology* **15**, 413–419.
[2]   Pearl, J. (1995). Causal diagrams for empirical research (with discussion), *Biometrika* **82**, 669–710.

M.H. GAIL

Confounder Summary Score

Consider an analysis of the effect of an "exposure" variable X on an outcome variable Y in which multiple **confounders** must be controlled (*see* **Confounding**). Simultaneous **stratification** on all observed confounder combinations may lead to many uninformative strata (i.e. strata in which there is either no variation in the exposure or no variation in the outcome). The usual method of coping with this problem is to estimate exposure effects from a regression model for the dependence of the outcome on the exposure and confounders.

Parametric modeling raises concerns about the dependence of the resulting effect estimates on the model specification. In one analysis of the National Halothane Study (NHS), the outcome was regressed on confounders, and the data were then stratified on the fitted values from the regression model [2]. In this manner, the problem of multiple confounders was reduced to stratification on just one variable, the fitted outcome $\hat{Y}$. It was later noted that this scoring procedure produces **biased** effect estimates unless the resulting fitted values are modified by removing the estimated exposure effect [3, 4]. To illustrate these ideas, let X denote the treatment or exposure of interest and let $\mathbf{Z}$ denote the row vector of confounders. The NHS procedure involved fitting a model such as

$$g[E(Y|\mathbf{Z} = \mathbf{z})] = \alpha^* + \mathbf{z}\gamma^*,$$

and then stratifying subjects on their fitted values:

$$\hat{Y} = g^{-1}(\hat{\alpha}^* + \mathbf{z}\hat{\gamma}^*).$$

Miettinen instead fit

$$g[E(Y|X = x, \mathbf{Z} = \mathbf{z},)] = \alpha + x\beta + \mathbf{z}\gamma.$$

He then stratified subjects on the modified score $g^{-1}(\hat{\alpha} + \mathbf{z}\hat{\gamma})$ (or, equivalently, on $\hat{\alpha} + \mathbf{z}\hat{\gamma}$), the fitted value obtained by deleting the estimated exposure effect $x\hat{\beta}$. The exposure effect $x\hat{\beta}$ is left out of the scoring to ensure that the strata are not defined in part by exposure. The inclusion of exposure when fitting the model also serves this purpose: note that the confounder coefficient, γ^*, in the model without exposure may carry some of the exposure effects unless X and $\mathbf{Z}$ are independent.

Miettinen termed these modified fitted values or linear predictors *confounder scores*, and called the scoring process *confounder summarization*. Assuming the fitted model was correct, Pike et al. [4] showed that adjustments using these modified scores could lead to unbiased effect estimates, as Miettinen claimed, but could also overstate significance (i.e. yield downwardly biased P values) for testing the null hypothesis of no exposure effect ($\beta = 0$). Pike et al. further showed that the original NHS approach would generally yield biased estimates but could yield valid significance levels for testing the null.

An alternative approach is to control confounding by stratifying on the fitted exposure values obtained by regressing exposure X on the confounders $\mathbf{Z}$. For binary X, Rosenbaum & Rubin [6] termed the resulting fitted values ($\hat{X}$) **propensity scores** and showed that these scores have a number of desirable properties. In particular, Rosenbaum & Rubin showed that, by stratifying on propensity scores, one could obtain valid effect estimates and significance levels from the same model. Scores based on outcome regression are sometimes referred to as *risk scores* or *prognostic scores*. Propensity scores are sometimes referred to as *balancing scores*, reflecting their use in creating strata such that covariate distributions are "balanced" across exposure groups.

Confounder summarization methods have seen relatively little use since their initial development. This disuse may be attributable to a number of factors. One problem is that these methods are not as insensitive to model misspecification as was hoped [1]. As an extreme but transparent example, suppose there is but one confounder, Z, that X given Z has a standard normal distribution, that Z has a standard normal marginal distribution, and that the regression of X on Z is

$$E(X|Z = z) = z^2.$$

If the model fitted for exposure scoring is

$$E(X|Z = z) = \alpha + \beta z,$$

then the ordinary least squares estimate β will have zero expectation and the resulting exposure scores will stratify subjects randomly, with little confounder control achieved by the stratification. Similarly discouraging examples can be constructed for risk scores.

Of course, careful modeling should detect misspecification as gross as just illustrated. Nonetheless, the example points out that confounder summarization may require as much modeling effort as ordinary analysis. Even more effort may be needed if multiple exposures are studied, for then separate propensity scores must be constructed for each exposure. Thus, there may be no convenience and little robustness advantage of confounder summarization over direct model-based estimation. Any robustness advantage may be further diminished when nonparametric regression methods can be used to estimate exposure effects.

The interpretation of strata and estimates constructed from confounder scores can also be difficult. While the confounder distributions may be balanced within strata, the strata will usually contain subjects with a heterogeneous mix of confounder profiles, the comparability of which may not be immediately obvious to a clinical reader. When the exposure effect varies across strata, it may be necessary to return to standard methods to identify the source of the variation.

Exposure regression can be used directly as part of a system of models for control of confounding in effect estimation [5]. This use, however, is distinct from its use in confounder summarization.

References

[1]   Drake, C. (1993). Effects of misspecification of the propensity score on estimators of treatment effect, *Biometrics* **49**, 1231–1236.

[2]   Halpern, J., Moses, L.E. & Bishop, Y.M.M. (1969). Analysis by regression methods, in *The National Halothane Study*, J.P. Bunker, W.H. Forrest & F. Mosteller, eds. National Institute of General Medical Sciences, Bethesda, Chapter IV-5.

[3]   Miettinen, O.S. (1976). Stratification by a multivariate confounder score, *American Journal of Epidemiology* **104**, 609–620.

[4]   Pike, M.C., Anderson, J. & Day, N.E. (1979). Some insights into Miettinen's multivariate confounder score approach to case–control study analysis, *Journal of Epidemiology and Community Health* **33**, 104–106.

[5]   Robins, J.M. & Greenland, S. (1994). Adjusting for differential rates of prophylaxis therapy for PCP in high- versus low-dose AZT treatment arms in an AIDS randomized trial, *Journal of the American Statistical Association* **89**, 737–749.

[6]   Rosenbaum, P.R. & Rubin, D.B. (1983). The central role of the propensity score in observational studies for causal effects, *Biometrika* **70**, 41–55.

SANDER GREENLAND

Confounding

The word *confounding* has been used to refer to at least three distinct concepts. In the oldest usage, confounding is a **bias** in estimating causal effects (*see* **Causation**). This bias is sometimes informally described as a mixing of effects of extraneous factors (called **confounders**) with the effect of interest. This usage predominates in nonexperimental research, especially in epidemiology and sociology. In a second and more recent usage, confounding is a synonym for noncollapsibility (*see* **Collapsibility**), although this usage is often limited to situations in which the parameter of interest is a causal effect. In a third usage, originating in the experimental-design literature, confounding refers to inseparability of main effects and **interactions** under a particular design. The term *aliasing* is also sometimes used to refer to the latter concept; this usage is common in the analysis of variance literature.

The three concepts are closely related and are not always distinguished from one another. In particular,

the concepts of confounding as a bias in effect estimation and as noncollapsibility are often treated as identical, although below we provide an example in which the two concepts diverge.

Confounding as a Bias in Effect Estimation

Confounding

A classic discussion of confounding in which explicit reference is made to "confounded effects" is Mill [14, Chapter X] (although in Chapter III Mill lays out the primary issues and acknowledges Francis Bacon as a forerunner in dealing with them). There, he lists a requirement for an experiment intended to determine causal relations:

> ... none of the circumstances [of the experiment] that we do know shall have effects susceptible of being *confounded with* those of the agents whose properties we wish to study (emphasis added).

It should be noted that, in Mill's time, the word "experiment" referred to an observation in which some circumstances were under the control of the observer, as it still is used in ordinary English, rather than to the notion of a comparative trial. Nonetheless, Mill's requirement suggests that a comparison is to be made between the outcome of his experiment (which is, essentially, an uncontrolled trial) and what we would expect the outcome to be if the agents we wish to study had been absent. If the outcomes is not as one would expect in the absence of the study agents, then his requirement ensures that the unexpected outcome was not brought about by extraneous circumstances. If, however, those circumstances do bring about the unexpected outcome, and that outcome is mistakenly attributed to effects of the study agents, then the mistake is one of confounding (or confusion) of the extraneous effects with the agent effects.

Much of the modern literature follows the same informal conceptualization given by Mill. Terminology is now more specific, with "treatment" used to refer to an agent administered by the investigator and "exposure" often used to denote an unmanipulated agent. The chief development beyond Mill is that the expectation for the outcome in the absence of the study exposure is now almost always explicitly derived from observation of a **control** group that is untreated or unexposed. For example, Clayton & Hills [2] state of **observational studies**,

> ... there is always the possibility that an important influence on the outcome ... differs systematically between the comparison [exposed and unexposed] groups. It is then possible [that] part of the apparent effect of exposure is due to these differences, [in which case] the comparison of the exposure groups is said to be *confounded* (emphasis in the original).

In fact, confounding is also possible in randomized experiments, owing to systematic improprieties in treatment allocation, administration, and compliance. A further and somewhat controversial point is that confounding (as per Mill's original definition) can also occur in perfect randomized trials due to *random* differences between comparison groups [6].

Various mathematical formalizations of confounding have been proposed. Perhaps the one closest to Mill's concept is based on the formal counterfactual model for causal effects. Suppose our objective is to determine the effect of applying a treatment or exposure x_1 on a population parameter μ of population A, relative to applying treatment or exposure x_0. For example, A could be a cohort of breast-cancer patients, treatment x_1 could be a new hormone therapy, x_0 could be a placebo therapy, and the parameter μ could be the 5-year survival probability. The population A is sometimes called the **target population** or *index population*; the treatment x_1 is sometimes called the *index* treatment; and the treatment x_0 is sometimes called the *control* or *reference* treatment (which is often a standard or placebo treatment).

The counterfactual model assumes that μ will equal μ_{A1} if x_1 is applied, μ_{A0} if x_0 is applied; the causal effect of x_1 relative to x_0 is defined as the change from μ_{A0} to μ_{A1}, which might be measured as $\mu_{A1} - \mu_{A0}$ or μ_{A1}/μ_{A0}. If A is observed under treatment x_1, then μ will equal μ_{A1}, which is observable or estimable, but μ_{A0} will be unobservable. Suppose, however, we expect μ_{A0} to equal μ_{B0}, where μ_{B0} is the value of the outcome μ observed or estimated for a population B that was administered treatment x_0. The latter population is sometimes called the *control* or *reference* population. *Confounding* is said to be present if in fact $\mu_{A0} \neq \mu_{B0}$, for then there must be some difference between populations A and B (other than treatment) that is affecting μ.

If confounding is present, a naive (crude) association measure obtained by substituting μ_{B0} for μ_{A0}

in an effect measure will not equal the effect measure, and the association measure is said to be *confounded*. For example, if $\mu_{B0} \neq \mu_{A0}$, then $\mu_{A1} - \mu_{B0}$, which measures the *association* of treatments with outcomes *across* the populations, is confounded for $\mu_{A1} - \mu_{A0}$, which measures the *effect* of treatment x_1 on population A. Thus, saying a measure of association such as $\mu_{A1} - \mu_{B0}$ is confounded for a measure of effect such as $\mu_{A1} - \mu_{A0}$ is synonymous with saying the two measures are not equal.

The preceding formalization of confounding gradually emerged through attempts to separate effect measures into a component due to the effect of interest and a component due to extraneous effects [1, 4, 9, 11, 12]. These decompositions will be discussed below.

One noteworthy aspect of the above formalization is that confounding depends on the outcome parameter. For example, suppose populations A and B have a different 5-year survival probability μ under placebo treatment x_0; that is, suppose $\mu_{B0} \neq \mu_{A0}$, so that $\mu_{A1} - \mu_{B0}$ is confounded for the actual effect $\mu_{A1} - \mu_{A0}$ of treatment on 5-year survival. It is then still possible that 10-year survival, v, under the placebo would be identical in both populations; that is, v_{A0} could still equal v_{B0}, so that $v_{A1} - v_{B0}$ is not confounded for the actual effect of treatment on 10-year survival. (We should generally expect no confounding for 200-year survival, since no treatment is likely to raise the 200-year survival probability of human patients above zero.)

A second noteworthy point is that confounding depends on the target population of inference. The preceding example, with A as the target, had different 5-year survivals μ_{A0} and μ_{B0} for A and B under placebo therapy, and hence $\mu_{A1} - \mu_{B0}$ was confounded for the effect $\mu_{A1} - \mu_{A0}$ of treatment on population A. A lawyer or ethicist may also be interested in what effect the hormone treatment would have had on population B. Writing μ_{B1} for the (unobserved) outcome of B under treatment, this effect on B may be measured by $\mu_{B1} - \mu_{B0}$. Substituting μ_{A1} for the unobserved μ_{B1} yields $\mu_{A1} - \mu_{B0}$. This measure of association is confounded for $\mu_{B1} - \mu_{B0}$ (the effect of treatment x_1 on 5-year survival in population B) if and only if $\mu_{A1} \neq \mu_{B1}$. Thus, the same measure of association, $\mu_{A1} - \mu_{B0}$, may be confounded for the effect of treatment on neither, one, or both of populations A and B.

Confounders

A third noteworthy aspect of the counterfactual formalization of confounding is that it invokes no explicit differences (imbalances) between populations A and B with respect to circumstances or covariates that might influence μ [8]. Clearly, if μ_{A0} and μ_{B0} differ, then A and B must differ with respect to factors that influence μ. This observation has led some authors to define confounding as the presence of such covariate differences between the compared populations. Nonetheless, confounding is only a consequence of these covariate differences. In fact, A and B may differ profoundly with respect to covariates that influence μ, and yet confounding may be absent. In other words, a covariate difference between A and B is a necessary but not sufficient condition for confounding. This point will be illustrated below.

Suppose now that populations A and B differ with respect to certain covariates, and that these differences have led to confounding of an association measure for the effect measure of interest. The responsible covariates are then termed *confounders* of the association measure. In the above example, with $\mu_{A1} - \mu_{B0}$ confounded for the effect $\mu_{A1} - \mu_{A0}$, the factors responsible for the confounding (i.e. the factors that led to $\mu_{A0} \neq \mu_{B0}$) are the confounders. It can be deduced that a variable cannot be a confounder unless it can affect the outcome parameter μ within treatment groups and it is distributed differently among the compared populations (e.g. see Yule [22], who however uses terms such as "fictitious association" rather than confounding). These two necessary conditions are sometimes offered together as a definition of a confounder. Nonetheless, counterexamples show that the two conditions are not sufficient for a variable with more than two levels to be a confounder as defined above; one such counterexample is given in the next section.

Prevention of Confounding

Perhaps the most obvious way to avoid confounding in estimating $\mu_{A1} - \mu_{A0}$ is to obtain a reference population B for which μ_{B0} is known to equal μ_{A0}. Among epidemiologists, such a population is sometimes said to be *comparable to* or *exchangeable with* A with respect to the outcome under the reference treatment. In practice, such a population may be difficult or impossible to find. Thus, an investigator may attempt to construct such a population, or to construct

exchangeable index and reference populations. These constructions may be viewed as *design-based* methods for the control of confounding.

Perhaps no approach is more effective for preventing confounding by a known factor than *restriction*. For example, gender imbalances cannot confound a study restricted to women. However, there are several drawbacks: restriction on enough factors can reduce the number of available subjects to unacceptably low levels, and may greatly reduce the generalizability of results as well. **Matching** the treatment populations on confounders overcomes these drawbacks and, if successful, can be as effective as restriction. For example, gender imbalances cannot confound a study in which the compared groups have identical proportions of women. Unfortunately, differential losses to observation may undo the initial covariate balances produced by matching.

Neither restriction nor matching prevents (although it may diminish) imbalances on unrestricted, unmatched, or unmeasured covariates. In contrast, randomization offers a means of dealing with confounding by covariates not accounted for by the design. It must be emphasized, however, that this solution is only probabilistic and subject to severe constraints in practice. Randomization is not always feasible, and (as mentioned earlier) many practical problems, such as differential loss and noncompliance, can lead to confounding in comparisons of the groups actually receiving treatments x_1 and x_0. One somewhat controversial solution to noncompliance problems is intention-to-treat analysis, which *defines* the comparison groups A and B by treatment assigned rather than treatment received. Confounding may, however, affect even intention-to-treat analyses. For example, the assignments may not always be random, as when blinding is insufficient to prevent the treatment providers from protocol violations. And, purely by bad luck, randomization may itself produce allocations with severe covariate imbalances between the groups (and consequent confounding), especially if the study size is small [6, 18]. Block randomization can help ensure that random imbalances on the blocking factors will not occur, but it does not guarantee balance of unblocked factors.

Adjustment for Confounding

Design-based methods are often infeasible or insufficient to prevent confounding. Thus there has been an enormous amount of work devoted to analytic adjustments for confounding. With a few exceptions, these methods are based on observed covariate distributions in the compared populations. Such methods can successfully control confounding only to the extent that enough confounders are adequately measured. Then, too, many methods employ parametric models at some stage, and their success may thus depend on the faithfulness of the model to reality. These issues cannot be covered in depth here, but a few basic points are worth noting.

The simplest and most widely trusted methods of adjustment begin with **stratification** on confounders. A covariate cannot be responsible for confounding within internally homogeneous strata of the covariate. For example, gender imbalances cannot confound observations within a stratum composed solely of women. More generally, comparisons within strata cannot be confounded by a covariate that is constant (homogeneous) within strata. This is so regardless of whether the covariate was used to define the strata. Generalizing this observation to a regression context, we find that any covariate with a residual variance of zero conditional on the regressors cannot confound regression estimates of effect (assuming that the regression model is correct). A broader and more useful observation is that any covariate that is unassociated with treatment conditional on the regressors cannot confound the effect estimates; this insight leads directly to adjustments using a **propensity score**. Sets of covariates sufficient for control of confounding may be easily characterized using graphical methods [16].

Some controversy has existed about adjustment for covariates in randomized trials. Although Fisher asserted that randomized comparisons were unbiased, he also pointed out that they could be confounded in the sense used here (e.g. see Fisher [6, p. 49]). Fisher's use of the word "unbiased" was unconditional on allocation, and therefore of little guidance for analysis of a given trial. The ancillarity of the allocation naturally leads to conditioning on the observed distribution of any pretreatment covariate that can influence the outcome parameter. Conditional on this distribution, the unadjusted treatment–effect estimate will be biased if the covariate is associated with treatment; this conditional bias can be removed by adjustment for the confounders [8, 17]. Note that the adjusted estimate is also unconditionally unbiased,

and thus is a reasonable alternative to the unadjusted estimate even without conditioning.

Measures of Confounding

The parameter estimated by a direct unadjusted comparison of cohorts A and B is $\mu_{A1} - \mu_{A0}$. A number of authors have measured the bias (confounding) of the unadjusted comparison by [9, 11]

$$(\mu_{A1} - \mu_{B0}) - (\mu_{A1} - \mu_{A0}) = \mu_{A0} - \mu_{B0}.$$

When the outcome parameters, μ, are **risks** (probabilities), epidemiologists use instead the analogous ratio

$$\frac{\mu_{A1}/\mu_{B0}}{\mu_{A1}/\mu_{A0}} = \frac{\mu_{A0}}{\mu_{B0}}$$

as a measure of bias [1, 4, 12, 20]; μ_{A0}/μ_{B0} is sometimes called the *confounding risk ratio*. The latter term is somewhat confusing because it is sometimes misunderstood to refer to the effect of a particular confounder on risk. This is not so, although the ratio does reflect the net effect of the differences in the confounder distributions of A and B.

Residual Confounding

Suppose now that adjustment for confounding is done by subdividing the total study population $(A + B)$ into K strata indexed by k. Let μ_{A1k} be the parameter of interest in stratum k of populations A and B under treatment x_0. The effect of treatment x_1 relative to x_0 in stratum k may be defined as $\mu_{A1k} - \mu_{A0k}$ or μ_{A1k}/μ_{A0k}. The confounding that remains in stratum K is called the *residual confounding* in the stratum, and is measured by $\mu_{A0k} - \mu_{B0k}$ or $\mu_{A1}k/\mu_{B0k}$.

Like effects, stratum-specific residual confounding may be summarized across the strata in a number of ways, for example by **standardization methods** or by other weighted-averaging methods. As an illustration, suppose we are given a standard distribution $p_1, \ldots, p_K$ for the stratum index k. In ratio terms, the standardized effect of x_1 vs. x_0 on A under this distribution is

$$R_{AA} = \frac{\sum\limits_{k} p_k \mu_{A1k}}{\sum\limits_{k} p_k \mu_{A0k}},$$

whereas the standardized ratio comparing A with B is

$$R_{AB} = \frac{\sum_{k} p_k \mu_{A1k}}{\sum_{k} p_k \mu_{B0k}}.$$

The overall residual confounding in R_{AB} is thus

$$\frac{R_{AB}}{R_{AA}} = \frac{\sum_{k} p_k \mu_{A0k}}{\sum_{k} p_k \mu_{B0k}},$$

which may be recognized as the standardized ratio comparing A and B when both are given treatment x_0, using $p_1, \ldots, p_K$ as the standard distribution.

Regression Formulations

For simplicity, the above presentation has focused on comparing two populations and two treatments. The basic concepts extend immediately to the consideration of multiple populations and treatments. Paired comparisons may be represented using the above formalization without modification. Parametric models for these comparisons then provide a connection to more familiar regression models.

As an illustration, suppose population differences and treatment effects follow the model

$$\mu_k(x) = \alpha_k + x\beta,$$

where the treatment level x may range over a continuum, and k indexes populations. Suppose population k is given treatment x_k, even though it could have been given some other treatment. The absolute effect of x_1 vs. x_2 on μ in population 1 is

$$\mu_1(x_1) - \mu_1(x_2) = (x_1 - x_2)\beta.$$

Substitution of $\mu_2(x_2)$, the value of μ in population 2 under treatment x_2, for $\mu_1(x_2)$ yields

$$\mu_1(x_1) - \mu_2(x_2) = \alpha_1 - \alpha_2 + (x_1 - x_2)\beta,$$

which is biased by the amount

$$\mu_1(x_2) - \mu_2(x_2) = \alpha_1 - \alpha_2.$$

Thus, under this model no confounding will occur if the intercepts α_k equal a constant α across populations, so that $\mu_k(x) = \alpha + \beta x$.

When constant intercepts cannot be assumed and nothing else is known about the intercept magnitudes, it may be possible to represent our uncertainty about α_k via the following mixed-effects model:

$$\mu_k(x) = \alpha + x\beta + \varepsilon_k.$$

Here, α_k has been decomposed into $\alpha + \varepsilon_k$, where ε_k has mean zero, and the confounding in $\mu_1(x_1) - \mu_2(x_2)$ has become an unobserved random variable, $\varepsilon_1 - \varepsilon_2$. Correlation of population membership k with x_k leads to a correlation of ε_k with x_k, which in turn leads to bias in estimating β. This bias may be attributed to or interpreted as confounding for β in the regression analysis. Confounders are now covariates that causally "explain" the correlation between ε_k and x_k. In particular, confounders normally reduce the correlation of x_k and ε_k when entered in the model. The converse is false, however: a variable that reduces the correlation of x_k and ε_k when entered need not be a confounder; it may, for example, be a variable affected by both the treatment and the exposure.

Confounding and Noncollapsibility

Much of the statistics literature does not distinguish between the concept of confounding as described above and the concept of noncollapsibility. It is increasingly recognized, however, that the two concepts are distinct: for certain outcome parameters, confounding may occur with or without noncollapsibility and noncollapsibility may occur with or without confounding [8, 13, 21]. Mathematically identical conclusions have been reached by other authors, albeit with different terminology in which noncollapsibility corresponds to bias and confounding corresponds to covariate imbalance [7, 10].

As an example of no **collapsibility** with no confounding, consider the response distributions under treatments x_1 and x_0 given in Table 1 for a hypothetical index population A, and the response distribution under treatment x_0 given in Table 2 for a hypothetical reference population B. If we take the odds of response as the outcome parameter μ, we get

$$\mu_{A1} = 1460/540 = 2.70$$

and

$$\mu_{A0} = \mu_{B0} = 1000/1000 = 1.00.$$

Table 1 Distribution of responses for population A, within strata of Z and ignoring Z, under treatments x_1 and x_0

Subpopulation	Number of responses under		Subpopulation size
	x_1	x_0	
$Z = 1$	200	100	400
$Z = 2$	900	600	1200
$Z = 3$	360	300	400
Totals	1460	1000	2000

Table 2 Distribution of responses for population B, within strata of Z and ignoring Z, under treatment x_0

Subpopulation	Number of responses under x_0	Subpopulation size
$Z = 1$	200	800
$Z = 2$	200	400
$Z = 3$	600	800
Totals	1000	2000

There is thus no confounding of the **odds ratio**: $\mu_{A1}/\mu_{A0} = \mu_{A1}/\mu_{B0} = 2.70/1.00 = 2.70$. Nonetheless, the covariate Z is associated with response and is distributed differently in A and B. Furthermore, the odds ratio is not collapsible: within levels of Z, the odds ratios comparing A under treatment x_1 with either A or B under x_0 are $(200/200)/(200/600) = (900/300)/(200/200) = (360/40)/(600/200) = 3.00$, a bit higher than the odds ratio of 2.70 obtained when Z is ignored.

The preceding example illustrates a peculiar property of the odds ratio as an effect measure: treatment x_1 (relative to x_0) elevates the odds of response by 170% in population A, yet within each stratum of Z it raises the odds by 200%. When Z is associated with response conditional on treatment but unconditionally unassociated with treatment, the stratum-specific effects on odds ratios will be further from the null than the overall effect if the latter is not null [7]. This phenomenon is often interpreted as a "bias" in the overall odds ratio, but in fact there is no bias if one does not interpret the overall effect as an estimate of the stratum-specific effects.

The example also shows that, when μ is the odds, the "confounding odds ratio" $(\mu_{A1}/\mu_{B0})/(\mu_{A1}/\mu_{A0}) = \mu_{A0}/\mu_{B0}$ may be 1 even when the odds ratio is not collapsible over the confounders. Conversely, we may have $\mu_{A0}/\mu_{B0} \neq 1$ even when the odds ratio

is collapsible. More generally, the ratio of crude and stratum-specific odds ratios does not equal μ_{A0}/μ_{B0} except in some special cases. When the odds are low, however, the odds will be close to the corresponding risks, and so the two ratios will approximate one another.

The phenomenon illustrated in the example corresponds to the differences between cluster-specific and population-averaged (marginal) effects in nonlinear mixed-effects regression [15]. Specifically, the clusters of correlated outcomes correspond to the strata, the cluster effects correspond to covariate effects, the cluster-specific treatment effects correspond to the stratum-specific log odds ratios, and the population-averaged treatment effect corresponds to the crude log odds ratio.

Results of Gail [7] imply that if the effect measure is the difference or ratio of response proportions and there is no confounding within levels of Z, then the above phenomenon – noncollapsibility without confounding – cannot occur. More generally, when the effect measure is an expectation over population units and there is no confounding conditional on the covariates at issue, then nonconfounding and collapsibility are algebraically equivalent. This equivalence may explain why the two concepts are often not distinguished.

Confounding in Experimental Design

Like the bias definition, the third usage of confounding stems from the notion of mixing of effects. However, the effects that are mixed are main (block) effects and interactions (or different interactions) in a linear model, rather than effects in the nonparametric sense of a counterfactual model. This definition of confounding differs even more markedly from other definitions in that it refers to an intentional design feature of certain experimental studies, rather than a bias.

The topic of confounded designs is extensive; some classic references are Fisher [6], Cochran & Cox [3], Cox [5], and Scheffé [19]. Confounding can serve to improve efficiency in estimation of certain contrasts and can reduce the number of treatment groups that must be considered. The price paid for these benefits is a loss of identifiability of certain parameters, as reflected by aliasing of those parameters.

As a simple example, consider a situation in which we wish to estimate three effects in a single experiment: that of treatments x_1 vs. x_0, y_1 vs. y_0, and z_1 vs. z_0. For example, in a smoking cessation trial these treatments may represent active and placebo versions of the nicotine patch, nicotine gum, and buspirone. With no restrictions on number or size of groups, a fully crossed design would be reasonable. By allocating subjects to each of the $2^3 = 8$ possible treatment combinations, one could estimate all three main effects, all three two-way interactions, and the three-way interaction of the treatments.

Suppose, however, that we were restricted to use of only four treatment groups (e.g. because of cost or complexity considerations). A naive approach would be to use groups of equal size, assigning one group to placebos only (x_0, y_0, z_0) and the remaining three groups to one active treatment each: (x_1, y_0, z_0), (x_0, y_1, z_0), and (x_0, y_0, z_1). Unfortunately, with a fixed number N of subjects available, this design would provide only $N/4$ subjects under each active treatment.

As an alternative, consider the design with four groups of equal size with treatments (x_0, y_0, z_0), (x_1, y_1, z_0), (x_1, y_0, z_1), and (x_0, y_1, z_1). This fractional factorial design would provide $N/2$ subjects under each active treatment, at the cost of confounding main effects and interactions. For example, no linear combination of group means containing the main effect of x_1 vs. x_0 would be free of interactions. If one could assume that all interactions were negligible, however, this design could provide considerably more precise estimates of the main effects than the naive four-group design.

To see these points, consider the following linear model:

$$\mu_{XYZ} = \alpha + \beta_1 X + \beta_2 Y + \beta_3 Z + \gamma_1 XY$$
$$+ \gamma_2 XZ + \gamma_3 YZ + \delta XYZ,$$

where X, Y, and Z equal 1 for x_1, y_1, and z_1, and 0 for x_0, y_0, and z_0, respectively. The group means are then

$$\mu_{000} = \alpha,$$
$$\mu_{110} = \alpha + \beta_1 + \beta_2 + \gamma_1,$$
$$\mu_{101} = \alpha + \beta_1 + \beta_3 + \gamma_2,$$
$$\mu_{011} = \alpha + \beta_2 + \beta_3 + \gamma_3.$$

Treating the means as observed and the coefficients as unknown, the above system is underidentified. In particular, there is no solution for any main effect β_j in terms of the means μ_{ijk}. Nonetheless, assuming all $\gamma_j = 0 = \delta$ yields immediate solutions for all the β_j. Additionally assuming a variance of σ^2 for each estimated group mean yields that the main-effect estimates under this design would have variances of σ^2, as opposed to $2\sigma^2$ for the main-effect estimates from the naive four-group design of the same size. For example, under the confounded fractional factorial design (assuming no interactions)

$$\hat{\beta}_1 = (\hat{\mu}_{110} + \hat{\mu}_{101} - \hat{\mu}_{000} - \hat{\mu}_{011})/2,$$

so $\text{var}(\hat{\beta}_1) = 4\sigma^2/4 = \sigma^2$, whereas under the naive design, $\hat{\beta} = \hat{\mu}_{100} - \hat{\mu}_{000}$ so $\text{var}(\hat{\beta}_1) = 2\sigma^2$. Of course, the precision advantage of the confounded design is purchased by the assumption of no interaction, which is not needed by the naive design.

References

[1]   Bross, I.D.J. (1967). Pertinency of an extraneous variable, *Journal of Chronic Diseases* **20**, 487–495.

[2]   Clayton, D. & Hills, M. (1993). *Statistical Models in Epidemiology*. Oxford University Press, New York.

[3]   Cochran, W.G. & Cox, G.M. (1957). *Experimental Designs*, 2nd Ed. Wiley, New York.

[4]   Cornfield, J., Haenszel, W., Hammond, W.C., Lilienfeld, A.M., Shimkin, M.B. & Wynder, E.L. (1959). Smoking and lung cancer: recent evidence and a discussion of some questions, *Journal of the National Cancer Institute* **22**, 173–203.

[5]   Cox, D.R. (1958). *The Planning of Experiments*. Wiley, New York.

[6]   Fisher, R.A. (1935). *The Design of Experiments*. Oliver & Boyd, Edinburgh.

[7]   Gail, M.H. (1986). Adjusting for covariates that have the same distribution in exposed and unexposed cohorts, in *Modern Statistical Methods in Chronic Disease Epidemiology*, S.H. Moolgavkar & R.L. Prentice, eds. Wiley, New York.

[8]   Greenland, S. & Robins, J.M. (1986). Identifiability, exchangeability, and epidemiological confounding, *International Journal of Epidemiology* **15**, 413–419.

[9]   Groves, E.R. & Ogburn, W.F. (1928). *American Marriage and Family Relationships*. Henry Holt & Company, New York, pp. 160–164.

[10]   Hauck, W.W., Neuhas, J.M., Kalbfleisch, J.D. & Anderson, S. (1991). A consequence of omitted covariates when estimating odds ratios, *Journal of Clinical Epidemiology* **44**, 77–81.

[11]   Kitagawa, E.M. (1955), Components of a difference between two rates, *Journal of the American Statistical Association* **50**, 1168–1194.

[12]   Miettinen, O.S. (1972). Components of the crude risk ratio, *American Journal of Epidemiology* **96**, 168–172,

[13]   Miettinen, O.S. & Cook, E.F. (1981). Confounding: essence and detection, *American Journal of Epidemiology* **114**, 593–603.

[14]   Mill, J.S. (1843). *A System of Logic, Ratiocinative and Inductive*. Reprinted by Longmans, Green & Company, London, 1956.

[15]   Neuhaus, J.M., Kalbfleisch, J.D. & Hauck, W.W. (1991). A comparison of cluster-specific and population-averaged approaches for analyzing correlated binary data, *International Statistical Review* **59**, 25–35.

[16]   Pearl, J. (1995). Causal diagrams for empirical research, *Biometrika* **82**, 669–710.

[17]   Robins, J.M. & Morgenstern, H. (1987). The mathematical foundations of confounding in epidemiology, *Computers and Mathematics with Applications* **14**, 869–916.

[18]   Rothman K.J. (1977). Epidemiologic methods in clinical trials, *Cancer* **39**, 1771–1775.

[19]   Scheffé, H.A. (1959). *The Analysis of Variance*. Wiley, New York.

[20]   Schlesselman, J.J. (1978). Assessing effect of confounding variables, *American Journal of Epidemiology* **108**, 3–8.

[21]   Wickramaratne, P. & Holford, T. (1987). Confounding in epidemiologic studies: the adequacy of the control groups as a measure of confounding, *Biometrics* **43**, 751–765.

[22]   Yule, G.U. (1903). Notes on the theory of association of attributes in statistics, *Biometrika* **2**, 121–134.

SANDER GREENLAND

Contact Rate in Disease Transmission *see* Communicable Diseases

Contamination in Community Trials *see* Nutritional Epidemiology

Control Drift *see* Nutritional Epidemiology

Control of Confounding, Design-Based *see* Confounding

Controlled Variable Error Model *see* Measurement Error in Epidemiologic Studies

Controls

Controls are subjects against whom a comparison is made in experimental or **observational studies**. In randomized clinical trials, the control group may receive no treatment, a placebo treatment, or the best currently accepted active treatment. This group is used as a basis of comparison against the group that receives the new experimental treatment. Sometimes the study subjects are stratified into risk groups and are allocated into experimental or control groups in such as way as to assure roughly equal numbers of subjects in the experimental and control groups within each stratum. In observational **cohort studies**, a comparison may be drawn with unexposed or less exposed members of the cohort ("internal" controls). If all members of a cohort are exposed, however, as in some studies of occupational risk (*see* **Occupational Epidemiology**), then an external unexposed or only slightly exposed control population, such as the general population of the US, may be taken as a basis of comparison (*see* **Standardization Methods**).

Controls chosen for comparison with cases in **case–control studies** may be selected from the general population (*see* **Case–Control Study, Population-Based**; **Case–Control Study, Prevalent**) or from a selected source, as in **hospital-based case–control studies**. Controls may also be matched to cases on characteristics that may **confound** the association between exposure and disease status (*see* **Matching**).

M.H. GAIL

Cornfield's Inequality

In response to claims that the relationship between smoking and lung cancer could be explained by a genetic or other omitted variable (OV), Cornfield et al. [6] developed an inequality linking the observed risk ratio (*see* **Relative Risk**) to the **prevalence** of the omitted variable in smoking and nonsmoking groups. They wrote:

> If an agent, A, with no causal effect upon the risk of a disease, nevertheless, because of a positive correlation with some other causal agent, B, shows an apparent risk, r, for those exposed to A relative to those not so exposed, then the prevalence of B, among those exposed to A, relative to the prevalence among those not so exposed, must be greater than r. Thus, if cigarette smokers have 9 times the risk of nonsmokers for developing lung cancer, and this is not because cigarette smoke is a causal agent, but only because cigarette smokers produce hormone X, then the proportion of hormone X-producers among cigarette smokers must be at least 9 times greater than among nonsmokers. If the relative prevalence of hormone X-producers is considerably less than ninefold, then hormone X cannot account for the magnitude of the apparent effect.

See [14, p. 40] for a discussion of the origins of the inequality.

Formally, the analysis involves three binary variables: (i) $Z = 1$ for treatment (smoker) and $Z = 0$ for control (nonsmoker), (ii) $D = 1$ for positive response (lung cancer) and $D = 0$ for negative response, (iii) $U = 1$ for presence of the unobserved omitted variable and $U = 0$ for its absence. We observe the joint distribution of Z and D, specifically $\pi = \Pr(Z = 1)$, $p_1 = \Pr(D = 1 | Z = 1)$ and $p_0 = \Pr(D = 1 | Z = 0)$, from which we calculate the observed risk ratio $R_O = p_1/p_0$. Could the observed risk ratio R_O deviate from one solely because of the unobserved variable, U? If this were the case, then D would be independent of Z given U. Hence,

$$p \equiv \Pr(D = 1 | Z = 1, U = 0)$$
$$= \Pr(D = 1 | Z = 0, U = 0)$$
$$= \Pr(D = 1 | U = 0)$$

and

$$PR_U = \Pr(D = 1 | Z = 1, U = 1)$$
$$= \Pr(D = 1 | Z = 0, U = 1)$$
$$= \Pr(D = 1 | U = 1),$$

where

$$R_U = \frac{\Pr(D = 1 | U = 1)}{\Pr(D = 1 | U = 0)}.$$

Here, R_U is the unobserved risk ratio linking the response, D, with the unobserved variable, U. We may assume that the two categories of the variable U, $U = 1$, and $U = 0$, have been labeled so that $R_U \geq 1$. Writing $f_1 = \Pr(U = 1 | Z = 1)$ and $f_0 = \Pr(U = 1 | Z = 0)$ gives

$$R_O = \frac{p_1}{p_0} = \frac{p(1 - f_1) + pR_U f_1}{p(1 - f_0) + pR_U f_0}$$
$$= \frac{f_1 R_U + 1 - f_1}{f_0 R_U + 1 - f_0}. \tag{1}$$

For a fixed $R_U \geq 1$, expression (1) is maximized when $f_1 = 1$ and $f_0 = 0$, leading to the inequality

$$R_O \leq R_U. \tag{2}$$

Similarly, for fixed values of f_0 and f_1, expression (1) is maximized by letting $R_U \to \infty$, yielding the inequality

$$R_O \leq \frac{f_1}{f_0} = \theta, \text{ say.} \tag{3}$$

Eqs. (2) and (3) say that the unobserved risk ratio, R_U, must exceed both the observed risk ratio, R_O, and the unobserved prevalence ratio, θ, if U is to explain away the association between treatment Z and response D. Expressions (2) and (3) are the inequalities of Cornfield et al. [6], and (3) is described in the quotation above.

Gastwirth [9] gave a sharper version of (3) by solving (1) for θ to obtain

$$\theta = R_O + \frac{R_O - 1}{R_U - 1} \frac{1}{f_0}, \tag{4}$$

or, equivalently,

$$f_1 = R_O f_0 + \frac{R_O - 1}{R_U - 1}. \tag{5}$$

We illustrate the result on data from the cohort study [37] of lung cancer in asbestos workers, as described in [9, p. 807]. Over the entire period of the study, the relative risk of exposed workers dying from lung cancer was 6.8 times their expected number, assuming workers had the rate of lung cancer in the general male population. As smoking is another risk factor for lung cancer, we apply Cornfield's inequality to see whether smoking could explain the asbestos–lung cancer association. It is known that blue-collar workers have a greater prevalence of smoking than in the general male population. At the time of the study, 60% of all males smoked, in contrast to about 80% of males in asbestos-related occupations. The prevalence ratio, $\theta = 0.8/0.6 = 1.33$, is much less than $R_O = 6.8$, so Cornfield's inequality implies that smoking cannot explain the entire association between asbestos and lung cancer.

When information about R_U is available, (4) can provide a substantially stronger statement. Suppose that a large study of workers exposed to chemical A found a relative risk of three for lung cancer. While smoking was controlled for in this imagined study, prior substantial exposure to asbestos, U, was not, although the literature indicates that R_U is, at most, 10. The original inequality (3) implies that the prevalence of asbestos exposure (U) in the exposed workers needs to be at least three times its prevalence among workers not exposed to chemical A. From the job histories of the workers one might estimate that the prevalence, f_0, of U among the unexposed group was 0.05, say. Then (5) implies that the prevalence of U among workers exposed to chemical A would need to reach 0.374 in order for the observed association between lung cancer and chemical A to be explained by prior substantial exposure to asbestos. This is much larger than $3 \times 0.05 = 0.15$ implied by the original inequality. Indeed, inequality (3) is obtained from (4) by letting R_U become arbitrarily large.

While Cornfield et al. [6] preferred the relative risk measure for assessing causality, the difference in proportions, or the absolute risk difference, is useful in public health. Write $\Delta_U = \Pr(D = 1|U = 1) - \Pr(D = 1|U = 0)$ for the difference in mortality rates associated with the unobserved variable, and write $\Delta_Z = \Pr(D = 1|Z = 1) - \Pr(D = 1|Z = 0)$ for the difference in mortality associated with the exposure. The corresponding inequality is given in the following lemma.

Lemma. If U is to explain entirely the observed difference Δ_Z, then one must have $(f_1 - f_0)\Delta_U \geq \Delta_Z$, and, in particular, one must have both $\Delta_U \geq \Delta_Z$ and $f_1 - f_0 \geq \Delta_Z$.

Inequalities closely related to Cornfield's inequality have been proposed by Bross [3, 4] and Schlesselmann [36]. Related equalities are discussed by Miettinen [24], Breslow & Day [2, p. 96], and Gail et al. [7], and the equalities might be used to calculate adjusted risk ratios. Gastwirth [10] suggests that the inequalities (2) and (3) be used in conjunction with Koopman's [16] one-sided confidence interval for the risk ratio $\Pr(D = 1|Z = 1)/\Pr(D = 1|Z = 0)$ to account for sampling error. Gastwirth [11] uses the reasoning underlying the inequality of Cornfield et al. [6] to examine the potential effect of **nonresponse** or **missing data**. Gail et al. [8] discuss the effect of failing to adjust for a covariate in a clinical trial.

Cornfield's inequality was the first formal method of sensitivity analysis in **observational studies** or nonrandomized experiments. The inequality may be viewed as asking how the conclusions of an observational study might be altered by departures of various magnitudes from the random assignment of treatments, where the departure is measured by the prevalence ratio, θ. Viewed in this way, sensitivity analysis based on Cornfield's inequality is identical in purpose, similar in spirit, though different in technical detail, to the method of permutational sensitivity analysis proposed later by Rosenbaum [27–31] and Rosenbaum & Krieger, [34]. The latter approach applies not only to binary responses, but also to continuous responses, discrete scores, censored survival times and multivariate outcomes. It permits sensitivity analysis for quantiles, Wilcoxon's [39] rank sum test and signed rank test, the logrank test and Gehan test [13] for survival times, the Hodges–Lehmann [15] point estimates of an additive effect, McNemar test [23], the **Mantel–Haenszel method** [20], and Mantel's extension for discrete scores [19], among others. In one very special case, Cornfield's inequality and Rosenbaum's sensitivity analysis give identical results. Specifically, with a binary response in a **case–control study** that approximates the relative risk by the **odds ratio**, the lower endpoint of the $1 - \alpha$ confidence interval for the relative risk in Cornfield's inequality occurs at the value of the sensitivity parameter yielding an upper bound of α for the significance level for testing no treatment effect; see Rosenbaum [28] for specifics. Other methods of sensitivity analysis are discussed in [1], [5], [26], and [35].

References

[1] Angrist, J.D., Imbens, G.W. & Rubin, D.B. (1996). Identification of causal effects using instrumental variables (with discussion), *Journal of the American Statistical Association* **91**, 444–472.

[2] Breslow, N. & Day, N. (1980). *The Analysis of Case–Control Studies*, Vol. 1: *Statistical Methods in Cancer Research*. International Agency for Research on Cancer of the World Health Organization, Lyon.

[3] Bross, I.D.J. (1966). Spurious effects from an extraneous variable, *Journal of Chronic Diseases* **19**, 637–647.

[4] Bross, I.D.J. (1967). Pertinency of an extraneous variable, *Journal of Chronic Diseases* **20**, 487–495.

[5] Copas, J.B. & Li, H.G. (1997). Inference in nonrandom samples (with discussion), *Journal of the Royal Statistical Society, Series B* **59**, 55–95.

[6] Cornfield, J., Haenszel, W., Hammond, E., Lilienfeld, A., Shimkin, M. & Wynder, E. (1959). Smoking and lung cancer: Recent evidence and a discussion of some questions, *Journal of the National Cancer Institute* **22**, 173–203.

[7] Gail, M., Wacholder, S. & Lubin, J. (1988). Indirect corrections for confounding under multiplicative and additive risk models, *American Journal of Industrial Medicine* **13**, 119–130.

[8] Gail, M., Wieand, S. & Piantadosi, S. (1984). Biased estimates of treatment effect in randomized experiments with nonlinear regressions and missing covariates, *Biometrika* **71**, 431–444.

[9] Gastwirth, J. (1988). *Statistical Reasoning in Law and Public Policy*. Academic Press, New York.

[10] Gastwirth, J. (1992). Method for assessing the sensitivity of statistical comparisons used in Title VII cases to omitted variables, *Jurimetrics* **33**, 19–34.

[11] Gastwirth, J. (1992). Employment discrimination: a statistician's look at analysis of disparate impact claims, *Law and Inequality* **11**, 151–179.

[12] Gastwirth, J.L., Krieger, A.M. & Rosenbaum, P.R. (1998). Dual and simultaneous sensitivity analysis for matched pairs, *Biometrics* **85**(4), 907–920.

[13] Gehan, E. (1965). A generalized Wilcoxon test for comparing arbitrarily singly-censored samples, *Biometrika* **52**, 203–223.

[14] Greenhouse, S. (1982). Jerome Cornfield's contributions to epidemiology, *Biometrics* **28**, Supplement, 33–46.

[15] Hodges, J. & Lehmann, E. (1963). Estimates of location based on rank tests, *Annals of Mathematical Statistics* **34**, 598–611.

[16] Koopman, P.A.R. (1984). Confidence intervals for the ratio of two binomials, *Biometrics* **40**, 513–517.

[17] Lin, D.Y., Psaty, B.M. & Kronmal R.A. (1998). Assessing the sensitivity of regression results to unmeasured confounders in observational studies, *Biometrics* **54**, 948–963.

[18] Manski, C. (1995). *Identification Problems in the Social Sciences*. Harvard University Press, Cambridge, Mass.

[19] Mantel, N. (1963). Chi-square tests with one degree of freedom: extensions of the Mantel–Haenszel procedure, *Journal of the American Statistical Association* **58**, 690–700.

[20] Mantel, N. & Haenszel, W. (1959). Statistical aspects of retrospective studies of disease, *Journal of the National Cancer Institute* **22**, 719–748.

[21] Marcus, S. (1997). Assessing non-constant bias with parallel randomized and nonrandomized clinical trials, *Journal of Clinical Epidemiology* **50**, 823–828.

[22] Marcus, S. (1997). Using omitted variable bias to assess uncertainty in an AIDS education treatment effect, *Journal of Educational and Behavioral Statistics* **22**, 193–201.

[23] McNemar, Q. (1947). Note on the sampling error of the differences between correlated proportions or percentages, *Psychometrika* **12**, 153–157.

[24] Miettinen, O. (1972). Components of the crude risk ratio, *American Journal of Epidemiology* **96**, 168–172.

[25] Pearl, J.C. (1995). Causal diagrams for empirical research (with discussion), *Biometrics* **82**, 669–710.

[26] Rosenbaum, P. (1986). Dropping out of high school in the United States: an observational study, *Journal of Educational Statistics* **11**, 207–224.

[27] Rosenbaum, P.R. (1987). Sensitivity analysis for certain permutation inferences in matched observational studies, *Biometrika* **74**, 13–26.

[28] Rosenbaum, P.R. (1991). Sensitivity analysis for matched case–control studies, *Biometrics* **47**, 87–100.

[29] Rosenbaum, P.R. (1993). Hodges–Lehmann point estimates of treatment effect in observational studies, *Journal of the American Statistical Association* **88**, 1250–1253.

[30] Rosenbaum, P.R. (1995). Quantiles in nonrandom samples and observational studies, *Journal of the American Statistical Association* **90**, 1424–1431.

[31] Rosenbaum, P.R. (1995). *Observational Studies*. Springer-Verlag, New York.

[32] Rosenbaum, P.R. (1997). Signed rank statistics for coherent predictions, *Biometrics* **53**, 556–566.

[33] Rosenbaum, P.R. (1999). Using quantile averages in matched observational studies, *Applied Statistics* **48**, 63–78.

[34] Rosenbaum, P. & Krieger, A. (1990). Sensitivity analysis for two-sample permutation inferences in observational studies, *Journal of the American Statistical Association* **85**, 493–498.

[35] Rosenbaum, P. & Rubin, D. (1983). Assessing sensitivity to an unobserved binary covariate in an observational study with binary outcome, *Journal of the Royal Statistical Society, Series B* **45**, 212–218.

[36] Schlesselmann, J.J. (1978). Assessing the effects of confounding variables, *American Journal of Epidemiology* **108**, 3–8.

[37] Selikoff, I., Hammond, E. & Churg, J. (1964). Asbestos exposure, smoking and neoplasia, *Journal of the American Statistical Association* **188**, 22–26.

[38]   Sobel, M.E. (1990). Effect analysis and causation in linear structural models, *Psychometrika* **55**, 495–515.

[39]   Wilcoxon, F. (1945). Individual comparisons by ranking methods, *Biometrics* **1**, 80–83.

(*See also* **Confounding**)

JOSEPH L. GASTWIRTH, ABBA M. KRIEGER & PAUL R. ROSENBAUM

Corrected Score Measures *see* Measurement Error in Epidemiologic Studies

Correction for Attenuation *see* Measurement Error in Epidemiologic Studies

Correlational Study

A correlational study is an **ecologic study** in which rates of disease in populations are correlated with average exposures or other features of such populations. The populations may be defined by geographic regions of residence, for example. Such correlations are useful for generating etiologic hypotheses, but because individual-level information is not available on exposure, disease outcome, and potential **confounders**, such correlations are subject to the **ecologic fallacy** and may be misleading.

M.H. GAIL

Cox Regression Model

The Cox or **proportional hazards** regression model [21] is used to analyze **survival** or failure time data. It is now perhaps the most widely used statistical model in medical research. Whenever the outcome of a clinical trial is the time to an event, the Cox model is the first method considered by most researchers. The model has also inspired an enormous statistical literature, ranging from the mathematical study of estimating the model parameters, to applied techniques for validating the model assumptions.

This article is divided into sections touching on some of the vast literature that has developed around the model:

1. model definition
2. history
3. using the Cox model–the basics
4. estimators and algorithms
5. asymptotic properties
6. time-dependent explanatory variables
7. model checking
8. alternatives and extensions.

Several books have now been published on survival analysis that devote major sections to the Cox model. The first of these appeared in the early 1980s [50, 23]. Of the more recent books some are mathematically rigorous [29, 6], while others are more applied [20, 60, 53]. The book by Andersen et al. [6] is the most comprehensive.

Model Definition

Cox's essential novelty was to model the hazard function (*see* **Hazard Rate**) rather than the mean or some other measure of location. Let X denote a random failure time and $\mathbf{Z}$ a vector of explanatory variables. The conditional hazard of X given $\mathbf{Z} = \mathbf{z}$ at time t is defined as

$$\lambda(t|\mathbf{z}) = \lim_{\Delta t \downarrow 0} \frac{\Pr(X \le t + \Delta t | X \ge t, \mathbf{z})}{\Delta t}. \quad (1)$$

The hazard function is sometimes called the intensity function or the force of mortality. Roughly, the hazard function is the probability that someone who is alive now will die in the next small unit of time. Cox proposed that the conditional hazard be modeled as the product of an arbitrary baseline hazard $\lambda_0(t)$ and an exponential form that is linear in $\mathbf{z}$:

$$\lambda(t|\mathbf{z}) = \lambda_0(t)\exp(\boldsymbol{\beta}'\mathbf{z}). \quad (2)$$

Here $\boldsymbol{\beta}$ is a vector of regression parameters and the infinite-dimensional parameter $\lambda_0(\cdot)$ is the hazard function for an individual with $\mathbf{Z} = \mathbf{0}$. The model in

(2) forces the hazard ratio between two individuals to be constant over time:

$$\frac{\lambda(t|\mathbf{z}_2)}{\lambda(t|\mathbf{z}_1)} = \exp[\boldsymbol{\beta}'(\mathbf{z}_2 - \mathbf{z}_1)].$$

The exponential form of the relative risk function has become standard and is the most stable computationally, but it is not the only possibility. The more general model,

$$\lambda(t|\mathbf{z}) = \lambda_0(t)r(\boldsymbol{\beta}'\mathbf{z}),$$

for some known function r has also been considered [82, 67].

History

A distinguishing feature of survival data is that it is subject to censoring. Very often one does not observe the survival time for all individuals in a study. One may only know that a certain individual was still alive at some time T^*. If T_i^* is the last time at which individual i is known to be alive, it is called a censoring time – the individual's follow-up was censored at T_i^*. In 1958, Kaplan & Meier [51] studied the product-limit estimator of a survival function based on censored data. The key concept of viewing the data as a process that reveals itself over time can be seen in their paper. Test statistics for censored data were considered a few years later [31, 59], and the Cox model may be viewed as the natural generalization to a regression setting of ideas present in Mantel's writing [59]. At about the same time, Feigl & Zelen [28] considered various exponential regression models. One of their models is equivalent to the Cox model with the baseline hazard constrained to be constant for all time, so that $\lambda(t|\mathbf{z})$ is a function of $\mathbf{z}$ but not t. However, unlike Cox [21], they formulate the model in terms of a parameterization of the mean survival time, even though they use the exponential assumption to predict the entire survival distribution.

Cox's 1972 paper [21] was instantly acclaimed as a breakthrough in the analysis of right censored data, as can been seen from the enthusiastic discussion published together with the article. The model was rapidly adopted by applied statisticians, particularly in clinical trials. Its use became widespread once user-friendly software became readily available. Today, one can hardly open a leading medical or statistical journal without finding at least one reference

to Cox (1972)! It is one of the most widely cited papers in scientific literature.

The original paper introduced a model that was to revolutionize the field, and provided the estimator that is today programmed into many statistical software packages. There were, however, several issues that were to challenge the statistical community. Some of these, such as how to deal with ties (two or more individuals with the same failure time) [63], and the basis for the proposed estimator, were addressed at the Royal Statistical Society meeting. Cox provided justification for the estimator himself by introducing the concept of a partial likelihood [22]. But it was not until later that the estimators were shown to be efficient [27, 11]. Formal proofs of consistency and asymptotic normality took nearly a decade [83, 5]. Another topic of considerable interest to statisticians is the effect of misspecification on the estimates [80], and model interpretation. Various types of misspecification have been considered: explanatory variables measured with error [65]; omission of important explanatory variables [54, 78, 16]; and rare but gross data contamination [9, 72].

Parallel with the theoretical progress was work on model building and model checking. The results were less satisfactory than the elegant theory that developed around counting processes and martingales, but a variety of tools are now available. These included goodness of fit tests, as well as residuals and other diagnostics. Andersen [4] and others have discussed the quality of presentation of Cox regression analyses in the medical literature. Despite their constructive suggestions, the "Methods" sections of many papers are still no more informative than "we used the Cox model".

The basic model, (2), has been generalized in various directions. Even the original paper [21] considered time-dependent covariates, but these still cause a variety of difficulties [3]. A simple generalization is to permit different baseline hazard functions in each of a number of strata (see **Stratification**). The stratified Cox model assumes that, within each stratum, the proportional hazards assumption is justified and that the effect of the variable $\mathbf{Z}$ is the same in all strata:

$$\lambda_j(t|\mathbf{z}) := \lambda(t|\mathbf{z}, \text{ stratum } j) = \lambda_{0j}(t)\exp(\boldsymbol{\beta}'\mathbf{z}). \quad (3)$$

By incorporating constructed variables, that are equal to an explanatory variable in some strata and constant in others, the stratified model, (3), can be used to model interactions between explanatory variables and strata. Suppose, for example, that one is stratifying by sex and including age as an explanatory variable. Let $z_1 = (\text{age} - 50)$ for men, $= 0$ for women; and let $z_2 = (\text{age} - 50)$ for women, $= 0$ for men. Then a model stratified on sex that includes z_1, z_2, and a treatment indicator z_3 permits interactions between age and sex, but assumes that the treatment acts proportionally on the hazards for any age–sex combination.

Many models used for analysis of multivariate survival data are generalizations of the Cox model, but they are not discussed here.

Using the Cox Model – the Basics

Before using the Cox model, or even attempting to interpret a published analysis, one must have some understanding of the assumptions that underlie the analysis. This section discusses those assumptions and explains a typical output from fitting the model in a statistical package.

There are three components to the data on each individual: the possibly censored failure time T; an indicator δ equal to 1 if T is a true failure time, 0 if it is censored; and $\mathbf{Z}$, the vector of explanatory variables. The model is flexible enough to incorporate explanatory variables that change value over the course of the study, but in this section we assume that $\mathbf{Z}$ is fixed and measured at time $t = 0$. The key censoring assumption is that conditional on $\mathbf{Z}$, the observation $(T = t, \delta = 0)$ tells us nothing more than that the true failure time X is greater than t.

In a clinical trial, the time origin for each individual will usually be his or her time of entry into the trial. If the trial ends at a particular calendar time, censoring all individuals who are not yet dead, then the censoring times are the times from entry until the

end of the trial and will vary from one individual to another. This is called administrative (or progressive type I) censoring. In such situations, it is necessary for survival to be independent of entry time for the above condition to be satisfied. To some extent this can be examined by including entry time as a covariate or by stratifying on the date of entry. Other forms of censoring are more problematic. If, for instance, a patient emigrates, one needs to consider whether this implies that the patient had in fact recovered. Conversely, a patient who fails to attend a follow-up clinic might be too sick to get out of bed. In such cases, the fact that the patient was censored at t tells us rather more than that she was alive at t.

The Cox model itself makes three assumptions: first, that the ratio of the hazards of two individuals is the same at all times; secondly, that the explanatory variables act multiplicatively on the hazard; and thirdly, that, conditionally on $\mathbf{Z}_i$ and $\mathbf{Z}_j$, the failure times of individuals i and j are independent. As with all regression models, one also assumes that the explanatory variables have been transformed so that they may be entered without further transformation and that all interactions have been included explicitly. We will see in the section on asymptotics that the independence assumption can be relaxed.

Table 1 presents the results of fitting a Cox model to data from 216 patients with primary biliary cirrhosis in a clinical trial of azathioprine vs. placebo [18]. The six variables were selected from an initial set of 25 partly using forward stepwise selection. An additional 32 patients were excluded because they had missing values of one or more of the six variables. Recruitment was over 6 years and follow-up a further 6 years. Of the 216 patients, 113 had censored survival times. The regression coefficients may be combined with their standard errors to obtain confidence intervals that rely on the asymptotic normality of the estimates.

Table 1 Cox model fitted to data from a clinical trial comparing the effects of azathioprine and placebo on the survival of 216 patients with primary biliary cirrhosis [18]. The six variables shown were selected, partly by a forward stepwise procedure, from 25 candidate variables

Variable	Coding	Coeff. $\hat{\beta}$	se($\hat{\beta}$)	exp($\hat{\beta}$)
Serum bilirubin	$\log_{10}$ (value in μmol/l)	2.51	0.316	12.3
Age	$\exp[(\text{age in years} - 20)/10]$	0.0069	0.0016	1.0
Cirrhosis	$0 = \text{No}; 1 = \text{Yes}$	0.88	0.216	2.4
Serum albumin	value in g/l	-0.0504	0.018	0.95
Central cholestasis	$0 = \text{No}; 1 = \text{Yes}$	0.68	0.275	2.0
Therapy	$0 = \text{azathioprine}; 1 = \text{placebo}$	0.52	0.201	1.7

The positive coefficient associated with treatment implies that patients on the placebo ($Z = 1$) had poorer prognosis than those on azathioprine ($Z = 0$): the hazard of those on placebo is about 1.7 times greater than that of those on active treatment. Similarly, older patients had poorer prognosis. The hazard ratio associated with two patients aged 50 and 30 is $\exp[0.0069(\exp 3 - \exp 1)] = 1.13$. Notice, however, that the effect on survival is not fully described by the information in Table 1 because, without estimating the baseline hazard, one cannot translate the regression coefficients into effects on 5-years survival nor on median survival.

Most statistical software for Cox regression will also estimate the cumulative baseline hazard function

$$\Lambda_0(t) = \int_0^t \lambda_0(u)\mathrm{d}u \qquad (4)$$

and from this one can calculate the estimated survival function for a given $\mathbf{z}$:

$$\Pr(X > t|\mathbf{z}) = \prod_{\{i:T_i \leq t\}} [1 - \mathrm{d}\hat{\Lambda}_0(T_i)\exp(\boldsymbol{\beta}'\mathbf{z})].$$

Plots of the estimated survival function can be made for various $\mathbf{z}$s, and these can be viewed like Kaplan–Meier graphs. Alternatively, the estimated survival function can be used to estimate 5-year survival, say, as a function of the prognostic index $\boldsymbol{\beta}'\mathbf{z}$.

Estimators and Algorithms

The regression coefficients $\boldsymbol{\beta}$ are estimated by maximizing the so-called partial likelihood $L(\boldsymbol{\beta})$ [22]. An individual is said to be at risk at t if he has not yet failed nor been censored. This concept can be generalized to allow for individuals who do not enter the study at time 0. Such delayed entry, or left truncation, as it is called, often arises when t is the age of a patient or the time from infection, so that patients enter the study at some time $T_i^0 > 0$. Consider $L_i(\boldsymbol{\beta})$, the conditional probability that individual i fails at time T_i given that exactly one individual fails at T_i and knowing the values of $\mathbf{Z}$ for all individuals at risk at T_i:

$$L_i(\boldsymbol{\beta}) = \frac{\lambda(T_i|\mathbf{Z}_i)}{\sum_{j \in R_i}\lambda(T_i|\mathbf{Z}_j)} = \frac{\exp(\boldsymbol{\beta}'\mathbf{Z}_i)}{\sum_{j \in R_i}\exp(\boldsymbol{\beta}'\mathbf{Z}_j)}, \qquad (5)$$

where $R_i = \{j : T_j^0 < T_i \leq T_j\}$ is the risk set just prior to T_i. The partial likelihood is the product of these conditional probabilities over all failure times: $L(\boldsymbol{\beta}) = \prod_i L_i(\boldsymbol{\beta})$. Notice that the partial likelihood is a function of $\boldsymbol{\beta}$ only – it does not depend on the baseline hazard $\lambda_0(\cdot)$. With certain types of censoring (or no censoring) the partial likelihood is just the marginal likelihood of the ranks of the failure times. If there are ties in the data (two or more individuals failing at the same time), then both the partial likelihood and the marginal likelihood become difficult computationally [50, pp. 74–78]. Instead, most packages use an approximation [63, 13]:

$$L_i(\boldsymbol{\beta}) = \frac{\exp(\boldsymbol{\beta}'\mathbf{S}_i)}{\left[\sum_{j \in R_i}\exp(\boldsymbol{\beta}'\mathbf{Z}_j)\right]^{d_i}}, \qquad (6)$$

where d_i is the number of individuals failing at T_i and $\mathbf{S}_i$ is the sum of the $\mathbf{Z}_j$ for these d_i individuals. The approximation is reasonable provided the number of ties at any failure time is small compared to the number in the risk set. Note that i indexes the N distinct failure times, whereas j indexes the n individuals ($n \geq N$).

It is standard practice to maximize the partial likelihood using Newton–Raphson to find a $\boldsymbol{\beta}$ at which the derivative of its logarithm is zero. Indeed, Jacobsen [47] has shown that, when the relative risk function $r(\boldsymbol{\beta}'\mathbf{z}) = \exp(\boldsymbol{\beta}'\mathbf{z})$, $l(\boldsymbol{\beta}) = \log L(\boldsymbol{\beta})$ is concave. (It is strictly concave provided there is no exact collinearity among the explanatory variables and that no linear combination of the variables is a perfect predictor of failure. The latter would imply an infinite observed hazard ratio.)

We use the following notation: let

$$\mathbf{S}^{(k)}(\boldsymbol{\beta}, T_i) = \sum_{j \in R_i} \mathbf{Z}^{\otimes k} \exp(\boldsymbol{\beta}'\mathbf{Z}_j),$$

where $\mathbf{Z}^{\otimes 0} = 1$, $\mathbf{Z}^{\otimes 1} = \mathbf{Z}$, and $\mathbf{Z}^{\otimes 2} = \mathbf{Z}\mathbf{Z}'$. Let $\mathbf{U}(\boldsymbol{\beta})$ denote the score

$$\mathbf{U}(\boldsymbol{\beta}) = \sum_i \frac{\mathrm{d}\log L_i(\boldsymbol{\beta})}{\mathrm{d}\boldsymbol{\beta}}$$

$$= \sum_i \left[\mathbf{S}_i - d_i\frac{\mathbf{S}^{(1)}(\boldsymbol{\beta}, T_i)}{\mathbf{S}^{(0)}(\boldsymbol{\beta}, T_i)}\right], \qquad (7)$$

and $\mathbf{I}(\boldsymbol{\beta})$ minus the Hessian:

$$\mathbf{I}(\boldsymbol{\beta}) = -\frac{\mathrm{d}U(\boldsymbol{\beta})}{\mathrm{d}\boldsymbol{\beta}} = \sum_i d_i$$

$$\times \left\{ \frac{\mathbf{S}^{(2)}(\boldsymbol{\beta}, T_i)}{\mathbf{S}^{(0)}(\boldsymbol{\beta}, T_i)} - \left[\frac{\mathbf{S}^{(1)}(\boldsymbol{\beta}, T_i)}{\mathbf{S}^{(0)}(\boldsymbol{\beta}, T_i)} \right]^{\otimes 2} \right\}. \quad (8)$$

Given an estimate $\boldsymbol{\beta}^{(m)}$, one step of the algorithm gives

$$\boldsymbol{\beta}^{(m+1)} = \boldsymbol{\beta}^{(m)} + \mathbf{I}(\boldsymbol{\beta}^{(m)})^{-1} U(\boldsymbol{\beta}^{(m)}).$$

The algorithm is generally started from $\boldsymbol{\beta}^{(0)} = \mathbf{0}$ and convergence is determined by the magnitude of $|\boldsymbol{\beta}^{(m+1)} - \boldsymbol{\beta}^{(m)}|$.

When there are S strata, one considers those at risk in each stratum separately. Let R_{si} denote the set of indices of individuals in stratum s at risk at time T_i, and let $L_{si}(\boldsymbol{\beta})$ be the partial likelihood contribution from stratum s and time T_i. Note that $\mathbf{S}_{si}$ is the sum of the $\mathbf{Z}_j$ of the d_{si} individuals in stratum s who fail at time T_i. The partial likelihood is then simply the product of the stratum specific partial likelihoods:

$$L(\boldsymbol{\beta}) = \prod_{s=1}^{S} \prod_i L_{si}(\boldsymbol{\beta}).$$

Although the partial likelihood is not in general a likelihood, it is usually treated as such. It is standard practice to report the value of the logarithm of the partial likelihood and to compare the partial likelihood ratio statistic to a chi-square distribution for testing between nested regression models. Similarly, the covariance of $\hat{\boldsymbol{\beta}}$ is estimated by $\mathbf{I}(\hat{\boldsymbol{\beta}})^{-1}$ and score tests are based on $\mathbf{U}(\mathbf{0})'\mathbf{I}(\mathbf{0})^{-1}\mathbf{U}(\mathbf{0})$. Indeed, in the absence of ties ($d_{si} = 1$ for all s and i), the score test from the Cox model with $K - 1$ dummy variables corresponding to a factor with K levels is identical to the K-sample log rank test. Further, the stratified log rank test is identical to the score test from the stratified Cox model.

Having computed $\hat{\boldsymbol{\beta}}$, the estimated regression coefficients, one can calculate the Breslow estimate of the cumulative baseline hazard [13] explicitly. The estimator for stratum s is

$$\hat{\Lambda}_{s0}(t) = \sum_{i:T_i \leq t} \frac{d_{si}}{\sum_{j \in R_{si}} \exp(\hat{\boldsymbol{\beta}}' \mathbf{Z}_j)}. \quad (9)$$

Estimation of the hazard function itself can be done by taking a smooth derivative of the cumulative hazard. This is usually achieved by the kernel method [68]. The jumps in the Breslow estimate should not be used without smoothing. The jump at T_i crudely approximates $\lambda_0(T_i)(T_i - T_{i-1})$ not $\lambda_0(T_i)$. Breslow [13] also showed that the maximum partial likelihood estimate of $\boldsymbol{\beta}$ and the estimated cumulative baseline hazard, (5), can also be obtained by maximizing the full likelihood for $\boldsymbol{\beta}$ and Λ_0 simultaneously, assuming that Λ_0 is piecewise linear spline, i.e. the hazard $\lambda_0(t)$ is constant between each pair of ordered failure times. This heuristic argument was made precise by Johansen [48]. He showed that, in certain circumstances, the partial likelihood is formally the profile likelihood for $\boldsymbol{\beta}$. He permitted Λ_0 to be a step function and assumed that at the jumps $\mathrm{d}\Lambda(t|\mathbf{z}) = \exp(\boldsymbol{\beta}'\mathbf{z})\mathrm{d}\Lambda_0(t)$.

During the 1970s anyone wishing to fit a Cox model had to use a stand-alone computer program such as the FORTRAN code provided in the book by Kalbfleisch & Prentice [50]. Today, however, the situation is very different and there are many commercially available general statistical packages that will fit a Cox model to large data sets (*see* **Software, Biostatistical**).

Asymptotic Properties

The large sample properties of the maximum partial likelihood estimator of $\boldsymbol{\beta}$ and of the Breslow estimator of Λ_0 are unsurprising, but proofs of these results took some time. When the Cox model holds with parameters $\boldsymbol{\beta}_0$ (and Λ_0), the distribution of $\hat{\boldsymbol{\beta}}$ can be approximated by multivariate normal with mean $\boldsymbol{\beta}_0$ and a covariance matrix that can be estimated by $\mathbf{I}^{-1}(\hat{\boldsymbol{\beta}})$.

Two quite different approaches were successful. The first due to Tsiatis [83] was to consider independent and identically distributed triples $(X_i, \mathbf{Z}_i, C_i)$, where X_i is the failure time and C_i is the censoring time. It is assumed that the X_i are generated from a Cox model with covariates $\mathbf{Z}_i$ and that X_i are conditionally independent of C_i given $\mathbf{Z}_i$. The observed data are $(T_i, \mathbf{Z}_i, D_i)$, $i = 1, \ldots, n$, where $T_i = \min(X_i, C_i)$ and $D_i = 1$ if $T_i = X_i$ (the event is observed), and $D_i = 0$ otherwise (the event is censored). The estimators are functionals of the observed data, and classical large sample theory is applied.

Under this model it can be shown that

$$\frac{\mathbf{S}^{(1)}(\hat{\boldsymbol{\beta}}, t)}{\mathbf{S}^{(0)}(\hat{\boldsymbol{\beta}}, t)} \to \mathbf{E}(\mathbf{Z}|T = t, D = 1)$$

and that $\mathbf{I}(\hat{\boldsymbol{\beta}})/n \to \mathbf{E}[D \operatorname{var}(\mathbf{Z}|T, D)]$ [70]. By viewing the estimators as functionals of the empirical distribution of the unobserved triples and using results from the theory of empirical processes, it is possible to study the large sample properties of the Cox estimators even when the data come from some other model [72].

The other approach to large sample theory using a martingale central limit theory requires reformulating the model. This approach adds much insight to the model and will be outlined here. The counting process view of survival analysis is due to Aalen [1]. Andersen & Gill [5] redefined the Cox model and provided elegant proofs of its large-sample properties under mild regularity conditions.

Counting Process Formulation

A multivariate counting process

$$N = \{N_i(t) : 0 \le t < \infty; i = 1, \dots, n\}$$

is a nondecreasing integer-valued stochastic process with n components. It is assumed that $N_i(0) = 0$ for all i and that the jumps are all of size $+1$. The process may count the number of events that have occurred in each of n individuals by time t. If the event is the death of a person, then $N_i(t) \in \{0, 1\}$ since people only die once! For technical reasons, N_i is taken to be right continuous (so that $N_i(t)$ represents the number of events in $[0, t]$) and no two components of N jump at the same time.

Associated with such a counting process is a cumulative intensity process A with components defined by

$$A_i(t + dt) - A_i(t)$$
$$= \Pr\{N_i(t + dt) - N_i(t) = 1 | \mathcal{F}_{t-}\},$$

where $\mathcal{F}_{t-}$ represents everything that has happened until just before t. The history $\mathcal{F}_{t-}$ will certainly include the paths of $N_j(\cdot)$ on $[0, t), j = 1, \dots, n$, and may include other information such as censoring or explanatory variables from $[0, t)$. $M = N - A$ is a multivariate martingale with respect to the history (filtration) $\{\mathcal{F}_t : t \ge 0\}$. The Andersen & Gill [7]

generalization of the Cox model is that

$$A_i(t + dt) - A_i(t) = \alpha_i(t)dt = Y_i(t)\lambda_0(t)$$
$$\times \exp[\boldsymbol{\beta}_0' \mathbf{Z}_i(t)]dt,$$

where $Y_i(t)$ is equal to 1 if individual i is under observation just before time t, and is equal to 0 otherwise. $Y_i(\cdot)$ is called the ith "at-risk" indicator process. Here we are assuming that the process A is absolutely continuous with derivative α. Note that we have written the explanatory variables as processes depending on t, and that the definition of the intensity process requires $\{\mathbf{Z}_i(u) : 0 \le u \le t, i = 1, \dots, n\}$ to be in the history $\mathcal{F}_{t-}$. This means that the value of $\mathbf{Z}(t)$ should be known just before t.

The classical Cox model corresponds to a very simple counting process, each component of which jumps at most once. We have

$$N_i(t) = I\{T_i \le t, T_i \le C_i\}$$

and

$$Y_i(t) = I\{X_i \ge t, C_i \ge t\} = I\{T_i \ge t\}.$$

N_i starts at 0 and jumps to one when individual i is observed to die. If individual i is censored, N_i remains 0 for ever. Recall that $\alpha_i(t)dt$ is the probability of N_i jumping in the interval $[t, t + dt]$. If individual i has died or been censored before time t, then there is no chance of observing a death in the interval $[t, t + dt]$, so $\alpha_i(t) = 0$. Otherwise $\alpha_i(t) = \lambda(t|\mathbf{Z}_i)$ by the definition of the hazard function. Hence in general $\alpha_i(t) = Y_i(t)\lambda(t|\mathbf{Z}_i)$.

Using the new notation, we define the log partial likelihood using information up to time u as

$$l(\boldsymbol{\beta}, u) = \int_0^u \sum_{i=1}^n \left(\boldsymbol{\beta}' \mathbf{Z}_i(t) dN_i(t) \right.$$

$$\left. - \log \left\{ \sum_{j=1}^n Y_j(t) \exp[\boldsymbol{\beta}' \mathbf{Z}_j(t)] \right\} dN_i(t) \right).$$

Note that $dN_i(t)$ is equal to either 0 or 1, because N_i is a counting process. Thus integration with respect to $dN_i(t)$ is simple: in the classical Cox model $\int f(t)dN_i(t) = D_i f(T_i)$. Differentiate l with respect to $\boldsymbol{\beta}$ to get the score process

$$\mathbf{U}(\boldsymbol{\beta}, u) = \int_0^u \sum_{i=1}^n [\mathbf{Z}_i(t) - \mathbf{E}(\boldsymbol{\beta}, t)]dN_i(t),$$

where

$$\mathbf{E}(\boldsymbol{\beta}, t) = \frac{\sum_{j=1}^{n} Y_j(t) \mathbf{Z}_j(t) \exp[\boldsymbol{\beta}' \mathbf{Z}_j(t)]}{\sum_{j=1}^{n} Y_j(t) \exp[\boldsymbol{\beta}' \mathbf{Z}_j(t)]}. \tag{10}$$

It is easy to show that at the true $\boldsymbol{\beta}$, integration of this integrand with respect to the intensity process is identically zero (for all u). Hence, at $\boldsymbol{\beta}_0$, one may replace $dN_i(t)$ by $dM_i(t)$:

$$\mathbf{U}(\boldsymbol{\beta}_0, t) = \int_0^u \sum_{i=1}^{n} [\mathbf{Z}_i(t) - \mathbf{E}(\boldsymbol{\beta}_0, t)] dM_i(t).$$

It follows from the theory of martingale transforms that $\mathbf{U}(\boldsymbol{\beta}_0, \cdot)$ is a martingale since the integrand $[\mathbf{Z}_i(t) - \mathbf{E}(\boldsymbol{\beta}_0, t)]$ is predictable (i.e. its value is known just prior to t). Under mild regularity conditions [5] one can apply a martingale central limit theorem to show that $n^{-1/2} \mathbf{U}(\boldsymbol{\beta}_0, \cdot)$ converges in distribution to a Gaussian process.

Extending the counting process notation in the obvious way to permit strata, so that, for instance, $Y_{si}(u)$ indicates whether individual i is at risk in stratum s at time u, the Breslow estimator is

$$\hat{\Lambda}_{s0}(t) = \int_0^t \frac{\sum_{i=1}^{n} dN_{si}(u)}{\sum_{i=1}^{n} Y_{si}(u) \exp[\hat{\boldsymbol{\beta}}' \mathbf{Z}_i(u)]}$$

$$= \int_0^t \sum_{i=1}^{n} dN_{si}(u) / S_s^{(0)}(\hat{\boldsymbol{\beta}}, u)$$

Let $J_s(t) = I\{\sum_{i=1}^{n} Y_{si}(t)\} > 0$. Then

$$\int_0^t J_s(u) d[\hat{\Lambda}_{s0}(u) - \Lambda_{s0}(u)] = \int_0^t \frac{J_s(u)}{S_s^{(0)}(\hat{\boldsymbol{\beta}}, u)}$$

$$\times \sum_{i=1}^{n} \{dN_{si}(u) - Y_{si}(u) \exp[\boldsymbol{\beta}_0' \mathbf{Z}_i(u)] d\Lambda_{s0}(u)\}$$

$$= \int_0^t \frac{J_s(u)}{S_s^{(0)}(\hat{\boldsymbol{\beta}}, u)} \sum_{i=1}^{n} dM_{si}(u).$$

Thus, once again, the asymptotics can be proved using a martingale central limit theorem.

Time-Dependent Explanatory Variables

The possibility of including explanatory variables that change with time was realized by Cox in his original article [21]. There it is suggested that the inclusion of a user-defined variable $Z_2(t) = tZ_1$ might be used as a test of the proportional hazards assumption. Other authors have included explanatory variables that change value at possibly random times. The classical example of this sort of covariate is one that indicates whether a patient has received a heart transplant before time t [25]. The uses and interpretations of these two types of time-dependent variables are quite different. In this section they will be discussed relying heavily on the ideas presented by Kalbfleisch & Prentice [50].

External or Ancillary Variables

An external variable is one that is not affected by the failure process. The simplest sort of external variable is a fixed or time-independent one. A second type is a defined variable such as $Z_2(t) = tZ_1$. Although Z_2 is not fixed, its entire path is known from the outset. A more general example of an external variable is a measure of air pollution as a predictor of severe asthma attacks. Although the level of air pollution is not known in advance, it is "external" to the individuals in the study. Furthermore, the marginal distribution of the variable does not involve the parameters of the failure time model. The whole history of an external variable can be included in $\mathcal{F}_0$ and the hazard or intensity process can be related to the survival function $\Pr(T \geq t | \mathcal{F}_0)$ in the usual way.

Internal Variables

An internal explanatory variable is the output of a stochastic process that is generated by the individual under study and so is observed only so long as the individual survives and is uncensored [50]. An example might be the level of β-2 microglobulin in a patient's sera. In practice, the actual level at any given time will be unknown. Instead one uses the level as measured in the most recent blood sample. Typically blood will be taken at most a dozen times during a trial. In such circumstances, the term "updated" may be preferred to "time-dependent".

The key point is that although one may include the history of an internal process up to time t in the filtration $\mathcal{F}_t$ and so define the hazard or intensity function, the intensity function is itself a random process and is not simply a function of the survival function. In general survival from u to t depends on $\{Z(s) : u \leq s \leq t\}$ and this is unknown at u. Furthermore, if Z is only observed when an individual is alive, then $\Pr(T \geq t | Z(t)$ is not missing$) = 1$. Thus it is not possible to make predictions of survival from models that include internal explanatory variables. To do that one must jointly model the survival process and the explanatory variable trajectory.

In a clinical trial with primary focus on a treatment which is fixed by randomization at time 0, internal variables may change in response to treatment. If the effect of treatment is predominantly reflected in the changing value of the explanatory variable, a Cox model of survival that includes both treatment and the updated measurements of the explanatory variable will show little or no treatment differences. Clearly, then, one must be very careful when interpreting the output of a Cox model that includes an internal explanatory variable. Treatment differences in a model that includes the values of explanatory variables only at time 0 may be inferred to be causative (because of randomization). When a large treatment difference is attenuated by inclusion of updated measurements of an internal variable, one may gain useful insights into the mechanism through which the treatment is effective. In such circumstances, it is sensible to also explore the effect of treatment on the internal variable directly.

As with censoring, the value of a variable may depend on the history of the trial so far, without depending on the history of a given individual. Thus, for instance, one might decide to change the environment of a controlled experiment after every 15 deaths. Such a variable is neither internal nor external, but for the purpose of making inference it is closer to an external process.

Computing with Time-Dependent Variables

There are many practical issues in fitting models using time-varying regressors, such as how to deal with missing values, that are not discussed here [3].

The Cox model does not distinguish between a single individual who enters a trial at time 0 and dies at time T_i with fixed regressors $\mathbf{Z}_i$, from two individuals both with regressors $\mathbf{Z}_i$ one of whom enters at time 0 and is censored at time u and one of whom enters at u and dies at T_i. This may sound surprising, but it is true; the likelihood contributions from $[0, u]$ and $(u, T_i]$ are $\Pr(X > u | \mathbf{Z}_i)$, and

$$\Pr(T_i \leq X < T_i + dt | X > u, \mathbf{Z}_i)/dt$$
$$= \frac{\Pr(T_i \leq X < T_i + dt | \mathbf{Z}_i)/dt}{\Pr(X > u | \mathbf{Z}_i)},$$

respectively. Furthermore, in the partial likelihood, all that matters is the $\mathbf{Z}$ values of the members of the risk set at each failure time, not whether a given individual happens to appear in several different risk sets. Thus, if $\mathbf{Z}(t)$ is only updated at a few times per person, it is simplest to treat each person as several "individuals" each with a time fixed covariate. Let the vector $(T_0, T, D, \mathbf{Z})$ denote the entry and exit times, the censoring indicator, and the value of $\mathbf{Z}(t)$ for $t \in (T_0, T]$, respectively. Then an individual who enters a trial at time 0 with $Z(t) = -2$ for $0 \leq t \leq 1, Z(t) = -3$ for $1 < t \leq 2, Z(t) = 2.5$ for $2 < t \leq 3$, and $Z(t) = 2$ for $3 < t \leq 3.6$ and dies at $T = 3.6$ is represented by the four data points $(0, 1, 0, -2)$, $(1, 2, 0, -3)$, $(2, 3, 0, 2.5)$, and $(3, 3.6, 1, 2)$.

When computing the likelihood with fixed regressors, it makes sense to use an updating formula. As one moves from one time point to the next, the risk set changes slightly due to the entry or the exit (due to death or censoring) of "individuals". The values for those "individuals" who remain in the risk set do not change and need not be recalculated. In this way the calculation is kept to order n (albeit $4n$ if each individual is treated as four because of changing covariate values).

By contrast, when using continuously varying regressors, one has no choice but to recalculate the partial likelihood contribution from each time point from scratch. This makes the calculation order n^2.

Many software packages that will handle updated regressors will not (easily) handle continuously varying regressors. It is difficult to fit models with user-defined variables such as $Z_2(t) = tZ_1$ using such packages. One might wish to compare the models with hazards $\lambda_0(t) \exp(\beta_1 Z_1)$ and $\lambda_0(t) \exp(\beta_1 Z_1 + \beta_2 t Z_1)$. Of course, for the purpose of testing $\beta_2 = 0$, it is not necessary to fit the latter model. Instead, one may calculate the score statistic for $\beta_2 = 0$ evaluated at the maximum partial likelihood estimate of β_1 from the model with the single (fixed) regressor.

Model Checking

An important aspect of modeling any set of data is assessing the adequacy of the fit and checking to see that the resulting inference is not unduly influenced by a few observations. In general the iterative process of model building and checking may be considered an art rather than a science. Here we review some of the tools available to the statistical artisan analyzing survival data by means of a Cox model.

The simplest form of graphical check comes from dividing the data into groups based on some explanatory variable and fitting a stratified Cox model. If the explanatory variable "$Z = s$" is well modeled by the Cox model, one has $\Lambda_{s0} = \Lambda_0 \exp(\gamma s)$, say. Thus, plotting the logarithm of the cumulative hazard estimate from each strata should reveal parallel curves. That is, the vertical distance between the two curves $\log \Lambda_{r0}(t)$ and $\log \Lambda_{s0}(t)$ should be the same for all t. The common distance should be $\gamma(r - s)$. In practice, such graphics, while intuitively appealing, are not particularly useful.

A closely related, but rather more useful, graph for two strata is obtained by plotting one cumulative hazard $\Lambda_{r0}(t)$ against the other $\Lambda_{s0}(t)$ for all or some selected values of t. Under proportional hazards, such an H–H plot should approximate a straight line through the origin with slope $\exp(\gamma s)$ [6, Section VII.3.1]. The method is easily extended to multiple strata. The disadvantages of the H–H plot are that they do not record the actual time t, and that, if the proportional hazards assumption is seen to be violated, it is difficult to know how to modify the proportional hazards model other than by using a stratified model. Hess [42] reviews a number of variants on these two simple graphical checks of proportional hazards and compares eight graphical methods on each of three data sets. He recommends smoothed plots of scaled Schoenfeld residuals. These are described in the subsection on residuals.

Goodness-of-Fit Tests

Several authors have developed formal goodness-of-fit tests. These can be divided into those designed to be able to detect global alternatives and those with greater power at detecting some specified alternative. Virtually all the tests are asymptotically equivalent to tests based on a defined time-dependent explanatory variable. We saw earlier that the first such tests were proposed by Cox himself [21]. One may add an additional regressor $Z_*(t) = Zg(t)$ for some function $g(t)$. Common choices for g included the identity function $g(t) = t$ and its logarithmic transform $g(t) = \log t$. Other authors use step functions that may jump at either a fixed or a random (but predictable) time. If the partial likelihood is maximized with $Z(t)$, then the partial likelihood ratio test is the statistic of choice. But for testing the goodness of fit, the score test is simpler to compute because it does not require fitting a model with a time-dependent regressor.

Gill & Schumacher [34] proposed a family of tests of the proportional hazards assumption between two samples, A and B. Their tests are motivated by comparing two different estimates of the relative hazard between the two samples. Under proportional hazards the two estimates will be similar, but they need not be in general. The estimates of relative hazard used are derived from linear rank tests, which are themselves equivalent to score tests from the Cox partial likelihood with specially defined time-dependent regressors [33]. The family of tests proposed by Gill & Schumacher [34] are thus similar in spirit to those proposed by Breslow et al. [14]. The latter consider the score test for $\beta_2 = 0$ in the model

$$\lambda_B(t) = \lambda_A(t) \exp[\beta_1 + \beta_2 g(t)],$$

corresponding to covariates $Z_1 = I(B)$ and $Z_2(t) = I(B)g(t)$. A popular choice is $g(t) = \hat{S}(t)$, the Kaplan–Meier estimate of survival in the combined sample at t. O'Quigley & Pessione [62] suggest using a step function for $g(t)$. For a one degree of freedom test, one must choose both the cut points and the values of the step function. For a more general alternative hypothesis, one could partition the time axis into J intervals. The null hypothesis is that the relative hazards $\exp \beta_j$ in all $j = 1, \ldots, J$ intervals are the same, and this can be tested with $J - 1$ degrees of freedom. Wei [85] proposes an omnibus goodness-of-fit test for the two-sample problem based on the supremum of the score statistic $\sup_t |U(\hat{\beta}, t)|$.

Schoenfeld [75] was interested in a more general goodness-of-fit test for the Cox model. He suggested embedding a Cox model with regressor Z in a much larger model with regressors Z and $\mathbf{Z}_*(t)$, where the $\mathbf{Z}_*(t)$ are a set of indicator variables that partition the regressor–time space. Thus, for instance, one might divide the time axis into three parts and the covariate space into four, and form the Cartesian product with 12 cells. In addition to the score test for the coefficients of $\mathbf{Z}_*$ being all zero, one can examine the "residuals", i.e. the difference between the observed and expected (under the basic model with covariate Z) number of events in each of the 12 cells. Lin et al. [58] avoid the need for an arbitrary partition of the space by deriving a supremum test based on the cumulative sum

$$W(t, z) = \sum_{Z_i \leq z} [O_i(t) - E_i(t)],$$

where $O_i(t) = N_i(t)$ and $E_i(t) = \int_0^t Y_i(u) \mathrm{d}\hat{\Lambda}_i(t)$ are, respectively, the observed and expected number of events in individual i, by time t.

Residuals

There have been numerous attempts to define residuals and to propose diagnostic plots for the Cox model. The situation is complicated by both the semiparametric model and the presence of censoring. Some of the proposed techniques are decidedly less useful than one might have hoped. In particular, attempts to define residuals that (under the Cox model) look like a random sample from a specified distribution, so that Q–Q plots can be drawn, have failed. Graphical assessment of the functional form of a covariate and of the constancy of the regression parameters over time have been more successful.

An early definition of residual for the Cox model was the estimated cumulative intensity for each individual:

$$\hat{A}_i(\infty) = \int_0^\infty Y_i(u) \mathrm{d}\hat{\Lambda}_i(u)$$

$$= \int_0^\infty Y_i(u) \exp[\hat{\boldsymbol{\beta}}' \mathbf{z}_i(u)] \mathrm{d}\hat{\Lambda}_0(u) \quad (11)$$

[if $Y_i(u) = I(T_i \geq u)$ and $\mathbf{z}_i(u) = \mathbf{z}_i$, then $\hat{A}_i(\infty) = \hat{\Lambda}_i(T_i) = \exp(\hat{\boldsymbol{\beta}}' \mathbf{z}_i) \hat{\Lambda}_0(T_i)]$ [24, 52]. Later authors made an adjustment to the residual depending on whether the individual was censored or not. The resulting residual $r_i = D_i - \hat{A}_i(\infty)$ is called the martingale residual and is a special case of the general family of residual processes defined by

$$\int_0^t H_i(u) \mathrm{d}\hat{M}_i(t), \quad (12)$$

where $\hat{M}_i(t) = N_i(t) - \int_0^t Y_i(u) \mathrm{d}\hat{\Lambda}_i(u)$ and H_i is a predictable process [8, 81]. Thus r_i is the estimated martingale transform, (12), with $H_i = 1$ and $t = \infty$. The martingale residual may be thought of as the difference between the observed and the expected number of events for the ith individual. The distribution of martingale residuals in a survival setting is very skewed since they have mean zero (under the true model) but range from 1 (for someone who fails at time 0) to minus a very large number (for someone who survives much longer than "expected"). Summing over individuals with similar covariate values $\{i : \mathbf{z}_i \in \mathcal{Z}\}$, say, one obtains the residual number of events for individuals with $\mathbf{z} \in \mathcal{Z}$. Thus, smoothing the martingale residuals against a regressor (or a potential regressor) gives an indication as to how well the model fits the data. Systematic departures from zero indicate that there is an excess (or deficit) in the modeled hazard for that group of individuals. Heuristically one has

$$\mathbf{E}\{N_i(\infty)|\mathbf{z}, z^*\} = A(\infty|\mathbf{z}, z^*) \approx \hat{A}(\infty|\mathbf{z})$$
$$+ \text{smooth}(r_i|z^*).$$

More recently, Grambsch et al. [36] have considered the model

$$\lambda(t|\mathbf{z}, z^*) = \lambda_0(t) \exp[\boldsymbol{\beta}' \mathbf{z} + f(z^*)]. \quad (13)$$

They propose fitting the Cox model with prognostic index $\boldsymbol{\beta}' \mathbf{z} + \gamma z^*$ and plotting $\log\{\text{smooth}[N_i(\infty)]\} - \log\{\text{smooth}[\hat{A}_i(\infty)]\} + \hat{\gamma} z^*$ vs. z^*. The smooth curve will approximate $f(z^*)$ to first order. In practice, the approximation seems to work well even when Z^* is correlated with the other regressors $\mathbf{Z}$.

The martingale residuals were defined by integrating the martingale difference array $\mathrm{d}\hat{M}_i(t)$ over the time axis to give a single residual per individual. To examine the proportional hazards assumption, one is more interested in obtaining a separate residual for each failure time. This can be done by summing the martingale differences, at a given time, over all individuals. Now $\Sigma_i \mathrm{d}\hat{M}_i(t) = 0$ for all t by the definition of the Breslow estimator $\hat{\Lambda}_0$. Nevertheless, one can use the martingale transform, (12), with $\mathbf{H}_i = \mathbf{Z}_i$. Then at each failure time one is comparing the observed value of $\mathbf{Z}$ in the individual that fails with its expected value. Such a residual,

$$\mathbf{r}^*(T_j) = \sum_i \mathbf{Z}_i(T_j)[dN_i(T_j) - Y_i(T_j)d\hat{\Lambda}_i(T_j)]$$

$$= \mathbf{S}_j - d_j \frac{\mathbf{S}^{(1)}(\hat{\boldsymbol{\beta}}, T_j)}{\mathbf{S}^{(0)}(\hat{\boldsymbol{\beta}}, T_j)},$$

was first proposed by Schoenfeld [76]. It is seen that the sum of the Schoenfeld residuals evaluated at $\boldsymbol{\beta}$ is equal to the score $\mathbf{U}(\boldsymbol{\beta})$. It is not difficult to show that, even under the model

$$\lambda(t|\mathbf{z}) = \lambda_0(t)\exp[\boldsymbol{\beta}(t)'\mathbf{z}], \qquad (14)$$

$\mathbf{S}^{(1)}[\boldsymbol{\beta}(t), t]/\mathbf{S}^{(0)}[\boldsymbol{\beta}(t), t] \to \mathbf{E}(\mathbf{Z}|T=t, D=1)$. Thus, using a one-step Taylor series expansion about $\boldsymbol{\beta}(t) = \hat{\boldsymbol{\beta}}$, one has

$$\boldsymbol{\beta}(t) \approx \hat{\boldsymbol{\beta}} + \hat{\mathbf{V}}(t)^{-1}\mathbf{r}^*(t),$$

where

$$\hat{\mathbf{V}}(t) = \frac{\mathbf{S}^{(2)}(\hat{\boldsymbol{\beta}}, t)}{\mathbf{S}^{(0)}(\hat{\boldsymbol{\beta}}, t)} - \left(\frac{\mathbf{S}^{(1)}(\hat{\boldsymbol{\beta}}, t)}{\mathbf{S}^{(0)}(\hat{\boldsymbol{\beta}}, t)}\right)^{\otimes 2}.$$

Hence, Grambsch & Therneau [35] have proposed plotting a smooth of $\hat{\boldsymbol{\beta}} + \hat{\mathbf{V}}(t)^{-1}\mathbf{r}^*(t)$ against t in order to get a feel of $\boldsymbol{\beta}(t)$. Often $\mathbf{V}(t) = \lim_{n\to\infty} \hat{\mathbf{V}}(t)$ does not vary much as a function of t, so for exploratory purposes it may be enough to use $\mathbf{I}(\hat{\boldsymbol{\beta}})/\Sigma N_i(\infty)$ in place of $\hat{\mathbf{V}}(t)$. This has the advantage of not having to store and invert a different covariance matrix at each failure time. In practice, $\mathbf{V}(t)$ will vary most when a variable Z has a skewed distribution and those in the tail are at greatest risk. In all cases it will be difficult to estimate $\hat{\mathbf{V}}(t)$ if the risk set is small at time t, and it is also for large values of t that the $V(t)$ is most likely to be substantially different from its average value.

Influence Diagnostics

Various measures of influential observations have been suggested for the Cox model. The influence diagnostic is intended to approximate the amount by which the regression estimate $\hat{\boldsymbol{\beta}}$ would change if the ith individual were removed from the data set [69]. One such approximation is the infinitesimal jackknife, first proposed by Cain & Lange [17]. Their residuals are equal to the components of the scaled efficient score statistic. This can be written as a martingale

transform residual with $\mathbf{H}_i(t) = \mathbf{Z}_i - \mathbf{E}(\hat{\boldsymbol{\beta}}, t)$. The scaling is done by $\mathbf{I}(\hat{\boldsymbol{\beta}})^{-1}$. One has

$$\tilde{\mathbf{r}}_i = I(\hat{\boldsymbol{\beta}})^{-1} \int_0^\infty [\mathbf{z}_i - \mathbf{E}(\hat{\boldsymbol{\beta}}, t)]d\hat{M}_i(t).$$

An alternative estimate of the influence of an individual is given by Storer & Crowley [79].

Alternatives and Extensions

We have already discussed many extensions of the basic Cox model. We have permitted nonproportional hazards through the stratified Cox model and through user-defined time-dependent variables. We have considered diagnostics to detect data that appear to come from more nonparametric models, such as the additive Cox model $\lambda(t|\mathbf{z}) = \lambda_0(t)\exp[\sum_k f_k(z_k)]$, in which some of the functions f_k may be assumed to be linear while others are left unspecified [39, 32, 37, 70], and the multiplicative hazards model $\lambda(t|\mathbf{z}) = \lambda_0(t)\exp[\boldsymbol{\beta}(t)'\mathbf{z}]$ [86, 30, 40, 41, 84].

We have also seen how the model that was originally perceived for survival data can be generalized quite naturally to event data in which a single individual may have multiple events. The events need not even all be of the same type. They may represent competing risks or more generally the various states in a multistate model. In the classic heart transplant situation, for example, one might use Cox regression to model the transition from identification as a potential recipient (state 0) to transplant (state 1); from state 0 to death (state 2); and from state 1 to death [26]. Three state models in which transitions from state 1 (diseased) back to state 0 (healthy) are possible are also common (see, for example, Andersen et al. [6, Example VII.2.10]). The study of (i) acute graft-vs.-host disease, (ii) chronic graft-vs.-host disease, (iii) leukemia relapse, and (iv) death following bone marrow transplantation (state 0) is also considered by Andersen et al. [6, Example VII.2.18].

We briefly mention a few alternatives to the semiparametric Cox model for regression analysis of censored survival data. Naturally one can try to adapt estimation in any parametric regression model to cope with right censored data. Loglinear models with Weibull or Gamma errors [50, Section 3.6] tend to be more popular in reliability (engineering) than in biostatistics. Particularly in epidemiology, one sometimes has a known population mortality rate that one wants to use in place of the baseline hazard function. The hazard for individual i is given by

$$\lambda_i(t) = \mu_i(t) \exp[\boldsymbol{\beta}' \mathbf{Z}_i(t)],$$

where μ_i is the population mortality corresponding to individual i [15, 7]. Fully parametric models have been studied using counting process techniques by Borgan [12]. Another Cox-like model that uses a known rate is the proportional excess hazards model [73] (*see* **Excess Risk**),

$$\lambda_i(t) = \mu_i(t) + \lambda_0(t) \exp[\boldsymbol{\beta}' \mathbf{Z}_i(t)],$$

in which the excess mortality is modeled by a Cox model.

A general family, known as the accelerated failure-time model, is a linear regression model for the logarithm of the survival time,

$$\log X = \boldsymbol{\beta}' \mathbf{Z} + \varepsilon,$$

where the error ε may be either from a specified distribution or from an unknown distribution. Gaussian errors and no censoring simply correspond to linear regression of $\log X$. If the errors are Weibull, then the model is also a proportional hazards model. Theoretical attention has focused on the semiparametric model with unknown error distribution. Another family of models that include the Cox model as a special case are the transformation models in which an unknown monotone transformation of the survival time is assumed to have a linear regression:

$$\psi(X) = \boldsymbol{\beta}' \mathbf{Z} + \varepsilon.$$

If the error distribution is extreme value ($\exp \varepsilon$ distributed exponential with mean 1), then the transformation model is a Cox model with cumulative baseline hazard given by $\exp[\psi(t)]$ and regression parameters $-\boldsymbol{\beta}$.

The Cox model is a multiplicative hazards model. Aalen [2] introduced an additive hazards model. A semiparametric version of the model [61] is given by

$$\lambda(t|\mathbf{Z}_1, \mathbf{Z}_2) = \boldsymbol{\alpha}_1(t)' \mathbf{Z}_1(t) + \boldsymbol{\alpha}_2' \mathbf{Z}_2(t).$$

If the variables $\mathbf{Z}_1$ include a constant, then we may pull out a baseline hazard and write the first term on the right of the equation as $\lambda_0(t) + \alpha_{11}(t)Z_{11}(t) + \cdots + \alpha_{1p}(t)Z_{1p}(t)$. The cumulative components of hazard $A_{1j}(t) = \int_0^t \alpha_{1j}(u)\mathrm{d}u$ can be estimated at parametric rates, and these must be smoothed to estimate the $\alpha_{1j}(u)$. The model extends naturally to the more general counting process formulation.

Several authors have considered "special" Cox models. These include models for matched pairs [44, 38] (*see* **Matching**), and for interval censored survival data [46], a model for periodic data [64], and a model for **case–cohort** data [66, 77]. Bayesian analysis of the Cox model was first considered by Kalbfleisch [49; 50, Section 8.4] and later by Hjort [43].

There has been relatively little written about robust estimation in the Cox model. Estimators that maximize a weighted partial likelihood have been proposed independently at least three times [56, 74, 71, 72]. The weights may be random and may depend on the regressors $\mathbf{Z}$, but they should be predictable (or at least asymptotically equivalent to predictable weights). A slightly different estimator which essentially corresponds to the efficient score function from a weighted full likelihood has also been studied [10].

Consideration of the Cox estimator for $\hat{\boldsymbol{\beta}}$ when the data do not come from a Cox model leads naturally to adoption of the sandwich estimator of the variance of $\hat{\boldsymbol{\beta}}$ [69, 57]. This is the usual infinitesimal jackknife estimator that can be obtained from the influence residuals

$$\widetilde{\mathrm{var}}(\hat{\boldsymbol{\beta}}) = \sum_i \tilde{r}_i \tilde{r}_i'.$$

The estimator is perhaps most useful when the data are clustered (*see* **Clustering**). Suppose that $\tilde{r}_{ki}$ is the influence residual from individual i in cluster k. Then define $\tilde{r}_k = \Sigma_i \tilde{r}_{ki}$ and estimate the variance of $\hat{\boldsymbol{\beta}}$ by $\Sigma_k \tilde{r}_k^{\otimes 2}$ [55]. This may be a simple technique for adjusting inference when using the Cox model with multivariate survival data. For instance, if each person could have several events, then one might wish to treat the person as a cluster. In another example, the clusters might be formed from survival data on individuals within families.

Another approach adapting the Cox model to multivariate data is through latent variables or frailties. The idea is that, conditionally on an unobserved variable or frailty, the survival times follow a Cox model. The value of the frailty W_i is assumed to be the same for all survival times within a cluster. Two frailty distributions have received the most attention: Clayton & Cuzick [19] considered the hazard model $\lambda_0(t) \exp(\boldsymbol{\beta}' \mathbf{Z} + W)$ in which $\exp W$ has a gamma distribution; Hougaard [45] favors using the positive stable distribution, as this is the only choice that yields proportional hazards both marginally (integrating over the unobserved variable) and conditionally.

References

[1] Aalen, O.O. (1978). Nonparametric inference for a family of counting processes, *Annals of Statistics* **6**, 701–726.

[2] Aalen, O.O. (1980). A Model for Nonparametric Regression Analysis of Counting Processes, *Springer Lecture Notes in Statistics*, Vol. 2. Springer-Verlag, New York, pp. 1–25.

[3] Altman, D.G. & De Stavola, B.L. (1994). Practical problems in fitting a proportional hazards model to data with updated measurements of the covariates, *Statistics in Medicine* **13**, 301–341.

[4] Andersen, P.K. (1991). Survival analysis 1982–1991: the second decade of the proportional hazards regression model, *Statistics in Medicine* **10**, 1931–1941.

[5] Andersen, P.K. & Gill, R.D. (1982). Cox's regression model for counting processes: a large sample study, *Annals of Statistics* **10**, 1100–1120.

[6] Andersen, P.K., Borgan, Ø., Gill, R.D. & Keiding, N. (1993). *Statistical Models Based on Counting Processes*. Springer-Verlag, New York.

[7] Andersen, P.K., Borch-Johnsen, K., Deckert, T., Green, A., Hougaard, P., Keiding, N. & Kreiner, S. (1985). A Cox regression model for the relative mortality and its application to diabetes mellitus survival data, *Biometrics* **41**, 921–932.

[8] Barlow, W.E. & Prentice, R. (1988). Residuals for relative risk regression, *Biometrika* **75**, 65–74.

[9] Bednarski, T. (1989). On sensitivity of Cox's estimator, *Statistics and Decisions* **7**, 215–228.

[10] Bednarski, T. (1993). Robust estimation in Cox's regression model, *Scandinavian Journal of Statistics* **20**, 213–225.

[11] Begun, J.M., Hall, W.J., Huang, W.M. & Wellner, J.A. (1983). Information and asymptotic efficiency in parametric–nonparametric models, *Annals of Statistics* **11**, 432–452.

[12] Borgan, Ø. (1984). Maximum likelihood estimation in parametric counting process models, with applications to censored failure time data, *Scandinavian Journal of Statistics* **11**, 1–16. Correction **11** (1984) 275.

[13] Breslow, N. (1974). Covariance analysis of censored survival data, *Biometrics* **30**, 89–99.

[14] Breslow, N.E., Edler, L. & Berger, J. (1984). A two-sample censored-data rank test for acceleration, *Biometrics* **40**, 1049–1062.

[15] Breslow, N.E., Lubin, J.H., Marek, P. & Langholz, B. (1983). Multiplicative models and cohort analysis, *Journal of the American Statistical Association* **78**, 1–12.

[16] Bretagnolle, J. & Huber-Carol, C. (1988). Effects of omitting covariates in Cox's regression model for survival data, *Scandinavian Journal of Statistics* **15**, 125–138.

[17] Cain, K.C. & Lange, N.T. (1984). Approximate case influence for the proportional hazards regression model with censored data, *Biometrics* **40**, 493–499.

[18] Christensen, E., Neuberger, J., Crowe, J., Altman, D.G., Popper, H., Portmann, B., Doniach, D., Ranek, L., Tygstrup, N. & Williams, R. (1985). Beneficial effect of azathioprine and prediction of prognosis in primary biliary cirrhosis: final results of an international trial, *Gastroenterology* **89**, 1084–1091.

[19] Clayton, D. & Cuzick, J. (1985). Multivariate generalizations of the proportional hazards model (with discussion), *Journal of the Royal Statistical Society, Series A* **148**, 82–117.

[20] Collett, D. (1994). *Modelling Survival Data in Medical Research*. Chapman & Hall, London.

[21] Cox, D.R. (1972). Regression models and life tables (with discussion), *Journal of the Royal Statistical Society, Series B* **34**, 187–220.

[22] Cox, D.R. (1975). Partial likelihood, *Biometrika* **62**, 269–276.

[23] Cox, D.R. & Oakes, D. (1984). *Analysis of Survival Data*. Chapman & Hall, London.

[24] Cox, D.R. & Snell, E.J. (1968). A general definition of residuals (with discussion), *Journal of the Royal Statistical Society, Series B* **30**, 248–275.

[25] Crowley, J. & Hu, M. (1977). Covariance analysis of heart transplant survival data, *Journal of the American Statistical Association* **72**, 27–36.

[26] Crowley, J. & Storer, B.E. (1983). Comment on "A reanalysis of the Stanford heart transplant data", by Aitkin, Laird and Francis, *Journal of the American Statistical Association* **78**, 277–281.

[27] Efron, B. (1977). The efficiency of Cox's likelihood function for censored data, *Journal of the American Statistical Association* **72**, 557–565.

[28] Feigl, P. & Zelen, M. (1965). Estimation of exponential survival probabilities with concomitant information, *Biometrics* **21**, 826–838.

[29] Fleming, T.R. & Harrington, D.P. (1991). *Counting Processes and Survival Analysis*. Wiley, New York.

[30] Gamerman, D. (1991). Dynamic Bayesian models for survival data, *Applied Statistics* **40**, 63–79.

[31] Gehan, E.A. (1965). A generalized Wilcoxon test for comparing arbitrarily single-censored samples, *Biometrika* **52**, 203–223.

[32] Gentleman, R. & Crowley, J. (1991). Local full likelihood estimation for the proportional hazards model, *Biometrics* **47**, 1283–1296.

[33] Gill, R.D. (1984). Understanding Cox's Regression Model: a martingale approach, *Journal of the American Statistical Association* **79**, 441–447.

[34] Gill, R.D. & Schumacher, M. (1987). A simple test for the proportional hazards assumption, *Biometrika* **74**, 289–300.

[35] Grambsch, P.M. & Therneau, T.M. (1994). Proportional hazards tests and diagnostics based on weighted residuals, *Biometrika* **81**, 515–526.

[36] Grambsch, P.M., Therneau, T.M. & Fleming, T.R. (1995). Diagnostic plots to reveal functional form for covariates in multiplicative intensity models, *Biometrics* **51**, 1469–1482.

[37] Gray, R.J. (1992). Flexible methods for analysing survival data using splines, with applications to breast cancer prognosis, *Journal of the American Statistical Association* **87**, 942–951.

[38] Gross, S.T. & Huber, C. (1987). Matched pair experiments: Cox and maximum likelihood estimation, *Scandinavian Journal of Statistics* **14**, 27–41.

[39] Hastie, T. & Tibshirani, R. (1990). Exploring the nature of covariate effects in the proportional hazards model, *Biometrics* **46**, 1005–1016.

[40] Hastie, T. & Tibshirani, R. (1993). Varying coefficient models (with discussion), *Journal of the Royal Statistical Society, Series B* **55**, 757–797.

[41] Hess, K.R. (1994). Assessing time-by-covariate interactions in proportional hazards regression models using cubic spline functions, *Statistics in Medicine* **13**, 1045–1062.

[42] Hess, K.R. (1995). Graphical methods for assessing violations of the proportional hazards assumption in Cox regression, *Statistics in Medicine* **14**, 1707–1723.

[43] Hjort, N.L. (1990). Nonparametric Bayes estimators based on beta processes in models for life history data, *Annals of Statistics* **18**, 1259–1294.

[44] Holt, J.D. & Prentice, R.L. (1974). Survival analysis in twin studies and matched pair experiments, *Biometrika* **65**, 159–166.

[45] Hougaard, P. (1984). Life table methods for heterogeneous populations: distributions describing the heterogeneity, *Biometrika* **71**, 75–83.

[46] Huang, J. (1996). Efficient estimation for the proportional hazards model with interval censoring, *Annals of Statistics* **24**, 540–568.

[47] Jacobsen, M. (1989). Existence and unicity of MLEs in discrete exponential family distributions, *Scandinavian Journal of Statistics* **16**, 335–349.

[48] Johansen, S. (1983). An extension of Cox's regression model, *International Statistical Review* **51**, 165–174.

[49] Kalbfleisch, J.D. (1978). Nonparametric Bayes analysis of survival data, *Journal of the Royal Statistical Society, Series B* **40**, 214–221.

[50] Kalbfleisch, J.D. & Prentice, R.L. (1980). *The Statistical Analysis of Failure Time Data*. Wiley, New York.

[51] Kaplan, E.L. & Meier, P. (1958). Nonparametric estimation from incomplete observations, *Journal of the American Statistical Association* **53**, 457–481.

[52] Kay, R. (1977). Proportional hazards regression models and the analysis of censored survival data, *Applied Statistics* **26**, 227–237.

[53] Kleinbaum, D.G. (1995). *Survival Analysis: A Self-Learning Text*. Springer-Verlag, New York.

[54] Lagakos, S. & Schoenfeld, D. (1984). Properties of proportional hazards score tests under misspecified regression models, *Biometrics* **40**, 1037–1048.

[55] Lee, E.W., Wei, L.J. & Amato, D.A. (1992). Cox-type regression analysis for large numbers of small groups of correlated failure time observations, in *Survival Analysis: State of the Art*, J.P. Klein, & P.K. Goel, eds. Kluwer, Dordrecht, pp. 237–247.

[56] Lin, D.Y. (1991). Goodness-of-fit analysis for the Cox regression model based on a class of parameter estimators, *Journal of the American Statistical Association* **86**, 725–728.

[57] Lin, D.Y. & Wei, L.J. (1989). The robust inference for the Cox proportional hazards model, *Journal of the American Statistical Association* **84**, 1074–1078.

[58] Lin, D.Y., Wei, L.J. & Ying, Z. (1993). Checking the Cox model with cumulative sums of martingale-based residual, *Biometrika* **80**, 557–572.

[59] Mantel, N. (1966). Evaluation of survival data and two new rank order statistics arising in its consideration, *Cancer and Chemotherapy Reports* **50**, 163–170.

[60] Marubini, E. & Valsecchi, M.G. (1995). *Analysing Survival Data from Clinical Trials and Observational Studies*. Wiley, Chichester.

[61] McKeague, I. & Sasieni, P. (1994). A partly parametric additive risk model, *Biometrika* **81**, 501–514.

[62] O'Quigley J. & Pessione F. (1989). Score tests for homogeneity of regression effects in the proportional hazards model, *Biometrics* **45**, 135–144.

[63] Peto, R. (1972). Contribution to the discussion of paper by D.R. Cox, *Journal of the Royal Statistical Society, Series B* **34**, 205–207.

[64] Pons, O. & de Turckheim, E. (1988). Cox's periodic regression model, *Annals of Statistics* **16**, 678–693.

[65] Prentice, R.L. (1982). Covariate measurement errors and parameter estimation in a failure time regression model, *Biometrika* **69**, 331–342.

[66] Prentice, R.L. (1986). A case-cohort design for epidemiologic cohort studies and disease prevention trials, *Biometrika* **73**, 1–11.

[67] Prentice, R. & Self, S. (1983). Asymptotic distribution theory for Cox-type regression models with general risk form, *Annals of Statistics* **11**, 804–813.

[68] Ramlau-Hansen, H. (1983). Smoothing counting process intensities by means of kernel functions, *Annals of Statistics* **11**, 453–466.

[69] Reid, N. & Crépeau, H. (1985). Influence functions for proportional hazards regression, *Biometrika* **72**, 1–9.

[70] Sasieni, P. (1992). Information bounds for the conditional hazard ratio in a nested family of regression models, *Journal of the Royal Statistical Society, Series B* **54**, 617–635.

[71] Sasieni, P.D. (1993). Maximum weighted partial likelihood estimates for the Cox model, *Journal of the American Statistical Association* **88**, 144–152.

[72] Sasieni, P.D. (1993). Some new estimates for Cox regression, *Annals of Statistics* **21**, 1721–1759.

[73] Sasieni, P.D. (1996). Proportional excess hazards, *Biometrika* **83**, 127–141.

[74] Schemper, M. (1992). Cox analysis of survival data with non proportional hazards functions, *Statistician* **41**, 455–465.

[75] Schoenfeld, D. (1980). Chi-squared goodness of fit tests for the proportional hazards regression model, *Biometrika* **67**, 145–153.

[76] Schoenfeld, D. (1982). Partial residuals for the proportional hazards regression model, *Biometrika* **69**, 239–241.

[77] Self, S.G. & Prentice, R.L. (1988). Asymptotic distribution theory and efficiency results for case-cohort studies, *Annals of Statistics* **16**, 64–81.

[78] Solomon, P.J. (1984). Effect of misspecification of regression models in the analysis of survival data, *Biometrika* **71**, 291–298. Amendment. **73** (1986) 245.

[79] Storer, B.E. & Crowley, J. (1985). A diagnostic for Cox regression and general conditional likelihoods, *Journal of the American Statistical Association* **80**, 139–147.

[80] Struthers, C.A. & Kalbfleisch, J.D. (1986). Misspecified proportional hazards models, *Biometrika* **73**, 363–369.

[81] Therneau, T.M., Grambsch, P.M. & Fleming, T.R. (1990). Martingale-based residuals for survival models, *Biometrika* **77**, 147–160.

[82] Thomas, D.C. (1981). General relative risk models for survival time and matched case-control analysis, *Biometrics* **37**, 673–686.

[83] Tsiatis, A.A. (1981). A large sample study of Cox's regression model, *Annals of Statistics* **9**, 93–108.

[84] Verweij, P.J.M. & van Houwelingen, H.C. (1995). Time-dependent effects of fixed covariates in Cox regression, *Biometrics* **51**, 1550–1556.

[85] Wei, L.J. (1984). Testing goodness of fit for the proportional hazards model with censored observations, *Journal of the American Statistical Association* **80**, 139–147.

[86] Zucker, D.M. & Karr, A.F. (1990). Nonparametric survival analysis with time-dependent covariate effects: a penalized partial likelihood approach, *Annals of Statistics* **18**, 329–353.

PETER SASIENI

Cross Level Bias *see* Ecologic Fallacy

Cross-Sectional Study

A cross-sectional study is a study to estimate the distribution of a quantity of interest (or joint distribution of several quantities) in a **target population**, at a certain moment in time. Ideally, this is accomplished by measurements from a random or stratified random sample of the target population, although convenience samples may also be used. A cross-sectional study is characterized by the fact that only one set of observations is taken from each subject, as opposed to a longitudinal study in which study participants provide observations at more than one point in time (*see* **Cohort Study**). Even if repeated or serial cross-sectional studies are conducted in the same population, the same individuals generally will not be sampled again except by chance.

Cross-sectional studies often have a binary variable as the quantity of primary interest, such as estimating the **prevalence** of a certain disease, risk factor, or health behavior. Continuous variables may also be of interest, for example the subject's weight or blood cholesterol level, although such data are often grouped or categorized in epidemiologic studies. One use of a cross-sectional study is to determine the association between an outcome variable and some explanatory variables, for example to estimate the prevalence of a disease, perhaps as a function of some explanatory variables. An association between outcomes and explanatory variables may suggest causality, although a causal link usually cannot be established from a single cross-sectional survey (*see* **Causation**; **Hill's Criteria for Causality**), because such studies give no information on the temporal ordering of possibly causal events. A second use of cross-sectional studies is to monitor changes in a population over time using a series of cross-sectional surveys; for example, the Monitoring the Future surveys [7] track drug use by teenagers over time in this way. Sometimes a better case for a causal link can be made with serial cross-sectional data; for example, Pirkle et al. [9] analyzed blood lead measurements from the second and third National Health and Nutrition Examination Surveys (NHANES), conducted in 1976–1980 and 1988–1991, respectively, to document a decline in blood lead levels in the US population that resulted from the gradual removal, since 1976, of most lead from gasoline. A third use of cross-sectional studies is to make some inference about disease incidence; this is harder to achieve, although some techniques for estimating incidence from a cross-sectional survey are discussed below.

As the distribution that is being estimated may be changing over time, the ideal cross-sectional study would be conducted instantaneously. However, a real study typically requires some time to conduct. In practice, the primary requirement is that the target distribution changes negligibly over the course of the study. In some situations this requirement is easily met: for example, a study of the prevalence of carpal tunnel syndrome can safely be conducted over an entire year; a study of the prevalence of varicella (chicken-pox) probably should be conducted within a week or two. In some situations cross-sectional surveys are conducted over a long period as a surveillance system (*see* **Surveillance of Diseases**). For example, the Centers for Disease Control (CDC), use ongoing **telephone surveys** to assess the prevalence of several chronic disease risk factors and tracks these over time [11]. These studies should be distinguished from incidence studies in which all new occurrences of a disease arising in a certain population in a given period are recorded; a defining characteristic of a cross-sectional survey is that subjects are sampled solely on the basis of their membership in a target population, not on the basis of a change in status. This distinction is somewhat blurred, however, in cross-sectional surveys that also collect retrospective data on duration of disease, since this type of data would allow identification of new cases.

Although a cross-sectional study can only measure a distribution at a single time point, interest is often centered on dynamic or time-dependent quantities; disease incidence is often the quantity of interest. One circumstance in which disease incidence can be measured from a cross-sectional survey occurs when an ephemeral state associated with recent onset can be identified. If the mean duration, w, of this state is known, then the prevalence of individuals in the ephemeral state can be converted into disease incidence using the relation prevalence/w = incidence. For a disease of short duration, the ephemeral state can be the entire course of the disease. For this method to be valid, the time-scale over which the disease incidence changes must be longer than w. For example, Brookmeyer & Quinn [2] estimated the incidence of human immunodeficiency virus (HIV) infection in a population of commercial sex workers in India by identifying the proportion of individuals who tested negative for HIV on a standard screening assay but who already had detectable levels of p24 antigen, one of the core proteins of HIV. See also Janssen et al. [6] for related work. Note that although this method is sensitive to the value of w,

it is possible to test for or estimate trends in incidence in serial cross-sectional surveys by comparing the prevalence of individuals in the ephemeral state over time. For such a comparison to provide valid inference on trends in incidence, it is not necessary to know w; we need know only that it is small compared with the time between the surveys.

The methods described above are appropriate for situations in which the incidence is changing over time. In many situations the population may be considered homogeneous over time; in these situations, interest may focus on the age of onset or on age-specific incidences. Keiding [8] discussed a variety of assumptions that allow estimation of these quantities from a cross-sectional survey, and also discussed methods to estimate disease prevalence from incidence data (*see* **Incidence–Prevalence Relationships**). Some of these methods require either retrospective data or external data such as age-specific mortality for the general population or for people with the specific disease of interest. Additional information about population dynamics can sometimes be obtained if two or more cross-sectional studies are conducted in the same population at different times. For example, it is possible to estimate the incidence of a disease by comparing two measurements of disease prevalence taken at different times and accounting for the aging of the population. By comparing the proportion of 15-year-olds with 19-year-olds who have a positive ppd (purified protein derivative) TB test with the proportion five years later among 20- to 24-year-olds, one could estimate rates of infection with *M. tuberculosis*, in essence treating these two groups as members of the same "pseudo-cohort". Techniques are available for converting these "cohort infection rates" to age-specific period rates [10]. However, the validity of this calculation depends on the assumption that there is no differential loss of people with disease (i.e. mortality or migration caused by the disease); otherwise, external data on the these effects are necessary. In addition, for different age groups to be treated as members of the same pseudo-cohort, the distribution of important covariates must be the same across age groups, a condition that may pose a special challenge for **observational studies**. For example, in a study of childbearing women, the women aged 15–20 years may have markedly different demographic characteristics than those aged 20–25 years.

Conclusions about incidence can sometimes be drawn by comparing crude (i.e. not age-specific) prevalences from successive cross-sectional surveys. For example, HIV prevalence among injection drug-users in Bangkok, Thailand, jumped from 1% at the start of 1988 to 32%–43% by August–September 1988 [12], implying a remarkable incidence of HIV infection over this period, as well as illustrating the usefulness of cross-sectional surveys as a surveillance tool. However, in less dramatic situations, trends in prevalence may be difficult to interpret because they are the net result of new cases and death or the loss of old cases. As with analyses of age pseudo-cohorts, knowledge of or assumptions on the nature of the death or loss of prevalent cases are required before inference on incidence can be made. An unchanging crude prevalence also does not necessarily imply steady-state conditions; Batter et al. [1] report an example where crude prevalence was steady over time but the distribution of cases by age had shifted.

The line between cross-sectional studies and a wide variety of **retrospective studies** is blurred when retrospective longitudinal data are collected in a cross-sectional survey. Examples of such data include age at menarche, the number of months breast-fed, prevalence of diarrhea in the last two weeks, or conditions surrounding the death of a child. The validity of such retrospective data is dependent on the respondent's ability to recall accurately the events of interest for the time-period considered. For example, to examine the association between short birth intervals and the survival of the subsequent child, it is possible to use birth history reports of mothers [5]. This same type of data can also be used to estimate fertility and mortality patterns many years before the study for analysis of long-term trends.

Several major differences between cross-sectional studies and longitudinal (or cohort) studies determine when either should be used. **Cohort studies** measure the effect of risk factors on disease incidence in a defined population, whereas cross-sectional studies measure the effects of risk factors on disease prevalence. As a result, differences may arise when the same associations are studied by the two methods. Factors that affect both disease incidence and mortality after disease will show a different association when measured cross-sectionally than when measured longitudinally. For example, a risk factor that is associated with both increased incidence and

increased mortality among individuals with disease will show a smaller association with disease prevalence in a cross-sectional survey than with disease incidence in a longitudinal study, because the persons with the risk factor will be less likely to survive until the time of the cross-sectional study (*see* **Case–Control Study, Prevalent**). Even factors unrelated to disease incidence may show an association with disease prevalence if they affect the survival of individuals with disease differentially. Thus, if disease etiology is of primary interest, cohort studies or incident **case–control studies** are usually preferable, whereas prevalence studies may provide more useful information for characterization of a population for public health purposes.

Cross-sectional studies sample prevalent, rather than incident, cases; the selection requirement of survival to the date at which the survey is conducted results in differences between the population of prevalent cases and the population obtained by following incident cases over time. The likelihood of being observed in a certain transient stage in a cross-sectional survey is proportional to the time spent in that stage (*see* **Length Bias**). As a result of heterogeneity in the course of disease, individuals with longer survival times are more likely to be sampled in a cross-sectional study than those with shorter survival times. Similarly, the population of prevalent cases who have a given characteristic may differ from the population of those who have ever developed that characteristic. A cross-sectional estimate of the relative prevalence of two types of cancer (one virulent, the other less so) would not be equal to the relative incidences, as the relative incidence of the virulent type would be greater than its relative prevalence. Although the results of the cross-sectional study may properly reflect the distribution of survival times or disease subtypes among those individuals currently living with disease, these quantities must be interpreted as instantaneous pictures of a dynamic, open population and not necessarily as reflective of some other population, such as those with incident disease (*see* **Biased Sampling of Cohorts in Epidemiology**).

Another distinction between cross-sectional and longitudinal studies is that a cross-sectional study or series of cross-sectional studies can only address aggregate changes in the population; unless the appropriate retrospective data are available, it is not possible to measure change at the individual level. For example, two cross-sectional surveys may find approximately the same proportion of respondents used a condom during their last sexual contact; to plan a public health campaign to increase condom usage, we may want to know additionally whether some respondents always use condoms and some never do, or if all individuals sometimes use condoms. Such data are most reliably obtained from a longitudinal study. In some cases, however, the closed nature of the longitudinal study is a disadvantage. For example, studies of HIV incidence conducted longitudinally often find a decreasing incidence of new HIV infections which may not represent the trend in the general population but instead represent a depletion of high-risk individuals in the cohort, as well as a change in behavior among study participants, who receive counseling on how to reduce their risk of acquiring HIV infection.

Cost is often a deciding factor that favors cross-sectional studies over longitudinal studies. This is especially true for studies of rare diseases, where very large cohorts or long follow-up may be required to observe enough cases to obtain statistically significant results. A variety of split-panel designs combine elements of both cross-sectional and longitudinal studies. Further discussion of these designs, as well as a general discussion of what types of questions can be answered with a cross-sectional study and what questions require a longitudinal study, can be found in Curtin & Feinleib [3] and Dwyer & Feinleib [4].

References

[1]   Batter, V., Matela, B., Nsuami, M., Manzila, T., Kamenga, M., Behets, F., Ryder, R.W., Heyward, W.L., Karon, J.M. & St Louis, M.E. (1994). High HIV-1 incidence in young women masked by stable overall seroprevalence among childbearing women in Kinshasa, Zaire: estimating incidence from serial seroprevalence data, *Journal of Acquired Immune Deficiency Syndrome* **8**, 811–817.

[2]   Brookmeyer, R. & Quinn, T.C. (1995). Estimation of current human immunodeficiency virus incidence rates from a cross-sectional survey using early diagnostic tests, *American Journal of Epidemiology* **141**, 166–172.

[3]   Curtin, L. & Feinleib, M. (1992). Considerations in the design of longitudinal surveys of health, in *Statistical Models for Longitudinal Studies of Health*, J.H. Dwyer, M. Feinleib, P. Lippert & H. Hoffmeister, eds. Oxford University Press, New York.

[4]   Dwyer, J. & Feinleib, M. (1992). Introduction to statistical models for longitudinal observation, in *Statistical Models for Longitudinal Studies of Health*, J.H. Dwyer,

M Feinleib, P. Lippert & H. Hoffmeister, eds. Oxford University Press, New York.

[5]   Hobcraft, J., McDonald, J. & Rutstein, S. (1985). Demographic determinants of infant and early child mortality, *Population Studies* **39**, 363–385.

[6]   Janssen, R.S., Satten, G.A., Stramer, S., Rawal, B.D., O'Brien, T.R., Weiblen, B.J., Hecht, F.M., Jack, N., Cleghorn, F.R., Kahn, J.O., Chesney, M.A. & Busch, M.P. (1998). New testing strategy to detect early HIV-1 infection for use in incidence estimates and for clinical and prevention purposes, *Journal of the American Medical Association* **280**, 42–48.

[7]   Johnston, L.D., O'Malley, P.M. & Bachman, J.G. (1996). *National Survey Results On Drug Use From the Monitoring the Future Study, 1975–1995. Vol. 1: Secondary School Students*, NIH Pub. No. 97–4139. National Institute on Drug Abuse, Rockville.

[8]   Keiding, N. (1991). Age-specific incidence and prevalence: a statistical perspective (with discussion), *Journal of the Royal Statistical Society, Series A* **154**, 371–412.

[9]   Pirkle, J.L., Brody, D., Gunter, E.W., Paschal, D.C., Flegal, K.M. & Matte, T.D. (1994). The decline in blood lead levels in the United States: The National Health and Nutrition Examination Surveys, *Journal of the American Medical Association* **272**, 284–291.

[10]   Preston, S. & Coale, A. (1982). Age structure, growth, attrition and accession: a new synthesis, *Population Index* **48**, 217–259.

[11]   Remington, P.C., Smith, M.Y., Williamson, D.F., Anda, R.F., Gentry, E.M. & Hogelin, G.C. (1988). Design, characteristics and usefulness of state-based behavioural risk factor surveillance: 1981–1987, *Public Health Reports* **103**, 366–375.

[12]   Weniger, B.G., Limpakarnjanarat, K., Ungchusak, K., Thanprasertsuk, S., Choopanya, K., Vanichseni, S., Uneklabh, T., Thongcharoen, P. & Wasi, C. (1991). The epidemiology of HIV infection and AIDS in Thailand, *Journal of Acquired Immune Deficiency Syndrome* **5**, Supplement 2, S71–S85.

GLEN A. SATTEN &
LAURENCE GRUMMER-STRAWN

Crude Incidence or Probability *see* Absolute Risk

Crude Probability of Death from a Cause *see* Competing Risks

Crude Risk

Crude risk is the probability that an individual will develop a particular disease in a given time interval in the presence of other **competing risks** of death. For example, the probability that a 30 year old woman will develop breast cancer between the ages of 30 and 60 is a crude risk. The crude risk is reduced by the fact that she may die of other diseases before she develops breast cancer. The term **absolute risk** is used synonymously with crude risk. Crude risk can be estimated without making special assumptions, such as the "independence" assumption used in competing risk analysis. Crude risk can be contrasted with the net risk in the theory of competing risks. Net risk refers to the probability of developing a particular disease if other competing risks are eliminated.

Crude risk is also used to describe the risk of disease in a heterogeneous population composed of different genders and age groups, for example. Crude risk is differentiated, in this context, from gender- and age-specific risks.

M.H. GAIL

Cumulative Hazard

The cumulative hazard on the interval $[0,\ t)$ is $\int_0^t \lambda(u)\mathrm{d}u$, where $\lambda(u)$ is the **hazard rate**. If $\lambda(u)$ is the hazard for total mortality, then the cumulative hazard is related to cumulative probability of death, $1 - \exp\left(-\int_0^t \lambda(u)\mathrm{d}u\right)$. If $\lambda(u)$ is a disease-specific **incidence rate** and if $\int_0^t \lambda(u)\mathrm{d}u$ is small, then the cumulative hazard approximates the "pure" probability of developing disease in the absence of other competing causes of death, provided that those other causes act independently of the cause of interest.

(*See also* **Competing Risks**).

M.H. GAIL

Cumulative Incidence

Cumulative incidence is the proportion of individuals in a cohort initially free of a given disease who develop that disease in a defined age or time interval. Cumulative incidence is a **crude risk** and is synonymous with the terms cumulative risk, **risk**, and **absolute risk**. Sometimes cumulative incidence refers to the number, rather than the proportion, of individuals in a cohort initially free of a given disease who develop the disease in a given age or time interval.

M.H. GAIL

Cumulative Incidence Rate

The cumulative **incidence rate** is a **cumulative hazard** and corresponds to the special case in which the hazard refers to the incidence rate for a specific disease. For small incidence rates, the cumulative incidence rate approximates the "pure" probability of developing the disease in the absence of competing causes of death (*see* **Competing Risks**) and should be distinguished from the crude probability of developing the disease in the presence of competing causes of death (*see* **Absolute Risk**; **Crude Risk**).

M.H. GAIL

Cumulative Incidence Ratio

The cumulative incidence ratio is the ratio of the **cumulative incidence** in an exposed cohort to that in an unexposed cohort over the same time period. The cumulative incidence ratio is the same as the **relative risk**.

(*See also* **Cohort Study**)

M.H. GAIL

Cumulative Incidence Risk *see* Absolute Risk

Cuzick–Edwards Test *see* Clustering

Cumulative Incidence Sampling for Controls *see* Case–Control Study

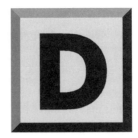

Darroch's Measure of Distinguish-ability *see* Agreement, Measurement of

Data Quality in Vital and Health Statistics

Data quality is not intrinsically interesting, but it is important. According to Greenwood writing about this in 1948,

> Most statistics can be used and are used for propaganda; hardly any are used more frequently for this purpose than medical statistics, so the student is once again urged to scrutinize the medical-statistical arguments of very important persons with great care and to verify the statistics used [7].

Analyses can only be as good as the data that underlie them: as the computing aphorism puts it, more succinctly if less elegantly than Greenwood's stricture, "Garbage in, garbage out".

To some extent quality, like beauty, is in the eye of the beholder – assessment of it is dependent on the purpose to which the data are to be put. Nevertheless, there are some general points that need to be considered when using routinely collected vital and health data (termed "routine data" hereafter, for brevity). Before discussing these, however, it is worth considering the particular ways in

which data quality is of importance for routine data analyses.

Data Quality in Routine Statistics Compared with *ad hoc* Studies

Data quality is of course not solely an issue for routine data analyses – it is important too in *ad hoc* studies in which data are collected specifically for research. The issues present somewhat differently for routine data, however, for several reasons.

First, routine data sets are often extremely large – this is one of their attractions for scientific analysis, but also potentially one of their drawbacks. Files containing many thousands or even millions of events will inevitably have involved data collection by a very large number of people, often with less-close supervision, or at least less-uniform supervision, than can be achieved in smaller research studies.

Secondly, the data have often not been collected primarily for the purpose to which the research investigator may put them. They may have been collected to fulfill legal obligations, or to supply aggregated large-scale statistics for governmental or administrative purposes, and often it is only secondarily that they are utilized for scientific investigation. As a consequence, the data collection methods and quality controls have usually been organized by individuals who will not use the data for the purposes to which the statistician wishes to put them. In comparison, in an *ad hoc* study, the data collection has usually been targeted deliberately to collect the information the analyst requires. Because of this "second-hand" aspect of routine data, the assessment of quality by the user often has also to be a second-hand process. Information on quality may never have been collected, and often the details of how the data were collected, with what constraints and instructions, may be known only to those working within the data-gathering organization, whose advice and knowledge may need to be sought.

Assessment of Data Quality

The following subsections discuss issues that need to be taken into account when assessing quality.

Quality of Information in the Underlying Data Sources, Especially with Respect to Diagnosis

Routine data are dependent on the quality of the underlying information from which they are compiled. Thus, for instance, it is likely that advances in diagnostic methods have greatly increased the proportion of leukemias and myelomas that are diagnosed now compared with 60 or 70 years ago. Past routine data on these malignancies were highly incomplete, not because of inadequate data collection, but because the cases were often not diagnosed. Similarly, geographical differences in apparent incidence of conditions may reflect better diagnosis in one place than another (*see* **Geographic Patterns of Disease**; **Mortality, International Comparisons**).

Incompleteness and inaccuracy of diagnosis may arise at several stages in the process from disease incidence to diagnostic labelling, and each needs to be considered when deciding whether apparent variations in rates are an artefact. There may be variation in whether subjects with illness realize they are ill, and whether they present to a doctor for diagnosis, depending, for instance, on social, financial, and educational factors. If patients present to a doctor, the diagnosis will depend on factors such as the propensity of the doctor to investigate, his or her diagnostic acumen, whether referral is made to a specialist, and the diagnostic methods and technologies employed, including, for fatal conditions, the extent to which autopsies are performed. Thus, for instance, incidence rates of prostatic cancer have been found to be much greater in Malmö, where "the autopsy service is superb" than in other cities in Sweden, but when

cases found "accidentally" at autopsy were excluded, the incidence rates in Malmö and other cities were similar [20]. If screening for a disease is introduced (*see* **Screening, Overview**), then asymptomatic cases will be detected that either would never otherwise have been diagnosed, or would have been diagnosed at a later date after they had become symptomatic; the former detection would be expected to lead to a permanent artefactual increase in rates, the latter to a temporary increase.

For mortality, when a diagnosis has been reached, the quality of the eventual statistics will also depend on how well the person certifying the cause of death (*see* **Death Certification**) (usually a doctor, but not always – see below) knows the patient's past medical history, which diagnosis he or she considers to have caused death (*see* **Cause of Death, Underlying and Multiple**), and the way in which he or she completes the death certificate, since the positioning of causes there can affect the underlying cause selected by the coding agency [8]. Studies requesting different practitioners to complete "dummy" death certificates for the same case history have been used to try to ascertain the extent to which, for instance, international differences in certification practice can affect apparent mortality rates [11], and similarly by requesting national statistical offices to code the certificates, to investigate how this coding affects rates [11, 17].

One method frequently used to check the quality of clinical or death certificate diagnostic information is to compare the diagnoses from this source with those reached by autopsy [6, 10]. An often-used general marker of quality of death certificate information in a population is the proportion of deaths recorded as due to senility: a high percentage of deaths certified to this cause suggests a poor quality of diagnostic information, at older ages at least. Quality of diagnostic data is also suggested by its source or basis – for instance, for mortality data, whether the diagnosis is supplied by a doctor or not, and for cancer registrations, the proportion of cases with histological verification, (although new diagnostic technologies, for instance, ultrasound imaging plus serum alpha-fetoprotein estimation for diagnosis of liver cancer [16], can sometimes lead to a reduced percentage histologically verified without reduced quality). For mortality, Alderson [1] gives tables of the extent to which deaths have been certified to ill-defined causes and the percentage of death certificates signed by doctors, in 31 countries (Japan and Western) since early in the twentieth century, and a description of the death registration system in each of these countries over time. For cancer registration (*see* **Disease Registers**), tables of the proportion of cases histologically verified, and other quality indicators – the proportion of cases registered from a death certificate only, the ratio of mortality to incidence, the percentage of cancers for which the primary site is unknown or ill-defined, and the proportion of cases with age unknown – for over 100 cancer registries worldwide, are given in *Cancer Incidence in Five Continents* [16].

As well as differences in diagnostic completeness and capability, routine data will also be affected by medical definitions of diseases, which may vary greatly by place or time, and can lead artefactually to apparent large differences in rates. Thus, for instance, great differences in diagnosis between countries have been shown for psychiatric conditions [3], and substantial apparent secular changes in bladder cancer rates can occur as a result of changes in pathological nomenclature for classifying papillomas (e.g. as "grade O carcinomas") [20].

The above discussion has related to the quality of diagnostic data, but the quality of the source data for other variables such as age, sex, and country of birth, which may be used in analysis, is also important and needs to be considered (see below).

Completeness of Data Collection

For legal reasons, certification of births and deaths is normally virtually complete in Western countries, although there can be exceptions, for instance during wartime [1]. Completeness may be deficient in a particular area within a country: for instance, a study in the West of Ireland, found that in 1966–69, 7.5% of deaths were not registered, and in 1974–77, 6.1% [13]. In the US, satisfactory levels of registration were achieved by different states in different years (the last, of the then-existent states, Texas, reached the level required to be admitted to the "National Death Registration Area", for which the federal government publishes data, in 1933) [12]. One stratagem to overcome quality deficiencies in particular geographical areas is to analyze only a geographical subset of the overall data set (e.g. particular states), for which good quality data are available.

Registration of morbidity is more often incomplete, and when comparing morbidity rates between places or over time, one must consider whether differences in completeness may explain apparent differences in incidence. Multiple data sources (e.g. death certificates, hospital admissions lists, pathologists' reports) may be needed to gain a high level of completeness, and addition of a new data source, for instance adding death certificates as a source for cancer registration, can lead to an abrupt increase in recorded rates [22]. For cancer registrations [18] and infectious disease notifications [24], countries differ as to whether reporting is legally compulsory, but it is uncertain whether in practice this affects completeness. In several countries a fee is paid to the notifying doctor for each infectious disease notification [24], but again it is not clear that this provides high completeness.

Often, completeness is better for more-serious than for less-serious conditions, if only because the most serious lead to death. Thus, for instance, non-melanoma skin cancers (which are rarely fatal) tend to be the worst registered of the common cancers, and notification of infections such as acute poliomyelitis and diphtheria is likely to be far more complete than that for dysentery [21]. For most purposes, substantially incomplete data are very difficult to interpret, especially since the missing data may be biased, but for certain uses they may be serviceable: for instance, if an infectious disease notification system is used primarily to detect epidemics, then it would not in principle invalidate its use if it was substantially incomplete, provided that the percentage incompleteness remained approximately constant over time. Nevertheless, greater confidence can be had in analyses based on reasonably complete data, because one can rarely be sure that the degree of incompleteness has remained unchanged; for example, for measles there is evidence that completeness can differ between epidemic and nonepidemic years, being greater during epidemics [5]. (Of course, if this was reliably the case, then it would actually improve detection of epidemics, although still diminishing the value of the data for scientific uses.)

Assessment of completeness is ideally carried out by comparison with a "gold standard" complete dataset collected by independent means, either by an *ad hoc* survey or in another routine data system – for instance, comparison of registration data with death certificates for anencephaly has been used to check completeness of congenital malformation notification [25]. Failing this, however, capture–recapture techniques can be used to assess completeness by comparing the data with those collected by other incomplete methods. For cancers, a frequently used but imperfect measure of completeness is the mortality to incidence ratio, comparing the numbers of cancers in mortality and cancer registration data for the same year(s): this can give an approximate guide to completeness, particularly for rapidly fatal cancers, but it is imperfect because it depends on comparable accuracy and precision in identification of cancer site and comparable definitions of place of residence in the two data sets, and on case-fatality and secular trends in incidence and mortality rates as well as completeness, and also because death certificates are often used as a source of cancer registration, so that incidence and mortality datasets are not independent. Another often-used indicator of completeness of cancer registration is the percentage of cases registered from a death certificate only: a high percentage indicates likely incompleteness, since equivalent nonfatal cases would probably never be registered.

Duplication

Like incompleteness, this should not be a problem for mortality and births data in Western countries, but it can be a substantial one for morbidity data. To avoid duplication, the data collection agency must first link multiple notifications that refer to the same person (*see* **Record Linkage**), and then differentiate between genuine double occurrence of the disease or event of interest in the same individual – for instance, two primary cancers incident in the same person, or a particular infectious disease caught on more than one occasion – and inadvertent duplicate recording of the same morbid event, often because it has been reported from more than one source.

Much less tends to be published about the extent of duplication within routine datasets than about their completeness, and this makes it particularly difficult for the user to be sure to what extent duplication has occurred. One issue that the user may need to clarify is the rules used by data coders to decide what should count as a duplicate – for instance, whether two primary cancers of the same site but different histologies, or two contralateral tumors in paired organs such as kidneys or testes, should count as one or two malignancies; the effect on recorded incidence rates can be appreciable. As another example, for tuberculosis statistics one needs to ascertain whether the

data refer to new cases only or to all cases (new and relapses); for some countries the former are not readily available, so that international comparisons may need to use the latter [19]. On a broader question, the user will also need to note whether the dataset is based on persons, disease occurrences, or events.

Having determined the basis of the data set and the rules used for decisions on duplicates, the user needs to compare these with the purpose of the study. Thus, rates of cancer incidence in an analysis including second and subsequent primary cancers will be greater than rates restricted to first primaries; neither is of lower quality for the purpose for which it was intended, but either is inappropriate or of deficient quality if intended for the opposite purpose. Similarly, rates of hospital admission from a hospital in-patient data system, counting two admissions of the same person for the same incident disease as two records, can give useful information for health care planning, but will generally be unsatisfactory for epidemiology.

Late Registrations, Alterations, and Deletions

Whereas birth and mortality data are normally collected within a few days of occurrence of the event, and will tend to produce complete statistics within a few months, complete collection of morbidity statistics may take several years. For instance, cancer registration inevitably takes a year or two to become reasonably complete: data must be obtained from several sources (such as clinical records, pathology records, and death certificates), cross-matched and duplicates eliminated. Furthermore, diagnostic confirmation of an initially suspected cancer may take weeks or months, and cancers initially identified by a registry at death may prove in retrospect to have been incident months or years earlier, and will then need to be registered as having occurred at that date of incidence. Because of these delays, plus the time taken to compile statistics and publish them, cancer registration statistics may differ appreciably depending on how long after the incidence date they were published. If data are analyzed too soon after incidence, then apparent decreases in rates may prove to be artefacts. Similarly, assessments of completeness of cancer registration need to be conducted sufficient years after incidence, if they are not to confuse lack of timeliness with eventual incompleteness: an apparent recent decline in completeness may be a consequence of premature assessment.

As well as leading to late registration of an event not previously registered, late information may also alter a diagnosis or other variable already recorded – for instance, an autopsy may reveal that a cancer registered years earlier at initial diagnosis was in fact of a different site from that registered, or indeed was not a cancer at all.

Some data systems incorporate a specific facility to improve quality after initial data collection, by taking account of new information from subsequent diagnostic investigation: for instance, to amend a death certificate diagnosis on the basis of autopsy findings [23] or to correct (or delete) an infectious disease notification on the basis of laboratory reports [24].

Validity and Precision of Data Collection

Data extraction from original sources, often by clerks, needs to be conducted accurately and without, for instance, miscategorization of adjacent anatomical sites or similar sounding diseases (*see* **Misclassification Error**). Accuracy can be measured by comparison with data re-collected from original sources [2], or by searching the files for the frequency of impossible or unlikely values or combinations, suggestive of inaccuracy – for instance prostate operations on women. It should be noted, however, that this will only provide a proxy for general quality if the data-collecting agency has not already conducted range and consistency checks to rid the data of these particular errors, and that if they have conducted these checks, this will not in itself produce a completely "clean" dataset, since it will leave all those errors that are not illogical or outside plausible ranges.

Less obviously, but also importantly, apparent rates of a disease will be affected by the extent to which information on diagnosis, even when correct, is sufficiently precise to identify that particular disease, rather than a more vague or general category that includes the disease. Thus, for instance, malignant melanoma of the conjunctiva is coded in the **International Classification of Diseases** (ICD) to "malignant neoplasm of the conjunctiva" (ICD-9 code 190.3), but the same tumor described as

a melanoma of the eye would be coded in a different 4-digit code (190.9), and if stated simply as "melanoma" would be coded within a different 3-digit category (172.9). In more extreme circumstances, if the tumor were simply known to be an eye disorder, unspecified, it would be coded in a different ICD chapter (379.9), and if it caused a death that was certified as of unknown cause, it would be coded in another chapter again (799.9). All of these codes are therefore locations where melanomas of the conjunctiva could be allocated, depending on the precision of data available, and the extent to which conjunctival melanoma statistics are valid depends on the extent to which such tumors are precisely specified and coded.

When procedures are introduced to improve precision of information, artefactual increases will occur in rates of precise diagnostic categories. Conversely, discontinuation of such procedures will tend to reduce apparent rates. For instance, in England and Wales from 1881 to 1992, "medical enquiries" were sent to certifying medical practitioners, requesting more precise diagnostic information when a death certificate diagnosis was deemed to be too vague. When this enquiry procedure has been discontinued, for instance, in 1981–82 due to a strike of Registrars, large changes in apparent rates of precise diagnostic categories occurred [23]. The data user can attempt to take account of such changes, first by asking the data collecting agency whether they have used such procedures and when these have changed; secondly by calculating and assessing rates for relevant imprecise ("dustbin") categories in parallel with consideration of the precise category under investigation; and thirdly, by tabulating data by single calendar year and looking for step-changes in rates, which are likely to indicate artefacts (of many types).

As well as the quality of diagnostic data, and of denominators (see below), it is also important to consider data quality, both in source material and in data collection, for variables by which **stratification** or adjustment (*see* **Standardization Methods**) will be made in analysis; for instance, age, sex, and occupation. The percentage of individuals with missing data for such variables (especially age and sex) can provide a useful overall quality indicator, and the extent to which digit preference is present for age (i.e. an excess of ages ending in 0 or 5) can indicate the quality of the age information.

*Coding, Bridge-Coding, and Assignment of
Underlying Cause*

Interpretation of routine datasets is dependent on
understanding of the coding system used. This may
be an internationally accepted and accessible system,
such as the ICD [26], or, for instance often for operations or occupations, it may be a locally derived
classification, which may be difficult to access outside the country. Even when the coding system is
internationally agreed, there may be superimposed
upon it local interpretations and deliberate deviations.
Thus, in England and Wales, mortality coders use in
addition to the ICD, a large locally derived manual
with numerous instructions on actions to take for particular descriptions of disease where the ICD does
not give sufficient guidance, or the Registrar General
has decided that the ICD should not be followed.
Similarly, routine data agencies sometimes convert
data coded under one revision of a coding system to
another, and may not subsequently keep the originally coded data. Interpretation is then dependent on
the methods for, and quality of, the conversion as
well as the original coding. For instance, for disease
coding, since there is not an internationally agreed
ICD conversion system, local judgements will have
been made in the conversion, and these may be different from those that the investigator might have
chosen.

For underlying cause mortality statistics, the statistical agency must, as well as coding diseases, select
the "underlying cause" of death when more than
one disease is mentioned on the death certificate
(*see* **Cause of Death, Underlying and Multiple**).
Again, although there are internationally agreed rules
in the ICD for making this choice, local decisions are
likely to have been superimposed, and occasionally
the ICD rules may deliberately have been broken. For
instance, in England and Wales from 1984 to 1992,
Rule 3 of the ICD, concerning selection of the underlying cause of death, was deliberately set aside for
individuals with a "major cause" of death such as cancer in part II of the death certificate, but whose cause
of death under Rule 3 would have been a "terminal
event" such as heart failure or unspecified pneumonia. This change greatly increased apparent mortality
from several conditions – for instance a 44% increase
occurred in deaths from diabetes and a 22% increase
in deaths from multiple sclerosis [15].

The above issues will be compounded when a
data set has been formed by aggregation of records
collected and coded by several different agencies,
rather than only one: for instance, when data for a
national morbidity registration system are collected
and coded regionally, and then brought together to
form a national data set. Artefacts may then occur
from each coding source, and also secular disconti-
nuities may occur when there is a change in the level
of the hierarchy, e.g. regional vs. national, at which
coding is undertaken.

Data Processing and Editing Errors

Clerical processing may produce individual errors or
repeated ones. Computers offer the opportunity to
create large-scale errors in data at high speed. Often
the data have been processed in batches through several stages, and errors may arise if a particular batch
is incorrectly processed through a stage, or has a stage
omitted. Thus, for instance, cancer registration data
from registries using the International Classification
of Diseases for Oncology (ICD-O) coding system will
need to be re-coded if aggregate data from several
registries are to be held and analyzed in ICD-9. Since
most codes are the same in these two systems, it may
not be immediately obvious if a batch of data has not
been re-coded, but the presence of a code that exists
in ICD-O but is impossible in ICD-9 (ICD code 169)
should alert the user to a likely failure in re-coding.

Computer editing of data can also lead to artefacts.
Thus, unknown to the user, default values may have
been substituted for missing information. In analyses
of seasonality, for instance, such default coding for
month and day of birth can lead to an apparent
large peak of incidence in people born on June 30!
Similarly, many editing systems do not allow entry
of records with variables missing, and data coders
or processors may then invent values, when these
cannot be ascertained, to enable records to be entered
into the system. One should be suspicious that this
has occurred when large datasets, for instance on
national mortality, are published with apparently no
individuals with missing values.

Denominators

Rates calculated from routine data sources are
dependent on the quality of denominators, frequently
but not always derived from the census, as well as

on that of the numerators, to which more attention is often paid. Census data will tend to be reasonably accurate in Western countries, although for groups who are particularly difficult to count, e.g. vagrants, the very old, or immigrants, the quality of these data may be a more serious problem.

Inaccuracy may be a greater problem in population estimates for intercensal years, which need to take account of estimated migration, births and deaths since the last census count. Thus, for instance, Draper et al. [4] found apparent secular increases in childhood leukemia rates of 50% in non-Hispanic whites and 53% in blacks in Los Angeles based on population estimates relating to a previous census, but when the rates were recalculated with denominators that took account of a subsequent census, the increases became only 22% and 24%, respectively.

Numerator/Denominator Discrepancies

A greater problem than the completeness and accuracy of the denominator data is frequently their appropriateness and comparability with the numerator. When denominator data originate (as they usually do) from a different source to that used for the numerator, differences in quality, definitions, and data collection methods between these sources may lead to **bias**. For instance, a census might count university students at their term-time place of residence, but when ill they may return to their parental home for treatment, and hence rates for serious disease in young adults might be underestimated for university towns, especially those where a large proportion of the young population are students. Similarly, the occupational data recorded at the census for a man will usually be his own statement of his occupation, whereas on his death certificate the occupational description will inevitably have been given by someone other than himself, usually a relative. The relative may view the past career of the deceased in a flattering light, such that electricians may become electrical engineers, and nursing assistants become nurses, or the relative may report a more prestigious occupation that the deceased left many years ago by early retirement (for instance, military officer or aircraft pilot), rather than a current, less prestigious occupation that might have been reported at the census [14]. In studies of disease risk by country of birth, the census report of an individual's birthplace may be different from that in a relative's statement, and discrepancies can also arise because these two variables are collected at different times, and boundaries of countries can change over time.

Special Issues for Analysis of Clusters and Other Rare Events

As well as the general considerations above, some further issues apply mainly, or with more force, to analyses of spatial or temporal clusters and other rare events (*see* **Clustering**). One is that rates of rare events may be far more disrupted by occasional, random errors or duplications in a dataset than are statistics for the data overall. For instance, a low level of duplication of records can produce an apparently highly significant cluster of cases in a particular small area which is due simply to records for one or two individuals being recorded two or three times, even though overall rates of disease in the dataset will have been little affected by the duplication rate. Similarly, small rates of random **misclassification** between a common and a rare category will have a far greater impact on the rate in the rare category than the common one. For instance, breast cancer is about 100 times more common in women than men. If there is a 1% random error rate in categorization of sex in cancer registration data, this will approximately double the apparent number of breast cancers in men but have a negligible effect on the number in women. Similarly, small random error rates in coding (or data entry) of diagnosis may greatly inflate apparent rates of rare diseases, while having little impact on rates of common diseases.

These considerations suggest that a higher level of data quality is needed for valid analysis of rare categories or clusters than for common categories, and that an effort should be made to verify the original individual records before coming to conclusions on the presence of clusters of small numbers of cases, or rates of rare diseases, within routine datasets.

Record linkage

Many of the most interesting uses of routine statistics relate to linkage between datasets – for instance, linking a births file with a childhood or adult morbidity file to determine whether prenatal risk factors are associated with risk of later disease (*see* **Record Linkage**). It should be noted that the validity of the analyses will be dependent on both the quality of the two datasets to be linked, and the quality of the linkage. Such problems will be cumulated where the data for analysis are derived by successive linkage, in stages, through several data sets. For instance, in England and Wales notification of incident cancers in study cohorts can be obtained from the National Health Service Central Register (NHSCR); for childhood cancers it has been found that this is 12.5% incomplete, because of the cumulation of shortfalls of a few percent at each of the several stages at which the data are gained, transmitted or linked, starting from initial cancer registration by a regional cancer registry and ending with identification by NHSCR that the cancer occurred in a cohort member, and notification of this information to the investigator [9].

Conclusion

Most epidemiologists have had the disappointing experience of making an apparent discovery in a dataset, only to find on more careful examination that it was in fact due to a deficiency of quality in the data, or to a misunderstanding of the way in which the data were compiled. It is worth paying great heed to data quality, if only to try to ensure that as far as possible one's publications are not similarly in error. As Greenwood noted half a century ago in his discourse on this subject, "This may involve a little trouble – which is worth taking. One should *never* believe that a disease is becoming more, or less, deadly until all other explanations have been excluded" [7].

References

[1] Alderson, M. (1981). *International Mortality Statistics.* Macmillan, London.
[2] Brewster, D., Crichton. J. & Muir, C. (1994). How accurate are Scottish cancer registration data?, *British Journal of Cancer* **70**, 954–959.
[3] Cooper, J., Kendall, R., Gurland, B.J., Sharpe, L., Copeland, J.R.M. & Simon, R. (1972). *Psychiatric diagnoses in New York and London. A Comparative Study of Mental Health Admissions.* Maudsley Monograph No. 20. Maudsley, London.
[4] Draper, G.J., Kroll, M.E. & Stiller, C.A. (1994). Childhood cancer, in *Trends in Cancer Incidence and Mortality*. R. Doll, J.F. Fraumeni Jr & C.S. Muir, eds. Cancer Surveys, Vol. 19/20. Cold Spring Harbor Laboratory Press, New York, pp. 493–517.
[5] Fine, P.E.M. & Clarkson, J.A. (1982). Measles in England and Wales – II: The impact of the measles vaccination programme on the distribution of immunity in the population, *International Journal of Epidemiology* **11**, 15–25.
[6] Goldman, L., Sayson, R., Robbins, S., Cohn, L.H., Bettmann, M. & Weisberg, M. (1983). The value of the autopsy in three medical eras, *New England Journal of Medicine* **308**, 1000–1005.
[7] Greenwood, M. (1948). The sources and nature of statistical information in special fields of statistics. Medical statistics. *Journal of the Royal Statistical Society, Series A* **111**, 230–234.
[8] Grulich, A.E., Swerdlow, A.J. dos Santos Silva, I. & Beral, V. (1995). Is the apparent rise in cancer mortality in the elderly real? Analysis of changes in certification and coding of cause of death in England and Wales, 1970–1990, *International Journal of Cancer* **63**, 164–168.
[9] Hawkins, M.M. & Swerdlow, A.J. (1992). Completeness of cancer and death follow-up obtained through the National Health Service Central Register for England and Wales, *British Journal of Cancer* **66**, 408–413.
[10] Heasman, M.A. & Lipworth, L. (1966). *Accuracy of Certification of Cause of Death*, General Register Office SMPS no. 20. HMSO, London.
[11] Kelson, M.C. & Heller, R.F. on behalf of the EEC Working Party (1983). The effect of death certification and coding practices on observed differences in respiratory disease mortality in 8 EEC countries, *Revue d'Épidémiologie et de Santé Publique* **31**, 423–432.
[12] MacMahon, B. & Pugh, T.F. (1970). *Epidemiology. Principles and Methods.* Little, Brown & Company, Boston.
[13] Medico-Social Research Board (1979). The registration and certification of deaths in the West of Ireland, in *Annual Report 1979*. Medico-Social Research Board, Dublin, pp. 13–17.
[14] Office of Population Censuses and Surveys (1978). *Occupational Mortality. The Registrar General's Decennial Supplement for England and Wales, 1970–72.* Series DS no. 1. HMSO, London.
[15] Office of Population Censuses and Surveys (1985). *Mortality Statistics, Cause, England and Wales 1984.* Series DH2 no. 11. HMSO, London.
[16] Parkin, D.M. & Muir, C.S. (1992). Comparability and quality of data, in *Cancer Incidence in Five Continents*, Vol. VI, D.M. Parkin, C.S. Muir, S.L. Whelan, Y.T. Gao, J. Ferlay & J. Powell, eds. IARC Scientific Publication no 120. IARC Lyon, pp. 45–173.
[17] Percy, C. & Dolman, A. (1978). Comparison of the coding of death certificates related to cancer in seven countries, *Public Health Reports* **93**, 335–350.
[18] Powell, J. (1992). Techniques of registration, in *Cancer Incidence in Five Continents*. Vol. VI. D.M. Parkin, C.S. Muir, S.L. Whelan, Y.T. Gao, J. Ferlay & J. Powell, eds. IARC Scientific Publication no. 120. IARC, Lyon, pp. 3–24.

[19]   Raviglione, M.C., Snider, D.E. Jr & Kochi, A. (1995). Global epidemiology of tuberculosis. Morbidity and mortality of a worldwide epidemic, *Journal of the American Medical Association* **273**, 220–226.

[20]   Saxén, E.A. (1982). Trends: facts or fallacy, in *Trends in Cancer Incidence. Causes and Practical Implications*, K. Magnus, ed. Hemisphere, Washington, pp. 5–16.

[21]   Stocks, P. (1949). *Sickness in the Population of England and Wales in 1944–1947*. SMPS no. 2. HMSO, London.

[22]   Swerdlow, A.J. (1986). Cancer registration in England and Wales: some aspects relevant to interpretation of the data, *Journal of the Royal Statistical Society, Series A* **149**, 146–160.

[23]   Swerdlow, A.J. (1989). Interpretation of England and Wales cancer mortality data: the effect of enquiries to certifiers for further information, *British Journal of Cancer* **59**, 787–791.

[24]   Taylor, I. (1965). *The Notification of Infectious Diseases in Various Countries*. Public Health Papers 27. WHO, Geneva, pp. 17–68.

[25]   Weatherall, J.A.C. (1969). An assessment of the efficiency of notification of congenital malformations, *Medical Officer* **121**, 65–68.

[26]   World Health Organization (1977). *Manual of the International Statistical Classification of Diseases, Injuries, and Causes of Death*. WHO, Geneva.

A.J. Swerdlow

Day's Cumulative Rate *see* Standardization Methods

Death Certificate Studies *see* Occupational Mortality

Death Certification

The processes through which a civil registration and **vital statistics** system is informed of the facts about each death occurring within its coverage area may involve information supplied by several different informants. Relatives or friends may supply personal particulars of the deceased either directly to the civil registration authorities or indirectly through a funeral director or other intermediary who then gives the information to a civil registrar. However, the legal determination of the fact of death and the statement of the medical **causes of death** are usually the responsibility of an attending physician. In the absence of an attending physician or in the case of death resulting from actual or suspected violence (e.g. accident, suicide, homicide), a medical/legal officer usually investigates to determine the medical and legal facts of the case. In many civil registration systems, the medical/legal officer is known as a "coroner" or "medical examiner" whose specific responsibilities are prescribed by law. The physician or medical/legal officer is required to certify, to the best of his or her knowledge, that the death took place at the time and place specified and was due to the causes recorded on the death certificate. In some countries a shortage of trained medical personnel makes this process impossible or impractical to carry out, but in those vital statistics systems where deaths are attended just prior to death or reviewed after death by qualified medical practitioners, the World Health Organization (WHO) recommends a specific format and procedure for the certification of cause of death. The WHO recommendations are based on the concept that for each death occurring, one and only one "underlying cause of death" is to be determined, counted, and statistically analyzed (*see* **Cause of Death, Underlying and Multiple**). WHO defines the underlying cause of death as "(a) the disease or injury which initiated the train of morbid events leading directly to death, or (b) the circumstances of the accident or violence which produced the fatal injury". WHO further recommends the use of the International Form of Medical Certificate of Cause of Death (Figure 1), which is designed to facilitate the selection of the underlying cause of death based on the sequence of morbid events reported by the medical practitioner [1].

The medical certificate shown in Figure 1 provides a uniform format for the medical practitioner signing the death certificate to indicate which condition led directly to death and to report any antecedent conditions which gave rise to that condition. The medical certificate is designed to facilitate the selection of the underlying cause of death when two or more conditions are recorded. If only one condition is reported by the certifier, this single condition should be recorded on line (a) of Part I of the Medical Certificate of Cause of Death and is considered as the "originating antecedent cause". If there is more than

Cause of death		Approximate interval between onset and death
I Disease or condition directly leading to death*	(a) . . . . due to (or as a consequence of)	. . . .
Antecedent causes Morbid conditions, if any, giving rise to the above cause, stating the underlying condition last	(b) . . . . due to (or as a consequence of)	. . . .
	(c) . . . . due to (or as a consequence of)	. . . .
	(d)	. . . .
II Other significant conditions contributing to the death, but not related to the disease or condition causing it	. . . .	. . . .
This does not mean the mode of dying, e.g. heart failure, respiratory failure. It means the disease, injury, or complication that caused death.		

Figure 1 International Form of Medical Certificate of Cause of Death

one condition involved in the train of events leading to death, the direct cause is entered on line (a) and antecedent causes are entered on lines (b), and, if needed, (c) and (d). The lowest used line reflects the originating cause, and the causes entered on the other lines reflect, in sequence, the train of events leading to death. Therefore, in a properly completed Medical Certificate, the lowest used line in Part I is considered to be the originating antecedent cause. Usually, the originating antecedent cause corresponds to the underlying cause of death, the condition used for statistical tabulation and analysis. However, in some circumstances the originating antecedent cause may be superseded by a condition more suitable for use as the underlying cause of death. In cases where the certificate does not appear to be properly filled out (e.g. the reported sequence does not make medical sense, or the originating cause is a vague or nonspecific condition and there are other more specific conditions reported elsewhere on the certificate), there is a set of international rules promulgated by WHO for selecting an underlying cause

of death. The selected underlying cause may then be modified by additional rules to make it more useful for statistical and epidemiologic purposes. These rules are particularly useful when it is impractical or impossible to query the medical practitioner who completed the certificate in order to obtain clarification or a more definitive description of the conditions leading to the death. While the rules may, in individual cases, appear to be arbitrary, they are intended to yield improved mortality statistics overall.

When determining the underlying cause of death from conditions recorded on a medical certificate, the international rules and guidelines first call for the application of the General Principle, which states, "... when more than one condition is entered on the certificate, the condition entered alone on the lowest used line of Part I should be selected only if it could have given rise to all of the conditions entered above it". If the General Principle does not apply, there are three Selection Rules that are to be applied sequentially until an originating antecedent cause is identified. However, that originating cause may not be the most useful and informative condition for statistical tabulation and analysis. For example, if senility or a generalized disease such as hypertension has been selected, this is less useful than if a reported manifestation of the aging process or of the hypertension had been chosen. Further, it might be necessary to modify the selected condition to conform with the requirements of the **International Classification of Diseases (ICD)**, either because a single code in the classification might represent two or more conditions that were both reported, or because the classification may give priority to a particular cause when it is reported with certain other conditions. Accordingly, there are six Modification Rules intended to improve the utility of mortality data. The Modification Rules are applied after the selection of the originating antecedent condition. Some Modification Rules require further application of the Selection Rules, resulting in an iterative process of selection, modification, and, if necessary, reselection before an underlying cause of death is determined [2].

In the case of perinatal deaths, WHO recommends a special Certificate of Cause of Perinatal Death. This certificate provides a section for the medical certifier to list diseases or conditions in the fetus or infant as well as maternal diseases or conditions which affected the fetus or infant. In the 10th Revision of the International Classification of Diseases (ICD-10), the perinatal period is defined as the period beginning at 22 completed weeks of gestation and ending at seven completed days after birth. WHO provides a special set of rules for the certification of deaths occurring during this period [3].

References

[1] World Health Organization (1967). *WHO Nomenclature Regulations*. World Health Organization, Geneva.

[2] World Health Organization (1992). *International Statistical Classification of Diseases and Related Health Problems*, 10th rev., Vol. 2. World Health Organization, Geneva, pp. 30–88.

[3] World Health Organization (1992). *International Statistical Classification of Diseases and Related Health Problems*, 10th rev., Vol. 2. World Health Organization, Geneva, pp. 89–96.

ROBERT A. ISRAEL

Death Indexes

An important aspect of follow-up studies (*see* **Cohort Study**) is the ability to determine which members of the original study cohort have been lost to follow-up because of death, and for many such studies, in addition to the fact of death, the **cause of death** is an essential piece of information. In places where a central register of all deaths is compiled (e.g. population register, or civil registration system) and is available for research use, the identification of individuals in a study who have died during some time period can be accomplished, provided that the necessary identifying information is available. However, even under relatively ideal circumstances, it is sometimes difficult to match study individuals against lists of deaths with 100% certainty that a correct match has been achieved. Most follow-up studies try to match on several variables (e.g. surname, given name, date of birth, mother's maiden name, etc.) and develop algorithms to establish "presumptive matches".

While the fact of death is, in most jurisdictions, considered public information, the cause of death may in some places be considered confidential and not releasable to researchers without the expressed permission of a next of kin or legal representative of the deceased. Because of confidentiality provisions, some custodians of death files require study protocols to be reviewed for adequate privacy safeguards before authorizing the release of cause of death data.

In a few countries, the problem of adequate follow-up for deaths occurring amongst a cohort is further complicated by the existence of only decentralized death files. A notable example of this is the US where the primary responsibility for registration of vital events rests with the individual states. For many years it was necessary for "death clearance" of study cohorts for researchers to send their list of study participants to each of the more than 50 registration areas to determine if any of their subjects had died there during some stated period of time. This was a costly and time-consuming process and tended to stifle certain kinds of epidemiologic research. In addition, each state has its own laws and procedures regarding confidentiality and release of information. Therefore, in spite of the fact that there was a central statistical file for national **vital statistics** purposes located at the US National

Center for Health Statistics, the states provided their data with the restriction that the Center not release individual record information without the consent of the states. After lengthy negotiations, an agreement between the states and the National Center for Health Statistics resulted in a US National Death Index which was designed to address these issues. To utilize this index, researchers submit their study protocol to a committee comprising selected state registration officials, federal officials, and representatives of the health research community. If this committee determines that the proposed study is bona fide research and not a commercial activity, and includes appropriate steps to protect confidential information and privacy, the protocol is approved and sent to the Director, National Center for Health Statistics, for final approval. Once the study has been approved, the National Center receives annual lists of study participants from researchers containing the required variables for computer matching against the statistical file of deaths (*see* **Record Linkage**). For each "presumptive match", the researcher receives information about the date, place of death, and death certificate registration number along with some details of the degree of agreement between the required variables. If the study requires cause of death information or other information from the death certificates, the researcher receives enough information to contact the appropriate State Registration Officials to request copies of the pertinent death certificates.

The US National Death Index has been in operation since data year 1979 and has significantly improved follow-up procedures for studies conducted in the US. It has reduced the necessary time and costs of efficient identification of deaths occurring in national follow-up study cohorts.

ROBERT A. ISRAEL

Deconfounding Principle in Control Selection *see* Case–Control Study

Decrement Function *see* Life Table

Deep Models for Screening *see* Screening, Models of

Demography

Demography is the study of human populations with respect to their size, structure, and dynamics. For demographers, a population is a group of individuals that coexist at a point in time and share a defining characteristic such as residence in the same geographical area. The structure or composition of a population refers to the distribution of its members by age, sex, and other characteristics, such as place of residence and marital or health status. The age and sex structure of a population results from past trends in fertility, mortality, and migration. Thus, these processes comprise the components of demographic change. The age and sex structure of a population, in turn, affects birth rates, death rates, and rates of migration. Changes in status such as getting married or divorced interact with population structure in a similar way.

Some authorities reserve the term demography for the mathematical and statistical study of the interrelationships between population size and structure and the components of demographic change. According to this terminology, demography can be contrasted with population studies, which investigate the determinants and consequences of demographic phenomena drawing on the concepts and theories of disciplines such as the social sciences, health sciences, and history. Others encompass population studies within demography and use the term *formal demography* to distinguish the statistical core of the discipline. Demography (according to this wider definition) is a multidisciplinary field: subdisciplines such as economic demography, historical demography, anthropological demography, and mathematical demography exist. They differ not only in their subject of study but also in their theoretical orientation and methods.

The term demography has been ascribed to a Belgian statistician, Achille Guillard, who coined it in 1855. However, the origins of modern demography are usually traced back to John Graunt's quantitative analyses of the "Bills of Mortality" published in 1662 [5]. The "Bills of Mortality" provided weekly lists of burials and baptisms in the parishes of London. Graunt used these data to examine the sex ratio at birth and to estimate the population of London. He showed that more deaths than births occurred in London, implying that the growth of the capital was due to in-migration from the countryside. He also estimated the proportion of births surviving to a range of ages, thereby developing the basic concept of the **life table**. Graunt's research prefigures modern applications of demographic science: information on fertility and mortality and population estimates for small areas remain the fundamental results of demographic analysis required by those engaged in policy formulation and planning.

Demographic Data

In most developed countries, civil registration of births and deaths is the primary source of fertility and mortality data. Government agencies routinely collect demographic information when births and deaths are certified for administrative purposes (*see* **Vital Statistics, Overview**). The primary source of data on the size, structure and distribution of national populations is the population census. Censuses aim to enumerate the whole population of a defined geographical area. They collect individual-level data on the population's characteristics that refer to a single point in time. As well as collecting data on the size and composition of the population, most censuses also ask about moves in a fixed period of time before the enumeration. In countries where vital statistics data are incomplete, questions may also be asked about fertility and mortality. Countries that issue identity numbers and require their population to report their place of residence can maintain continuous population registers. In a few European countries these registers now fuse the functions of the registration system with those of the census.

The evolution of demographic analysis and of routine collection of data on populations by the government were interlinked. Standard demographic measures and techniques of analysis were developed largely for the study of vital statistics with census-based denominators. In recent decades, however, demographers have relied increasingly on survey data to supplement those from traditional sources. In particular, in countries where registration of vital events is incomplete national **sample surveys** are the main source of vital statistics. One of the first subjects to be investigated in demographic surveys was family planning. Other early surveys collected women-based fertility histories to supplement the event-based data generated by birth registration. Fertility history and family planning data remain the focus of many demographic surveys, including the two major international programs of surveys conducted since the 1970s, namely the World Fertility Survey and the Demographic and Health Surveys.

Issues

Between the mid-nineteenth and mid-twentieth centuries the more developed regions of the world went through a *demographic transition* from a high-fertility, high-mortality, and low-growth demographic regime to a low-fertility, low-mortality, and low-growth demographic regime. As mortality tended to fall before fertility, this transition was marked by rapid population growth. Since 1945, a similar transition has begun in most less developed countries. As a result, the world's population has grown from about 2.5 billion to about 6 billion in the second half of the twentieth century. It is expected to grow to between 9 and 16 billion by 2100.

Efforts to understand the determinants of the transition of fertility and mortality to low levels are a central concern of demography. Many demographers now believe that explanations that focus on economic factors and the provision of health and family planning programs are inadequate and need to be supplemented by accounts that take into account the ideational and cultural determinants of demographic behavior.

Thomas Malthus was the first author to develop a systematic argument that high fertility leading to population growth could have adverse effects on economic welfare [7]. He argued that a growing population must eventually outstrip its subsistence base, bringing about rising mortality from famine, pestilence, and war. Although the past two centuries of human history have followed a very different path from that envisaged by Malthus, concern still exists about the impact of population growth on economic development and the environment. Today, however, economic demographers tend to be more sanguine about the consequences of population growth than those with a background in ecology [3].

Many demographic outcomes are of concern to policy makers and much demographic research has an avowedly applied intent. Demography bears on the efforts of international agencies and national governments to promote family planning and improve health in the developing world. In the developed world, population growth has slowed but low fertility and the reduction in death rates in old age are producing an increasingly aged population. Recent changes in patterns of marriage and divorce and of childbearing inside and outside marriage also have major implications for the family and public policy.

Demographic studies of mortality tend to focus on the analysis of routine data. Demographers' research into health and mortality cannot be distinguished clearly from that of epidemiologists. However, demographers tend to be concerned with the distribution of disease and premature death (*see* **Descriptive Epidemiology**) across social groups and their implications for other aspects of social life, rather than with measuring risk factors for specific conditions.

Demographic Analysis

The aim of formal demographic analysis is to isolate the components of demographic patterns by dividing a population into relatively homogeneous subgroups. Analysis by age and sex has primacy over analysis by other compositional factors. Human biology causes the propensity to die and to give birth to be differentiated by age and sex everywhere. It imposes a degree of uniformity on age patterns of mortality and fertility in all human populations.

Classical demographic analysis is based on a fairly small set of measures and techniques. Most of these are also used in cognate disciplines. Calculation of **rates**, ratios, and proportions represent the basic way for controlling for population size. In demography, rates calculated for the whole population that make no allowance for the influence of population structure on the phenomenon of interest are referred to as *crude rates*. Examples are the crude birth rate and crude death rate (*see* **Vital Statistics, Overview**).

Calculation of age-specific rates and rates specific to other subgroups of the population allow the analyst to isolate the propensity to experience the event being studied from the influence of population structure. A range of methods of standardization are used

to produce synthetic indices that summarize such specific rates (*see* **Standardization Methods**). The distinction between cohort analysis and **cross-sectional** or period analysis is fundamental to demography. Demographers use the term *cohort* to refer to groups of individuals who experience a defining event at the same time. Examples include **birth cohorts** and marriage cohorts. Cohort analysis studies the subsequent experience of such groups. This contrasts with epidemiologic usage, which refers to all those eligible for recruitment into a longitudinal study as a **cohort**.

Period measures are often treated as referring to a synthetic or hypothetical cohort, so that summary indices can be calculated that indicate what would happen to a cohort that went through life experiencing the specific rates of the period under study. For example, the most widely used index of period fertility is the *total fertility rate*. This measures how many children women would bear on average if they went through life with the fertility of a specific period. It is calculated by summing the age-specific fertility rates of a particular year, usually for five-year age groups, over all ages at which women bear children. The total fertility rate is thus a form of directly standardized rate, calculated using a uniform age distribution as the standard.

Two basic aspects of any demographic process are its intensity, or quantum, and its timing, or tempo. The intensity of a nonrenewable event such as death or first marriage can be measured by the proportion of a cohort who eventually experience the event. Both the expected timing of any nonrenewable process and the distribution of times of its occurrence can be studied using **life table** methods. The intensity of a renewable process such as birth or disease incidence can be measured by the mean number of events per person, and their tempo by the characteristics of the distribution of the events in time. Renewable events can be categorized by the order of their occurrence, and events of a particular order can be analyzed as a nonrenewable process. For example, the proportion of women who have had a birth of order i that go on to bear a child of order $i + 1$ is known as a *parity progression ratio*.

Investigation of the determinants of fertility and mortality has been facilitated by making a distinction between proximate and distal determinants. The approach is most developed with respect to fertility. A proximate determinant is one that has a direct impact on the outcome of interest while a distal determinant can only affect the outcome via a proximate determinant. The proximate determinants of fertility are those factors that determine a woman's exposure to sexual intercourse, her probability of conceiving, and the probability that a pregnancy ends in a live birth. The strength of the approach is that only a few of the proximate determinants of individuals' fertility differ between populations in their impact at the aggregate level. Thus, the four main proximate determinants of fertility differences between groups and over time are the proportion of women in sexual unions, postpartum infecundity associated with breast-feeding, contraception, and abortion. Socioeconomic determinants of fertility must operate through these few proximate factors and a single characteristic may have countervailing effects on fertility via different proximate determinants.

Demographic Models

Analysis of data on actual populations is paralleled by mathematical models of the interrelationship between population size and structure and the components of demographic change. Stable population theory as developed by Lotka in the 1920s and 1930s demonstrates that any closed single-sex population subject to constant fertility and mortality rates converges on an unchanging age structure and a constant rate of growth. This stable outcome is independent of the initial age structure of the population. The special case of a stable population that is unchanging in size is termed a *stationary population*. Its age structure is a function of the life table. Recent developments, known as generalized stable population theory, demonstrate that the mathematics of stable populations can be extended to populations in which growth rates vary by age because of a history of fertility and mortality change and to populations subject to decrements other than mortality [8].

One crucial application of demography is to the forecasting of future population change. This is usually undertaken using cohort-component methods of population projection [2]. These methods provide a precise way of controlling for the influence of population structure and of working out the implications of any scenario postulated for future vital rates. Despite this, population forecasts have often proved wide of the mark. Fertility, mortality, and migration remain difficult to predict. Forecasts informed by a theoretical understanding of the determinants of these components of population change often perform little better than the simple extrapolation of past trends in vital rates.

The increasing availability of survey data and information technology that makes it practicable to undertake individual-level analysis of data on large samples, have facilitated convergence between demographic methods and other forms of statistical analysis. Thus, many of the developments in demographic analysis during the past few decades have been closely linked to those in statistical methods more generally. Demographers have both adopted and contributed to the development of methods such as event history analysis [10], the modeling of unobserved heterogeneity, and random-effects models [4]. Other fields of methodologic research in recent years include the extension of life table methods into multistate models that allow for increments as well as decrements from each state [6] and methods and models for the study of families and households [1].

One particularly successful field has been the development of indirect methods for estimating vital rates in populations with limited and defective vital statistics [9]. Indirect methods use stable population theory and its extensions to describe the relationship between conventional indices of fertility, mortality, and migration and items of information that can be collected more reliably in single-round surveys and censuses in less developed countries. For example, it is possible to estimate life table indices of child mortality from data on the proportion of women's children ever-born who have died, tabulated by the age of the women concerned [9].

References

[1]   Bongaarts, J., Burch, T. & Wachter, K., eds. (1987). *Family Demography: Methods and their Applications.* Clarendon Press, Oxford.

[2]   Brass, W. (1974). Perspectives in population prediction, *Journal of the Royal Statistical Society, Series A,* **137**, 532–583.

[3]   Cassen, R. (1994). Overview, in *Population and Development: Old Debates, New Conclusions*, R. Cassen and contributors. Transaction, Oxford.

[4]   Goldstein, H. (1995). *Multilevel Statistical Models.* Edward Arnold, London.

[5]   Graunt, J. (1964). *Natural and Political Observations Mentioned in a Following Index, and Made upon the*

Bills of Mortality. London, 1662. Reprinted, with an introduction by B. Benjamin, in *Journal of the Institute of Actuaries* **90**, 1–61.

[6]   Land, K.C. & Rogers, A., eds (1982). *Multidimensional Mathematical Demography*. Academic Press, New York.

[7]   Malthus, T.R. (1970). *An Essay on the Principle of Population* (London, 1798), A. Flew, ed. Penguin, Harmondsworth.

[8]   Preston, S.H. & Coale, A.J. (1982). Age structure, growth, attrition, and accession: a new synthesis, *Population Index* **48**, 217–259.

[9]   United Nations (1983). *Indirect Techniques for Demographic Estimation*. ST/ESA/Series A/81. United Nations, New York.

[10]   Yamaguchi, K. (1991). *Event History Analysis*. Sage, London.

IAN M. TIMÆUS

Density Sampling

Density sampling is a method of sampling **controls** in a **case–control study**. Controls are sampled from the population at risk at the times of incidence of each case or, as is more common in practice, over the period of accrual of the cases. Time-matched analysis of such case–control data yields unbiased estimates of the **relative hazard** (or **incidence density ratio**), even when the disease is common [1–4]. An advantage of density sampling is that it can reduce **bias** from secular changes in the **prevalence** of exposure during the course of the study [1].

References

[1]   Greenland, S. & Thomas, D.C. (1982). On the need for the rare disease assumption in case–control studies, *American Journal of Epidemiology* **116**, 547–553.

[2]   Miettinen, O.S. (1976). Estimability and estimation in case-reference studies, *American Journal of Epidemiology* **103**, 226–235.

[3]   Prentice, R.L. & Breslow, N.E. (1978). Retrospective studies and failure time models, *Biometrika* **65**, 153–158.

[4]   Sheehe, P.R. (1962). Dynamic risk analysis in retrospective matched pair studies of disease, *Biometrics* **18**, 323–341.

M.H. GAIL

Descriptive Epidemiology

Descriptive epidemiology is the study of the incidence and **prevalence** of diseases and associated mortality in populations. Unlike **analytic epidemiology**, descriptive epidemiologic studies usually do not rely on individual-level data, for example on exposures, disease outcome, and potential **confounders**. Instead, descriptive studies estimate the risk of disease in various groups defined by age, gender, and ethnicity, evaluate time trends in disease rates, identify geographic localization of populations with high rates of disease (*see* **Geographic Patterns of Disease**), and attempt to correlate disease rates in populations with features of the population, such as the average level of exposure to a potential carcinogen. Descriptive studies are used to determine the effectiveness of programs to control disease, and descriptive studies are used to generate etiologic hypotheses that are then tested in analytic studies (*see* **Age–Period–Cohort Analysis**; **Correlational Study**; **Ecologic Study**).

M.H. GAIL

Detection Bias

Detection (also called diagnostic or unmasking) bias results from closer follow-up or more intense scrutiny of one comparison group than another. In a **case–control study**, the detection of a higher proportion of subclinical outcomes among the exposed leads to an overrepresentation of exposed cases relative to exposed controls in the study population. In a **cohort study**, as subjects are followed over time for the occurrence of a disease, subjects who develop unrecognized subclinical disease would be misclassified as nondiseased. If exposed subjects are under greater scrutiny than the unexposed, then they may be less likely to have such undiagnosed subclinical disease. This implies that detection bias can lead to **selection bias** in a case–control study, and can also be a source of differential misclassification in a follow-up study (*see* **Misclassification Error**).

HOLLY A. HILL & DAVID G. KLEINBAUM

Diagnostic Bias *see* Validity and Generalizability in Epidemiologic Studies

Diagnostic Test Evaluation Without a Gold Standard

Diagnostic tests are an important part of medical decision making. In daily clinical practice many tests are performed to obtain diagnoses. To interpret a test it is important to realize that a negative answer does not always mean that the disease is absent, because false negative results may occur. Also, a positive result does not always mean that disease is present. A finding usually associated with a disease sometimes occurs in patients who do not have the disease: a false positive result.

A perfect test is positive in all patients with the disease and negative in all patients who do not have the disease. Usually this test is referred to as the gold standard. After applying the gold standard test one knows which patients have the disease and which patients are free of it. However, most tests are imperfect. Measures to assess the performance of a diagnostic test are **sensitivity** and **specificity**. The sensitivity of a test is defined as the proportion of positive test results in those with the disease. The specificity is defined as the proportion of negative test results in those without the disease. To measure the sensitivity and specificity of a test for a disease, the test's results are compared with those on a gold standard test, as shown in Table 1. The sensitivity is the ratio of the number of patients with true positive tests and the number of diseased patients. The specificity is the ratio of the number of patients with false negative tests and the number of nondiseased patients.

Problems arise when the sensitivity and the specificity of the reference test are unknown. The 2×2 table of test vs. reference test contains too little information to estimate all unknown parameters, even if the **prevalence** of the disease is known.

Hui & Walter [4] pointed out that the parameters can still be estimated for two tests if data can be collected from populations with different prevalences and it can be assumed that the test errors are conditionally independent given the disease status. A general discussion can be found in the paper of Faraone & Tsuang [3].

Notation

Let D stand for disease status; $D = 1$ if diseased and $D = 0$ if not. Let T_i stand for the result of test i, $i = 1$ or 2; $T_i = 1$ if the test is positive and $T_i = 0$ if the test is negative. The sensitivity of test i is denoted by SENS_i and the specificity by SPEC_i, i.e. $\text{SENS}_i = \Pr(T_i = 1 | D = 1)$ and $\text{SPEC}_i = \Pr(T_i = 0 | D = 0)$. Let there be G subpopulations (groups) indexed by g with prevalences $\pi_g = \Pr(D = 1 | \text{group } g)$. Under conditional independence of T_1 and T_2 given D, the probabilities in the $T_1 \times T_2$ contingency table in group g are given by

$$
\begin{aligned}
\Pr(T_1 &= t_1, T_2 = t_2 | \text{group } g) \\
&= \pi_g \times \text{SENS}_1^{t_1} \times (1 - \text{SENS}_1)^{1-t_1} \\
&\quad \times \text{SENS}_2^{t_2} \times (1 - \text{SENS}_2)^{1-t_2} \\
&\quad + (1 - \pi_g) \times (1 - \text{SPEC}_1)^{t_1} \times \text{SPEC}_1^{1-t_1} \\
&\quad \times (1 - \text{SPEC}_2)^{t_2} \times \text{SPEC}_2^{1-t_2}.
\end{aligned}
\tag{1}
$$

Estimation

The n_g observations in group g follow a 4-nomial distribution with these probabilities for the four cells.

Table 1 The relationship between the results of a test and gold standard

Results of test for disease under study	Results of gold standard		Total
	Disease present	Disease absent	
Positive	True positive	False positive	Positive tests
Negative	False negative	True negative	Negative tests
Total	Diseased patients	Nondiseased patients	

The number of parameters is $G + 4$ (G prevalences, two sensitivities, and two specificities). The number of degrees of freedom is $3G$, so the minimal requirement for identifiability of the model is that $G \geq 2$. If at least two prevalences are different, identifiability is indeed obtained, provided that it is assumed that SENS + SPEC > 1. (See [4] for the invariance of the problem under "reflection with respect to 1/2".) The parameters can be obtained by direct maximum likelihood applied to the joint likelihood of the G tables, as proposed by Hui & Walter [4] for the case when $G = 2$.

In de Bock et al. [1] it is shown that the estimation problem can be solved elegantly by the expectation-maximization (EM) algorithm [2]. Multinomial distributions with amalgamated cells is one of the examples given in that paper. The EM algorithm considers the true disease status D of all individuals as the missing observation. If this information were available, the data for each group could be conveyed in the $2 \times 2 \times 2$ table of $T_1 \times T_2 \times D$.

The M-step of the EM algorithm estimates all parameters in a straightforward way. Let $X_{g,ijk}$ be the number in the ijk-cell of the gth $2 \times 2 \times 2$ table. The index i (0, 1) corresponds to T_1, index j to test T_2, and k to disease D. Let "+" stand for summation; then the estimates are given by

$$\hat{\pi}_g = X_{g,++1} / X_{g,+++}, \qquad (2)$$

$$\widehat{\text{SENS}}_1 = \sum_g X_{g,1+1} \Big/ \sum_g X_{g,++1},$$

i.e.
$$\frac{\text{number positive on } T_1 \text{ and diseased}}{\text{number diseased}}, \qquad (3)$$

and

$$\widehat{\text{SPEC}}_1 = \sum_g X_{g,0+0} \Big/ \sum_g X_{g,++0},$$

i.e.
$$\frac{\text{number negative on } T_1 \text{ and not diseased}}{\text{number not diseased}}, \qquad (4)$$

and similarly for SENS$_2$ and SPEC$_2$.

In the E-step, the full table $X_{g,ijk}$ is reconstructed from the available table $X_{g,ij+}$ by

$$\hat{X}_{g,ijk} = \hat{P}(D = k | T_1 = i, T_2 = j, \text{ group} = g)$$
$$\times X_{g,ij+}. \qquad (5)$$

In the estimated probabilities $\hat{P}$ the parameter estimates from the previous step are used.

For example,

$$\hat{P}(D = 1 | T_1 = 1, T_2 = 1, \text{group} = g)$$

$$= \frac{\hat{\pi}_g \times \widehat{\text{SENS}}_1 \times \widehat{\text{SENS}}_2}{\left\{ \begin{array}{l} \hat{\pi}_g \times \widehat{\text{SENS}}_1 \times \widehat{\text{SENS}}_2 + (1 - \hat{\pi}_g) \\ \times (1 - \widehat{\text{SPEC}}_1) \times (1 - \widehat{\text{SPEC}}_2) \end{array} \right\}} . \qquad (6)$$

The EM algorithm converges in a slow but sure way to the maximum likelihood estimator (MLE). The process can be stopped if the increase in total log likelihood is smaller than some prespecified ε. To compute the standard errors of the estimated parameter, second derivatives of log likelihood have to be used as in Hui & Walter [4]. The advantages of EM are that it is very easy to program, and that the estimates never exceed the boundaries of the parameter space.

Generalizations

De Bock et al. [1] generalized the situation sketched above to the case where there are more than two tests, and in each group test results are available for precisely two tests. The generalization of the EM algorithm is straightforward.

A second generalization can be made by relaxing the condition of conditional independence. The model can be extended by introducing **odds ratios** lambda (λ) in the conditional 2×2 tables to model the dependency. The simplest model is when λ is constant. An extension would be to have different λs for diseased ($D = 1$) and not diseased ($D = 0$). See LeCessie & van Houwelingen [5] for a general discussion on modeling dependence in 2×2 tables.

References

[1] de Bock, G.H., Houwing-Duistermaat, J.J., Springer, M.P., Kievit, J. & van Houwelingen, J.C. (1994). Sensitivity and specificity of diagnostics tests in acute maxillary sinusitis determined by maximum likelihood in the absence of an external standard, *Journal of Clinical Epidemiology* **47**, 1343–1352.

[2] Dempster, A.P., Laird, N.M. & Rubin, D.B. (1977). Maximum likelihood for incomplete data via the EM-algorithm, *Journal of the Royal Statistical Society, Series B* **39**, 1–38.

[3] Faraone, S.V. & Tsuang, M.T. (1994). Measuring diagnostic accuracy in the absence of a gold standard, *American Journal of Psychiatry* **151**, 650–657.

[4]   Hui, S.L., & Walter, S.D. (1980). Estimating error rates of diagnostic tests, *Biometrics* **36**, 167–171.
[5]   LeCessie, S. & van Houwelingen, J.C. (1994). Logistic regression for correlated binary data, *Applied Statistics* **43**, 95–108.

(*See also* **Diagnostic Tests, Evaluation of**)

G.H. DE BOCK & J.C. VAN HOUWELINGEN

Diagnostic Tests, Evaluation of

The field of diagnostic medicine is complex. In part, this is due to the fact that the process of medical diagnosis is dynamic, and it is difficult to formulate straightforward scientific questions amenable to simple study designs. For example, in interpreting the result of an individual test the doctor must consider the context in which it is applied. Has it been selected to rule-in or rule-out a diagnosis? What other tests have already been performed and what were their results? What options are available for performing subsequent tests? What are the characteristics of the patient that might predispose to the diagnosis under consideration? The evaluation of a test in the context of other tests is addressed elsewhere. In this article, discussion is limited to evaluation studies of individual tests, or comparisons of two alternative tests. Furthermore, we consider only *diagnostic* tests, i.e. tests of symptomatic patients in which we wish to rule-in or rule-out a candidate diagnosis. This contrasts with *screening* tests, performed on asymptomatic normal subjects, e.g. the use of mammography on a population at risk of breast cancer (*see* **Screening, Models of**; **Screening, Overview**).

Many diagnostic tests, especially radiologic and psychometric tests, are evaluated subjectively, leading typically to test results that are classified in ordinal categories which are defined verbally. This contrasts with tests which possess quantitative results, as is the case for most laboratory tests. In either case, a useful conceptual device is to consider the test as having an underlying continuous scale, which may be discretized into ordinal categories either by judgment or by arithmetic rounding. The underlying continuous scale provides a metric for trading off the two different kinds of errors of diagnosis, false positives and false negatives, and thus for establishing a scale on which to calibrate the results of alternate tests for the purposes of comparison. The notation defined below reflects this assumption. There are various outcomes that can in principle be used to evaluate and compare the utility of medical diagnostic tests. The ultimate outcome involves evaluating whether use of the test, and the subsequent impact on medical therapy, leads to improvements in the natural history of the disease, e.g. lower mortality from the disease. It is rare for tests to be evaluated against this standard. Even studies of the impact of individual diagnostic tests on patient management are unusual. Overwhelmingly, medical researchers have been satisfied with evaluating tests on the basis of measures of diagnostic accuracy. In the following we thus limit attention to the issue of diagnostic accuracy.

Measures of Accuracy

Consider a diagnostic test result denoted x, and let D be a binary indicator of the "true" disease status, where $D = 1$ represents disease and $D = 0$ represents absence of disease. Let $F_x(x) = \Pr(X \leq x | D = 1)$ be the distribution of the test result in diseased cases, and let $G_x(x) = \Pr(X \leq x | D = 0)$ be the corresponding distribution in "control" subjects, i.e. patients suspected of having the disease who are candidates for testing in the relevant medical context. The most commonly used measures of accuracy are based on a binary classification of the test result. Suppose that the classification point is x, i.e. the test is positive if $X > x$ and negative otherwise. Then the **sensitivity** of the test is defined to be the proportion of diseased patients who are classified as diseased, i.e. $1 - F_x(x)$. The **specificity** is the corresponding proportion of control patients who are classified as normal, i.e. $G_x(x)$ [28]. High values of the sensitivity and the specificity indicate an accurate test.

There are several other measures in common usage related to the sensitivity and specificity. The *false positive ratio* is the specificity subtracted from 1, i.e. $1 - G_x(x)$. The *false negative ratio* is the sensitivity subtracted from 1, i.e. $1 - F_x(x)$. "Prospective" measures of accuracy are defined in terms of the conditional probabilities that the patient is diseased given the test results [25]. Thus the **positive predictive value** is

$$
\begin{aligned}
&\Pr(D = 1 | X \geq x) \\
&= \frac{\pi(1 - F_x(x))}{\pi[1 - F_x(x)] + (1 - \pi)[1 - G_x(x)]},
\end{aligned}
$$

where $\pi = \Pr(D = 1)$ is the "prior" probability of disease, i.e. the **prevalence** of disease in the population under study. Likewise the negative predictive value is defined to be

$$
\Pr(D = 0 | X \leq x) = \frac{(1 - \pi)G_x(x)}{(1 - \pi)G_x(x) + \pi F_x(x)}.
$$

In fact, the term "accuracy" is often used in medical circles to mean the overall relative frequency of correct diagnosis in a study. That is, if $A(x)$ is the accuracy, then

$$
A(x) = \pi[1 - F_x(x)] + (1 - \pi)G_x(x).
$$

Finally, the likelihood ratio can be used to represent the extent to which the odds of disease is altered as a result of the test, via Bayes' Theorem [21]. In the context of a binary test there are two likelihood ratios, corresponding to a negative and a positive test result, $F_x(x)/G_x(x)$ and $[1 - F_x(x)]/[1 - G_x(x)]$, respectively.

Clearly, all of these measures are limited by the fact that they correspond to a specific, and possibly arbitrary, classification point, x. For the likelihood ratio in particular, knowledge of the actual test result, X, leads obviously to a more appropriate factor for updating using Bayes Theorem, i.e. $f_X(X)/g_X(X)$, where $f_X(\cdot)$ and $g_X(\cdot)$ are the corresponding density functions of the test result. Likewise, changing the classification point will either increase the sensitivity at the expense of the specificity, or vice versa, with corresponding effects on the error rates and the predictive values. The arbitrariness of the classification point is especially a problem when diagnostic tests are being compared, or when the same test is used in different studies with different classification points since the classifications for the two tests are unlikely to be "calibrated" in practice (see later discussion). For this reason receiver operating characteristic (ROC) curve analysis has become a preferred method for evaluating and comparing tests. The ROC curve is a plot of $F_x(x)$ vs. $G_x(x)$. If the ROC plot lies along the 45° line, then the test is random and hence uninformative. The higher the curve lies above the 45° line, the more accurate is the test. Thus the area under the curve is often used as a measure of accuracy that does not require a specific classification point. The area, A, is given by

$$
A = 1 - \int_0^1 F_x(x) \mathrm{d}G_x(x). \tag{1}
$$

The area can be interpreted as the probability that a randomly chosen diseased subject has a test result that is greater than that of a randomly chosen control subject [12].

Biases

Despite the availability of the various measures of accuracy described in the previous Section, diagnostic tests are characterized predominantly by their sensitivities and specificities in the literature. These are often reported on the basis of a **retrospective** analysis of a series of patients treated in a hospital or clinic, and may suffer from incomplete reporting of study details, especially the factors affecting selection of patients for inclusion in the analysis. However, regardless of the quality of the studies, it is empirically evident that the ranges of values reported for the sensitivity and specificity of any important diagnostic test are usually very wide. A typical example is presented in the meta-analysis of the use of myelography for the detection of lumbar disk herniation, where the sensitivity estimates ranged from 75% to 98%, and the specificity estimates ranged from 20% to 100% [15]. Wide variation in reported estimates is due to the fact that studies of diagnostic test accuracy are plagued by a number of common **biases** [3]. These have been studied extensively in recent years, and various methods have been proposed for providing bias corrections.

Perhaps the most important factor causing variation in reported estimates of sensitivities and specificities is the fact that the classification point for the test may differ dramatically from study to study. This is, of course, not really a bias, but merely a definitional problem, and one that can be resolved in the meta-analytic context by plotting the pairs of sensitivity/specificity estimates in an ROC format [14]. Usually this will demonstrate the fact that sensitivities and specificities are inversely related, due to the fact that the classification point varies from study to study. Ideally, the classification points used would be defined in the individual studies, but often this is not the case. Indeed, for subjectively interpreted tests, the classification point (or points) cannot be defined precisely, and can only be inferred empirically. If variation in the reported sensitivities and specificities is due only to variation in the classification points used, then the plotted values should lie on a single ROC curve, except for random variation in the estimates. However, a much wider scatter is common, and this can be due to a number of possible biases.

Perhaps the most common biases are those due to problems with the "gold standard" reference test. These fall into two major categories: the problem of verification bias in which only a selected subset of patients receive the reference test and where unverified patients are ignored, and the problem in which the reference test is recognized to be an imperfect standard.

Verification bias is an especially serious problem since it has a counterintuitive aspect (*see* **Bias in Observational Studies**). The bias is caused if the selection of patients to receive the reference test is influenced by the result of the test under investigation [20]. If the study is restricted to patients who receive the reference test, say biopsy proven cases, then the study is biased, yet many investigators will believe that such a restriction follows sound scientific practice. It is often impossible to design an unbiased study since application of the possibly invasive reference test may be unethical when the test under investigation is negative. That is, the risks or inconvenience of the reference test may be considered to be medically inappropriate in the absence of a positive test. The standard bias correction method is based on the assumption that selection of a patient for the reference test is a conscious decision, and must therefore be based on available clinical factors, such as the test result, x, and the results of other relevant tests or patient factors, denoted collectively by z [5]. Consequently, the predictive values, conditional on x and z, can be estimated without bias from the verified sample, denoted $v+$, i.e.

$$\Pr(D = 1|x, z, v+) = \Pr(D = 1|x, z),$$

and so unbiased estimates of the distributions $F_x(\cdot)$ and $G_x(\cdot)$ can be obtained by combining these unbiased predictive values with the distribution of the test result unconditional on disease status, denoted $h_{x|z}(x)$, estimated from all subjects, both verified and

unverified, using

$$f_{x|z}(x) \propto h_{x|z}(x)\Pr(D = 1|x, z, v+)$$

and

$$g_{x|z}(x) \propto h_{x|z}(x)\Pr(D = 0|x, z, v+).$$

Clearly, such an approach requires that data be collected on the test results and covariates of all patients in the series on whom the test is applied, regardless of whether the reference test is performed subsequently.

All of the accuracy measures described earlier are defined in relation to a "gold standard" reference test. Inaccuracy in the reference test will invariably lead to bias in the estimated characteristics of the test under consideration. If conditional independence between the two tests can be assumed, then bias corrections are possible. However, this assumption is usually untenable since most tests of the same phenomenon are likely to be positively correlated, even after conditioning on true disease status [27]. In these circumstances, the effect of the bias will be to inflate the sensitivity and specificity estimates artificially. Recently, a technique known as "discrepant analysis" has been popularized, primarily for the evaluation of tests for infectious diseases, where deoxyribonucleic acid (DNA) amplification techniques have the capacity to detect very small quantities of the organism in settings where cell culture, the conventional reference test, is frequently false negative [22]. This technique involves performing a third adjudicatory test, and possibly others, in patients for whom there is disagreement between the result of the test under consideration and the reference test. Unfortunately, this approach has been shown to be seriously biased [11, 18].

In evaluating the reported accuracy of diagnostic tests there are a number of other issues that can adversely affect the validity of the estimates, or cause further between-study variation in accuracy measures. Frequently, a test may produce an uninterpretable result. For example, for abdominal examinations bowel gas may obscure the result of ultrasound [19]. Barium in the gastrointestinal tract may obscure the result of computed tomography. A needle aspirate for the diagnosis of hepatic cancer may produce fragments which are inadequate for histological examination [23]. These problems are frequently not reported, the uninterpretable tests being simply removed from the analysis [19]. For subjectively interpreted tests, interobserver variation can have a substantial impact.

This may be reflected by variation in the empirical classification points used, or by genuine variation in accuracy, or both, and only ROC analysis can resolve these issues. Finally, the accuracy of a test may change over time, due to improvements in the ability of the readers to make use of the technology, or due to technological enhancements. For example, it is widely accepted that the quality and resolution of mammograms has improved markedly during the three decades since they became available, and the published accuracy results reflect this trend [9].

Comparisons of Tests

Consider two diagnostic tests, with results denoted by x and y. Parameters of test y have corresponding notation to those of test x, as defined earlier. Comparison of the two tests on the basis of accuracy requires that we calibrate the classification points used, otherwise, for example, the sensitivity of test x may be larger than that of test y merely because the classification rule was more strict for test x. ROC analysis is a natural way of calibrating the comparison, and this is the reason for its use as the definitive analytic tool.

Calibration of the comparison at a specific classification point is achieved by equating the marginal distributions of the two tests, where the prevalence of disease is standardized. Let the marginal distributions be defined by

$$M_x(x) = \pi F_x(x) + (1 - \pi)G_x(x),$$

and

$$M_y(y) = \pi F_y(y) + (1 - \pi)G_y(y). \tag{2}$$

Let $x_z = M_x^{-1}(z)$ and $y_z = M_y^{-1}(z)$. Then x_z and y_z represent the classification points corresponding to the zth quantile of these marginal distributions, i.e. $M_x(x_z) = M_y(y_z)$, for all z. It is easily seen from Eq. (2) that if the sensitivity of test x is greater than the sensitivity of test y at this quantile, then the specificity of test x is also greater than the specificity of test y, i.e.

$$1 - F_x(x_z) > 1 - F_y(y_z) \iff G_x(x_z) > G_y(y_z).$$

Thus the tests are fully equivalent if and only if $1 - F_x(x_z) = 1 - F_y(y_z)$ and $G_x(x_z) = G_y(y_z)$, for every value of z, i.e. throughout the entire ROC curve. The preceding theory relies on π being common to

the two tests. In a comparison study this is necessarily true in the paired-sample design, and indeed this design is the common design in comparison studies for reasons of efficiency [13].

The widely used methods developed for ROC analysis have mostly focused on comparing the areas under the ROC curves rather than comparisons at different calibrated quantiles. In fact, if one constructs the combined ranked sample of test results for a given test, i.e. combining diseased and normal subjects, and then evaluates the Wilcoxon statistic for comparing diseased and normal subjects, then this statistic is the area under the nonparametric trapezoidal ROC curve [2]. The asymptotic variance of this statistic is well known under the null hypothesis that the test is uninformative, i.e. the area is 0.5, and can be modified easily for the more common circumstance in which the area is substantially greater than 0.5 [12]. In the paired-sample setting, i.e. where both diagnostic tests are applied to each subject, the correlation between the test results within each subject must be taken into account, and methods have been developed specifically for this purpose [7].

Parametric methods are also widely used, primarily based on the binormal model. In this model it is assumed that if the distribution of tests results in normal (control) subjects is transformed to a standard normal distribution, then the same transformation on the diseased subjects will also lead to a normal distribution, with mean μ_x and variance σ_x^2, say, for test x [8]. In this case the area under the ROC curve is given by

$$A = \Phi\left(\frac{\mu_x}{(1 + \sigma_x^2)^{1/2}}\right),$$

where $\Phi(\cdot)$ is the standard normal distribution function. However, it is conventional to test for equivalence of the ROC curves by simultaneously testing that $\mu_x = \mu_y$ and $\sigma_x^2 = \sigma_y^2$, rather than simply testing for equality of the areas. In the paired sample setting the two test results are assumed to have corresponding bivariate normal distributions in the diseased and nondiseased populations, with correlation parameters to account for the within-patient dependencies [17]. Widely distributed noncommercial software is available for performing these analyses [16].

Finally, methods have recently been proposed for testing the equivalence of the two tests at all possible classification points in a nonparametric fashion, using bootstrapping techniques [6]. This can be accomplished for continuous paired data by permuting within pairs the ranks of the marginal rank order statistic, and obtaining a permutation test [26]. Such an analysis does not rely on the comparison of a summarized (parametric) measure of accuracy, such as the area or the binormal parameters as outlined above.

Study Design

In designing a study to evaluate or compare diagnostic tests, great care is necessary to ensure that the data are collected in a format suitable for resolving the problems and biases outlined in the previous Section. A source of detailed practical advice, with an emphasis on radiologic imaging studies, is the text by Swets & Pickett [24]. A recent trend has been the development of multi-institutional field studies, which parallel the early development of multicenter trials, and which have provided guidance on the organizational and methodologic challenges of large-scale accuracy studies [10].

There are five general issues pertinent to comparative studies of diagnostic tests: representativeness of the sample; completeness of data reporting; recording of test results; mapping of test results to "truth" data; and control of the comparison. First, representativeness is especially important since the ease with which a patient can be diagnosed accurately varies widely from patient to patient, and so a nonrepresentative sample of patients could substantially bias the estimates of accuracy. Secondly, completeness of data recording and reporting is important in the context of verification bias and the problems of uninterpretable test results. In cases where verification bias might be a problem, the ideal study is one in which we can be sure that all patients are scheduled for the definitive reference test (e.g. surgery) prior to the conduct of the tests under evaluation, otherwise the **missing data** are likely to be selective, i.e. not missing at random. Thirdly, as we have seen, valid comparison of tests is only possible if a "calibrated" analysis is achievable, i.e. using ROC analysis. Therefore, the test data must be collected in sufficient detail to facilitate such an analysis. That is, binary reporting of test results (positive or negative) is inadequate, and a minimum requirement is several ordinal classifications. Fourthly, it is critical that the data from the experimental tests and from the reference test are

recorded in a manner that permits meaningful correlation. In medical imaging studies, this means that a precise anatomical mapping of the results is possible. For example, if the purpose of the study is not only to detect disease, but to localize it, each of the test results, including the reference test, needs to be recorded for each of the anatomic regions of interest. Thus, careful form design and data collection is essential. Fifthly, if the tests under evaluation are interpreted subjectively, it is critical that evaluation of the second test is accomplished without knowledge of the first. Thus, blinding the test readers, or randomization of the test order, is necessary to prevent bias.

Finally, as is the case for all research studies, an adequate sample size is necessary to reduce statistical variation in the accuracy estimates to a level that permits meaningful interpretation of the data. Various methods for calculating study power are available [12, 16, 24].

Current Developments

There has been a substantial recent increase in research activity in the biostatistical literature on methods pertaining to the evaluation of diagnostic tests. The major themes of this work were summarized in a recent review article [4]. Even more recently, an issue of *Academic Radiology* was devoted to statistical developments in this field pertinent to medical imaging studies [1]. All of the articles addressed either one of two topics: covariate analysis of ROC curves, including models for accommodating random effects, such as test readers; and meta-analysis of diagnostic tests. Interest in covariate modeling stems from recognition of the fact that studies of the accuracy of diagnostic tests can be influenced by multiple factors. Meta-analysis is important in recognition of the fact that there exists a vast literature of published diagnostic accuracy studies, and we need methods that can synthesize these results reliably, in recognition of the limitations and biases that may be present in the individual studies. The field promises to continue to be an active area of biostatistical research in the foreseeable future.

References

[1]   Advances in statistical methods for diagnostic radiology: a symposium (1995). *Academic Radiology* **2**, S1–S84.

[2] Bamber, D. (1975). The area above the ordinal dominance graph and the area below the receiver operating characteristic graph, *Journal of Mathematical Psychology* **12**, 387–415.

[3] Begg, C.B. (1987). Biases in the assessment of diagnostic tests, *Statistics in Medicine* **6**, 411–423.

[4] Begg, C.B. (1991). Advances in statistical methodology for diagnostic medicine in the 1980's, *Statistics in Medicine* **10**, 1887–1895.

[5] Begg, C.B. & Greenes, R.A. (1983). Assessment of diagnostic tests when disease verification is subject to selection bias, *Biometrics* **39**, 207–215.

[6] Campbell, G. (1994). Advances in statistical methodology for the evaluation of diagnostic and laboratory tests, *Statistics in Medicine* **13**, 499–508.

[7] DeLong, E.R., DeLong, D.M. & Clarke-Pearson, D.L. (1988). Comparing the areas under two or more correlated receiver operating characteristic curves: a nonparametric approach, *Biometrics* **44**, 837–846.

[8] Dorfman, D.D. & Alf, E. (1969). Maximum likelihood estimation of parameters of signal detection theory and determination of confidence intervals: rating method data, *Journal of Mathematical Psychology* **6**, 487–496.

[9] Fletcher, S.W., Black, W., Harris, R., Rimer, B.K. & Shapiro, S. (1993). Report on the international workshop on screening for breast cancer, *Journal of the National Cancer Institute* **85**, 1644–1656.

[10] Gatsonis, C. & McNeil, B.J. (1990). Collaborative evaluations of diagnostic tests: experience of the Radiation Diagnostic Oncology Group, *Radiology* **175**, 571–575.

[11] Hadgu, A. (1996). The discrepancy in discrepant analysis, *Lancet* **348**, 592–593.

[12] Hanley, J.A. & McNeil, B.J. (1982). The meaning and use of the area under a receiver operating characteristic curve, *Radiology* **143**, 29–36.

[13] Hanley, J.A. & McNeil, B.J. (1983). A method of comparing the area under two ROC curves derived from the same cases, *Radiology* **148**, 839–843.

[14] Irwig, L., Tosteson, A.N.A., Gatsonis, C., Lau, J., Colditz, G., Chalmers, T.C. & Mosteller, F. (1994). Guidelines for meta-analyses evaluating diagnostic tests, *Annals of Internal Medicine* **120**, 667–676.

[15] Kardaun, J.W. & Kardaun, O.J. (1990). Comparative diagnostic performance of three radiologic procedures for the detection of lumbar disc herniation, *Methods of Information in Medicine* **29**, 12–22.

[16] Metz, C.E. Fortran programs ROCFIT, CORROC, LABROC, CLABROC. Department of Radiology, University of Chicago, 5841 South Maryland Avenue.

[17] Metz, C.E., Wang, P.L. & Kronman, H.B. (1984). A new approach for testing the significance of differences between ROC curves for correlated data, in *Information Processing in Medical Imaging*, F. Deconick, ed. Nijhoff, The Hague, pp. 432–445.

[18] Miller, W.C. (1998). Bias in discrepant analysis: when two wrongs don't make a right, *Journal of Clinical Epidemiology* **51**, 219–231.

[19] Poynard, T., Chaput, J.C. & Etienne, J.P. (1982). Relations between effectiveness of a diagnostic test, prevalence of the disease and percentages of uninterpretable results, *Medical Decision Making* **2**, 285–302.

[20] Ransohoff, D.F. & Feinstein, A.R. (1978). Problems of spectrum and bias in evaluating the efficacy of diagnostic tests, *New England Journal of Medicine* **299**, 926–930.

[21] Sackett, D.L., Haynes, R.B. & Tugwell, P. (1985). *Clinical Epidemiology: A Basic Science for Clinical Medicine*, Little Brown & Company, Boston.

[22] Schachter, J., Stamm, W.E., Quinn, T.C., Andrews, W.W., Burczak, J.D. & Lee, H.H. (1994). Ligase chain reaction to detect Chlamydia trachomatis infection of the cervix, *Journal of Clinical Microbiology* **32**, 2540–2543.

[23] Schwerk, W.B., Durr, H.K. & Schmitz-Moorman, P. (1983). Ultrasound guided fine-needle biopsies in pancreatic and hepatic neoplasms, *Gastrointestinal Radiology* **8**, 219–229.

[24] Swets, J.A. & Pickett, R.M. (1982). *Evaluation of Diagnostic Systems: Methods from Signal Detection Theory.* Academic Press, New York.

[25] Vecchio, T.J. (1966). Predictive value of a single diagnostic test in an unselected population, *New England Journal of Medicine* **274**, 1171–1173.

[26] Venkatraman, E.S. & Begg, C.B. (1996). A distribution-free procedure for comparing receiver operating characteristic curves from a paired experiment, *Biometrika* **83**, 835–848.

[27] Walter, S.D. & Irwig, L.M. (1988). Estimation of test error rates, disease prevalence and relative risk from misclassified data: a review, *Journal of Clinical Epidemiology* **41**, 923–938.

[28] Yerushalmy, J. (1947). Statistical problems in assessing methods of medical diagnosis with special reference to X-ray techniques, *Public Health Reports* **62**, 1432–1449.

(*See also* **Diagnostic Test Evaluation Without a Gold Standard**)

Colin B. Begg

Differential Error

Suppose a response variable Y has a conditional distribution $F(y|x)$ given a true exposure measurement $X = x$. Suppose that an error process yields Z instead of X. Then the error process is differential if $F(y|x,z) \neq F(y|x)$; namely, if it is not **nondifferential error**. Naive use of Z in place of X in the model $F(y|x)$ leads to estimates of **exposure** effect that can be **biased** in any direction (*see* **Bias in Observational Studies**; **Bias, Overview**; **Measurement Error in Epidemiologic Studies**; **Misclassification Error**; **Validity and Generalizability in Epidemiologic Studies**).

The term differential error can also be applied to errors in the outcome measure, Y. Suppose that one measures the error-prone version W of Y, instead of Y itself. Then the error process is differential if $F(w|x, y) \neq F(w|y)$. Such differential error can also result in bias in any direction if W is simply substituted for Y in the model $F(y|x)$.

M.H. GAIL

Differential Length Biased Sampling *see* Biased Sampling of Cohorts in Epidemiology

Differential Measurement Error *see* Measurement Error in Epidemiologic Studies

Direct Standardization *see* Standardization Methods

Directory Sampling *see* Random Digit Dialing Sampling for Case–Control Studies

Disease Registers

Disease registers are an important tool for clinicians, epidemiologists, and health service planners. Their nature will vary according to the functions they are serving, but all relate to individuals with, or at high risk of, a specified chronic disease. Often registers are used for more than one purpose.

The following sections describe: examples and objectives of registers of different types; problems of case definition, ascertainment, and **biases**; validity checks; and possibilities created by **record linkage**.

Types of Disease Registers

Registers Contributing to the Organization and Quality of Clinical Care

Patient Registers Held by Clinicians. The simplest form of disease register is one set up by individual clinicians relating to their own patients. The conditions registered are usually those that require either regular maintenance therapy or **screening** for early signs of preventable complications. Such registers are essentially part of the normal process of clinical care. They are generally designed for **prevalent cases**, i.e. patients who are alive, have not moved away, and whose condition is clinically important.

One of the most common conditions for which disease registers are used is diabetes mellitus. This is typical in that most patients have an ongoing need of insulin or another prescribable drug. They are also at high risk of future complications, particularly problems of the feet, or eyes, and of the cardiovascular system. Many of these complications have been shown to be either preventable, or less serious if diagnosed and treated early.

In recent years the holding of disease registers has extended from one held by a clinician of his/her own patients, with a special interest in a particular condition, to the sharing of registers by groups of clinicians working in general or hospital practice. Moreover, for an increasing number of conditions, including diabetes [6] and coronary artery disease [11], there are now internationally shared registers, with all the necessary confidentiality constraints.

Registers of Relatives of Patients with Genetic Conditions. A more recent development is to extend registration to blood relatives of individuals known to have a serious genetic condition. An example of this is the condition of familial adenomatous polyposis. Persons with this condition have numbers of colonic polyps, initially benign but at high risk of becoming malignant.

One method of management is to screen teenage members of affected families and to remove the colon of those found to have polyps at the age of 18–20 as a prophylactic measure [2]. Another approach under investigation is to treat those at high risk with low-dose aspirin, which may be protective against malignancy. Implementation of such programs on a population scale, and their audit, is greatly assisted by the existence of registers of those at risk.

Registers of Individuals at Risk because of Hazardous Exposure.   Where specific hazards are known to increase the risk of subsequent serious disorders, registration of those who have been exposed may be a useful clinical tool. This has been done for babies who were born extremely immature, or who have had severe asphyxial episodes. These babies are at high risk of neurologic damage which may not manifest itself for some years. Early diagnosis of sensory or neurologic problems in children on such registers allows prompt action, although it is mostly in visual and hearing disorders that it has been shown to be effective [5]. Parents of children at risk because of stormy births are normally aware of such risks and appreciate the **surveillance**.

Registers Held for the Implementation of Public Health Functions

Registers of serious common conditions may be held for the purpose of monitoring and improving the health of populations as opposed to that of individuals. They are usually held at the level of residents of an administrative area. Questions of exclusion or inclusion may arise when residents of one area are treated, move into, or are born or die, in another area.

In contrast to most registers held for clinical purposes which need only include *prevalent* cases, registers held for public health functions may need to include all **incident cases** regardless of severity or survival. Moreover, for most public health functions the measures used will be **incidence** or **prevalence rates** rather than absolute numbers of cases.

The calculation of rates implies that the number of individuals at risk is known. In some registers, for instance those of congenital anomalies, this implies the inclusion of cases lost as late prenatal or postnatal death amongst the numerator and denominator. This is possible where there is a definitive diagnostic test which can be used prenatally or in the early postnatal period, e.g. the detection of a chromosomal anomaly, of a specific genetic defect, or ultrasound visualization of malformations visible during or after pregnancy [10].

The aims of such registers include:

1. the ascertainment of environmental hazards to health (*see* **Environmental Epidemiology**)
2. the provision of current and projected prevalence and severity data for health care planners
3. the monitoring of survival, or quality of life, of affected individuals
4. the monitoring of the efficacy, implementation and acceptance of preventive measures.

Important examples are cancer, diabetes, ischemic heart disease, or congenital anomaly registers, which may be held at regional, national, or international levels.

Ascertainment of Environmental Hazards to Health.   New environmental causes of ill-health may be suspected when trends in registration rates of specific conditions change over time, in different places or in persons of different characteristics, or occupations. New patterns of incidence, such as clusters over time and space, may also draw attention to possible causes (*see* **Clustering**). When the conditions concerned are rapidly lethal, or lethal prenatally, it is important to ascertain all incident cases as far as possible, as well as prevalent cases. Where evidence is found that there has been a real change in incidence, registered cases may act as a sampling frame to set up **case–control studies** to investigate possible causes.

Negative findings from such studies are as important as positive findings if they can rule out putative associations with environmental exposures.

Provision of Current and Projected Prevalence and Severity Data for Health Care Planners. Health care planners require information to allow them to project future needs of individuals with specific conditions, in terms of prevalence and severity. This requires good quality prevalent disease registers, which include clinical and survival data.

Monitoring of Outcome of Affected Individuals. Registers which provide information on survival, quality of life, and treatment given, are important sources of clinical audit, allowing the comparison of survival after different treatments or treatment in different places. Such audit will, however, also require basic demographic data such as age, sex, place of residence and, if possible, socioeconomic circumstances, which could **confound** comparisons of survival. Such comparisons, although not so rigorous as randomized controlled trials, may point to differences that should be further explored.

Monitoring of the Efficacy, Implementation, and Acceptance of Preventive Measures. Preventive measures of disease may include primary prevention, namely the abolition of the cause. In the case of cancers or heart disease, these include smoking or alcohol abuse. Preventable serious congenital disorders include neural tube defects, in part preventable by periconceptional folic acid supplementation, and rubella embryopathy, preventable by preconceptional rubella immunization. Where registers exist of incident cases of such conditions, trends over time, place, or in different population groups will act as an audit of the extent to which the preventive action is being implemented.

In conditions where secondary preventive action may follow the screening out of asymptomatic or prenatal cases, the use of a disease register to monitor the prevalence of symptomatic cases, or births with specific congenital anomalies, will allow the auditing of the efficacy and effectiveness of specific screening programs. Examples are where cervical or breast cancer screening is on offer, and how this affects the mortality due to such cancers; or where prenatal screening programs are available, whether there is a change in ratio of legally terminated pregnancies with Down's syndrome or neural tube defects to registered affected births.

Registers Held for Research Purposes. Registers may be held purely for etiologic research. They typically require the inclusion of incident rather than prevalent cases. Their design and maintenance must take account of, or may reveal, the natural history of the condition registered.

How the Natural History of a Disease may Affect Registration

Congenital Anomalies

Many congenital conditions which lead to permanent impairment are ascertainable and therefore registerable at birth, e.g. spina bifida. Others may not be visible or do not lead to symptoms until some time after birth. These include congenital heart defects, cerebral palsy, or mental retardation. For such conditions it is impossible to estimate true incidence rates since many affected children may have died before ascertainment, and only age-specific prevalence rates can be calculated. Other congenital conditions, e.g. gastrointestinal atresias, are curable by surgery shortly after birth. Such conditions may need to be considered in the ascertainment of incident cases, but not in ascertaining prevalent cases.

The advent of prenatal diagnosis of some conditions, often leading to termination of pregnancy, raises other questions. Had they not been prenatally diagnosed, many fetuses with conditions such as chromosomal anomalies would have been lost as spontaneous miscarriages, and the cause would not have been ascertained. This is an important point in registers of Down's syndrome, where in recent years in England and Wales about half of all affected pregnancies are diagnosed prenatally, leading to an apparent increase in incident cases, although the numbers of affected births are falling [1].

Acquired Diseases

Acquired chronic conditions may lead to permanent impairment which cannot be cured, or they may be "curable", at least in the sense of not recurring. The course of the disease may be variable, as in multiple sclerosis, with attacks and remissions, the patient sometimes having no symptoms or clinical signs in remission. Alternatively, in conditions such as ischemic heart disease, minor symptoms and signs of the disease may persist, but this may be punctuated by acute episodes of myocardial infarction. Tunstall–Pedoe [11] gives a full account of the methodologic problems raised in the registration of ischemic heart disease, stemming from the notification of heart attacks as acute episodes instead of as "abstractions from a chronic disease". He shows that such registration, which has been used for international comparisons, is the only way to measure the burden of chronic heart disease.

Case Definition

The nature and quality of a register is crucially dependent upon the ascertainment of individuals meeting a clear and unambiguous case definition. Case definition must include guidance on which cases should be included and which excluded, including the cutoff points in terms of level of severity or objective test results. Where relevant, it is helpful if registration forms include diagrams which indicate the parts of the body that are affected, or scales which indicate severity.

Sometimes researchers may choose to use a very broad definition on the assumption that they can select specific subgroups from the information requested.

One question that commonly arises is how to handle cases with multiple pathology, e.g. multiple apparently unrelated malformations or cancers. Particularly for research purposes, the setting up of a register must include a protocol which deals with these questions and the method of ascertainment to be used. For clinical registers held by one practitioner this may be less important, but as soon as clinical registers are shared with others (and this often implies a new use as a research tool also), such a protocol is equally important.

Ascertainment

The completeness of registers varies with the methods used for ascertainment and diagnosis.

Methods of Ascertainment

Ascertainment may depend on clinical presentation and the recognition of the defined condition, or it may be the result of a process of screening where this is clinically possible. Both the severity of the condition and the characteristics of the individuals ascertained will usually vary sharply depending on the methods used. Examples are the marked differences between numbers of cases on registers of individuals with diabetes mellitus who presented for medical care, and those registers which resulted from population

screening of urine and glucose tolerance testing [3]. The ease and completeness with which cases are found may be helped if the treatment is standard and unique, as in the case of insulin, where monitoring of prescriptions is a method of ascertainment of cases.

Methods of Diagnosis

Particularly where the register is shared with others, the diagnostic process must be based on a formal protocol. There are many different methods of diagnosis. For those conditions where a definitive diagnostic test is available e.g. an identifiable single gene defect or a chromosome anomaly, or the results of bacterial or viral culture, the easiest and most complete ascertainment may be obtained from laboratory results. Where diagnosis is largely based on clinical findings its success may depend on the personal acumen of the physician, but is usually backed up by objective blood, urine, or imaging investigations. Such methods may lead to full, or nearly full, ascertainment where the condition is such that self-referral is the rule. For lethal conditions clinical ascertainment can be backed up by searching for relevant details on **death certificates**.

Multiple Sources of Ascertainment

It is now increasingly common to use multiple sources of ascertainment. This can be particularly useful for chronic conditions of low lethality which may not always require medical care. For instance, individuals with conditions such as cerebral palsy or mental retardation may present to a variety of services – medical, paramedical (such as physiotherapy), educational, or social. Moreover, it has been shown that even the ascertainment of diabetes or cancer can be improved by the use of multiple sources. For diabetes, multiple sources that have been used include prescriptions, family practitioner registers, hospital diabetic clinic records, and, where relevant, health insurance data. For cancer registrations, sources include hospital records or death certificates with a mention of cancer, histology reports, and oncology clinic records.

Multiple ascertainment is designed to lead to duplication of notification, and the information gathered and the design of the register must be such that duplicates can be identified and eliminated.

Duplicate Notification. Duplicate notification will also occur where affected individuals already registered in one place move to another place which keeps a related register, and precautions must be taken to eliminate these. Clerical errors in recording dates, spelling mistakes in recording names, or name changes are all difficulties which must be taken account of in seeking for duplicates. Record linkage techniques can be used to check for duplicates, including phonetic name matching [7].

Case Identification

The degree to which registered cases need personal identification will vary according to the aims of the register. Clinical registers are often part of family practitioner or hospital records, and named identification is essential for their use.

Registers kept for public health or research purposes often do not need to be named except where a follow-up of registered individuals is planned. On the other hand the recording of some personal identifiers is essential, if only to allow the finding and elimination of duplicates, and to have such basic epidemiologic information as date of birth and sex.

If the aims of the register include an investigation of changes in incidence, prevalence, or survival, other dates must be collected, such as at first presentation and, where relevant, of death. Similarly, to seek for evidence of clustering, place of residence, and sometimes of birth or occupation, will be needed, usually recorded in the form of post- or zip-code data. When personal identifiers are kept there must be meticulous care to preserve patient confidentiality.

Record Linkage

The growth of computerized health information has led to opportunities to link records from different sources, and thus to enhance register information.

For instance, in the UK it is possible to access information from death registration. Given Ethics Committee permission, bona fide researchers are permitted to arrange for the linkage of this information with their own register data, thus providing the necessary data to calculate the survival of the individuals on a register, and to find their causes of death. Similarly, linkage with nonconfidential items from birth records may provide valuable information linking birth events with health in later life [9].

Such linkage is an essential part of cancer registration in the UK, since recording of cancer as a **cause of death** is an important method of ascertainment for the regional cancer registers. Moreover, the linkage at national level of data from all regional cancer registers allows for identification and elimination of duplicate records due to patient movements [8].

Validation

An important aspect of maintaining the quality of disease registers is the validation of the data at regular intervals. Validation can include an assessment of completeness of registration and of data on each record, the success with which duplicates are eliminated, and most importantly the rigor to which the given case definition is adhered.

There is a growing literature on methods of examining the likely completeness of ascertainment. Where there are different but independent methods, "capture–recapture" techniques can be used [4].

The examination of the validity of case registration can be a difficult task. An area where this has received particular attention is in the World Health Organization monitoring of trends and determinants in cardiovascular disease (MONICA) study, which was the registration in a number of different countries of heart attacks. This is well described by Tunstall-Pedoe [11], who discusses problems arising from different standards of record keeping, the use of coding rules for clinical history, symptoms and diagnostic tests, and validity checks of the clinical data, coding, and laboratory or other tests.

Conclusions

Disease registers are becoming an increasingly powerful clinical and epidemiologic tool, particularly for international comparisons. Their use predicates clear aims, good design, coverage, complete and accurate recording of validated data, and rigorous methods of preserving confidentiality.

References

[1]   Alberman, E.D., Mutton, D.E., Ide, R., Nicholson, A. & Bobrow, M. (1995). Down's syndrome births and pregnancy terminations in 1989–1993: preliminary findings, *British Journal of Obstetrics and Gynaecology* **102**, 445–447.

[2]   Bulow, S., Bulow, C., Nielsen, T.F., Karlsen, L. & Moesgard, F. (1995). Centralized registration, prophylactic examination, and treatment results in improved prognosis in familial adenatomatous polyposis. Results from the Finnish Polyposis Register, *Scandinavian Journal of Gastroenterology* **30**, 989–993.

[3]   Butterfield, J. (1964). Summary of results of the Bedford Diabetes Survey, *Proceedings of the Royal Society of Medicine* **57**, 196–200.

[4]   Hook, E. & Regal, R.R. (1992). The value of capture-recapture methods even for apparent exhaustive surveys, *American Journal of Epidemiology* **135**, 1060–1067.

[5]   Johnson, A. (1995). Use of registers in child health, *Archives of Disease in Childhood* **72**, 474–477.

[6]   Krans, H.M.J., Porta, M., Keen, H. & Staehr Johansen, K. (1995). *Diabetes Care and Research in Europe: The St. Vincent Declaration Action Programme.* International Diabetes Federation European Region, World Health Organization, Regional Office for Europe, Copenhagen, Chapter 14.

[7]   Langley, J.D. & Botha, J.L. (1994). Use of record linkage techniques to maintain the Leicestershire Diabetes Register. Computer Methods Programs, *Biomedicine* **41**, 287–295.

[8]   Office of Population Censuses and Surveys (now Office of National Statistics) (1990). *Review of the National Cancer Registration System in England and Wales.* HMSO, London.

[9]   Office of Population Censuses and Surveys (now Office of National Statistics) (1993). Uses of OPCS Records for Medical Research, *Occasional Paper 41.* HMSO, London.

[10]   Office of Population Censuses and Surveys (now Office of National Statistics) (1995). The OPCS Monitoring Scheme for Congenital Malformations, *Occasional Paper 43.* HMSO, London.

[11]   Tunstall-Pedoe, H. (1989). Diagnosis, measurement, and surveillance of coronary events, *International Journal of Epidemiology* **18**, Supplement 1, 169–173.

(*See also* **Birth Cohort Studies**; **Death Indexes**)

EVA ALBERMAN

Dispersion Test *see* Clustering

Distance Methods for Clustering *see* Clustering

Dose–Response

Dose–response refers to a relationship between an amount of exposure or treatment and the degree or probability of an outcome in an individual or population. The dose may represent the amount, duration or intensity of exposure or treatment, and the outcome may represent a favorable effect, such as lowering of elevated blood pressure, or an unfavorable effect, such as increased risk of developing cancer. For example, the risk of lung cancer is known to increase with the number of cigarettes smoked each day and with the duration of smoking. A monotonic relationship of increasing disease risk with increasing exposure is often taken as one indication of a causal relationship between exposure and risk (*see* **Hill's Criteria for Causality**).

M.H. GAIL

Doubly Censored Data *see* Incubation Period of Infectious Diseases

Dynamic Population

A dynamic population is a population that gains and loses members, unlike a fixed population. A dynamic population is stable or in the steady state if the sizes of all subgroups (e.g. age and gender subgroups) remain constant. **Relative hazards** can be estimated in a dynamic population from **case–control studies** based on **density sampling**. The well-known relationship, disease **prevalence** = disease incidence × average disease duration, which holds when a dynamic population is stationary, requires modification for nonstationary dynamic populations (*see* **Incidence–Prevalence Relationships**).

M.H. GAIL

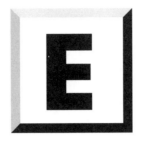

Ecologic Fallacy

The ecologic fallacy is the mistaken assumption that a statistical association observed between two ecologic (group-level) variables (*see* **Ecologic Study**) is equal to the association between the corresponding variables at the individual level. This assumption is often made implicitly or explicitly when using ecologic data to make inferences about the biologic (individual-level) effect of an exposure on the **risk** of a disease or other health outcome. Suppose, for example, we observe a positive ecologic association between exposure **prevalence** and the rate of a disease across many regions (groups). The magnitude and direction of the association between exposure status and disease risk within regions (at the individual level) could be different from the ecologic association, even if there is no error in measuring either ecologic variable. Just because the disease rate is higher in regions with a larger exposure prevalence does not mean that exposed individuals are at greater risk of disease than are unexposed individuals. It is possible that the risk is particularly high for unexposed individuals living in regions with a relatively high exposure prevalence. The underlying problem of the ecologic fallacy, therefore, is that each group is not entirely homogeneous with respect to the exposure. If every region were made up entirely of exposed individuals or unexposed individuals, then there would be no ecologic fallacy because information on the joint distribution of exposure and disease within groups would not be missing.

From a statistical perspective, the ecologic fallacy is due to *cross-level bias* in estimating the biologic effect of an exposure on disease risk on the basis of ecologic data. Thus, the fundamental problem of cross-level inference is not an all-or-none phenomenon, but rather a continuum of **systematic error** in effect estimation. In an ecologic analysis involving simple linear regression, cross-level bias arises when the disease rate in the unexposed (reference) population is correlated with exposure prevalence across groups or when the difference in rates between exposed and unexposed populations (biologic effect) varies across groups. (*see* **Ecologic Study** for a contemporary interpretation of "ecologic fallacy" and for a discussion of cross-level bias.)

HAL MORGENSTERN

Ecologic Study

An ecologic or aggregate study focuses on the comparison of groups, rather than individuals. The underlying reason for this focus is that individual-level data are missing on the joint distribution of at least two and perhaps all variables within each group; in this sense, an ecologic study is an "incomplete" design [48]. Ecologic studies have been conducted by social scientists for more than a century [18] and have been used extensively by epidemiologists in many research areas. Nevertheless, the distinction between individual-level and group-level (ecologic) studies and the inferential implications are far more complicated and subtle than they first appear. Before 1980, ecologic studies were usually presented in the first part of epidemiology textbooks as simple "descriptive" analyses in which disease rates are stratified by place or time to test hypotheses preliminarily; little attention was given to statistical methods or inference (for example [56]). The purpose of this article is to provide a methodologic overview of ecologic studies, which emphasizes study design, statistical methods, and causal inference. Although ecologic studies are easily and inexpensively conducted, the results are often difficult to interpret.

Concepts and Rationale

Before discussing the design and interpretation of ecologic studies, we must first define the concepts of ecologic measurement, analysis, and inference.

Levels of Measurement

The sources of data used in epidemiologic studies typically involve direct observations of individuals (e.g. age and blood pressure); they may also involve observations of groups, organizations, or places (e.g. social disorganization and air pollution). These observations are then organized to measure specific variables in the study population: individual-level variables are properties of individuals, and ecologic variables are properties of groups, organizations, or places. To be more specific, ecologic measures may be classified into three types:

1. *Aggregate measures* are summaries (e.g. means or proportions) of observations derived from individuals in each group, e.g. the proportion of smokers and median family income.
2. *Environmental measures* are physical characteristics of the place in which members of each group live or work, e.g. air-pollution level and hours of sunlight. Note that each environmental measure has an analog at the individual level, and these individual exposures (or doses) usually vary among members of each group (though they may remain unmeasured).
3. *Global measures* are attributes of groups, organizations, or places for which there is no distinct analog at the individual level (unlike aggregate

and environmental measures), e.g. population density, level of social disorganization, the existence of a specific law, or type of health-care system.

Levels of Analysis

The unit of analysis is the common level for which the data on all variables are reduced and analyzed. In an *individual-level analysis*, a value for each variable is assigned to every subject in the study. It is possible, even common in **environmental epidemiology**, for one or more predictor variables to be ecologic measures. For example, the average pollution level of each county might be assigned to every subject who is a resident of that county.

In a *completely ecologic analysis*, all variables (exposure, disease, and covariates) are ecologic measures so that the unit of analysis is the group, e.g. region (*see* **Geographical Analysis**), worksite, school, health-care facility, demographic stratum, or time interval. Thus, within each group, we do not know the joint distribution of any combination of variables at the individual level (e.g. the frequencies of exposed cases, unexposed cases, exposed noncases, and unexposed noncases); all we know is the marginal distribution of each variable, e.g. the proportion exposed and the disease rate (i.e. the T frequencies in Figure 1).

In a *partially ecologic analysis* of three or more variables, we have additional information on certain joint distributions (the M, N, or A/B frequencies in Figure 1); but we still do not know the full joint distribution of all variables within each group (i.e.

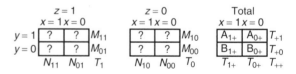

Figure 1 Joint distribution of exposure status ($x = 1$ vs. 0), disease status ($y = 1$ vs. 0), and covariate status ($z = 1$ vs. 0) in each group of a simple ecologic analysis: T frequencies are the only data available in a completely ecologic analysis of all three variables; M frequencies require additional data on the joint distribution of z and y within each group; N frequencies require additional data on the joint distribution of x and z within each group; A and B frequencies require additional data on the joint distribution of x and y within each group; and ? cells are always missing in an ecologic analysis

the ? cells in Figure 1 are missing). For example, in an ecologic study of cancer incidence by county, the joint distribution of age (a covariate) and disease status within each county (the *M* frequencies in Figure 1) might be obtained from the census and a population tumor registry (*see* **Disease Registers**). From these sources, the investigator would be able to estimate age-specific cancer rates for each county.

Multilevel analysis is a special type of modeling technique that combines analyses conducted at two (or more) levels [7, 27, 100, 101]. For example, an individual-level analysis might be conducted in each group, followed by an ecologic analysis of all groups using the results from the individual-level analyses. This approach will be described in a later section.

Levels of Inference

The underlying goal of a given epidemiologic study or analysis may be to make *biologic* (or biobehavioral) *inferences* about effects on individual *risks* or to make *ecologic inferences* about effects on group *rates* [62]. The target level of causal inference, however, does not always match the level of analysis. For example, the purpose of an ecologic analysis may be to make a biologic inference about the effect of a specific exposure on disease risk. As discussed later in this article, such *cross-level inferences* are particularly vulnerable to bias.

If the objective of a study is to estimate the *biologic effect* of wearing a motorcycle helmet on the risk of motorcycle-related mortality among motorcycle riders, the target level of causal inference is biologic. On the other hand, if the objective is to estimate the *ecologic effect* of helmet-use laws on the motorcycle-related mortality rate of riders in different states, the target level of causal inference is ecologic. Note that the magnitude of this ecologic effect depends not only on the biologic effect of helmet use, but also on the degree and pattern of compliance with the law in each state. Furthermore, the validity of the ecologic effect estimate depends on our ability to control for differences among states in the joint distribution of **confounders**, including individual-level variables such as age and amount of motorcycle riding.

We might also be interested in estimating the *contextual effect* of an ecologic exposure on individual risk, which is also a form of biologic inference [3, 92]. If the ecologic exposure is an aggregate measure,

we would generally want to separate its effect from the effect of its individual-level analog. For example, we might estimate the contextual effect of living in a poor area on the risk of disease, controlling for individual poverty level [45]. Contextual effects can be profound in infectious-disease epidemiology, where the risk of disease depends on the **prevalence** of the disease in others with whom the individual has contact [50, 93] (*see* **Communicable Diseases**).

In evaluating motorcycle-helmet laws in the US, we would probably not expect a contextual *effect* of living in a state that mandates helmet use on the risk of motorcycle-related mortality in riders, controlling for individual helmet use. If a rider's helmet use does not change after the helmet law takes effect, we would not expect his risk of motorcycle-related mortality to change. Nevertheless, we might expect to observe a contextual *association* between the same variables after the law because of differential compliance with the law within states. That is, those riders who comply with the law, but who would not have worn helmets without the law, may be at lower risk than are riders who do not comply with the law. Consequently, the risk of motorcycle-related mortality among riders who do not wear helmets will be higher in states with the helmet law than in states without the law.

Rationale for Ecologic Studies

There are several reasons for the widespread use of ecologic studies in epidemiology, despite frequent cautions about their methodologic limitations:

1. *Low cost and convenience.* Ecologic studies are inexpensive and take little time because various secondary data sources, each involving different information needed for the analysis, can easily be linked at the aggregate level. For example, data obtained from population registries, **vital statistics** records, large **sample surveys**, and the census are often linked at the state, county, or census-tract level.

2. *Measurement limitations of individual-level studies.* In environmental epidemiology and other research areas, we often cannot accurately measure relevant exposures or doses at the individual level for large numbers of subjects – at least not with available time and resources. Thus, the only practical way to measure the exposure may be

ecologically [62, 63]. This advantage is especially true when investigating apparent clusters of disease in small areas [94] (*see* **Clustering**). Sometimes individual-level exposures, such as dietary factors, cannot be measured accurately because of substantial within-person variability; yet ecologic measures might accurately reflect group averages [41, 76].

3. *Design limitations of individual-level studies.* Individual-level studies may not be practical for estimating exposure effects if the exposure varies little within the study area. Ecologic studies covering a much wider area, however, might be able to achieve substantial variation in mean exposure across groups (for example [68], [72], and [81]).

4. *Interest in ecologic effects.* As noted above, the stated purpose of a study may be to assess an ecologic effect; i.e. the target level of inference may be ecologic rather than biologic – to understand differences in disease rates among populations [60, 81]. Ecologic effects are particularly relevant when evaluating the impacts of social processes or population interventions such as new programs, policies, or legislation. As discussed later in this article, however, an interest in ecologic effects does not necessarily obviate the need for individual-level data.

5. *Simplicity of analysis and presentation.* In large complex studies conducted at the individual level, it may be conceptually and statistically simpler to perform ecologic analyses and to present ecologic results than to do individual-level analyses. For example, data from large periodic surveys, such as the National Health Interview Survey, are often analyzed ecologically by treating some combination of year, region, and demographic group as the unit of analysis. As discussed later in this article, however, such simplicity of analysis and presentation often conceals methodologic problems.

Study Designs

In an ecologic study design, the planned unit of analysis is the group. Ecologic designs may be classified on two dimensions: the method of exposure measurement and the method of grouping [48, 62]. Regarding the first dimension, an ecologic design is called *exploratory* if there is no specific exposure of interest or the exposure of potential interest is not measured, and it is called *analytic* if the primary exposure variable is measured and included in the analysis. (This use of the term "analytic" is not to be confused with **analytic epidemiology**, which refers to **cohort** and **case–control** studies conducted at the individual level.) In practice, this dimension is a continuum, since most ecologic studies are not conducted to test a single hypothesis. Regarding the second dimension, the groups of an ecologic study may be identified by place (multiple-group design), by time (time-trend design), or by a combination of place and time (mixed design).

Multiple-Group Designs

Exploratory Study. In an exploratory multiple-group study, we compare the rate of disease among many regions during the same period. The purpose is to search for spatial patterns that might suggest an environmental etiology or more specific etiologic hypotheses. For example, the National Cancer Institute (NCI) mapped the age-adjusted cancer mortality rates in the US by county for the period 1950–69 [58]. For oral cancers, they found a striking difference in geographic patterns by sex: among men, the mortality rates were greatest in the urban Northeast; but among women, the rates were greatest in the Southeast. These findings led to the hypothesis that snuff dipping, which is common among rural southern women, is a risk factor for oral cancers [2]. The results of a subsequent case–control study supported this hypothesis [99].

Exploratory ecologic studies may also involve the comparison of rates between migrants and their offspring and residents of their countries of emigration and immigration [41, 56] (*see* **Migrant Studies**). If the rates differ appreciably between the countries of emigration and immigration, migrant studies often yield results suggesting the influence of certain types of risk factors for the disease under study. For example, if US immigrants from Japan have rates of a disease similar to US whites but much lower than Japanese residents, the difference may be due to environmental or behavioral risk factors operating during adulthood. On the other hand, if US immigrants from Japan and their offspring have rates much lower than US whites but similar to Japanese residents, the difference may be due to genetic risk factors.

Such interpretations, however, especially in the first instance, are often limited by differences between countries in the classification and detection of disease or cause of death.

In mapping studies (*see* **Mapping Disease Patterns**), such as the NCI investigation, a simple comparison of rates across regions is often complicated by two statistical problems. First, regions with smaller numbers of observed cases show greater variability in the estimated rate; thus, the most extreme rates tend to be observed for those regions with the fewest cases. Second, nearby regions tend to have more similar rates than do distant regions (i.e. autocorrelation) because unmeasured risk factors tend to cluster in space. Statistical methods for dealing with both problems have been developed by fitting an autoregressive spatial model to the data and using empirical Bayes techniques to estimate the smoothed rate for each region [12, 17, 61, 64] (*see* **Geographical Analysis**). The degree of spatial autocorrelation or clustering can be measured to reflect environmental effects on the rate of disease [96, 97]. The empirical Bayes approach can also be applied to data from analytic multiple-group studies (described below) by including covariates in the model (for example [11], and [15]).

Analytic Study.   In an analytic multiple-group study, we assess the ecologic association between the average exposure level or prevalence and the rate of disease among many groups. This is the most common ecologic design; typically, the unit of analysis is a geopolitical region. For example, Hatch & Susser [38] examined the association between background gamma radiation and the incidence of childhood cancers between 1975 and 1985 in the region surrounding a nuclear plant. Average radiation levels for each of 69 tracts in the region were estimated from a 1976 areal survey. The authors found positive associations between radiation level and the incidence of leukemia (an expected finding) as well as solid tumors (an unexpected finding).

Data analysis in this type of multiple-group study usually involves fitting a mathematical model to the data. Ordinary least squares procedures, however, may be inadequate because the groups typically vary in size and much of the unexplained variability in rates across groups cannot be attributed to sampling error alone. To address these concerns, Pocock et al. [69] proposed a linear model in which the

unexplained variation is treated as random effects. Model parameters were estimated by an iteratively reweighted least squares procedure. A similar procedure was used by Breslow [6] to fit loglinear models. Prentice & Sheppard [73] proposed a linear **relative risk model**, which leads readily to the estimation of rate ratios (assuming the model is properly specified). Prentice & Thomas [77] considered an exponential relative risk model, which they argue may be more parsimonious than the linear-form model for specifying covariates. These methods can be applied to data aggregated by place and/or time (to be discussed below). Use of ecologic modeling to estimate exposure effects (rate ratios and differences) will be described in the next section.

Time-Trend Designs

Exploratory Study.   An exploratory time-trend or time-series study involves a comparison of the disease rates over time in one geographically defined population. In addition to providing graphical displays of temporal trends, time-series data can also be used to forecast future rates and trends. This latter application, which is more common in the social sciences than in epidemiology, usually involves fitting autoregressive integrated moving average (ARIMA) models to the outcome data [39, 66]. The method of ARIMA modeling can also be extended to evaluate the impact of a population intervention [59], to estimate associations between two or more time-series variables [9, 66], and to estimate associations in a mixed ecologic design ([85]; see below).

A special type of exploratory time-trend analysis often used by epidemiologists is **age–period–cohort analysis**. This approach typically involves the collection of retrospective data from a large population over a period of 20 or more years. Through graphical or tabular displays (for example [23] and [25]) or formal modeling techniques (for example [42] and [57]), the objective is to estimate the separate effects of three time-related variables on the rate of disease: age, period (calendar time), and birth cohort (year of birth). By describing the occurrence of disease in this way, the investigator attempts to gain insight about temporal trends, which might lead to new hypotheses.

Lee et al. [54] conducted an age–period–cohort analysis of melanoma mortality among white males in the US between 1951 and 1975. They concluded that the apparent increase in the melanoma mortality rate was due primarily to a cohort effect. That is, persons born in more recent years experienced throughout their lives a higher rate than did persons born earlier. In a subsequent paper, Lee [53] speculated that this cohort effect might reflect increases in sunlight exposure or sunburning during youth, which he hypothesized is a risk factor for melanoma.

From a purely statistical perspective, there is an inherent problem in making inferences from the results of age–period–cohort analyses because of the linear dependency among the three time-related variables [25, 26, 42]. Thus, we cannot allow the value of one variable to change when the values of the other two variables are held constant. As a result of this identifiability problem, each data set has alternative interpretations with respect to the combination of age, period, and cohort effects; there is no unique set of effect parameters when all three variables are modeled simultaneously. The only way to decide which interpretation should be accepted is to consider the findings in light of prior knowledge and, possibly, to constrain the model by ignoring one effect.

Analytic Study. In an analytic time-trend study, we assess the ecologic association between change in average exposure level or prevalence and change in disease rate in one geographically defined population. As with exploratory designs, this type of assessment can be done by simple graphical displays or by time-series regression modeling (for example [66]).

In their analytic time-trend study, Darby & Doll [16] examined the associations between average annual absorbed dose of radiation fallout from weapons testing and the incidence rate of childhood leukemia in three European countries between 1945 and 1985. Although the leukemia rate varied over time in each country, they found no convincing evidence that these changes were attributable to changes in fallout radiation.

Causal inference from analytic time-trend studies is often complicated by two problems. First, changes in disease classification and diagnostic criteria can produce distorted trends in the observed rate of disease, which can lead to substantial **bias** in estimating exposure effects. Second, there may be an appreciable induction/**latent period** between first exposure to a risk factor and disease detection. To deal with the latter issue in an ecologic time-trend study, the investigator can lag observations between average exposure and disease rate by a duration assumed to reflect the average induction/latent period of exposure-induced cases. There are two approaches for selecting the lag: (i) an a priori method based on knowledge of the disease; and (ii) empirical methods that maximize the observed association of interest or optimize the fit of the model that includes a lag parameter. Unfortunately, the first method is often problematic because adequate prior knowledge is lacking, and the second method can produce results that are biologically meaningless and very misleading [37].

Mixed Designs

Exploratory Study. The exploratory mixed design combines the basic features of the exploratory multiple-group study and the exploratory time-trend study. Time-series (ARIMA) modeling or age–period–cohort analysis can be used to describe or predict trends in the disease rate for multiple populations. For example, to test Lee's [53] hypothesis that changes in sunlight exposure during youth can explain the observed increase in melanoma mortality in the US, we might conduct an age–period–cohort analysis, stratifying on region according to approximate sunlight exposure (without measuring the exposure). Assuming the amount of sunlight in the regions has not changed differentially over the study period, we might expect the cohort effect described earlier to be stronger for sunnier regions.

Analytic Study. In an analytic mixed design, we assess the association between change in average exposure level or prevalence and change in disease rate among many groups. Thus, the interpretation of estimated effects is enhanced because two types of comparisons are made simultaneously: change over time within groups and differences among groups. For example, Crawford et al. [14] evaluated the hypothesis that hard drinking water (i.e. water with a high concentration of calcium and magnesium) is a protective risk factor for cardiovascular disease (CVD) mortality. They compared the absolute change in CVD mortality rate between 1948 and 1964 in 83 British towns, by water-hardness change, age, and sex. In all sex–age groups, especially for men, the authors found an inverse association between trends in water hardness and CVD mortality. In middle-aged men, for example, the increase in CVD mortality was less in towns that made their water harder than in towns that made their water softer.

Effect Estimation

A major quantitative objective of most epidemiologic studies is to estimate the effect of one or more exposures on disease occurrence in a well-defined population at risk. A measure of effect in this context is not just any measure of association such as a correlation coefficient; rather, it reflects a particular causal parameter, i.e. a counterfactual contrast in disease occurrence [30, 33, 36, 63, 83]. In studies conducted at the individual level, effects are usually estimated by comparing the rate or risk of disease, in the form of a ratio or difference, for exposed and unexposed populations. In multiple-group ecologic studies, however, we cannot estimate effects directly in this way because of the missing information on the joint distribution within groups. Instead, we regress the group-specific disease rates, Y, on the group-specific exposure prevalences, X. (Note that throughout this article uppercase letters will be used to represent ecologic variables and their estimated regression coefficients; lowercase letters will be used to represent individual-level variables and their estimated regression coefficients.)

The most common model form for analyzing ecologic data is the linear model. Ordinary least-squares methods can be used to produce the following prediction equation: $\hat{Y} = B_0 + B_1X$, where B_0 and B_1 are the estimated intercept and slope. An estimate of the biologic effect of the exposure (at the individual level) can be derived from the regression results [1, 28]. The predicted disease rate ($\hat{Y}_{x=1}$) in a group that is entirely exposed is $B_0 + B_1(1) = B_0 + B_1$, and the predicted rate ($\hat{Y}_{x=0}$) in a group that is entirely unexposed is $B_0 + B_1(0) = B_0$. Therefore, the estimated rate difference is $B_0 + B_1 - B_0 = B_1$, and the estimated rate ratio is $(B_0 + B_1)/B_0 = 1 + B_1/B_0$.

Alternatively, fitting a loglinear (exponential) model to the data yields the following prediction equation: $\ln[\hat{Y}] = B_0 + B_1X$ or $\hat{Y} = \exp[B_0 + B_1X]$. Applying the same method used above for linear models, the estimated rate ratio is $\hat{Y}_{x=1}/\hat{Y}_{x=0} = \exp[B_1]$.

Note that the ecologic method of effect estimation requires rate predictions be extrapolated to both extreme values of the exposure variable (i.e. $X = 0$ and 1), which are likely to lie well beyond the observed range of the data. It is not surprising, therefore, that different model forms (e.g. loglinear vs. linear) can lead to very different estimates of effect [31]. Fitting a linear model, in fact, may lead to negative, and thus meaningless, estimates of the rate ratio.

As an illustration of rate-ratio estimation in an ecologic study, consider Durkheim's [20] examination of religion and suicide in four groups of Prussian provinces between 1883 and 1890 (see Figure 2). The groups were formed by ranking 13 provinces according to the proportion (X) of the population that was Protestant. Using ordinary least-squares linear regression, we estimate the suicide rate ($\hat{Y}$, per 10^5/year) in each group to be $3.66 + 24.0(X)$. Therefore, the estimated rate ratio, comparing Protestants with other religions, is $1 + (24.0/3.66) = 7.6$. Note in Figure 2 that the fit of the linear model appears excellent ($R^2 = 0.97$). In general, however, ecologic tests of fit can be misleading about the underlying model at the individual level that generated the ecologic data [35].

Confounders and Effect Modifiers

There are two methods used to control for **confounders** in multiple-group ecologic analyses. The first is to treat ecologic measures of the confounders as covariates ($\mathbf{Z}$) in the model, e.g. percent male and percent white in each group. If the individual-level effects of the exposure and covariates

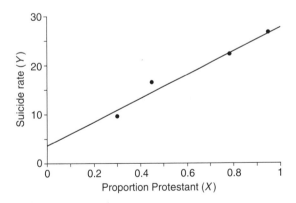

Figure 2 Suicide rate (Y, per 10^5/year) by proportion Protestant (X) for four groups of Prussian provinces, 1883–90. The four observed points (X, Y) are (0.30, 9.56), (0.45, 16.36), (0.785, 22.00), and (0.95, 26.46); the fitted line is based on unweighted least-squares regression. Adapted from Durkheim [20]

are additive (i.e. if the disease rates follow a linear model), then the ecologic regression of Y on X and $\mathbf{Z}$ will also be linear with the same coefficients [31, 52] (see **Additive Model**). That is, the estimated coefficient for the exposure variable in a linear model can be interpreted as the rate difference adjusted for the covariates, provided the effects are truly additive and there are no other sources of bias. To estimate the adjusted rate ratio for the exposure effect, we must first specify values for all covariates ($\mathbf{Z}$) in the model, because the effects of X and $\mathbf{Z}$ are assumed to be additive – not multiplicative. Thus, the estimated rate ratio, conditional on covariate levels ($\mathbf{Z}$), is the predicted rate in a group that is entirely exposed ($\hat{Y}_{x=1|\mathbf{Z}}$) divided by the predicted rate in a group that is entirely unexposed ($\hat{Y}_{x=0|\mathbf{Z}}$).

Fitting an additive loglinear model to the ecologic data yields an estimate of the adjusted rate ratio that is independent of covariates – i.e. $\hat{Y}_{x=1|\mathbf{Z}}/\hat{Y}_{x=0|\mathbf{Z}} = \exp[B_1]$, where B_1 is the estimated coefficient for the exposure. Thus, the effects of X and $\mathbf{Z}$ are assumed to be multiplicative (see **Multiplicative Model**). Unfortunately, this ecologic estimate is a biased estimate of the individual-level rate ratio, even if the effects are multiplicative at the individual level and no other sources of bias are present [31, 79].

The second method used to control for confounders in ecologic analyses is rate standardization for these confounders, followed by regression of the standardized rates as the outcome variable (see **Standardization Methods**). Note that this method requires additional data on the joint distribution of the covariate and disease within each group (i.e. the M frequencies in Figure 1). Nevertheless, it cannot be expected to reduce bias unless all predictors in the model (X and $\mathbf{Z}$) are also mutually standardized for the same confounders [31, 34, 82]. Standardization of the exposure prevalences, for example, requires data on the joint distribution of the covariate and exposure within groups (i.e. the N frequencies in Figure 1); unfortunately, this information is not usually available in ecologic studies.

As in individual-level analyses, product terms (e.g. XZ) are often used in ecologic analyses to model **interaction** effects, i.e. to assess **effect modification**. In ecologic analyses, however, the product of X and Z (both group averages) is not, in general, equal to the average product of the exposure, x, and covariate, z, at the individual level within groups. Assuming a linear model, XZ will be equal to the mean xz in each

group only if x and z are uncorrelated within groups [31]. Thus, as pointed out in the next section, interaction (nonadditive) effects at the individual level complicate the interpretation of ecologic results.

Methodologic Problems

Despite the many practical advantages of ecologic studies mentioned previously, there are several methodologic problems that may severely limit causal inference, especially biologic inference.

Ecologic Bias

The major limitation of ecologic analysis for making causal inferences is ecologic bias, which is the failure of expected ecologic effect estimates to reflect the biologic effect at the individual level [22, 28, 34, 35, 62, 79]. In addition to the usual sources of bias that threaten individual-level analyses, the underlying problem of ecologic analyses for estimating biologic effects is heterogeneity of exposure level and covariate levels within groups. As noted earlier, this heterogeneity is not fully captured with ecologic data because of missing information on joint distributions (see Figure 1). Although researchers have long recognized the discrepancy between individual- and group-level associations (for example [24] and [91]), Robinson [80] was the first to describe mathematically how ecologic associations could differ from the corresponding associations at the individual level within groups of the same population. He expressed this relationship in terms of correlation coefficients, which was later extended by Duncan et al. [19] to regression coefficients in a linear model. The phenomenon became widely known as the **ecologic fallacy** [86], and researchers came to recognize that the magnitude of the ecologic bias may be severe in practice [13, 21, 79, 87, 89].

As an illustration of ecologic bias, consider again Durkheim's data on religion and suicide (Figure 2). The estimated rate ratio of 7.6 in the ecologic analysis may not mean that the suicide rate was nearly 8 times greater in Protestants than in non-Protestants. Rather, since none of the regions was entirely Protestant or non-Protestant, it may have been non-Protestants (primarily Catholics) who were committing suicide in predominantly Protestant provinces. It is certainly plausible that members of a religious minority might have been more likely to take their own lives than were members of the majority. The implication of this alternative explanation is that living in a predominantly Protestant area has a contextual effect on suicide risk among non-Protestants, i.e. there is an interaction effect at the individual level between religion and religious composition of one's area of residence.

Interestingly, Durkheim [20] compared the suicide rates (at the individual level) for Protestants, Catholics, and Jews living in Prussia. From his data, we find that the rate was about twice as great in Protestants as in other religious groups. Thus, there appears to be substantial ecologic bias (i.e. comparing rate-ratio estimates of about 2 vs. 8). Durkheim, however, failed to notice this quantitative difference because he did not actually estimate the magnitude of the effect in either analysis.

Greenland & Morgenstern [34] showed that ecologic bias can arise from three sources when using simple linear regression to estimate the crude exposure effect: the first may operate in any type of study; the latter two are unique to ecologic studies (i.e. *cross-level bias*) but are defined in terms of individual-level parameters.

1. *Within-group bias*: ecologic bias may result from bias within groups due to **confounding**, **selection** methods, or **misclassification**, even though within-group effects are not estimated. Thus, for example, if there is positive confounding of the crude effect parameter in every group, we would expect the crude ecologic estimate to be biased as well.
2. *Confounding by group*: ecologic bias may result if the background rate of disease in the unexposed population varies across groups, specifically, if there is a nonzero ecologic correlation between mean exposure level and the background rate.
3. *Effect modification by group* (on an additive scale): ecologic bias may also result if the rate difference for the exposure effect at the individual level varies across groups.

Confounding and effect modification by group (the sources of cross-level bias) can arise in three ways: (i) extraneous risk factors (confounders or modifiers) are differentially distributed across groups; (ii) the ecologic exposure variable has a contextual effect on

risk separate from the biologic effect of its individual-level analog, e.g. living in a predominantly Protestant area vs. being Protestant (in the suicide example); or (iii) disease risk depends on the prevalence of that disease in other members of the group, which is true of many infectious diseases [50].

To appreciate the sources of cross-level bias, it is helpful to consider simple numerical illustrations involving both individual-level and ecologic analyses with the same population. The hypothetical example in Table 1 involves a dichotomous exposure, x, and three groups. At the individual level, both the rate difference and rate ratio vary somewhat across the groups, but the effect is positive in all groups; the crude and group-standardized rate ratio is 2.0. Fitting a linear model to the ecologic data, however, we find that the slope for the exposure variable, X, is negative and the rate ratio is 0.50, suggesting a protective effect. The reason for such large ecologic bias is heterogeneity of the rate difference across groups (effect modification by group). In this example, there is no confounding by group because the unexposed rate is the same (100 per 10^5/year) in all three groups.

The example in Table 2 illustrates the conditions for no cross-level bias. First, group is not a modifier of the exposure effect at the individual level because the rate difference (100 per 10^5/year) is uniform across groups (even though the rate ratio varies). Second, group is not a confounder of the exposure effect because there is no ecologic correlation between the percent exposed ($100X$) and the unexposed rate. Thus, the individual-level and ecologic estimates of the rate ratio are the same (1.8) and unbiased, even though the R^2 for the fitted model is very low (0.029).

Unfortunately, the two conditions that produce cross-level bias cannot be checked with ecologic data because those conditions are defined in terms of individual-level associations. This inability to check the validity of ecologic results seriously limits biologic inference. Furthermore, the fit of the ecologic regression model, in general, gives no indication of the presence, direction, or magnitude of ecologic bias. Thus, a model with excellent fit may yield substantial bias, and one model with a better fit than another model may yield more bias. For example, there was substantial bias when fitting a linear model to Durkheim's suicide data in Figure 2, despite an excellent fitting model ($R^2 = 0.97$). Recall that the

Table 1 Number of new cases, person-years (P-Y) of follow-up, and disease rate (Y, per 100 000/year), by group and exposure status (x) (top panel); summary parameters for each group (middle panel); and results of individual-level and ecologic analyses (bottom panel): hypothetical example of ecologic bias due to effect modification by group

Exposure status (x)	Group 1			Group 2			Group 3		
	Cases	P-Y	Rate	Cases	P-Y	Rate	Cases	P-Y	Rate
Exposed ($x = 1$)	20	7 000	286	20	10 000	200	20	13 000	154
Unexposed ($x = 0$)	13	13 000	100	10	10 000	100	7	7 000	100
Total	33	20 000	165	30	20 000	150	27	20 000	135
% exposed ($100X$)			35			50			65
Rate difference (per 10^5/year)			186			100			54
Rate ratio			2.9			2.0			1.5

Individual-level analysis: *Ecologic analysis*: Linear model
    Crude rate ratio[a] = 2.0 $\hat{Y} = 200 - 100X$ ($R^2 = 1$)
    Adjusted rate ratio (SMR)[b] = 2.0   Rate ratio = 0.50

[a]Rate ratio for the total population, unadjusted for group.
[b]Rate ratio standardized for group, using the exposed population as the standard.

Table 2 Number of new cases, person-years (P-Y) of follow-up, and disease rate (Y, per 100 000/year), by group and exposure status, x, (top panel); summary parameters for each group (middle panel); and results of individual-level and ecologic analyses (bottom panel): hypothetical example of no ecologic bias

Exposure status (x)	Group 1			Group 2			Group 3		
	Cases	P-Y	Rate	Cases	P-Y	Rate	Cases	P-Y	Rate
Exposed ($x = 1$)	16	8 000	200	30	10 000	300	24	12 000	200
Unexposed ($x = 0$)	12	12 000	100	20	10 000	200	8	8 000	100
Total	28	20 000	140	50	20 000	250	32	20 000	160
% exposed ($100X$)			40			50			60
Rate difference (per 10^5/year)			100			100			100
Rate ratio			2.0			1.5			2.0

Individual-level analysis: *Ecologic analysis:* Linear model
    Crude rate ratio[a] = 1.8 $\hat{Y} = 133 + 100X (R^2 = 0.029)$
    Adjusted rate ratio (SMR)[b] = 1.8   Rate ratio = 1.8

[a]Rate ratio for the total population, unadjusted for group.
[b]Rate ratio standardized for group, using the exposed population as the standard.

estimated rate ratio was 7.6, compared with a "true" rate ratio of approximately 2 (see section "Effect Estimation" above). If we fit a loglinear model to the same data, we get $\hat{Y} = \exp[1.974 + 1.418X]$ and $R^2 = 0.91$; therefore, the estimated rate ratio is $\exp[1.418] = 4.1$. Thus, the loglinear model produces less bias even though it has a smaller R^2 than does the linear model. In general, we cannot expect to reduce bias by using better-fitting models in ecologic analysis.

A potential strategy for reducing ecologic bias is to use smaller units in an ecologic study (e.g. counties instead of states) to make the groups more homogeneous with respect to the exposure. On the other hand, this strategy might not be feasible owing to the lack of available data aggregated at the same level, and it can lead to another problem: greater migration between groups (see the section "Other Problems", subsection "Migration Across Groups") [62, 95].

Problems of Confounder Control

As indicated in a previous section, covariates are included in ecologic analyses to control for confounding, but the conditions for a covariate being a confounder are different at the ecologic and individual levels [34, 35]. At the individual level, a risk factor must be associated with the exposure to be a confounder. In a multiple-group ecologic study, in contrast, a risk factor may produce ecologic bias (i.e. it may be an ecologic confounder) even if it is unassociated with the exposure in every group, especially if the risk factor is ecologically associated with the exposure across groups [31, 34]. Conversely, a risk factor that is a confounder within groups may not produce ecologic bias if it is ecologically unassociated with the exposure across groups.

Control for confounders is more problematic in ecologic analyses than in individual-level analyses [31, 34, 35]. Even when all variables are accurately measured for all groups, adjustment for extraneous risk factors may not reduce the ecologic bias produced by these risk factors. In fact, it is possible for such ecologic adjustment to increase bias [34, 35].

It follows from the principles presented in the previous section that there will be no ecologic bias in a multiple linear regression analysis if all the following conditions are met:

1. There is no residual within-group bias in exposure effect in any group due to confounding by unmeasured risk factors, selection methods, or misclassification.
2. There is no ecologic correlation between the mean value of each predictor (exposure and covariate) and the background rate of disease in the joint reference (unexposed) level of all predictors (so that group does not confound the predictor effects).
3. The rate difference for each predictor is uniform across levels of the other predictors within groups (i.e. the effects are additive).
4. The rate difference for each predictor, conditional on other predictors in the model, is uniform across groups (i.e. group does not modify the effect of each predictor on the additive scale at the individual level).

These conditions are sufficient, but not necessary, for the ecologic estimate to be unbiased, i.e. there might be little or no bias even if none of these conditions is met. On the other hand, minor deviations from the latter three conditions can produce substantial cross-level bias [31]. Since the sufficient conditions for no cross-level bias cannot be checked with ecologic data

alone, the unpredictable and potentially severe nature of such bias makes biologic inference from ecologic analyses particularly problematic.

The conditions for no cross-level bias with covariate adjustment are illustrated in the hypothetical example in Table 3. Both the exposure, x, and covariate, z, are dichotomous variables, and there are three groups. At the individual level, the covariate is not a confounder of the exposure effect because there is no exposure–covariate association within any of the groups. Thus, the crude and adjusted estimates of the rate ratio are nearly the same (1.3). In the ecologic analysis, however, the covariate is a confounder because there is an inverse association between the exposure, X, and the covariate, Z, across groups. Thus, although the crude ecologic estimate of the rate ratio (0.32) is severely biased, the adjusted estimate (1.3) is unbiased. The reasons for no cross-level bias with covariate adjustment are: (i) the rate (100 per 10^5/year) in the joint reference group ($x = z = 0$) does not vary across groups, i.e. condition 2 is met; and (ii) the rate difference (100 per 10^5/year) is uniform within groups and across groups, i.e. conditions 3 and 4 are met.

The example in Table 4 illustrates cross-level bias when the null hypothesis is true. At the individual level, the covariate (z) is a strong confounder because it is a predictor of the disease in the unexposed population and it is associated with exposure status, x, within groups. Thus, the crude rate ratio (2.1) is biased. At the ecologic level, however, there is no association between the exposure, X, and the covariate, Z, so that the covariate is not an ecologic confounder. Nevertheless, both the crude and adjusted rate ratios (8.6) are strongly biased because the rate in the joint reference category ($x = z = 0$) is ecologically correlated with both the exposure, X, and the covariate, Z – i.e. condition 2 is not met.

Lack of additivity at the individual level (refer to condition 3) is common in epidemiology, but unmeasured modifiers do not bias results at the individual level if they are unrelated to the exposure [30]. Furthermore, interactions may be handled readily at the individual level by including product terms as predictors in the model (e.g. xz). In ecologic analyses, however, lack of additivity within groups is a source of ecologic bias, and this bias cannot be eliminated by the inclusion of product terms (e.g. XZ) unless the effects are exactly multiplicative and the two variables are uncorrelated within groups [78]. If x and z

Table 3 Number of new cases, person-years (P-Y) of follow-up, and disease rate (Y, per 100 000/year), by group, covariate status, z, and exposure status, x (top panel); summary parameters for each group (middle panel); and results of individual-level and ecologic analyses (bottom panel): hypothetical example of no ecologic bias; covariate is an ecologic confounder but not a within-group confounder

Covariate status (z)	Exposure status (x)	Group 1			Group 2			Group 3		
		Cases	P-Y	Rate	Cases	P-Y	Rate	Cases	P-Y	Rate
1	Exposed	18	3 000	600	24	4 000	600	24	4 000	600
	Unexposed	60	12 000	500	40	8 000	500	30	6 000	500
	Total	78	15 000	520	64	12 000	533	54	10 000	540
0	Exposed	4	2 000	200	8	4 000	200	12	6 000	200
	Unexposed	8	8 000	100	8	8 000	100	9	9 000	100
	Total	12	10 000	120	16	12 000	133	21	15 000	140
Total	Exposed	22	5 000	440	32	8 000	400	36	10 000	360
	Unexposed	68	20 000	340	48	16 000	300	39	15 000	260
	Total	90	25 000	360	80	24 000	333	75	25 000	300

% exposed ($100X$)				20			33		40
% with $z = 1$ ($100Z$)				60			50		40

Individual-level analysis:
    Crude rate ratio[a] = 1.3
    Adjusted rate ratio (SMR)[b] = 1.3

Ecologic analysis: Linear models
    Crude: $\hat{Y} = 420 - 286X$ ($R^2 = 0.94$); rate ratio = 0.32
    Adjusted: $\hat{Y} = 100 + 100X + 400Z$ ($R^2 = 1$); rate ratio[c] = 1.3

[a]Rate ratio for the total population, unadjusted for group or the covariate.
[b]Rate ratio standardized for group and the covariate, using the exposed population as the standard.
[c]Setting $Z = 0.50$ (the mean for all three groups).

Table 4 Number of new cases, person-years (P-Y) of follow-up, and disease rate (Y, per 100 000/year), by group, covariate status, z, and exposure status, x (top panel); summary parameters for each group (middle panel); and results of individual-level and ecologic analyses (bottom panel): hypothetical example of ecologic bias due to confounding by group; covariate is a within-group confounder but not an ecologic confounder

Covariate status (z)	Exposure status (x)	Group 1			Group 2			Group 3		
		Cases	P-Y	Rate	Cases	P-Y	Rate	Cases	P-Y	Rate
1	Exposed	40	8 000	500	195	13 000	1500	140	14 000	1 000
	Unexposed	60	12 000	500	180	12 000	1500	60	6 000	1 000
	Total	100	20 000	500	375	25 000	1500	200	20 000	1 000
0	Exposed	2	2 000	100	6	2 000	300	12	6 000	200
	Unexposed	28	28 000	100	69	23 000	300	48	24 000	200
	Total	30	30 000	100	75	25 000	300	60	30 000	200
Total	Exposed	42	10 000	420	201	15 000	1340	152	20 000	760
	Unexposed	88	40 000	220	249	35 000	711	108	30 000	360
	Total	130	50 000	260	450	50 000	900	260	50 000	520

% exposed ($100X$)				20			30		40
% with $z = 1$ ($100Z$)				40			50		40

Individual-level analysis:
    Crude rate ratio[a] = 2.1
    Adjusted rate ratio (SMR)[b] = 1.0

Ecologic analysis: Linear models
    Crude: $\hat{Y} = 170 + 1300X$ ($R^2 = 0.16$); rate ratio = 8.6
    Adjusted: $\hat{Y} = -2040 + 1300X + 5100Z$ ($R^2 = 1$); rate ratio[c] = 8.6

[a]Rate ratio for the total population, unadjusted for group or the covariate.
[b]Rate ratio standardized for group and the covariate, using the exposed population as the standard; also the common rate ratio within each group.
[c]Setting $Z = 0.433$ (the mean for all three groups).

are correlated within groups, additional data on the $x–z$ associations (the N frequencies in Figure 1) can be used to improve the ecologic estimate of each predictor controlling for the other [68, 76].

Another source of ecologic bias is misspecification of confounders [35]. Although this problem can also arise in individual-level analyses, it is more difficult to avoid in ecologic analyses because the relevant confounder may be the distribution of covariate histories for all individuals within each group. In ecologic studies, therefore, adjustment for covariates derived from available data (e.g. proportion of current smokers) may be inadequate to control confounding. It is preferable, whenever possible, to control for more than a single summary measure of the covariate distribution (e.g. the proportions of the group in each of several smoking categories), provided the outcome rate is not standardized (see section "Effect Estimation" above). In addition, since it is usually necessary to control for several confounders (among which the effects may not be linear and additive), the best approach for reducing ecologic bias is to include covariates for categories of their joint distribution within groups. For example, to control ecologically for race and sex, the investigator might adjust for the proportions of white women, nonwhite men, and nonwhite women (treating white men as the referent), rather than the conventional approach of adjusting for the proportions of men (or women) and whites (or nonwhites).

Within-Group Misclassification

The principles of misclassification bias with which epidemiologists are familiar when interpreting the results of analyses conducted at the individual level do not apply to ecologic analyses. At the individual level, for example, nondifferential misclassification of exposure nearly always leads to **bias toward the null**. In multiple-group ecologic studies, however, this principle does not hold when the exposure variable is an aggregate measure. Brenner et al. [5] have shown that nondifferential misclassification of a dichotomous exposure within groups usually leads to bias away from the null and that the bias may be severe.

As an illustration of this distinct feature of ecologic analysis, consider the two-group example in Table 5, which contrasts analyses with correctly classified and misclassified exposure data at both the individual and ecologic levels. The **sensitivity** and **specificity** of exposure classification are assumed to be 0.9 for both cases and noncases in the population. The correct rate ratio at the individual level is 5.0; with nondifferential exposure misclassification,

Table 5 Number of new cases, person-years (P-Y) of follow-up, and disease rate (Y, per 100 000/year), by group, type of exposure classification (correct vs. misclassified[a]), and exposure status (top panel); % exposed by group (middle panel); and results of individual-level and ecologic analyses (bottom panel): hypothetical example of ecologic bias away from the null due to nondifferential exposure misclassification within groups

Exposure classification	Exposure status	Group 1			Group 2		
		Cases	P-Y	Rate	Cases	P-Y	Rate
Correctly classified	Exposed ($x = 1$)	50	20 000	250	100	40 000	250
	Unexposed ($x = 0$)	40	80 000	50	30	60 000	50
	Total	100	100 000	100	130	100 000	130
Misclassified[a]	Exposed ($x' = 1$)	49	26 000	188	93	42 000	221
	Unexposed ($x' = 0$)	41	74 000	55	37	58 000	64
	Total	100	100 000	100	130	100 000	130
% exposed – correctly classified (100X)				20			40
% exposed – misclassified (100X')				26			42

Individual-level analysis:
   Correct: rate ratio[b] = 5.0
   Misclassified: rate ratio[c] = 3.4

Ecologic analysis: Linear models
   Correct: $\hat{Y} = 50 + 200X$; rate ratio = 5.0
   Misclassified: $\hat{Y} = 25 + 250X'$; rate ratio = 11.0

[a]Sensitivity = specificity = 0.9 for both cases and noncases (nondifferential misclassification).
[b]Common rate ratio within each group.
[c]Common rate ratio, using the Mantel-Haenszel method.

the observed rate ratio would be 3.4, which is biased toward the null. Although an ecologic analysis of the correctly classified data yields an unbiased estimate of the rate ratio (5.0), an analysis with misclassified data would yield an observed rate ratio of 11.0, which is strongly biased away from the null. To appreciate the direction of the misclassification bias in this ecologic analysis, notice that the difference in the percent exposed ($100X$) between the two groups decreases from $40\% - 20\% = 20\%$ to $42\% - 26\% = 16\%$ when the exposure is misclassified (see Table 5). Thus, the slope in the misclassified analysis increases from 200 to 250 per 10^5/year. In addition, the intercept decreases from 50 to 25 per 10^5/year. Each of these changes causes the observed rate ratio with the misclassified data to increase (away from the null).

It is possible to correct for nondifferential misclassification of a dichotomous exposure or disease in ecologic analyses, based on prior specifications of sensitivity and specificity [4, Appendix 1; 32]. Suppose, for example, we wish to correct for nondifferential exposure misclassification when using simple linear regression (no covariates) to estimate the exposure effect. The corrected estimator of the rate ratio derived from the model results is $(B_0 + B_1 \text{Se})/[B_0 + B_1(1 - \text{Sp})]$, where B_0 and B_1 are the estimated intercept and slope from the misclassified data, Se is the sensitivity of exposure classification, and Sp is the specificity. Greenland & Brenner [32] also derived a corrected estimator for the variance of the estimated rate ratio.

In studies conducted at the individual level, misclassification of a covariate, if nondifferential with respect to both exposure and disease, will usually reduce our ability to control for that confounder [29, 84]. That is, adjustment will not completely eliminate the bias due to the confounder. In ecologic studies, however, nondifferential misclassification of a dichotomous confounder within groups does not affect our ability to control for that confounder, provided there is no cross-level bias [4].

If the outcome and all but one predictor (i.e. the exposure or a covariate) in a given analysis are measured at the individual level, then this partially ecologic analysis may also be regarded as nonecologic with the ecologic variable misclassified. Thus, the resulting bias may be understood in terms of misclassification bias operating at the individual level.

Other Problems

Lack of Adequate Data.   Certain types of data, such as medical histories, may not be available in aggregate form; or available data may be too crude, incomplete, or unreliable, such as sales data for measuring behaviors [62, 95]. In addition, secondary sources of data from different administrative areas or from different periods may not be comparable. For example, disease rates may vary across countries because of differences in disease classification or case detection. Furthermore, since many ecologic analyses are based on mortality rather than incidence data, causal inference is further limited because mortality reflects the course of disease as well as its occurrence [48].

Temporal Ambiguity.   In a well-designed cohort study of disease incidence, we can usually be confident that disease occurrence did not precede the exposure. In ecologic studies, however, use of incidence data provides no such assurance against this temporal ambiguity [62]. The problem is most troublesome when the disease can influence exposure status in individuals or when the disease rate can influence the mean exposure in groups (through the impact of population interventions designed to change exposure levels in areas with high disease rates).

The problem of temporal ambiguity in ecologic studies (especially time-trend studies) is further complicated by an unknown or variable induction and **latent periods** between exposure and disease detection [37, 95]. The investigator can only attempt to deal with this problem in the analysis by examining associations for which there is a specified lag between observations of average exposure and disease rate. Unfortunately, there may be little prior information about induction and latency on which to base the lag, or appropriate data may not be available to accommodate the desired lag.

Collinearity.   Another problem with ecologic analyses is that certain predictors, such as sociodemographic and environmental factors, tend to be more highly correlated with each other than they are at the individual level [13, 87]. The implication of such collinearities is that it is very difficult to separate the effects of these variables statistically; analyses yield model coefficients with very large variances so that effect estimates may be highly unstable. In general, collinearity is most problematic in multiple-group ecologic analyses involving a small number of large, heterogeneous regions [19, 92].

Migration Across Groups.   Migration of individuals into or out of the source population can produce **selection bias** in a study conducted at the individual level because migrants and nonmigrants may differ on both exposure prevalence and disease risk. Although it is clear that migration can also cause ecologic bias [49, 70], little is known about the magnitude of this bias or how it can be reduced in ecologic studies [63].

Ecologic Results and Epidemiologic Controversy

Contemporary epidemiologists take a conservative view of ecologic studies. Knowing that ecologic estimates of effect may be severely biased because of problems discussed in the previous section, epidemiologists tend to trust ecologic findings only if such findings agree with the results of other studies conducted at the individual level, particularly **case–control** and **cohort studies**. Nevertheless, this conservative view ignores the possibility that in certain situations ecologic results might be less biased than are results from case–control and cohort studies, which may, for example, involve appreciable error in measuring exposures (*see* **Measurement Error in Epidemiologic Studies**). Inconsistencies between the results of ecologic and other studies, therefore, can generate controversy about risk-factor effects and the potential for prevention.

One such controversy involving ecologic evidence concerns the possible effect of dietary fat on the risk of breast-cancer. In 1990, Prentice & Sheppard [74] reported results from three types of ecologic studies: (i) an international comparison of breast-cancer incidence during the period 1978–82 in 21 countries (analytic multiple-group design); (ii) a comparison of trends in breast-cancer incidence between the 1960s and 1978–82 among 10 of the 21 countries in the previous analysis (analytic mixed design); and (iii) a comparison of breast-cancer incidence in US residents of Japanese descent vs. Japanese residents (exploratory multiple-group design). Using data from the 21-country study, the authors found that a 50% reduction in the supply (disappearance) of total fat is associated with a 60% reduction in the

incidence of breast cancer among post-menopausal women (ages 55–69). The magnitude of this association did not change appreciably when controlling for gross national product, per capita supply of non-fat calories, and other ecologic variables available to the investigators. The results were similar when the exposure was measured as grams of fat per day and percent of calories from fat [75]. In addition, the association between fat and breast cancer observed in the 21-country analysis was consistent with the results of the two other ecologic analyses.

Despite the large effect and the consistency of these ecologic findings, causal inference is limited for several reasons (for example [40], [43], [75], and [98]): First, because of food wastage, nonhuman consumption, and poor reporting, the per capita *supply* of fat may not be proportional to the per capita *consumption* of fat across countries. Furthermore, the ecologic analyses were conducted within age–sex strata, but per capita fat supply was obtained only for the total population of each country. Second, there may have been systematic differences in breast-cancer detection across countries. Third, Prentice & Sheppard did not have data to control for certain breast-cancer risk factors, such as reproductive history and energy restriction or physical activity early in life. Fourth, the ecologic estimates of effect are susceptible to cross-level bias for other reasons discussed in the previous section.

Although Prentice & Sheppard [74] could not address the above limitations directly, they conducted additional analyses to demonstrate that their ecologic findings were consistent with the results of a pooled analysis of raw data from 12 case–control studies of fat and breast cancer [44]. Using the effect estimate from the 21-country study, they projected the rate ratios (**"relative risks"**) that would be expected in the pooled analysis of case–control studies, assuming random nondifferential error in measuring dietary fat – i.e. assuming the amount of measurement error does not depend on other variables in the analysis. To estimate the amount of measurement error, Prentice & Sheppard used the results of a **validation study** in which food-frequency data (the type used in the case–control studies) were compared with food-record data for the same subjects. They found, for example, that the projected rate ratio for the highest quintile of fat consumption vs. the lowest quintile was 1.46, compared with an observed rate ratio of 1.53 in the pooled analysis of case–control studies [74].

Reactions to the results of Prentice & Sheppard varied considerably. While Hiller & McMichael [40] called their work "a revitalization of ecological studies", Willett & Stampfer [98] maintained that "virtually all the analyses presented by Prentice and Sheppard are irrelevant to etiologic relationships between fat intake and risk of cancer".

One possible problem with the method of Prentice & Sheppard is their assumption that error in measuring fat intake is **nondifferential** with respect to disease status. Since dietary fat is measured after cases are detected in case–control studies, it is possible that cases were more likely to exaggerate their past consumption of fat or that controls were more likely to underestimate it; thus, the rate ratio would be positively biased. To address this concern, Hunter et al. [46] conducted a pooled analysis of raw data from seven cohort studies in which error in measuring fat intake at baseline would be expected to be nondifferential with respect to subsequent disease status. The estimated rate ratio for the highest quintile of (energy-adjusted) fat intake versus the lowest quintile was 1.05, and this estimate did not change much when correcting for random nondifferential error in measuring fat intake. Thus, Hunter et al. [46] concluded that there was no evidence of a positive effect of dietary fat on breast-cancer risk. The implication is that effect estimates from the case–control studies were positively biased by differential recall of fat intake and/or selection methods (*see* **Recall Bias**) and that effect estimates from ecologic studies were also positively biased due to the problems mentioned above.

As coherent as these interpretations may appear, they still depend on rather strong assumptions about the error in measuring fat intake at the individual level. It is possible, for example, that the amount of measurement error depends on relevant variables other than disease status. This possibility was evaluated in a recent study by Prentice [71], who used the fat-effect estimate from the 21-country study to project the rate ratios expected in cohort studies under more realistic assumptions of measurement error. To assess the amount of measurement error, Prentice used the results of another validation study in which food-frequency data were compared with 4-day food-record data at two times, one year apart. In this way, he allowed the amount of error in measuring fat intake to depend on body mass index; and he allowed for measurement errors for the two assessment instruments to be correlated. Under these conditions, he found that the projected rate ratio for the effect of total fat, comparing the highest and lowest quintiles, is approximately 1.1. Prentice concluded, therefore, that the results of Hunter et al.'s [46] pooled analysis of cohort studies is consistent with an effect of fat intake estimated from the international ecologic study.

It is not likely that these recent findings of Prentice will settle disagreements about the possible effect of dietary fat on the risk of breast cancer. Whether ecologic or nonecologic studies provide more accurate estimates of diet effects on cancer incidence remains controversial.

Multilevel Analyses and Designs

Knowing the severe methodologic limitations of ecologic analysis for making biologic inferences, many epidemiologists who report ecologic results argue that there can be no cross-level bias when their primary objective is to estimate an ecologic effect (for example [8], [10] and [88]). For example, we might want to estimate the ecologic effect (effectiveness) of state laws requiring smoke detectors by comparing the fire-related mortality rate in those states with the law vs. other states without the law [62]. Although this is a reasonable objective, the interpretation of observed ecologic effects is complicated by two related issues.

First, disease occurs in individuals; thus, the disease rate in a population is an aggregate, not a global, measure. Consequently, biologic inference may be implicit to the objectives of an ecologic study unless the underlying biologic and contextual effects are already known from previous research. Can smoke detectors placed appropriately in homes reduce the risk of fire-related mortality in those homes by providing an early warning of smoke? Does living in an area where most homes are properly equipped with smoke detectors reduce the risk of fire-related mortality in homes with and without smoke detectors? The first question refers to a possible biologic (biobehavioral) effect; the second question refers to a possible contextual effect. The ecologic effect of smoke-detector laws depends on these biologic and contextual effects as well as other factors, e.g. the level of enforcement, the quality of smoke-detector design and construction, the cost and availability of smoke detectors, and their proper placement, installation, operation, and maintenance. In an ecologic study without additional information, the ecologic effect is completely confounded with related biologic and contextual effects.

The second complicating issue in interpreting observed ecologic effects is the need to control for confounders measured at the individual level. Even if the exposure is a global measure, such as a law, groups are seldom completely homogeneous or comparable with respect to confounders. To make a valid comparison between states with and without smoke-detector laws, for example, we would need to control for differences among states in the joint distribution of extraneous risk factors, such as socioeconomic status of residents, firefighter availability and access, building design and construction (see also the earlier section "Problems of Confounder Control").

Perhaps the best solution to these problems is to incorporate both individual-level and ecologic measures in the same analysis. This approach might include different measures of the same factor; for example, each subject would be characterized by his or her own exposure level as well as the average exposure level for all members of the group to which he or she belongs (aggregate measure). Not only would this approach help to clarify the sources and magnitude of ecologic and cross-level bias, but it would also allow us to separate biologic, contextual, and ecologic effects. It is especially appropriate in social epidemiology, infectious-disease epidemiology, and the evaluation of population interventions.

There are various statistical methods for including both individual-level and ecologic measures in the same analysis; two will be discussed here. The first method, often called *contextual analysis* in the social sciences, is a simple extension of conventional (generalized linear) modeling such as multiple linear regression and logistic regression [3, 47]. The model, which is fit to the data at the individual level, includes both individual-level and ecologic predictors. For example, suppose we wanted to estimate the effect of "herd immunity" on the risk of an infectious disease. The risk, y, of disease might be modeled as a function of the following linear component: $\beta_0 + \beta_1 x + \beta_2 X + \beta_3 xX$, where x is the individual's immunity status and X is the prevalence of immunity in the group to which that individual belongs [93]. Therefore, β_1 represents the biologic effect of individual immunity, β_2 represents the contextual effect of herd immunity, and β_3 represents the interaction effect, which allows the herd-immunity effect to depend on the individual's immune status. The interaction term is needed in this application, since we would expect no herd immunity effect among immune individuals. Note, however, that the interpretation of the interaction effect depends on the form of the model.

An important limitation of contextual analysis is that outcomes of individuals within groups are treated as independent. In practice, however, the outcome of an individual in one group often depends on the outcomes of other individuals in that group. Ignoring such within-group dependence ("clustering") generally results in estimated variances of contextual effects that are biased downward, making confidence intervals too narrow. To handle this problem of within-group dependence, we can add random effects to the conventional (contextual) model described above; this approach is called *mixed-effects modeling, multilevel modeling*, or *hierarchical regression* [7, 27, 100, 101]. Multilevel modeling is a powerful technique with many applications. It can be used to estimate contextual and ecologic effects and to derive improved (empirical Bayes) estimates of biologic effects. It can also be used to determine how much of the difference in outcome rates across groups (ecologic effect) can be explained by differences in the distribution of individual-level risk factors (biologic effects).

As an illustration, suppose that we want to estimate the biologic and contextual effects of income level on a continuous measure of health status (ignoring other potential confounders). Let y_{ij} = the health status of the ith individual living in the jth census tract (group), and x_{ij} = the annual income of the ith individual living in the jth census tract. At the first level of analysis, we model the individual's health status within each census tract as a function of income level – i.e.

$$y_{ij} = \beta_{0j} + \beta_{1j} x_{ij} + \varepsilon_{ij}, \qquad (1)$$

where ε_{ij} is the error term representing the unique (residual) effect associated with the ith individual in the jth census tract. At the second (ecologic) level, we model the census tract-specific intercepts (β_{0j}) and slopes, β_{1j}, from the first level as a function of average census-tract income, X_j – i.e.

$$\beta_{0j} = B_{00} + B_{01} X_j + E_{0j}, \qquad (2)$$

$$\beta_{1j} = B_{10} + B_{11} X_j + E_{1j}, \qquad (3)$$

where E_{0j} and E_{1j} are error terms representing the random effects associated with the jth census tract. The underlying assumption is that the census tract-specific regression parameters are random samples from a population of such parameters. By substituting (2) and (3) into (1), we obtain the following combined two-level model:

$$y_{ij} = B_{00} + B_{01}X_j + B_{10}x_{ij} + B_{11}x_{ij}X_j$$
$$+ E_{0j} + E_{1j}x_{ij} + \varepsilon_{ij}, \qquad (4)$$

where B_{10} represents the biologic effect of individual income on health status, B_{01} represents the contextual effect of average census-tract income on health status, and B_{11} represents the interaction effect of individual income and average census-tract income. Using an empirical Bayes procedure, we can also derive an improved estimate of the individual-income effect (β_{1j}) for each census tract. This is accomplished by computing a weighted average of the estimated slope for census tract j in level 1 (1) and the predicted value of this slope using all census tracts in level 2 (3).

Applying multilevel analysis to survey data collected in the UK, Humphreys & Carr-Hill [45] found that living in a poor area (electoral ward) had a detrimental effect on several health outcomes, controlling for socioeconomic status and other individual-level covariates. In a conventional ecologic analysis, the effects of living in a poor area and being poor (low socioeconomic status) would be confounded, and ecologic estimates of effect would be susceptible to cross-level bias.

Multilevel analysis can also be extended to more than two levels. For example, we might want to predict certain health outcomes in nursing-home residents as a function of characteristics of the residents (e.g. age and health status), their physicians (e.g. type of specialty and country of medical training), and the nursing homes (e.g. size and doctor-to-patient ratio). In this type of analysis, residents are grouped by their physician (who might provide care to many residents in one home) and by their nursing-home affiliation.

The simplest design for generating multilevel analyses is a single survey of a population that is large and diverse enough so that multiple groups (e.g. counties or ethnic groups) can be defined for ecologic measurement and analysis. In addition to environmental and global variables for regions or organizations, ecologic measures are derived by aggregating all subjects in each group. An alternative, more efficient, approach is a *multilevel* or *hybrid design* in which a two-stage sampling scheme is used first to select groups (stage 1), followed by the selection of individuals within groups (stage 2) (for example [45] and [65]). A hybrid design might involve conducting a conventional multiple-group ecologic study by linking different data sources, then obtaining supplemental data from individuals randomly sampled from each group (*see* **Record Linkage**). For example, by estimating the exposure–covariate association in each subsample, this approach can be used to improve the control of confounders in an ecologic analysis [65, 68, 73]. A variation of this hybrid design might involve a case–control study as the second stage. Cases would be identified in the first (ecologic) stage, and controls would be matched to cases on group affiliation and possibly other factors (*see* **Matching**).

Conclusions

There are several practical advantages of ecologic studies, which make them especially appealing for doing various types of epidemiologic research. Despite these advantages, however, ecologic analysis poses major problems of interpretation when making ecologic inferences and especially when making biologic inferences. From a methodologic perspective, it is best to have individual-level data on as many relevant nonglobal measures as possible. Just because the exposure variable is measured ecologically, for example, does not mean that other variables should be as well. The accuracy of effect estimates from ecologic studies can often be improved by obtaining additional data on the within-group associations between covariates, between the exposure and covariates, or between the disease and covariates.

Several epidemiologists have recently called for greater emphasis on understanding differences in health status between populations – a return to a public-health orientation, in contrast to the individual (reductionist) orientation of modern epidemiology [51, 55, 60, 67, 81, 90]. This recommendation represents an important challenge for the future of epidemiology, but it cannot be met simply by conducting ecologic studies; multiple levels of measurement and analysis are needed. Even when the purpose of the study is to estimate ecologic effects, individual-level information is often essential for drawing valid inferences about these effects. Thus, to address the underlying research questions, we typically would want to estimate and control for biologic and contextual effects, preferably using multilevel analysis. In contemporary epidemiology, the "ecologic fallacy" reflects the failure of the investigator to recognize the need for biologic inference and thus for individual-level data. This need arises even when the primary exposure of interest is an ecologic measure and the outcome of interest is the health status of entire populations.

Acknowledgments

Parts of this articles have been reproduced with permission from the *Annual Review of Public Health*, volume 16, pp. 61–81. © 1995 Annual Reviews, Inc.

References

[1] Beral, V., Chilvers, C. & Fraser, P. (1979). On the estimation of relative risk from vital statistical data, *Journal of Epidemiology and Community Health* **33**, 159–162.

[2] Blot, W.J. & Fraumeni, J.F., Jr (1977). Geographic patterns of oral cancer in the United States: etiologic implications, *Journal of Chronic Diseases* **30**, 745–757.

[3] Boyd, L.H., Jr & Iversen, G.R. (1979). *Contextual Analysis: Concepts and Statistical Techniques*. Wadsworth, Belmont.

[4] Brenner, H., Greenland, S. & Savitz, D.A. (1992). The effects of nondifferential confounder misclassification in ecologic studies, *Epidemiology* **3**, 456–459.

[5] Brenner, H., Savitz, D.A., Jöckel, K.-H. & Greenland, S. (1992). Effects of nondifferential exposure misclassification in ecologic studies, *American Journal of Epidemiology* **135**, 85–95.

[6] Breslow, N.E. (1984). Extra-Poisson variation in log-linear models, *Applied Statistics* **33**, 38–44.

[7] Bryk, A.S. & Raudenbush, S.W. (1992). *Hierarchical Linear Models: Applications and Data Analysis Methods*. Sage, Thousand Oaks.

[8] Casper, M., Wing, S., Strogatz, D., Davis, C.E. & Tyroler, H.A. (1992). Antihypertensive treatment and US trends in smoking mortality, 1962 to 1980, *American Journal of Public Health* **82**, 1600–1606.

[9] Catalano, R. & Serxner, S. (1987). Time series designs of potential interest to epidemiologists, *American Journal of Epidemiology* **126**, 724–731.

[10] Centerwall, B.S. (1989). Exposure to television as a risk factor for violence, *American Journal of Epidemiology* **129**, 643–652.

[11] Clayton, D.G., Bernardinelli, L. & Montomoli, C. (1993). Spatial correlation in ecological analysis, *International Journal of Epidemiology* **22**, 1193–1202.

[12] Clayton, D. & Kaldor, J. (1987). Empirical Bayes estimates of age-standardized relative risks for use in disease mapping, *Biometrics* **43**, 671–681.

[13] Connor, M.J. & Gillings, D. (1984). An empiric study of ecological inference, *American Journal of Public Health* **74**, 555–559.

[14] Crawford, M.D., Gardner, M.J. & Morris, J.N. (1971). Changes in water hardness and local death-rates, *Lancet* **2**, 327–329.

[15] Cressie, N. (1993). Regional mapping of incidence rates using spatial Bayesian models, *Medical Care* **31**, Supplement, YS60–YS65.

[16] Darby, S.C. & Doll, R. (1987). Fallout, radiation doses near Dounreay, and childhood leukaemia, *British Medical Journal* **294**, 603–607.

[17] Devine, O.J., Louis, T.A. & Halloran, M.E. (1994). Empirical Bayes methods for stabilizing incidence rates before mapping, *Epidemiology* **5**, 622–630.

[18] Dogan, M. & Rokkan, S. (1969). Introduction, in *Social Ecology*, M. Dogan & S. Rokkan, eds. MIT Press, Cambridge, Mass., pp. 1–15.

[19] Duncan, O.D., Cuzzort, R.P. & Duncan, B. (1961). *Statistical Geography: Problems in Analyzing Areal Data*. Greenwood Press, Westport, pp. 64–67.

[20] Durkheim, E. (1951). *Suicide: A Study in Sociology*. Free Press, New York, pp. 153–154.

[21] Feinleib, M. & Leaverton, P.E. (1984). Ecological fallacies in epidemiology, in *Health Information Systems*, P.E. Leaverton & L. Massé, eds. Praeger, New York, pp. 33–61.

[22] Firebaugh, G. (1978). A rule for inferring individual-level relationships from aggregate data, *American Sociological Review* **43**, 557–572.

[23] Frost, W.H. (1939). The age selection of mortality from tuberculosis in successive decades, *American Journal of Hygiene* **30**, 91–96.

[24] Gehlke, C.E. & Biehl, K. (1934). Certain effects of grouping upon the size of the correlation coefficient in census tract material, *Journal of the American Statistical Association* **29**, Supplement, 169–170.

[25] Glenn, N.D. (1977). *Cohort Analysis*, Series/No. 07-005. Sage, Thousand Oaks.

[26] Goldstein, H. (1979). Age, period and cohort effects – a confounded confusion, *Bias* **6**, 19–24.

[27] Goldstein, H. (1995). *Multilevel Statistical Models*, 2nd Ed. Edward Arnold, London.

[28] Goodman, L.A. (1959). Some alternatives to ecological correlation, *American Journal of Sociology* **64**, 610–625.

[29] Greenland, S. (1980). The effect of misclassification in the presence of covariates, *American Journal of Epidemiology* **112**, 564–569.

[30] Greenland, S. (1987). Interpretation and choice of effect measures in epidemiologic analysis, *American Journal of Epidemiology* **125**, 761–768.

[31] Greenland, S. (1992). Divergent biases in ecologic and individual-level studies, *Statistics in Medicine* **11**, 1209–1223.

[32] Greenland, S. & Brenner, H. (1993). Correcting for non-differential misclassification in ecologic analyses, *Applied Statistics* **42**, 117–126.

[33] Greenland, S., Maclure, M., Schlesselman, J.J., Poole, C. & Morgenstern, H. (1991). Standardized regression coefficients: a further critique and review of some alternatives, *Epidemiology* **2**, 387–392.

[34] Greenland, S. & Morgenstern, H. (1989). Ecological bias, confounding, and effect modification, *International Journal of Epidemiology* **18**, 269–274.

[35] Greenland, S. & Robins, J. (1994). Invited commentary: ecologic studies – biases, misconceptions, and counterexamples, *American Journal of Epidemiology* **139**, 747–760.

[36] Greenland, S., Schlesselman, J.J. & Criqui, M.H. (1986). The fallacy of employing standardized regression coefficients and correlations as measures of effect, *American Journal of Epidemiology* **123**, 203–208.

[37] Gruchow, H.W., Rimm, A.A. & Hoffman, R.G. (1983). Alcohol consumption and ischemic heart disease mortality: are time-series correlations meaningful?, *American Journal of Epidemiology* **118**, 641–650.

[38] Hatch, M. & Susser, M. (1990). Background gamma radiation and childhood cancers within ten miles of a US nuclear plant, *International Journal of Epidemiology* **19**, 546–552.

[39] Helfenstein, U. (1991). The use of transfer function models, intervention analysis and related time series methods in epidemiology, *International Journal of Epidemiology* **20**, 808–815.

[40] Hiller, J.E. & McMichael, A.J. (1990). Dietary fat and cancer: a comeback for ecological studies?, *Cancer Causes and Control* **1**, 101–102.

[41] Hiller, J.E. & McMichael, A.J. (1991). Ecological studies, in *Design Concepts in Nutritional Epidemiology*, B.M. Margetts & M. Nelson, eds. Oxford University Press, Oxford, pp. 323–353.

[42] Holford, T.R. (1991). Understanding the effects of age, period, and cohort on incidence and mortality rates, *Annual Review of Public Health* **12**, 425–457.

[43] Howe, G.R. (1990). Dietary fat and cancer, *Cancer Causes and Control* **1**, 99–100.

[44] Howe, G.R., Hirohata, T., Hislop, T.G., Iscovich, J.M., Yuan J.-M., Katsonyanni, K., Lubin, F., Marubini, E., Modan, B., Rohan, T., Toniolo, P. & Shunzhang, Y. (1990). Dietary factors and risk of breast cancer: combined analysis of 12 case–control studies, *Journal of the National Cancer Institute* **82**, 561–569.

[45] Humphreys, K. & Carr-Hill, R. (1991). Area variations in health outcomes: artefact or ecology, *International Journal of Epidemiology* **20**, 251–258.

[46] Hunter, D.J., Spiegelman, D., Adami, H.O., Beeson, L., van den Brandt, P.A., Folsom, A.R., Fraser, G.E., Goldbohm, A., Graham, S., Howe, G.R., Kushi, L.H., Marshall, J.R., McDermott, A., Miller, A.B., Speizer, F.E., Wolk, A., Yaun, S.-S. & Willett, W. (1996). Cohort studies of fat intake and the risk of breast cancer – a pooled analysis, *New England Journal of Medicine* **334**, 356–361.

[47] Iversen, G.R. (1991). *Contextual Analysis*. Sage, Thousand Oaks.

[48] Kleinbaum, D.G., Kupper, L.L. & Morgenstern, H. (1982). *Epidemiologic Research: Principles and Quantitative Methods*. Van Nostrand Reinhold, New York, pp. 77–81, 130–134, 184–280.

[49] Kliewer, E.V. (1992). Influence of migrants on regional variations of stomach and colon cancer mortality in the western United States, *International Journal of Epidemiology* **21**, 442–449.

[50] Koopman, J.S. & Longini, I.M., Jr (1994). The ecological effects of individual exposures and nonlinear disease dynamics in populations, *American Journal of Public Health* **84**, 836–842.

[51] Krieger, N. (1994). Epidemiology and the web of causation: has anyone seen the spider? *American Journal of Epidemiology* **39**, 887–903.

[52] Langbein, L.I. & Lichtman, A.J. (1978). *Ecological Inference*, Series/No. 07–010. Sage, Thousand Oaks.

[53] Lee, J.A.H. (1982). Melanoma and exposure to sunlight, *Epidemiologic Reviews* **4**, 110–136.

[54] Lee, J.A.H., Petersen, G.R., Stevens, R.G. & Vesanen, K. (1979). The influence of age, year of birth, and date on mortality from malignant melanoma in the populations of England and Wales, Canada, and the white population of the United States, *American Journal of Epidemiology* **110**, 734–739.

[55] Link, B.G. & Phelan, J. (1995). Social conditions as fundamental causes of disease, *Journal of Health and Social Behavior* **5** (extra issue), 80–94.

[56] MacMahon, B. & Pugh, T.F. (1970). *Epidemiology: Principles and Methods*. Little, Brown, & Company, Boston, pp. 137–198, 175–184.

[57] Mason, K.O., Mason, W., Winsborough, H.H. & Poole, W.K. (1973). Some methodological issues in the cohort analysis of archival data, *American Sociological Review* **38**, 242–258.

[58] Mason, T.J., McKay, F.W., Hoover, R., Blot, W.J. & Fraumeni, J.F., Jr. (1975). *Atlas of Cancer Mortality for US Counties: 1950–1969*, DHEW Publ. No. (NIH) 75–780. US Government Printing Office, Washington, pp. 36–37.

[59] McDowall, D., McCleary, R., Meidinger, E.E. & Hay, R.A., Jr (1980). *Interrupted Time Series Analysis*. Sage, Beverly Hills.

[60] McMichael, A.J. (1995). The health of persons, populations, and planets: epidemiology comes full circle, *Epidemiology* **6**, 633–636.

[61] Mollie, A. & Richardson, S. (1991). Empirical Bayes estimation of cancer mortality rates using spatial models, *Statistics in Medicine* **10**, 95–112.

[62] Morgenstern, H. (1982). Uses of ecologic analysis in epidemiologic research, *American Journal of Public Health* **72**, 1336–1344.

[63] Morgenstern, H. & Thomas, D. (1993). Principles of study design in environmental epidemiology, *Environmental Health Perspectives* **101**, Supplement 4, 23–38.

[64] Moulton, L.H., Foxman, B., Wolfe, R.A. & Port, F.K. (1994). Potential pitfalls in interpreting maps of stabilized rates, *Epidemiology* **5**, 297–301.

[65] Navidi, W., Thomas, D., Stram, D. & Peters, J. (1994). Design and analysis of multilevel analytic studies with applications to a study of air pollution, *Environmental Health Perspectives* **102**, Supplement 8, 25–32.

[66] Ostrom, C.W., Jr (1990). *Time Series Analysis: Regression Techniques*, 2nd Ed. Sage, Newbury Park.

[67] Pearce, N. (1996). Traditional epidemiology, modern epidemiology, and public health, *American Journal of Public Health* **86**, 678–683.

[68] Plummer, M. & Clayton, D. (1996). Estimation of population exposure in ecological studies, *Journal of the Royal Statistical Society, Series B* **58**, 113–126.

[69] Pocock, S.J., Cook, D.G. & Beresford, S.A.A. (1981). Regression of area mortality rates on explanatory variables: what weighting is appropriate?, *Applied Statistics* **30**, 286–295.

[70] Polissar, L. (1980). The effect of migration on comparison of disease rates in geographic studies in the United States, *American Journal of Epidemiology* **111**, 175–182.

[71] Prentice, R.L. (1996). Measurement error and results from analytic epidemiology: dietary fat and breast cancer, *Journal of the National Cancer Institute* **88**, 1738–1747.

[72] Prentice, R.L., Kakar, F., Hursting, S., Sheppart, L., Klein, R. & Kushi, L.H. (1988). Aspects of the rationale for the Women's Health Trial, *Journal of the National Cancer Institute* **80**, 802–814.

[73] Prentice, R.L. & Sheppard, L. (1989). Validity of international, time trend, and migrant studies of dietary factors and disease risk, *Preventive Medicine* **18**, 167–179.

[74] Prentice, R.L. & Sheppard, L. (1990). Dietary fat and cancer: consistency of the epidemiologic data, and disease prevention that may follow from a practical reduction in fat consumption, *Cancer Causes and Control* **1**, 81–97.

[75] Prentice, R.L. & Sheppard, L. (1991). Dietary fat and cancer: rejoinder and discussion of research strategies, *Cancer Causes and Control* **2**, 53–58.

[76] Prentice, R.L. & Sheppard, L. (1995). Aggregate data studies of disease risk factors, *Biometrika* **82**, 113–125.

[77] Prentice, R.L. & Thomas, D. (1993). Methodologic research needs in environmental epidemiology: data analysis, *Environmental Health Perspectives* **101**, Supplement 4, 39–48.

[78] Richardson, S. & Hémon, D. (1990). Ecological bias and confounding (letter), *International Journal of Epidemiology* **19**, 764–766.

[79] Richardson, S., Stücher, I. & Hémon, D. (1987). Comparison of relative risks obtained in ecological and individual studies: some methodological considerations, *International Journal of Epidemiology* **16**, 111–120.

[80] Robinson, W.S. (1950). Ecological correlations and the behavior of individuals, *American Sociological Review* **15**, 351–357.

[81] Rose, G. (1985). Sick individuals and sick populations *International Journal of Epidemiology* **14**, 32–38.

[82] Rosenbaum, P.R. & Rubin, D.B. (1984). Difficulties with regression analyses of age-adjusted rates, *Biometrics* **40**, 437–443.

[83] Rubin, D.B. (1978). Bayesian inference for causal effects: the role of randomization, *Annals of Statistics* **6**, 34–58.

[84] Savitz, D.A. & Baron, A.E. (1989). Estimating and correcting for confounder misclassification, *American Journal of Epidemiology* **129**, 1062–1071.

[85] Sayrs, L.W. (1989). *Pooled Time Series Analysis*. Sage, Newbury Park.

[86] Selvin, H.C. (1958). Durkheim's *Suicide* and problems of empirical research, *American Journal of Sociology* **63**, 607–619.

[87] Stavraky, K.M. (1976). The role of ecologic analysis in studies of the etiology of disease: a discussion with reference to large bowel cancer, *Journal of Chronic Diseases* **29**, 435–444.

[88] Stewart, A.W., Kuulasmaa, K. & Beaglehole, R. (1994). Ecological analysis of the association between mortality and major risk factors of cardiovascular disease, *International Journal of Epidemiology* **23**, 505–516.

[89] Stidley, C. & Samet, J.M. (1994). Assessment of ecologic regression in the study of lung cancer and indoor radon, *American Journal of Epidemiology* **139**, 312–322.

[90] Susser, M. & Susser, E. (1996). Choosing a future for epidemiology: II. From black box to Chinese boxes and eco-epidemiology, *American Journal of Public Health* **86**, 674–677.

[91] Thorndike, E.L. (1939). On the fallacy of imputing the correlations found for groups to the individuals or smaller groups composing them, *American Journal of Psychology* **52**, 122–124.

[92] Valkonen, T. (1969). Individual and structural effects in ecological research, in *Social Ecology*, M. Dogan & S. Rokkan, eds. MIT Press, Cambridge, Mass., pp. 53–68.

[93] Von Korff, M., Koepsell, T., Curry, S. & Diehr, P. (1992). Multilevel analysis in epidemiologic research on health behaviors and outcomes, *American Journal of Epidemiology* **135**, 1077–1082.

[94] Walter, S.D. (1991). The ecologic method in the study of environmental health. I. Overview of the method, *Environmental Health Perspectives* **94**, 61–65.

[95] Walter, S.D. (1991). The ecologic method in the study of environmental health. II. Methodologic issues and feasibility, *Environmental Health Perspectives* **94**, 67–73.

[96] Walter, S.D. (1992). The analysis of regional patterns in health data: I. Distributional considerations, *American Journal of Epidemiology* **136**, 730–741.

[97] Walter, S.D. (1992). The analysis of regional patterns in health data: II. The power to detect environmental effects, *American Journal of Epidemiology* **136**, 742–759.

[98] Willett, W.C. & Stampfer, M.J. (1990). Dietary fat and cancer: another view, *Cancer Causes and Control* **1**, 103–109.

[99] Winn, D.M., Blot, W.J., Shy, C.M., Pickle, L.W., Toledo, A. & Fraumeni, J.F., Jr (1981). Snuff dipping and oral cancer among women in the southern United States, *New England Journal of Medicine* **304**, 745–749.

[100] Wong, G.Y. & Mason, W.M. (1985). The hierarchical logistic regression model for multilevel analysis, *Journal of the American Statistical Association* **80**, 513–524.

[101] Wong, G.Y. & Mason, W.M. (1991). Contextually specific effects and other generalizations for the hierarchical linear model for comparative analysis, *Journal of the American Statistical Association* **86**, 487–503.

HAL MORGENSTERN

Eddy Models for Screening *see* Screening, Models of

Ederer–Myers–Mantel Test *see* Clustering

Effect Modification

The term *effect modification* is due to Miettinen [5], and is closely related to the concept of **interaction**. When we analyze the association of an exposure with disease incidence, an effect modifier is a variable over which the effect of exposure on disease risk varies. For example, we might use the **relative risk** to describe the association of cigarette smoking to lung cancer risk. If the relative risk associated with cigarette smoking differs statistically between asbestos-exposed subjects and subjects with no asbestos exposure, then we say that asbestos exposure modifies the effect of cigarette smoking on lung cancer risk, and we call asbestos exposure an effect modifier.

We study effect modification for a variety of reasons. We might be interested in effect modification for its public health implications: if the effects of certain modifiable risk factors for breast cancer are confined to a subgroup of women, for example, efforts to modify these risk factors or increase **screening** could be targeted only at subpopulations where the intervention will prevent the most women from developing advanced disease.

We might also look for effect modification to support a hypothesis that the joint biologic effect of two exposures is to inhibit or enhance each others' individual effects. Effect modification supports this hypothesis unequivocally when the exposure decreases risk for one value of the effect modifier and increases risk for another value of the effect modifier (Siemiatycki & Thomas [7]; Thompson [8]), a situation Thompson calls "crossover" (*see* **Synergy of Exposure Effects**).

Relationship to Interaction

Effect modification is closely related to statistical interaction in regression models. In relative risk regression models, where regression coefficients for main effect exposure variables have the interpretation of log relative risks, a significant interaction between exposure and a second variable means that the second variable is an effect modifier (*see* **Relative Risk Modeling**). This is true because the model with interaction says the relative risk associated with exposure will be different depending on the value of the effect modifier.

However, the relationship between statistical interaction and effect modification depends on the correspondence between what measure we choose for the effect of exposure on disease risk and the form of the regression model we use to assess interaction. To see this, we examine three possible regression models and their corresponding measures of effect.

Multiplicative Models and Relative Risks

Logistic regression, Poisson regression with a log link function, and multiplicative **Cox regression** are all examples of **multiplicative models** for which the relative risk is the implicit measure of effect [1, 2].

For example, if we applied the logistic regression model to data from a **case–control study** of smoking and asbestos exposure as risk factors for mesothelioma, then for

$$X_A = \begin{cases} 0, & \text{no occupational asbestos exposure,} \\ 1, & \text{occupational asbestos exposure,} \end{cases}$$

$$X_S = \begin{cases} 0, & \text{never smoked,} \\ 1, & \text{ever smoked,} \end{cases}$$

and $p =$ the probability of being a case in the case–control sample, a simple logistic model without interaction is

$$\text{logit } p = \ln \frac{p}{1-p} = \beta_0 + \beta_A X_A + \beta_S X_S.$$

In a **cohort study**, a similar model would hold with $p =$ the population probability of developing the disease during the study period.

This model implies that the **odds ratio** associated with ever having smoked, e^{β_S}, is the same whether or not an individual has had occupational exposure to asbestos. To allow the odds ratios associated with smoking to differ according to whether or not the subject had been exposed to asbestos, we add the interaction term $\beta_{AS} X_A X_S$ to the model. Thus, if we use the logistic regression model, the presence or absence of interaction corresponds to presence or absence of effect modification when the measure of effect we use is the odds ratio, or the relative risk, which it approximates. This correspondence also holds for the following Poisson regression model:

$$\ln \lambda = \beta_0 + \beta_A X_A + \beta_S X_S,$$

where λ is the disease incidence rate for a time interval/covariate combination, and for the multiplicative Cox regression model

$$\ln \lambda(t) = \ln \lambda_0(t) + \beta_0 + \beta_A X_A + \beta_S X_S,$$

where $\lambda(t)$ is the hazard function. If we are interested in whether the relative risk difference (see below) associated with smoking is different among asbestos-exposed individuals from what it is among non-asbestos-exposed individuals, the presence or absence of an interaction term in a multiplicative model will not give us this information except in the case of crossover. Instead, we need to look for interaction in an additive relative risk regression model.

Additive Relative Risk Models and Relative Risk Differences

Most investigators would agree that when they are considering public health implications of some exposure, additive measures of the effect of exposure on risk are more useful than multiplicative measures for identifying subgroups where interventions should be targeted. In addition, Rothman has argued that the additive scale is better for assessing whether there is biological interaction, and that **additive models** should be used instead of the multiplicative models when assessing whether there is effect modification [6]. This has been disputed by Siemiatycki & Thomas [7] and Thompson [8], however, who show that, depending on the biologic model for how exposure affects disease risk, biologic interaction may or may not manifest itself as a statistical interaction on either the additive or multiplicative scales.

In a case–control study, the additive measure of effect that can be estimated is the additive relative risk or relative risk difference. The relative risk difference measures the difference in risk of disease for different exposure combinations relative to the disease risk in a baseline group where all the covariates have the value zero. For example, in a case–control study of lung cancer like the one described above, let $p(0,0)$ be the probability of being a case among those exposed to neither smoking nor asbestos, and $p(X_A, X_S)$ the probability of being a case among those with asbestos and smoking exposure given by X_A and X_S. Then the relative risk difference comparing combinations of exposure (X_A, X_S) and (X'_A, X'_S) is

$$RRD = \frac{p(X_A, X_S) - p(X'_A, X'_S)}{p(0,0)}.$$

When the relative risk difference is the measure of the effect of exposure (X_A, X_S) compared with exposure (X'_A, X'_S), we say that asbestos exposure modifies the effect of smoking if the relative risk difference associated with smoking differs between those occupationally exposed to asbestos and those without occupational asbestos exposure. Whether or not this type of effect modification exists depends on whether or not there is an interaction term in the additive relative risk regression model:

$$\frac{p}{1-p} = e^{\beta_0}(1 + \beta_A X_A + \beta_S X_S).$$

Table 1   History of having given birth, family history of breast cancer, and breast cancer risk, from Colditz et al. [3]

	No family history				Family history			
	Cases	Person-years	Relative risk	95% CI	Cases	Person-years	Relative risk	95% CI
Never given birth	150	69 666	1.0^a	–	16	5 816	1.0^a	–
Ever given birth	1788	994 628	0.83	(0.71, 0.99)	5816	78 559	1.4	(0.83, 2.3)

[a]Reference group

Similar correspondences hold for the additive relative risk versions of the Poisson regression model

$$\lambda = e^{\beta_0}(1 + \beta_A X_A + \beta_S X_S),$$

and the Cox regression model

$$\lambda(t) = \lambda_0(t)(1 + \beta_A X_A + \beta_S X_S).$$

The relative risk difference can be estimated using data from both case–control and cohort studies. See Breslow & Day [2] for more details.

Additive Risk Models and Risk Differences

Using data from a cohort study, it is also possible to estimate absolute differences in the risk of disease or the disease **incidence rate**. Letting $p(x_A, x_S)$ denote the disease risk or probability of developing disease during the study period for those with asbestos exposure given by X_A and smoking exposure given by X_S, then the risk difference comparing combinations of exposure (X_A, X_S) and (X'_A, X'_S) is

$$RD = p(X_A, X_S) - p(X'_A, X'_S).$$

If the risk difference is the measure of the effect of exposure (X_A, X_S) compared with (X'_A, X_S), then we say asbestos exposure modifies the effect of smoking if the risk difference associated with smoking differs between those occupationally exposed to asbestos and those without occupational asbestos exposure. Whether or not this type of effect modification exists depends on whether or not there is an interaction term in the additive risk model:

$$p = \beta_0 + \beta_A X_A + \beta_S X_S.$$

Similar correspondences hold for additive versions of the Poisson regression model

$$\lambda = \beta_0 + \beta_A X_A + \beta_S X_S,$$

and incidence rate regression models

$$\lambda(t) = \lambda_0(t) + \beta_A X_A + \beta_S X_S.$$

See Lin & Ying [4] for inference under the additive incidence rate model.

Example

Colditz et al. [3] studied how a variety of known risk factors for breast cancer were modified by family history of breast cancer. Data abstracted from the article are given in Table 1, broken down by whether the woman had ever given birth and whether she had a family history of breast cancer in a mother or sister. Crude relative risks based on a Poisson regression model are also given in Table 1.

From these results we see that without adjustment for other factors, among women without a history of breast cancer in their mother or sisters, the birth of a child appears to confer protection from breast cancer. However, among women with a history of breast cancer in the mother or a sister, the birth of a child is associated with, if anything, an increase in risk. If these differences are also seen in other studies, they might argue that screening schedules should be the most frequent in parous women with a family history of breast cancer. If the relative risk associated with parity among women with a family history were statistically different from one, these data would satisfy Thompson's [8] criteria for crossover, from which some interaction in the biological mechanisms might be inferred.

References

[1]   Breslow, N.E. & Day, N.E. (1980). *Statistical Methods in Cancer Research*, Vol. I: *The Analysis of Case–Control Studies*. Oxford University Press, Oxford.

[2]   Breslow, N.E. & Day, N.E. (1987). *Statistical Methods in Cancer Research*, Vol. II: *The Design and Analysis of Cohort Studies*. Oxford University Press, Oxford.

[3]   Colditz, G.A., Rosner, B.A. & Speizer, F.E. (1996). Risk factors for breast cancer according to family history of breast cancer, *Journal of the National Cancer Institute* **88**, 365–371.

[4] Lin, D.Y. & Ying, Z. (1994). Semiparametric analysis of the additive risk model, *Biometrika* **81**, 61–71.

[5] Miettinen, O. (1974). Confounding and effect modification, *American Journal of Epidemiology* **100**, 350–353.

[6] Rothman, K.J. (1976). Causes, *American Journal of Epidemiology* **104**, 587–593.

[7] Siemiatycki, J. & Thomas, D.C. (1981). Biological models and statistical interactions: an example from multistage carcinogenesis, *International Journal of Epidemiology* **10**, 383–387.

[8] Thompson, W.D. (1991). Effect modification and the limits of biological inference from epidemiologic data, *Journal of Clinical Epidemiology* **44**, 221–232.

BARBARA MCKNIGHT

Egret *see* Software, Biostatistical

Eligibility Restriction

Eligibility restriction, or simply restriction, is a design strategy used to control for a potential **confounder**. For example, if gender is a potential confounder in a study of heart disease and diet, then one might choose to restrict the study to females. This design would eliminate gender as a potential confounder, but it would yield no direct information on the effect of diet on heart disease risk in males (*see* **Matching**).

Eligibility restrictions are also used in clinical trials for various other purposes, such as eliminating individuals not thought to benefit from the treatments under study or eliminating subjects not thought to be healthy enough to comply with protocol requirements.

M.H. GAIL

Environmental Epidemiology

Environmental epidemiology encompasses a wide array of topics related to the study and evaluation of the determinants of diseases in human populations.

The term "environmental" as used here is general in scope, and pertains to all aspects of our environment that may influence disease **risk**. Environmental exposures include substances that might affect our immediate surroundings, such as pollutants in the air we breathe or water we drink, as well as factors related to our occupation, recreation, and lifestyle that might influence probabilities of disease occurrence. Thus, for example, the dominant environmental determinant of lung cancer in nearly all populations around the world is cigarette smoking, while diet and nutrition contribute to risk of several other cancers and cardiovascular and other diseases. Since molecular and genetic traits may predispose individuals to the adverse effects of exposure to specific environmental factors, environmental epidemiology can be considered to include the entire spectrum of research into the etiology and prevention of human diseases.

In this article we describe methods for and examples of epidemiologic studies of the environmental determinants of chronic diseases, the major killers in human populations today. Emphasis is placed upon epidemiologic and statistical methodologic tools for the detection and evaluation of risks associated with environmental exposures. Acute diseases are not considered, although some of the basic techniques for assessing environmental factors have arisen from principles developed in tracking outbreaks of infectious diseases.

The article is divided according to method of study of environmental factors in disease risk. First are **descriptive epidemiologic** studies. These investigations, which study patterns of disease in general populations and their correlations with environmental indices of the populations, are useful primarily for generating hypotheses about disease etiology. More important are **case–control** and **cohort studies**, which are **analytic epidemiologic** studies that evaluate risk of disease in individuals characterized by presence and level of exposure to environmental variables of interest. These **observational** (nonexperimental) epidemiologic studies form the basis for most of what is known about the causes of chronic diseases. Finally, are randomized trials, whereby agents or procedures that are thought to have potential for reduction in disease risk are evaluated experimentally with random assignment of individuals to various exposure groups. The credibility of evidence from these clinical intervention trials is usually higher than from observational studies, but for practical reasons only a limited number of such trials have been undertaken.

Providing Clues to Environmental Factors

Clues to environmental causes of disease are often uncovered by examining patterns of disease mortality and incidence. For extremely rare diseases, even occurrence of a few cases within a short period of time and at a particular space can raise suspicion. Such "clusters" of disease (*see* **Clustering**), often detected by alert clinicians, can in some situations lead to the eventual discovery of the causal agents. For instance, the development of hepatic angiosarcoma among three workers in a single manufacturing plant in Kentucky led to the identification of vinyl chloride as the likely causal agent [24], and the observation of vaginal adenocarcinoma in several young women in Boston was traced to synthetic estrogens taken by their mothers during pregnancy [38]. The large majority of clusters of a few cases of a disease, however, have proven to be uninformative with respect to discovering or evaluating a causal agent. Heath [36], for example, described investigations by the Centers for Disease Control of clusters of childhood cancer in a number of communities in the US, none of which conclusively linked the leukemia or other cancer cases with environmental exposures. Leukemia clusters around nuclear power facilities have also failed to be causally related to radiation exposures from the plants [46]. Similarly, clusters of birth defects and other abnormalities have been assessed among residents near hazardous waste sites with potential for exposure to solvents, metals, and other compounds, but firm conclusions have been difficult to achieve [55, 65]. Although some clusters may be due to environmental determinants, it seems likely that many apparent clusters have resulted from **selection bias**, limitations of geographic boundaries or time periods, or chance [46, 56].

The play of chance is sometimes underestimated in assessment of clusters of small numbers of disease events, especially when the clusters occur in one of many arbitrarily and narrowly defined space-time units. Occurrence of a cluster of two events when 0.2 are "expected", for example, can result in a "significant" ($P = 0.02$ for a one-sided test under Poisson assumption) excess. If the boundaries of the cluster were drawn specifically to encompass the cases, however, the statistical significance loses its nominal meaning. Furthermore, if the cluster was in one of many time–space units evaluated, the multiple comparisons may generate at least one with a "significant" excess. Sometimes investigators are tempted to include the index cluster (that is, the cases that generated the cluster) in determining whether the disease excess occurs in other time–space units, but this fundamental violation of principles of independence invalidates such an evaluation. Finally, the existence of a cluster *per se* of a small number of disease events in a time–space unit conveys no information about the causes of the cluster.

Geographic clustering can also occur for more common chronic diseases, and be based on fairly large numbers of disease events. Excess occurrences of more common diseases are not so obvious to the practicing physician, but broad clustering may be uncovered through a systematic monitoring of disease morbidity and mortality (*see* **Surveillance of Diseases**). These clusters, typically based on large enough numbers of cases for the calculation of stable rates across time and space, may more often prove to be useful in generating productive leads to disease **causation**. Primary examples are the clusterings of high rates of certain diseases in contiguous areas seen in national atlases, which depict the distribution of mortality rates across small geographic units, such as counties in the US [47, 62] (*see* **Geographical Analysis; Mapping Disease Patterns**).

Geographic variation suggestive of environmental determinants can be particularly useful for leads to cancer studies. The US cancer maps have shown distinctive patterns of clearly nonrandom distributions of various cancers [47, 62]. Sharply elevated rates of oral cancer mortality among women, for example, have clustered in the southeastern part of the country. The finding led to several hypotheses, including one concerning occupational exposures in the textile industry, an industry employing large numbers of southern women, and one concerning smokeless tobacco, used by some women in rural areas of the South [8]. Subsequent analytic epidemiologic studies generated by the patterns seen in the cancer maps identified the use of oral snuff as the key risk factor and the cause of the large majority of cheek and gum cancers, tumors occurring where the tobacco powder was typically placed [70].

Mortality records have generally been the primary source of health data for generating clues to environmental factors for chronic diseases. In most countries of the world, systematic recording of all deaths is conducted by local governments (*see* **Death Certification**) and used for the compilation of national death rates by **causes of death**. Using population estimates generated from the national censuses as denominators, mortality **rates** by age, sex, and race can be computed for deaths due to various causes across time and for various geographic units. The ascertainment of deaths is nearly 100% complete in most populations, but inaccurate determination of the cause of death and certain other limitations may affect routinely collected mortality data. Cancer deaths are generally properly identified on death certificates, although the accuracy and completeness in recording cancer deaths vary by the type of cancer [59], but **misclassification** can be problematic for some other causes of death. Changes in recording practices and the coding of cause of death (*see* **International Classification of Diseases (ICD)**) also may contribute to the apparent changes in secular trends of cause-specific mortality [33]. Mortality data are of limited use for diseases with low fatality, and disease-specific death rates can be influenced by nonenvironmental factors such as improved survival due to changes in treatment modalities or early detection (*see* **Vital Statistics, Overview**).

Some limitations that may affect mortality patterns can be circumvented by using incidence data. Registries sometimes exist for various diseases, most notably cancer, with population-based registries in many parts of the world [58] (*see* **Disease Registers**). In the US, registries participating in the Surveillance, Epidemiology, and End Results (SEER) Program supported by the National Cancer Institute have been collecting diagnostic, treatment, and survival information on newly diagnosed cancer cases in about 10% of the population across the country since 1973 [43]. These data have been used for monitoring cancer incidence trends and patterns of cancer occurrence by demographic and geographic subgroups [27]. For instance, it has been observed recently that adenocarcinomas of the esophagus and gastric cardia are among the cancers with the most rapid rise in incidence during the past two decades in the US, particularly among white men [12]. This striking trend has led to the generation of multiple hypotheses about environmental factors. One hypothesis is that the increasing use of exposures that promote reflux, particularly obesity and pharmaceutical agents that relax the lower esophageal sphincter, may contribute to the rising incidence trends [20, 69].

Registries of incident cases of nonmalignant diseases are more limited in number and tend not be national in scope. If the population base from which the cases arise is well defined, however, these too can provide the basis for the calculation of rates and trends which may trigger hypotheses about environmental causes. Thus, for example, in Sweden and Denmark, all hospitalizations are registered, so that national patterns of various diseases requiring hospitalizations can be routinely monitored [1]. Illnesses not resulting in hospitalization will be missed, but the incidence and **prevalence** of serious conditions can be ascertained for the entire country.

Information on births is usually routinely collected in populations throughout the world. In addition to sociodemographic variables such as maternal age, race and occupation, information on birthweight, Apgar score and method of delivery is often collected. In the US birth certificates were standardized nationally in 1989 to include a checkbox for congenital abnormalities and medical risk factors, including tobacco and alcohol use, medical history, and prenatal care [19, 71]. The birth certificate data therefore can be used not only for monitoring disease occurrence among newborns [49], but also as a research tool to identify potential risk factors for these newborn illnesses, such as maternal sociodemographic characteristics in relation to congenital syphilis [26] and maternal smoking, ethnicity, and birthweight in relation to sudden infant death syndrome [45].

Systematically ascertained data on exposure to environmental agents are less readily available than data on measures of disease mortality or incidence. Thus, for example, the prevalence of cigarette smoking – the single most important environmental cause of disease in the US – is not known for counties across the country. National probability **sample surveys**, such as the National Health Interview Surveys conducted periodically beginning in 1960 and the series of National Health and Nutrition Examination Surveys (NHANES) starting from NHANESI in 1971–75 to the NHANESIII in 1988–94 have estimated smoking prevalences by broad, but not small-area, geographic regions. These National Center for Health Statistics (NCHS) surveys can be useful for monitoring national estimates of prevalence of a number of environmental exposures classified by demographic subgroups and over time

[23, 42, 63]. The exposures include not only tobacco consumption, but also diet and nutrition, medical variables, occupation, and other characteristics measured over time and by geographic areas.

Census data often provide a rich source of exposure data for generating clues to environmental risk factors. In addition to population counts by age, sex, and race, the census yields information on income, education, urbanization, occupation, and other factors for various geographic units, the smallest in the US being census tracts and postal zip codes. Usually this information is provided every 10 years. In some countries special censuses of manufacturing provide detailed industrial data at the small-area level, enabling calculation of indices of the percent of the population employed in hundreds of industrial categories. Although small-area data are generally not routinely available on average levels of general population exposures to chemical or physical agents, some registries of environmental exposures (e.g. to radon) exist in selected areas. In Sweden, a number of registries of exposure to chemical substances have been established for **record linkage** with national registries of cancer and mortality [1].

Statistical analyses of correlations of mortality or other aggregate health data with measures of average environmental exposures for the populations can help generate and refine hypotheses about disease causation. The correlations can assess not only concordance across geographic areas but also across time, and can be useful in helping to refute as well as refine hypotheses. Thus, rising then recently declining trends in lung cancer mortality correlate well with the rise and decline in smoking prevalence among American men [11, 31]. However, mortality rates of all cancers combined in the US have been relatively steady since the 1930s once lung cancer is removed [3, 21, 43], a pattern not consistent with the theory that increases in environmental exposures from pesticides or other chemicals are causing large-scale increases in cancer. Rising incidence of breast and prostate cancers, the major cancers among women and men, respectively, has been reported recently, but the increases seem related to changes in diagnostic techniques rather than environmental influences [27]. Furthermore, complete explanations for the rising incidence of non-Hodgkin's lymphoma are not clear. Geographic correlations have indicated that rates of lymphoma were highest in the north central part of the country, and have led to case–control studies evaluating workplace and environmental exposures associated with farming and other occupations [72] (*see* **Occupational Epidemiology**). Similarly, rates of lung cancer in US counties among workers employed in the chemical, petroleum, paper/pulp, and shipbuilding industries, adjusted for urbanization and other demographic factors (but not cigarette smoking), suggested that exposures associated with these industries may be contributing to lung cancer in the affected counties [9]. As described later, some of these hypotheses have been confirmed and some dismissed through subsequent analytic epidemiologic studies.

One of the reasons the descriptive studies linking rates of disease and exposure for groups may generate spurious leads is that correlation can occur among group averages in the absence of associations between disease and exposure at the individual level, the so-called "**ecologic fallacy**" (*see* **Ecologic Study**). Thus, studies of individual patients and their exposures typically are required to evaluate adequately hypotheses about the environmental determinants of disease. Such investigations are described in the next section.

Testing Hypotheses About Environmental Risk Factors

There are many environmental substances for which sufficient exposure is known to increase risk of certain chronic diseases. Foremost is cigarette smoking, believed to result in premature death in nearly half of all individuals who smoke and to account for more than one in every six deaths in the US [68]. Table 1 lists a number of substances besides cigarette smoke which have been classified as causes of cancer in humans [16, 40]. Many are drugs used to treat some cancers that can subsequently increase risk of other cancers, but also included are environmental substances to which certain occupational groups or certain segments of the general population may be exposed. Almost all of these substances have been identified by means of epidemiologic studies, although supporting evidence from experimental studies in animals generally exists. There are other compounds for which carcinogenicity is suspected because the compounds (often at very high doses) have induced tumors in one or more species of non-human animals, but evidence from environmental

Table 1 Agents classified by the International Agency for Research on Cancer as carcinogenic to humans

Aflatoxins
Aluminum production
4-Aminobiphenyl
Analgesic mixtures containing phenacetin
Arsenic and arsenic compounds
Asbestos
Auramine, manufacture of
Azathioprine
Benzene
Benzidine
Beryllium and beryllium compounds
Betel quid with tobacco
N, N-Bis(2-chloroethyl)-2-naphthylamine
   (Chlornaphazine)
Bis(chloromethyl)ether and chloromethyl methyl
   ether (technical-grade)
Boot and shoe manufacture and repair
1, 4-Butanediol dimethanesulphonate
   (Myleran)
Cadmium and cadmium compounds
Chlorambucil
1-(2-Chloroethyl)-3-(4-methylcyclohexyl)-1-
   nitrosourea (Methyl-CCNU)
Chromium compounds, hexavalent
Chronic infection with hepatitis B virus
Chronic infection with hepatitis C virus
Coal gasification
Coal-tar pitches
Coal-tars
Coke production
Cyclophosphamide
Diethylstilbestrol
Erionite
Estrogen replacement therapy
Estrogens, nonsteroidal
Estrogens, steroidal
Ethylene oxide
Furniture and cabinet making
Hematite mining, underground, with exposure to
   radon
Human papilloma virus
Infection with schistosoma haematobium
Iron and steel founding
Isopropyl alcohol manufacture, strong-acid
   process
Magenta, manufacture of
Melphalan
8-Methoxypsoralen (Methoxsalen) plus ultraviolet
   radiation
Mineral oils, untreated and mildly treated
MOPP (combined therapy with nitrogen mustard,
   vincristine, procarbazine, and prednisone) and
   other combined chemotherapy including
   alkylating agents

Table 1 *Continued*

Mustard gas (sulfur mustard)
2-Naphthylamine
Nickel and nickel compounds
Oral contraceptives, combined
Oral contraceptives, sequential
Radon
Rubber industry
Shale-oils
Solar radiation
Soots
Strong inorganic acid mists containing sulfuric
   acid
Talc containing asbestiform fibers
Tobacco products, smokeless
Tobacco smoke
Treosulphan
Vinyl chloride
Wood dust

epidemiology is required before a substance can be considered a known human carcinogen.

Determining whether an environmental exposure has caused an increased risk of disease is generally not easy. A series of criteria need be satisfied before an association between the exposure and the disease can be considered causal in nature (*see* **Hill's Criteria for Causality**), and evidence regarding whether they are met is not always clear. The primary tools for making such an assessment are epidemiologic case–control and cohort studies; their utility in environmental epidemiology is described below.

Case–Control Studies

The most common epidemiologic study design for evaluating the environmental determinants of chronic diseases is the case–control study. This approach provides the advantage of the ability to assemble relatively large numbers of patients with the disease of interest (often not feasible via cohort studies) whose exposure histories can then be ascertained. These histories are then compared with those obtained in a similar manner from appropriately selected **controls**, and **odds ratios** calculated as the measure of association between the environmental exposure of interest and the risk of the disease. The case–control approach typically enables the collection of information not only on the key exposure, but also on other factors that may influence risk, so that **confounding** by these other disease determinants can be controlled.

Methods for the appropriate selection of controls, a key concern in case–control studies, are described in detail in the article on **case–control studies**. The essential feature is that the controls be selected from the same base population (study base) from which the cases arise. Thus, if cases arise, say, from among patients with lung function impairment detected by screening employees in a particular industrial facility, whereas controls are selected from the general population of the area where the facility is located, it is possible that case–control differences could be influenced by nonenvironmental determinants that led to employment in the facility. Some of these confounding factors (e.g. age, sex, education) might be controlled for in the statistical analysis, but differences in unmeasured factors may exist.

This fundamental requirement of the same study base for cases and controls is sometimes violated in studies of environmental risk factors because the underlying population from which the cases arose is not always well defined. For example, in studies of rare diseases, specialty treatment centers are often sought for the ascertainment of cases. Selecting controls from other patients is generally advantageous when cases are restricted to a particular one or several hospitals, but in this situation the case patients come not only from the surrounding areas, but also from far distances to receive the specialized care. Patients admitted to the same facility for other conditions might not have the same referral patterns, and thus selecting the most appropriate controls is problematic.

The method of ascertainment of information should also be similar for cases and controls. Suppose the cases with lung function abnormalities mentioned above and the controls were both drawn from employees of similar characteristics (except for their disease) at the industrial facility. Suppose also that information on exposure to silica, the environmental factor of interest, and on presence of concomitant silicosis, was obtained for the cases as part of their evaluation of lung abnormalities. Then if information for the controls came not from a review of personnel or radiographic information as for the cases, but from questionnaires about silica exposures and about diagnoses of silicosis, differences between cases and controls could be due to the way the information was ascertained rather than to the presence of silica exposure or silicosis *per se* (see **Bias in Case–Control Studies**).

Issues regarding **selection**, information or other biases must be considered in all case–control studies. When evaluating certain environmental exposures, additional concerns need be addressed. One is **recall bias**. Individuals afflicted with a disease, particularly if life threatening in themselves or in a close relative, often tend to wonder about what may have caused the illness, or may have been prompted to examine past events during medical work-up and treatment. Sometimes this involves attempts at reconstructing events that may have taken place many years before, and can involve a process of speculating as to possible critical initiating "environmental" events. Controls, on the other hand, will typically have not gone through such prompting or soul searching. Thus, when cases and controls are interviewed, the responses may be different in part because the cases may have thought more about their illness (see **Bias in Observational Studies**).

Such recall biases can be mitigated in part by asking structured and specific as opposed to open-ended questions. At one time it was thought that exposure to chicken pox and the Varicella virus during pregnancy might increase the risk of cancer in the offspring. The suggestion came from a case–control study in which mothers were asked to list illnesses occurring during pregnancy, and mothers of the cancer patients more often listed chicken pox than mothers of the controls [7]. When prenatal medical records were examined for mention of chicken pox, however, no case–control differences were found. Furthermore, when the questionnaire for the mothers was changed to ask specially about chicken pox during pregnancy, again no case–control difference was apparent [13]. The main effect of medical record review and specific questioning was to raise the reported prevalence of chicken pox among the controls to match that among the cases. The controls had underreported the infection when asked the nonspecific open-ended question about illnesses during pregnancy, probably because they had not thought about and recalled antecedent conditions to the extent of the mothers whose children had developed cancer.

Despite the potential problems with the case–control approach, if conducted properly these studies can provide crucial information about environmental determinants of disease. Case–control studies are often the most appropriate mechanism to test hypotheses generated by the ecologic studies of grouped cancer rates and their correlates described in the previous section. Thus, the US cancer maps spawned a series of case–control studies in areas of the country where rates of particular cancers were elevated. The case–control studies obtained detailed information on the lifestyle, occupational, medical, and other characteristics of the subjects. These studies determined, for example, that although cigarette smoking was the dominant risk factor for lung cancer, employment in shipyards during World War II (and presumed exposure to asbestos) contributed to the clustering of excess rates of this cancer in the 1960s–1980s in southern coastal areas [10, 14]. Other case–control studies showed that use of herbicides in farming was associated with the higher rates of non-Hodgkin's lymphoma in the plains states [66], factors associated with northern European ancestry contributed to the clustering of excess kidney cancer mortality in north central states [52], and use of moonshine whiskies was largely responsible for the excess of esophageal cancer among black men in coastal South Carolina [18].

Case–control studies have also helped elucidate environmental factors for other diseases, especially when used to test etiologic hypotheses. The studies also have been used for hypothesis generation. An advantage of the case–control approach is the ability to look at many different antecedent exposures simultaneously. Often multiple associations are examined in case–control studies with a tendency to report in separate articles those associations based on odds ratios whose confidence limits exclude the value 1.0. The inherent multiple comparison problem is sometimes masked by the splitting of findings into multiple publications, especially when *ex post facto* explanations of the findings emerge as if they were a priori hypotheses, which can lead to undue emphasis of their importance. The case–control study, however has proven to be the key tool of environmental epidemiology, and its strengths generally outweigh its disadvantages. Some of the problems that beset case–control studies of environmental factors can be overcome in cohort studies, as described below.

Cohort Studies

Cohort studies involve the identification of individuals characterized by exposure status and followed for the occurrence of disease after exposure. The studies tend to be much larger, and often more expensive than case–control studies, because sizeable numbers of participants must be enrolled and followed to generate sufficient numbers of cases for meaningful analysis.

Cohort studies are especially useful in tracking occupational groups exposed to chemical or physical substances hypothesized to increase risk of cancer or other diseases. The hypotheses about potential risks can best be tested among groups of people with the widest range of exposure to the substance, typically workers involved in the manufacture or use of the agent. Of the over 50 compounds or processes classified as capable of causing cancer in humans following sufficient exposure (Table 1), more than half are found in occupational settings. Hence studies, typically cohort studies, among occupational groups have provided key evidence regarding whether human exposure might increase risk of cancer.

Occupational cohort studies also are of direct relevance to assessing effects of general environmental exposures. If no excess risk is seen among workers handling or otherwise heavily exposed to the agents, then it is highly unlikely that off-site exposures, generally at much lower doses, would increase risk. If an occupational excess is found, detailed study would be undertaken to characterize the risk as a function of level, timing and duration of exposure. The resultant **dose–response** trends would then be informative in predicting risks at low environmental levels. Hence, much of the information on potential effects of general environmental exposures arises from occupational studies, typically cohort studies (*see* **Occupational Mortality**).

In evaluating environmental agents with cohort studies, a key element is the measurement and classification of exposure status of cohort members. One of the strengths of a cohort study, besides its ability to ascertain a broad spectrum of health outcomes, is its ability to characterize all participants by exposure level prior to disease outcome. In principle, a prospective cohort study (where current cohort members are followed forward in time) should generally be able to obtain more reliable exposure data than a case–control study. Special problems may arise in **historical cohort studies** (where cohort members identified in the past are traced to the present) and in difficult settings where there may be imprecision of exposure assessment, including misclassification of categorical levels of exposure. In occupational studies of potentially hazardous substances, especially retrospective or historical cohort surveys where rosters of past employees are assembled, complete knowledge of levels and duration of exposure to individual workers is seldom known, even for relatively heavily studied substances. For example, asbestos is a well-known carcinogen, substantially increasing risk of lung cancer and mesothelioma when exposure levels are sufficiently high, but in nearly 50 cohort studies of various groups of asbestos-exposed workers, estimates of cumulative exposures to individual workers are available in less than a dozen, and even in those the individual estimates are based on rough approximations of presumed average airborne asbestos exposure concentrations associated with specific jobs across broad time periods [39]. Thus, some level of misclassification of exposure is bound to occur. For dichotomous categorization of exposure, if misclassification is random (nondifferential), then *on average* the **relative risks** associated with the exposure will be dampened and pulled towards the null (*see* **Bias Toward the Null**), although this is not necessarily the case when multiple categories are involved (*see* **Measurement Error in Epidemiologic Studies**). Of course, in any particular investigation, chance errors in classification could result in exaggerated as well as attenuated **relative risk** estimates.

One cohort study with relatively precise exposure estimates is the study of survivors of the atomic bombs of Hiroshima and Nagasaki. Since the early 1950s, a cohort of nearly 100 000 individuals has been tracked for mortality, and subsets have been tracked for other health outcomes [41]. Each cohort member at enrollment into the study was questioned about his/her whereabouts at the time of explosion. The event was so traumatic that nearly all individuals could recall exactly where they were and even what position they were standing in when the blast occurred. The radiation from the bombs was released almost instantaneously, so that exposure occurred within seconds (there was little radioactive fallout). Experimental models had demonstrated that levels of gamma and neutron radiation declined exponentially as distance from the hypocenter increased and provided the basis, after taking into account shielding from metal, wooden, brick, and other structures, for estimates of radiation received for almost all cohort members. Subsequent statistical analyses have shown that rates of mortality from leukemia, breast,

and several other cancers, but not nonmalignant disease, varied in proportion to radiation dose [66], and have provided a valuable base of information for the establishment of radiation safety standards worldwide.

Cohort studies of nonoccupational population groups exposed to environmental chemicals or other pollutants seldom are able to measure exposure very precisely. For example, in 1976 an explosion in a plant near Seveso, Italy, resulted in 2,3,7,8-tetrachlorodibenzo-p-dioxin contamination in surrounding neighborhoods. Chloracne and other reversible acute effects of exposure were observed in some residents closest to the plant, and a long-term monitoring for mortality, cancer, and other health outcomes was established. Cohorts of over 50 000 residents, classified in residential zones according to degree of potential for dioxin exposure, have been followed since. Results have been mixed, with little departure from expectations in mortality, suggested excesses of certain types of cancer, and no evidence of birth abnormalities following the contamination [4–6, 48, 60]. There have been difficulties in estimating exposure, but average exposure levels may have been below the limits of epidemiology as a tool for detecting and quantifying risks of chronic diseases in this population [17].

Other prospective cohort studies also may enable precise exposure classification for exposures occurring at the start of or during follow-up. In the Framingham [25, 30] and other cohorts where heart disease was the primary endpoint, measurement of blood pressure, serologic indicators, and other exposure markers could be assessed using best available methodology, and participants could be classified by baseline levels of these variables. Many of the markers are measured with error, sometimes with the particular measured value being a realization from an underlying probabilistic distribution with a large variance, so that even in these investigations perturbations in exposure classification can occur. Nevertheless, cohort studies have provided key information on the environmental determinants, including lifestyle factors, and disease risk. In the Framingham study, follow-up of approximately 5000 residents beginning in 1948 has demonstrated the predictive value of serum cholesterol (originally total and subsequently LDL and HDL fractions), hypertension, smoking, and dietary factors in cardiovascular disease risk [32, 64]. Other cohorts established from the 1950s classified individuals by tobacco smoking status. Reports from the US Surgeon General in a series of comprehensive US governmental monographs which unequivocally declared that cigarette smoking increases risk of lung cancer, relied heavily on results from cohorts of British physicians [28], American Cancer Society volunteers [34], US veterans [51], and other groups in reaching this conclusion.

One of the problems facing case–control studies, the potential for recall bias associated with the differential recollection of events because of the disease, is eliminated in cohort studies since the environmental exposure is determined prior to and independent of the disease occurrence.

Cohort studies also are less likely than case–control studies to be affected with selection or information biases, because the study base can often be unambiguously defined and data on all cohort members may be more readily collected in a standardized fashion (*see* **Bias in Cohort Studies**). Potential study base problems can arise, however, in situations where the cohort consists of exposed individuals whose disease experience is compared with that of an external population, for example with national rates of disease. Such comparisons are common in occupational and other cohort studies, but the resulting indices of risk (e.g. relative and **absolute risks**, standardized incidence or mortality ratios; *see* **Standardization Methods**) can be influenced by differences between the cohort and external populations other than the exposure itself. Among the 50 cohort studies of asbestos-exposed workers, for example, only a minority involved comparisons of disease rates among heavy vs. light vs. nonexposed workers, but instead usually compared the overall occupational group vs. national or local populations [39]. It is known that employed populations tend to have a somewhat more favorable mortality experience than the general population because ill and less fit individuals are less likely to be employed (see discussion of the "healthy worker effect" in **Occupational Epidemiology**). On the other hand, some groups, especially of blue collar workers, may have higher prevalences of cigarette smokers (this is the case for heavily asbestos exposed insulation workers [35]) or have other attributes which could increase risk relative to general population norms. This problem is mitigated by use of internal comparisons by level of exposure,

but even here nonexposure-related differences could confound comparisons. Thus, for example, neurologic and behavioral differences of production workers in the same facility could be related to social or other traits rather than to exposure to solvents or other chemicals.

Hence, cohort studies, like case–control studies, must take care to control for confounding in evaluations of potential adverse effects of environmental exposures. Cohort studies, however, are often at a disadvantage compared to case–control studies with respect to control for confounding. With their smaller size, case–control studies usually seek information on all known or suspected risk factors for the disease being studied. Cohort studies, on the other hand, typically with multiple disease endpoints and large number of participants, generally do not have this luxury and must limit the amount of information obtained per subject. A solution to this problem is offered by conducting case–control studies nested within cohort studies (*see* **Case–Control Study, Nested**). This approach enables detailed exposure and confounding variable assessment in samples of cohort members rather than in the entire cohort. In a cohort study of over 35 000 workers in mines and factories in Southern China, for example, broad classification of exposure to silica was obtained for all cohort members, but detailed occupational exposure, smoking, and other histories were obtained only for the nearly 300 persons with lung cancer plus about twice as many matched controls [29, 50]. The study found mixed results, suggesting a small increase in lung cancer among those with silicosis but not with silica exposure *per se*.

Cohort studies, particularly those involving a large number of lifestyle variables, can also suffer from the tendency to report on one variable at a time in a publication, as mentioned earlier when discussing case–control studies. Thus, the multiple comparison problem can arise in cohort studies when results are divided and described according to the least publishable unit.

Together, cohort and case–control studies provide the basis for most of what is known about the environmental determinants of human illness. Nevertheless, because of methodologic limitations these nonexperimental studies often fall short of providing sufficient evidence to determine whether exposure to a particular environmental agent can increase risk of disease. The most definitive epidemiologic evidence for determining a cause-and-effect relation can come from an experimental trial, whereby random assignment of individuals to exposed and unexposed groups mitigates against the biases that can afflict observational studies (*see* **Bias in Observational Studies**; **Bias, Overview**). Such trials are described below.

Randomized Trials

Trials involving exposure of individuals to environmental substances are ethical only when there is sufficient suspicion that the substance may lower risk of disease. Trials involving the evaluation of new drugs, for example, have been common and have provided the mechanism for the discovery and/or confirmation of the effectiveness of various treatments for human illness. The principles of these clinical trials also apply to the evaluation of a variety of agents that offer potential for the prevention of disease.

A number of randomized prevention trials have been launched, many within the past decade or so. The largest investigations have involved nutritional interventions, randomly assigning participants into groups receiving vs. not receiving certain vitamins, minerals or dietary modifications. Follow-up has typically been concurrent with the intervention, with cancer and heart disease generally the primary endpoints. In some instances the randomization unit is not the individual, but rather a group, for example, as in the one trial where communities were randomized to receive intense vs. routine educational programs aimed at smoking cessation [22]. In this trial the direct endpoint was not a health outcome, but rather an exposure (cigarette smoking), which if reduced would lower subsequent disease risk. Some of the key trials in cardiovascular disease research also have involved interventions to lower exposure markers. The Multiple Risk Factor Intervention Trial, a large trial enrolling nearly 13 000 males age 35–57 at high risk of heart disease, sought to alter several exposure (e.g. smoking), biomarker (e.g. serum cholesterol), and precursor conditions (e.g. hypertension) that increase risk of cardiovascular disease [53, 54]. Thus, intervention trials can be used to provide experimental tests both of whether increasing exposure to an environmental agent thought to reduce disease risk or decreasing exposure to an agent thought to be hazardous results in a lower risk.

The primary advantage of clinical/intervention trials over observational studies arises from randomization. The random assignment of persons to treatment groups tends to reduce differences between the groups with respect to all variables except the intervention or variables correlated with the intervention. Thus two of the main afflictions of case–control and cohort studies, namely bias and confounding, are removed. Chance is still an issue, but by choosing a sufficiently large study size for the trial, the effects of random errors can be minimized. One of the largest intervention trials involved random assignment, within strata defined by age and sex, of nearly 30 000 individuals in Linxian, China, into one of eight treatment groups [15]. The groups were defined by a one-half replicate of a 2^4 factorial experimental design, whereby four types of vitamin/mineral supplements were being assessed as potential inhibitors of esophageal and stomach cancer in a population with one of the world's highest rates of these cancers. Cigarette smoking status, a risk factor for these cancers, was not matched for in the design, but the randomization accomplished this task. After randomization, the prevalence of smoking across the eight intervention groups varied by less than 1% [44]. Similarly, other measured differences across the treatments were all uniformly small, providing confidence that unmeasured variables were also likely to be evenly distributed by treatment, and thus bias and confounding were unlikely to affect study results.

The large vitamin/mineral intervention trials thus far have shown mixed results for the effects of supplementation on subsequent cancer or heart disease risk, despite the consistent demonstration from both case–control and cohort studies of lowered risks among persons with high intakes of foods (especially fruits and vegetables) with high contents of carotenoids, vitamin C, and other nutrients. The Linxian trial [15] found a small (13%) but significant reduction in cancer mortality following 5 years of supplements with a combination of beta carotene, vitamin E, and selenium. Large trials in Finland [2] and the US [57], however, found significantly increased, rather than decreased, risks of lung cancer among smokers supplemented with beta carotene or beta carotene plus retinol, respectively, while a 12-year follow-up of among 22 000 US physicians, few of whom smoked, found no effect of beta carotene supplementation on cancer or heart disease [37].

The beta carotene results from these trials provide a stark reminder of the limitations of the observational (case–control and cohort) studies. The vast majority of observational studies have shown lowered cancer risks, with reductions typically of 30%–50% among heavy compared with light consumers of foods rich in beta carotene [67]. Limited evidence of cancer inhibition from beta carotene studies in experimental animals provided a biologic basis for the hypothesis, and even a potential mechanism of action, in particular beta carotene's ability to quench singlet oxygen radicals. Publication in 1981 of a prominent review article [61] helped to stimulate enthusiasm for the beta carotene hypothesis and to lead to the incorporation of beta carotene in several randomized trials. The results of these trials now indicate that the enthusiasm may have been misplaced, and that correlates of beta carotene rather than beta carotene *per se* may have been responsible for the reduced risks associated with intake of beta carotene-containing foods seen in the case–control and cohort studies. This unfolding of events suggests that caution be applied in the interpretation of case–control or cohort studies linking various environmental exposures with disease risk, and heightens the necessity for careful assessment of bias, confounding, and chance before etiologic interpretations are offered, especially since few environmental exposures will be able to be evaluated via randomized intervention trials.

References

[1] Adami, H.-O. (1996). Sweden: a paradise for epidemiologists?, *Lancet* **347**, 588–589.

[2] Alpha-Tocopherol, Beta Carotene Cancer Prevention Study Group. (1994). The effect of vitamin E and beta carotene on the incidence of lung cancer and other cancers in male smokers, *New England Journal of Medicine* **330**, 1029–1035.

[3] American Cancer Society (1995). *Cancer Facts and Figures, 1995.* American Cancer Society, Atlanta.

[4] Bertazzi, P.A., Pesatori, A.C., Consonni, D., Tironi, A., Landi, M.T. & Zocchetti, C. (1993). Cancer incidence in a population accidentally exposed to 2,3,7,8-tetrachlorodibenzo-para-dioxin, *Epidemiology* **4**, 398–406.

[5] Bertazzi, P.A., Zocchetti, C., Pesatori, A.C., Guercilina, S., Consuinni, D., Tironi, A. & Landi, M.T. (1992). Mortality of a young population after accidental exposure to 2,3,7,8-tetracholorodibenzodioxin, *International Journal of Epidemiology* **21**, 118–123.

[6] Bertazzi, P.A., Zocchetti, C., Pesatori, A.C., Guercilena, S, Sanarico, M. & Radice, L. (1989). Ten-year mortality study of the population involved in the Seveso incident in 1976, *American Journal of Epidemiology* **129**, 1187–1200.

[7] Bithell, J.F., Draper, G. & Gerbach, P. (1973). Association between malignant disease in children and maternal virus infections, *British Medical Journal* **2**, 706–710.

[8] Blot, W.J. & Fraumeni, J.F., Jr (1977). Geographic patterns of oral cancer in the United States: etiologic implications, *Journal of Chronic Diseases* **30**, 745–757.

[9] Blot, W.J. & Fraumeni, J.F. Jr (1979). Studies of respiratory cancer in high risk communities, *Journal of Occupational Medicine* **21**, 276–278.

[10] Blot, W.J. & Fraumeni, J.F., Jr (1981). Cancer among shipyard workers, in *Banbury Report*, Vol. 9. Cold Spring Harbor Laboratory, New York, pp. 37–50.

[11] Blot, W.J. & Fraumeni, J.F., Jr (1996). Cancers of the lung and pleura, in *Cancer Epidemiology and Prevention*, 2nd Ed., D. Schottenfeld & J. Fraumeni, eds. Oxford University Press, New York, pp. 637–665.

[12] Blot, W.J., Devesa, S.S., Kneller, R.W. & Fraumeni, J.F., Jr (1991). Rising incidence of adenocarcinoma of the esophagus and gastric cardia, *Journal of the American Medical Association* **265**, 1287–1289.

[13] Blot W.J., Draper, G., Kinlen, L. & Kinnier-Wilson, M. (1980). Childhood cancer in relation to prenatal exposure to chicken pox, *British Journal of Cancer* **42**, 342–344.

[14] Blot, W.J., Harrington, J.M., Toledo, A., Hoover, R., Heath, C.W., Jr & Fraumeni, J.F., Jr (1978). Lung cancer after employment in shipyards during World War II, *New England Journal of Medicine* **299**, 620–624.

[15] Blot, W.J., Li, J.-Y., Taylor, P.R., Guo, W., Dawsey, S., Wang, G.-Q., Yang, C.S., Zheng, S.-F., Gail, M., Lit, G.-Y., Yu, Y., Liu, B.-Q., Tangrea, J., Sun, Y.-H., Lin, F., Fraumeni, J.F., Jr, Zhang, Y.-H. & Li, B. (1993). Nutrition intervention trials in Linxian, China: supplementation with specific vitamin/mineral combination, cancer incidence, and disease-specific mortality in the general population, *Journal of the National Cancer Institute* **85**, 1483–1492.

[16] Boffetta, P., Kogevinas, M., Simonato, L., Wilbourn, J. & Saracci, R. (1995). Current perspectives on occupational cancer risks, *International Journal of Occupational and Environmental Health* **1**, 315–325.

[17] Boroush, M. & Gough, M. (1994). Can cohort studies detect any human cancers that may result from exposure to dioxin? Maybe, *Regulatory Toxicology and Pharmacology* **20**, 198–210.

[18] Brown, L.M., Blot, W.J., Schuman, S.H., Smith, V.M., Ershow, A.G., Marks, R.D. & Fraumeni, J.F., Jr (1988). Environmental factors and high risk of esophageal cancer among men in coastal South Carolina, *Journal of the National Cancer Institute* **80**, 1620–1625.

[19] Buescher, P.A., Taylor, K.P., Davis, M.H. & Bowling, J.M. (1993). The quality of the new birth certificate data: a validation study in North Carolina, *American Journal of Public Health* **83**, 1163–1165.

[20] Chow, W.H., Finkle, W.D., McLaughlin, J.K., Frankl, H., Ziel, H.K. & Fraumeni, J.F., Jr (1995). The relation of gastroesophageal reflux disease and its treatment to adenocarcinomas of the esophagus and gastric cardia, *Journal of the American Medical Association* **274**, 474–477.

[21] Cole, P. & Rodu, B. (1996). Declining cancer mortality in the United States, *Cancer* **78**, 2045–2048.

[22] COMMIT Research Group (1995). Community Interventional Trial for smoking cessation (COMMIT): I. Cohort results from a four-year community intervention, *American Journal of Public Health* **85**, 183–192.

[23] Cooper, R.S., Liao, Y. & Rotimi, C. (1996). Is hypertension more severe among U.S. blacks, or is severe hypertension more common?, *Annals of Epidemiology* **6**, 173–180.

[24] Creech, J.L. & Johnson, M.N. (1974). Angiosarcoma of the liver in the manufacture of polyvinyl chloride, *Journal of Occupational Medicine* **16**, 150.

[25] Dawber, T.R., Meadors, G.F. & Moore, F.E. (1951). Epidemiological approaches to heart disease: the Framingham study, *American Journal of Public Health* **41**, 279–286.

[26] Desenclos, J.C., Scaggs, M. & Wroten, J.E. (1992). Characteristics of mothers of live infants with congenital syphilis in Florida, 1987–1989, *American Journal of Epidemiology* **136**, 657–661.

[27] Devesa, S.S., Blot, W.J., Stone, B.J., Miller, B.A., Tarone, R.E. & Fraumeni, J.F., Jr (1995). Recent cancer trends in the United States, *Journal of the National Cancer Institute* **87**, 175–182.

[28] Doll, R., Peto, R., Wheatly, K., Gray, R. & Sutherland, I. (1994). Mortality in relation to smoking: 40 years' observations on male British doctors, *British Medical Journal* **309**, 901–911.

[29] Dosemeci, M., Chen, J.Q., Hearl, F.J., Wu, Z., McCawley, M.A., Chen, R.A., McLaughlin, J.K., Peng, K., Cheng, A.L., Rexing, S.H. & Blot, W.J. (1993). Estimating historical exposure to silica for mine and pottery workers in the People's Republic of China, *American Journal of Industrial Medicine* **24**, 55–66.

[30] Feinlieb, M. (1985). The Framingham Study: sample selection, follow-up, and methods of analyses, in *Selection, Follow-up, and Analysis in Prospective Studies: A Workshop*, NIH Publication No. 85–2713, L. Garfinkel, O. Ochs & M. Mushinski, eds. US Department of Health and Human Services, National Institutes of Health, Bethesda, pp. 59–64.

[31] Fiore, M.C., Novotny, T.E., Pierce, J.P., Hatziandreu, E.J., Patel, K.M. & Davis, R.M. (1989). Trends in cigarette smoking in the United States: the changing influence of gender and race, *Journal of the American Medical Association* **261**, 49–55.

[32] Gordon, T., Castelli, W., Hjortland, M.C., Rannel, W.B. & Dawber, T.R. (1977). High density lipoprotein as a protective factor against coronary heart disease, *American Journal of Medicine* **62**, 707–714.

[33] Grulich, A.E., Swerdlow, A.J., Dos Santos Silva, I. & Beral, V. (1995). Is the apparent rise in cancer mortality in the elderly real? Analysis of changes in certification and coding of cause of death in England and Wales, 1970–1990, *International Journal of Cancer* **63**, 164–168.

[34] Hammond, E.C. (1996). Smoking in relation to the death rates of one million men and women, *National Cancer Institute Monograph* **19**, 127–204.

[35] Hammond, E.C., Selikoff, I.J. & Seidman, H. (1979). Asbestos exposure, cigarette smoking, and death rates, *Annals of the New York Academy of Science* **330**, 473–490.

[36] Heath, C.W. (1988). Investigation of cancer case clusters: possibilities and limitations, in *Unusual Occurrences as Clues to Cancer Etiology*, R.W. Miller, et al., eds. Japan Scientific Press, Tokyo, p. 27–38.

[37] Hennekens, C.H., Buring, J.E., Manson, J.E., Stampfer, M., Rosner, B., Cook, N.R., Belanger, C., LaMotte, F., Gaziano, J.M., Ridker, P.M., Willett, W. & Peto, R. (1996). Lack of effect of long-term supplementation with beta carotene on the incidence of malignant neoplasms and cardiovascular disease, *New England Journal of Medicine* **334**, 1145–1149.

[38] Herbst, A.L., Ulfelder, H. & Poskanzer, D.C. (1971). Adenocarcinoma of the vagina: association of maternal stilbesterol therapy with tumor appearance in young women, *New England Journal of Medicine* **284**, 878–881.

[39] Hughes, J.M. & Weill, H. (1994). Asbestos and man-made fibers, in *Epidemiology of Lung Cancer*, J.M. Samet, ed. Marcel Dekker, New York, pp. 185–205.

[40] International Agency for Cancer Research (1987). *IARC Monographs on the Evaluation of Carcinogenic Risks to Humans. Overall Evaluations of Carcinogenicity: An Updating of IARC Monographs Vols. 1 to 42*. IARC, Lyon.

[41] Jablon, S. (1985). Selection, followup and analysis in the Atomic Bomb Casualty Commission Study, *National Cancer Institute Monograph* **67**, 53–58.

[42] Johnson, C.L., Rifkind, B.M., Sempos, C.T., Carroll, M.D., Bachorik, P.S., Briefel, R.R., Gordon, D.J., Burt, V.L., Brown, C.D., Lippel, K. & Cleeman, J.I. (1993). Declining serum total cholesterol levels among US adults. The National Health and Nutrition Examination Surveys, *Journal of the American Medical Association* **269**, 3002–3008.

[43] Kosary, C.L., Ries, L.A.G., Miller, B.A., Hankey, B.F., Harras, A. & Edwards, B.K., eds (1995). *SEER Cancer Statistics Review, 1973–1992: Tables and Graphs*, NIH Publication No. 96–2789. National Cancer Institute, Bethesda.

[44] Li, B., Taylor, P.R., Li, J.-Y., Dawsey, S.M., Wang, W., Tangrea, J.A., Lin, B.-Q., Ershow, A.G., Zheng, S.-F., Fraumeni, J.F., Jr., Yang, Q., Yu, Y., Sun, Y., Li, G., Zhang, D., Greenwald, P., Lian, G.-T., Yang, C.S. & Blot, W.J. (1993). Linxian nutrition intervention trials:

design, methods, participant characteristics, and compliance, *Annals of Epidemiology* **3**, 577–585.

[45] Li, D.K. & Daling, J.R. (1991). Maternal smoking, low birth weight, and ethnicity in relation to sudden infant death syndrome, *American Journal of Epidemiology* **134**, 958–964.

[46] MacMahon, B. (1992). Leukemia clusters around nuclear facilities in Britain, *Cancer Causes and Control* **3**, 283–288.

[47] Mason, T.J., McKay, F.W., Hoover, R., Blot, W.J. & Fraumeni, J.F., Jr (1975). *Atlas of Cancer Mortality for U.S. Counties 1950–1969*, DHEW Publication No. (NIH) 75–780. US Department of Health Education and Welfare, National Institutes of Health, Bethesda.

[48] Mastroiacovo, P., Spagnolog, A., Marni, E., Meazza, L., Bertollini, R., Segni, G. & Burgna-Pignatti, C. (1998). Birth defects in the Seveso area after TCDD contamination, *Journal of the American Medical Association* **259**, 1668–1672.

[49] Mathis, M.P., Lavoie, M., Hadley, C. & Toomey, K.V. (1995). Birth certificates as a source for fetal alcohol syndrome case ascertainment – Georgia, 1989–1992, *Morbidity and Mortality Weekly Reports* **44**, 251–253.

[50] McLaughlin, J.K., Chen, J.Q., Dosemeci, M., Chen, R.A., Rexing, S.H., Wu, Z., Hearl, F.J., McCawley, M.A. & Blot, W.J. (1992). A nested case–control study of lung cancer among silica exposed workers in China, *British Journal of Industrial Medicine* **49**, 167–171.

[51] McLaughlin, J.K., Hrubec, Z., Blot, W.J. & Fraumeni, J.F., Jr (1995). Smoking and cancer mortality among U.S. veterans: a 26-year followup, *International Journal of Cancer* **60**, 190–193.

[52] McLaughlin, J.K., Mandel, J.S., Blot, W.J., Schuman, L.M., Mehl, E.S. & Fraumeni, J.F., Jr (1984). A population-based case-control study of renal cell carcinoma, *Journal of the National Cancer Institute* **72**, 275–284.

[53] Multiple Risk Factor Intervention Trial Group (1977). Statistical design considerations in the NHLI Multiple Risk Factor Intervention Trial (MRFIT), *Journal of Chronic Diseases* **30**, 261–275.

[54] Multiple Risk Factor Intervention Trial Group (1982). Multiple risk factors intervention trial: risk factor changes and mortality results, *Journal of the American Medical Association* **248**, 1465–1477.

[55] National Research Council (1991). *Environmental Epidemiology*, Vol. 1: *Public Health and Hazardous Wastes*. National Academy Press, Washington.

[56] Olsen, S.F., Martuzzi, M. & Elliott, P. (1996). Cluster analysis and disease mapping – Why, when, and how?, *British Medical Journal* **313**, 863–866.

[57] Omenn, G.S., Goodman, G.E., Thornquist, M.D., Blames, J., Cullen, M.R., Glass, A., Keogh, J.P., Meyskens, F.L., Valanis, B., Williams, J.H., Barnhart, S. & Hammar, S. (1996) Effects of a combination of beta carotene and vitamin A on lung cancer and cardiovascular disease, *New England Journal of Medicine* **334**, 1150–1155.

[58] Parkin, D.M, Muir, C.S., Whelan, S.L., Gao, Y.-T., Ferlay, J. & Powell, J., eds (1992). *Cancer Incidence in Five Continents*, Vol. VI. IARC Scientific Publications, Lyon, France.

[59] Percy, C.L., Miller, B.A. & Ries, L.A.G. (1990). Effect of changes in cancer classification and the accuracy of cancer death certificates on trends in cancer mortality, *Annals of the New York Academy of Science* **609**, 87–97.

[60] Pesatori, A.C., Consonni, D., Tironi, A., Zocchetti, C., Fini, A. & Bertazzi, P.A. (1993). Cancer in a young population in a dioxin-contaminated area, *International Journal of Epidemiology* **22**, 1010–1013.

[61] Peto, R., Doll, R., Buckley, J.D. & Sporn, M.B. (1981). Can dietary beta-carotene materially reduce human cancer rates?, *Nature* **290**, 201–208.

[62] Pickle, L.W., Mason, T.J., Howard, N., Hoover, R. & Fraumeni, J.F., Jr (1987). *Atlas of U.S. Cancer Mortality Among Whites: 1950–1980*, DHHS Publication No. (NIH) 87–2900. US Department of Health and Human Services, National Institutes of Health, Bethesda.

[63] Pirkle, J.L., Flegal, K.M., Bernert, J.T., Brody, D.J., Etzel, R.A. & Maurer, K.R. (1996). Exposure of the US population to environmental tobacco smoke. The Third National Health and Nutrition Examination Survey, 1988 to 1991, *Journal of the American Medical Association* **275**, 1233–1240.

[64] Posner, B.M., Franz, M.M., Quatromoni, P.A., Gagnon, D.R., Sytkowski, P.A., D'Agostino, R.B. & Cupples, A. (1995). Secular trends in diet and risk factors for cardiovascular disease: The Framingham Study, *Journal of the American Dietetic Association* **95**, 171–179.

[65] Sever, L.E. (1995). Epidemiologic aspects of environmental hazards to reproduction, in *Introduction to Environmental Epidemiology*, E. Talbott & G. Graun, eds. CRC Press, Boca Raton, pp. 81–98.

[66] Shimizu, T., Kato, H. & Schull, W.J. (1990). Studies of the mortality of A-bomb survivors, *Radiation Research* **130**, 249–266.

[67] Steinmetz, K.A. & Potter, J.D. (1991). Vegetables, fruit and cancer. I. Epidemiology, *Cancer Causes and Control* **2**, 325–357.

[68] Surgeon General (1989). *Reducing the Health Consequences of Smoking: 25 Years of Progress*. US Department of Health and Human Services, Office of Smoking and Health, Rockville.

[69] Wang, H.H., Hsieh, C. & Antonioli, D.A. (1994). Rising incidence rate of esophageal adenocarcinoma and use of pharmaceutical agents that relax the lower esophageal sphincter, *Cancer Causes and Control* **5**, 573–578.

[70] Winn, D.M., Blot, W.J., Shy, C.M. & Fraumeni, J.F., Jr (1981). Snuff dipping, oral cancer and dentures, *New England Journal of Medicine* **305**, 230–231.

[71]   Woolbright, L.A. & Harshbarger, D.S. (1995). The revised standard certificate of live birth: analysis of medical risk factor data from birth certificates in Alabama, 1988–92, *Public Health Reports* **110**, 59–63.

[72]   Zahm, S.H., Weisenburger, D.D., Babbitt, P.A., Saal, R.C., Vaught, J.B., Cantor, K.P. & Blair, A. (1990). A case–control study of non-Hodgkin's lymphoma and the herbicide 2, 4-dichlorophenoxyacetic acid (2,4-D) in eastern Nebraska, *Epidemiology* **1**, 349–356.

WILLIAM J. BLOT, WONG-HO CHOW & JOSEPH K. MCLAUGHLIN

Epicure *see* Software, Biostatistical

Epidemic Curve

An epidemic curve is a plot of time trends in the occurrence of a disease or other health-related event for a defined population and time period. The epidemic curve can help to demonstrate that the events are in excess of what would be expected based on past experience [4]. Time intervals are indicated on the *x*-axis and the event rate is shown on the *y*-axis. The event rate may measure the number of cases per unit time (e.g. cases per day or year), or it may express the numbers of events relative to the number in the study population (cases per 100 000 person–years). The latter **incidence rates** may be age-adjusted (*see* **Standardization Methods**).

Historically, the epidemic curve has been widely used by infectious disease epidemiologists to document the scope and duration of an epidemic, to help determine the source of the infection and the modes of transmission or exposure, and to glean information about the **incubation period** of the disease [6]. Epidemic curves are used in other settings to document the scope of public health problems.

Example 1

An estimated 224 000 persons nationwide became ill with salmonellosis during 1994 after eating a nationally distributed brand of ice cream that was contaminated with *Salmonella enteritidis* [5]. Epidemic curves for Minnesota, an epicenter of the outbreak, and for the entire US helped to determine that the outbreak occurred during September and October of that year as a result of contamination that occurred between mid-August and mid-October.

Example 2

The number of acquired immune deficiency syndrome (AIDS) cases in the US exhibited exponential growth during the early 1980s, followed by a slowing of the rate of increase beginning in mid-1987 [2]. This pattern likely reflects a decline in the number of new human immunodeficiency virus (HIV) infections compared with peak infection rates in the mid-1980s.

Example 3

Age-adjusted lung cancer death rates per 100 000 men in the US climbed 15-fold between 1930 and 1990 [7], a result of trends in tobacco consumption during earlier decades [3]. The epidemic curve is expected to decline in the US as a result of smoking cessation [3]; but epidemiologists predict a rising epidemic curve for tobacco-related deaths in the next century among Chinese men, as a result of their recent increase in cigarette smoking [8].

While it is reasonable to speak of an "epidemic" of violent death or of specific neoplastic diseases (Example 3), analysis of the epidemic curve is currently most refined in the field of infectious disease epidemiology.

In a *common source outbreak*, susceptibles are exposed to a pathogen about the same point in time (Example 1). In this type of outbreak the resulting epidemic curve tends to be relatively short and sharp, as the cases distribute according to the incubation period of the disease. With food-borne outbreaks, a point source of exposure is sometimes identified from the case reports and the pathogen may be recognized from the observed incubation period. In a *propagated* or *progressive outbreak*, cases result from person-to-person transmission, often yielding a broader epidemic curve (Example 2).

Statistically, if the infection curve is known, one can estimate the distribution of the incubation period from the observed epidemic curve [1]. Conversely, if the incubation period is known, one can estimate the infection curve from the observed epidemic curve (*see* **Back-Calculation**). To avoid bias, it is essential that the epidemic curve be constructed using a well-defined case definition and that surveillance for the event is as complete and consistent as possible. In practice, the case definition may include both clinical and epidemiologic criteria [9].

References

[1] Bacchetti, P. & Moss, A.J. (1989). Incubation period of AIDS in San Francisco, *Nature* **338**, 251–253.

[2] Brookmeyer, R. (1991). Reconstruction and future trends of the AIDS epidemic in the United States, *Science* **253**, 37–42.

[3] Devesa, S.S., Blot, W.J. & Fraumeni, J.F. Jr (1989). Declining lung cancer rates among young men and women in the United States: a cohort analysis, *Journal of the National Cancer Institute* **81**, 1568–1571.

[4] Evans, A.S. (1989). Epidemiologic concepts and methods, in *Viral Infections of Humans: Epidemiology and Control*, A.S. Evans, ed., 3rd Ed. Plenum, New York.

[5] Hennessy, T.W., Hedberg, C.W., Slutsker, L., White, K.E., Besser-Wick, J.M., Moen, M.E., Feldman, J., Coleman, W.W., Edmonson, L.M., MacDonald, K.L. & Osterholm, M.T. (1996). A national outbreak of *Salmonella enteritidis* infection from ice cream, *New England Journal of Medicine* **334**, 1281–1286.

[6] Kelsey, J.L., Thompson, W.D. & Evans, A.S. (1986). *Methods in Observational Epidemiology*. Oxford University Press, New York, Chapter 9, pp. 212–253.

[7] Parker, S.L., Tong, T., Bolden, S. & Wingo, P.A. (1996). Cancer statistics, 1997, *CA–A Cancer Journal for Clinicians* **47**, 5–27; see Figure 4.

[8] Peto, R., Chen, Z. & Boreham, J. (1996). Tobacco – the growing epidemic in China, *Journal of the American Medical Association* **275**, 1683–1684.

[9] Sharrar, R.G. (1992). General principles of epidemiology, in *Preventive Medicine and Public Health*, B.J. Cassens, ed., 2nd Ed. Williams & Wilkins, Baltimore, pp. 1–21.

(*See also* **Communicable Diseases**; **Epidemic Models, Deterministic**; **Epidemic Models, Stochastic**; **Epidemic Thresholds**; **Infectious Disease Models**)

PHILIP S. ROSENBERG

Epidemic Models, Deterministic

In this article we review some of the approaches, both standard and recent, to the theory of deterministic epidemic models. By deterministic we mean that one considers populations consisting of sufficiently many well-mixed individuals. At the level of the individuals, however, we do consider processes such as infection and the individual course of infection to be stochastic events. What separates the deterministic models from the approach taken in stochastic epidemic models (*see* **Epidemic Models, Stochastic**) is that we invoke a law of large numbers argument to lift these individual stochasticities to population determinism.

There are many ways in which an article like this could be structured. We have chosen to use four concrete infections as stepping-stones to review current issues in epidemic modeling and the types of deterministic model employed and questions studied. These infections are measles, malaria, helminths, and human immunodeficiency virus (HIV), respectively, reflecting the order in which they were important historically in shaping epidemic theory. Of course, many of the models discussed under these headings are used in a great variety of settings and there is a certain degree of arbitrariness in the place in which they occur here. We do not intend to provide detailed mathematical results, but on the contrary stress the evolution of the subject and the practical problems faced. Our main aim is to point the interested reader to more advanced literature.

The current issues in epidemic modeling – both stochastic and deterministic – are illustrated in the recent review books by Mollison [40], Isham & Medley [31] and Grenfell & Dobson [19]. In these most of the issues touched on below are discussed and reviewed extensively. For a review of the recent mathematical deterministic theory, see [12].

Measles

As in stochastic epidemic modeling, the diseases that sparked the development of modern deterministic theory are the childhood infections, most notably measles. This arises predominantly from their large public health importance in the late nineteenth and early twentieth centuries. In late nineteenth century England a sophisticated system of **vital statistics** had been initiated by William Farr, and data series became available that were both reliable enough and long enough to generate hypotheses about the possible mechanisms underlying epidemic spread. It should be noted that the germ theory of infection became firmly established only after the 1880s. Germ theory is the notion that certain diseases are caused by living organisms multiplying within the host and capable of being transmitted between hosts.

The most striking aspect of measles epidemics, i.e. their regular cyclic behavior, was noticed first by Arthur Ransome around 1880. Speculation about the underlying cause centered around the availability of sufficiently many susceptible individuals of the right age-class in close enough proximity to each other. Early shimmers of the modern notion of critical community size for sustaining endemic measles [4, 5] were also present. Two factors that commonly occur in many current models to investigate epidemic spread of measles and other infections are the importance of age-structure and of periodicity in contacts. The age and school season were recognized as important as early as 1896 [24].

Against this background it was William Hamer who published a discrete time epidemic "model" for the transmission of measles [25]. The mathematical rendering was later given in [50]. Hamer's observation can be reformulated as stating that the incidence of new cases in a time interval is proportional to the product SI of the (spatial) density S of susceptibles and the (spatial) density I of infectives in the population. This assumption of mass action – in analogy to its origin in chemical reaction kinetics – is fundamental to the modern theory of deterministic epidemic modeling. When densities are constant and one would like to express the incidence in terms of numbers of individuals, the incidence is proportional to SI/N, where N is the total population size [9].

The popularity of mass action is explained because of its mathematical convenience and the fact that at low densities it is a reasonable approximation of a much more complex contact process. At higher densities it grossly overestimates contact opportunities. As a side remark we note that Frost and Reed in 1928 recognized for measles that although multiple contacts of infectives with the same susceptible can occur, this susceptible can become infected only once. This led them to develop the stochastic Reed–Frost model that does not have this particular problem. Incidentally, this problem with mass action had already been solved by P.D. En'ko long before it was introduced. He studied a model for measles transmission that is very similar to the Reed–Frost

approach (see [13]). For a comparison between all approaches, see Dietz & Schenzle [15].

Currently, expressions like $\beta C(N)SI/N$ are frequently used for the incidence, where $\beta C(N)$ gives the successful contacts per unit of time for a given infective. A fraction S/N of these contacts will be with a susceptible in a homogeneously mixing population. The function $C(N)$ is taken to saturate with increasing density, reflecting the fact that contacts take time and moreover satiation occurs (think of sexual contacts and insect vectors taking blood meals; see, for example, [27] and [51]). A standard compartment model for infection transmission with a **latent period** and lasting immunity (a so-called Susceptible $\rightarrow$ Exposed $\rightarrow$ Infective $\rightarrow$ Removed (SEIR) model) is

$$\frac{dS}{dt} = \mu N - \beta C(N)\frac{SI}{N} - \mu S, \qquad (1)$$

$$\frac{dE}{dt} = \beta C(N)\frac{SI}{N} - (\sigma + \mu)E, \qquad (2)$$

$$\frac{dI}{dt} = \sigma E - (\gamma + \mu)I. \qquad (3)$$

An equation for R is superfluous here since $N = S + E + I + R$ is constant in this model. A very large number of variants of this model – usually denoted by strings of S, E, I, and R – are studied in the literature for a large number of different infections. In most cases this entails analysis of the dynamic behavior with practical applications to problems concerning control of the infection (see [29] for a brief review of this area). Examples of important extensions are introducing an additional death rate due to the disease, loss of immunity with re-entering of the S-class, a birth rate directly into the infective class (vertical transmission) (see [7] for all of these), density-dependent demography, and of course heterogeneity which we will discuss later. In [32] a comprehensive treatment of the mathematical theory of compartmental systems is given. Whether certain possible additions matter depends partly on the time scale of the phenomenon one is interested in. For example, on the time scale of individual epidemic outbreaks, the population can often be regarded as being in a demographic steady state (see [12]), and the inflow of new susceptibles can often be neglected in a short enough period (closed population). Useful results include the so-called final size equations for closed populations. These relate the initial size S_0 of the susceptible population to the basic reproduction number R_0 (see below) and the size $S(\infty)$ of the susceptible population that remains after the epidemic has come to an end. Both S_0 and $S(\infty)$ might be observable in practical situations or estimated from population data. Estimates of R_0 can then be obtained from a final-size relation. In the case of system (1)–(3), with $C(N) = N$ (mass action) and disregarding latency (i.e. $\sigma \to \infty$), we obtain

$$\ln \frac{S(\infty)}{S_0} = R_0 \left[\frac{S(\infty)}{S_0} - 1 \right]. \qquad (4)$$

One of the many present-day approaches towards understanding the dynamics of measles epidemics (see [6] for a review) is to include a periodic forcing $\beta(t) = b_0[1 + b_1 cos(2\pi t)]$ in the contact rate of compartmental models to mimic the increase in successful contact opportunities during school seasons (see [20]). The dynamics of these models have been extensively studied (see, for example, [47] and [49]) and compared with data. Detecting nonlinearity and chaos from stochastic effects in data of recurrent epidemics is an important theme in this area [16].

In contrast to seasonal contact rates – that are studied in only a few other settings (see malaria section below) – the incorporation of age structure is relevant to almost all important human infections (see [3] and [7]). Age-structured models come in discrete age-class systems of differential equations and continuous age systems of partial differential equations [52]:

$$\frac{\partial S}{\partial t} + \frac{\partial S}{\partial a} = -\mu S - \lambda S, \qquad (5)$$

$$\frac{\partial I}{\partial t} + \frac{\partial I}{\partial a} = -\mu I + \lambda S - \gamma I, \qquad (6)$$

$$\frac{\partial R}{\partial t} + \frac{\partial R}{\partial a} = -\mu R + \gamma I, \qquad (7)$$

with

$$S(t, 0) = \int_0^\infty b(a)N(t, a)\,da, \quad I(t, 0) = R(t, 0) = 0, \qquad (8)$$

and appropriate initial conditions. The so-called *force of infection* $\lambda(t)$ is defined by

$$\lambda(t) = \int_0^\infty k(a')I(t, a')\,da'. \qquad (9)$$

Often the force of infection depends on the age a of the susceptible with the kernel $k(a')$ replaced by

$k(a, a')$ to reflect the different mixing patterns of individuals of different ages. Extensions of models like this have been compared with data for measles, notably by Schenzle [48], and showed remarkable accuracy even in following the shift in trend after vaccination was implemented. Mathematical theory centers around dynamic behavior and stability criteria for endemic steady states for various variants of this model (see [30]).

One of the applied issues in studying age-structured models is to predict the effects of changes in vaccination strategies [17]. For childhood infections not all strategies of vaccinating children at various ages can result in eradication of the infectious agent from the population. For this to occur the basic reproduction number R_0 has to be less than 1 in a population where the distribution with respect to age and vaccination status is in a demographic steady state. The basic reproduction number is one of the central notions of epidemic theory. It is defined as the expected number of secondary cases caused by a single infective in a susceptible population that is in a demographic steady state. For modern theory of calculating R_0 for infections in heterogeneous populations, see [11] and [26]. Consider system (5)–(9). Let the stable age distribution be given by $S(a) = S_0 e^{-ra} \mathcal{F}_d(a)$, where r is the intrinsic population growth rate and $\mathcal{F}_d$ is the survival function. One can show that

$$R_0 = S_0 \int_0^\infty k(a)e^{-ra}\mathcal{F}_d(a)\,da. \qquad (10)$$

In the article on Reproduction Number a relation is given for the fraction of the population that needs to be vaccinated in order to assure eradication:

$$v > 1 - \frac{1}{R_0}. \qquad (11)$$

If we vaccinate a fraction v at birth, then we have a susceptible population of size $S_0(1 - v)$ and the relation is the same as above with R_0 given by (10).

Optimal vaccination policies can also take economic considerations into account using similar methods (see, for example, [23] and [41]).

These models have shown that some vaccination strategies in use can have unforeseen detrimental effects in a population (see [3], for exposition and review). If fewer susceptibles are around in certain age-classes as a result of vaccination, then the average age at acquiring infection will rise. For infections such as rubella, complications can arise when the infection is contracted for the first time during pregnancy. This leads to the situation where even though rubella prevalence can decrease due to vaccination, the number of serious complications can increase as a result. It is in this type of application for childhood infections that age-structured models and their analysis have provided important epidemiologic insight that might otherwise have been difficult to obtain.

Malaria

Independently from Hamer, Ronald Ross in 1911 introduced the mass action idea in continuous time in his study of the transmission of malaria [44]. Ross's work in subsequent years (see [45]) qualify him as the true founding father of modern epidemic theory. It was partly under his influence that Anderson McKendrick started his own studies into the mathematical modeling of epidemic phenomena, initially also in the context of malaria and other tropical infections. His series of papers with Kermack from 1927 onwards, see below, is regarded as the foundation upon which much of modern theory rests. The papers have recently been reprinted [34].

One of the distinguishing characteristics of malaria is that the protozoan parasite is indirectly transmitted between humans by mosquitoes. Several important human infections depend on similar vectors for their transmission. For modeling this brings about a new problem in that the population dynamics of the vector have to be described. A simple model capturing the essentials is (see [3])

$$\frac{dx}{dt} = ab\frac{M}{N}y(1-x) - \gamma x, \tag{12}$$

$$\frac{dy}{dt} = acx(1-y) - \mu y, \tag{13}$$

where x and y are the fractions of infected humans and mosquitoes, respectively, and where M/N is the number of (female) mosquitoes per human host in an infection free steady state. Common extensions in a similar vein are seasonality in vector emergence and the incorporation of heterogeneity in the human population. The basic reproduction number for the above model is given by

$$R_0 = \frac{M}{N}\frac{a^2bc}{\gamma\mu}. \tag{14}$$

Since the work of Ross and notably Macdonald [36], eradication campaigns have been aimed at controlling the mosquito population strongly enough to achieve $R_0 < 1$. With the emergence of both vector resistance to chemical control and parasite resistance to drug treatment malaria is regaining its strength as arguably the most severe infectious disease of man.

There has been much debate over the possibility of eradicating malaria by vaccination. We have seen that the minimum proportion of hosts that must be vaccinated to prevent a disease from establishing, or to eradicate it when present in the population, is $1 - 1/R_0$. Estimates of $R_0 > 80$ based on the age at first infection would then imply that eradication by vaccine would be a hopeless task. However, Gupta & Day [21] have suggested that malaria could be composed of several strains, each of which confers strain-specific lifelong immunity. This observation is consistent with sero prevalence data obtained from the Gambia. The age at first infection would then be

$$A = \frac{L}{\sum_j R_0^j}, \tag{15}$$

where the R_0^j are the basic reproduction numbers of the individual strains, and L is the life expectancy of the host. The proportion that must be vaccinated is then $1 - 1/\max(R_0^j)$. As $\max(R_0^j)$ could be in the range 5–10 this analysis implies that the eradication of malaria by vaccination could be a feasible proposition. See Saul [46] for a critique of this theory.

One of the most important outstanding issues in malaria and in many other infections is to understand the phenomenon of acquired immunity. Here, an individual's immune level to disease rises with frequent reinfection. It is unclear how this should be modeled mathematically. An infection pressure in the vector population gives rise to a distribution of initial doses of infection that a human receives. The infectious output towards biting mosquitoes of a given infected human is the result of a complex battle with the immune system. This output distribution then feeds back into the population. Currently the word immunoepidemiology is used to signify an area of modeling that tries to link both immunologic processes within individual hosts with epidemiologic processes of transmission between hosts. Given the implications that this interaction between immunity and epidemiology has for control strategies that affect the build-up of natural immunity, this area is likely to see much activity by epidemic modelers in the near future.

Helminths

Chronologically speaking, the tropical helminth infections such as schistosomiasis are the next step in the genesis of epidemic theory. Early work by Kostitzin in 1934 was followed 30 years later by Macdonald's study of schistosomiasis [37] and a flourishing of activity in the 1970s and 1980s (see [3] for a review).

A major difference between microparasites and macroparasites is that the former reproduce rapidly within the host, whereas the latter reproduce by releasing infective stages into the environment, which eventually complete a life cycle and (re)infect hosts. Hence, for infections caused by parasitic helminths the compartment models that classify a host as susceptible, infectious, etc. become inappropriate, and a model that allows multiple infections is required. A second problem then presents itself. The notion that the pool of susceptibles diminishes during the course of an epidemic does not necessarily hold, differential equation models no longer have a negative feedback mechanism that is automatically incorporated, and careful attention must be paid to the mechanisms that regulate the parasite population. Early models for parasites of wild animals [1] included increased mortality of the host due to parasitic infection, therefore heavily parasitized hosts had a short life expectancy, and upon dying removed large numbers of parasites from the system. For many helminth infections of humans this would not be the case, and cognisance must be taken of regulatory mechanisms such as acquired immunity.

A simple model for the dynamics of a parasitic helminth in a population of constant size would be

$$\frac{dM}{dt} = \mu(Q(M) - 1)M, \qquad (16)$$

where M is the mean number of parasites per host, μ is the loss rate of parasites from the system and $Q(M)$ is the ratio of parasite transmission rate to loss rate. This model could stand as a prototype for many similar formulations to be found in [3] and other sources, and would be appropriate where host immunity was a function of current mean parasite burden. Hence Q is a positive nonincreasing function

of M, at steady state $Q(M) = 1$, and the parasite population can persist whenever $Q(0) > 1$.

The number $Q(0)$ is the basic reproduction number (ratio, quotient) for the parasite population. It may be defined as the expected number of offspring of a typical parasite that reach reproductive maturity, in a completely susceptible host population [2]. Hence, whereas for microparasites the reproduction number is defined in terms of secondary infections of hosts, for macroparasites it is defined in terms of the parasite population dynamics. This definition has been formalized in Heesterbeek & Roberts [28].

The model presented above incorporates simplistic expressions for parasite transmission and host immunity. Many helminth parasites have complicated development stages outside the definitive host that must be modeled explicitly. For example, cestode parasites are tapeworms, with an obligatory intermediate host and transmission maintained by a carnivore–herbivore relationship (see [43]). The dominant feedback is provided by immunity to the larval stage acquired by the intermediate host. For trematodes, such as the parasites that cause schistosomiasis, there is an obligatory two host cycle (for example human/snail) with a free-living stage, and immunity to superinfection is acquired by the definitive host.

Immunity acquired against adult helminth parasites may be stimulated by larvae (hence challenge) or adult parasites, and may act against larvae by protecting the host from further infection, against adult parasites by increasing their rate of mortality, or against continued transmission by reducing their egg output. A theoretical framework for these mechanisms has been developed by Woolhouse [53]. Essentially, the model presented above was extended to include the age structure of the host to obtain

$$\frac{\partial M}{\partial t} + \frac{\partial M}{\partial a} = \mu(Q(M) - 1)M(a, t), \qquad (17)$$

where, for fixed time t, $M(a, t)$ is the density of mean parasite burden over host age a. Woolhouse [53] remarks that the function Q (in our notation) "represents the entire process of transmission between hosts, incorporating the dynamics of any free-living or vector-born stages, host exposure and innate susceptibility to infection". The inclusion of an age structure in the model was motivated by the fact that host–parasite data are often presented via age–intensity curves, and age-structured models may be used to analyze these. Assuming that the epidemiology of the parasite has remained constant for some time we set $\partial M / \partial t = 0$ and obtain predicted age–intensity relationships.

Acquired immunity may be included in a variety of ways, for example if Q were also a function of past worm burden we could have $Q(M, H)$ with $\partial Q / \partial H < 0$ and, when $\partial M / \partial t = 0$, write

$$\frac{dH}{da} = M - \sigma H, \qquad (18)$$

where σ is the rate of fade of immunity. Woolhouse [54] used this framework to compare the age–intensity and age–egg output curves generated by four assumed mechanisms with data from studies of schistosomiasis infections. See [8] for the incorporation in a more comprehensive model for schistosomiasis control. For a review of the epidemiology and modeling of schistosomiasis, see [55].

Since parasite numbers within hosts are frequently too low to warrant a deterministic description at that level, models have been developed that allow for stochasticity within individuals but continue to treat the host population deterministically with an age-structured model (see [22] and [35]). In addition, these models incorporate the fact that as a rule there is large variation in individual parasite burden. This implies that a description using only mean burdens is often less appropriate.

HIV/AIDS

The infection that has sparked off a tremendous increase in epidemic modeling activity is undoubtedly HIV, starting with seminal papers by Anderson and May (e.g. [38]). The effect has been that in the past 10 years more different infections of humans and animals have been studied with more realistic models than ever before. Progress of the whole area of epidemic modeling is no longer attached to specific classes of infections as it was in the early days. There is now much progress not only on the applied front, but also in mathematical advances necessary to cope with the more involved models that aim to take relevant heterogeneity in the population into account. One of the reasons could be that sexually transmitted diseases, and certainly acquired immune deficiency syndrome (AIDS), call for the incorporation of much structure combined. Examples are age structure for differences in infectivity, susceptibility,

and certainly also contact structure and discrete characteristics such as sex, sexual preferences, and sexual activity. Two complications are particularly important: varying infectivity as a function of time elapsed since infection and long-lasting partnerships. The first complication is relevant to almost all infectious diseases, the second is related to sexual transmission. We deal with both below. One of the key notions to come out of HIV modeling is that of a core-group of infecteds. This is a small group that is very active in contacts and can keep the epidemic going in a much larger group where the internal contacts alone cannot sustain it [33].

It was realized early on in the modeling of HIV that humans generally form (sexual) partnerships that last longer than individual sexual contacts. Let us assume monogamous partnerships. During such a partnership two susceptible partners are not at risk to infection, and an infective can only cause a single new case until the partnership dissolves. This has consequences for the spread of infection. This observation has given rise to pair formation models where the formation and breaking up of partnerships is explicitly taken into account [14]. These models differentiate in the most basic case between single susceptibles and infectives and three types of pairs. If one lets partnership duration tend to zero while keeping the infection potential during a partnership constant, then one obtains the mass action models we discussed previously. In recent years progress has turned to more complicated contact structures such as circles of friends [10] and beyond deterministic theory to random graphs that reflect an underlying dynamic social contact structure in a population.

We now turn to variable infectivity. Chronologically this important aspect of deterministic epidemic theory was introduced by Kermack and McKendrick in 1927 after McKendrick's ventures into epidemiology had broadened beyond tropical infections. Their integral equation model incorporates – in modern notation – a function $A(\tau)$ to describe the average infectivity of an individual at a time τ since this individual became infected. For childhood infections, influenza, and other infections with long-lasting immunity $A(\tau)$ is a one-humped curve with narrow support. Usually the function does not rise away from zero immediately since many infections have a nonnegligible latency period between infection and becoming infectious. The latency period should not be confused with the **incubation period** which separates infection from the occurrence of symptoms. We consider incubation periods below. For HIV, the function $A(\tau)$ is typically a two-humped function. There is a peak in the early months of infection, followed by a long period of very low but probably nonzero infectivity (typically lasting several years), and ending in a second rise to high levels as the infection progresses to full-blown AIDS and ultimately death.

One striking feature of infection with the HIV virus is the long (>8 year) incubation period of AIDS. A proposed explanation is that the virus mutates within the host, with each strain stimulating both strain-specific and nonspecific immune responses; and although each strain is able to multiply in the presence of specific responses, it is regulated by the combination of specific and nonspecific responses. A simple mathematical model then shows that initially the individual virus strains are suppressed at a low level by the immune system of the host, but eventually the number of strains exceeds a "viral diversity threshold". When this occurs the nonspecific responses can no longer contain the virus population, and all viral strains are able to multiply [42]. Here a mathematical model has generated a hypothesis for the within-host dynamics of a disease that has yet to be tested against observation.

Now imagine an infection that results in complete immunity or death, in a population that is closed (i.e. inflow of new susceptibles is negligible on the time scale of the epidemic), where contacts are described by mass action. Let $S(t)$ be the density of susceptibles in the population at time t. Assume that a single infection triggers an autonomous process within the host. This allows an age representation for the infectivity. We can describe the infection process by the following integral equation:

$$\frac{dS}{dt}(t) = S(t) \int_0^\infty A(\tau) \frac{dS}{dt}(t-\tau)d\tau. \quad (19)$$

The incidence of new infecteds $i(t,0) = -dS/dt(t)$ and we can reformulate the above in terms of the incidence $i(t,\tau)$ as

$$i(t,0) = S(t) \int_0^\infty A(\tau)i(t-\tau,0)d\tau, \quad (20)$$

where the latter integral is the force of infection. This equation can be understood by noting that the infected individuals of infection age τ that are infecting susceptibles at time t are doing so with infectivity $A(\tau)$. These infecteds are precisely those

who became infected at time $t-\tau$. Only if we choose $C(N) = N$ (mass action) and the unrealistic $A(\tau) = \beta \exp(-\gamma\tau)$, and if we neglect latency, can we reduce the above to the system of ordinary differential equations (1)–(3) by calculating $I(t) = \int_{-\infty}^t \exp[-\gamma(t-\tau)](dS/dt)(\tau)d\tau$ and differentiating. Kermack and McKendrick already showed that the disease will spread in the population of constant density S_0 if and only if $R_0 > 1$ with

$$R_0 = S_0 \int_0^\infty A(\tau)d\tau. \quad (21)$$

This basic result of deterministic epidemic theory can be extended to populations with arbitrary heterogeneity. Consider the individuals labeled with a variable ξ, say, taking values in some state space $\Omega \subset \mathbb{R}^m$. Now, both S and A can depend on the type of individual. The general integral equation formulation for a closed population is

$$i(t,\xi) = S(t,\xi) \int_\Omega \int_0^\infty A(\tau,\xi,\eta)i(t-\tau,\eta)d\tau d\eta. \quad (22)$$

The compartmental ordinary differential equation models, with and without heterogeneity, and the age-structured model above are special cases of this equation for specific choices of A. One can show that R_0 generalizes naturally to the spectral radius of the so-called *next generation operator* associated with the integral equation [11, 26].

To show the connection with age-structured models let $\Omega = [0,\infty)$ and $\xi = a$ and disregard demography. Under the condition

$$A(\tau,a,b) = k(a,b+\tau)\exp\left[-\int_b^{b+\tau}\gamma(c)dc\right] \quad (23)$$

define

$$I(t,a) = \int_0^a i(t-\tau,a-\tau)\exp\left[-\int_{a-\tau}^a \gamma(c)dc\right]d\tau. \quad (24)$$

Differentiating I leads to the system (5)–(6) (with $\mu = 0$).

In the HIV/AIDS context questions relate again to evaluating effects of control measures (including behavior change). In an age-structured setting the possible demographic impact of HIV in developing countries is an important issue [39]. In Heesterbeek & Dietz [26] it is shown how models with continuous age structure in the form (22) relate to models with discrete age-classes and the so-called Who Acquires

Infection From Whom (WAIFW) matrices. These matrices are studied as an approach to link theory to population data [3, 18]. One can also give a final size relation for (22) in a closed population.

The modeling process within the deterministic frame of model (22) has shifted to specifying the infectivity kernel A. The modeling depends of course on the type of question to be studied. Often the modeling will make use of stochastic processes – notably Markov processes – to describe change in an individual's set of characteristics. Many models are in some sense special cases of (22). In a way, these models have already made a choice for A, as we have seen in the age-structured and compartmental model for measles. The modeling of A for more realistic (measurable) situations combining heterogeneity (in individual traits, individual behavior and space) and immunologic and evolutionary processes is one of the major challenges in the near future. This modeling will draw on deterministic but increasingly also on stochastic techniques and theory. It is likely that the days are numbered for realistic progress in theory that is only deterministic. The theory has reached a stage where progress on current issues of epidemiologic importance (e.g. understanding persistence and critical community size) can only be achieved if deterministic and stochastic theory go hand in hand.

References

[1] Anderson, R.M. & May, R.M. (1978). Regulation and stability of host–parasite population interactions. 1. Regulatory processes, *Journal of Animal Ecology* **47**, 219–247.

[2] Anderson, R.M. & May, R.M. (1982). *Population Biology of Infectious Diseases*. Springer-Verlag, Berlin.

[3] Anderson, R.M. & May, R.M. (1991). *Infectious Diseases of Humans: Dynamics and Control*. Oxford University Press, Oxford.

[4] Bartlett, M.S. (1957). Measles periodicity and community size, *Journal of the Royal Statistical Society, Series A* **120**, 48–70.

[5] Bartlett, M.S. (1960). *Stochastic Population Models in Ecology and Epidemiology*. Methuen, London.

[6] Bolker, B. & Grenfell, B.T. (1995). Space, persistence and the dynamics of measles, *Philosophical Transactions of the Royal Society, Series B* **348**, 309–320.

[7] Busenberg, S. & Cooke, K. (1993). *Vertically Transmitted Diseases, Models and Dynamics*. Springer-Verlag, Berlin.

[8] Chan, M.S., Guyatt, H.L., Bundy, D.A.P., Booth, M., Fulford, A.J.C. & Medley, G.F. (1995). The development of an age structured model for schistosomiasis transmission dynamics and control and its validation for *Schistosoma mansoni, Epidemiology and Infection* **115**, 325–344.

[9] De Jong, M.C.M., Diekmann, O. & Heesterbeek, J.A.P. (1995). How does transmission of infection depend on population size?, in *Epidemic Models, their Structure and Relation to Data*, D. Mollison, ed. Cambridge University Press, Cambridge, pp. 84–94.

[10] Diekmann, O., De Jong, M.C.M. & Metz, J.A.J. (1998). A deterministic epidemic model taking account of repeated contacts between the same individuals, *Journal of Applied Probability* **35**, 448–462.

[11] Diekmann, O., Heesterbeek, J.A.P. & Metz, J.A.J. (1990). On the definition and the computation of the basic reproduction ratio R_0 in models for infectious diseases in heterogeneous populations, *Journal of Mathematical Biology* **28**, 365–382.

[12] Diekmann, O., Heesterbeek, J.A.P. & Metz, J.A.J. (1995). The legacy of Kermack and McKendrick, in *Epidemic Models, their Structure and Relation to Data*, D. Mollison, ed. Cambridge University Press, Cambridge, pp. 95–115.

[13] Dietz, K. (1988). The first epidemic model: A historical note on P.D. En'ko, *Australian Journal of Statistics* **30A**, 56–65.

[14] Dietz, K. & Hadeler, K.P. (1988). Epidemiological models for sexually transmitted diseases, *Journal of Mathematical Biology* **26**, 1–25.

[15] Dietz, K. & Schenzle, D. (1985). Mathematical models for infectious disease statistics, in *A Celebration of Statistics: the ISI Centenary Volume*, A.C. Atkinson, & S.E. Feinberg, eds. Springer-Verlag New York, pp. 167–204.

[16] Ellner, S., Gallant, R. & Theiler, J. (1995). Detecting nonlinearity and chaos in epidemic data, in *Epidemic Models, their Structure and Relation to Data*, D. Mollison, ed. Cambridge University Press, Cambridge, pp. 229–247.

[17] Greenhalgh, D. (1990). Vaccination campaigns for common childhood diseases, *Mathematical Biosciences* **100**, 201–240.

[18] Greenhalgh, D. & Dietz, K. (1994). Some bounds on estimates for reproductive ratios derived from the age-specific force of infection, *Mathematical Biosciences* **124**, 9–57.

[19] Grenfell, B.T. & Dobson, A.P., eds (1995). *Ecology of Infectious Diseases in Natural Populations*, Cambridge University Press, Cambridge.

[20] Grenfell, B.T., Bolker, B. & Kleczkowski, A. (1995). Seasonality, demography and the dynamics of measles in developed countries, in *Epidemic Models, their Structure and Relation to Data*, D. Mollison, ed. Cambridge University Press, Cambridge.

[21] Gupta, S. & Day, K.P. (1994). A strain theory of malaria transmission, *Parasitology Today* **10**, 476–481.

[22] Hadeler, K.P. & Dietz, K. (1984). Population dynamics of killing parasites which reproduce in the host, *Journal of Mathematical Biology* **21**, 45–65.

[23] Hadeler, K.P. & Müller, J. (1996). Optimal vaccination patterns in age-structured populations, in *Models for Infectious Human Diseases, Their Structure and Relation to Data.* V. Isham & G. Medley, eds. Cambridge University Press, Cambridge, pp. 90–104.

[24] Hamer, W.H. (1896). Age-incidence in relation with cycles of disease-prevalence, *Transactions of the Epidemiological Society of London* **XVI**(1896-97), 64–77.

[25] Hamer, W.H. (1906). Epidemic disease in England, the evidence of variability and of persistency of type, *Lancet* **i**, 733–739.

[26] Heesterbeek, J.A.P. & Dietz, K. (1996). The concept of R_0 in epidemic models, *Statistica Neerlandica* **50**, 89–110.

[27] Heesterbeek, J.A.P. & Metz, J.A.J. (1993). The saturating contact rate in marriage and epidemic models, *Journal of Mathematical Biology* **31**, 529–539.

[28] Heesterbeek, J.A.P. & Roberts, M.G. (1995). Threshold quantities for helminth infections, *Journal of Mathematical Biology* **33**, 415–434.

[29] Hethcote, H.W. (1994). A thousand and one epidemic models, in *Frontiers in Theoretical Biology*, S.A. Levin, ed. Lecture Notes in Biomathematics, Vol. 100, Springer-Verlag, New York, pp. 504–515.

[30] Inaba, H. (1990). Thresholds and stability results for an age-structured epidemic model, *Journal of Mathematical Biology* **28**, 411–434.

[31] Isham, V. & Medley, G., eds (1996). *Models for Infectious Human Diseases, Their Structure and Relation to Data.* Cambridge University Press, Cambridge.

[32] Jacquez, J.A. (1997). *Compartmental Models.* BioMedware, Ann Arbor.

[33] Jacquez, J., Simon, C. & Koopman, J. (1995). Core groups and the R_0's for subgroups in heterogeneous SIS and SI models, in *Epidemic Models, their Structure and Relation to Data*, D. Mollison, ed. Cambridge University Press, Cambridge, pp. 279–301.

[34] Kermack, W.O. & McKendrick, A.G. (1927). Contributions to the mathematical theory of epidemics, part I, *Proceedings of the Royal Society, Series A* **115**, 700–721. Reprinted (along with parts II and III), *Bulletin of Mathematical Biology* **53**(1991) 33–55.

[35] Kretzschmar, M. (1989). A renewal equation with a birth–death process as a model for parasitic infections, *Journal of Mathematical Biology* **27**, 191–221.

[36] Macdonald, G. (1957). *The Epidemiology and Control of Malaria.* Oxford University Press, Oxford.

[37] Macdonald, G. (1965). The dynamics of helminth infections, with special reference to schistosomes, *Transactions of the Royal Society for Tropical Medicine* **59**, 489–506.

[38] May, R.M. & Anderson, R.M. (1988). The transmission dynamics of human immunodeficiency virus (HIV), *Philosophical Transactions of the Royal Society, Series B* **321**, 565–607.

[39] May, R.M., Anderson, R.M. & McLean, A. (1988). Possible demographic consequences of HIV/AIDS epidemics: I. Assuming HIV infection always leads to AIDS, *Mathematical Biosciences* **90**, 475–505.

[40] Mollison, D. (ed.) (1995). *Epidemic Models, their Structure and Relation to Data.* Cambridge University Press, Cambridge.

[41] Müller, J. (1994). *Optimal Vaccination Patterns in Age-structured Populations.* PhD Thesis, University of Tübingen.

[42] Nowak, M.A. & May, R.M. (1991). Mathematical biology of HIV infections: antigenic variation and diversity threshold, *Mathematical Biosciences* **106**, 1–21.

[43] Roberts, M.G. (1994). Modelling of parasitic populations: Cestodes, *Veterinary Parasitology* **54**, 145–160.

[44] Ross, R. (1911). *The Prevention of Malaria*, 2nd Ed. John Murray, London.

[45] Ross, R. & Hudson, H.P. (1917). An application of the theory of probabilities to the study of a priori pathometry, part III *Proceedings of the Royal Society of London, Series A* **43**, 225–240.

[46] Saul, A. (1996). Transmission dynamics of Plasmodium falciparam, *Parasitology Today* **12**, 74–79.

[47] Schaffer, W.M. (1985). Can nonlinear dynamics elucidate mechanisms in ecology and epidemiology?, *IMA Journal of Mathematics Applied to Medicine and Biology* **2**, 221–252.

[48] Schenzle, D. (1984). An age-structured model of pre- and post vaccination measles transmission, *IMA Journal of Mathematics Applied to Medicine and Biology* **1**, 169–191.

[49] Schwarz, I.B. (1985). Multiple stable recurrent outbreaks and predictability in seasonally forced nonlinear epidemic models, *Journal of Mathematical Biology* **21**, 347–361.

[50] Soper, M.A. (1929). The interpretation of periodicity in disease prevalence, *Journal of the Royal Statistical Society, Series A* **92**, 34–61.

[51] Thieme, H. (1992). Epidemic and demographic interaction in the spread of potentially fatal diseases in growing populations, *Mathematical Biosciences* **111**, 99–130.

[52] Webb, G.F. (1985). *Theory of Nonlinear Age-dependent Population Dynamics.* Marcel Dekker, New York.

[53] Woolhouse, M.E.J. (1992). A theoretical framework for the immunoepidemiology of helminth infection. *Parasite Immunology* **14**, 563–578.

[54] Woolhouse, M.E.J. (1994). Immunoepidemiology of human schistosomes: taking the theory into the field, *Parasitology Today* **10**, 196–202.

[55] Woolhouse, M.E.J. (1994). Epidemiology of human Schistosomes, in *Parasitic and Infectious Diseases: Epidemiology and Ecology.* M.E. Scott & G. Smith, eds. Academic Press, San Diego, pp. 197–217.

(*See also* **Epidemic Models, Spatial**; **Epidemic Thresholds**; **Infectious Disease Models**)

J.A.P. HEESTERBEEK & M.G. ROBERTS

Epidemic Models, Spatial

If we are to gain proper understanding of the dispersal and control of diseases such as malaria, rabies, and acquired immune deficiency syndrome (AIDS), then we have to recognize that they develop within a truly spatial framework. The common assumption that individuals mix homogeneously over the whole region available to them stems mainly from mathematical convenience; in real life we have to accept that both individuals and disease often develop within separate subregions. Classic examples of such spatial catastrophes include: 25 million deaths in fourteenth century Europe from Black Death out of a population of 100 million; the Aztecs lost half their population of 3.5 million from smallpox; around 20 million died in the world influenza pandemic in 1919; whilst millions of people are believed to be currently affected by human immunodeficiency virus (HIV)/AIDS. A particularly interesting case is the spread of one of the world's greatest cholera pandemics, the El Tor strain. It was first identified outside Mecca in 1905, and was later recognized in the 1930s as being endemic in the Celebes. Little was heard of it until 1961, when it suddenly exploded out of the Celebes, reaching India in 1964, and advancing into central Africa, Russia and Europe by the early 1970s. The total burden of misery and suffering that results from such disease is clearly immense, and any understanding that modeling techniques can bring to alleviate this terrible state of affairs *has* to invoke spatial transmission properties.

Disease is spread through two different mechanisms. First, infected individuals may *migrate* to a different location, thereby infecting susceptibles at this new site. Migration patterns can be truly local (spread of HIV in "shooting galleries"), mid-range (sexual transmission between neighboring cities), or global (spread of human disease through intercontinental travel). Secondly, the disease itself may spread through *cross-infection*, either locally (between neighboring trees) or globally (aerosol dispersal of plant disease). Some situations may involve both mechanisms, such as the UK outbreaks of foot-and-mouth disease. Hengeveld's account [5] of documented invasion scenarios contains many varied examples, including cholera in North America, stripe rust in wheat, the expansion of cattle egret in North and South America, and rabies in Central Europe.

If migration or cross-infection is highly localized, then infectives/infection may *diffuse* over a continuous region. In contrast, if it results in substantive changes in location then we either have a *spatial jump* process (plants infected by wind-blown spores), or a *stepping-stone* process if infection can only occur at specific sites (influenza epidemics in Icelandic coastal settlements).

Given that many populations develop within reasonably well-defined subregions, the stepping-stone approach is a sensible one to consider first. We envisage the process as being spatially distributed amongst n sites, with migration and/or cross-infection being allowed between them. This may involve nearest neighbors, all sites with a common transmission rate, or all sites but with the transmission rate changing with intersite distance (called the contact distribution). Such migration scenarios were first posed by Kimura [7] in a genetics context, but substantive theoretical development really began following Bailey's simple birth–death–migration process [1]. In this model the population develops on an infinite set of colonies (thereby avoiding edge-effect problems), all individuals undergo a simple birth–death process with rates λ and μ, respectively, and individuals in colony i can migrate at rate ν_1, ν_2 to the two nearest neighbors $i + 1$ and $i - 1$. For the equivalent general epidemic process, with $X_i(t)$ susceptibles and $Y_i(t)$ infectives in colony i at time t, the infective population at i increases at rate $\beta X_i(t) Y_i(t)$. In the opening stages $\beta X_i(t) \simeq \beta X_i(0) = \lambda$ (say), so there the two processes are roughly equivalent. Unfortunately, even Bailey's process teeters on the edge of mathematical intractability, so the prospects for making substantial theoretical progress with more complicated spatial epidemic processes are remote. Replacing migration with cross-infection (at rate α_1, α_2) makes this situation even worse, since the infective population birth rate changes to $X_i(t)[\beta Y_i(t) + \alpha_1 Y_{i-1}(t) + \alpha_2 Y_{i+1}(t)]$.

Consider, for example, the recent (nonspatial) upsurge of interest in modeling the population dynamics of the AIDS epidemic. Much of the mathematical development is deterministic, though this does facilitate the allowance of many sources of change (see [6]). One surprisingly tractable nonlinear model is that of Ball & O'Neill [2], and to place this within a spatial nearest-neighbor setting let $x_i(t)$, $y_i(t)$ and $z_i(t)$ denote the number of susceptible, HIV-infected and removed (i.e. full-blown AIDS or dead) individuals at site i. Then allowing for the migration of infectives gives rise to the deterministic representation

$$dx_i/dt = -\beta x_i y_i/(x_i + y_i),$$

$$dy_i/dt = \beta x_i y_i/(x_i + y_i)$$
$$- (\nu_1 + \nu_2)y_i + \nu_1 y_{i-1} + \nu_2 y_{i+1},$$

$$dz_i/dt = \gamma y_i.$$

This situation is in marked contrast to the spatial general epidemic model with cross-infection, with

$$dx_i/dt = -x_i[\beta y_i + \alpha_1 y_{i-1} + \alpha_2 y_{i+1}],$$

$$dy_i/dt = x_i[\beta y_i + \alpha_1 y_{i-1} + \alpha_2 y_{i+1}] - \gamma y_i,$$

$$dz_i/dt = \gamma y_i.$$

Such equations are easily modified to enable general migration at rate ν_{ij} from site i to site j, and cross-infection at rate α_{ij} between infectives in site i and susceptibles at site j. Exact solution is usually not possible, though approximate results may be obtained using careful linearization procedures; for numerical solutions use MATLAB, etc. Often we are interested in qualitative, rather than quantitative, behavior, and visual inspection of graphical output over a range of parameter settings is usually sufficient to highlight the most important aspects of the process.

Although the propagation of an epidemic through towns or villages is easily visualized in terms of a stepping-stone process, for disease dispersal in animals or plants a diffusion model may be more appropriate. Near the wavefront itself the number of susceptibles may be assumed to be fairly constant, and so there the process reduces to a simple birth–death process amenable to Skellam's diffusion approach [17]. On describing the infective density at position (u, v) by Brownian motion with zero drift and displacement variances $\mathrm{var}[u(1)] = \mathrm{var}[v(1)] = D^2$, we have the polar normal probability density function (pdf),

$$\phi(r, \theta; t) = (2\pi D^2 t)^{-1} r \exp[-r^2/(2D^2 t)].$$

Since there is no drift this pdf spreads out in ever-expanding circles, and for an infective population of final size N the radial velocity $R(t)/t$ is $D\{[2\ln(N)]/t\}^{1/2}$, which decreases as $t^{-1/2}$. For a long time scale, say several decades, which is the case for fox rabies in Europe and the El Tor cholera

strain, we might assume exponential growth at rate ψ, whence N is replaced by $N\exp(\psi t)$ and the velocity now remains constant at $D\{[2\psi \ln(N)]\}^{1/2}$. The combination of population growth and diffusion is essential if spatial expansion is not to fade out.

The diffusion approach involves a poor Taylor series expansion, and so the two scenarios can give rise to substantially different results. For example, with Bailey's birth–death process the wavefront velocities (for $\lambda > \mu$) are the solutions to the equation [12]

$$\nu_1 + \nu_2 + \mu - \lambda = (c^2 + 4\nu_1 \nu_2)^{1/2} - c\ln\{[c$$
$$+ (c^2 + 4\nu_1 \nu_2)^{1/2}]/(2\nu_1)\},$$

while the equivalent diffusion velocities take the much simpler form

$$c_{\mathrm{diff}} = (\nu_1 - \nu_2) \pm \{2(\lambda - \mu)(\nu_1 + \nu_2)\}^{1/2}.$$

These two results are compatible only if $\lambda - \mu \ll \nu_1 + \nu_2$.

Given that substantial behavioral differences can occur between deterministic and stochastic analyses of the same process, ideally a deterministic approach should always be performed in parallel with a stochastic analysis. Unfortunately, even the simplest stochastic spatial scenario of a two-site birth–death–migration process produces intractable mathematics. Some degree of success is possible using approximation techniques, such as regarding $\{x_i(t), y_i(t), z_i(t)\}$ as a multivariate normal distribution with moments obtained from the cumulant equations by replacing third- and higher-order cumulants by zero. However, this will quite likely require use of a computer algebra package, and direct numerical computation of the original population probability equations may be the best option.

The problem with probability "solutions" is that they usually convey information only on population values at a fixed time t. What we really require is the full history of process development. Simulation provides the answer, for given the rapidly expanding nature of affordable computer power, moments and probabilities may be obtained using standard Monte Carlo procedures. Detailed examples of how to construct simulation code for space–time stochastic models are contained in Renshaw [13], and these are easily modified to cope with any spatial epidemic construction. No matter how complicated, a process can always be described as a series of events

$E_1, E_2, \ldots$ occurring at times $t_1, t_2, \ldots$. First detail all possible infection, removal, migration, and cross-infection changes. Then in essence:

1. evaluate the corresponding rates $r_1, r_2, \ldots$ and put $R = r_1 + r_2 + \cdots$;
2. generate two uniform U(0, 1) random variables U_1 and U_2;
3. select the jth event if $r_1 + \cdots + r_{j-1} \le U_1 R < r_1 + \cdots + r_j$;
4. evaluate the inter-event time $s = -\ln(U_2)/R$;
5. update population sizes and time $t \to t + s$, and return to point 1.

Figure 1 shows two simulations of a two-colony Ball & O'Neill process under both migration and cross-infection regimes. At time $t = 0$ there are 100 susceptibles in each colony, with one infective in colony 1 and none in colony 2. For illustration, only one-way spatial rates are used, namely from colony 1 to 2. Thus an epidemic in colony 2 has to be kick-started from colony 1 before all the infectives there have been removed. Whilst the deterministic and stochastic developments for cross-infection are broadly comparable, under migration substantial time-shift differences occur between them, especially in colony 2. Though rough agreement between stochastic and deterministic realizations will usually occur, the problem is one of consistency. Unlike cross-infection, with migration total colony sizes are not fixed, so individual sites may pass through their threshold population values and thereby undergo considerable behavioral change.

Such differences can become even more marked when the system comprises three or more sites, and susceptibles may both migrate and give birth. For with appropriate parameter values, susceptibles can move ahead of epidemic flare-ups and grow to above the local threshold population value before either a migrating infective or cross-infection starts a fresh

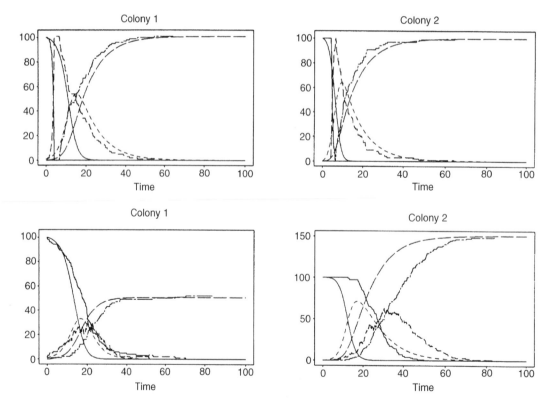

Figure 1   Deterministic (smooth) and stochastic (rough) realizations of a two-colony Ball & O'Neill model under cross-infection (upper) and migration (lower) showing the number of susceptibles (———), infectives (- - - - - -) and removals (– – – –): parameter values are $\beta = 0.5, \gamma = 0.1, \nu_1 = 0.1, \nu_2 = 0, \alpha_1 = 0.01, \alpha_2 = 0$ (produced by Ian Hirsch)

epidemic outbreak (*see* **Epidemic Thresholds**). Persistence occurs through a *stochastic dynamic:* it is precisely the ability of susceptibles to be constantly on the move recolonizing empty sites, and infectives to pursue them, that keeps the whole process alive. In such situations we have to rely on simulating individual stochastic realizations. For even if exact probability expressions could be constructed they would tell us little, being an average over all possible realizations. Moreover, if the behavioral variability between realizations is considerable, then even using a basic deterministic approach can be risky, especially when it relates to epidemic control. Mollison [8] provides a striking example of this, in which he challenges Murray et al.'s deterministic study [11] of how fox rabies might invade a new country: they predict a roughly circular expanding wave of advance, followed after a quiet phase of about seven years by another wave originating from the same starting point. First, European evidence suggests that after a short while the rabies invasion could break back across the devastated territory immediately behind it and induce an epidemic equilibrium there. Secondly, the later wave is an artifact of modeling population size as continuous, rather than discrete. For the model has fox density declining not to zero, but to 10^{-18} of a fox per square kilometer, and this "atto-fox" restarts the epidemic wave as soon as the susceptible population has grown sufficiently large. Though such numerical nonsense may be easily eliminated, the discrepancies between the overall predictions and reality are a serious cause for concern.

The mathematics surrounding spatial stochastic processes is notoriously difficult, and where deterministic solutions can be of considerable help is in determining *qualitative* behavior when there exists an underlying endemic equilibrium level $\{X^*, Y^*\}$ of susceptibles and infectives. In a brilliant pioneering paper Turing [19] developed elegant deterministic solutions which predict the types of behavior likely to be encountered when N colonies lie on a ring. In general, let $f(X_i, Y_i)$ and $g(X_i, Y_i)$ denote the rates of change at colony i in susceptibles, $X_i(t)$, and infectives, $Y_i(t)$, respectively. Then if susceptibles and infectives migrate to neighboring sites at rates μ and ν,

$$\mathrm{d}X_i/\mathrm{d}t = f(X_i, Y_i) + \mu(X_{i+1} - 2X_i + X_{i-1}),$$

$$\mathrm{d}Y_i/\mathrm{d}t = g(X_i, Y_i) + \nu(Y_{i+1} - 2Y_i + Y_{i-1}).$$

On considering local departures from equilibrium by writing $X_i(t) = X^* + x_i(t)$ and $Y_i(t) = Y^* + y_i(t)$, the functions f and g may be approximated by linear forms in x_i and y_i (see [13] and [15]). The resulting equations are amenable to Laplace transform solution, while adding white noise to the linearized deterministic equations allows the construction of second-order moments and spectra [14]. Cross-infection may be treated similarly. Turing's aim was to examine whether it is feasible to generate *spatially* stable waves, and his idea is simple but profound. For if in the absence of diffusion X_i and Y_i tend to a *linearly stable* uniform state, then under certain conditions spatially inhomogeneous patterns can evolve through *diffusion-driven instability*. Since diffusion is usually considered to be a stabilizing process, care is clearly needed when 'guessing' how nonspatial models will behave when they are placed in a spatial environment.

Although the spread of infectives/infection through local migration/contact is commonplace, propagation will often occur between nonnearest colonies. Provided the colonies lie on a regular grid, such as a Turing ring, spatial measures of autocorrelation and frequency may be obtained by using time series techniques [16]. However, sites will often not be regularly spaced; for example, cities, towns, and villages connected by air, road, and rail, and we need to use weighted measures based upon local population size, area of location, extent of links with other areas, etc. [4]. We therefore have a space–time bivariate marked point process $\{(X_{u,v}, Y_{u,v}); (u, v) \in R\}$ with association between the locations (u, v) in a region R, local epidemic reactions at each location, and spatial epidemic migration/infection between different locations. The study of such complexity is still in its infancy, and stochastic modeling has to proceed through simulation. Appropriate measures of spatial correlation that are applicable to both marks (X, Y) and points (u, v) can be found in Stoyan & Stoyan's excellent overview [18].

For the purpose of illustration we have concentrated on purely homogeneous scenarios. However, recent interest in AIDS has stimulated much progress in diverse areas of epidemic modeling, particularly with regard to the treatment of heterogeneity, both between individuals and in mixing of subgroups of the population. The study of epidemics is an exciting, active, and rapidly expanding field, and the review papers of Mollison et al. [10] and Bolker, et al. [3] provide excellent starting points for investigating the dynamics of diseases in human, animal, marine, and plant populations. Key theoretical issues are addressed in Mollison [9]. Moreover, improved computer technology has led to the availability of better databases and computationally intensive methods in the analysis of data: it has also allowed the simulation of more detailed and realistic models. We can therefore now tackle major challenges to our understanding of spatial epidemics, including the effects of: heterogeneity due to differences between both individuals and mixing; the dependence of persistence on chaotic behavior and spatial patchiness; nonstationarity due to weather, demographic variables and evolution; varying migration and cross-infection scenarios; and boundary edge effects.

References

[1]   Bailey, N.T.J. (1968). Stochastic birth, death and migration processes for spatially distributed populations, *Biometrika* **55**, 189–198.

[2]   Ball, F. & O'Neill, P. (1993). A modification of the general epidemic motivated by AIDS modelling, *Advances in Applied Probability* **25**, 39–62.

[3]   Bolker, B.M., Altmann, M., Aubert, M., Ball, F., Barlow, N.D., Bowers, R.G., Dobson, A.P., Elkington, J.S., Garnett, G.P., Gilligan, C.A., Hassell, M.P., Isham, V., Jacquez, J.A., Kleczkowski, A., Levin, S.A., May, R.M., Metz, J.A.J., Mollison, D., Morris, M., Real, L.A., Sattenspiel, L., Swinton, J., White, P. & Williams, B.G. (1995). Group report: spatial dynamics of infectious diseases in natural population, in *Ecology of Infectious Diseases in Natural Populations*, B.T. Grenfell & A.P. Dobson, eds. Cambridge University Press, Cambridge, pp. 399–420.

[4]   Cliff, A.D. & Ord, J.K. (1981). *Spatial Processes: Models and Applications*. Pion, London.

[5]   Hengeveld, R. (1989). *Dynamics of Biological Populations*. Chapman & Hall, London.

[6]   Isham, V. (1988). Mathematical modelling of the transmission dynamics of HIV infection and AIDS: a review, *Journal of the Royal Statistical Society, Series A* **151**, 5–30.

[7]   Kimura, M. (1953). "Stepping stone" model of population, *Annual Report of the National Institute of Genetics, Japan* **3**, 62–63.

[8]   Mollison, D. (1991). Dependence of epidemic and population velocities on basic parameters, *Mathematical Biosciences* **107**, 255–287.

[9]   Mollison, D., ed. (1995). *Epidemic Models: Their Structure and Relation to Data*. Cambridge University Press, Cambridge.

[10]   Mollison, D., Isham, V. & Grenfell, B. (1994). Epidemics: models and data, *Journal of the Royal Statistical Society, Series A* **157**, 115–149.

[11]   Murray, J.D., Stanley, E.A. & Brown, D.L. (1986). On the spatial spread of rabies among foxes, *Proceedings of the Royal Society of London, Series B* **229**, 111–150.

[12]   Renshaw, E. (1977). Velocities of propagation for stepping-stone models of population growth, *Journal of Applied Probability* **14**, 591–597.

[13]   Renshaw, E. (1991). *Modelling Biological Populations in Space and Time*. Cambridge University Press, Cambridge.

[14]   Renshaw, E. (1994). The linear spatial-temporal interaction process and its relation to $1/\omega$-noise, *Journal of the Royal Statistical Society, Series B* **56**, 75–91.

[15]   Renshaw, E. (1994). Non-linear waves on the Turing ring, *Mathematical Scientist* **19**, 22–46.

[16]   Renshaw, E. & Ford, E.D. (1983). The interpretation of process from pattern using two-dimensional spectral analysis: methods and problems of interpretation, *Applied Statistics* **32**, 51–63.

[17]   Skellam, J.G. (1951). Random dispersal in theoretical populations, *Biometrika* **38**, 196–218.

[18]   Stoyan, D. & Stoyan, H. (1994) *Fractals, Random Shapes and Point Fields: Methods of Geometrical Statistics*. Wiley, New York.

[19]   Turing, A.M. (1952). The chemical basis of morphogenesis, *Philosophical Transactions of the Royal Society of London, Series B* **237**, 37–72.

(*See also* **Epidemic Models, Deterministic**; **Epidemic Models, Stochastic**; **Infectious Disease Models**)

ERIC RENSHAW

Epidemic Models, Stochastic

Although the development of an epidemic in a population susceptible to disease is a stochastic (random) **process**, it can often be described with reasonable accuracy by a deterministic model, provided the initial number of susceptibles is sufficiently large (*see* **Epidemic Models, Deterministic**). The deterministic results for the numbers of susceptibles and infectives in the population at time $t \geq 0$, are taken to represent the equivalent means of the more accurate stochastic process.

When the initial number of susceptibles is moderate or small, as in a school or a household, the deterministic model is inadequate and it becomes necessary to rely on a stochastic model. Such a model can be constructed in discrete time $t = 0, 1, 2, \ldots$, with the unit being the latent period of infection, or possibly a day or a week. It may also be constructed in continuous time $t \geq 0$; in both cases the models are usually Markovian. Most of the models assume homogeneous mixing (law of mass action), which states that the probability of a susceptible becoming infected is proportional to the number of possible contacts between susceptibles and infectives, or the product of these in the population at the instant of infection.

Explicit solutions can be found for some of the main stochastic models in use, but, however intractable the problem may be analytically, one can always describe the development of an epidemic by simulation methods. In this article we give a brief outline of the most common discrete- and continuous-time stochastic epidemic models.

Stochastic Models in Discrete Time

The most commonly used models in discrete time are the chain binomial models; these are due to Reed & Frost (see [1]), and Greenwood [12]. Since the Greenwood model is simpler, we consider it first.

The Greenwood Chain Binomial

In this model, we assume that at time $t = 0$, there are $X(0) = n$ susceptibles subject to an infection which is not dependent on the existing number of infectives in the population. We follow the progress of the epidemic at times $t = 1, 2, \ldots$, the epochs at which the number of infectives and surviving susceptibles are recorded. Suppose that the probability of instantaneous infection of a susceptible at time $t = 0$ is $p < 1$. If each susceptible is infected independently, then the distribution of the remaining susceptibles at time $t = 1$ will be binomial, with the probability $q = 1 - p$ of noninfection, so that

$$\Pr\{X(1) = x_1 | X(0) = n\}$$
$$= \binom{n}{x_1} q^{x_1} p^{n-x_1}, \quad x_1 = 0, 1, 2, \ldots, n. \quad (1)$$

The infectives $Y(1) = n - x_1$ are now removed, and the infection process is repeated for $t = 1, 2, \ldots$, T until either no further infectives are produced at T, $Y(T) = 0$, or all the susceptibles have been infected, $X(T) = 0$. The infection process then ceases, and T is referred to as the duration of the epidemic. The evolution of the epidemic is dictated by the sequence of binomial distributions, whence the name "chain binomial" for the model. Gani & Jerwood [10] noted that the process $\{X(t); t = 0, 1, \ldots, T\}$ was in fact a simple Markov chain with transition probability matrix

$$
\mathbf{P} = \begin{array}{c} \\ 0 \\ 1 \\ \vdots \\ n \end{array}
\begin{array}{c} \nearrow \ \ 0 \quad\quad\ 1 \quad\ \ \cdot\ \cdots\ \ n \\
\left[
\begin{array}{ccccc}
1 & 0 & \cdot & \cdots & 0 \\
p & q & 0 & \cdots & 0 \\
\vdots & \vdots & \vdots & & \vdots \\
p^n & \binom{n}{1} p^{n-1} q & \cdot & \cdots & q^n
\end{array}
\right].
\end{array} \quad (2)
$$

This formulation allows one to carry out simple calculations on the probabilities of such quantities as the number of infectives generated up to time t, or the duration of the epidemic, within the Markov chain framework. For example, the probability of the duration T of the epidemic is given by

$$\Pr\{t = T\}$$
$$= E' \begin{bmatrix} 0 & \cdot & \cdots & 0 \\ p & 0 & \cdots & 0 \\ \vdots & \vdots & & \vdots \\ p^n & \binom{n}{1} p^{n-1} q & \cdots & 0 \end{bmatrix}^{T-1} \begin{bmatrix} 1 \\ q \\ \vdots \\ q^n \end{bmatrix},$$
$$(3)$$

where the $1 \times (n+1)$ row vector $E' = \{0 \ldots 0 \ 1\}$ indicates that $X(0) = n$, the $(n+1) \times 1$ column vector $\{1 \ q \ldots q^n\}'$ gives the probabilities that $Y(t) = 0$ at any time t, and the central matrix is the $\mathbf{P}$ of (2) with its diagonal elements replaced by zeros. This matrix geometric distribution states that $X(t)$ circulates among the states $0, 1, 2, \ldots, n$ for the first $T - 1$ epochs, before $Y(T) = 0$ at T.

The Reed–Frost Chain Binomial

In this slightly more complex model, we assume that at time $t = 0$ there are $X(0) = n$ susceptibles and $Y(0) = y_0$ infectives. Infection is now dependent on the *number* of infectives y_0. The probability of contact of each susceptible with an infective is $p < 1$, with a contact resulting in infection; $q = 1 - p$ is the probability of no contact. If each infective is independent of all other infectives, then the probability of at least one infectious contact will be $(1 - q^{y_0})$. If the susceptibles are also independent, then at time $t = 1$, with $x_1 + y_1 = n$,

$$\Pr\{X(1) = x_1, Y(1) = y_1 | X(0) = n, Y(0) = y_0\}$$

$$= \binom{n}{x_1} (q^{y_0})^{x_1} (1 - q^{y_0})^{y_1}. \quad (4)$$

Note that if q^{y_0} is replaced by q, then (4) reduces to the Greenwood formula (1).

We see that we now have a bivariate Markov chain $\{X(t), Y(t); t = 0, 1, 2, \ldots\}$ which provides us with standard methods for calculating probabilities related to the epidemic. We also remark that for small values of p, the probability of at least one infective contact is $1 - q^{y_0} \sim p y_0$, so that the mean number of new infectives is $p y_0 n$, as for the law of mass action. At $t = 1$, the infectives y_1 are again removed, but not before they can infect the remaining susceptibles, which they are assumed to do instantaneously. The process is now repeated for $t = 2, 3, \ldots, T$ until either $Y(T) = 0, X(T) > 0$, or $X(T) = 0$, when the epidemic terminates.

An example for $X(0) = 3$, with $Y(0) = 1, 2$, or 3 may help to visualize the Markov chain more clearly. The transition probability matrix $\mathbf{P}$ takes the form

$Y(t)$	$X(t)$	$Y(t{+}1)=0$				$Y(t{+}1)=1$				$Y(t{+}1)=2$				$Y(t{+}1)=3$			
		$X(t{+}1)=0$	1	2	3	0	1	2	3	0	1	2	3	0	1	2	3
0	0	1															
	1		1														
	2			1													
	3				1												
1	0	1															
	1		q			p	0			0	0			0	0		
	2			q^2		0	$2pq$	0		p^2	0	0		0	0	0	
	3				q^3	0	0	$3pq^2$	0	0	$3p^2q$	0	0	p^3	0	0	0
2	0	1															
	1		q^2			$1-q^2$	0			0	0			0	0		
	2			q^4		0	$2(1-q^2)q^2$	0		$(1-q^2)^2$	0	0		0	0	0	
	3				q^6	0	0	$3(1-q^2)q^4$	0	0	$3(1-q^2)^2q^2$	0	0	$(1-q^2)^3$	0	0	0
3	0	1															
	1		q^3			$1-q^3$	0			0	0			0	0		
	2			q^6		0	$2(1-q^3)q^3$	0		$(1-q^3)^2$	0	0		0	0	0	
	3				q^9	0	0	$3(1-q^3)q^6$	0	0	$3(1-q^3)^2q^3$	0	0	$(1-q^3)^3$	0	0	0

or, in abridged form

$$\mathbf{P} = \begin{bmatrix} \mathbf{I} & \mathbf{0} & \mathbf{0} & \mathbf{0} \\ \mathbf{Q} & \mathbf{A}_{11} & \mathbf{A}_{12} & \mathbf{A}_{13} \\ \mathbf{Q}^2 & \mathbf{A}_{21} & \mathbf{A}_{22} & \mathbf{A}_{23} \\ \mathbf{Q}^3 & \mathbf{A}_{31} & \mathbf{A}_{32} & \mathbf{A}_{33} \end{bmatrix}, \quad (5)$$

One can carry out Markov chain calculations with $\mathbf{P}$ in much the same way as for the Greenwood model. The structure of larger matrices for $n > 3$ is similar, with probabilities of the form (4).

In the present example, the duration T of the epidemic with $X(0) = 3$ and $Y(0) = 1$, will have the distribution

$$\Pr\{t = T\} = \{\, 0000, \quad 0001, \quad 0000, \quad 0000 \,\}$$

$$\times \begin{bmatrix} 0 & 0 & 0 & 0 \\ 0 & \mathbf{A}_{11} & \mathbf{A}_{12} & \mathbf{A}_{13} \\ 0 & \mathbf{A}_{21} & \mathbf{A}_{22} & \mathbf{A}_{23} \\ 0 & \mathbf{A}_{31} & \mathbf{A}_{32} & \mathbf{A}_{33} \end{bmatrix}^{T-1} \begin{bmatrix} \mathbf{I} \\ \mathbf{Q} \\ \mathbf{Q}^2 \\ \mathbf{Q}^3 \end{bmatrix}. \quad (6)$$

Here, the initial 1×16 row vector records the values $X(0) = 3$ and $Y(0) = 1$ at $t = 0$, the final 16×4 matrix gives the probabilities that $Y(t)$ is zero at any time t, and the central matrix indicates that $X(t)$ circulates among the states 0, 1, 2, 3, for $T - 1$ epochs before $Y(T) = 0$ at time T.

While the structure of the bivariate Markov chain in the Reed–Frost model is more complex than that of the simple Markov chain in the Greenwood model, both follow the same basic principles. It should be pointed out that for $X(0) = 2$ and $Y(0) = 1$, the two models yield exactly the same probabilities, but this is not the case for larger values of $X(0)$ or $Y(0)$. For further details of these models, the reader is referred to Bailey's treatise [3] and Daley & Gani's monograph [5]. It may be worth mentioning that the models can be modified to allow for immigration into and emigration out of the population subject to infection; for such an example on the spread of human immunodeficiency virus (HIV) among intravenous drug users, see [11].

Stochastic Models in Continuous Time

There are many continuous time models in use, of which three are the most common. The first is the simple epidemic (SI model) in which the population is subdivided into two categories, susceptibles (S) and infectives (I). This is not entirely realistic, but may hold approximately over a short period of time. The second is the general epidemic (SIR model) where there are three categories, susceptibles (S), infectives (I) and removals (R), that is individuals who have recovered and are immune, or who have died from the disease. This is a more realistic model for a population of fixed size. The third is the carrier-borne epidemic (CSR model) consisting of infective carriers (C) of the disease who may not know that they are infectious and are gradually dying off, and a separate category of susceptibles (S) subject to infection by the carriers, who are then removed (R) directly after they become infected. We consider each of these in turn.

The Simple SI Epidemic

In this model, we shall consider an initial population consisting of $X(0) = n$ susceptibles, and $Y(0) = 1$ infective for simplicity, subject to homogeneous mixing. At any time $t > 0$, we assume that in any

time interval $(t, t + \delta t)$, the infinitesimal transition probability of a further infection is given by

$$\Pr\{X(t + \delta t) = x - 1, \ Y(t + \delta t) = y + 1 | X(t) = x,$$
$$Y(t) = y\} = \beta x y \delta t + o(\delta t), \tag{7}$$

where $y = n + 1 - x$, and β is the infection rate. Note that the infectives remain infectious for all time, and $X(t) + Y(t) = X(0) + Y(0) = n + 1$, so that we need keep track of only one quantity, say $X(t)$ at $t \geq 0$. The equation (7) indicates that $\{X(t); t \geq 0\}$ is a Markov chain in continuous time, namely a death process with the state-dependent death parameter

$$\mu_x = \beta x(n + 1 - x).$$

It is readily shown that the state probabilities $p_x(t) = \Pr\{X(t) = x | X(0) = n\}$ satisfy the system of Kolmogorov forward differential equations

$$\frac{dp_x}{dt} = \beta(x + 1)(n - x)p_{x+1} - \beta x(n + 1 - x)p_x,$$
$$0 \leq x \leq n - 1,$$

$$\frac{dp_n}{dt} = -\beta n \, p_n, \tag{8}$$

subject to the initial condition $p_n(0) = 1$. Bailey [2] has shown that an explicit solution of these equations is possible by solving the partial differential equation for the moment generating function (or the probability generating function) of the process, in terms of hypergeometric functions, but these prove rather difficult to handle.

A simpler method relies on the use of the Laplace transforms

$$p_x^*(s) = \int_0^\infty \exp(-st)p_x(t)dt, \quad \mathrm{Re}(s) > 0,$$

of the state probabilities. From (8), it is easily seen that

$$p_n^*(s) = \frac{1}{s + \beta n}, \tag{9}$$

or $p_n(t) = \exp(-\beta n t)$, and

$$p_x^*(s) = \frac{\beta(x + 1)(n - x)}{s + \beta x(n + 1 - x)} p_{x+1}^*(s),$$
$$0 \leq x \leq n - 1. \tag{10}$$

Thus, in principle, the transform $p_x^*(s)$ can be found as

$$p_x^*(s) = \frac{n!(n-x)!}{x!}\beta^{n-x}\prod_{j=x}^{n}\frac{1}{s+\beta j(n+1-j)}, \tag{11}$$

so that $p_x(t)$ may be derived explicitly. Unfortunately, the values $s + \beta j(n+1-j)$ are repeated for $j = n$ and $j = 1$, $j = n-1$ and $j = 2$, and so on, with the result that $p_x(t)$ is rather more complicated than a simple sum of exponentials.

The problem can be overcome by an approximation which replaces the integer n by the number $N = n + e$, where $e > 0$ is some small positive quantity. Then, the Laplace transforms $p_x^*(s)$ of (11) are replaced by the approximate $q_x^*(s)$ of the form

$$q_x^*(s) = \frac{n!(n-x)!}{x!}\beta^{n-x}\prod_{j=x}^{n}\frac{1}{s+\beta j(N+1-j)}, \tag{12}$$

where the values $s + \beta j(N+1-j)$ are now distinct for all values of j. It follows that $q_x(t)$ is a sum of exponentials of the form

$$q_x(t) = \sum_{j=x}^{n} c_{xj}\exp[-\beta j(N+1-j)t], \tag{13}$$

for which the coefficients c_{xj} can be readily evaluated (see [3]). Letting $e \to 0$ in (13) allows us to derive the exact values $p_x(t)$.

Since the random intervals between each infection have negative exponential density functions

$$\beta j(n+1-j)\exp[-\beta j(n+1-j)t], \quad 1 \le j \le n,$$

the mean duration of the epidemic has the form

$$E(T) = \sum_{j=1}^{n}\frac{1}{\beta j(n+1-j)}. \tag{14}$$

This can be approximated by

$$\frac{1}{\beta(n+1)}\int_1^n\left(\frac{1}{x}+\frac{1}{n+1-x}\right)dx = \frac{2\ln n}{\beta(n+1)}. \tag{15}$$

Kendall [16] has obtained the elegant result that for large values of n, the distribution of $W = (n+1)T - 2\ln n$ can be approximated explicitly by a modified Bessel function of the second kind.

The General SIR Epidemic

This is possibly the most frequently used continuous-time epidemic model; it was foreshadowed in a paper by McKendrick [18] and analyzed in more detail by Bartlett [4]. Here the closed population is subdivided into three categories: susceptibles (S), infectives (I) and removals (R), with their initial values being respectively $X(0) = n$, $Y(0) = 1$ for simplicity, and $Z(0) = 0$, the total population remaining fixed at $n + 1$.

We assume that in any time interval $(t, t + \delta t)$, the infinitesimal transition probabilities of the process are given by the probability of a further infection

$$\Pr\{X(t+\delta t) = x - 1, \ Y(t+\delta t) = y+1 | X(t) = x,$$
$$Y(t) = y\} = \beta xy\delta t + o(\delta t), \tag{16}$$

precisely as for the SI epidemic in (7), and the probability of a removal

$$\Pr\{X(t+\delta t) = x, Y(t+\delta t) = y - 1 | X(t) = x,$$
$$Y(t) = y\} = \gamma y\delta t + o(\delta t). \tag{17}$$

These hold for all $0 \le x \le n, 0 \le y \le n+1-x$, with β as the infection rate and γ as the removal rate, except when the values of $X(t)$ or $Y(t)$ are outside their permissible ranges. Note that $x + y \le n + 1$ for all $t \ge 0$; we do not need to keep track of the value of $Z(t)$, since $X(t) + Y(t) + Z(t) = n + 1$ for all $t \ge 0$.

In this model, $\{X(t), Y(t); t \ge 0\}$ is a bivariate Markov chain in continuous time. $X(t)$ is a death process with parameter $\mu_{xy} = \beta xy$, dependent on both the number of susceptibles x and the number of infectives y, while $Y(t)$ is a birth and death process with birth parameter $\mu_{xy} = \beta xy$ and death parameter γy.

The state probabilities $p_{xy}(t) = \Pr\{X(t) = x, Y(t) = y | X(0) = n, Y(0) = 1\}$ satisfy the forward Kolmogorov differential equations

$$\frac{dp_{xy}}{dt} = \beta(x+1)(y-1)p_{x+1,y-1}$$
$$- (\beta x + \gamma)yp_{xy} + \gamma(y+1)p_{x,y+1},$$
$$0 \le x \le n, \quad 0 \le y \le n+1-x, \tag{18}$$

with $p_{xy}(t) = 0$ when x or y is outside the permissible range, and $p_{n1}(0) = 1$. Gani [9] was able to obtain an explicit solution for the Laplace transforms of the $p_{xy}(t)$ based on a matrix formulation of the problem, but this is rather complicated, and a simpler approach such as that of Griffiths et al. [13] may prove more suitable in practice.

Quantities of interest are the final size of the epidemic, apart from the initial $Y(0) = 1$, and its distribution for varying parameters β and γ. Bailey [3] lists the probabilities of this final size for $X(0) = 1, 2, 3, 4, 5$, and $Y(0) = 1$, and exhibits graphs for the cases $X(0) = 10, 20, 40$ for increasing values of $\rho = \gamma/\beta$. But perhaps the most illuminating result about the final size of the epidemic is the Threshold Theorem of Whittle [23] (*see* **Epidemic Thresholds**). This is obtained by bounding the stochastic process for the number $Y(t)$ of infectives above and below by birth and death processes with a simpler birth parameter than the actual value βxy. We shall simply quote Whittle's results, which the reader can study in greater depth by reference to his paper.

Assuming an intensity i for the epidemic, so that the final number of infectives other than the initial $Y(0) = 1$ is ni, and writing $\rho = \gamma/\beta$ and

$$\pi_i = \sum_{w=0}^{ni} P_w,$$

where the $P_w = \Pr\{X(\infty) = n - w\}$, $0 \le w \le n$, are the probabilities of a final size w of the epidemic, Whittle [23] proves that for large n

$$\frac{\rho}{n} \le \pi_i \le \frac{\rho}{n(1-i)}, \quad \text{for } \rho < n(1-i),$$

$$\frac{\rho}{n} \le \pi_i \le 1, \qquad \text{for } n(1-i) \le \rho < n, \quad (19)$$

$$\pi_i = 1, \qquad \text{for } n \le \rho.$$

This may be interpreted as stating that if $\rho \ge n$, then there is a zero probability that the epidemic exceeds any preassigned intensity i, while if $\rho < n$, then the probability of an epidemic is approximately $1 - \rho/n$ for small i. Similar results hold for the case where $Y(0) = a > 1$ with ρ/n and $\rho/n(1-i)$ now raised to the power a in the inequalities (19). This threshold theorem is the stochastic analog of Kermack & McKendrick's threshold theorem [17] for the deterministic general epidemic.

The Carrier-Borne CSR Epidemic

In this model, the carriers $U(t)$, $t \ge 0$, form a separate category, with an initial number $U(0) = b \ge 1$.

The process $\{U(t); t \ge 0\}$ is a pure death process with parameter $\mu_u = \mu u$, such that the infinitesimal probability of a carrier dying in $(t, t + \delta t)$ is

$$\Pr\{U(t + \delta t) = u - 1 | U(t) = u\} = \mu u \delta t + o(\delta t),$$

$$1 \le u \le b,$$

independent of the number of susceptibles in the population. The state probabilities of this process at any time $t \ge 0$ are known to be of the binomial form

$$\Pr\{U(t) = u | U(0) = b\}$$

$$= \binom{b}{u} [\exp(-\mu u t)][1 - \exp(-\mu t)]^{b-u},$$

$$0 \le u \le b. \quad (20)$$

The susceptibles $X(t)$ are infected by homogeneous mixing with the carriers $U(t)$, and the infinitesimal probability of such an infection in any interval $(t, t + \delta t)$ when $U(t) = u \ge 1$, is

$$\Pr\{X(t + \delta t) = x - 1, U(t + \delta t) = u | X(t) = x,$$

$$U(t) = u\} = \beta x u \delta t + o(\delta t), \quad 1 \le x \le n,$$

where β is the infection parameter. After becoming infected, a susceptible is removed directly from the population.

The process $\{X(t), U(t); t \ge 0\}$ is a bivariate Markov chain in continuous time, in which $U(t)$ is itself an independent Markov chain which influences the process $X(t)$. If we denote the state probabilities at time $t \ge 0$ by

$$p_{xu}(t) = \Pr\{X(t) = x, U(t) = u | X(0) = n,$$

$$U(0) = b\}, \quad 0 \le u \le b, \quad 0 \le x \le n,$$

we can derive the forward Kolmogorov differential equations of the process as

$$\frac{\mathrm{d}p_{xu}}{\mathrm{d}t} = \beta(x+1)u p_{x+1,u} - (\beta x + \mu)u p_{xu}$$

$$+ \mu(u+1)p_{x,u+1}, \quad (21)$$

with $p_{xu}(t) = 0$ when x or u are outside their permissible ranges, and $p_{nb}(0) = 1$.

The model was originally formulated by Weiss [22], and solved by him, Dietz [7] and Downton [8]. A straightforward method of solution, also outlined in Bailey [3], involves the derivation of the partial differential equation of the probability generating function obtained from (21). Its solution is found by the method of separation of variables. An alternative method relies on the more general approach presented by Puri [21]. The probabilities $p_{xu}(t)$ are found explicitly as

$$p_{xu}(t) = \binom{n}{x} \binom{b}{u} \sum_{j=x}^{n} (-1)^{j-x} \binom{n-x}{j-x}$$

$$\times \left(\frac{\mu}{\mu + j\beta} \right)^{b-u} (\exp -u(\mu + j\beta)t)$$

$$\times [1 - \exp -(\mu + j\beta)t]^{b-u}, \qquad (22)$$

with the expectation of $X(t)$ given by

$$E[X(t)] = n \left(\frac{\mu + \beta \exp -(\mu + \beta)t}{\mu + \beta} \right)^b. \qquad (23)$$

The distribution of the duration time T of the epidemic, which ends when either $U(t) = 0$ or $X(t) = 0$, can also be derived explicitly. The model can be made more complex by making the parameters time-dependent, and also allowing emigration and immigration of both the susceptibles and carriers.

Concluding Remarks

A very large number of stochastic models have been developed for a variety of diseases, including most recently acquired immune deficiency syndrome (AIDS). These include spatial models for the geographic spread of infections (*see* **Epidemic Models, Spatial**), models for parasitic or host–vector diseases such as malaria and schistosomiasis, and models for sexually transmitted diseases. While each disease may require a slightly different model in order to approximate realism, the principles used in constructing them are similar to those displayed in the small range of examples above.

There is a wealth of recent literature on stochastic epidemic research, and the reader may wish to refer to the recent review paper by Mollison et al. [20], the book of papers on AIDS epidemiology edited by Jewell et al. [15], or the books on more general epidemic models edited by Mollison [19] and Isham & Medley [14] and that recently authored by Diekman & Heesterbeek [6].

References

[1]   Abbey, H. (1952). An examination of the Reed–Frost theory of epidemics, *Human Biology* **24**, 201–233.

[2]   Bailey, N.T.J. (1963). The simple stochastic epidemic: a complete solution in terms of known functions, *Biometrika* **50**, 235–240.

[3]   Bailey, N.T.J. (1975). *The Mathematical Theory of Infectious Diseases*. Griffin, London.

[4]   Bartlett, M.S. (1949). Some evolutionary stochastic processes, *Journal of the Royal Statistical Society, Series B* **11**, 211–229.

[5]   Daley, D.J. & Gani, J. (1999). *Epidemic Modelling: An Introduction*. Cambridge University Press, Cambridge.

[6]   Diekman, O. & Heesterbeek, H.J. (1999). *Mathematical Epidemiology of Infections Diseases*. Wiley, New York.

[7]   Dietz, K. (1966). On the model of Weiss for the spread of epidemics by carriers, *Journal of Applied Probability* **3**, 375–382.

[8]   Downton, F. (1967). Epidemics with carriers: a note on a paper of Dietz. *Journal of Applied Probability* **4**, 264–270.

[9]   Gani, J. (1967). On the general stochastic epidemic, in *Proceedings of the Fifth Berkeley Symposium on Mathematical Statistics and Probability*, Vol. 4. University of California Press, Berkeley, pp. 271–279.

[10]   Gani, J. & Jerwood, D. (1971). Markov chain methods in chain binomial epidemic models, *Biometrics* **27**, 591–604.

[11]   Gani, J. & Yakowitz, S. (1993). Modelling the spread of HIV among intravenous drug users, *IMA Journal of Mathematics Applied in Medicine and Biology* **10**, 51–65.

[12]   Greenwood, M. (1931). On the statistical measure of infectiousness, *Journal of Hygiene* **31**, 336–351.

[13]   Griffiths, J.D., Smedley, J.K. & Weale, T.G. (1987). Terminal distributions along a "Knight's Line" for a stochastic epidemic, *IMA Journal of Mathematics Applied in Medicine and Biology* **4**, 69–79.

[14]   Isham, V. & Grenfell, B.T., eds (1996). *Models for Infectious Human Diseases: Their Structure and Relation to Data*. Cambridge University Press, Cambridge.

[15]   Jewell, N.P., Dietz, K. & Farewell, V.T., eds (1992). *AIDS Epidemiology: Methodological Issues*. Birkhauser, Boston.

[16]   Kendall, D.G. (1957). La propagation d'une épidémie ou d'un bruit dans une population limitée, *Publications de l'Institut de Statistique de l'Université de Paris* **6**, 307–311.

[17]   Kermack, W.O. & McKendrick, A.G. (1927). A contribution to the mathematical theory of epidemics I, *Proceedings of the Royal Society, Series A* **115**, 700–721.

[18]   McKendrick, A.G. (1926). Applications of mathematics to medical problems. *Proceedings of the Edinburgh Mathematical Society* **44**, 98–130.

[19] Mollison, D. (ed.) (1995). *Epidemic Models: Their Structure and Relation to Data.* Cambridge University Press, Cambridge.

[20] Mollison, D., Isham, V. & Grenfell, B.T. (1994). Epidemics: models and data (with discussion), *Journal of the Royal Statistical Society, Series A* **157**, 115–149.

[21] Puri, P.S. (1975). A linear birth and death process under the influence of another process, *Journal of Applied Probability* **12**, 1–17.

[22] Weiss, G.H. (1965). On the spread of epidemics by carriers, *Biometrics* **21**, 481–490.

[23] Whittle, P. (1955). The outcome of a stochastic epidemic – a note on Bailey's paper, *Biometrika* **42**, 116–122.

(*See also* **Infectious Disease Models**)

J. GANI

Epidemic Thresholds

The practically most important result to come out of the mathematical theory of epidemics is the threshold theorem, which broadly states that an epidemic can only become established in a population if the initial susceptible population size is larger than some critical value, which depends on the parameters governing the spread of disease. The threshold theorem is important because it immediately tells us what proportion of susceptibles need to be vaccinated in order to prevent an epidemic occurring.

Two broad classes of epidemic models are considered in this article. The majority of the article is devoted to *closed population* epidemic models, which assume that the timescale of the epidemic is sufficiently short so that demographic changes in the population can be ignored. The models considered are of the susceptible → infective → removed (SIR) type, in which a susceptible individual becomes infected by having "adequate contact" with an infective. It then remains infectious for a while before being removed, by either death, the termination of its infectious period or public health measures. Removed individuals are assumed to be immune to further infection and thus play no further role in the epidemic. The threshold behaviors of a homogeneously mixing deterministic model and its stochastic counterpart, the so-called deterministic and stochastic general epidemics, are

considered first, before moving on to more general stochastic models incorporating, for example, more realistic infection mechanisms, heterogeneous populations, and spatial effects. The article closes with a brief description of the threshold behavior of *open population* models, which incorporate demographic effects.

Closed Population Epidemics

General Deterministic Epidemic

The general deterministic epidemic is defined by the following system of differential equations:

$$\frac{dx}{dt} = -\beta xy, \qquad \frac{dy}{dt} = \beta xy - \gamma y, \qquad \frac{dz}{dt} = \gamma y, \tag{1}$$

where $x(t)$, $y(t)$, and $z(t)$ denote, respectively, the numbers of susceptible, infectious, and removed individuals at time t, and the parameters β and γ are known as the infection and removal rates (*see* **Epidemic Models, Deterministic**). The model assumes a homogeneously mixing population, with adequate contacts between two given individuals occurring at rate β. Thus if there are x susceptibles and y infectives at time t, there are xy possible contacts, each occurring at rate β, that will result in a new infection occurring; hence the term βxy in (1). The model also assumes that infectious individuals are each removed at rate γ, giving rise to the term γy in (1).

Suppose that at time $t = 0$ there are a infectives, n susceptibles, and no removed cases. It follows from the second formula in (1) that, provided that $y > 0$, $dy/dt > 0$ if and only if $x > \rho$, where $\rho = \gamma/\beta$.

Thus a build-up of infection will occur in the population if and only if $n > \rho$. This is part of the celebrated threshold theorem of Kermack & McKendrick [15].

General Stochastic Epidemic

The general stochastic epidemic is obtained by replacing the infinitesimal transition rates governing (1) by infinitesimal transition probabilities (*see* **Epidemic Models, Stochastic**). For $t \geq 0$, let $X(t)$, $Y(t)$, and $Z(t)$ be, respectively, the numbers of infective, susceptible, and removed individuals at time t. Suppose that $(X(0), Y(0), Z(0)) = (n, a, 0)$, so that $X(t) + Y(t) + Z(t) = n + a$ ($t \geq 0$). Then the epidemic is completely specified by $\{(X(t), Y(t)); t \geq 0\}$, which is a continuous time Markov chain with infinitesimal transition probabilities

$$\Pr\{[X(t+h), Y(t+h)] = (i-1, j+1) | [X(t), Y(t)]$$
$$= (i, j)\} = \beta i j h + o(h)$$

for an infection, and

$$\Pr\{[X(t+h), Y(t+h)] = (i, j-1) | [X(t), Y(t)]$$
$$= (i, j)\} = \gamma j + o(h)$$

for a removal.

The epidemic terminates as soon as the number of infectives becomes zero. Let $T = n - X(\infty)$ be the total size of the epidemic; that is, the number of initial susceptibles that are ultimately infected. Note that rescaling the time axis so that the infection rate β is one shows that the distribution of T depends on β and γ only through $\rho = \gamma/\beta$. A system of linear equations governing the distribution of T is given in Bailey [2, p. 94], in which diagrams illustrating the distribution for various values of n and ρ are also given [2, pp. 98–99]. When $n < \rho$ the distribution of T is unimodal, with the mode at some small argument value (often zero), while if $n > \rho$ the distribution of T is bimodal, with a second mode at a large argument value. Thus again there is a threshold at $n \approx \rho$, although, because of the presence of chance effects, the change in behavior at the threshold is less sharp than in the deterministic model. Also, the value of n at which the distribution of T changes from being unimodal to bimodal is slightly larger than ρ [18].

To understand its threshold behavior it is fruitful to give a more detailed, but equivalent, description of the general stochastic epidemic. The assumptions underlying the general stochastic epidemic are consistent with a model in which infectives behave independently, making contacts at the points of a Poisson process with rate $n\beta$ throughout an infectious period that follows a negative exponential distribution with mean γ^{-1}. For each contact, the individual contacted is chosen independently and uniformly from the n initial susceptibles. If a contacted individual is susceptible then it becomes infected; otherwise, nothing happens. Clearly, the rate at which an infective is removed is γ, and if there are x susceptibles and y infectives at time t the rate at which infectious contacts are being made is $yn\beta$. However, the probability

that a given contact is with a susceptible is x/n. Hence, the rate at which new infections occur is $yn\beta \times x/n = \beta xy$, as required by the general stochastic epidemic.

Note that if all the contacts in the above epidemic were to result in the spread of infection, then the process of infectives would follow a birth-and-death process (see for example, [11, pp. 251–254]) with birth rate $n\beta$ and death rate γ. Of course, it is unlikely that all the contacts made in the epidemic are with susceptibles, so the birth-and-death process is usually only an upper bound to the process of infectives. However, if n is large the probability of contacting a previously contacted individual will be small, particularly in the early stages of the epidemic. Thus, for large n, the early stage of the epidemic is well approximated by the above birth-and-death process and occurrence of a minor/major epidemic may be associated with extinction/nonextinction of the birth-and-death process. Hence, by standard results for birth-and-death processes, the probability that a major epidemic occurs is given by

$$p_{\text{MAJ}} = \begin{cases} 0, & \text{if } n\beta \leq \gamma, \\ 1 - (\gamma/n\beta)^a, & \text{if } n\beta > \gamma, \end{cases}$$

so major epidemics can occur only if $n > \rho$.

The above threshold behavior can be made mathematically precise in several ways: see, for example, Whittle [20], who gave the first stochastic epidemic threshold theorem, Williams [21] and Ball [3].

Although the deterministic and stochastic general epidemics both have the same threshold value of $n = \rho$, the interpretation of the threshold behavior is quite different in the two models. In the deterministic model, if $n \leq \rho$ $(n > \rho)$ minor (major) epidemics will always occur. In the stochastic model, for large n, if $n \leq \rho$ minor epidemics always occur, while if $n > \rho$ a major epidemic occurs with a probability lying strictly between 0 and 1.

R_0 and Vaccination Strategies

A unifying concept in the analysis of the threshold behavior of epidemic models is the reproduction number (or ratio) R_0 of the epidemic, which is usually defined informally as the expected number of infectious contacts made by a typical infective during its entire infectious period, in a population consisting of susceptibles only (see, for example, [12]).

The difficulty in applying this definition for complex models is in determining what is a typical infective. Diekmann et al. [9] show that, for a very broad class of deterministic models, R_0 is given by the maximal eigenvalue of an appropriate "next generation" linear operator, thus providing a formal definition. However, in the general stochastic epidemic, it is clear that a typical infective makes infectious contacts at the points of a Poisson process with rate $n\beta$ throughout an infectious period that follows a negative exponential distribution with mean γ^{-1}. Thus, $R_0 = n\beta/\gamma$ and from the previous section major epidemics can only occur if $R_0 > 1$.

Now consider a general epidemic that is above threshold and suppose that a proportion θ of initial susceptibles are vaccinated against the disease being modeled. After vaccination, the initial number of susceptibles is reduced to $n' = (1 - \theta)n$ and hence R_0 is reduced to $R_0' = (1 - \theta)R_0$. Thus major epidemics will be prevented if $R_0' \leq 1$; that is if

$$\theta \geq 1 - \frac{1}{R_0}.$$

This formula, which gives the critical level of vaccination coverage to prevent an epidemic occurring, holds quite generally for single population epidemic models.

General Single Population Epidemic

The approximation of the process of infectives by a birth-and-death process holds for a very wide class of epidemic models, although the approximating process is generally a branching process. Now consider an epidemic, initiated by a infectives among n susceptibles, in which infectious individuals have independent and identically distributed life histories, $H = (T_I, \eta)$, where T_I is the time elapsing between an individual's infection and its eventual removal or death, and η is a point process of times, relative to an individual's infection, at which infectious contacts are made. As before, for each contact, the individual contacted is chosen independently and uniformly from the n initial susceptibles and an infection occurs only if the contacted individual is still susceptible.

If the initial number of susceptibles n is large, the process of infectives can be approximated by a branching process (corresponding to the case in which all contacts result in new infections), in which

a typical individual lives until age T_I and reproduces at ages according to η. Moreover, the approximation can be made precise in the limit as $n \to \infty$ (see [5]). Let R be the number of contacts made by a typical infective in the epidemic model, let $R_0 = \mathrm{E}(R)$, and let $f(s) = \mathrm{E}(s^R)$ be the probability generating function of R. Then, by standard branching process theory (see, for example, [14]), a major epidemic occurs with nonzero probability if and only if $R_0 > 1$ and the probability of a major epidemic is $1 - p^a$, where p is the smallest solution of $f(s) = s$ in $[0, 1]$.

A few examples illustrate the generality of the model:

1. Suppose that η is a Poisson process with rate β. Then R follows a Poisson distribution with random mean βT_I, so $R_0 = \beta\mathrm{E}(T_I)$. Note that if T_I follows a negative exponential distribution with mean γ^{-1}, then the general stochastic epidemic is obtained.

2. In most, if not all, real-life epidemics the infectious period of an infective is preceded by a **latent period** during which a recently infected individual is unable to infect other susceptibles. Let T_L and T_I be random variables describing the lengths of typical latent and infectious periods, respectively. Suppose that η is a Poisson process with rate $\beta(t)$, where

$$\beta(t) = \begin{cases} \beta, & \text{if } T_L < t < T_L + T_I, \\ 0, & \text{otherwise.} \end{cases}$$

Then, again, $R_0 = \beta\mathrm{E}(T_I)$. Note that the introduction of a latent period does not change R_0.

3. Suppose that η is a Poisson process with random rate $\Lambda(t)$ $(0 \leq t < \infty)$. Then R is Poisson with random mean $\int_0^\infty \Lambda(t)\,dt$, so $R_0 = \int_0^\infty \mathrm{E}[\Lambda(t)]\,dt$. Such a model might be appropriate for the spread of acquired immune deficiency syndrome (AIDS), as it is known that the infectiousness of an infective varies considerably throughout the long **incubation period** (see, for example, [1]).

General Multipopulation Epidemic

Now consider the spread of an epidemic among a population that is partitioned into m groups, labeled $1, 2, \ldots, m$, with group i consisting initially of a_i infectives and n_i susceptibles. The partitioning of the population into groups could reflect important heterogeneities (such as owing to age, sex, and genotype), geographic location, or a multispecies population, as in host–vector epidemics such as malaria. Infectious individuals have independent life histories, with life histories of infectives in the same group being identically distributed. For $i = 1, 2, \ldots, m$, the life history of a typical group i infective is $H_i = (T_I^{(i)}, \eta_{i1}, \eta_{i2}, \ldots, \eta_{im})$, where $T_I^{(i)}$ denotes the infectious period and, for $j = 1, 2, \ldots, m$, η_{ij} is a point process governing times when infectious contacts are made with group j individuals. For each contact, the individual contacted is chosen independently and uniformly from the initial susceptibles in the contacted group.

If the initial numbers of susceptibles in every group are all large, then the process of infectives approximately follows a multitype branching process, and the approximation can be made precise in the limit as $n_i \to \infty$ ($i = 1, 2, \ldots, m$) [4]. For $i, j = 1, 2, \ldots, m$ let R_{ij} be the total number of group j contacts made by a typical group i infective throughout its infectious period. Let $\mathbf{M} = (m_{ij})$ be the $m \times m$ matrix with elements $m_{ij} = \mathrm{E}(R_{ij})$ and let R_0 be the eigenvalue of $\mathbf{M}$ having maximum modulus. Then, by standard multitype branching process theory [16], subject to mild regularity conditions, a major epidemic occurs with nonzero probability if and only if $R_0 > 1$.

The models of the last two sections can be extended to allow for some or all previously infected individuals to become susceptible again, either immediately following their infectious period or at some later time. The process of infectives for such models can be sandwiched between that of the corresponding SIR model and its branching process approximation, so the two models have identical threshold behavior. Models in which all infectives become susceptible immediately following their infectious period are known as susceptible $\to$ infective $\to$ susceptible (SIS) models.

Deterministic versions of the models of the last two sections can usually be written down, although they will often involve a continuous partitioning of the population; for example, to incorporate nonexponential infectious periods. The framework of Diekmann et al. [9] can be used to determine R_0 for such a deterministic model. The value of R_0 will be the same as for the corresponding stochastic model.

Structured Populations

The threshold behavior of the above multipopulation epidemic assumes that all the group sizes are large. Although this may be reasonable in some practical situations, in others it clearly is not. Two such cases are now outlined.

Epidemics Among Households

Consider the spread of an epidemic among a population consisting of m households, each of size n. Suppose that infectives have independent and identically distributed life histories, $H = (T_I, \eta_L, \eta_G)$, where T_I denotes the infectious period of a typical infective, and η_L and η_G are point processes governing times at which *local* and *global* contacts are made, respectively. Each local (global) contact of a given infective is with an individual chosen independently and uniformly from the $n\,(nm)$ initial individuals in its household (the population).

Becker & Dietz [8] consider the case of highly infectious diseases, and assume that if one individual in a household becomes infected then the whole household becomes infected. Let $\tilde{R}$ be the total number of global contacts emanating from a typical infectious household. Then, provided that the number of households, m is large, the process of infected households can be approximated by a branching process with offspring distribution the distribution of $\tilde{R}$. Thus a major epidemic (one affecting a large number of households) can only occur if $\tilde{R}_0 = \mathrm{E}(\tilde{R}) > 1$. Note that under the above "highly infectious" assumption $\tilde{R}_0 = nR_0$, where now R_0 is the expected number of global contacts made by a typical infective. In general, $\tilde{R}_0 = \mu R_0$, where μ is the expected total size (including the initial infective) of a single household epidemic initiated by one infective, in which global infections are ignored; see Ball et al. [6], where extensions – for example, to unequal household sizes – are discussed.

Spatial Epidemics

A spatial model is often appropriate for plant diseases and also for animal diseases, such as fox rabies (*see* **Epidemic Models, Spatial**). The simplest spatial models usually assume that individuals are located one to each point of a regular lattice and that successive contacts of an infective are with individuals at locations (relative to the infective) chosen independently from a *contact distribution* (see, for example, [17]). The threshold behavior of such epidemics is usually obtained by taking the lattice to be infinite and determining conditions under which a finite initial number of infectives can give rise to an infinite epidemic.

Let R_0 be the expected number of contacts made by a typical infective. For one-dimensional lattices, the epidemic goes extinct with probability one, so no threshold exists. For two-dimensional lattices, there is a critical (CRIT) value of R_0, R_0^{CRIT} say, such that the probability of an infinite epidemic is zero if $R_0 < R_0^{CRIT}$ and strictly positive if $R_0 > R_0^{CRIT}$. The existence of R_0^{CRIT} is usually shown by comparing the epidemic with an appropriate percolation process. The value of R_0^{CRIT} depends on the contact distribution. It is known only in a few very special cases. However, $R_0^{CRIT} > 1$ and for nearest-neighbor infection models simulations show that $R_0^{CRIT} \approx 2$.

Note that for both epidemics among a community of households and spatial epidemics, the deterministic and stochastic models will have *different* threshold values, essentially because a deterministic model implicitly assumes that all the group sizes are large. For stochastic models, the threshold values of SIR and corresponding SIS models are now different.

Open Population Epidemics

Consider the general deterministic epidemic, and suppose that susceptibles are recruited into the population at rate ν and all individuals die from natural causes at rate μ. Then the differential expressions in (1) become

$$\frac{dx}{dt} = -\beta xy - \mu x + \nu,$$

$$\frac{dy}{dt} = \beta xy - (\gamma + \mu)y,$$

$$\frac{dz}{dt} = \gamma y - \mu z. \tag{2}$$

Setting $dx/dt = 0$ and $\beta = 0$ shows that the disease-free equilibrium population size is $x_0 = \nu/\mu$. Thus the expected number of infectious contacts made by an infective in an otherwise susceptible population is given by $R_0 = \beta\nu/(\gamma + \mu)\mu$, since now infectives are effectively removed at rate $\gamma + \mu$.

Setting $dx/dt = dy/dt = 0$ in (2) gives the equilibrium numbers of susceptibles and infectives. When $R_0 \le 1$, the only equilibrium point is the *disease-free* one $(x^*, y^*) = (\nu/\mu, 0)$. Moreover, this equilibrium is globally asymptotically stable, in the sense that $(x(t), y(t)) \to (x^*, y^*)$ as $t \to \infty$, irrespective of the initial values $(x(0), y(0))$. When $R_0 > 1$, there is a second *endemic* equilibrium point $(x^*, y^*) = (\beta^{-1}(\gamma + \mu), (\gamma + \mu)^{-1}\nu - \beta^{-1}\mu)$, and this too is globally asymptotically stable (unless, of course, $y(0) = 0$); see, for example, Hethcote [13] for details. Thus, if $R_0 \le 1$ the disease cannot become established in the population, while if $R_0 > 1$ it will become established and remain endemic. A similar conclusion holds for a very broad range of open population deterministic epidemic models, including multipopulation models.

The stochastic version of the above model is far more difficult to analyze. Suppose that the disease is introduced into a susceptible population, which is at its disease-free equilibrium level $x_0 = \nu/\mu$. Then, provided that x_0 is sufficiently large, the early stages of the epidemic can still be approximated by a birth-and-death process. Hence, the epidemic will only have a nonzero probability of taking off if $R_0 > 1$. However, even if it does take off, the epidemic will ultimately go extinct with probability one (cf. [19]), although it may take a very long time to do so. Thus, for practical purposes, endemic behavior is possible. However, simulations and observed data on epidemics show that long-term persistence of infection can only occur if the population is larger than some critical level. This has a long history, going back to the pioneering work of Bartlett [7]. The problem of determining the critical community size, for endemic outbreaks to occur, in terms of the parameters of the underlying model still awaits a satisfactory solution [10].

References

[1] Anderson, R.M. (1988). The epidemiology of HIV infection: variable incubation plus infectious periods and heterogeneity in sexual activity, *Journal of the Royal Statistical Society, Series A* **151**, 66–93.

[2] Bailey, N.T.J. (1975). *The Mathematical Theory of Infectious Diseases and its Applications*. Griffin, London.

[3] Ball, F.G. (1983). The threshold behaviour of epidemic models, *Journal of Applied Probability* **20**, 227–241.

[4] Ball, F.G. (1997). The threshold behaviour of stochastic epidemics, in *Proceedings of the Fourth International*

Conference on Mathematical Population Dynamics, to appear.

[5]   Ball, F.G. & Donnelly, P.J. (1995). Strong approximations for epidemic models, *Stochastic Processes and Their Applications* **55**, 1–21.

[6]   Ball, F.G., Mollison, D. & Scalia-Tomba, G. (1997). Epidemics with two levels of mixing, *Annals of Applied Probability* **7**, 46–89.

[7]   Bartlett, M.S. (1956). Deterministic and stochastic models for recurrent epidemics, in *Proceedings of the Third Berkeley Symposium on Mathematical Statistics and Probability* Vol. 4. University of California Press, Berkeley, pp. 81–109.

[8]   Becker, N.G. & Dietz, K. (1995). The effect of the household distribution on transmission and control of highly infectious diseases, *Mathematical Biosciences* **127**, 207–219.

[9]   Diekmann, O., Heesterbeek, J.A.P. & Metz, J.A.J. (1990). On the definition and the computation of the basic reproduction ratio R_0 in models for infectious diseases in heterogeneous populations, *Journal of Mathematical Biology* **28**, 365–382.

[10]   Dietz, K. (1995). Some problems in the theory of infectious disease transmission and control, in *Epidemic Models: Their Structure and Relation to Data*, D. Mollison, ed. Cambridge University Press, Cambridge, pp. 3–16.

[11]   Grimmett, G.R. & Strizaker, D.R. (1992). *Probability and Random Processes*, 2nd Ed. Clarendon Press, Oxford.

[12]   Heesterbeek, J.A.P. & Dietz, K. (1996). The concept of R_0 in epidemic theory, *Statistica Neerlandica* **50**, 89–110.

[13]   Hethcote, H.W. (1976). Qualitative analyses of communicable disease models, *Mathematical Biosciences* **28**, 335–356.

[14]   Jagers, P. (1975). *Branching Processes with Biological Applications*. Wiley, Chichester.

[15]   Kermack, W.O. & McKendrick, A.G. (1927). A contribution to the mathematical theory of epidemics, *Proceedings of the Royal Society of London, Series A* **115**, 700–721.

[16]   Mode, C.J. (1971). *Multitype Branching Processes: Theory and Application*. Elsevier, New York.

[17]   Mollison, D. (1977). Spatial contact models for ecological and epidemic spread, *Journal of the Royal Statistical Society, Series B* **39**, 283–326.

[18]   Nåsell, I. (1995). The threshold concept in stochastic epidemic and endemic models, in *Epidemic Models: Their Structure and Relation to Data*, D. Mollison, ed. Cambridge University Press, Cambridge pp. 71–83.

[19]   Ridler-Rowe, C.J. (1967). On a stochastic model of an epidemic, *Journal of Applied Probability* **4**, 19–33.

[20]   Whittle, P. (1955). The outcome of a stochastic epidemic – a note on Bailey's paper, *Biometrika* **42**, 116–122.

[21]   Williams, T. (1971). An algebraic proof of the threshold theorem for the general stochastic epidemic, *Advances in Applied Probability* **3**, 223.

F.G. BALL

Epidemiology, Overview

Epidemiology and biostatistics together constitute the quantitative foundation for public health and clinical research. Epidemiology has been variably defined [20, 25], but all definitions have as essential components the collection and use of data from populations or groups. Epidemiology might be viewed as formulating study designs to provide unbiased evidence for testing hypotheses by applying methods for gathering and using data from populations or groups of people. The domain of epidemiology includes both observation and experiment, although, ethically, the study of injurious factors is limited to observation. The consequences of exposure to potentially injurious agents can only be assessed by comparing disease risks in persons exposed through natural circumstances, including personal choice, with disease risks in those not exposed. Potentially beneficial agents, like chemopreventive micronutrients, might be evaluated using the same observational approaches or, in a clinical trial, by randomly assigning participants to the agent to be tested or to a placebo or other comparison therapy.

The principles of epidemiologic research are not unique to epidemiology and, in fact, permeate other branches of science concerned with human health and well-being: health services research, psychology, sociology and anthropology. Nor can a sharp point of demarcation be drawn between biostatistics and epidemiology. The most basic distinction places statistical aspects of design and data analysis in the domain of biostatistics and overall design and data collection in epidemiology, but the conducting of contemporary epidemiologic research needs integrated efforts from biostatisticians and epidemiologists, and often from clinicians and basic scientists. In addition, since the findings of much epidemiologic research often have immediate applications to clinical and public health policy, considerable media and public attention is directed to epidemiologic studies, frequently before they have been replicated and their results confirmed.

This article provides an overview of the field of epidemiology, setting a context for the more specific articles in this volume. It addresses the history of epidemiology, the purposes of epidemiologic research, the pathways for using epidemiologic evidence to further public health, and the current scope of the field, which is increasingly fragmented into specific areas of inquiry. The other articles in this book provide detailed reviews of different study designs, analytic methods and specifically focused areas of epidemiology.

History of Epidemiology

The beginning of contemporary epidemiology is often dated to the mid-twentieth century, when many large-scale studies were initiated to assess the causes of the shifting pattern of disease in the developed world observed during the preceding decades: rising mortality from seemingly new chronic diseases, like coronary heart disease and lung cancer, even as mortality from infectious diseases declined [39]. The many landmark studies on this theme that gave rise to current approaches are well known to biostatisticians and epidemiologists alike; for example, the Framingham Heart Study initiated in 1949 [11], and the British physicians' study initiated in 1951 [13]. In addition to these cohort studies, case–control studies were also carried out to characterize more quickly and efficiently the causes of the emerging chronic diseases. For example, the first convincing evidence on smoking and lung cancer was derived from case–control studies reported in the 1940s and early 1950s [52]. Cohort studies were also initiated to characterize the consequences of unique exposures, like the study of Japanese atomic-bomb survivors, which still continues today [43].

The origins of epidemiology, however, can be traced back centuries. Society has continually attempted to find the causes of epidemics of disease, whether the plague centuries ago or the sudden appearance of acquired immune deficiency syndrome, (AIDS), only two decades ago [46]. The search for causes, discussed in the third section, is intrinsically linked to the search for cures and avenues for prevention, and now as in the past, epidemiologic evidence remains central to the development of policies to protect and improve the public's health. An epidemiologic perspective is also central to the provision of care for individual patients who need to be cared for in a population context that recognizes the many factors determining their health and disease status. While "evidence-based" medicine and clinical epidemiology have been only recently touted [18, 40], the role of quantitative inference in clinical medicine was recognized in the nineteenth century by the French physician, Pierre Louis [28, 46].

One element of epidemiology is the description of the occurrence of disease, generally by person, place and time. The counting of disease events can be traced to Graunt who published his book, *Natural and Political Observations Made Upon the Bills Of Mortality*, in 1662 [6]. In this volume, he analyzed the bills of mortality for London, which included the weekly numbers of deaths and their causes, and the numbers of children christened. From these data, he inferred a lifetable for survival in London at the time. His acquaintance, Sir William Petty, also saw the relevance of counting to medicine and he too attempted to estimate life expectancy at birth [6, 46]. Thirty years after the publication of Graunt's book, Edmund Halley, better known for the comet bearing his name, described a lifetable for Breslau and in doing so he showed a clear understanding of population dynamics.

In the nineteenth century, major developments again took place in London. Wlliam Farr advanced counting to a new level through his work at the General Register Office [15, 46]. Farr held responsibility for health statistics for England and Wales and in that capacity he systematically collected and analyzed data, developing new methods and showing the insights into population health that could be gained from valid descriptive data (*see* **Vital Statistics, Overview**). Farr's contemporary, John Snow, undertook investigations of cholera epidemics in London and also practiced anesthesia, giving chloroform to Queen Victoria for childbirth [44]. Snow's investigations of cholera in London, undertaken by the newly founded London Epidemiological Society, led to the determination that cholera was transmitted via contaminated drinking water. Proof of this hypothesis prompted preventive interventions, including the recommendation to remove the handle of the Broad Street pump, a source of contaminated drinking water.

The further rise of epidemiology to the modern era was based in a scientific framework grounded in the emerging recognition of the role of microorganisms in causing disease and the rise of infectious disease epidemiology. In fact, the first principles for evaluating research findings for evidence of causality are often attributed to Robert Koch, although he had benefited from his teacher, Jacob Henle [14]. Koch applied these principles in his identification of the tubercle bacillus as the cause of tuberculosis.

Epidemiology has also used experimental methods. Early eighteenth-century examples include Lind's small trial of fresh fruit to prevent scurvy and Jenner's experimental use of cowpox vaccination to prevent smallpox. Early in the twentieth century, Goldberger conducted experiments that showed pellagra to result from a dietary deficiency, subsequently shown to be a lack of niacin [2, 32]. The contemporary clinical trial originated in the twentieth century as the concept of randomization of participants was introduced and the power of the design was shown in studies of streptomycin for tuberculosis and of vaccination for polio, for example [27, 31].

The first academic department of epidemiology was founded at the Johns Hopkins University School of Hygiene and Public Health in Baltimore in 1919 with the appointment of Wade Hampton Frost [16]. Frost combined interests in infectious diseases and research methods [30] and he saw the relevance of epidemiology to solving problems in public health. His department and its problem-oriented teaching methods became a model for institutions worldwide. Now, schools of public health throughout the world grant master's and doctoral degrees in epidemiology, as do some medical schools.

By the mid-twentieth century, the stage was set for the rise of modern epidemiology: academic departments were established and the new epidemics of coronary heart disease, chronic lung disease, and cancer motivated new research approaches that could address multicaused diseases with lengthy incubation periods and long natural histories. The prospective cohort study was initially the central design for investigating these diseases. Prospectively conducted cohort studies afforded the opportunity to collect data to test multiple hypotheses concerning disease etiology and the strength of this design was quickly shown by the success of the Framingham and other studies in identifying causes of heart disease and through the rapid confirmation that smoking caused lung cancer

and other diseases by the studies of British physicians and other groups, including the one million persons enrolled in the American Cancer Society's Cancer Prevention Study (CPS) [41].

The Framingham study is still considered a model for community-based research. Dawber [11] has chronicled the origins of the study, which was implemented in the late 1940s to address the rising occurrence of cardiovascular disease. The long-term success of the study can be attributed to the selection of a small and cooperative community, sustained support from the National Institutes of Health (NIH), and to the prescience of the original investigators who established rigorous and standardized protocols for data collection. Data were collected relevant to testing the principal extant hypotheses concerning etiology, which were listed at the study's beginning. As a result, much of our initial understanding of risk factors for cardiovascular diseases was based on evidence from this study. Supplementary studies of other diseases capitalized on the opportunity afforded by having the Framingham population under followup, and offspring of the original cohort have now been enrolled in a new cohort study that should be informative on familial factors affecting cardiovascular disease risk. The longitudinal data on multiple risk factors necessitated methodologic advances, since appropriate multivariate methods had not been available. For example, Gordon and colleagues [21] described application of discriminant analysis in a 1959 paper.

The cohort design (*see* **Cohort Study**) remains central to observational epidemiologic research, although elaborations of the design have been made to enhance feasibility while reducing costs. For example, large cohorts, like the Nurses' Health Study participants, have been followed primarily by using mailed questionnaires and matching against central registries to determine vital status. It has even been possible to obtain biologic specimens, including toenails for trace metal analysis and blood for DNA, using this approach. In the US, the NIH has taken the lead in establishing multicenter prospective cohort studies, particularly in the area of cardiovascular disease – for example, the Atherosclerosis Risk in Communities (ARIC) study, the Community Heart Study (CHS), and the Strong Heart Study of heart disease in Native Americans. These multisite studies gain external validity by drawing participants from communities across the US. Data collection is standardized and data are accumulated, evaluated and managed at central coordinating centers.

Opportunities for data linkage have now facilitated the conduct of cohort studies. Using record linkage approaches, lists of exposed individuals can be matched for outcome against death indexes and disease registries (*see* **Record Linkage**). Pioneering cohort studies based on this approach were conducted in Canada, where a mortality register of deaths back to 1950 has been available for matching and establishing vital status and cause of death [36]. The National Health and Nutrition Examination Survey (NHANES) conducted by the National Center for Health Statistics has been given a longitudinal component by linkage against death certificates and additional follow-up data collection [10].

The **case–control** design, discussed in detail elsewhere in this volume, is the other principal observational design for testing hypotheses and has also evolved over the same 50 years. Inherent limitations of this design have led some epidemiologists to consider it inferior to the cohort study [2, 17]. Information obtained by interview from cases and controls may be affected by bias; differential bias across cases and controls may create confusing patterns of association. The results of case–control studies conducted among persons selected through a particular institution, e.g. a hospital or clinic, may also be subject to selection bias [4]. Control selection may also be problematic [46] and design principles and feasibility may be in conflict.

There is now substantial understanding of these problems, however, and a methodologic foundation for the case–control design has been firmly established [1]. Cornfield [9] proposed the odds ratio as an estimate of the relative risk for case–control data and Mantel & Haenszel [29] described methods of stratified analyses in their 1959 paper: "Statistical aspects of the analysis of data from retrospective studies of disease". Miettinen further elaborated the underlying principles and analytic methods [33, 34] as did others [7, 42]. More generally, the links between cohort and case–control designs were noted and case-based sampling designs for cohort studies were proposed that unified the two approaches [26, 38].

The case–control design has proved effective for identifying strong causes of disease, such as smoking and lung cancer, diethylstilbestrol and adenocarcinoma of the vagina, and vinyl chloride and angiosarcoma of the liver. The design has been widely applied in research on the etiology of cancer, primarily by using population-based registries to identify cases and sampling to select representative controls. This design is conceptually equivalent to a case–control study nested within a cohort representing all residents of the registry's catchment area. One landmark study of this design addressed artificial sweeteners and bladder cancer; the study included 3010 cases and 5783 controls [23]. The case–control approach has now also been applied to assess screening and the risks and benefits of therapy.

The randomized trial, an experimental design, is widely held to be the gold standard of population studies. While experimental designs have been used to test therapeutic interventions for several centuries, the modern clinical trial originated in the twentieth century [27]. The use of randomization was advocated in the late 1940s by Austin Bradford Hill and applied in two seminal trials: a test of the pertussis vaccine and an assessment of the efficacy of streptomycin in treating tuberculosis [12]. The clinical trial has since rapidly evolved to include variations in the design and the development of multicenter approaches that make extremely large trials possible.

The core element is the random assignment of subjects to different therapeutic or preventive options. While randomization does not guarantee comparability of the study groups, it does eliminate the potential bias that may result from an investigator's preconceptions. Randomization makes it impossible to predict the assignment of the next person enrolled in the study. While in observational studies we will often match on variables that are known to influence outcomes, the advantage of randomization over matching is that randomization increases the likelihood of comparability of the groups even for factors that influence prognosis but of which we may be unaware or may be unable to measure. Ideally, randomized trials are conducted "blindly" – that is, the subject is unaware of which regimen he is receiving, and the physician or other health care provider does not know to which therapy the individual has been assigned. This is often accomplished by using a placebo, an inert material that looks and tastes like the active drug. At times, however, blinding may be difficult or impossible to implement, a problem that is most significant when the outcome being studied is a subjective one such as pain. In recent years considerable attention has focused on ethical issues pertaining to the use of placebos since using placebos may often involve not offering a currently available agent that is at least partially effective.

The randomized trial has most often been applied to clinical therapies, but has found increasing value for studying the benefits of community-wide interventions with public health measures.

The Specialization of Epidemiology

With the increasing complexity of epidemiologic research, epidemiologists and their areas of inquiry have become increasingly focused and specific. The bifurcation of the field into "infectious disease epidemiology" and "chronic disease epidemiology" no longer holds. The field has become multidimensional with cells defined by disease (e.g. cancer or heart disease), exposure (e.g. environment or nutrition), methods (e.g. genetic or molecular) and problem domain (clinical or outcome). Increasingly, genetics overlays all lines of inquiry, particularly those directed at disease etiology.

The core methods and principles are comparable across these areas of epidemiology, but each has its own special aspects. Of course, in each area there is a specific biomedical substrate, reflecting the exposures and outcomes of interest and the underlying biological phenomena. Additionally, methods for exposure and outcome assessment may be specific to an area. In studying occupation and health there are specific measurement methods for characterizing workplace exposures and the job itself may be used as an exposure surrogate, sometimes with the application of a job-by-exposure matrix [8]. Studies in the domain of genetic epidemiology use specific study designs, often family-based, and analytic methods that characterize patterns of association of disease risk with genetic markers. Other articles in this volume cover **clinical epidemiology**, **environmental epidemiology**, **genetic epidemiology**, **nutritional epidemiology**, **occupational epidemiology**, **pharmacoepidemiology** and **risk assessment**.

Epidemiology, Policy and Public Health

The direct linkage of epidemiologic evidence to making policy intended to advance public health is widely acknowledged. Almost universally, epidemiologists tell the story of John Snow and the Broad Street pump as an illustration of the immediacy of observational findings for solving public health problems. This example is particularly compelling because Snow demonstrated the waterborne transmission of cholera before there was knowledge of the existence of the *Vibrio cholerae* organism. There are numerous other examples, also considered as triumphs of epidemiologic inquiry: establishing cigarette smoking as a cause of lung cancer and other diseases, identifying powerful and remediable causes of cancer like asbestos exposure and diethylstilbestrol administration during pregnancy, and the characterization of risk factors for AIDS.

As a core discipline of biomedical research, epidemiology is not unique in generating evidence relevant to policy. After all, the ultimate goal of all biomedical research is to advance the health of people. Epidemiology, as a scientific method applied directly in the population context, brings evidence that directly bears on the health of the population and this direct linkage is what distinguishes epidemiology from other branches of biomedical research. As a consequence, epidemiologic findings generally have immediate relevance to setting policies pertinent to health and this relevance often gives prominence to epidemiologic evidence in the diverse processes by which policies are made. This prominence has occasioned targeted review and criticism of specific epidemiologic findings and of epidemiology generally. As epidemiologic research has addressed increasingly complex questions concerning the causes of disease, the risks of environmental factors and the benefits of interventions, the resulting evidence may be subject to uncertainties that cloud decision-making, leading some to question the utility of epidemiologic data.

The community of epidemiologic researchers is divided in its view of epidemiology and policy. At one extreme, some would consider epidemiology as being no different from other branches of science where the rationale for research is often given as advancing knowledge; at the other, epidemiologic research would be construed as justified only if the evidence were to be relevant to advancing public health. Epidemiologists are similarly divided in their view of the role of epidemiologists in policy-making processes. Some eschew such involvement and one respected journal, *Epidemiology*, does not allow authors to offer policy recommendations. Others have called for renewed

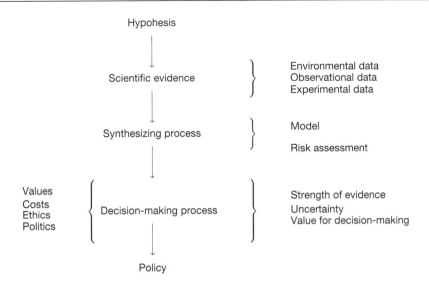

Hypohesis

↓

Scientific evidence } Environmental data
                        Observational data
                        Experimental data

↓

Synthesizing process } Model

                         Risk assessment

↓

Values
Costs   } Decision-making process } Strength of evidence
Ethics   Uncertainty
Politics   Value for decision-making

↓

Policy

Figure 1 Science/policy interface

Table 1 Some pathways and examples for translation of epidemiologic evidence into policy

Regulatory
• Occupational health and safety
• Environmental quality
• Drug safety

Public health recommendations
• Vaccination
• Diet
• Smoking

Legal system
• Causation of injury

Health care delivery
• Practice guidelines
• Outcome assessment

activism by epidemiologists and engagement with the sweeping social problems that underlie many of the increased risks that epidemiologists have elegantly and repetitively described [37, 45]. Even as debate continues, the use of epidemiology for policy purposes is burgeoning with the rise of the outcomes movement and calls for evidence-based medicine, and the need to apply the explosively expanding knowledge of the human genome in clinical and population contexts.

The paths and processes leading from hypothesis to policy are diverse and often lengthy and ill-defined (see Figure 1 and Table 1). In the area of infectious diseases, findings may lead quickly to action; John Snow acted immediately in response to his own findings on the waterborne transmission of cholera. Continuing in this tradition, investigators addressing infectious disease problems make policy recommendations more often than investigators working in other areas [24]. For some areas of inquiry, evidence may accumulate slowly, e.g. diet and cancer, and only reach a level of certainty sufficient for policy-making after decades of research. Of course, research and policy-making are interactive and iterative, and policies may change as evidence evolves.

Some of the routes for translating epidemiologic and other data into policy are listed in Table 1. They range from formal and structured, as in the requirements of specific regulations, to informal and unstructured, as in the choices that individuals take for their own lifestyles. For example, the 1996 draft cancer policy guidelines of the US Environmental Protection Agency [51] offer instruction for evaluating and interpreting epidemiologic data. Criteria for causality have been rigorously applied in the reports of the Surgeon General on smoking and health [49, 50]. Gail [19] traced the application of these criteria to the evidence on smoking and lung cancer and showed their utility for organizing the relevant lines of evidence and making certain that alternatives to the causal hypothesis could be satisfactorily addressed. Specific actions

Table 2 Some processes for translation of epidemiologic evidence into policy

Application of causal criteria
   Expert opinion
   Consensus methods
   Committee review
   Quantitative synthesis
   Risk assessment
   Jury evaluation

may be invoked if the evidence reaches a threshold of certainty, e.g. a causal association is found or a target level of risk is reached. Embedded within these translation routes are processes for identifying and evaluating the relevant evidence (Table 2).

New tools for conducting epidemiologic research, together with the increasing capacity to manage and analyze large databases, have made epidemiologic evidence more informative for answering policymaker's questions. Large administrative databases, such as the Health Care Financing Administration's Medicare files, can be explored to test hypotheses with immediate policy relevance – outcome of myocardial infarction in relation to hospital volume [47] and patterns of care by race and gender [22, 35], for example. Increasingly powerful multivariable methods for data analysis can detect policy-relevant patterns of association with the confidence that the associations are not spurious, while new models for longitudinal data analysis facilitate the capacity to describe disease and its development in time [48].

For many policy issues, the evidence comes from numerous and sometimes heterogeneous studies. Synthesis of such data for policy purposes has often been accomplished by expert review and consensus, tabular summary, or the application of criteria for causality. These processes have proved effective, particularly for strong associations, but uncertainties in the evidence have undermined conclusions, particularly if conclusions weighted by policy are reached. An example is the epidemiologic evidence on passive smoking, which has been the scientific basis for programs to reduce smoking in public places and repeatedly questioned by the tobacco industry and its consultant scientists. Combining evidence from multiple studies, whether experimental or observational, has proved to be an efficacious approach for synthesis. This combination can be accomplished by meta-analysis, combining summary estimates from individual studies, and pooled analysis, analyzing data jointly from individual

participants in multiple studies (*see* **Meta-Analysis in Epidemiology**). While the use of meta-analysis has been questioned [3], properly conducted meta-analyses have yielded useful and sometimes unexpected findings [5]. Pooled analysis is a more powerful approach, offering the possibility of controlling, confounding and exploring effect modification at the individual level, but requiring the effort of creating the pooled data set for analysis. The array of alternative approaches for synthesis, ranging from expert opinion to quantitative summary, has not been rigorously evaluated, but more recent approaches, involving a systematic evaluation and quantitative summary of data, seem preferable.

Summary

The twentieth century has seen a remarkable evolution of epidemiology and also of biostatistics, the companion quantitative science of public health and medicine. Epidemiology has moved from being a problem-solving approach used in the field to a core scientific method of biomedical research. As scientific questions around the public's health have become more complex, the field of epidemiology has itself become more complex with speciation into subareas defined by exposures, outcomes, and the methods and domains of inquiry. Evidence forthcoming from epidemiologic research is given weight in policy development for health care and public health, attesting to the immediacy and relevance of epidemiologic data.

References

[1]   Armenian, H. & Lilienfeld, D.E. (1994). Overview and historical perspective, *Epidemiologic Reviews* **16**, 1–5.

[2]   Austin, H., Hill, H.A., Flanders, W.D. & Greenberg, R.S. (1994). Limitations in the application of case–control methodology, *Epidemiologic Reviews* **16**, 65–76.

[3]   Bailar, J.C., III. (1997). The promise and problems of meta-analysis, *New England Journal of Medicine* **337**, 559–561.

[4]   Berkson, J. (1946). Limitations of the application of fourfold table analysis to hospital data, *Biometrics* **2**, 47–53.

[5]   Berlin, J.A. & Colditz, G.A. (1999). The role of meta-analysis in the regulatory process for foods, drugs, and devices, *Journal of the American Medical Association* **281**, 841–844.

[6]   Bernstein, P.L. (1996). *Against the Gods. The Remarkable Story of Risk*. Wiley, New York.

[7] Breslow, N.E. & Day, N.E. (1980). *Statistical Methods in Cancer Research*. International Agency for Research on Cancer, Lyon.

[8] Checkoway, H., Pearce, N.E. & Crawford, D.J. (1989). *Research Methods in Occupational Epidemiology*. Oxford University Press, New York.

[9] Cornfield, J. (1951). A method of estimating comparative rates from clinical data. Applications to cancer of the lung, breast, and cervix, *Journal of the National Cancer Institute* 1269–1275.

[10] Cox, C.S., Rothwell, S.T. & Madans, J.H. et al. (1992). Plan and operation of the NHANES I Epidemiologic Follow-up Study, 1987. National Center for Health Statistics, *Vital and Health Statistics* 27, 1–190.

[11] Dawber, T.R. (1980). *The Framingham Study. The Epidemiology of Atherosclerotic Disease*. Harvard University Press, Cambridge, Mass.

[12] Doll, R. (1992). Sir Austin Bradford Hill and the progress of medical science, *British Medical Journal* 305, 1521–1526.

[13] Doll, R. & Hill, A.B. (1954). The mortality of doctors in relation to their smoking habits. A preliminary report, *British Medical Journal* 1, 1451–1455.

[14] Evans, A.S. (1993). *Causation and Disease: A Chronological Journey*. Plenum Medical Books, New York.

[15] Eyler, J.M. (1978). The conceptual origins of William Farr's epidemiology: numerical methods and social thought in the 1830s, in *Times, Places, and Persons. Aspects of the History of Epidemiology*, A.M. Lilienfeld, ed. Johns Hopkins University Press, Baltimore, pp. 1–21.

[16] Fee, E. (1987). *Disease and Discovery. A History of the Johns Hopkins School of Hygiene and Public Health*. Johns Hopkins University Press, Baltimore.

[17] Feinstein, A.R. (1973). Clinical biostatistics. XX. The epidemiologic trohoc, the ablative risk ratio, and "retrospective" research, *Clinical Pharmacology and Therapeutics* 14, 291–307.

[18] Fletcher, R.H. (1996). *Clinical Epidemiology: The Essentials*. Williams & Wilkins, Baltimore.

[19] Gail, M.H. (1996). Statistics in action, *Journal of the American Statistical Association* 91, 1–13.

[20] Gordis, L. (1996). *Epidemiology*. W.B. Saunders, Philadelphia.

[21] Gordon, T., Moore, F.E., Shurtleff, D. & Dawber, T.R. (1959). Some methodologic problems in the long-term study of cardiovascular disease: observations on the Framingham study, *Journal of Chronic Diseases* 10, 186–206.

[22] Gornick, M.E., Eggers, P.W., Reilly, T.W., Mentnech, R.M., Fitterman, L.K., Kucken, L.E. & Vladeck, B.C. (1996). Effects of race and income on mortality and use of services among Medicare beneficiaries, *New England Journal of Medicine* 335, 791.

[23] Hoover, R.N. & Strasser, P.H. (1980). Artificial sweeteners and human bladder cancer preliminary results, *Lancet* 1, 837–840.

[24] Jackson, L.W., Lee, N.L. & Samet, J.M. (1999). Frequency of policy recommendations in epidemiologic publications, *American Journal of Public Health* 89, 1206–1211.

[25] Last, J.M. (1995). *A Dictionary of Epidemiology*. Oxford University Press, New York.

[26] Liddell, F.D.K., McDonald, J.C. & Thomas, D.C. (1977). Methods of cohort analysis: appraisal by application to asbestos mining, *Journal of the Royal Statistical Society* 140, 469–491.

[27] Lilienfeld, A.M. (1982). *Ceteris paribus*: the evolution of the clinical trial, *Bulletin of the History of Medicine* 56, 1–18.

[28] Lilienfeld, A.M. & Lilienfeld, D.E. (1980). *Foundations of Epidemiology, 2nd Ed*. Oxford University Press, New York.

[29] Mantel, N. & Haenszel, W. (1959). Statistical aspects of the analysis of data from retrospective studies of disease, *Journal of the National Cancer Institute* 22, 719–748.

[30] Maxcy, K.F. (1941). *The Papers of Wade Hampton Frost. A Contribution to the Epidemiological Method*. Commonwealth Fund, New York.

[31] Meinert, C.L. & Tonascia, S. (1986). *Controlled Clinical Trials: Design, Conduct, and Analysis*. Oxford University Press, New York.

[32] Middleton, J. (1999). The blues and pellagra: a public health detective story, *British Medical Journal* 319, 1209.

[33] Miettinen, O.S. (1970). Matching and design efficiency in retrospective studies, *American Journal of Epidemiology* 91, 111–118.

[34] Miettinen, O.S. (1985). The "case–control" study: valid selection of subjects, *Journal of Chronic Diseases* 38, 543–548.

[35] Mustard, C.A., Kaufert, P., Kozyrskyj, A. & Mayer, T. (1998). Sex differences in the use of health care services, *New England Journal of Medicine* 338, 1678–1683.

[36] Newcombe, H.B. (1988). *Handbook of Record Linkage: Methods for Health and Statistical Studies, Administration and Business*. Oxford University Press, Oxford.

[37] Pearce, N. (1996). Traditional epidemiology, modern epidemiology, and public health, *American Journal of Public Health* 86, 678–683.

[38] Prentice, R.L. (1986). A case–cohort design for epidemiologic cohort studies and disease prevention trials, *Biometrika* 73, 1–11.

[39] Rothman, K.J. & Greenland, S. (1998). *Modern Epidemiology*. Lippincott-Raven, Philadelphia.

[40] Sackett, D.L., Richardson, W.S., Rosenberg, W. & Haynes, R.B. (1997). *Evidence-Based Medicine. How to Practice and Teach EBM*. Churchill Livingstone, New York.

[41] Samet, J.M. & Muñoz, A. (1998). Evolution of the cohort study, *Epidemiologic Reviews* 20, 1–14.

[42] Schlesselman, J.J. (1982). *Case Control Studies*. Oxford University Press, New York.

[43] Schull, W.J. (1997). Brain damage among individuals exposed prenatally to ionizing radiation: a 1993 review, *Stem Cells* **15**, 129–133.

[44] Shephard, D.A.E. (1995). *John Snow. Anesthetist to a Queen and Epidemiologist to a Nation. A Biography.* York Point Publishing, Cornwall, Prince Edward Island, Canada.

[45] Shy, C.M. (1997). The failure of academic epidemiology: witness for the prosecution, *American Journal of Epidemiology* **145**, 479–484.

[46] Stolley, P.L. & Lasky, T. (1995). *Investigating Disease Patterns: The Science of Epidemiology.* W.H. Freeman, San Francisco.

[47] Thiemann, D.R., Coresh, J., Oetgen, W.J. & Powe, N.R. (1999). The association between hospital volume and survival after acute myocardial infarction in elderly patients, *New England Journal of Medicine* **340**, 1640–1648.

[48] Thomas, D. (1998). New techniques for the analysis of cohort studies, *Epidemiologic Reviews* **20**, 122–134.

[49] US Department of Health and Human Services (USDHHS) (1989). *Reducing the Health Consequences of Smoking. 25 Years of Progress. A Report of the Surgeon General.* US Government Printing Office, Washington.

[50] US Department of Health Education and Welfare (DHEW) (1964). *Smoking and Health. Report of the Advisory Committee to the Surgeon General,* DHEW Publication No. (PHS) 1103. US Government Printing Office, Washington.

[51] US Environmental Protection Agency (EPA) (1996). *Proposed Guidelines for Carcinogen Risk Assessment,* EPA/600/P-92/003C. Office of Research and Development, Washington.

[52] White, C. (1990). Research on smoking and lung cancer: a landmark in the history of chronic disease epidemiology, *Yale Journal of Biology and Medicine* **63**, 29–46.

Jonathan M. Samet & Leon Gordis

Epidemiology as Legal Evidence

In tort cases concerned with diseases resulting from exposure to a toxic chemical or drug, epidemiologic studies are used to assist courts in determining whether the disease of a particular person, typically the plaintiff, was a result of his or her exposure. This may seem puzzling to scientists, because whenever there is a natural or background rate of an illness one cannot be certain that its manifestation in a specific individual who was exposed to a toxic agent actually arose from that exposure. Indeed, the probability of causation in a specific individual is nonidentifiable [15]. The standard of proof courts utilize in civil cases, however, is the preponderance of the evidence or the "more likely than not" criterion. Thus, scientific evidence that a particular agent can cause a specific disease or set of related diseases in the general population supports an individual's claim that his or her disease came from their exposure. Conversely, scientific studies indicating no increased risk of a specific disease amongst exposed individuals are relied on by defendants, typically producers of the chemical or drug, to support the safety of their product. Similar questions of **causation** arise in cases alleging harm from exposure to hazardous wastes, although the issue in these cases is often whether the exposure was sufficient in magnitude and duration to cause the disease.

Epidemiologic studies are also used to determine eligibility for Workers' Compensation, where the issue is whether the employee's disease arose from exposure to an agent in the course of employment [5, p. 831], in regulatory hearings to determine safe exposure levels in the workplace (*see* **Occupational Health and Medicine**), and have even been submitted as evidence in criminal cases [4, p. 153]. We emphasize scientific evidence in tort law, which includes product liability and mass chemical exposure cases, because it is the major area of the law utilizing epidemiologic studies as evidence.

Tort Law

Tort law generally concerns suits for wrongful injury that do not arise from a contract between the parties. Thus, remedies to compensate for injuries from a wide variety of accidents resulting from someone's negligence, e.g. professional malpractice, assault and battery, environmentally induced injury, and fraud can be obtained by a successful plaintiff. Product liability is a special area of tort law dealing with the obligations of manufacturers of products to consumers who may suffer personal injury arising from the use of the product.

In any tort claim the plaintiff needs to establish a *prima facie* case by showing that the defendant has a legal duty of care due to the plaintiff and that the defendant breached that duty. In addition, a plaintiff needs to show that (i) she suffered an injury and that the defendant's failure to fulfill its duty of care was the (ii) factual and (iii) legal cause of the injury in question. The law also recognizes defenses that relieve the defendant of liability. The two most prominent ones in tort suits are contributory negligence by the plaintiff and statutes of limitations, which bar suits that are brought after a specified period of time has elapsed from either the time of the injury or the time when the relationship between the injury and the use of the product was known to the plaintiff [7]. In some jurisdictions, especially in Europe [10, p. 834], if the injury results from a defect arising from the product's compliance with a mandatory legal provision at the time it was put on the market, then the manufacturer is not liable. There are substantial differences between jurisdictions as to whether a plaintiff's contributory negligence totally absolves the defendant from liability, reduces it in proportion to the relative fault of the parties, or has no effect on the liability of a defendant whose contribution to the injury was small. In the US, the plaintiff's fault is rarely a complete bar to recovery when the defendant's negligence had a significant role. Similarly, the effective starting date of the limitations period varies among nations and among the states in the US.

When reading actual legal cases that rely on scientific evidence one needs to be aware of the relevant legal rules. For example, although the epidemiologic evidence linking the appearance of a rare form of vaginal cancer in a young woman to her mother's use of diethylstilbestrol during pregnancy is quite strong [1], some states barred plaintiffs from suing because the statute of limitations had expired. Since the cancers were recognized only when the young women passed puberty, typically in the late teens or early twenties, a number of injured women could not receive compensation. Other states, however, interpreted the limitations period as beginning at the time the plaintiff should have been aware of the connection. In Europe, the European Economic Community (EEC) directive of 1985 provides for a 10-year statute of limitations and allows plaintiffs to file claims within three years after discovering the relationship. Markesinis [10] summarizes the directive and the relevant English and German laws.

Epidemiologic evidence is most useful in resolving the issue of cause in fact, i.e. whether exposure to the product made by the manufacturer, or chemicals spilled onto one's land by a nearby company, can cause the injury suffered by the plaintiff. An alternate formulation of the factual cause issue is whether exposure increases the probability of contracting the disease in question to an appreciable degree. **Case–control studies** were used for this purpose in the litigation surrounding Rely and other highly absorbent tampons [5, p. 840]. Within a year or two after these products were introduced, the incidence of toxic shock syndrome (TSS) amongst women who were menstruating at the time of the illness began to rise sharply. Several studies, cited in Gastwirth [5, p. 918], indicated that the estimated **relative risk** of contracting the disease for users of these tampons was at least 10, which was statistically significant.

In light of the sharp decline in the incidence of TSS after the major brand, Rely, was taken off the market, the causal relationship seems well established and plaintiffs successfully used the studies to establish that their disease was most likely a result of using the product. When only one case–control study, however, indicates an association between exposure and a disease, courts are less receptive. Inskip [9] describes the problems that arose in a British case concerning radiation exposure of workers and leukemia in their children.

There is a rough rule relating the magnitude of the relative risk, R, of a disease related to exposure and the legal standard of preponderance of the evidence, i.e. at least half of the cases occurring amongst individuals exposed to the product in question should be attributable to exposure. As the **attributable risk** is $(R - 1)/R$, this is equivalent to requiring a relative risk of at least 2.0. While a substantial literature discusses this requirement (see [16, pp. 1050–1054], [5, Chapters 13 and 14], [20], and [2, pp. 167–170] for discussion and references), courts have been reluctant to adopt it formally, since it would allow the public to be exposed to agents with relative risks just below 2.0 without recourse. The lowest value of R accepted by a court the writer has seen is 1.5, in a case concerning the health effects of asbestos exposure. Courts usually require that the estimated R be statistically significantly greater than 1.0 and have required a confidence interval for R but also consider the role of other error rates [2, pp. 153–154]. When a decision must be based on sparse evidence, courts implicitly consider the power of a test and may not strictly adhere to significance at the 0.05 level.

The relative risk estimated from typical case–control studies is taken as an average for the overall population. Courts also consider the special circumstances of individual cases and have combined knowledge of the prior health of a plaintiff, the time sequence of the relevant events, the time and duration of exposure, as well as the **latent period** of the disease, with epidemiologic evidence to decide whether or not exposure was the legal cause of a particular plaintiff's disease.

So far, our discussion has dealt with the criteria for factual causality where an injury has already occurred. In some cases concerning exposure to a toxic chemical, plaintiffs have asked for medical monitoring, such as periodic individual exams or a follow-up study. As this is a new development, a specific minimal value of R has not been established.

In product liability law, a subclass of tort, in addition to negligence claims, sometimes one can assert that the manufacturer is subject to strict liability [11, 14]. In strict liability the test is whether the product is unreasonably dangerous, not whether the manufacturer exercised appropriate care in producing the product. Epidemiologic studies indicating a substantial increased risk of a disease can be used to demonstrate that the product is "unreasonably dangerous" from the viewpoint of the consumer.

Some product liability cases concern the manufacturer's duty to warn of dangers that were either known to the manufacturer or could reasonably have been foreseen at the time the product was marketed. In the US, producers are also expected to keep abreast of developments after the product is sold and to issue a warning and possibly recall the product if postmarketing studies show an increased risk of serious disease or injury.

One rationale underlying the duty to warn is informed consent [13, p. 209]. Because asbestos was linked to lung cancer by a major study [19] published in the 1960s, the plaintiff in *Borel vs. Fibreboard Paper Products Corp.*, 493 F. 2d 1076 (5th Cir. 1973) prevailed on his warning claim. The opinion observed that a duty to warn arises whenever a reasonable person would want to be informed of the risk in order to decide whether to be exposed to it.

The time when the risk is known or knowable to the manufacturer is relevant. In *Young vs. Key Pharmaceuticals*, 922 P.2d 59 (Wash. 1996) the plaintiff alleged that the defendant should have warned about the risk of seizure from the drug given him for asthma. The firm argued that the studies existing in 1979, when the child was injured, were not clinically reliable. Even though subsequent research confirmed those early studies that suggested an increased risk, the court found that the defendant did not have a duty to warn in 1979.

The reverse situation may have occurred in the *Wells* case, 788 F.2d 741 (11th Cir. 1986). At the time the mother of the plaintiff used the spermicide made by the defendant, two studies had shown an increased risk of limb defects and the court found the firm liable for failing to warn. Subsequent studies, which still may not be definitive, did not confirm the earlier ones, and in a later case the defendant was found not to be liable. While this seems inconsistent from a scientific point of view, from a legal perspective both decisions may be reasonable because the information available at the two times differed.

Government Regulation

Epidemiologic studies are used by regulatory agencies such as the Food and Drug Administration (FDA) and Occupational Safety and Health Administration (OSHA) to get manufacturers to recall harmful products or give an appropriate warning. Indeed, the manufacturer of Rely tampons recalled the product after the fourth case–control study linked it to TSS. More recently, case–control studies supported a warning campaign.

In 1982, after a fourth study indicated an association between aspirin use and Reye's syndrome, the FDA proposed a warning label on aspirin containers. The industry challenged the original studies, and the Office of Management and Budget (OMB) asked the FDA [12, 18] to wait for another study. The industry suggested that caretakers of cases would be under stress and might guess aspirin, especially if they had heard of an association, so two new control groups (children hospitalized for other reasons and children who went to an emergency room) were included in the follow-up study [21]. The **odds ratios** (OR) for cases compared with each of these two control groups were about 50, far exceeding those of the school (OR = 9.5) and neighborhood controls (OR = 12.6).

In late 1984 the government, aware of these results, asked for a voluntary warning campaign; a warning was mandatory as of June 1986. The following are the Reye's syndrome cases and fatalities from 1978 to 1989: 1978 (236, 68); 1979 (389, 124); 1980 (555, 128); 1981 (297, 89); 1982 (213, 75); 1983 (198, 61); 1984 (204, 53); 1985 (93, 29); 1986

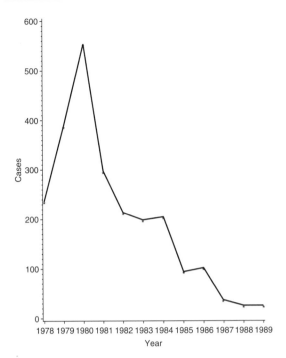

Figure 1 The number of cases of Reye's syndrome for the years 1978–1989

(101, 27); 1987 (36, 10); 1988 (25, 11); 1989 (25, 11). The cases are graphed in Figure 1. Notice the sharp decline between 1983–84 and 1985–86, reflecting the effect of the warning campaign.

Criteria for Admissibility of Studies as Evidence

Courts are concerned with the reliability of scientific evidence, especially as it is believed that lay people may give substantial weight to scientific evidence. In the US, the *Daubert* decision, 113 US 2786 (1993), set forth criteria that courts may use to screen scientific evidence before it goes to a jury. The case concerned whether a drug, Bendectin, prescribed for morning sickness caused birth defects, especially in the limbs. Related cases and the studies are described at length in Green [8]. The *Daubert* decision replaced the *Frye* 293 F. 1013 (DC Cir. 1923) standard, which stated that the methodology used by an expert should be "generally accepted" in the field by the criteria in the Federal Rules of Evidence. The court gave the trial judge a gatekeeping role to ensure

that scientific evidence is reliable. Now judges may examine the methodology used and inquire as to whether experts are basing their testimony on peer reviewed studies and methods of analysis before admitting the evidence at trial.

The US Supreme Court decision in *Daubert* remanded the case for reconsideration under the new guidelines for scientific evidence. The lower court, 43 F. 3d (9th Cir. 1995), decided that the expert's testimony did not satisfy the *Daubert* guidelines for admissibility in part because the plaintiff's expert never submitted the meta-analysis of several studies, which was claimed to indicate an increased relative risk, for peer review. Similarly, in *Rosen vs. Ciba-Geigy*, 78 F.3d 316 (7th Cir. 1996), the court excluded expert testimony that a man's smoking while wearing a nicotine patch for three days caused a heart attack. The appeals court said that the expert's opinion lacked the scientific support required by *Daubert* because no study supported the alleged link between short-term use of the patch and heart disease caused by a sudden nicotine overdose. The *Rosen* opinion notes that the trial judge is not to do science but to ensure that when scientists testify in court they adhere to the same standards of intellectual rigor they use in their professional work. If they do so and their evidence is relevant to an issue in the case, then their testimony is admissible, even though the methods used are not yet accepted as canonical in their branch of science.

The basic features of *Daubert* were reinforced and extended by the US Supreme Court in *General Electric Co. vs. Joiner*, 5 22 US 136 (1997) and *Kumho Tire vs. Carmichael*, 119 S. Ct. 1167 (1997). *Joiner* concerned the potential effect of exposure to polychlorinated biphenyls (PCBs) and the development of small-cell lung cancer in a worker with a family history of lung cancer who had smoked for eight years. The trial court, 864 F. Supp. 1310 (N.D. Ga. 1994), did not accept the opinions of the plaintiff's experts as scientific, but the Court of Appeals reversed applying a "stringent standard of review". The Supreme Court reinstated the original decision of the trial judge noting that admissibility of scientific evidence should be reviewed under the usual "abuse of discretion" standard. After discussing the original studies and four epidemiologic studies mentioned by the plaintiff's experts the Court observed that a trial judge "may conclude that there is simply too great an analytical gap between the data and the opinion proferred".

In the *Kumho* case the US Supreme Court extended the trial court's duty to ensure that expert evidence is relevant and reliable before it is admitted as testimony based on technical or specialized knowledge.

Medical Monitoring

Traditionally, courts have awarded damages to plaintiffs only when a physical injury occurs. Recently, individuals exposed to agents increasing one's risk of a serious illness, e.g. cancer, in the future have sued for the cost of periodic medical monitoring. The US Supreme Court in *Metro-North Commuter R.R. vs. Buckley*, 117 S. Ct. 2113 (1997) did not allow ordinary tort law liability with its lump-sum remedy to apply to asbestos-exposed workers under the federal law covering railroad employees. The opinion left open alternative "more finely tailored" medical cost recovery rules.

Subsequently, the Louisiana Supreme Court in *Bourgeois vs. A.P. Green Ind.*, 716 So 2d 355 (La. 1998), did allow asymptomatic plaintiffs who had been exposed to asbestos to often periodic medical exams through a judicially supervised fund. The opinion stated seven criteria plaintiffs need to satisfy. Epidemiologic evidence is relevant to demonstrating the following ones:

1. The plaintiff must show significant exposure to a proven hazardous substance.
2. As a result of this exposure the plaintiff suffers a significantly increased risk of contracting a serious latent disease.
3. The plaintiff's risk of the serious disease is greater than that of the general public.

References

[1]   Apfel, R.J. & Fisher, S.M. (1984). *To Do No Harm; DES and the Dilemmas of Modern Medicine*. Yale University Press, New Haven.

[2]   Bailey, L.A., Gordis, L. & Green, M. (1994). Reference guide on epidemiology, in *Reference Manual on Scientific Evidence*. Federal Judicial Center, Washington, pp. 122–178.

[3]   Ferguson, P.R. (1996). *Drug Injuries and the Pursuit of Compensation*. Sweet and Maxwell, London.

[4]   Finkelstein, M.O. & Levin, B. (1990). *Statistics for Lawyers*. Springer-Verlag, New York.

[5]   Gastwirth, J.L. (1988). *Statistical Reasoning in Law and Public Policy*. Academic Press, San Diego,

[6]   Gastwirth, J.L. (1999). Suggestions for reconciling the values of statistical science with the goals and needs of the legal and regulatory processes, *Proceedings of the Section on Epidemiology at the 1998 Meeting of the American Statistical Association*.

[7]   Green, M.D. (1988). The paradox of statutes of limitations in toxic substances litigation, *California Law Review* **76**, 965–1014.

[8]   Green, M.D. (1996). *Bendectin and Birth Defects*. University of Pennsylvania Press, Philadelphia.

[9]   Inskip, H.M. (1996). Reay and Hope *versus* British Nuclear Fuels plc: issues faced when a research project formed the basis of litigation, *Journal of the Royal Statistical Society, Series A* **159**, 41–47.

[10] Markesinis, B. (1994). *German Tort Law*, 3rd Ed. Clarendon Press, Oxford.

[11] Markesinis, B. & Deakin, S.F. (1994). *Tort Law*, 3rd Ed. Clarendon Press, Oxford.

[12] Novick, J. (1987). Use of epidemiological studies to prove legal causation: asprin and Reye's syndrome, a case in point, *Tort and Insurance Law Journal* **23**, 536–557.

[13] Phillips, J.J. (1988). *Products Liability*, 3rd Ed. West, St Paul.

[14] Robertson, D.W., Powers, W. Jr & Anderson, D.A. (1988). *Cases and Materials on Torts*. West, St Paul.

[15] Robins, J. & Greenland, S. (1989). The probability of causation under a stochastic model for individual risk *Biometrics* **45**, 1125–1138.

[16] Rubinfeld, D.L. (1985). Econometrics in the courtroom, *Columbia Law Review* **85**, 1048–1097.

[17] Sanders, J. & Kaye, D.H. (1997). Expert advice on silicone implants: *Hall vs. Baxter Healthcare, Inc., Jurimetrics* **37**, 113–128.

[18] Schwartz, T.M. (1988). The role of federal safety regulations in products liability actions, *Vanderbilt Law Review* **41**, 1121–1169.

[19] Selikoff, I.J., Hammond, E.C. & Churg, J. (1964). Asbestos exposure, smoking and neoplasia, *Journal of the American Medical Association* **188**, 22–26.

[20] Thompson, M.M. (1992). Causal inference in epidemiology: implications for toxic tort litigation, *North Carolina Law Review* **71**, 247–291.

[21] US Public Health Service (1985). Public health service study on Reye's syndrome and medications, *New England Journal of Medicine* **313**, 847–849.

[22] Wagner, W.E. (1997). Choosing ignorance in the manufacture of toxic products, *Cornell Law Review* **82**, 773–855.

[23] Wolf, E.S. (1998). A selective bibliography: standards for admissibility of scientific evidence, *The Record* **53**, 201–212.

JOSEPH L. GASTWIRTH

Error-Prone Predictor *see* Measurement Error in Epidemiologic Studies

Etiologic Fraction *see* Attributable Risk

Evidentiary Populations *see* Target Population

Excess Fraction; Excess Incidence *see* Attributable Risk

Excess Mortality

In the modeling of mortality in clinical or epidemiologic studies, it is sometimes relevant to use the mortality of the general population as a reference for comparisons. Rather than establishing a reference sample of the general population from which the study sample is drawn, one usually relies on published life tables and includes the population mortality rate as a known function in the model for the survival times in the study group. Two classes of hazard rate models have been studied in some detail: *multiplicative hazard rate* models, in which the mortality of the study group is described by multiplying the reference rate by some parameter, *the relative mortality*, which may further depend on specific risk factors or follow-up time; and additive hazard rate *models*, in which the reference rate is modified by adding a parameter, *the excess mortality*, which again may depend on specific risk factors or follow-up time. Multiplicative models are related to calculation of *standardized mortality ratios* (SMR), a technique that has been employed by epidemiologists for many years (*see* **Standardization Methods**).

However, additive models may be viewed as the theoretical basis for calculation of *relative survival* and the *corrected survival curve*.

In a simple additive hazard rate model, the mortality rate $\lambda_i(t)$ of an individual i, $i = 1, \ldots, n$, in the sample satisfies

$$\lambda_i(t) = \mu_i(t) + \gamma(t),$$

where $\mu_i(t)$ is the *known* population rate at time t for an individual of the same sex and born in the same year as individual i. The excess mortality $\gamma(t)$ is assumed common for all individuals in the sample. The integrated excess mortality is defined as

$$\Gamma(t) = \int_0^t \gamma(u) \mathrm{d}u.$$

Unlike the multiplicative model, which is mainly a descriptive means for relating the observed mortality in a sample to population mortality rates, the additive model may be given an interpretation in a **competing risk** framework when the excess mortality rate is positive. If the sample consists of individuals suffering from a given disease, one may consider using the population mortality rate for all other causes of deaths as the known rate $\mu_i(t)$ and the excess rate $\gamma(t)$ will then represent mortality due to the disease. In this situation, the model may therefore permit estimation of *cause-specific mortality* without relying on information about cause of death.

For a sample of individuals $i = 1, \ldots, n$, let x_i denote the time of entry and $X_i \geq x_t$ the survival time (in which case $D_i = 1$) or censoring time (in which case $D_i = 0$). In a clinical setting the time t would usually be time since treatment and x_i is typically zero, but the model could also be used with age as the underlying time scale and then left truncation, i.e. $x_i > 0$, will often be present. Define $N(t)$ to be the observed number of deaths in $[0, t]$ and let $Y(t)$ denote the number at risk at time t:

$$Y(t) = \sum_{i=1}^n Y_i(t) = \sum_{i=1}^n I(x_i < t \leq X_i).$$

Following Andersen & Væth [2], the integrated excess mortality may be estimated by

$$\hat{\Gamma}(t) = \sum_{X_i \leq t} \frac{D_i}{Y(X_i)} - \int_0^t \mu^*(u) \mathrm{d}u.$$

The first term is the ordinary Nelson–Aalen estimate, and the second term is the integral of the average population mortality rate, $\mu^*(u)$, defined for each u as the average of the population mortality rates corresponding to the individuals at risk at time u

$$\mu^*(u) = \frac{1}{Y(u)} \sum_{i=1}^{n} \mu_i(u) Y_t(u).$$

The variance of $\hat{\Gamma}(t)$ can be estimated by

$$\sum_{X_i \leq t} \frac{D_i}{[Y(X_i)]^2}$$

An estimate of the excess mortality rate $\gamma(t)$ can be obtained by kernel smoothing techniques (see, for example, Andersen et al. [3, Section IV.4.2]). The survival function

$$S^*(t) = \exp\left(-\int_0^t \mu^*(u)\mathrm{d}u\right)$$

derived from the hazard rate $\mu^*(t)$ may be viewed as a continuous time generalization of the so-called Ederer Method II for calculation of the *expected survival curve*, which, unlike Ederer Method I, adjusts for deaths and censoring during follow-up (see [7] or [11]). Furthermore, an estimate of the "survival" function

$$\exp\left(-\int_0^t \gamma(u)\mathrm{d}u\right)$$

for the excess mortality is obtained as the *relative survival function* $\hat{S}(t)/S^*(t)$.

A *parametric* version of the simple additive hazard rate model above has been studied by Buckley [5], who considered maximum likelihood estimation in a model *with piecewise constant excess mortality rate*. An iterative procedure is required to solve the likelihood equations, but simple, explicit moment estimates are also available. For the special case with a constant excess mortality rate γ for all $t \in [0, \tau]$, $\tau < \infty$ denoting an upper limit for the observed survival times, one may show [2, 5] that the maximum likelihood estimate is the solution to

$$\sum_{i=1}^{n} \frac{D_i}{\hat{\gamma} + \mu_i(X_i)} = T(\tau),$$

where

$$T(\tau) = \int_0^\tau Y(u)\mathrm{d}u = \sum_{i=1}^{n}(X_i - x_i)$$

is the total number of *person–years at risk* during follow-up (i.e. the total time on test). The moment estimate is simply

$$\tilde{\gamma} = \frac{N(\tau) - E(\tau)}{T(\tau)},$$

where

$$E(\tau) = \sum_{i=1}^{n} \int_0^\tau \mu_i(u) Y_i(u)\mathrm{d}u$$

may be interpreted as the expected number of deaths during follow-up, and the moment estimate is therefore the excess number of deaths divided by the total time at risk. The variance of the estimate $\tilde{\gamma}$ can be estimated by

$$\frac{N(\tau)}{[T(\tau)]^2}.$$

Within the framework of parametric models, standard large-sample methods provide goodness of fit tests for the constant excess mortality model relative to a piecewise constant excess mortality. Alternatively, generalized *total time on test procedures* are available for assessing the goodness of fit of a constant excess mortality rate (see [2] and [3, Section VI.3.2–3]).

Both parametric and nonparametric regression models generalizing the simple, additive excess mortality model have been developed. The parametric models for the excess mortality rate include, among others, loglinear regression models studied by Pocock et al. [9] and Hakulinen & Tenkanen [8], and a linear regression model considered by Campbell [6]. A semiparametric **proportional hazards** regression model for the excess rate has been proposed and studied by Sasieni [10], and Zahl [12] has introduced a linear nonparametric regression model for the excess rate, generalizing Aalen's linear hazard regression model [1]. Finally, one may group the time scale(s) and the risk factors and represent the data as a multidimensional table of number of deaths and person-years at risk. Additive hazard rate models and more general regression models can than be analyzed within the framework of **Poisson regression** (see, for example, Breslow & Day [4, Chapter 4]).

References

[1]   Aalen, O.O. (1989). A linear regression model for the analysis of life times, *Statistics in Medicine* **8**, 907–925.

[2]   Andersen, P.K. & Væth, M. (1989). Simple parametric and nonparametric models for excess and relative mortality, *Biometrics* **45**, 523–535.

[3]   Andersen, P.K., Borgan, Ø., Gill, R.D. & Keiding, N. (1993). *Statistical Models Based on Counting Processes.* Springer-Verlag, New York.

[4]   Breslow, N.E. & Day, N.E. (1987). *Statistical Methods in Cancer Research, Vol. II, The Design and Analysis of Cohort Studies.* International Agency for Research on Cancer, Lyon.

[5]   Buckley, J.D. (1984). Additive and multiplicative models for relative survival rates, *Biometrics* **40**, 51–62.

[6]   Campbell, M.J. (1985). Multiplicative and additive models with external controls in a cohort study of cancer mortality, *Statistics in Medicine* **4**, 353–360.

[7]   Ederer, F., Axtell, L.M. & Cutler, S.J. (1961). The relative survival rate: a statistical methodology, *National Cancer Institute Monographs* **6**, 101–121.

[8]   Hakulinen, T. & Tenkanen, L. (1987). Regression analysis of relative survival rates, *Applied Statistics* **36**, 309–317.

[9]   Pocock, S.J., Gore, S.M. & Kerr, G.R. (1982). Long term survival analysis: the curability of breast cancer, *Statistics in Medicine* **1**, 93–104.

[10] Sasieni, P.D. (1996). Proportional excess hazards, *Biometrika* **83**, 127–141.

[11] Zahl, P.H. (1995). A proportional regression model for 20 year survival of colon cancer in Norway, *Statistics in Medicine* **14**, 1249–1261.

[12] Zahl, P.H. (1996). A linear non-parametric regression model for the excess intensity, *Scandinavian Journal of Statistics* **23**, 353–364.

(*See also* **Survival Analysis, Overview**)

MICHAEL VÆTH

Excess Relative Risk

Relative risks are commonly used to describe the relationship between the **risks** or rates in different populations. For populations with risks R_0 and R_1, the relative risk is $RR = R_1/R_0$. In many situations, it is useful to describe R_1 as $R_0 + E$, where E is the excess risk. In this case we have $RR = (R_0 + E)/R_0 = 1 + ERR$, where ERR represents the excess relative risk. The most commonly used approach to modeling relative risks involves loglinear models of the form $RR = e^{\beta z}$. But it is often useful, especially in **dose–response** analyses, to model the ERR directly.

When exposures vary over a broad range, simple ERR models (e.g. linear in dose) can provide a clearer, and in many cases better, description of the exposure effect on the risk than loglinear risk models. Ratios of ERRs are more appropriate than ratios of RRs as a summary of the impact of exposure. **Effect modification** and analyses of the joint effects of multiple exposures (*see* **Synergy of Exposure Effects**) are often expressed more naturally in terms of effects on the ERR rather than as **interactions** in **multiplicative** relative risk models. For additional details about specific ERR models and issues related to the use of these models (*See* **Poisson Regression for Survival Data in Epidemiology**).

DALE PRESTON

Excess Risk

The excess risk or rate in a population is the difference between the **risk** (rate) R_1 for a population exposed to some risk factor (e.g. radiation or smoking) and the risk R_0 in an otherwise identical population without the exposure. In simple terms the excess risk E is defined as $E = R_1 - R_0$. The excess risk is closely related to the **attributable risk** $AR = E/R_1$ and the **excess relative risk** $ERR = E/R_0$.

Since excess risk models involve the sum of background and excess risks, they are intrinsically additive, and it is common, though potentially confusing, to refer to them as **additive models**. The development of adequate excess risk models generally requires that the risk be modeled as a sum of nonlinear functions describing the background and excess risks. Models for both the background and excess risks often involve multiplicative functions of risk-modifying factors. In contrast to **relative risk models**, for which it is possible to use semiparametric **Cox regression models**, fitting excess risk models generally requires explicit parametric modeling of R_0 or specification of R_0 with external rates.

It is both feasible and useful, however, to model background rates directly for problems involving either excess or relative risk by using modern statistical methods, such as **Poisson regression**.

Relative risk models have come to dominate discussion of risk in epidemiologic studies. However, description in terms of excess risks and rates is important for: understanding the impact of an exposure on risk in a population; developing exposure standards to limit risks to the general public or to special groups; and developing and assessing mechanistic models of the effect of exposure on risk.

Historically, attention has focused on the comparison of simple (usually time-constant) excess and relative risk models [3]. However, when one makes use of more general classes of excess and relative risk models, it is best to view these models as complementary, rather than competing, descriptions of risk.

Excess risk and attributable risk can also be estimated from **population-based case–control studies** [1, 2].

References

[1]   Benichou, J. (1991). Methods of adjustment for estimating the attributable risk in case–control studies: a review, *Statistics in Medicine* **10**, 1753–1773.

[2]   Benichou, J. & Wacholder, S. (1994). A comparison of three approaches to estimate exposure-specific incidence rates from population-based case-control studies, *Statistics in Medicine* **13**, 651–661.

[3]   Breslow, N.E. & Day, N.E. (1987). *Statistical Methods in Cancer Research*. Vol. II. *The Design and Analysis of Cohort Studies*. IARC Scientific Publication No. 82, Oxford University Press, New York.

DALE PRESTON

Expected Number of Deaths

Several procedures are available if the mortality in a study group is to be compared with the mortality of the general population from which the sample is drawn. In a clinical setting calculation of an *expected survival curve* is often performed, and in epidemiologic studies of geographic or occupational variations of mortality the observed number of deaths is usually compared with *the expected number of deaths* based on published mortality rates for the general population. Calculation of expected number of deaths is an integral part of the **standardization** of vital rates, which is one of the oldest statistical techniques; see Keiding [10] for a review of early

applications of the method. Standardization of rates is closely related to **multiplicative** *hazard rate models* and the use of *relative mortality* to describe deviations from the expected mortality (see, for example, Breslow [5], Breslow & Day [6] or Hoem [9]).

Two methods have been developed for the calculation of expected number of deaths. The classical approach, *the person-years method*, is derived as a sum of products of age- and sex-specific rates and the corresponding time at risk, whereas *the prospective method* involves calculation of a sum of conditional survival probabilities. For a further description the following setup is introduced.

Consider a sample of n independent individuals. Individual i is followed from time u_i to time t_i if death does not occur prior to t_i. Let T_i denote the time of death and define $X_i = \min(t_i, T_i)$. The mortality rate at time t, assuming that the individual is subject to the same risks as a person from the external reference population having the same demographic description, is denoted $\lambda_i(t)$. The corresponding survival function is denoted $S_i(t)$. The reference population is usually taken to be the general population, and the mortality rate and the survival function may be determined from published data taking into account the sex, date of birth, and age at entry of the person.

Set D_i to 1 if death occurs during follow-up and to 0 otherwise, i.e. $D_i = I(u_i < T_i \le t_i)$. The observed number of deaths is then $D = \sum D_i$. Introduce

$$A_i = \int_{u_i}^{X_i} \lambda_i(s)\mathrm{d}s,$$

and let $A = \sum A_i$ denote the *total exposure to death*. The probability of dying during follow-up is obtained as

$$p_i = \frac{S_i(u_i) - S(t_i)}{S_i(u_i)}.$$

It is easily seen that $\mathrm{E}(D_i | T_i > u_i) = p_i$. Moreover, one may show (see, for example Breslow [4] or Berry [2]) that also $\mathrm{E}(A_i | T_i > u_i) = p_i$.

These results suggest two different ways of calculating the expected number of deaths, $\mathrm{E}(D)$, on the assumptions that mortality in the study group is identical to that of the reference population.

The prospective method [8, 11] utilizes the relationship $\mathrm{E}(D) = \sum p_i$ directly; the expected number of deaths is simply obtained as $\sum p_i$. Note, however, that the potential follow-up time, t_i, must be known for *all* individuals in order to compute the expected number of deaths by this method. Such knowledge is not available for many censoring schemes, and this requirement therefore severely limits the applicability of the prospective method.

Deviations from the expected number of deaths may be assessed by computing

$$X_P^2 = \frac{\left(D - \sum p_i\right)^2}{V},$$

where $V = \sum \mathrm{var}(D_i) = \sum p_i(1 - p_i)$. The distribution of the test statistic is approximately a chi-square distribution on one degree of freedom.

The **person-years** method (see, for example, Case & Lea [7] or Berry [2]) relies on the relationship $E(A) = \sum p_i$, which shows that A is an unbiased estimate of the expected number of deaths on the hypothesis that the mortality in the study group is identical to that of the reference population. The total exposure to death, A, is therefore used as *an estimate* of the expected number of deaths. Usually the distinction between "total exposure to death" and "expected number of deaths" is not done and the random variable A simply denotes the expected number of deaths. Note, however, that for extended follow-up of old individuals the contribution A_i to the total exposure to death may exceed 1. Consequently, one may encounter situations where the expected number of deaths is larger than the number of individuals in the sample (see Smith [12] for one such example) suggesting that this terminology is misleading. Note, moreover, that A is not an unbiased estimate of the expected number of deaths if the mortality in the sample differs from that of the reference population. The size of the bias has been studied by Keiding & Væth [11] within the framework of the multiplicative hazard rate model.

With this method the hypothesis of no difference between observed and expected number of deaths may be tested by computing

$$X_{PY}^2 = \frac{(D - A)^2}{A}.$$

On the null hypothesis the distribution of the test statistic is approximately a χ^2 distribution on one degree of freedom. Calculations of asymptotic relative efficiency by Anderson & Anderson [1] indicate that the person-years method is more efficient than the prospective method for **proportional hazards** alternatives and that the efficiency gain increases as the proportion of individuals dying during follow-up goes up.

The person-year method is easily adapted to studies of cause-specific mortality (*see* **Competing Risks**). The total mortality rate in the reference population is simply replaced by the relevant cause-specific mortality rate and deaths from other causes are treated as censoring. This solution is not applicable for the prospective method as it would require knowledge of when an individual who dies of the cause in question would have died from one of the other causes. One may instead extend the above model by introducing cause-specific mortality probabilities for each individual taking all causes of mortality into account. Interpretation of deviations from the expected number of deaths is, however, complicated by the fact that excess death for one cause will necessarily imply a deficit for some of the other causes [12].

In application of the person-years method one usually assumes that the mortality rate $\lambda_i(t)$ is constant in one-year (or five-year) intervals, and the contribution A_i is then the sum of products of the age-specific rates and the time spent in the corresponding age category during follow-up. Interchanging the order of summation one obtains the standard formula for the expected number of deaths, $A = \sum \lambda_{as} Y_{as}$, where λ_{as} is the sex- and age-specific mortality rate of the reference population and Y_{as} is the total person-years at risk in the corresponding sex and age category. From this formulation it is seen that D/A is the *standardized mortality ratio* (SMR) (see, for example, Breslow and Day [6, Chapter 2]), which is used extensively in the analysis of epidemiologic data on occupational hazards for comparing mortality in a study population with mortality in a standard population (*see* **Standardization Methods**).

The classical approach of indirect standardization and calculation of a SMR follows from a simple, multiplicative model relating the mortality rate $\lambda_i(t)$ of an individual in the study population to the known mortality rate $\lambda_i^*(t)$ for the reference population

$$\lambda_i = \theta \lambda_i^*(t).$$

For this model one may show [3] that the standardized mortality ratio, D/A, is the maximum likelihood estimate of the relative mortality θ and that the test statistic, X_{PY}^2, given above is a score test for testing the hypothesis $\theta = 1$. The simple, multiplicative model has been developed further to deal with regression problems using **proportional hazards** regression models of the form

$$\lambda_i(t; \mathbf{z}_i) = \exp(\beta' \mathbf{z}_i) \lambda_i^*(t),$$

where $\mathbf{z}_i$ is a vector of independent variables and β the corresponding vector of regression parameters. With grouped data such models are often referred to as **Poisson regression** models (see, for example, Berry [2] or Breslow & Day [6, Chapter 4]).

References

[1]   Anderson, J.R. & Anderson, K.M. (1984). Letter to the editor re Hartz et al. (1983), *Statistics in Medicine* **4**, 107–108.
[2]   Berry, G. (1983). The analysis of mortality by the subject-year method, *Biometrics* **39**, 173–184.
[3]   Breslow, N.E. (1975). Analysis of survival data under the proportional hazards model, *International Statistical Review* **43**, 45–58.
[4]   Breslow, N.E. (1978). The proportional hazards model: applications in epidemiology, *Communications in Statistics – Theory and Methods* **7**, 315–332.
[5]   Breslow, N.E. (1985). Cohort analysis in epidemiology, in *A Celebration of Statistics: The ISI Centenary Volume*, A.C. Atkinson & S.E. Fienberg, eds. Springer-Verlag, Heidelberg, pp. 109–143.
[6]   Breslow, N.E. & Day, N.E. (1987). *Statistical Methods in Cancer Research*. Vol. II. *The Design and Analysis of Cohort Studies*. International Agency for Research on Cancer, Lyon.
[7]   Case, R.M. & Lea, A.J. (1955). Mustard gas poisoning, chronic bronchitis and lung cancer, *British Journal of Preventive and Social Medicine* **9**, 62–72.
[8]   Hartz, A.J., Giefer, E.E. & Hoffmann, R.G. (1983). A comparison of two methods for calculating expected mortality, *Statistics in Medicine* **2**, 381–386.
[9]   Hoem, J.M. (1987). Statistical analysis of a multiplicative model and its application to the standardization of vital rates: a review, *International Statistical Review* **55**, 119–152.
[10]   Keiding, N. (1987). The method of expected number of deaths, 1786–1886–1986, *International Statistical Review* **55**, 1–20.
[11]   Keiding, N. & Væth, M. (1986). Calculating expected mortality, *Statistics in Medicine* **5**, 327–334.
[12]   Smith, P.G. (1984). Letter to the editor re Hartz et al. (1983), *Statistics in Medicine* **3**, 301.

(*See also* **Cohort Study**; **Occupational Epidemiology**; **Survival Analysis, Overview**)

MICHAEL VÆTH

Expected Survival Curve *see* Excess Mortality

Experimental Study

An experimental study is a study in which conditions are controlled and manipulated by the experimenter. For example, in a comparative clinical trial the method of assigning treatments to subjects is determined by the investigator. Often, randomized treatment assignment is employed to assure that the innumerable potential **confounding** factors not controlled by the experimental design have similar distributions in the various treatment groups. Special design features are used to improve the efficiency of an experimental study, including **stratification**, **matching**, and factorial experiments to study several treatments simultaneously. Experimental studies afford good opportunities to reduce the possibility of confounding, to obtain good measurements on various factors that might influence outcomes (*see* **Effect Modification**), to avoid **biases** in measuring outcomes, and to limit the obfuscating impact of other controllable factors that influence outcomes.

An experimental study is distinguished from an **observational study** in which the investigator does not control the treatment or exposure assignment, nor many other aspects of the process under study. An observational study is thus more subject to problems of confounding, **measurement error**, and bias than an experimental study, but many of these issues must also be carefully considered and controlled in the design, conduct, and interpretation of experimental studies.

(*See also* **Bias from Nonresponse**; **Bias in Observational Studies**)

M.H. GAIL

Exposure Effect

An exposure effect is a quantitative measure of the impact of exposure on an outcome measure.

Estimates of exposure effects are derived by contrasting the outcomes in an exposed population with outcomes in an unexposed population or in a population with a different level of exposure. **Relative risk, excess risk**, and **relative odds** are examples of exposure effects used in connection with dichotomous outcomes, whereas **relative hazards** are used to characterize exposure effects when the outcome is time-to-response or the event rate per **person–year** exposure time. Mean differences are often used to characterize exposure effects for quantitative outcomes.

When regression models are used, exposure effects correspond to model parameters. For example, consider a model with multiple linear regression $\beta_0 + \beta_1 E + \beta_2 X$, where E indicates a level of exposure and X some other factors influencing outcome. The exposure effect, β_1, measures the effect on outcome of a unit increase in exposure, with other factors, X, held constant. If E only takes on values 1 for exposed and 0 for unexposed, β_1 is the adjusted mean difference between exposed and unexposed; and if, in addition, the outcome is dichotomous, β_1 is the adjusted risk difference. If the effect of exposure depends on levels of another factor, say X_1, an **interaction** term involving $X_1 E$ is needed in the previous regression. Then no single number characterizes the exposure effect, and **effect modification** is said to occur.

In the theory of **causation**, each individual or study unit is hypothesized to have two responses, the response if exposed and the response if unexposed. Only one such response is observed on each individual, but hypothesized individual-level effects can be defined, such as the difference in responses the individual would have if exposed and if unexposed. In the context of this "counterfactual" theory of causal effects, the exposure effects described in the previous paragraph can be regarded as summary measures of individual-level causal exposure effects.

(*See also* **Cox Regression Model**; **Logistic Regression**; **Poisson Regression**; **Relative Risk Modeling**)

M.H. GAIL

External Validity *see* Validity and Generalizability in Epidemiologic Studies

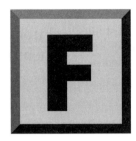

Failure-Time Analysis *see* Survival Analysis, Overview

Fixed Cohort *see* Fixed Population

Fixed Population

A fixed population or fixed cohort is a group of individuals defined by a common fixed characteristic, such as all men in the US born in 1941. Membership in a fixed population does not change over time by immigration or emigration, unlike a **dynamic population**, although members of a fixed cohort may experience the health event under study, or may die or be lost to follow-up.

M.H. Gail

Follow-Up Bias *see* Bias from Loss to Follow-Up

Force of Infection *see* Communicable Diseases

Force of Mortality *see* Hazard Rate

Fraction of Etiology *see* Attributable Risk

Frailty Selection *see* Biased Sampling of Cohorts in Epidemiology

Frequency Matching

Frequency matching, also known as category matching, is a sampling design used in **case–control studies** that yields **controls** with the same distribution over categories defining levels of potential **confounders** as is observed in the cases. For example, suppose that cases are classified into 20 categories defined by gender and by ten ten-year age intervals, and that the distribution of cases in these categories is observed. A frequency-matched sample of controls with this same distribution could be obtained by sampling as controls a constant multiple of the number of cases in each category. Sometimes, for convenience, one obtains frequency-matched controls that conform to the expected distribution of cases rather than wait to match the on actual distribution of cases.

Frequency matching is also used in **cohort studies** to assure that the control cohort has the same distribution over categorical levels of potential confounders as the exposed cohort.

(*See also* **Matching**)

M.H. GAIL

Functional Modeling *see* Measurement Error in Epidemiologic Studies

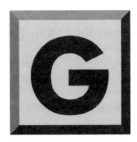

Geary–Moran Statistics *see* Clustering

General Epidemic *see* Epidemic Models, Stochastic

Generalizability *see* Validity and Generalizability in Epidemiologic Studies

Generalized Impact Fraction *see* Attributable Risk

GENESYS Sampling Systems and Survey Sampling Inc. *see* Random Digit Dialing Sampling for Case–Control Studies

Genetic Epidemiology, Overview

By 1967 discussions among researchers had led to the realization that the merger of methods to analyze family data from mathematical genetics and statistical tools from epidemiology was both inevitable and desirable [9]. This merger was designated *genetic epidemiology*, for which Morton [9] proposed the following definition:

> genetic epidemiology: A science that deals with etiology, distribution, and control of disease in groups of relatives and with inherited causes of disease in populations.

The formal definition of the new field followed two decades of discussion dating back to Neel & Schull [10] defining "epidemiological genetics" in 1954. This dynamic time period saw the emergence of genetic epidemiology from the broader field of population genetics and the synthesis of several parallel developments in mathematics and statistics as they applied to human disease. But to understand the role of this relatively new field, its impact on human genetics, and its evolving definition in the post Human Genome Project era, it is necessary to review its history.

In the beginning, genetics was "genetic epidemiology". By stating the observation that an offspring receives one of two factors from each parent and has a 50% chance of passing each factor to its offspring,

Gregor Mendel defined the probabilities that set the mathematical and statistical tone for the broad scientific discipline called genetics.

Mendel's original work also set the stage for the three characteristics that provide the cultural milieu for genetic epidemiology. First, scientists ignored Mendel's seminal discovery for nearly 50 years. The mathematical proofs, computational details, and statistical arguments required by genetic epidemiology leave most geneticists bored and/or frightened, preferring to ignore genetic epidemiology. Secondly, the question of whether Mendel's results were "too good" [5], foretold a field that relishes controversy over methods, interpretations, and applications. Such "family fights" prove stimulating to the investigators involved but have had the tendency to convince other geneticists that the field lacks focus and rigor. And finally, until very recently genetic epidemiology was a small field easily dominated by a few creative and powerful figures whose scientific differences and personal animosity made for exciting and stimulating arguments and intense scientific fads.

As genetics developed at the turn of the century, the research was concentrated in two areas:

1. defining phenotypes, which for humans is clinical genetics, at that time including rudimentary biochemical genetics; and
2. studying the mathematical properties of genes in populations, population genetics.

By the 1930s cytogenetics (the study of chromosomes) was flourishing, primarily in *Drosophila*, and has continued to develop as a major area of research. And most recently the field of molecular genetics has exploded in a wealth of research and knowledge leading to the initiation of the Human Genome Project in 1989.

Genetic epidemiology shares the use of mathematics and statistics as its primary tools with the field of population genetics, but its definition of a unique niche within genetics results from its interaction with all of the other areas. The history will be divided into three broad and, to some extent, overlapping categories:

1. population genetics;
2. Mendel's first law: segregation of alleles at one locus; and
3. Mendel's second law: independent assortment of two loci.

The Beginning (1): Population Genetics

The seminal beginning to population genetics was the definition of the Hardy-Weinberg Law in 1908. In 1932 Snyder [13] applied this law to demonstrate the mode of inheritance for tasting phenylthiocarbamide (PTC). Snyder not only provided a clear example of the appropriateness of the Hardy–Weinberg equilibrium for the human population but also demonstrated a mathematical method for testing that a phenotype was inherited. This was both useful and restricted by the fact that is was limited to traits sufficiently common to allow random sampling of a large number of families. This restriction of population genetic principles to common traits has limited their usefulness until recently.

Another significant issue addressed by early population genetic principles was the role of Mendelian factors in the inheritance of quantitative traits. Early investigators argued that segregating alleles could not possibly account for quantitative traits with Gaussian distributions. In 1918 Fisher [4] demonstrated conclusively that "many small, equal, and additive loci" would result in exactly the Gaussian distribution for a phenotype. From that finding grew the entire field of quantitative genetics, including heritability, breeding factors, and other crucial insights for plant and animal breeders. Eventually these quantitative genetic principles also contributed to our understanding of human inheritance.

Population genetics research continued to develop in several areas relevant to studies in genetic epidemiology, including describing the structure of populations. The principal distinction for these areas is that they apply to all populations and traits, thus providing insight for the study of human disease but are not restricted to the study of specific disease etiology.

The Beginning (2): Mendel's First Law

A second early and significant area of research developed to address statistical issues arising from the use of family data. Mendel began with pure breeding parents and tested the F1, F2, and backcross data. For human diseases that are *rare* in the population, the approach is to ascertain families where the disease is *known* to exist thereby avoiding a huge random sample which might capture little or no information.

However, the use of ascertainment introduces immediate bias into the sample, as recognized as early as 1912 by Weinberg [14]. Although numerous investigators have proposed solutions to this problem, it continues as a serious concern for genetic epidemiologists to this day.

Data were analyzed for the presence of genes using the Weinberg and a priori forms of ascertainment correction until 1958 when Morton [8] proposed a likelihood approach to segregation analysis. The use of likelihood scoring to estimate parameters permitted incorporation of an ascertainment probability, proportion of sporadic cases, and other concepts of interest. It also provided a direct estimate of the penetrance and a likelihood ratio test for whether it differed from 1.0. The likelihood model much more closely approximated reality than the simpler approaches and was fairly widely applied.

By the 1960s, sufficient numbers of genetic loci had been identified in humans to establish a need for other forms of statistical analysis. For example, the procedure for paternity exclusion was refined and applied both scientifically and in legal situations. Interest developed in models specifying the relationship among family members. Methods originally developed by the brilliant but not oft published Charles Cotterman [11] brought binary numbers and matrix algebra to the forefront. An elegant modeling system, path analysis, incorporated the relationships among relatives and the possibility of environmental factors in order to determine the etiology of more complex traits. Models were developed to utilize twin data as special cases in an attempt to estimate more rigorously the importance of environmental factors.

Also during the 1960s quantitative genetics made its presence felt in human genetics. Falconer [3] introduced the idea of a normally distributed, quantitative trait as the "liability" or "susceptibility" for a genetic disorder. This underlying trait was polygenic in nature, conforming to the work of Fisher cited above. When environmental factors were known to influence the trait, such as birth order effects, the model was called multifactorial to include both polygenic genetic effects and the environment. The disorder, however, was dichotomous in phenotype, such as the presence or absence of a birth defect, and the underlying quantitative trait led to the phenotype through theoretical "thresholds", leading to the multifactorial threshold (MF/T) models. This breakthrough in thinking was followed by a burst

of research and what amounted to a fad in genetic epidemiology, as every trait of unknown etiology was shown to be inherited in a multifactorial fashion. The bubble burst in 1972 when Reich et al. [12] pointed out the simple statistical fact that the model was indeterminate unless there were at least two thresholds. Fortunately for many human phenotypes, e.g. birth defects, the presence of at least two thresholds was a simple matter since the frequency of the disorder differed markedly in the two sexes.

The popularity of the multifactorial models helped genetic epidemiologists realize that many of the diseases and disorders of interest would have much more complex etiologies than single locus inheritance. But few if any traits survived a rigorous test of MF/T. The popularity of the MF/T model declined and was replaced by the concept of genetic heterogeneity.

The realization that etiologies were complex dictated the development of more mathematically sophisticated models and statistical tests. For example, until the development of the "mixed model", the presence of single locus inheritance and the presence of multifactorial inheritance were tested as separate hypotheses that did not contain the same parameter space, that of an overarching general model, and so were not *true* alternative hypotheses. The "mixed model" was so named because it defined that necessary general model and led directly to the more rigorous testing of the possible modes of inheritance.

A split had developed in the field, however, and a serious controversy raged over the question of whether to use nuclear family data (parents and their offspring) or larger extended pedigrees for testing genetic hypotheses. As with the other previous disputes, the field experienced a surge forward as models were developed both for nuclear families and for extended pedigrees. There were two primary developments in the area of pedigree analysis. First the publication of the Elston–Stewart algorithm [2] provided an efficient, recursive mathematical approach to evaluating the likelihood over an extended family. Its importance to all of genetics was recognized with the presentation of the William Allan Award by the American Society of Human Genetics to Elston in 1996. (The first William Allan Award was presented in 1962 to Newton Morton for segregation analysis and the introduction of lod scores to linkage analysis.) The second development was the introduction of *transmission probabilities*. The use of these parameters expanded the ability to test genetic models to determine whether they fit the data best while remaining within the constraints of Mendel's first law. Which form of data to use, nuclear families or pedigrees, was resolved methodologically by a reformulation of both approaches to incorporate the parameters of the other and the definition of a single "complex segregation" analysis approach.

Two additional major developments were to occur in the arena of Mendel's first law. The first of these was the introduction, through a series of papers, of regressive models by Bonney and his colleagues. These models, the most complex to date, incorporate numerous **confounding** factors, such a cohort effects (*see* **Age–Period–Cohort Analysis**). However, by virtue of their complexity and the number of parameters involved, they require huge data sets and are often applied in more restricted forms.

The second remaining development was the merger of segregation analysis with linkage analysis, but first it is necessary to discuss linkage analysis itself.

The Beginning (3): Mendel's Second Law

The phenomenon of linkage, i.e. the violation of the independent assortment of Mendel's second law, was first studied extensively in experimental organisms, primarily *Drosophila* and mouse. The concepts of linkage groups, recombination frequency, genetic distance, and mapping functions were all observed, defined, and/or analyzed throughout the first half of this century. Linkage has proven to be a powerful genetic tool. In spite of this power, very little was done in humans before 1950 because so few marker loci existed. The first linkage in humans was demonstrated by Mohr [6] in 1954. About this time, however, the use of new laboratory techniques to identify genes (for example, electrophoresis) began and is still going on with the molecular biology revolution.

The breakthrough in human linkage studies required not only the means to develop marker loci but also the statistical tools to analyze the data. Studies with experimental organisms are done by using fixed mating schemes and counting the recombinants in the offspring. For humans the two restricting factors were unknown phase (which of the two marker alleles was on the chromosome with the disease allele) of the parents and the small family size. To overcome these obstacles the data had to be pooled, but pooling matings of opposite phase

would result in apparent independent assortment. Therefore each small family had to be analyzed and *then* pooled. By extending the principles of sequential sampling, Morton [7] defined lod scores for linkage analysis in humans. Over the course of the past 40 years untold numbers of lod scores have been calculated – at the beginning by hand [7] and later by a plethora of computer algorithms.

The observation that insulin dependent diabetes mellitus (IDDM) type 1 showed a strong association with alleles of the human leukocyte antigen (HLA) system on chromosome 6 defined a new situation for linkage analysis. The question debated extensively was whether this association represented linkage disequilibrium between HLA markers and an IDDM locus or a susceptibility role for the HLA alleles. The problem was further complicated by the nature of the HLA multi-locus region which contained numerous haplotypes in disequilibrium. If IDDM were solely genetic, then reduced penetrance would have to be invoked when analyzing unaffected individuals. This problem stimulated the development of methods to detect linkage that were directed towards using only affected individuals. Recent publications have independently demonstrated that the "model-free" methods can be considered as subsets of the model-based methods and by doing so have raised a set of statistical questions for genetic epidemiologists to resolve regarding application and interpretation of the different methods.

The rapid explosion in the development of the human genome linkage map led to the necessity for methods that could analyze multiple loci simultaneously. These methods provide additional precision in determining the actual location of purported disease loci.

Likelihood models were derived for simultaneously estimating the segregation parameters and the linkage relationships for a disease locus (loci). More recently, alternative approaches of using linkage information alone to determine the mode of inheritance have been proposed.

In the End. . .

In summary, it is important to emphasize three points. First it is impossible in any overview to include all of the important factors that contributed to the development of a scientific discipline. Therefore, this discussion slighted some developments and emphasized others. The second point is to restate the long-term goal of genetic epidemiology: to understand the causes of genetic disease in humans. To this end, the research efforts must be translated into terms that can be discussed with patients in families at risk and that leads to the formulation of the next set of research questions. Neither of these end points is simple to derive from the often convoluted results of analyzing complex disorders in less-than-ideal data.

And finally, the field of genetic epidemiology has been responsive to the need for interaction and the exchange of ideas. The journal *Genetic Epidemiology* was established in 1984 and the International Genetic Epidemiology Society was founded in 1991, adopting the journal as its official publication. The depth of methodological disagreements and their effect on the genetic community led directly to the establishment of the Genetic Analysis Workshop (GAW) series, the most recent being GAW 10 in 1996 [1]. These workshops provide a unique atmosphere where methods are compared and evaluated in a controlled workshop format.

The next challenge for the field of genetic epidemiology is to develop new approaches to utilize the vast amounts of information that will become available as the human genome is sequenced and to apply these techniques to the most common and complex of disorders rigorously and imaginatively.

References

[1] Bailey-Wilson, J.E., Borecki, I.B., Falk, C.T., Goldstein, A.M., Suarez, B.K. & MacCluer, J.W. (1997). Proceedings of Genetic Analysis Workshop 10, *Genetic Epidemiology* **14**, to appear.

[2] Elston, R.C. & Stewart, J. (1971). A general model for the genetic analysis of pedigree data, *Human Heredity* **21**, 523–542.

[3] Falconer, D.S. (1965). The inheritance of liability of certain diseases, estimates from the incidence among relatives, *Annals of Human Genetics* **29**, 51–76.

[4] Fisher, R.A. (1918). The correlation between relatives on the supposition of Mendelian inheritance, *Transactions of the Royal Society of Edinburgh* **52**, 399–433.

[5] Fisher, R.A. (1936). Has Mendel's work been rediscovered?, *Annals of Science* **1**, 115–137.

[6] Mohr, J. (1954). *A study of Linkage in Man*. Munkegaard, Copenhagen.

[7] Morton, N.E. (1955). Sequential tests for the detection of linkage, *American Journal of Human Genetics* **7**, 277–318.

[8] Morton, N.E. (1958). Segregation analysis in human genetics, *Science* **127**, 79–80.

[9] Morton, N.E. (1982). *Outline of Genetic Epidemiology*. Karger, New York.

[10] Neel, J.V. & Schull, W.J. (1954). *Human Heredity*. University of Chicago Press, Chicago.

[11] Optiz, J.S. (1983). Cotterman and combinatorial genetics, *American Journal of Medical Genetics* **16**, 389–392.

[12] Reich, T., James, S.W. & Morris, C.A. (1972). The use of multiple thresholds in determining the mode of transmission of semi-continuous traits, *Annals of Human Genetics* **36**, 163–184.

[13] Snyder, L.H. (1932). Studies in human inheritance. IX. The inheritance of taste deficiency in man, *The Ohio Journal of Science* **32**, 436–440.

[14] Weinberg, J. (1912). Weitere Beitrage zur Theorie der Vererbung. 4. Uber Methode und Feglerquellen der Untersuchung auf Mendelsche Zahlen beim Menschen, *Arch. Rass. U. Geg. Biol.* **9**, 165–174.

M.A. SPENCE

GENMOD *see* Synergy of Exposure Effects

Geographic Patterns of Disease

The study of geographic patterns of disease is part of the classic triad in **descriptive epidemiology** of "time, person, place". Here, place is used as a surrogate for the mix of lifestyle, environmental, and possibly genetic factors that may underly variations in rates of disease across populations. The purpose is both to *describe* such variations and to identify possible *causes* that could explain them.

Of course, apparent geographic variations in disease rates may be artifactual rather than real. Problems may occur either with the enumeration of cases (numerator) or with the population at risk (denominator), or both. Thus spurious geographic variations in disease could reflect differences between populations in case definition, completeness of ascertainment, diagnostic accuracy, and coding or (for mortality) survival rates. Enumeration of the population (e.g. at census) may be incomplete, or recent migration may distort population estimates. Great care is therefore required in interpretation. Despite these difficulties, publications such as *Cancer Incidence in Five Continents* [23], and international mortality statistics (*see* **Mortality, International Comparisons**) compiled by the World Health Organization, have provided an invaluable starting point for epidemiologic enquiry.

The analysis of geographic patterns of disease depends crucially on *scale*. Whereas broad-scale patterns may be apparent at an international level, for example, differences between developed and developing countries in the incidence of infectious diseases such as malaria, and in cardiovascular diseases [38], other patterns may only be apparent at a *local* level. These will include, for example, clusters of disease (*see* **Clustering**) and possible variations in disease risk near putative point sources of environmental pollution.

In this article we briefly discuss disease variations both at the broader and at the local (small-area) scale. We review issues involved in disease mapping (the usual means of presenting descriptive geographic data on disease occurrence) and discuss some of the problems associated with geographic **correlational studies (ecologic studies)**. Here the aim is to explore geographic variation in disease in terms of underlying spatially varying "risk factors". The emphasis is on small-area applications, where a number of recent advances in methodology have been made.

International Variations in Disease

International differences in disease occurrence may give important clues as to etiology, which may then be further studied in individual-level studies (e.g. cohort–control or case–control). Thus, in the Seven Countries Study, Keys [20] described large differences in population saturated fat intakes, which were predictive of population differences in the occurrence of coronary heart disease. The INTERSALT Study found cross-population differences in average blood pressure levels, and difference in blood pressure with age, that were associated positively with average levels of salt intake (measured by urinary sodium excretion); a similar positive relationship was also found at individual level [15]. Other examples include the incidence of malignant melanoma and multiple sclerosis, both of which are strongly related to latitude. While this relationship is inverse for melanoma (i.e. a tendency for higher rates near the equator, reflecting

greater exposure to sunlight [16]), it is positive for multiple sclerosis (i.e. low incidence in countries near the equator [21]).

Migrant Studies

Migrant studies represent a special case of geographic study. Here, the disease experience of individuals or groups of people is examined as they move from one location or country to another. This affords a unique opportunity to examine the extent to which environmental or genetic influences might determine geographic variations in disease risk. Whereas genetic factors are important in determining which *individuals* become sick, at the population level, overwhelmingly, environmental and lifestyle factors predominate [29]. Thus, in the case of multiple sclerosis, migrants moving from a high risk to a low risk area retain their higher risk if migrating after the age of around 15 years, but attain the risk of the host country if migrating at younger ages [21]. These findings are compatible with an infectious etiology of multiple sclerosis, with infection acquired in childhood. Another example is the low levels of blood pressure, with little or no rise with age, found among remote and isolated population groups around the world [15, 27]. Blood pressures are found to increase rapidly with migration to an urban environment [27], again indicating the overwhelming importance of environmental factors in determining the unfavorable blood pressure pattern among populations.

Local Variations in Disease

Variations in disease incidence or mortality at national [19] or subnational [17] level have been described, usually in the form of a disease atlas (see the section on *Disease Mapping*, below). Here we briefly address the occurrence of disease at the local (small-area) scale. Although in this context no satisfactory definition of the term "small area" exists, Cuzick & Elliott [9] suggest a working definition as follows:

> As a rough guide, any region containing fewer than about 20 cases of disease can be considered a small area ... Many cancers have annual incidence rates of around 5 per 100 000, so for a collective period of 5 years a small area constitutes a population of around 100 000 or fewer. In some instances, such as a cluster of disease in a remote area or small village,

it could be much less, but usually populations of at least 10 000 are needed to form an aggregation of minimal size.

Of course, populations could be much smaller if the disease experience over many such areas is of primary interest – for example, in small-area disease mapping (see next section).

Disease Clusters and Clustering

A problem commonly facing public health authorities is how to deal with reports of apparent disease excess in their locality (i.e. disease "clusters"; *see* **Clustering**). These reports may subsequently be linked to a putative pollution source. This complicates interpretation since, for post hoc enquires of this type, formal statistical testing is no longer valid. Although there is little potential for isolated cluster investigations to yield new information on the cause of disease, nonetheless the public health authorities often feel compelled to respond. A careful review of cases, and selection of an appropriate denominator and time frame, may result in risk estimates (observed/expected ratios) that are close to 1. This is despite the potential for **bias** towards elevated risk ratios (*see* **Relative Risk**) – areas at apparently "low" risk do not come to the attention of the authorities! In some instances, replication of the study in other similarly polluted areas (if such can be found), or in a different time period, may be the only feasible way forward. It can also be helpful to place an alleged "cluster" in a wider context by carrying out small-area disease mapping across a larger region (see [37] for a recent example).

An alternative approach to the study of a single disease cluster is to examine more generally for evidence of clustering. Such evidence for Hodgkin's disease has been cited in support of ideas of an infectious etiology [1], although other explanations, including artifacts related to diagnostic coding, population mobility, or variations in birth rates, are also possible [9].

Small-area Studies Near Sources of Environmental Pollution

Recently, high-resolution geographically referenced routine health data (*see* **Vital Statistics, Overview**) have become available in certain countries. Together with advances in computing and in statistical methodology, this has led to the development of largely automated systems to examine the distribution of disease near point sources of environmental pollution. In the UK, the Small Area Health Statistics Unit (SAHSU) has been established specifically to: respond rapidly to reports of disease excess ("clusters") near sources of environmental pollution; carry out studies of health statistics more generally around sources of pollution; carry out descriptive geographic studies at small-area level; and develop the methodology. Recent studies include an investigation of cancer incidence and mortality near a pesticide factory following media reports of excess cancers in the vicinity [37], and a national study of cancer incidence near radio and television transmitters [10] following reports of a leukemia excess near one of the transmitters [11].

A major problem in the interpretation of such studies is the issue of socioeconomic **confounding**. Measures of social deprivation (calculated from the census statistics) have been shown to be powerful predictors of the occurrence of disease [18], including stomach and lung cancer (though not leukemia). Deprived areas do not occur randomly throughout a region, but tend to coincide with industrial sites and correlate with higher smoking rates. Failure to account for social deprivation could thus seriously bias investigation of other lifestyle or environmental risk factors and ill-health. This is illustrated by results of a national study of cancer risk near municipal solid waste incinerators in Great Britain [14]. **Excess risk** was found for a number of cancer sites, including stomach and lung, that persisted after adjustment for deprivation at the small-area scale. However, in the areas with available data, a similar excess was found also for the period before the incinerators were operational. This indicated the presence of residual **confounding** that had not been fully accounted for in the statistical analysis [14].

Disease Mapping

Maps have long been used to describe geographic patterns of disease (*see* **Mapping Disease Patterns**). For example, Stocks, in a series of atlases published in the 1930s, described the geographic variation in cancer mortality across counties in England and Wales (reproduced in [34]). A survey in 1991 [36] identified 49 international, national, and regional disease atlases;

more recent examples include those by Swerdlow & dos Santos Silva [34] and Bernardinelli et al. [4]. Such maps typically show standardized mortality or incidence ratios (*see* **Standardization Methods**) for geographic areas such as countries, counties, or districts. The rate in area i is estimated by O_i/E_i, where O_i is the observed number of deaths or incident cases of disease in the area (assumed to follow an independent Poisson distribution) and E_i is the expected number of cases (calculated by applying age- and sex-specific death or disease rates to the census population counts for the area).

Maps convey instant visual information on the spatial distribution of disease and can identify subtle patterns which may be missed in tabular presentations. Their purpose is usually to display variations in ill-health (for example, related to the underlying sociodemography), formulate etiologic hypotheses, aid **surveillance** to detect areas of high disease incidence, and help place specific disease clusters and point source studies in proper context.

While disease maps have both visual and intuitive appeal, considerable caution is required to avoid overinterpretation. Apparent geographic variation in rates may simply reflect between-area differences in the quality of reporting, diagnosis, and classification of disease, or confounding due to ethnic and socioeconomic factors. Furthermore, disease maps implicitly assume that risk is homogeneous within areas. This is unlikely for the large areas used in many national and international atlases, and may result in misleading inference about individual-level risk.

There is currently considerable scientific interest in exploring more *local* geographic variations in disease. For example, in the UK, we have been carrying out small-area mapping at the level of electoral ward (average 5000 people) and census enumeration district (400 people).

Disease mapping at the small-area level raises a number of statistical issues. For relatively rare events such as death and cancer incidence, the observed numbers of cases tend to be small in areas with low population, and typically exhibit extra-Poisson sampling variation. This may be assessed formally using the Pothoff–Whittinghill test [26] (*see* **Clustering**). The sparseness of population data results in unreliable estimates of the area-specific standardized rate ratios, which may create the impression of spurious geographic variation when displayed on a map. These considerations have led to the use of statistical

smoothing techniques which pool information across areas. Empirical Bayes [7, 13] and hierarchical Bayes [6, 22] estimates of area-specific relative risk represent a compromise between the area-specific standardized rate ratios (*see* **Standardization Methods**) and the overall mean for the whole map.

Small-area disease data often exhibit spatial correlation due to the influence of unmeasured or unknown risk factors which themselves vary smoothly in space. Various hypothesis tests are available to assess such spatial autocorrelation – for example, the rank-adjacency D-statistic [19] and Smans' test [31].

Figure 1 shows a map of "unsmoothed" (standardized incidence ratio, adjusted for age, sex, and deprivation) and smoothed (empirical Bayes) estimates of brain cancer incidence for 1974–1986 across electoral wards in the West Midlands region of England [12]. As can be seen, much of the random variability is removed by smoothing, especially the apparent high rates found in the large, sparsely populated rural areas. Overall, there is only weak evidence of heterogeneity across the map (Potthoff–Whittinghill test; $p = 0.04$), and no evidence of spatial autocorrelation [12].

Bayesian prior distributions for the area-specific relative risks which allow smoothing towards a local mean, rather than the overall map mean, are also used to model spatial interdependence in small-area studies [6, 7, 22]. Implementation of Bayesian hierachical–spatial models has been made feasible by recent computational [32] and *software* developments, namely Bayesian inference using Gibbs sampling (BUGS) [33] - involving Markov chain Monte Carlo simulation algorithms: this approach represents the current state of the art in small-area mapping of disease.

Technical Issues Concerning Presentation of Geographic Disease Data

Maps provide a succinct summary of geographic patterns in disease. However, visual perception may be influenced by various features of the map, such as the plotting symbols used (e.g. solid shading vs. hatching, color vs. gray scale) and the grouping of data into categories (e.g. percentiles of the distribution of risk, and numerically equidistant cutpoints) [31]. An empirical study [35] found that the manner of data display may have at least as much effect on observer perception of spatial variation as actual differences

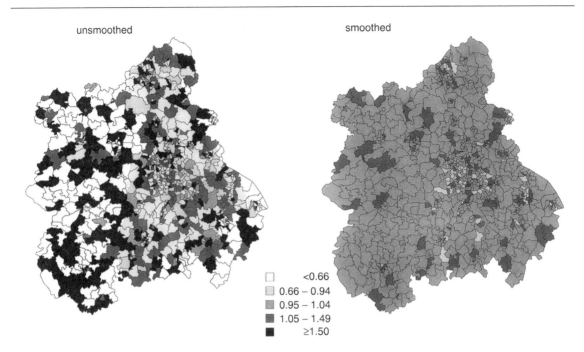

unsmoothed   smoothed

☐	<0.66
▨	0.66 – 0.94
▨	0.95 – 1.04
▨	1.05 – 1.49
■	≥1.50

Figure 1   Age-, sex-, and deprivation-adjusted relative risks of brain and central nervous system tumors for electoral wards in West Midlands region, England, age 15–64 years, 1974–1986. Unsmoothed risks (left) and after map smoothing (right) using empirical Bayes method. Reproduced from Eaton et al. [12] by permission of *British Journal of Cancer*

in the data. Recently, nonparametric mixture distributions have been used to model the underlying relative risk of disease in small geographic areas [30]. This approach facilitates more objective mapping of disease patterns, since areas are categorized according to statistically driven estimation of the mixture components.

The summary statistic used for presentation may also influence visual interpretation of disease maps. Common choices include standardized rate ratios, smoothed relative risks, or *P* values. The former tend to yield erratic maps which are visually dominated by extreme estimates of low precision in sparsely populated areas; the latter are criticized for confusing statistical significance with biological importance and tend to overemphasize areas of high population in which even small deviations from the expected disease rate may achieve statistical significance. Significance testing of standardized rate ratios also suffers from the multiple decision problem, as each ratio is considered independently of the others on the map.

In our view, maps showing Bayesian shrinkage estimates of relative risk represent the best compromise, although it is important to realize that

these estimates are not judgment-free. For example, they depend on the functions used to describe the distribution of relative risks across the map, and to define the local neighborhood over which spatial interdependence between the small areas is assumed. However, smoothing ensures that precision of the area-specific estimates is approximately comparable across the map, and Bayesian credible intervals are not subject to the constraints of multiple significance testing. Mapping of posterior functions of Bayesian risk estimates is also possible. For example, a map showing the posterior probability that the relative risk in each area ranks above the median [2] conveys information about the size *and* uncertainty associated with each area-specific estimate. Further advances in the application of Bayesian methods to disease mapping, and appropriate display methods, including measures of uncertainty, are to be expected.

Geographic Correlation Studies

Geographic correlation studies are a valuable means of formulating and testing etiologic hypotheses: disease patterns are compared with the geographic distribution of environmental and lifestyle exposures. They are particularly useful when individual-level measurements of exposure are either difficult or impossible to obtain for use in epidemiologic study (for example, air pollution) or are measured imprecisely (for example, diet, and sunlight exposure). (See [16] for further discussion and [28] for a review of the statistical methods.)

Examples of broad-scale **ecologic studies** are given in the section on *International Variations in Disease*. In some cases – for example, sunlight and melanoma, salt and blood pressure – the ecologic relationships have also been demonstrated at individual level. However, the potential for *bias* in such ecologic studies [16] should be recognized. Exposure *within* areas is often heterogeneous; thus the ecologic (average group-level) association between exposure and disease may not equate to the relationship in individuals. To assume otherwise is to commit the **ecologic fallacy** [24]. Small-area studies may be less prone than broad-scale geographic studies to ecologic bias since the group data are closer to the level of the individual. Nonetheless, positive findings arising from ecologic analyses usually require replication in other data sets and, where possible, at individual level.

As already noted, a major problem in small-area disease studies is the potential for confounding by socioeconomic variables. Adjustment may be made by including, say, a deprivation score such as the Carstairs [5] index (based on small-area census statistics) as a covariate in the ecologic regression analysis. Alternatively, indirect standardization of the expected small-area disease counts can be done by stratifying on the socioeconomic status of the areas as well as on age and sex (*see* **Stratification**). Modeling of spatial autocorrelation between small areas in an ecologic regression study also provides some control for the effect of confounding due to location [8], but further development of these methods is required, and in particular their application to "real" data sets.

Interest has focused on ecologic designs which combine data on the general population with individual-level survey data to improve estimation of group exposure [25]. Methods to adjust for random measurement error in exposure are also receiving attention [3]. Such techniques should enhance the ability of ecologic analyses to estimate the *size* of exposure–disease relationships, not merely to identify the possible presence of such associations.

Summary and Conclusions

The study of geographic patterns of disease plays a central role in descriptive epidemiology, and has led to some notable etiologic insights. However, geographic studies are associated with major problems of data quality, bias, confounding, and presentation which can seriously complicate their interpretation. The methodologic challenge is clear: to produce objective, statistically valid analyses of geographic variations in ill-health and its determinants, with particular emphasis on developments to combine the best features of individual-level and ecologic studies. Recent advances, particularly in methods for small-area studies, have begun to address these issues. As such techniques become routinely available, they should enhance our ability to quantify the effects of environmental pollution (*see* **Environmental Epidemiology**) and lifestyle characteristics on human health.

References

[1]   Alexander, F.E. (1990). Clustering and Hodgkin's disease, *British Journal of Cancer* **62**, 708–711.

[2]   Bernardinelli, L., Clayton, D.G. & Montomoli, C. (1995). Mapping disease risk: how important are priors?, *Statistics in Medicine* **14**, 2411–2431.

[3]   Bernardinelli, L., Pascutto, C., Best, N.G. & Gilks W.R. (1997). Disease mapping with errors in covariates, *Statistics in Medicine* **16**, 741–752.

[4]   Bernardinelli, L., Maida, A., Marinoni, A., Clayton, D.G., Romano, G., Montomoli, C., Fadda, D., Solinas, M.G., Castiglia, P., Cocco, P.L., Ghislandi, M., Berzuini, C., Pascutto, C., Nerini, M., Styles, B., Capocaccia, R., Lispi L. & Mallardo, E. (1994). *Atlas of Cancer Mortality in Sardinia, 1983–87*. FATMA-CNR.

[5]   Carstairs, V. & Morris, R. (1991). *Deprivation and Health in Scotland*. Aberdeen University Press, Aberdeen.

[6]   Clayton, D.G. & Bernardinelli, L. (1992). Bayesian methods for mapping disease risk, in *Geographical and Environmental Epidemiology: Methods for Small-Area Studies*, P. Elliott, J. Cuzick, D. English & R. Stern, eds. Oxford University Press, Oxford, pp. 205–220.

[7]   Clayton, D.G. & Kaldor, J. (1987). Empirical Bayes estimates of age-standardized relative risks for use in disease mapping, *Biometrics* **43**, 671–682.

[8]   Clayton, D.G., Bernardinelli, L. & Montomoli, C. (1993). Spatial correlation in ecological analysis, *International Journal of Epidemiology* **22**, 1193–1202.

[9]   Cuzick J. & Elliott, P. (1992). Small area studies: purpose and methods, in *Geographical and Environmental Epidemiology: Methods for Small-Area Studies*,

P. Elliott, J. Cuzick, D. English & R. Stern, eds. Oxford University Press, Oxford, pp. 14–21.

[10] Dolk, H., Elliott, P., Shaddick, G., Walls, P. & Thakrar, B. (1997). Cancer incidence near radio and television transmitters in Great Britain. II. All high power transmitters, *American Journal of Epidemiology* **145**, 10–17.

[11] Dolk, H., Shaddick, G., Walls, P., Grundy, C., Thakrar, B., Kleinschmidt, I. & Elliott, P. (1997). Cancer incidence near radio and television transmitters in Great Britain. I. Sutton Coldfield transmitter, *American Journal of Epidemiology* **145**, 1–9.

[12] Eaton, N., Shaddick, G., Dolk, H. & Elliott, P. (1997). Small-area study of the incidence of neoplasms of the brain and central nervous system among adults in the West Midlands Region, 1974–86, *British Journal of Cancer* **75**, 1080–1083.

[13] Efron, B. & Morris, C. (1975). Data analysis using Stein's estimation and its generalisation, *Journal of the American Statistical Association* **70**, 311–319.

[14] Elliott, P., Shaddick, G., Kleinschmidt, I., Jolley, D., Walls, P., Beresford, J. & Grundy, C. (1996). Cancer incidence near municipal solid waste incinerators in Great Britain, *British Journal of Cancer* **73**, 702–710.

[15] Elliott, P., Stamler, J., Nichols, R., Dyer, A.R., Stamler, R., Kesteloot, H. & Marmot, M. (1996). INTERSALT revisited: further analyses of 24 hour sodium excretion and blood pressure within and across populations, *British Medical Journal* **312**, 1249–1253.

[16] English, D. (1992). Geographical epidemiology and ecological studies, in *Geographical and Environmental Epidemiology: Methods for Small-Area studies*, P. Elliott, J. Cuzick, D. English & R. Stern, eds. Oxford University Press, Oxford, pp. 3–13.

[17] Gardner, M.J., Winter, P.D. & Barker, D.J.P. (1984). *Atlas of Mortality from Selected Diseases in England and Wales 1968–1978*. Wiley, Chichester.

[18] Jolley, D.J., Jarman, B. & Elliott, P. (1992). Socioeconomic confounding, in *Geographical and Environmental Epidemiology: Methods for Small-Area Studies*, P. Elliott, J. Cuzick, D. English & R. Stern, eds. Oxford University Press, Oxford, pp. 115–124.

[19] Kemp, I., Boyle, P., Smans, M. & Muir C. (1985). *Atlas of Cancer in Scotland, 1975–1980, Incidence and Epidemiologic Perspective*. IARC Scientific Publication No. 72, International Agency for Research on Cancer, Lyon.

[20] Keys, A., ed. (1970). *Coronary Heart Disease in Seven Countries*. American Heart Association Monograph no. 29. American Heart Association, New York.

[21] Kurtzke, J.F. (1985). Neurological system, in *Oxford Textbook of Public Health*, Vol. 4. Oxford University Press, Oxford, Chapter 12, pp. 203–249.

[22] Mollie, A. (1996). Bayesian mapping of disease, in *Markov Chain Monte Carlo in Practice*, W.R. Gilks, S. Richardson & D.J. Spiegelhalter, eds. Chapman & Hall, London, pp. 359–379.

[23] Muir, C., Waterhouse, J., Mack, T., Powell, J. & Whelan, S., eds. (1987). *Cancer Incidence in Five Continents*, Vol. V. IARC Scientific Publication No. 88, International Agency for Research on Cancer, Lyon.

[24] Piantadosi, S., Byar, D.P. & Green, S.B. (1988). The ecological fallacy, *American Journal of Epidemiology* **127**, 893–904.

[25] Plummer, M. & Clayton, D. (1996). Estimation of population exposure in ecological studies, *Journal of the Royal Statistical Society, Series B* **58**, 113–126.

[26] Pothoff R.F. & Whittinghill, M. (1966). Testing for homogeneity. II. The Poisson distribution, *Biometrika* **53**, 183–190.

[27] Poulter, N.R., Khaw, K.T., Hopwood, B.E.C., Mugambi, M., Peart, W.S., Rose, G. & Sever, P.S. (1990). The Kenyan Luo migration study: observations on the initiation of a rise in blood pressure, *British Medical Journal* **300**, 967–972.

[28] Richardson, S. (1992). Statistical methods for geographical correlation studies, in *Geographical and Environmental Epidemiology: Methods for Small-Area Studies*, P. Elliott, J. Cuzick, D. English & R. Stern, eds. Oxford University Press, Oxford, pp. 181–204.

[29] Rose, G. (1985). Sick individuals, sick populations, *International Journal of Epidemiology* **14**, 32–38.

[30] Schlattmann, P., Dietz, E. & Bohning, D. (1996). Covariate adjusted mixture models and disease mapping with the program DismapWin, *Statistics in Medicine* **15**, 919–929.

[31] Smans, M. & Esteve, J. (1992). Practical approaches to disease mapping, in *Geographical and Environmental Epidemiology: Methods for Small-Area Studies*, P. Elliott, J. Cuzick, D. English & R. Stern, eds. Oxford University Press, Oxford, pp. 141–157.

[32] Smith, A.F.M. & Roberts, G.O. (1993). Bayesian computation via the Gibbs sampler and related Markov chain Monte Carlo methods, *Journal of the Royal Statistical Society, Series B* **55**, 3–23

[33] Spiegelhalter, D.J., Thomas, A., Best, N.G. & Gilks, W.R. (1995). *BUGS: Bayesian Inference Using Gibbs Sampling, Version 0.50*. Medical Research Council Biostatistics Unit, Cambridge.

[34] Swerdlow, A. & dos Santos Silva, I. (1993). *Atlas of Cancer Incidence in England and Wales 1968–85*. Oxford University Press, Oxford.

[35] Walter, S.D. (1993). Visual and statistical assessment of spatial clustering in mapping data, *Statistics in Medicine* **12**, 1275–1291.

[36] Walter S.D. & Birnie, S.E. (1991). Mapping mortality and morbidity patterns: an international comparison, *International Journal of Epidemiology* **20**, 678–689.

[37] Wilkinson, P., Thakrar, B., Shaddick, G., Stevenson, S., Pattenden, S, Landon, M., Grundy, C. & Elliott, P. (1997). Cancer incidence and mortality around the Pan Britannica Industries pesticide factory, Waltham Abbey, *Occupational and Environmental Medicine* **54**, 101–107.

[38] World Bank (1993). *World Development Report 1993, Investing in Health.* Oxford University Press, Oxford.

PAUL ELLIOTT & NICOLA BEST

Geographical Analysis

The purpose of this article is to give an overview of methods of analyzing epidemiologic data in which geographic location is of primary importance. Methods may be distinguished by the purposes of the analyses, which include (i) modeling **risk** as a function of geographically referenced variables; (ii) hypothesis testing about specific sources of risk; (iii) **mapping disease patterns** to provide a visual representation of risk variation; (iv) identifying areas of apparently elevated risk deserving further epidemiologic investigation (*see* **Environmental Epidemiology**); and (v) detecting specific or generalized clusters, which may be indicative of unsuspected sources of risk or of a contagious disease mechanism (*see* **Clustering**). These methods are reflected in the central sections of the article, which are preceded by an overview of the underlying models and followed by a discussion of the issues involved in the choice of method.

Interest in geographic epidemiology has increased greatly in recent years and the number of methods proposed in the literature is very large. It would be quite impossible to review these methods comprehensively in this article; rather the object is to form a general classification according to their objectives and the underlying assumptions. Many proposed analyses will inevitably be omitted and an adverse judgment on them should not be inferred. On the face of it, geographic analysis is a topic in spatial statistics [26, 30, 35, 80], but there are special aspects which distinguish it from many of the other areas of application in the latter field.

It should be remarked at the outset that the likelihood of a geographic analysis revealing relationships of real scientific or clinical significance in a given case may be fairly low, for a number of reasons. First, in spite of considerable improvements in data availability over recent years, it is difficult to acquire accurate population sizes. A relatively high rate of individual migration and the development of new residential districts mean that population estimates can be seriously in error at the end of the intercensal period – 10 years in the UK, for example. Migration also implies that people are typically exposed to risks associated with different locations as they move around, which must inevitably dilute the sensitivity of any geographic analysis. Local mobility further confuses the picture: adults work and children go to school in areas which are often quite different from their place of residence, so that geographically mediated risks may be only weakly related to home address. It should also be remembered that most geographic observations – including those that have subsequently been found to be of real significance and value – have been anecdotal and the analyses have been executed *post hoc*. This inevitably adds to the difficulty of interpreting them.

Nevertheless, there have been notable triumphs of geographic epidemiology: the well-known story of John Snow and cholera [86]; the observations of Denis Burkitt leading to the recognition of a vector-related etiology of a human tumor [19, 20]; and more recently, the detection of the cause of an outbreak of epidemic asthma [3]; all are striking demonstrations of the epidemiologic potential of geographic observations. There is also a less positive but equally important reason for carrying out geographic analyses effectively. People are in practice very concerned about the impact of their environment on their health and it is important that anxieties are explored in a manner that inspires confidence, if only to provide reassurance in particular cases.

Underlying Models

Case-Independence and Other General Issues

It is important to distinguish at the outset mechanisms of disease in which cases are or are not intrinsically related. Examples of case-dependence include contagious and familial diseases (*see* **Communicable Diseases**); any tendency of such cases to be close geographically is unlikely to identify any component of risk which is essentially geographic. Rather, interest centers on establishing the case-dependence as an intrinsic phenomenon independent of geographic location.

For case-independent disease processes, however, we suppose that cases occur independently of one another, *conditional on the underlying risk factors*, which may include some aspect of geographic location.

On this assumption, any spatial autocorrelation, or general tendency of cases to be closer to one another than expected, will be inherited from the spatial structure of the underlying pattern of risk factors. Within the frequentist framework, at least, it is *unnecessary to model it by means of a spatially correlated error process*, except to the extent that this may be a convenient way of allowing for spatially varying risk factors that we cannot observe. We return to this point below.

Models for case-dependent processes are not well developed. Spatial modeling of epidemics [4, 67] is concerned with the dynamics of spatial spread and has rather little interaction with epidemiologic analysis in the sense of this article. Some authors [1, 5, 15] have proposed clustering models in which "parent" cases give rise to "offspring" cases according to a defined stochastic mechanism; it is much easier to postulate models of this kind than to handle them analytically. "Second-order" point processes, which model the tendency of points to be clustered, have been studied using Ripley's K functions [79] in the epidemiologic context by Diggle & Chetwynd [36] and applied also by Diggle & Morris [38]; they are not easily related to specific models of person–person interaction, however.

In practice, much geographic epidemiology is applied to diseases – notably malignant diseases – for which there is very little evidence of case-dependency. Although it may be the objective of some analyses to detect such dependency, the assumption of independence is a reasonable basis at least for a null hypothesis H_0 of spatial uniformity. It is therefore quite sensible to discuss most of the methods of geographic epidemiology against a modeling background which assumes case-independence and this will be the standpoint of this article. Once this position is accepted, the basic models for the spatial distribution of disease become relatively simple.

Two other general aspects of the models we discuss should be mentioned. In the first place, it may be argued that much of epidemiologic analysis reduces to considering the associations between observations on a disease $\mathcal{D}$, a variable of primary interest $\mathcal{E}$, such as an exposure variable, and a set of other variables $\mathcal{C}$, which may be thought of as covariates and which may include possible **confounding** variables. In many analyses the variables in $\mathcal{C}$ are regarded as being fixed, even though they may be subject to error or sampling variation. For many purposes this will suffice; although the analysis may not be strictly correct [40], it can be justified in terms of a conditional argument – i.e. it is valid in the subspace of all outcomes in which $\mathcal{C}$ is as observed; alternatively, we may argue that it is reliably assessing the importance of a *modified* variable incorporating the unobservable error. In **observational studies** $\mathcal{D}$ and $\mathcal{E}$ are intrinsically random, but even here it is quite usual to condition on one or the other rather than to model the full joint distribution. This gives rise to a duality of analysis corresponding to the **case–control** and **cohort** approaches [18]. In this respect, geographic analyses are no different from any other epidemiologic analyses: geographic location may be treated as a covariate $\mathcal{C}$ or as a primary interest variable $\mathcal{E}$; in the latter case, $\mathcal{E}$ may be regarded as fixed with $\mathcal{D}$ random, or vice versa. This "duality principle", that either form of conditioning leads to valid and useful analyses of epidemiologic data, permits us to employ analyses of either kind interchangeably, which we will do below without further comment.

Secondly, we emphasize that, however we choose to model location, it is imperative to build in a reference distribution (normally in the form of a population density) at a fundamental level; not least this is because of the implication for the underlying variation in local variance. Analyses which start by assuming a homogeneous spatial distribution of cases and "correct for" heterogeneity of population distribution are to be regarded with suspicion and may give misleading results.

Areal Data

Most geographic data are in areal form, i.e. counts Y_i, $i = 1, 2, \ldots, k$ of numbers of cases in areas A_i, nearly always administratively defined, within a study region $\mathcal{R}$. These will be accompanied by population information, initially in the form of the sizes of the populations at risk in different relevant groups; such groupings will usually include age and sex, and often other factors such as socioeconomic status and ethnic group. If the risk within a given area A_i is constant, the Y_i are clearly binomial. Variation of this risk upsets this assumption, but only slightly in practice, particularly if the risk is small (which it will be for a rare disease or when modeling annual rates). In the latter case we can use the Poisson approximation even if there is identifiable heterogeneity of risk within the A_i.

We can therefore simplify the account by adopting the Poisson model and supposing that the population sizes have already been used in conjunction with reference rates to construct "expected" numbers e_i of disease cases, either by a process of **standardization** or using a suitable regression model [10]. The case-independence assumption then implies that the Y_i are independently distributed with Poisson distributions having means $\theta_i e_i$, say, where we take θ_i as the **relative risk** (RR) in A_i – i.e. the risk relative to the assumptions under which the $\{e_i\}$ were computed. The factors θ_i may now be modeled in terms of possible explanatory variables using methods which are well understood, for example a **Poisson regression**; this employs a loglinear model, which is a particular case of a Generalized Linear Model (GLM) [61]. Such a model can be tested for goodness of fit; usually this may be satisfactorily accomplished using the residual deviance, though there are problems in interpreting this if the e_i are very small – say with appreciably many observations significantly less than around five. If there is evidence that the model does not fit well, this indicates that there is a component of risk that has not been incorporated into the model; it is said that there is "extra-Poisson" variation [16]. Modifications of the analysis in this case include postulating a distribution for θ over the A_i, for example from a gamma distribution, which leads to a negative binomial distribution for the Y_i [50]. The implications for model validity and inference do not depend on whether there is a geographic element to this variation; if there is, a richer model involving spatial autocorrelation may be fitted [27].

Continuous Data

The discrete structure of areal data, with the imposition of administrative boundaries, is not ideal either practically or mathematically. In principle, data may be available on a continuous basis, i.e. by the provision of the exact geographic coordinates of a sample of cases. The case-independence assumption and the duality principle then imply that these cases may be regarded as a random sample from a bivariate density function $\psi(x, y)$ of geographic location with coordinates (x, y). This density function determines the distribution of the place of residence of a randomly selected individual with the disease. Equivalently the case locations may be regarded as a realization of a Poisson process with intensity

$f(x, y)$ proportional to $\psi(x, y)$. As before, we need a reference group and this may be taken to be the population density $\pi(x, y)$, where we use this term to refer not so much to a general demographic concept, but to a second mathematical density function describing the probability that a randomly selected member of the population will reside at a given point (x, y). We are now in a position to define a *risk function* giving the risk of being affected by the disease incurred by a randomly selected individual at location (x, y), namely.

$$\mu(x, y) = f(x, y)/N\pi(x, y,),$$

where N is the aggregate of the population in $\mathcal{R}$, in the form of **person-years at risk** if appropriate.

In practice, of course, these mathematically defined risk functions must be estimated from the data, the problem being one of estimating the ratio of two densities. Methods of estimating a single density have recently been much studied and developed [83, 84] and, although ratios present certain rather special problems, they are not insuperable. For the distribution of cases, the general methods apply, with the proviso that population-related densities are extremely multimodal and in this respect atypical of most of the examples to which density estimation has been applied. The estimation of the population density raises rather special problems, in that published data will still be in areal form, but the normal methods of density estimation can be adapted; alternative methods are available [64, 89].

It should also be noted that the population density may be satisfactorily estimated from a sample of **controls** [9], which has the advantage that the geographic resolution of their locations will be equal to that of the cases. Use of controls also removes the need to ascertain the entire population, though in the absence of information about whole-population risk the risk function will be determined only up to an unknown factor. In this case it may be regarded as a "relative risk function" (RRF), defined by $\theta(x, y) = \psi(x, y)/\pi(x, y)$, giving the risk at a particular location relative to the average in the whole of $\mathcal{R}$ [9].

The continuous model of geographic risk is attractive mathematically and opens up a number of new possibilities for analysis. In practice, however, there are considerable difficulties with obtaining suitable sampling frames for the controls. Case–control analyses have not been much used in practice, though they may reasonably be expected to assume greater significance in the future, as the geographic accuracy of address data improves.

Spatial Autocorrelation

The rationale for taking account of spatial autocorrelation is attributed by Cook & Pocock [27] to Lazar [60] as being that "failure to allow for spatially correlated errors may result in serious overestimates of the significance of relationships". Lazar demonstrates that this is true when the relationships in question are assessed using correlation coefficients with precision estimated from the data.

As argued above, however, case-independence implies that any spatial autocorrelation in observed disease rates must be due to a similar autocorrelation in one or more associated factors that have not been taken into account in the model, i.e. it is not really the *error* mechanism that should be modified by taking account of autocorrelations. Of course, the word "error" in statistical parlance has come to be synonymous with anything not accounted for in an explanatory model. The point is not merely semantic, however; use of the word in this context has the unfortunate effect of distracting attention from the importance of case-independence and to the construction of methods which do not make use of the known variances of binomial and Poisson data.

Cook & Pocock propose, in a study of heart disease, a model for the Standardized Mortality Ratio (SMR) (*see* **Standardization Methods**) of the form:

$$\ln(Y_i/e_i) = \mathbf{X}\beta + \varepsilon,$$

where the linear predictor $\mathbf{X}\beta$ is in the usual form for a linear regression model and

$$\varepsilon \sim \mathrm{N}[0, \sigma^2 \mathbf{A}],$$

with $\mathbf{A}$ an autocovariance matrix. Exploratory analysis led them to propose an autocorrelation function decaying exponentially with distance. Estimation in this model did indeed lead to a reduction in the significance of the effect of water hardness, the regression coefficient being reduced by around 40% and its standardized value from -5.0 to -3.0.

Cook & Pocock conclude that failure to adjust for spatial autocorrelation leads us to overstate the significance of fitted regression coefficients. Although this is probably true in their example, it may not always be so, as may be seen more easily by considering a GLM in which terms may be assessed for significance in their own right, without recourse to an estimate of residual variance. It would be quite possible to have an unobserved covariate $\mathcal{C}$ which is spatially autocorrelated and which induces autocorrelations in the residuals, but which is independent of a fitted variable $\mathcal{E}$. Although taking account of $\mathcal{C}$ would improve the fit of the model, it would not necessarily reduce the contribution of $\mathcal{E}$ to the total deviance and need not, therefore, affect its significance. Nor is the reduction of the estimate of the regression coefficient conclusive, since $\mathcal{C}$ might be incidentally associated with $\mathcal{D}$ and $\mathcal{E}$; the latter could still be an important causative factor. Incorporation of autocorrelation is, nevertheless, a feature of many contributions to the field and it is generally supposed to be of considerable importance, both theoretically and practically. To some extent this view is encouraged by Bayesian modeling, where the emphasis is on the inclusion of terms to represent any unknown component of variation without consideration of model parsimony.

Bayesian Modeling

The models outlined above are essentially frequentist and assume the existence of unique but unknown parameters. The Bayesian alternative is becoming increasingly popular in statistics generally and particularly with the epidemiologic community [24, 31, 47, 52].

The seminal contribution by Clayton & Kaldor [25] distinguishes heterogeneity deriving from spatial and nonspatial sources. These give rise to corresponding methods of smoothing rates for disease mapping (see below) and were motivated primarily by this application. The methods have had considerable influence on geographic epidemiology and have been used to elaborate inferential modeling by numerous authors [59, 66] in the spirit of the frequentist approach outlined above. They are exemplified by the analysis by Richardson et al. [78] of childhood leukemia in relation to natural (background) radiation. These authors extend the standard Poisson regression to a Generalized Linear Mixed Model (GLMM) [17, 23], with random effect terms u_i, v_i specific to area A_i:

$$\ln \theta_i = \mathbf{X}_i \beta + u_i + v_i, \quad i = 1, 2, \ldots, k.$$

Here u_i models nonspatial heterogeneity through the assumption that

$$[u_i|u_j, j \neq i] \sim N[\bar{u}_i, \lambda_u^{-1}], \quad \text{where}$$

$$\bar{u}_i = \sum_{j \neq i} u_j/(k-1).$$

Spatial structure is modeled by v_i through the assumption that

$$[v_i|v_j, j \neq i] \sim N[\bar{v}_i, \lambda_v^{-1}], \quad \text{where}$$

$$\bar{v}_i = \sum_{j \neq i} W_{ij}v_j/(k_i - 1),$$

where the adjacency matrix element $W_{ij} = 1$ if areas i, j are adjacent, 0 otherwise, and k_i is the number of areas adjacent to A_i. We require $\sum u_i = \sum v_i = 0$ for identifiability.

The parameters λ_u, λ_v control the degree of variation in the dispersion terms. In an empirical Bayes treatment, these would be estimated; instead Richardson et al. pursue a "full Bayes" solution in which, together with β, they are given prior distributions. Choice of the "hyperparameters" in such prior distributions leads to the notion of a "hierarchical Bayes" model.

In the childhood leukemia analysis [78], the effect of radiation in a frequentist Poisson regression was very weak and was limited to acute nonlymphocytic leukemia and to one of three 5-year periods. It was reduced to the point of nonsignificance in the GLMM, and the variation in both the $\{u_i\}$ and the $\{v_i\}$ estimates appeared to be significant. Similar doubts attach to the interpretation of these results, however: to the extent that the random effects are independent of natural radiation, they should not affect inference for the latter. To the extent that they are associated with it, they may represent **confounders**, but the possibility that radiation is a primary and important effect cannot be excluded.

The models outlined above preserve the discreteness of areal data. A model for continuous data is more difficult mathematically. Typically it is assumed that the logarithm of the RRF is a realization of a spatial Gaussian process [58]. The mean of this process might be taken to be constant if the primary purpose is to model spatial relationship, which would be determined by an autocorrelation function; otherwise it could involve parameters designed to detect locational effects. The methods are comparatively new and untested.

The considerable computational difficulties with Bayesian methods have recently been facilitated by Markov chain Monte Carlo (MCMC) methods. These are computationally expensive and care needs to be taken to ensure that the chain is fully sampling the stationary distribution it is intended to estimate. It is also unclear how much the precision is affected by the need to estimate large numbers of parameters, though it should be remembered that the precision of classical frequentist methods incorporates information from the specification of the model and is therefore crucially dependent on its correctness. The book by Gilks [45] gives much technical detail about MCMC and available software, and includes a discussion of geographic applications, particularly issues affecting the choice of priors [65].

Analysis by Location

Areal Modeling

The simplest kind of geographic analysis merely attempts to model a disease rate at a particular location in relation to geographically defined variables associated with that location. Examples of such variables could include geographic variables such as altitude [19], possible measurable risk factors such as background radiation levels, and demographic characteristics of the population, such as socioeconomic status. The latter type of variable imputes to individuals at risk the average of some risk for the whole population in their immediate vicinity, giving rise to an "ecologic" analysis which is not without its dangers [37, 43] (*see* **Ecologic Fallacy**; **Ecologic Study**). Functions of location, such as distance from a specified point, also come into this category of analysis and are dealt with below.

Under the case-independence assumption discussed above, statistical analysis may proceed in an entirely classical way, for example using GLMs. As discussed above, a typical such model would be a Poisson regression with $\ln(e_i)$ as an offset. The residual deviance in this model may then be used to determine whether there is any extra-Poisson variation, which may be evidence of clustering (see below).

Continuous Analogs

Continuous data require an analogous method to analyze the risk function $\mu(x, y)$ or RRF $\theta(x, y)$. For case–control data with equal numbers of cases and controls, this can be achieved by a conditional **logistic regression**. We define

$$\rho(x, y) = \theta(x, y)/[1 + \theta(x, y)],$$

which gives the conditional probability that an individual sampled at (x, y) is a case rather than a control [9]. This probability can in principle be modeled logistically using any variable defined by location (x, y) as well as other attributes of the individual concerned [39]. As remarked, above, however, case–control analyses of this sort have not to date been used to anything like the same extent as areal data methods.

Focused Tests of Point Source Hypotheses

A particular kind of locational analysis involves the study of the relationship between disease incidence and the location of some putative source of risk S. Such an analysis imputes risk to geographic location or, equivalently, uses some function of location as a surrogate for risk. This inevitably requires the construction of a one-dimensional function of location. Distance from S is an obvious choice, though analyses can apply equally well to other measures, incorporating, for example, geographic characteristics such as altitude, bearing to prevailing wind, etc.

Most analyses of data in relation to point sources carried out to date are statistically elementary and consist in examining a single standardized incidence ratio (SIR) for a predefined region $\mathcal{R}$ around S, comparing it with one or more control rates which would typically be national (*see* **Standardization Methods**). Such analyses have the great merit that they are easily understood, but they suffer from the severe disadvantage that they are not at all powerful against any sensible alternative hypothesis. They are also particularly dependent on the size of the region $\mathcal{R}$, though this is an intrinsic difficulty with other analyses too.

It is almost certainly better to use a method that makes explicit use of distance or other risk surrogate. Suppose that the true RR at a distance d is $\theta(d)$. Then, whether the data are in areal or continuous form, it follows easily from the Neyman–Pearson lemma [28] that the most powerful test of the null hypothesis of constant risk (H_0) is based on a Linear Risk Score

(LRS) computed as the sum over n cases

$$T = \sum_j \ln(\theta(d_j)),$$

where d_j is the distance of the jth case from S [11]. It follows that the SIR test is only powerful against a hypothesis that supposes a dichotomization of risk inside and outside $\mathcal{R}$. Of course, the usefulness of the general result is limited by the fact that we do not know the true risk function $\theta(\cdot)$, but it provides a benchmark against which other methods may be calibrated. Moreover, it turns out that using a (canonical) risk score of $1/d$ or $1/\text{rank}(d)$ is quite powerful against a wide range of alternatives [13]. Locally most powerful tests have also been proposed by Waller [91] and others [57, 88, 92]; these score tests are clearly not "uniformly" most powerful against *all* alternatives and it is unclear how local their power properties might be.

The problem of our ignorance of the true risk function led Stone [8, 87] to propose a test designed to detect a general monotonic decreasing RRF. This test has recently become very popular in the UK. Known as Stone's (maximum) likelihood ratio (MLR) test, it is a test in which the alternative hypothesis is:

$$H_1 : \theta_1 \geq \theta_2 \geq \ldots \geq \theta_k (\geq 1),$$

i.e. the areas A_i, ordered by distance from S, have RRs θ_i estimated by maximizing the likelihood subject to the restriction that they are monotonic nonincreasing. The final constraint is optional though important, the issue being similar to the choice of a conditional or unconditional test discussed below [11]. This estimation problem is related to that of isotonic regression [81]; the computation required is nontrivial but feasible in practice. Stone also proposed the so-called "$P_{\max}$" test based on the first order-restricted RR estimate, $\hat{\theta}_1$. This turns out to be

$$\max_j \sum_{i=1}^{j} Y_i \Big/ \sum_{i=1}^{j} e_i,$$

i.e. the maximal cumulative RR as distance from S increases. These tests are undoubtedly important and in some situations very effective. The application of the Neyman–Pearson lemma referred to above, however, implies that Stone's test is never most powerful, and it is not hard to find alternatives for which it has low power compared with canonical LRS tests.

Whichever test statistic is used, it is crucially important to distinguish between the *conditional* and *unconditional* form of the test [11]. The former conditions on the total number of cases observed in $\mathcal{R}$ and is affected only by the spatial information in the data. It would be appropriate whenever the rates used to compute the $\{e_i\}$ may not be reliable in $\mathcal{R}$; if they are trustworthy, however, the conditional analysis ignores potentially valuable information and can even lead to the rejection of H_0 resulting from a *deficit* of cases in the outer parts of the region $\mathcal{R}$. The unconditional form uses the overall disease incidence information as well as the spatial information, but is appropriate only when the $\{e_i\}$ are reliable. In practice, conditional and unconditional tests may produce very different results, especially from small data sets, and it is very important to decide *a priori* which form of test will be used.

Disease Mapping

History and Atlases

The mapping of the incidence of disease and mortality has a long history, well summarized by Howe [48]. Early endeavors were concerned with depicting the epidemic spread of infectious disease, often represented by contours of first occurrence date. More recently, with the diminishing importance of infectious disease in the developed world, the emphasis has changed to representing mortality or incidence in an attempt to infer geographically related explanations of variation in rates. For example, the *Atlas of United States Mortality* [71] contains color maps for each of 18 major causes of death. The colors indicate the 10, 20, 40, 60, 80, and 90 percentiles of the age-standardized death rates in Health Service Areas (HSAs); for example, the top band includes all HSAs whose rates are in the top 10% for the US as a whole. Rates based on small numbers are distinguished by hatching. Cancer atlases, in particular, have been produced for countries all over the world, including the US, continental Europe, China, and the UK [14, 44].

Some maps depict cartograms, in which regions are drawn with areas proportional to their population sizes (*see* **Mapping Disease Patterns**). This may help to overcome the problem of unequal population distribution, but it has the disadvantage that the resulting maps are geographically unfamiliar. We will confine our attention in this section to representational maps in which the geometry is preserved.

Areal Mapping by RR and Other Measures

Most atlases attempt to depict data in discrete form, using administratively defined areas. One of the major concerns in such mapping is the question of what to map. Plotting rates in small areas tends to produce a misleading picture, in that apparently high rates may appear in low-density regions by chance. This problem is exacerbated by the negative correlation usually found between population density and the sizes of administrative areas. Because areas of similar population density are often adjacent, this can induce an apparent spatial pattern where none exists. Some authors [29, 44] have employed a measure of statistical significance instead of or as well as SIRs; with these, however, small values of P which are statistically but not scientifically significant may arise in areas with large populations. It is now generally regarded as preferable to plot **rates** rather than P values, controlling the influence of sampling variation by using a degree of smoothing [21]. The latter may be *empirical* or *model-based*.

Nonspatial Smoothing

The rationale for smoothing is that the maximum likelihood estimate of the disease rate in a particular small area is, because of its statistical variability, a poor indicator of the true rate in that area. If, for example, there was very little evidence of geographic variation, we would probably abandon an area-specific estimate and use the global rate for the whole region. Smoothing may be seen as an attempt to compromise between the two positions, using both local and global information.

An attractive method of combining this information is the Bayesian formulation referred to above [25, 52, 63]. In this, it is assumed that the underlying RRs $\{\theta_i\}$ in areas $\{A_i\}$ have a gamma prior distribution, with mean μ and variance σ^2. It follows that the mean of the posterior distribution of θ_i is

$$\tilde{\theta}_i = \frac{y_i + \mu^2/\sigma^2}{e_i + \mu/\sigma^2},$$

a formula that demonstrates how $\tilde{\theta}_i$ varies, according to the value of σ^2, between the area-specific maximum likelihood (ML) estimate Y_i/e_i and the global mean μ, whose ML estimate is $\sum_i Y_i / \sum_i e_i$. Unfortunately the ML estimation of σ^2 requires an iterative method, though a simpler moment-estimator is available [25].

Estimating the posterior mean in this way is the basis of the Empirical Bayes (EB) method of smoothing. It shrinks the local estimates towards the global mean, but does not take any account of the spatial relationship of one area to another.

Spatial Smoothing Using Bayesian Models

The Bayesian modeling of spatial structure described above can be used to produce estimates of the RR which are smoothed by reference to adjoining areas as well as the overall mean. The original paper by Clayton & Kaldor [25] describes a method that did not take account of the varying number of areas adjacent to a given A_i and consequently lacked internal consistency; developments by Besag et al. [6] have led to a version that meets this objection. The goal of making the rates in adjacent areas more similar to one another than identical rates in well-separated areas may seem very reasonable. It must be remembered, however, that it will inevitably give an appearance of spatial relationship even where none exists; it is therefore essential that maps produced using these methods are clearly indicated as such.

Empirical Smoothing

Although the Bayesian methodology is very attractive theoretically, it employs fairly sophisticated algorithms and is not easily related intuitively to the original data. Empirical methods of smoothing may be better in this respect and numerous methods have been proposed [14]. A particularly attractive method is described by Pukkala and applied to cancer in Finland [76]. At each point of a fine lattice, an estimated risk is computed as a weighted average of the rates in all the A_i whose centers are within a defined distance of the point. The weights take account of the distances of the A_i and also of their population sizes. The result is a map free of the original small area boundaries. A more elaborate method in which numerators and denominators of rates are smoothed separately is described by Kafadar [51].

Smoothing Based on the RRF

The formulation of a model for geographic data in terms of density functions discussed above suggests a simple, probability-based method of depicting risk continuously. All we need to do is to plot an estimate of the risk function or the RRF as the ratio of the densities for cases and controls [9, 53]. Although first used for continuous, case–control data, this method can in principle be extended to employ areal data, though no account has yet been published.

Degree of Smoothing and Other Issues

Whatever method of smoothing is employed, it is important to realize that determining the degree or scale of smoothing is intrinsic to any spatial method. For areal data, the sizes of the areas will be involved in this determination. Particular methods may offer choice at other levels of the analysis: for example, the bandwidth in the case of risk function estimation based on density estimates. The question of whether one may reasonably expect the data to determine how much smoothing should be applied is unclear. From a Bayesian standpoint, one should expect to build into the analysis a prior idea of the degree of risk variation. Estimating this degree from the data is akin to using empirical Bayes ideas and departs from the spirit of the "full Bayes" approach. Density estimation methods are certainly associated with data-driven methods of bandwidth determination, such as cross-validation [84]. However, these typically use criteria of doubtful relevance to the presentation of meaningful maps, and in practice may not produce satisfactory analyses.

The methods described above all incorporate information about the variation in the population density and this should be regarded as essential because of the variation in precision implied. Methods designed for homoscedastic continuous data, such as geophysical data, can give quite misleading results and should be avoided.

Clustering

Types of Clustering

Clustering may be defined as the tendency of observations to be situated closer to one another than would be expected; the role of chance in this expectation is crucial and much statistical effort is directed towards determining whether an observed cluster could easily be accounted for by chance. In the context of geographic analyses, the issue is that of whether people affected by a disease reside, work or otherwise congregate at places which are closer together than would be expected. From a mathematical point of view, the aggregation could be in any continuum and this gives rise to the notion of clustering in time, space or in the space–time product space. Mathematical considerations also suggest that the nature of the continuum should make rather little difference to the nature of the tests available, specifically that a test working in time, for example, should have an analog in space.

We remark also that it may be useful to distinguish various different types or modes of clustering. Cases may be close together because of a violation of the case-independence assumption; such clustering might provide evidence of a localized genetic effect or of a contagious process. Alternatively, aggregations might be due to variations in underlying risk. Either effect may be highly localized (as with a single familial cluster or a single environmental hazard) or may be widely disseminated. The statistical analysis is not capable of distinguishing these essentially different mechanisms, though different tests will be more sensitive to one rather than another.

We aim in this section to give a brief and relatively abstract overview of the methods available; further details of several of the methods may be found in **Clustering**.

Direct Methods

A set of rates or risk estimates, whether in discrete or continuous form, may be regarded as a risk function θ over geographic space and clustering should appear as some kind of nonuniformity of this function. Many functionals of θ suggest themselves as possible statistics to test for nonuniformity and to some extent the kind of alternative for which they should be powerful is intuitively obvious.

Thus, to detect a single isolated cluster, extremum statistics would be appropriate. These might include, for discrete areal data, occupancy statistics based on a large count in one or more areas [42], and for continuous case–control data, an analog in the form of the maximum height of the RRF estimated by density estimation [82] and tested under a permutation hypothesis. For continuous time, the **scan statistic**

[56, 68] counts the maximum number of cases within a fixed length window as it moves through the study period; the distribution theory is analytically difficult [46, 90].

One of the problems with tests based on discrete areal data is that a cluster straddling two or more adjacent areas may be completely missed. A geographic analog of the scan statistic would solve this problem, but is presumably even less tractable analytically than in time, partly because of the dimensionality difference and partly because it is essential to allow for variation in population density. This is of minor importance, however, given that Monte Carlo testing provides a way to execute even the most complicated of tests.

The Geographical Analysis Machine of Openshaw [70] is effectively a scan test, though it was derived more by empirical than theoretically well-founded considerations. By varying the size and location of the scanning window, it entails a considerable amount of computation; the criterion of clustering is based on statistical significance. More recently, Anderson & Titterington [2] have used a method based on observed frequencies and applied it to case–control cancer data in South Lancashire. It adjusts the size of the scanning window at each point of $\mathcal{R}$ to ensure that it contains a constant expected number of cases under H_0; this involves extensive numerical integration.

If interest is more in general heterogeneity of risk, it would be more appropriate to use a dispersion statistic of some sort. For areal data this entails determining whether there is "extra-Poisson variation", i.e. whether the Y_i are appreciably different from the e_i. The Potthoff–Whittinghill test has recently become very popular with epidemiologists [75]. As a likelihood score test it is asymptotically locally most powerful, but it is hard to see why it should be better than the deviance statistic $\sum\{e_i - y_i + y_i \ln(y_i/e_i)\}$ when the null hypothesis is not nearly true and the e_i are moderately large.

For continuous data we can compute a suitable measure of overall dispersion, such as the weighted variance of $\hat{\theta}(x, y)$:

$$T_{\text{var}} = \int \int_{\mathcal{R}} \pi(x, y)\{\hat{\theta}(x, y) - 1\}^2 \, dx \, dy.$$

This is similar to the "integrated squared difference statistic" used by Anderson & Titterington [2], with rather different weighting which reflects the extent to which population density relates to the local information.

Distance-Based Methods

For many problems in statistics, inverse sampling provides an alternative mode of analysis. In the clustering context, we may ask "What distance d from a given point P includes the nearest x cases?" rather than "What is the number x of cases within a distance d of P?". This gives rise to a class of tests based on nearest neighbor distances (NND) [32]. The simplest example, designed for case–control data, counts the number of individuals among the k nearest neighbors of each case that are cases (as opposed to controls). Cuzick & Edwards give analytical results for the null distributions of the different tests and evaluate their power. Further details are given in **Clustering**. The tests have been widely used in epidemiologic investigations. A related method for areal data, due to Besag & Newell [7], considers each case in turn and aggregates the areas around it that are necessary to include the xth nearest case. Tests of this kind have the feature that they adapt the scale on which they seek to detect clustering to varying population density; this may or may not be an advantage according to the clustering mechanism envisaged.

An historically earlier class of tests forms a kind of dual to the NND test in that they count the number of pairs of cases that are close in some sense. The original idea is due to Knox [55] and relates to space–time clustering. Because this is effectively detecting an **interaction** between the time and space variables, it can condition on the marginal distributions in time and space and so circumvent our ignorance about these distributions. To put it another way, the test uses the information on the marginal distributions already present in the data by asking the question "Given the number N_T of pairs of cases close in time and the number of pairs N_S close in space, what should be the number N_{TS} of pairs close in both time and space?" In fact, the distribution of N_{TS} depends on complex aspects of the configuration of the points in space and time, but Knox conjectured that N_{TS} should have approximately a Poisson distribution with mean

$$E[N_{TS}] = N_T N_S \bigg/ \binom{n}{2},$$

where the denominator is simply the number of pairs in the set of all n cases considered.

David & Barton [33] demonstrated that, in many situations, this conjecture is well-founded and derived expressions for the variance of N_{TS}. In a number of combinatorially impressive papers, the analysis has been extended (i) to allow for **latent periods** [74]; (ii) to permit a more general measure of closeness than the indicator function originally proposed by Knox [62]; (iii) to the analysis of cross-clustering of events of different types [54]; (iv) to a range of different distance categories [77]; and (v) to a permutation test for space-only clustering using a sample of controls [72, 73]. More recently, Jacquez [49] proposed a version in which closeness was defined in terms of belonging to the set of k nearest neighbors. The power advantages claimed for this may be practically important, though ultimately dependent on the form of the alternative.

Knox's original space–time test remains very popular, but most of these extensions have been used rather little. The space-only test (v) is particularly worthy of more attention, providing as it does an alternative to the Cuzick–Edwards test.

The power of the Knox-type tests is controversial. Barton et al. [5] demonstrated that the original space–time test is remarkably sensitive to the introduction of extra, "offspring" cases if $E[N_{ST}]$ is small under the null hypothesis. Chen et al. [22], however, concluded that the test was not very powerful, though this seems to have been due to latent periods that were not allowed for in the analysis. Bradshaw [15] performed extensive simulations to estimate the power under a similar alternative and concluded that using a general continuous, distance-based closeness measure offered rather little improvement over a well-chosen step-function.

Spatial Relationship

The modeling of spatial structure suggests a number of tests based on estimates of spatial similarity. Theoretical development is possible as long as rates are modeled using the multivariate normal distribution as an asymptotic approximation to frequency data; the normal family is the only one that has an analytically tractable multivariate form, so that attempts to extend analytical methods to other families inevitably make limited progress.

Under the normal model the distribution of the data is completely specified by the covariance matrix which, in the spatial context, will be constructed by reference to postulated autocorrelations. These may be expressed as functions of distance, adjacencies of neighboring areas, lengths of common area boundaries, or other measures. To some extent these will be chosen for mathematical convenience, but the scientific relevance should not be overlooked: Euclidean distance may be important in some contexts and to ignore it could be misleading; in other contexts a measure of degree of adjacency may better reflect the variation of risk with population density.

Different structures in a model for spatial data are reflected in the numerous different tests available. Cliff & Ord [26] give a comprehensive account, though epidemiologic application requires attention to the need to take account of differing population sizes in different areas. This can be done by suitable modifications using weights, or by applying the methods to rates which have been standardized in respect of their sampling variability. Walter [94] reports an empirical investigation of the power of three popular tests of this kind. Munasinghe & Morris [69] use (local) estimates of "regional spatial autocorrelation" to identify particular locations with suspected clustering.

Issues of Interpretation

Much has been written on the interpretation of clusters (*see* **Clustering**; **Geographic Patterns of Disease**). An essential problem is that clusters are mostly reported *post hoc* and it is therefore impossible to assess their statistical significance formally. To say that a cluster is unusual begs the question of the reference set: an extreme that would be unusually high in a single administrative district might well occur quite frequently in a national investigation. From a statistical point of view, it would seem to be desirable to investigate the tendency of a disease to cluster by systematic analysis of a case register (*see* **Disease Registers**). Opinions are divided as to whether this is a good idea [85]. Certainly the investigator should have some idea of what to do if a new cluster is detected and ideally should work to an appropriate protocol.

Choice of Statistical Procedure

It is clear, even from the brief overview in this article, that there is a plethora of different methods for addressing questions raised by geographical data in epidemiology. Even allowing for the multiplicity of these questions and the different types of practical situation arising, it must be the case that some of the methods are worse than others and should be discarded. Very few studies have attempted to assess the comparative characteristics of competing methods and new ones are often introduced without any justification, either theoretical or empirical. We may consider optimality of the relevant procedures at three levels.

Theoretical Considerations

Because the underlying models are complicated it is difficult to obtain theoretical results on power, for example. Nevertheless, there are some guiding principles that should indicate whether a method is likely to work well. As discussed above, the principal of these is that any sensible method should recognize the importance of population density variation. This is important not only in relation to a satisfactory control or comparison group, but also because of the great variation in local information. Thus the homoscedasticity assumptions of geophysical methods such as kriging, for example, make them unsuitable for epidemiologic data unless suitably modified. Epidemiology is concerned essentially with counting people rather than measuring continuous quantities.

Another general principle applies to distance-based methods. In essence it is closeness of individuals, not their distance, that is important, yet it is surprising how many analyses compute mean distances, which are inevitably heavily influenced by the least interesting, large values. It is essential that distance-based methods employ some inverse function to give most weight to the nearest individuals.

Many analyses are bad simply because they violate these principles and lose power or efficiency as a consequence. A smaller number are actually wrong as a result of serious statistical errors, perhaps concerned with sampling theory. This may occur, for example, when small areas are sampled randomly and assumed to be typical of areas in which index cases reside. This is almost certainly never the case, since the latter are sampled with probability proportional to size and administrative areas vary in size very considerably. Moreover, they do so in a way that is highly related to other geographic variables, such as population density. This can lead to artifactual associations which are highly misleading [12].

Statistical Performance

Frequently, it will be unclear which of a number of theoretically acceptable methods is best in the sense of having the best power or efficiency. It will very often be necessary to resort to simulation; this is a relatively straightforward way to address the issue, though it is not always easy to summarize the output from simulation experiments.

Some authors compare procedures by looking at the significance levels achieved in application to particular data sets, implicitly supposing that a smaller P value is evidence of a better test. Unfortunately, this is not so and it really is necessary to examine test performance on a large number of data sets simulated under a known alternative. Power is the usual performance characteristic considered, but it is worth remarking that the expected significance level (ESL) of Dempster & Schatzoff [34] has a number of advantages, including simplicity of simulation and the removal of type I error as a parameter of the experiment. Bithell & Dutton [13] follow Stone [87] in using the ESL in extensive simulations of methods for point source analyses.

There is a particular difficulty with Bayesian methods because of the essentially different philosophical standpoint involved. The Bayesian formulates a model on certain assumptions that are subjective, as with the choice of priors. Subject to these assumptions, the analysis will not only be optimal, but uniquely correct in some sense. Appropriate questions about method performance are therefore concerned more with issues of sensitivity than efficiency: how different would the answers be if the underlying assumptions were different in specified respects? On the whole, rather little of the literature on Bayesian methods in geographical epidemiology seems to address such issues.

Parameter Choice

Frequentist analyses also incur a problem of parameter choice, in that most analyses, even within a class known to work well in theory, will have one or more "tuning parameters". Probably the most important of these is the class of distance scale parameters: for example, how close is "close" in a clustering test? The distance scale parameter is intrinsic to every geographic analysis and appears in the guise of smoothing parameters, covariance functions, and so on. Other quantities which may have to be chosen in advance of the analysis include an analogous time scale parameter, study region size, age, and diagnostic groups. The practical choice of such parameters should ideally be informed by knowledge of the disease process under consideration. In practice this may be difficult and it will be tempting to do several analyses, with the obvious dangers of multiple testing. Allowance for multiple testing by parameter variation is always possible using Monte Carlo methods, but it does, of course, sacrifice power.

Some Studies to Date

There have been rather few systematic comparative studies of different methods of analysis to date. Chen et al. [22] and Walter [93] have carried out studies of the statistical properties of a limited number of tests. More general issues – involving the problems of parameter choice discussed above – are more difficult to study, involving as they do the decisions of the investigators.

In the spirit of comparative analysis, the Childhood Cancer Research Group in Oxford released a major set of childhood leukemia data in standard format to interested investigators, who reported the results of their differing analyses in a single volume [41]. There was no element of competition in this exercise, however, and, since the data were real, it was not possible to say which investigators had the "right" answers: simulated data sets are required to answer such questions.

The International Agency for Research Against Cancer have published the results of a "blind trial" in which investigators were presented with simulated data sets incorporating clustering known only to the organizers [1]. The results make it clear that the investigators' strategies and choice of test parameters are at least as important as the statistical properties of the procedures. This reflects real life, but makes it difficult to extrapolate conclusions to the way methods would perform in the hands of other investigators. Interestingly, no investigators in this experiment chose to use Bayesian methods, even though there was quite a lot of prior information about the distributions of the parameters governing the construction of the data sets.

Conclusion

We conclude from this discussion, as have others [95], that there is an urgent and widespread need, not for more elaborate statistical methods, but for clear principles by which existing methods should be judged, together with carefully designed simulation experiments where appropriate.

References

[1]   Alexander, F.E. & Boyle, P., eds (1996). *Methods for Investigating Localized Clustering of Disease*. IARC, Lyon.

[2]   Anderson, N.H. & Titterington, D.M. (1995). Some methods for investigating spatial clustering, with epidemiological applications, *Journal of the Royal Statistical Society, Series A* **160**, 87–105.

[3]   Antó, J.M. & Sunyer, J. (1992). Soya bean as a risk factor for epidemic asthma, in *Geographical Environmental Epidemiology: Methods for Small-Area Studies*, P. Elliott, J. Cuzick, D. English & R. Stern, eds. OUP for World Health Organization, Oxford, pp. 323–341.

[4]   Bailey, N.T.J. (1978). Spatial models in the epidemiology of infectious diseases, in *Biological Growth and Spread. Lecture Notes in Biomathematics, No. 38*, W. Jäger, H. Rost & P. Tautu, eds. Springer-Verlag, Heidelberg.

[5]   Barton, D.E., David, F.N., Fix, E., Merrington, M. & Mustacchi, P. (1966). Tests for space–time interaction and a power function, *Proceedings of the Fifth Berkeley Symposium on Mathematical Statistics and Probability*, Vol. 4. University of California Press, Berkeley, pp. 217–227.

[6]   Besag, J., York, J. & Mollié, A. (1991). Bayesian image restoration with applications in spatial statistics (with discussion), *Annals of the Institute of Statistical Mathematics* **43**, 1–59.

[7]   Besag, J. & Newell, J. (1991). The detection of clusters in rare diseases, *Journal of the Royal Statistical Society, Series A* **154**, 143–155.

[8]   Bithell, J.F. & Stone, R.A. (1989). On statistical methods for analyzing the geographical distribution of cancer cases near nuclear installations, *Journal of Epidemiology and Community Health* **43**, 79–85.

[9]   Bithell, J.F. (1990). An application of density estimation to geographical epidemiology, *Statistics in Medicine* **9**, 691–701.

[10] Bithell, J.F., Dutton, S.J., Neary, N.M. & Vincent, T.J. (1995). Use of regression methods for control of socioeconomic confounding, *Journal of Epidemiology and Community Health* **49**, Supplement 2, S15–S19.

[11] Bithell, J.F. (1995). The choice of test for detecting raised disease risk near a point source, *Statistics in Medicine*, **14**, 2309–2322.

[12] Bithell, J.F. & Draper, G.J. (1995). Apparent association between benzene and childhood leukaemia: methodological doubts concerning a report by Knox, *Journal of Epidemiology and Community Health* **49**, 437–439.

[13] Bithell, J.F. & Dutton, S.J. (1996). Optimal frequentist procedures for detecting raised disease risk near point sources, in *American Statistical Association Proceedings of the 1995 Joint Meetings of the Section on Epidemiology*. American Statistical Association, Alexandria, pp. 1–10.

[14] Boyle, P., Muir, C.S. & Grundmann, E., eds (1989). *Cancer Mapping*. Springer-Verlag, Berlin.

[15] Bradshaw D. (1982). A comparison of tests for space–time clustering of disease cases. *D.Phil. Thesis*, University of Oxford.

[16] Breslow, N.E. (1984). Extra-Poisson variation in log-linear models, *Applied Statistics* **33**, 1, 38–44.

[17] Breslow, N.E. & Clayton, D.G. (1993). Approximate inference in generalized linear mixed models, *Journal of the American Statistical Association* **88**, 421, 9–25.

[18] Breslow, N.E. & Powers, W. (1978). Are there two logistic regressions for retrospective studies?, *Biometrics* **34**, 1, 100–105.

[19] Burkitt, D. & Wright, D. (1966). Geographical and tribal distribution of the African lymphoma in Uganda, *British Medical Journal* **i**, 569–573.

[20] Burkitt, D.P. & Wright, D.H. (1970). *Burkitt's Lymphoma*. Churchill Livingstone, Edinburgh.

[21] Cartwright, R.A., Alexander, F.E., McKinney, P.A. & Ricketts, T.J. (1990). *Leukaemia and Lymphoma: An Atlas of Distribution within Areas of England and Wales 1984–1988*. Leukaemia Research Fund, Leeds.

[22] Chen, R., Mantel, N. & Klingberg, M.A. (1984). A study of three techniques for time–space clustering in Hodgkin's disease, *Statistics in Medicine* **3**, 173–184.

[23] Clayton, D.G. (1996). Generalized linear mixed models, in *Markov Chain Monte Carlo in Practice*, W.R. Gilks, S. Richardson & D.J. Spiegelhalter, eds. Chapman & Hall, London, pp. 275–301.

[24] Clayton, D. & Bernardinelli, L. (1992). Bayesian methods for mapping disease risk, in *Geographical Environmental Epidemiology: Methods for Small-Area Studies*, P. Elliott, J. Cuzick, D. English & R. Stern, eds. OUP for World Health Organization, Oxford, pp. 205–220.

[25] Clayton, D. & Kaldor, J. (1987). Empirical Bayes estimates of age-standardized relative risks for use in disease mapping, *Biometrics* **43**, 671–682.

[26] Cliff, A.D. & Ord, J.K. (1981). *Spatial Processes: Models and Applications*. Pion, London.

[27] Cook, D.G. & Pocock, S.J. (1983). Multiple regression in geographical mortality studies, with allowance for spatially correlated errors, *Biometrics* **39**, 361–372.

[28] Cox, D.R. & Hinkley, D.V. (1974). *Theoretical Statistics*. Chapman & Hall, London.

[29] Craft, A.W., Openshaw, S. & Birch, J.M. (1985). Childhood cancer in the Northern Region, 1968–82:

incidence in small geographical areas, *Journal of Epidemiology and Community Health* **39**, 53–57.

[30] Cressie, N.A.C. (1993). *Statistics for Spatial Data*, Revised Ed. Wiley, New York.

[31] Cressie, N.A.C. (1996). Bayesian and constrained inference for extremes in epidemiology, in *American Statistical Association Proceedings of the 1995 Joint Meetings of the Section on Epidemiology*. American Statistical Association, Alexandria, pp. 11–17.

[32] Cuzick, J. & Edwards, R. (1990). Spatial clustering for inhomogeneous populations (with discussion), *Journal of the Royal Statistical Society, Series B* **52**, 73–104.

[33] David, F.N. & Barton, D.E. (1966). Two space–time interaction tests for epidemicity, *British Journal of Preventive and Social Medicine* **20**, 44–48.

[34] Dempster, A.P. & Schatzoff, M. (1965). Expected significance levels as a sensitivity index for test statistics, *Journal of the American Statistical Association* **60**, 420–436.

[35] Diggle, P.J. (1983). *Statistical Analysis of Spatial Point Patterns*. Academic Press, London.

[36] Diggle, P.J. & Chetwynd A.G. (1991). Second order analysis of spatial clustering for inhomogeneous populations, *Biometrics* **47**, 1155–1163.

[37] Diggle P. & Elliott P. (1995). Disease risk near point sources: statistical issues for analyses using individual or spatially aggregated data, *Journal of Epidemiology and Community Health* **49**, S20–S27.

[38] Diggle, P.J. & Morris, S. (1996). Second-order analysis of spatial clustering, in *Methods for Investigating Localized Clustering of Disease*, F.E. Alexander & P. Boyle, eds. IARC, Lyon, pp. 207–214.

[39] Diggle, P.J. & Rowlington, B.S. (1994). A conditional approach to point process modelling of elevated risk, *Journal of the Royal Statistical Society, Series A* **157**, 433–440.

[40] Donnelly, C.A. (1995). The spatial analysis of covariates in a study of environmental epidemiology, *Statistics in Medicine* **14**, 2393–2409.

[41] Draper, G., ed. (1991). *The Geographical Epidemiology of Childhood Leukaemia and non-Hodgkin Lymphomas in Great Britain, 1966–83. Studies on Medical and Population Subjects, No. 53*. HMSO, London.

[42] Ederer, F., Myers, M.H. & Mantel, N. (1964). A statistical problem in space and time: do leukemia cases come in clusters?, *Biometrics* **20**, 626–638.

[43] English, D. (1992). Geographical epidemiology and ecological studies, in *Geographical Environmental Epidemiology: Methods for Small-Area Studies*, P. Elliott, J. Cuzick, D. English & R. Stern, eds. OUP for World Health Organization, Oxford, pp. 3–13.

[44] Gardner, M.J., Winter, P.G., Taylor, C.P. & Acheson, E.D. (1983). *Atlas of Cancer Mortality in England and Wales, 1968–1978*. Wiley, Chichester.

[45] Gilks, W.R., Richardson, S. & Spiegelhalter, D.J. (1996). *Markov Chain Monte Carlo in Practice*. Chapman & Hall, London.

[46] Glaz, J. (1993). Approximations for the tail probabilities and moments of the scan statistic, *Statistics in Medicine* **12**, 1845–1852.

[47] Heisterkamp, S.H., Doornbos, G. & Gankema, M. (1993). Disease mapping using empirical Bayes and Bayes methods on mortality statistics in the Netherlands, *Statistics in Medicine* **12**, 1895–1914.

[48] Howe, G.M. (1989). Historical evolution of disease mapping in general and specifically of cancer mapping, in *Cancer Mapping*, P. Boyle, C.S. Muir & E. Grundmann, eds. Springer-Verlag, Berlin, pp. 1–21.

[49] Jacquez, G.M. (1996). A *k* nearest neighbour test for space–time interaction, *Statistics in Medicine* **15**, 1935–1949.

[50] Johnson, N.L., Kotz S. & Kemp, A.W. (1992). *Univariate Discrete Distributions*, 2nd Ed. Wiley, New York.

[51] Kafadar, K. (1996). Smoothing geographical data, particularly rates of disease, *Statistics in Medicine* **15**, 2539–2560.

[52] Kaldor, J. & Clayton, D. (1989). Role of advanced statistical techniques in cancer mapping, in *Cancer Mapping*, P. Boyle, C.S. Muir & E. Grundmann, eds. Springer-Verlag, Berlin, pp. 87–98.

[53] Kelsall, J.E. & Diggle, P.J. (1995). Non-parametric estimation of spatial variation in relative risk, *Statistics in Medicine* **14**, 2335–2342.

[54] Klauber, M.R. (1971). Two-sample randomization tests for space–time clustering, *Biometrics* **27**, 129–142.

[55] Knox, E.G. (1964). The detection of space–time interactions, *Applied Statistics* **13**, 25–29.

[56] Knox, E.G. & Lancashire, P.J. (1982). Detection of minimal epidemics, *Statistics in Medicine* **1**, 183–189.

[57] Lawson, A.B. (1993). On the analysis of mortality events associated with a prespecified fixed-point, *Journal of the Royal Statistical Society, Series A* **156**, 363–377.

[58] Lawson, A.B. (1994). Using spatial Gaussian priors to model heterogeneity in environmental epidemiology, *Statistician* **43**, 69–76.

[59] Lawson, A.B. (1995). MCMC methods for putative pollution source problems in environmental epidemiology, *Statistics in Medicine* **14**, 2473–2485.

[60] Lazar, P. (1981). Geographical correlations between disease and environmental exposure, in *Perspectives in Medical Statistics*, J.F. Bithell & R. Coppi, eds. Academic Press, London.

[61] McCullagh, P. & Nelder, J.A. (1989). *Generalized Linear Models*, 2nd Ed. Chapman & Hall, London.

[62] Mantel N. (1967). The detection of disease clustering and a generalized regression approach, *Cancer Research* **27**, 209–220.

[63] Manton, K.G., Woodbury, M.A., Stallard, E., Riggan, W.B., Creason, J.P. & Pellom, A.C. (1989). Empirical Bayes procedures for stabilizing maps of U.S. cancer mortality rates, *Journal of the American Statistical Association* **84**, 637–650.

[64] Martin D. & Bracken I. (1991). Techniques for modelling population-related raster databases, *Environment & Planning A* **23**, 1069–1075.

[65] Mollié, A. (1996). Bayesian mapping of disease, in *Markov Chain Monte Carlo in Practice*, W.R. Gilks, S. Richardson & D.J. Spiegelhalter, eds. Chapman & Hall, London, pp. 359–379.

[66] Mollié, A. & Richardson, S. (1991). Empirical Bayes estimates of cancer mortality rates using spatial models, *Statistics in Medicine* **10**, 95–112.

[67] Mollison D. (1977). Spatial contact models for ecological and epidemic spread, *Journal of the Royal Statistical Society, Series B* **39**, 283–326.

[68] Naus J.I. (1965). The distribution of the size of the maximum cluster of points on a line, *Journal of the American Statistical Association* **60**, 532–538.

[69] Munasinghe, R.L. & Morris, R.D. (1996). Localization of disease clusters using regional measures of spatial autocorrelation, *Statistics in Medicine* **15**, 893–905.

[70] Openshaw, S. & Craft, A. (1991). Using Geographical Analysis Machines to search for evidence of clusters and clustering in childhood leukaemia and non-Hodgkin lymphomas in Britain, in *The Geographical Epidemiology of Childhood Leukaemia and non-Hodgkin Lymphomas in Great Britain, 1966–83. Studies on Medical and Population Subjects, No. 53*, G. Draper, ed. HMSO, London, pp. 109–122.

[71] Pickle, L.W., Mungiole, M., Jones, G.K. & White, A.A. (1996). *Atlas of United States Mortality*. National Center for Health Statistics, Hyattsville.

[72] Pike, M.C. & Smith, P.G. (1974). A note on a "close pairs" test for space clustering, *British Journal of Preventive and Social Medicine* **28**, 63–64.

[73] Pike, M.C. & Smith, P.G. (1974). A case–control approach to examine disease for evidence of contagion, including disease with long latent periods, *Biometrics* **30**, 263–279.

[74] Pike, M.C. & Smith, P.G. (1968). Disease clustering: a generalization of Knox's approach to the detection of space–time interactions, *Biometrics* **24**, 541–556.

[75] Potthoff, R.F. & Whittinghill, M. (1966). Testing for homogeneity. II. The Poisson distribution, *Biometrika* **53**, 183–190.

[76] Pukkala, E. (1989). Cancer maps of Finland: an example of small-area based mapping, in *Cancer Mapping*, P. Boyle, C.S. Muir & E. Grundmann, eds. Springer-Verlag, Berlin, pp. 208–215.

[77] Raubertas R.F. (1988). Spatial and temporal analysis of disease occurrence for detection of clustering, *Biometrics* **44**, 1121–1129.

[78] Richardson, S., Montfort, C., Green, M., Draper, G. & Muirhead, C. (1995). Spatial variation of natural radiation and childhood leukaemia incidence in Great Britain, *Statistics in Medicine* **14**, 2487–2501.

[79] Ripley, B.D. (1977). Modelling spatial patterns (with discussion), *Journal of the Royal Statistical Society, Series B* **39**, 172–212.

[80] Ripley, B.D. (1981). *Spatial Statistics*. Wiley, New York.

[81] Robertson, T., Wright F.T. & Dykstra R.L. (1988). *Order Restricted Statistical Inference*. Wiley, London.

[82] Rossiter, J.E. (1991). *Epidemiological applications of density estimation. D.Phil. thesis*, University of Oxford.

[83] Scott, D.W. (1992). *Multivariate Density Estimation*. Wiley, London.

[84] Silverman, B.W. (1986). *Density Estimation for Statistics and Data Analysis*. Chapman & Hall, London.

[85] Smith, D. & Neutra, R. (1993). Approaches to disease clustering investigations in a State Health Department, *Statistics in Medicine* **12**, 1757–1762.

[86] Snow, J. (1855). *On the Mode of Communication of Cholera*, 2nd Ed. Churchill Livingstone, London.

[87] Stone, R.A. (1988). Investigations of excess environmental risks around putative sources: statistical problems and a proposed test, *Statistics in Medicine* **7**, 649–660.

[88] Tango, T. (1995). A class of tests for detecting "General" and "Focused" clustering of rare diseases, *Statistics in Medicine* **14**, 2323–2334.

[89] Tobler, W.R. (1979). Smooth pycnophylactic interpolation for geographical regions, *Journal of the American Statistical Association* **74**, 519–535.

[90] Wallenstein, S., Naus, J. & Glaz, J. (1993). Power of the scan statistic for detection of clustering, *Statistics in Medicine* **12**, 1829–1844.

[91] Waller, L.A. (1996). Statistical power and design of focused clustering studies, *Statistics in Medicine* **15**, 765–782.

[92] Waller, L.A. & Lawson, A.B. (1995). The power of focused tests to detect disease clustering, *Statistics in Medicine* **14**, 2290–2308.

[93] Walter, S.D. (1992). The analysis of regional patterns in health data. II. The power to detect environmental effects, *American Journal of Epidemiology* **136**, 742–758.

[94] Walter, S.D. (1993). Assessing spatial patterns in disease rates, *Statistics in Medicine* **12**, 1885–1894.

[95] Wartenburg, D. & Greenberg, M. (1993). Solving the cluster puzzle: clues to follow and pitfalls to avoid, *Statistics in Medicine* **12**, 1763–1772.

JOHN F. BITHELL

Geographical Analysis Machine
see Geographical Analysis

GLIM *see* Software, Biostatistical

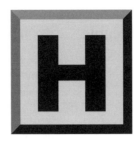

Hawthorne Effect

The Hawthorne effect is an effect on study participants that results from their knowing that they are being studied. For example, in a study of methods to promote smoking cessation, it might be necessary to contact study participants each year to determine smoking status. The Hawthorne effect could distort study results if this repeated annual contact affected smoking behavior or the reporting of smoking behavior.

M.H. GAIL

Hazard Rate

The hazard rate at time t of an event is the limit $\lambda(t) = \mathrm{limit}_{\Delta \downarrow 0} \Delta^{-1} \Pr(t \leq T \prec t + \Delta | t \leq T)$, where T is the exact time to the event. Special cases and synonyms of hazard rate, depending on the event in question, include force of mortality (where the event is death), instantaneous incidence rate, **incidence rate**, and **incidence density** (where the event is disease occurrence).

For events that can only occur once, such as death or first occurrence of an illness, the probability that the event occurs in the interval $[0, t)$ is given by $1 - \exp(-\int_0^t \lambda(u)\mathrm{d}u)$ (see **Survival Analysis, Overview**). The quantity $\int_0^t \lambda(u)\mathrm{d}u$ is known as the **cumulative hazard**.

Often, the theoretical hazard rate $\lambda(u)$ is estimated by dividing the number of events that arise in a population in a short time interval by the corresponding **person-years at risk**. The various terms, hazard rate, force of mortality, incidence density, person–years incidence rate, and incidence rate are often used to denote estimates of the corresponding theoretical hazard rate.

M.H. GAIL

Health Ratio *see* Synergy of Exposure Effects

Healthy Migrant Effect *see* Migrant Studies

Healthy Worker Effect *see* Occupational Epidemiology

Helminths *see* Epidemic Models, Deterministic

Herd Immunity *see* Communicable Diseases

***H–H* Plot** *see* Cox Regression Model

Hidden Bias *see* Propensity Score

Hill's Criteria for Causality

Despite philosophic criticisms of inductive inference, inductively oriented causal criteria have commonly been used to make such inferences. If a set of necessary and sufficient causal criteria could be used to distinguish causal from noncausal associations in **observational studies**, the job of the scientist would be eased considerably. With such criteria, all the concerns about the logic or lack thereof in causal inference could be forgotten: it would only be necessary to consult the checklist of criteria to see if a relation were causal. We know from philosophy that a set of sufficient criteria does not exist [3, 6]. Nevertheless, lists of causal criteria have become popular, possibly because they seem to provide a road map through complicated territory.

A commonly used set of criteria was proposed by Sir Austin Bradford Hill [1]; it was an expansion of a set of criteria offered previously in the landmark Surgeon General's report on Smoking and Health [11], which in turn were anticipated by the inductive canons of John Stuart Mill [5] and the rules of causal inference given by Hume [3]. Hill suggested that the following aspects of an association be considered in attempting to distinguish causal from noncausal associations: strength, consistency, specificity, temporality, biologic gradient, plausibility, coherence, experimental evidence, and analogy. The popular view that these criteria should be used for causal inference makes it necessary to examine them in detail:

Strength

Hill's argument is essentially that strong associations are more likely to be causal than weak associations because, if they could be explained by some other factor, the effect of that factor would have to be even stronger than the observed association and therefore would have become evident (*see* **Cornfield's Inequality**). Weak associations, on the other hand, are more easily explained by undetected **biases**. To some extent this is a reasonable argument, but, as Hill himself acknowledged, the fact that an association is weak does not rule out a causal connection. A commonly cited counterexample is the relation between cigarette smoking and cardiovascular disease.

Counterexamples of strong but noncausal associations are also not hard to find; any study with strong **confounding** illustrates the phenomenon. For example, consider the strong but noncausal relation between Down syndrome and birth rank, which is confounded by the relation between Down syndrome and maternal age. Of course, once the confounding factor is identified, the association is diminished by adjustment for the factor. These examples remind us that a strong association is neither necessary nor sufficient for causality, nor is weakness necessary nor sufficient for absence of causality. In addition to these counterexamples, we have to remember that neither **relative risk** nor any other measure of association is a biologically consistent feature of an association; as described by many authors [4, 7], it is a characteristic of a study population that depends on the relative **prevalence** of other causes. A strong association serves only to rule out hypotheses that the association is entirely due to one weak unmeasured **confounder** or other source of modest bias.

Consistency

Consistency refers to the repeated observation of an association in different populations under different circumstances. Lack of consistency, however, does not rule out a causal association, because some effects are produced by their causes only under unusual circumstances. More precisely, the effect of a causal agent cannot occur unless the complementary component causes act, or have already acted, to complete a sufficient cause. These conditions will not always be met. Thus, transfusions can cause human immunodeficiency virus (HIV) infection but they do not always do so: the virus must also be present. Tampon use can cause toxic shock syndrome, but only when other conditions are met, such as presence of certain bacteria. Consistency is apparent only after all the relevant details of a causal mechanism are understood, which is to say very seldom. Even studies of exactly the same phenomena can be expected to yield different results simply because they differ in their methods and **random errors**. Consistency serves only to rule out hypotheses that the association is attributable to some factor that varies across studies.

Specificity

The criterion of specificity requires that a cause leads to a single effect, not multiple effects. This argument has often been advanced to refute causal interpretations of exposures that appear to relate to myriad effects, especially by those seeking to exonerate smoking as a cause of lung cancer. The criterion is wholly invalid, however. Causes of a given effect cannot be expected to lack other effects on any logical grounds. In fact, everyday experience teaches us repeatedly that single events or conditions may have many effects. Smoking is an excellent example: it leads to many effects in the smoker. The existence of one effect does not detract from the possibility that another effect exists. Thus, specificity does not confer greater validity to any causal inference regarding the exposure effect. Hill's discussion of this criterion for inference is replete with reservations, and many authors regard this criterion as useless and misleading [8, 9].

Temporality

Temporality refers to the necessity that the cause precede the effect in time. This criterion is unarguable, insofar as any claimed observation of causation must involve the putative cause C preceding the putative effect D. It does *not*, however, follow that a reverse time order is evidence against the hypothesis that C can cause D. Rather, observations in which C followed D merely shows that C could not have caused D in these instances; they provide no evidence for or against the hypothesis that C can cause D in those instances in which it precedes D.

Biologic Gradient

Biologic gradient refers to the presence of a monotone (unidirectional) **dose–response** curve. We often expect such a monotonic relation to exist. For example, more smoking means more carcinogen exposure and more tissue damage, hence more carcinogenesis. Such an expectation is not always present, however. The somewhat controversial topic of alcohol consumption and mortality is an example. Death rates are higher among nondrinkers than among moderate drinkers, but ascend to the highest levels for heavy drinkers. Because modest alcohol consumption can have beneficial effects on serum lipid profiles, such a J-shaped dose–response curve is at least biologically plausible.

Conversely, associations that do show a monotonic trend in disease frequency with increasing levels of exposure are not necessarily causal; confounding can result in a monotonic relation between a noncausal risk factor and disease if the confounding factor itself demonstrates a biologic gradient in its relation with disease. The noncausal relation between birth rank and Down syndrome mentioned above shows a biologic gradient that merely reflects the progressive relation between maternal age and the occurrence of Down syndrome.

Thus the existence of a monotonic association is neither necessary nor sufficient for a causal relation. A nonmonotonic relation only conflicts with those causal hypotheses specific enough to predict a monotonic dose–response curve.

Plausibility

Plausibility refers to the biologic plausibility of the hypothesis, an important concern but one that is far from objective or absolute. Sartwell [9], emphasizing this point, cited the remarks of Cheever, in 1861, who was commenting on the etiology of typhus before its mode of transmission (via body lice) was known:

> It could be no more ridiculous for the stranger who passed the night in the steerage of an emigrant ship to ascribe the typhus, which he there contracted, to the vermin with which bodies of the sick might be infested. An adequate cause, one reasonable in itself, must correct the coincidences of simple experience.

What was to Cheever an implausible explanation turned out to be the correct explanation, since it was indeed the vermin that caused the typhus infection. Such is the problem with plausibility: it is too often not based on logic or data, but only on prior beliefs. This is not to say that biological knowledge should be discounted when evaluating a new hypothesis, but only to point out the difficulty in applying that knowledge.

The Bayesian approach to inference attempts to deal with this problem by requiring that one quantify, on a probability (0 to 1) scale, the certainty that one has in prior beliefs, as well as in new hypotheses. This quantification displays the dogmatism or open-mindedness of the analyst in a public fashion, with certainty values near 1 or 0 betraying a strong commitment of the analyst for or against a hypothesis. It can also provide a means of testing those quantified beliefs against new evidence [2]. Nevertheless, the Bayesian approach cannot transform plausibility into an objective causal criterion.

Coherence

Taken from the Surgeon General's report on Smoking and Health [11], the term *coherence* implies that a cause and effect interpretation for an association does not conflict with what is known of the natural history and biology of the disease. The examples Hill gave for coherence, such as the histopathologic effect of smoking on bronchial epithelium (in reference to the association between smoking and lung cancer) or the difference in lung cancer incidence by sex, could reasonably be considered examples of plausibility as well as coherence; the distinction appears to be a fine one. Hill emphasized that the absence of coherent information, as distinguished, apparently, from the presence of conflicting information, should not be taken as evidence against an association being considered causal. On the other hand, presence of conflicting information may indeed undermine a hypothesis, but one must always remember that the conflicting information may be mistaken or misinterpreted [12].

Experimental Evidence

It is not clear what Hill meant by experimental evidence. It might have referred to evidence from laboratory experiments on animals, or to evidence from human experiments. Evidence from human experiments, however, is seldom available for most epidemiologic research questions, and animal evidence relates to different species and usually to levels of exposure very different from those that humans experience. From Hill's examples, it seems that what he had in mind for experimental evidence was the result of removal of some harmful exposure in an intervention or prevention program, rather than the results of laboratory experiments [10]. The lack of availability of such evidence would at least be a pragmatic difficulty in making this a criterion for inference. Logically, however, experimental evidence is not a criterion but a test of the causal hypothesis, a test that is simply unavailable in most epidemiologic circumstances.

Although experimental tests can be much stronger than other tests, they are not as decisive as often thought, because of difficulties in interpretation. For example, one can attempt to test the hypothesis that malaria is caused by swamp gas by draining swamps in some areas and not in others to see if the malaria rates among residents are affected by the draining. As predicted by the hypothesis, the rates will drop in the areas where the swamps are drained. As Popper emphasized, however, there are always many alternative explanations for the outcome of every experiment. In this example, one alternative, which happens to be correct, is that mosquitoes are responsible for malaria transmission.

Analogy

Whatever insight might be derived from analogy is handicapped by the inventive imagination of scientists who can find analogies everywhere. At best, analogy provides a source of more elaborate hypotheses about the associations under study; absence of such analogies only reflects lack of imagination or experience, not falsity of the hypothesis.

Conclusion

As is evident, the standards of epidemiologic evidence offered by Hill are saddled with reservations and exceptions. Hill himself was ambivalent about the utility of these "standards" (he did not use the word *criteria* in the paper). On the one hand he asked "in what circumstances can we pass from this observed *association* to a verdict of *causation?*" (original emphasis). Yet, despite speaking of verdicts on causation, he disagreed that any "hard-and-fast rules of evidence" existed by which to judge causation:

> None of my nine viewpoints [criteria] can bring indisputable evidence for or against the cause-and-effect hypothesis and none can be required as a *sine qua non*.

Actually, the fourth criterion, temporality, is a *sine qua non* for causality: If the putative cause did not precede the effect, that indeed is indisputable evidence that the observed association is not causal (although this evidence does not rule out causality in other situations, for in other situations the putative cause may precede the effect). Other than this one condition, however, which may be viewed as part of the definition of causation, there is no necessary or sufficient criterion for determining whether an observed association is causal.

Acknowledgment

This article is adapted from Chapter 2 of *Modern Epidemiology* 2nd Ed. [8], with permission from the publisher.

References

[1] Hill, A.B. (1965). The environment and disease: association or causation?, *Proceedings of the Royal Society of Medicine* **58**, 295–300.

[2] Howson, C. & Urbach, P. (1993). *Scientific Reasoning. The Bayesian Approach*, 2nd Ed. Open Court, LaSalle.

[3] Hume, D. (1978). *A Treatise of Human Nature* (originally published in 1739). Oxford University Press edition, with an Analytical Index by L. A. Selby-Bigge, published 1888. 2nd Ed. with text revised and notes by P.H. Nidditch, published 1978.

[4] MacMahon, B. & Pugh, T.F. (1967). Causes and entities of disease, in *Preventive Medicine*, D.W. Clark & B. MacMahon, eds. Little, Brown & Company, Boston.

[5] Mill, J.S. (1862). *A System of Logic, Ratiocinative and Inductive*, 5th Ed. Parker, Son and Bowin, London.

[6] Popper, K.R. (1968). *The Logic of Scientific Discovery*. Harper & Row, New York.

[7] Rothman, K.J. (1976). Causes, *American Journal of Epidemiology* **104**, 587–592.

[8] Rothman, K.J. & Greenland, S. (1998). *Modern Epidemiology*, 2nd Ed. Lippincott, Philadelphia, Chapter 2.

[9] Sartwell, P. (1960). On the methodology of investigations of etiologic factors in chronic diseases – further comments, *Journal of Chronic Diseases* **11**, 61–63.

[10] Susser, M. (1988). Falsification, verification and causal inference in epidemiology: reconsiderations in the light of Sir Karl Popper's philosophy, in *Causal Inference*, K.J. Rothman, ed. Epidemiology Resources, Inc., Boston.

[11] US Department of Health, Education and Welfare (1964). Smoking and Health: Report of the Advisory Committee to the Surgeon General of the Public Health Service, *Public Health Service Publication No. 1103*. Government Printing Office, Washington.

[12] Wald, N.A. (1985). Smoking, in *Cancer Risks and Prevention*, M.P. Vessey & M. Gray, eds. Oxford University Press, New York, Chapter 3.

(*See also* **Causation**)

KENNETH J. ROTHMAN & SANDER GREENLAND

Incidence Density

An incidence density is an **incidence rate** and can be used to estimate a **hazard rate**.

M.H. GAIL

Incidence Density Ratio

The incidence density ratio is the ratio of the **incidence density** in one group to that in another group. The incidence density ratio approximates the hazard ratio if time intervals are small and can be estimated both from **cohort studies** and from **case–control studies** in which controls are selected by **density sampling**.

M.H. GAIL

Incidence Rate

The incidence rate is the number of persons who develop a disease of interest over a defined interval of time or age divided by the corresponding **person-years at risk** among members of the source population. Subjects are only "at risk" before they develop the disease of interest if, as is common, the incidence rate describes the rate of first occurrence of a disease. Usually, relatively short time intervals are used, compared with the timescale for development of disease, such as five-year intervals for a cancer incidence study. When individual follow-up data are not available to compute person-years at risk, the person-years are often estimated as the interval width times the population size at the midpoint of the interval. Synonyms for incidence rate include **incidence density** and person-years incidence rate. Incidence rate sometimes denotes a population **hazard rate**, rather than the estimate defined above. Sometimes the term incidence rate is used instead of **cumulative incidence rate**, but the concepts are distinct.

M.H. GAIL

Incidence–Prevalence Relationships

This article attempts a statistical view on the classical epidemiologic concepts of (age-specific) incidence and **prevalence**. Each individual's dynamics in the **Lexis diagram** is modeled by a simple three-state illness–death stochastic process in the age direction and individuals are recruited from a Poisson process in the time direction. Observable quantities are regarded as *estimators* of the *parameters* (incidence, prevalence, mortality, mean duration, etc.) of the statistical model.

The next section discusses increasingly complex versions of the classical epidemiologic relation

$$\text{prevalence} = \text{incidence} \times \text{duration},$$

and its generalization to age- and duration-specific incidence and mortality. Then some comments are provided on statistical techniques for estimating **incidence rates** from prevalence surveys, while the following section considers, conversely, the feasibility of estimating prevalence from information on incidence and mortality. The material is also relevant in the theory of **screening**, as briefly pointed out later.

A related topic *not* touched in this article is inference on mortality (or further morbidity) from follow-up of a **cross-sectional** sample, the so-called *prevalent cohort study*. This topic is treated in the article **Biased Sampling of Cohorts in Epidemiology**.

Prevalence, Incidence, and Duration

Most – even rather elementary – textbooks in epidemiology contain versions of the statement

$$\text{prevalence} = \text{incidence} \times \text{duration}, \qquad (1)$$

see, for example, [15, pp. 65–66] or [10, pp. 64–66]. In broad generality, (1) is a conservation equation called Little's equation in queuing theory:

time-average number of units in the system
   = arrival rule × average delay time per unit.

See Little [13] for the first general proof in the context of strictly stationary processes in steady state conditions and Ramalhoto et al. [21] for a comprehensive discussion.

In epidemiology, the archetypical situation concerns irreversible transitions between a healthy state H, a diseased state I, and the dead state D, simplest in the time- and age-homogeneous Markov illness–death process specified by intensities as follows:

$$H \xrightarrow{\alpha} I$$
$$\mu \searrow \qquad \swarrow \nu$$
$$D$$

and fed by a stationary homogeneous Poisson process with (birth) intensity β. Here α is disease intensity for

a healthy individual (the connection to the epidemiologic concept of disease incidence to be discussed below) and μ and ν are death intensities for healthy and diseased, respectively. Sometimes ν is called the **case fatality** rate or just lethality.

In this stochastic process our approach to prevalence is to imagine a **cross-sectional** sample taken at a particular time t, say $t = 0$. We may then calculate the expected number of healthy at $t = 0$ as

$$\int_0^\infty \beta \exp[-(\alpha + \mu)a]\mathrm{d}a = \frac{\beta}{\alpha + \mu}$$

since a person born at time $-a$ has probability $\exp[-(\alpha + \mu)a]$ of remaining alive and healthy until time 0; similarly the expected number of diseased at $t = 0$ is

$$\int_0^\infty \int_0^a \beta \exp[-(\alpha + \mu)y]\alpha \exp[-\alpha(a - y)]\mathrm{d}y\mathrm{d}a$$

$$= \frac{\alpha\beta}{(\alpha + \mu)\nu}.$$

Under the present assumptions, disease duration is exponentially distributed with mean ν^{-1}. Definition of disease incidence requires more care. The intensity α refers to the healthy only, while *disease incidence in the population* may be defined as the rate of occurrence of new disease in the whole population. This is

$$\beta \int_0^\infty \exp[-(\alpha + \mu)\alpha]\mathrm{d}a = \frac{\beta\alpha}{\alpha + \mu}$$

and we see that

$$\text{E(diseased)} = \frac{\beta\alpha}{\alpha + \mu}\nu^{-1}$$

$$= \text{disease incidence} \times \text{mean duration},$$

yielding (1) in the present interpretation of units of individuals (rather than the often used prevalence proportion in relative units).

Note, furthermore, that what we shall often term prevalence odds satisfies

$$\frac{\text{E(diseased)}}{\text{E(healthy)}} = \frac{\alpha\beta/[(\alpha + \mu)\nu]}{\beta/(\alpha + \mu)} = \frac{\alpha}{\nu},$$

that is,

$$\text{prevalence odds} = \text{incidence} \times \text{mean duration},$$

where incidence is now understood as *intensity of getting diseased for a healthy individual.*

Alho [5] viewed the above relations between prevalence, incidence, and duration in the macrodemographic context of stable population theory.

The above discussion may be generalized to *time-*, *age-* and disease *duration*-dependent intensities $\beta(t)$, $\alpha(t, a)$, $\mu(t, a)$, and $\nu(t, a, d)$, as documented by Keiding [11]. We may then also discuss such concepts as *age-specific prevalence*, expressing the probability of having the disease for a person at age a alive at time t. The general formulas become complicated and are not reproduced here, although some applications will be indicated below.

In the particular case of *time homogeneity*, which, though not very realistic nevertheless underlies most epidemiologic folklore, similar relations between prevalence, incidence, and duration result as above. In particular, the rate of occurrence of new cases in the population becomes

$$\beta \int_0^\infty \exp\{-[\alpha(a) + \mu(a)]\}\alpha(a)\mathrm{d}a,$$

and the expected number of diseased at $t = 0$ (prevalence on the population scale, "absolute" prevalence) becomes

$$\beta \int_0^\infty \int_0^a \exp\{-[\alpha(y) + \mu(y)]\}\alpha(y)$$
$$\times \exp[-\nu(a, a - y)]\mathrm{d}y\mathrm{d}a.$$

In the simple case where the case fatality rate $\nu(a, d)$ depends only on duration d but not age a, a change of order of integration yields

$$\int_0^\infty \beta \exp\{-[\alpha(y) + \mu(y)]\}\alpha(y)\mathrm{d}y$$
$$\times \int_0^\infty \exp[-\nu(v)]\mathrm{d}v,$$

where the first factor is incidence as just specified, while since $\exp[-\nu(v)]$ is the survival function of a diseased, the second factor is mean survival. This provides an interpretation of

$$\text{prevalence} = \text{incidence} \times \text{duration}$$

in the age-dependent case, and Keiding [11] specified how to obtain a similar interpretation when $\nu(a, d)$ depends also on a.

The relation *prevalence odds* = *disease intensity* × *mean duration* discussed in the time/age/duration homogeneous special case above, also generalizes to the age/duration inhomogeneous case, see again Keiding [11] and O'Neill et al. [19].

Inference on Incidence from Prevalence Data

As has been known in population statistics (**demography**) for hundreds of years, it is true under very restrictive stationarity assumptions (no dependence of birth and death rates on calendar time, no migration) that the age distribution of the living has density proportional to the survival function (= 1 − distribution function) of the mortality. Inference on mortality rates is therefore in principle available from the age distribution of the living.

The simplest generalization of this to morbidity (disease incidence) is analysis of *current status data* where age-specific incidence rates are estimated from the age distributions of diseased and healthy in a cross-sectional sample. Diamond & McDonald [8] gave a survey based on parametric models in discrete and continuous time while Keiding [11] and Keiding et al. [12] focused on variants of current nonparametric survival analysis techniques. Ades & Nokes [2] gave a useful practical discussion of the range and limitations of these ideas in modeling infectivity rates from seroprevalence studies; and Marschner [16] gave sample size calculations.

As emphasized by Preston [20], the crucial stationarity assumption may only be verified from at least two successive cross-sectional samples, which however might then be directly used for inference without the stationarity assumption. Recent work in this direction is due particularly to Marschner [17, 18] and Ades [1] as well as a series of papers by Brunet & Struchiner (for example [6]), in the pseudo-stochastic mathematical biology tradition.

Inference on Prevalence from Incidence and Mortality Data

It is not uncommon that disease incidence and mortality are more directly estimable (e.g. from a historically prospective incidence study with follow-up) than prevalence. In that case the relations between prevalence, incidence and duration may be used to estimate prevalence, possibly calendar time-and/or age-specifically, see Keiding [11]. Such calculations will often be variations of the nonparametric Aalen–Johansen estimator of a transition probability in a nonhomogeneous Markov illness–death process, and this link provides a methodology for derivation of standard errors.

Application of such ideas has been primarily in the context of cancer [7, 9, 23], although there are also examples from neuroepidemiology [22, 24], reference [22] containing counterfactual and predictive "what if" calculations under specified past or future structures in incidence and mortality.

Screening

There are strong relations between the above material and the mathematical theory of **screening** for chronic disease [25, 26], in the simplest but also most important case by having the three states *Healthy, Preclinical* (where the patient feels healthy but screening can identify the disease), and *Clinical*(ly manifest) diseased. The same relations are valid, properly interpreted, and Zelen & Feinleib [26] actually also obtained a *prevalence = incidence × mean duration* result. O'Neill et al. [19] formalized a concept of *initiation*, equivalent to subclinical disease onset. The comprehensive exposition of the theory of screening by Albert et al. [3, 4] and Louis et al. [14] is based on probability densities rather than intensities as in this article and most of the other references.

References

[1]   Ades, A.E. (1995). Serial HIV seroprevalence surveys: interpretation, design and role in HIV/AIDS prediction, *Journal of Acquired Immunodeficiency Syndrome* **9**, 490–499.

[2]   Ades, A.E. & Nokes, D.J. (1993). Modeling age- and time specific incidence from seroprevalence: toxoplasmosis, *American Journal of Epidemiology* **137**, 1022–1034.

[3]   Albert, A., Gertman, P.M. & Louis, T.A. (1978). Screening for the early detection of cancer – the temporal natural history of a progressive disease state, *Mathematical Biosciences* **40**, 1–59.

[4]   Albert, A., Gertman, P.M., Louis, T.A. & Liu, S.-I. (1978). Screening for the early detection of cancer – II. The impact of screening on the natural history of the disease, *Mathematical Biosciences* **40**, 61–109.

[5]   Alho, J.M. (1992). On prevalence, incidence and duration in general stable populations, *Biometrics* **48**, 587–592.

[6]   Brunet, R.C. & Struchiner, C.J. (1996). Rate estimation from prevalence information on a simple epidemiologic model for health interventions, *Theoretical Population Biology* **50**, 209–226.

[7]   Capocaccia, R. & de Angelis, R. (1997). Estimating the completeness of prevalence based on cancer registry data, *Statistics in Medicine* **16**, 425–440.

[8]   Diamond, I.D. & McDonald, J.W. (1992). Analysis of current status data, in *Demographic Applications of Event History Analysis*, J. Trussel, R. Ilankinson & J. Tilton, eds. Clarendon Press, Oxford, pp. 231–252.

[9]   Feldman, A.R., Kessler, L., Myers, M.H. & Naughton, M.D. (1986). The prevalence of cancer. Estimates based on the Connecticut Tumor Registry, *New England Journal of Medicine* **315**, 1394–1397.

[10] Ilennekens, C.H. & Buring, J.E. (1987). *Epidemiology in Medicine*. Little, Brown & Company, Boston.

[11] Keiding, N. (1991). Age specific incidence and prevalence: a statistical perspective (with discussion), *Journal of the Royal Statistical Society, Series A* **154**, 371–412.

[12] Keiding, N., Begtrup, K., Scheike, T.H. & Hasibeder, G. (1996). Estimation from current-status data in continuous time, *Lifetime Data Analysis* **2**, 119–129.

[13] Little, J.D.C. (1961). A proof for the queuing formula: $L = \lambda W$, *Operations Research* **9**, 383–387.

[14] Louis, T.A., Albert, A. & Heghinian, S. (1978). Screening for the early detection of cancer. III. Estimation of disease natural history, *Mathematical Biosciences* **40**, 111–144.

[15] MacMahon, B. & Pugh, T.F. (1970). *Epidemiology: Principles and Methods*. Little, Brown & Company, Boston.

[16] Marschner, I.C. (1994). Determining the size of a cross-sectional sample to estimate the age-specific incidence of an irreversible disease, *Statistics in Medicine* **13**, 2369–2381.

[17] Marschner, I.C. (1996). Fitting a multiplicative incidence model to age- and time-specific prevalence data, *Biometrics* **52**, 492–499.

[18] Marschner, I.C. (1997). A method for assessing age–time disease incidence using serial prevalence data, *Biometrics* **53**, 1384–1398.

[19] O'Neill, T.J., Tallis, C.M. & Leppard, P. (1985). The epidemiology of a disease using hazard functions, *Australian Journal of Statistics* **27**, 283–297.

[20] Preston, S.H. (1987). Relations among standard epidemiologic measures in a population, *American Journal of Epidemiology* **126**, 336–345.

[21] Ramalhoto, M.F., Amaral, J.A. & Cochito, M.T. (1983). A survey of J. Little's formula, *International Statistical Review* **51**, 255–278.

[22] Somnier, F.E., Keiding, N. & Paulson, O.B. (1991). Epidemiology of Myasthenia Gravis in Denmark: a longitudinal and comprehensive population survey, *Archives of Neurology* **48**, 733–739.

[23]   Verdecchia, A., Capocaccia, R., Egidi, V. & Colini, A. (1989). A method for the estimation of chronic disease morbidity and trends from mortality data, *Statistics in Medicine* **8**, 201–216.

[24]   Werdelin, L. & Keiding, N. (1990). Hereditary ataxias and associated disorders. Epidemiological aspects, *Neuroepidemiology* **9**, 321–331.

[25]   Zelen, M. (1986). A review of the theory of screening for chronic diseases: single exam and the scheduling of examinations, in *Statistical Design: Theory and Practice*. Cornell University Press, Ithaca, pp. 27–41.

[26]   Zelen, M. & Feinleib, M. (1969). On the theory of screening for chronic diseases, *Biometrika* **56**, 601–614.

NIELS KEIDING

Incident Case

An incident case is a subject who has just developed the disease or condition of interest for the first time. Incident cases of chronic diseases are particularly valuable for etiologic investigations because disease incidence, unlike disease **prevalence**, is determined by etiologic factors only and not by factors that influence survival following disease onset. To contrast incident with prevalent cases, *see* **Biased Sampling of Cohorts in Epidemiology**; **Case–Control Study, Prevalent**; **Cross-Sectional Study**; **Incidence–Prevalence Relationships**; **Prevalent Case**.

M.H. GAIL

Incubation Period *see* Latent Period

Incubation Period of Infectious Diseases

The incubation period is the time interval between exposure to a disease-causing agent and the onset of symptomatic disease. For example, the incubation period of an infectious disease refers to the time interval between infection or exposure to a viral or bacterial agent and the onset of symptomatic (clinical) disease. The incubation period is also called the clinical latency period (*see* **Latent Period**). The focus of this article is on modeling and estimating the incubation period of infectious diseases. However, some of the ideas may also be applicable to the incubation period of noninfectious disease, for example the incubation period of radiation-induced cancer that refers to the time interval from radiation exposure to cancer diagnosis.

The length of the incubation period depends on the disease and the infectious agent. It can be very short, perhaps only several days in the case of a streptococcal sore throat, or perhaps several weeks in the case of smallpox, or perhaps a decade in the case of the acquired immune deficiency syndrome (AIDS). After an individual is exposed to an infectious agent, the agent multiplies, and the host defenses are weakened. Eventually, the individual may experience the onset of clinical disease. Individuals may or may not be infectious (that is, capable of transmitting the infection to others) during the incubation period or subsequently.

The incubation period of a disease can be very variable among individuals [2, 21]. A single number, such as the mean or median incubation period, does not reveal the significant heterogeneity in incubation periods in a population for a given infectious diseases. The incubation period distribution, $F(t)$, is the probability that the incubation period is less than or equal to t time units. The probability density function of incubation periods usually is asymmetric and is skewed to the right. Sartwell [23, 24] suggested that the lognormal distribution adequately describes the incubation period distribution of a number of diseases. However, other parametric models for survival data may also adequately describe incubation period distributions, including the Weibull, gamma, log-logistic, and piecewise exponential models [9]. There is no requirement that all infected individuals eventually develop clinical disease. Thus, the distribution function, F, may not be proper. For example, one may postulate that a proportion, p, of infected individuals eventually develop clinical disease with incubation distribution, F_1, and the remaining proportion of infected individuals, $1 - p$, never develop disease; then we have the mixture model $F(t) = pF_1(t)$.

Studies of the incubation period distribution are important for several reasons. First, the incubation period distribution is important for forecasting the course of epidemics, and is used with either transmission models [1] or **back-calculation** approaches [9]. If the incubation period is long, then infected individuals may be silently and unknowingly spreading the infection to others. Secondly, identification of covariates or cofactors that may lengthen the incubation period may lead to the development of effective therapeutic interventions. Thirdly, knowledge of the incubation period is useful in counseling infected patients about their prognosis. Finally, the incubation period is a critical parameter in designing clinical trials of early interventions and vaccines (*see* **Communicable Diseases**; **Infectious Disease Models**).

The ideal study for estimating the incubation period is to monitor a **cohort** of uninfected individuals, determine the dates of infection, and then to follow the infected patients to determine the dates of the onset of clinical disease. The data for estimating the incubation period distribution would consist of the time interval between infection and disease for those patients who became infected. If an infected individual did not develop clinical disease at the time of last follow-up, then the data would be right censored at that time. Classical survival analysis techniques could be used to estimate the incubation period distribution from right-censored *data* [12]. Kaplan–Meier survival curves could be used to estimate $F(t)$ non-parametrically, the cumulative distribution function of incubation periods. Parametric models could also be fit to the right-censored incubation period data. A simple example is the case of a single point source epidemic, as might occur with salmonellosis where infection is transmitted from contaminated food or water [21]. In this example a cohort may be defined as all individuals who were exposed (e.g. individuals who are in a restaurant on the given day that contaminated food was served), in which case the date of exposure is known precisely. Another example of a point source epidemic for a noninfectious disease is the onset of leukemia associated with radiation exposure following the 1945 atomic bomb explosion in Hiroshima [11]. The incidence of leukemia appeared to peak about six years after exposure. Survival analyses could be performed on the time intervals from exposure to clinical disease, and of course some of these intervals may be right censored at the times of last follow-up (*see* **Epidemic Curve**).

Unfortunately, the ideal study of incubation periods can seldom be performed because of a number of

important complications. First, it may not be possible to identify a cohort of initially uninfected individuals, and to follow them over time. Instead, we may only have available a sample of cases who already have clinical disease (see the section "Retrospective ascertainment" below). Even if a cohort is assembled and followed over time, it may not be possible to ascertain either the exact dates of infection (exposure) or the onset of clinical disease (see the section "Cohort studies" below). For example, an individual may already be infected at the time of enrollment in a cohort study, but the time that incident infection occurred is unknown. Many of these problems have surfaced in studies of the incubation period of AIDS, and have been the subject of active methodologic research among statisticians in recent years. In the next sections we discuss more fully these complexities and the methodologic approaches to address them. The issues are illustrated with studies of AIDS, although the methods are applicable more generally to other infectious diseases.

Retrospective Ascertainment

The first data on the incubation period of AIDS (time from human immunodeficiency virus (HIV) infection to AIDS diagnosis) were based on transfusion-associated AIDS cases [22]. In that study, AIDS cases were identified who had become infected by receiving a transfusion of infected blood. The date of infection was estimated retrospectively as the date of blood transfusion. There was an important selection criterion to get into the study, namely that subjects had to have AIDS. Early in an epidemic of a new disease the only data about incubation periods that may be gathered rapidly may come from symptomatic cases of disease who have already been identified. These cases of disease are then retrospectively studied to determine dates of exposure to the infectious agent. Such studies have been referred to as having "retrospective ascertainment" because only individuals with symptomatic disease are included and then they are retrospectively studied. A naive analysis of this type of data, which did not account for the selection criteria, could lead to serious underestimation of the incubation period. This is because the data are right truncated. Individuals with long incubation periods may not yet have symptomatic disease, and thus could not possibly be included in the data set. To analyze such data properly, the analysis must condition properly on the selection criteria [18, 19].

There are other **biases** with studies based on retrospective ascertainment. For instance in the transfusion example, patients who receive blood transfusion are often elderly and sick with chronic diseases, and thus they may die from other causes of death before developing AIDS. This leads to length-biased sampling: we are more likely to observe patients with shorter incubation periods, because patients with long incubation periods may die first from another disease and thus are never included in the data set. In a series of papers, statisticians have developed methods to correct for these and other biases (see, for example, [18], [19], and [25]). However, none of these methods can correct for the fundamental limitation of this sort of data: they are retrospective and involve only cases of disease and so without strong parametric assumptions they provide essentially no information about the prospective probability of getting a disease once one is infected.

Cohort Studies

A second type of study involves identifying a cohort of uninfected individuals, ascertaining as best one can the subsequent dates of infection, and following the infected individuals to ascertain the date of onset of clinical disease. The first issue concerns the difficulty in identifying the date of infection. The usual method is to test individuals serially with a laboratory assay such as the test for antibodies to the infectious agent. In the case of AIDS, individuals may be serially tested with enzyme-linked immunosorbent assays (ELISAs) or Western Blot assays to identify the dates of seroconversion to HIV antibodies [16]. A complication is that the date of seroconversion does not correspond to the date of infection. Infected individuals will be seronegative for antibodies to the virus until they develop detectable antibodies, usually within several months. Although we define the incubation period as the time from infection to the clinical diagnosis of disease, many studies cannot identify the actual dates of infection but only the time of antibody seroconversion. However, in the case of AIDS, the time from infection to antibody seroconversion is relatively short (approximate median is two months) compared with the much longer period from seroconversion to the onset of disease. Accordingly,

many studies define the incubation period to be the time interval from antibody seroconversion (becoming antibody positive) to the onset of clinical disease. Nevertheless, this points out that the results of studies of incubation periods may depend on the choices of the assays that are used to ascertain infection or exposure to the infectious agent. Polymerase chain reaction (PCR) testing may identify evidence of infection considerably earlier than antibody testing [17].

If individuals are periodically screened by laboratory tests for evidence of infection, then the date of infection can at best be determined up to an interval (i.e. interval censored). This interval is defined by the time of the latest screening test that was negative for infection, L, and the earliest screening test that was positive for infection, R. The term *doubly censored data* refers to time to event data for which both the time origin and failure time are censored. In cohort studies of the incubation period the data are frequently doubly censored because the date of infection is interval censored and the date of onset of clinical disease is right censored for those individuals who have not developed clinical disease by the time of the last follow-up.

A popular *ad hoc* approach for analyzing doubly censored data on incubation periods is to estimate (impute) the calendar date of infection by the midpoint of the interval. The imputed midpoint calendar date of infection is $S = (L + R)/2$. Then, standard survival analysis techniques for right-censored data are used on the incubation periods with imputed dates of infection. However, such approaches will typically be biased and give incorrect variance estimates. The bias of the estimated incubation resulting from midpoint imputation depends critically on the width of the intervals, $R - L$, the incubation distribution, and the density of infection times. For example, in the exponential growth phase of simple epidemics, midpoint imputation will tend to underestimate the time of infection and thus overestimates the incubation period. Law & Brookmeyer [20] studied the impact of midpoint imputation, and concluded that with a median incubation period of 10 years in the case of AIDS, the bias resulting from midpoint imputation associated with intervals even as large as two years is relatively small.

A more formal parametric approach for analyzing the doubly censored data in studies of the incubation period involves specifying parametric models and joint estimation of both the probability densities of infection times and of incubation times. The likelihood function is maximized to obtain the maximum likelihood estimators. This approach was used by Brookmeyer & Goedert [10] to estimate the incubation period of HIV infection among hemophiliacs. Bacchetti & Jewell [4] used a weakly semiparametric approach. A discrete time scale was used with a separate parameter to represent the discrete **hazard** for each month. To avoid irregularities that result from trying to estimate a large number of parameters (e.g. wildly varying hazards from one month to the next with large variances), a penalized likelihood function was used that penalized for "roughness" in the estimated hazard function. A completely nonparametric approach to the problem has been given by De Gruttola & Lagakos [14]. However, the completely nonparametric estimate of the incubation period distribution, $F(t)$, is often numerically unstable, and it is not defined for all values of t.

Deconvolution Methods

Occasionally, population data may be available both about the incidence of clinical disease and infection rates in the population. The expected **cumulative incidence** of clinical disease up to calendar time t, $D(t)$, is related to infection rates $g(s)$ at calendar time s (numbers of new infections per unit time) and the incubation period distribution, by the convolution equation

$$D(t) = \int_0^t g(s)F(t-s)\,ds.$$

The basic idea is to use data on $D(t)$ and an estimate of $g(s)$ to glean information about F. This method was pioneered by Bacchetti & Moss [5] and Bacchetti [3] in connection with estimating the incubation period of HIV infection. The usefulness of the method depends on the availability of accurate information on the infection rates in the population, $g(s)$, and accurate disease **surveillance** data over time. For example, detailed information about historical infection rates was available in San Francisco on the basis of several epidemiologic surveys and cohort studies [5, 26]. The statistical framework is as follows. Let y_j represent the number of cases of disease in calendar interval I_j. Suppose that N, the cumulative number of infections that have occurred, is known.

Then the vector of counts of cases of disease, $\mathbf{y}$, has a multinomial distribution with sample size N and cell probabilities that involve the incubation distribution and the known infection rates. Maximum likelihood estimation methods are used to estimate the parameters of the incubation period distribution. The method is closely related to the back-calculation methodology which uses data on $D(t)$ and an estimate of F to estimate historical infection rates $g(s)$. Back-calculation is a method for estimating past infection rates from disease surveillance data. The method requires reliable counts of numbers of cases of disease diagnosed over time and a reliable estimate of the incubation period distribution. The method has been used to obtain short-term projects of disease incidence and to estimate **prevalence** of infection [6, 9]. Early references on back-calculation are [7] and [8]

Synthesis of Studies of the Incubation Period

The main complications in the analysis and interpretation of studies of the incubation period include uncertainty in the dates of infection and the sampling criteria by which individuals are included in the data set. Accordingly, it is important to synthesize and compare estimates across studies because the estimates may be used on different methodologies with different underlying assumptions.

In the case of AIDS, many different methodologies outlined in this article have been used to study the incubation period distribution. The results from several different methodologies have been compared [15] and a general picture emerges [9]. The probability of developing AIDS within the first two years of HIV antibody seroconversion is very small, less than 0.03. Then the hazard of progression to AIDS begins to rise rapidly so that the cumulative probability of developing AIDS within seven years of seroconversion is approximately 0.25 and the median incubation period is nearly 10 years. When comparing incubation period estimates from different studies, an important consideration is whether treatments were available to delay progression and thus alter the incubation period distribution. Treatments such as zidovudine (AZT) became available beginning in 1987 which may lengthen the incubation period. In the case of AIDS, the one covariate that has been shown to influence the length of the incubation period in multiple studies is the age at infection [13].

References

[1] Anderson, R.M. & May, R.M. (1992). *Infectious Diseases of Humans: Dynamics and Control.* Oxford University Press, Oxford.

[2] Armenian, H.K. & Lilienfeld, A.M. (1974). The distribution of incubations periods of neoplastic diseases, *American Journal of Epidemiology* **99**, 92–100.

[3] Bacchetti, P. (1990). Estimating the incubation period of AIDS by comparing population infection and diagnostic patterns, *Journal of the American Statistical Association* **85**, 1002–1008.

[4] Bacchetti, P. & Jewell, N.P. (1991). Nonparametric estimation of the incubation period of AIDS based on a prevalent cohort with unknown infection times, *Biometrics* **47**, 947–960.

[5] Bacchetti, P. & Moss, A.R. (1989). Incubation period of AIDS in San Francisco, *Nature* **338**, 251–253.

[6] Bacchetti, P., Segal, M. & Jewell, N.P. (1993). Back-calculation of HIV infection rates (with discussion), *Statistical Science* **8**, 82–119.

[7] Brookmeyer, R. & Gail, M.H. (1986). Minimum size of the acquired immunodeficiency syndrome (AIDS) epidemic in the United States, *Lancet* **2**, 1320–1322.

[8] Brookmeyer, R. & Gail, M.H. (1988). A method for obtaining short-term projections and lower bounds on the size of the AIDS epidemic, *Journal of the American Statistical Association* **83**, 301–308.

[9] Brookmeyer, R. & Gail, M.H. (1994). *AIDS Epidemiology: A Quantitative Approach.* Oxford University Press, New York.

[10] Brookmeyer, R. & Goedert, J. (1989). Censoring in an epidemic with an application to hemophilia-associated AIDS, *Biometrics* **45** 325–335.

[11] Cobb, S., Miller, M. & Wald, N. (1959). On the estimation of the incubation period in malignant disease, *Journal of Chronic Disease* **9**, 385–393.

[12] Cox, D.R. & Oakes, D. (1984). *Analysis of Survival Data.* Chapman & Hall, London.

[13] Darby, S.C., Doll, R. & Thakrar, R., Rizza, C. & Cox, D.R. (1990). Time from infection with HIV to onset of AIDS in patients with hemophilia in the United Kingdom, *Statistics in Medicine* **9**, 681–689.

[14] De Gruttola, V. & Lagakos, S.W. (1989). Analysis of doubly-censored survival data with applications to AIDS, *Biometrics* **45**, 1–11.

[15] Gail, M.H. & Rosenberg, P.S. (1992). in *AIDS Epidemiology: Methodologic Issues*, N. Jewell, K. Keietz, & V. Farewell, eds. Birkhauser, Boston, pp. 1–38.

[16] Haseltine, W.A. (1989). Silent HIV infections, *New England Journal of Medicine* **320**, 1487–1489.

[17] Horsborgh, C.R., Qu, C.Y., Jason, I.M., Holmberg, S., Longini, I., Schable, C., Mayer, K., Lifson, A., Schochetman, G., Ward, J., Rutherford, G., Evatt, B., Seage, G. & Jaffe, H. (1989). Duration of human immunodeficiency virus infection before detection of antibody, *Lancet* **2**, 637–640.

[18] Kalfbleisch, J.D. & Lawless, J.F. (1989). Inference based on retrospective ascertainment: an analysis of the data on transfusion related AIDS, *Journal of the American Statistical Association* **84**, 360–372.

[19] Lagakos, S., Barraj, L. & De Gruttola, V. (1988). Non-parametric analysis of truncated survival data with application to AIDS, *Biometrika* **75**, 515–523.

[20] Law, C.G. & Brookmeyer, R. (1992). Effects of mid-point imputation on the analysis of doubly censored data, *Statistics in Medicine* **11**, 1569–1578.

[21] Lilienfeld, A.M. & Lilienfeld, D.E. (1980). *Foundations of Epidemiology*, 2nd Ed. Oxford University Press, Oxford.

[22] Lui, K.J., Lawrence, D.N., Morgan, W.M., Peterman, T., Haverkos, H. & Bregman, D. (1986). A model based approach for estimating the mean incubation period of transfusion-associated acquired immunodeficiency syndrome, *Proceedings of the National Academy of Sciences* **83**, 3051–3055.

[23] Sartwell, P.E. (1950). The distribution of incubation periods of infectious disease, *American Journal of Hygiene* **51**, 310–318.

[24] Sartwell, P.E. (1966). The incubation period and the dynamics of infectious of disease, *American Journal of Epidemiology* **83**, 204–216.

[25] Wang, M.-C. (1992). The analysis of retrospectively ascertained data in the presence of reporting delays, *Journal of the American Statistical Association* **87**, 397–406.

[26] Winkelstein, W., Samuel, M., Padian, N.S., Wiley, J., Lang, W., Anderson, R. & Levy, J. (1987). The San Francisco Men's Health Study III. Reduction in human immunodeficiency virus transmission among homosexual/bisexual men, 1982–1986, *American Journal of Public Health* **77**, 685–689.

RON BROOKMEYER

Indirect Standardization *see* Standardization Methods

Individual(ized) Risk *see* Absolute Risk

Infant and Perinatal Mortality

An infant death is defined as the death of a live-born baby before a completed year after birth [26]. The concept of infant mortality did not emerge until the latter half of the nineteenth century, although data for much earlier periods have subsequently been used to construct infant mortality rates [3, 11]. Similarly, the idea that stillbirths and deaths in the first week of life could be grouped together and described as perinatal deaths was not put forward until 1948 [16], but perinatal mortality rates have been constructed retrospectively for earlier years.

The Emergence of the Concept of "Infantile Mortality"

In 1858, Sir John Simon, Medical Officer to the General Board of Health used the term "infantine death rate" for mortality among children under the age of five. In his introduction to *Papers Relating to the Sanitary State of the People of England* [18], he expressed the view that this rate was a proxy measure of the health of the population. Drawing attention to the wide differences between districts, he commented that these infantine death rates

> ... furnish a very sensitive test of sanitary circumstances; so that differences of infantine death-rate are, under certain circumstances, the best proof of differences of household condition in any number of compared districts. And, secondly, those places where infants are most apt to die are necessarily the places where survivors are most apt to be sickly ... [18].

He went on to suggest that, "Deaths which occur in excess within five years of birth are mainly due to two sets of causes; first to the common infectious diseases of childhood prevailing with unusual fatality; and secondly to the endemic prevalence of convulsive disorders, diarrhoea and pulmonary inflammation". A factor that he did not mention was differences in the completeness of registration of births. It was likely that some babies who died shortly after birth were not registered; in particular, babies born outside marriage in big cities.

William Farr first used the current definition of infant mortality indirectly when reporting deaths in 1875, although he did not explicitly use the term "infant", nor the word "infantile", which was more commonly used in the succeeding decades. He wrote, "I show that in 1000 infants born in 1875 no less than 158 died in the first year of life ..." [5].

Infantile Mortality and Stillbirth Registration

In the same report, William Farr commented on the implications of changes in the law that had made the registration of live births compulsory in 1875. He pointed out that, "In the case of children born alive – or who breathe – both the birth and death are registered, but still-born children are not registered in England" but "Under the provisions of the new Registration Act, no still-born children, however, should be buried without a certificate stating that they were still-born" [5]. There is good evidence that these certificates were also used to bury victims of infanticide [11].

An international survey undertaken for the Select Committee on Stillbirth Registration and published in 1893 showed that Britain and Ireland lagged behind many other countries in not having stillbirth registration [10]. Nearly 20 years later, a second and fuller survey was done by the "Special Committee on Infantile Mortality" set up by the Royal Statistical Society [17].

These surveys covered European countries, New Zealand, states of Australia and the US and provinces of Canada. The Royal Statistical Society's survey also covered other British colonies and some Latin American countries. It found that stillbirth registration was compulsory in most countries, but that, "The large majority of the countries where registration is not required are under the British Crown, and it may be concluded that the Registration Laws in force in such countries have been based on the English model." In contrast, Sweden had introduced registration of both live and still births and deaths as early as 1749, followed by Denmark and Norway in 1801.

The surveys found wide differences between the countries in their criteria for birth registration and for distinguishing between infant deaths and stillbirths. As William Farr had already pointed out, "In France, under the provisions of the Code Napoleon, children who die (either before or after birth) before registration, are recorded as still-born. Dr Bertillon estimates that twenty-two in 100 of the children registered in France as still-born breathed, and such children in England would be registered among the births and deaths" [5].

It was this problem that prompted the Royal Statistical Society's enquiry. When presenting the Committee's report to the Society, Reginald Dudfield focused his attention on the need for a definition of stillbirth, as none of the countries with stillbirth registration appeared to have one in their legislation [4]. He considered two sets of issues. The first was the question of "viability". This was linked to the gestational age after which the fetus should be considered a child capable of independent life. The second was how to establish whether the fetus or child was, or had been, alive at birth.

After asking the Obstetrical Section of the Royal Society of Medicine for a definition of stillbirth, he recommended the following slightly amended version:

> A "still-born child" means a child whose body at birth measures not less than 13 inches (32 centimetres) in length from the crown of the head to the sole of the heel and who, when completely born (the head, body and limbs of the child, but not necessarily the afterbirth being extruded from the body of the mother), exhibits no sign of life – that is to say whose heart has ceased to function, as demonstrated by the absence of pulsation in the cord at its attachment to the body of the child and the absence of any heart-sounds or impulses.
> NOTE: Crying and/or breathing – being secondary signs of life, manifested only when the heart is acting – can be relied upon as signs of life, but in the absence of either or both is not to be held to be proof of absence of life in the child [4].

When stillbirth registration was eventually introduced in England and Wales in 1927, a shorter definition based on gestational age was used:

> "Stillborn" and "stillbirth" shall apply to any child who has issued forth from its mother after the twenty-eighth week of pregnancy and which did not at any time after being completely expelled from its mother breathe or show any other signs of life [6].

Public Concern About Infantile Mortality and Developments in Analysis

The Royal Statistical Society's enquiry came at a time when there had been a growing concern about

infant mortality in a number of countries. In Britain, this had been prompted by the discovery that many potential recruits for the Boer War were unfit and by the campaign by the Women's Co-operative Guild for maternity services.

The Royal Statistical Society Committee also discussed the way in which the infantile mortality rate was calculated. It had defined this as the ratio of the deaths during the first year of life to births. Its enquiries had revealed, however, that some countries had used the estimated numbers alive under the age of one year instead. Given the relative inaccuracy of population estimates, the Committee recommended using births instead.

Having pointed out that some countries compiled their birth statistics by year of registration and others by year of occurrence, it recommended using occurrences. It also recommended that stillbirths should be tabulated separately and that in countries where live-born babies who died before registration were registered as stillbirths, they should actually be counted as infant deaths [17].

As a result of public concern about infant mortality, analyses of infant mortality by age at death in the Annual Reports of the Registrar General from 1904 were more detailed than in earlier years. In addition, a series of four reports on infant mortality was published by the Local Government Board, the government department responsible for public health. In the first of these, the Board's Chief Medical Officer, Arthur Newsholme reiterated John Simon's view in stating that, "Infant mortality is the most sensitive index we possess of social welfare and of sanitary administration, especially under urban conditions" [14]. These reports compared the infant mortality rates for different parts of England and Wales and discussed the comparisons and local data in relation to factors such as sex, legitimacy, family size, the quality of help available in childbirth, the ages of mothers, poverty, overcrowding and defective sanitation.

A similar concern about infant mortality in the US at the same period has been attributed to its emergence as a world power.

> The problem of infant mortality is one of the great social and economic problems of our day … A nation may waste its forests, its water power, its mines, and to some degree, even its lands, but if it is to hold its own in the struggle for supremacy, its children must be conserved at any cost. On

the physical, intellectual and moral strength of the children of today the future depends [9].

One response to this was the setting up of the Children's Bureau and its enquiry in 1913 into infant mortality in eight cities. This enquiry took a cohort approach, following up children born in a given year, and was analyzed by a statistician, Robert Morse Woodbury (*see* **Birth Cohort Studies**). Having considered the same broad range of factors as Arthur Newsholme, he concluded that the level of the father's earnings was the strongest "causal" factor associated with infant mortality [23].

These conclusions underpinned calls for political action to improve the conditions for young children and their parents, but these were not the only views held at the time. Followers of the eugenics movement took the view that heredity was the prime factor in infant mortality and that attempts to reduce it hindered natural selection by delaying or preventing the death of children who would survive as "weaklings" [15].

The introduction of new technology in the form of punched card equipment increased the extent to which infant mortality could be analyzed by cause, age at death, and other factors [3]. Peter McKinlay's analysis of the decline in infant mortality in England and Wales in the first quarter of the twentieth century showed that, "... all ages have not shared in this amelioration to the same extent ... as a general rule, the nearer to birth the less has the mortality been affected" [12].

In his analysis, he subdivided infant mortality into two categories, "(a) the death rate from 'congenital debility, malformation and premature birth' (number 28 of causes of death given for each separate district in the Annual Reports of the Registrar General), and (b) the remainder of the infant deaths under one year". He labeled these as "neo-natal" and "post-natal", respectively, and called stillbirths "ante-natal" deaths.

He concluded from his analysis of differences between areas of England and Wales that

only the provision of skilled assistance to mothers in childbed is of importance in connection with ante-natal mortality. ... The neo-natal death rate is related both to variations in external environment and in the obstetrical assistance available to mothers in childbed. ... The postnatal death rate seems to offer the greatest scope for administrative measures.

In this case the health of the mother would appear to come first in order of appearance, environment also is of some importance, whereas the effects of variations in obstetrical services have now ceased to be reflected on the mortality of infancy [12].

The term "neonatal" was also used a few years later in an international analysis for the League of Nations [19]. This had a demographic focus and started by looking at trends in countries' infant mortality in relation to their birth rates, population changes and overall death rates. It brought together the two streams of opinion on infant mortality in stating that, "It is evident that the causes of infant mortality may be divided into two distinct categories: (a) those depending on the fitness of the infant to live at all, and (b) those arising from the unfitness of the surroundings to support infant life" [19].

In comparing the death rates for different countries, the author grouped together deaths of live-born babies under the age of one month with stillbirths, partly to get over the differences in stillbirth registration referred to earlier. The term "birth mortality" was suggested for this combined rate. This rate varied far less between countries than that for older babies. The author commented that, "Infant mortality has repeatedly been stated to be the best measure of the sanitary state of a country ... if the infant mortality rate is employed for this purpose, it should clearly be only the part relating to infants over 1 month" [19].

The Establishment of Current Definitions

In the latter half of the twentieth century, the current definitions of fetal death, stillbirth, and the components of the infant mortality rate have become established. They are shown in Figure 1. Introducing these definitions, the Registrar General's Statistical Review for England and Wales for 1951 commented that the use of the term "neonatal period" was "now traditional among obstetricians and compilers of vital statistics" and its first use by writers of Annual Reviews had been in 1936 [7]. It also pointed out the term "perinatal mortality" had first been used in 1950. The term had been coined by a demographer Sigismund Peller, who took the view that time trends in early neonatal deaths had more in common with those in stillbirths than with those in the rest of the first year of life [16].

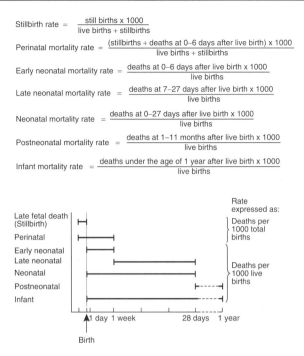

Stillbirth rate $=\dfrac{\text{still births} \times 1000}{\text{live births} + \text{stillbirths}}$

Perinatal mortality rate $=\dfrac{(\text{stillbirths} + \text{deaths at 0–6 days after live birth}) \times 1000}{\text{live births} + \text{stillbirths}}$

Early neonatal mortality rate $=\dfrac{\text{deaths at 0–6 days after live birth} \times 1000}{\text{live births}}$

Late neonatal mortality rate $=\dfrac{\text{deaths at 7–27 days after live birth} \times 1000}{\text{live births}}$

Neonatal mortality rate $=\dfrac{\text{deaths at 0–27 days after live birth} \times 1000}{\text{live births}}$

Postneonatal mortality rate $=\dfrac{\text{deaths at 1–11 months after live birth} \times 1000}{\text{live births}}$

Infant mortality rate $=\dfrac{\text{deaths under the age of 1 year after live birth} \times 1000}{\text{live births}}$

Figure 1   Definitions of stillbirth and infant morality rates. Reproduced from Macfarlane & Mugford [11] by permission of the Office for National Statistics. © Crown copyright 1984

In most developed countries, infant mortality rates have fallen persistently and dramatically in the latter half of the twentieth century to well below 10 infant deaths per 1000 live births. As the survival rates of preterm and immature babies have risen, the definitions used have been extended to include ever smaller babies and fetuses and countries still differ considerably in their criteria for registering live and still births. [8, 13].

The World Health Organization's Expert Committee on Vital Statistics recommended in 1950 that, as a minimum, all countries register and tabulate all fetal deaths after the 28th completed week of gestation [24]. This was endorsed in the seventh revision of the **International Classification of Diseases (ICD)**. This was the first to incorporate a definition of stillbirth that separates the definition of a dead-born fetus from the criteria for registration.

A quarter of a century later, a different approach was used in the ninth revision of the ICD. This recommended that *national* perinatal statistics should include all fetuses and babies delivered "weighing at least 500 g or, where birthweight is unavailable, the corresponding gestational age (22 weeks) or body

length (25 cm crown–heel), whether alive or dead" [25]. It went on to acknowledge that countries' legal requirements might have different criteria for registration purposes and that international comparisons should be restricted to fetuses and babies "weighing 1000 g or more (or, where birthweight is unavailable, the corresponding gestational age (28 weeks) or body length (35 cm crown–heel)" [25].

The tenth revision of the ICD took yet another approach and defined the perinatal period "which commences at 22 completed weeks (154 days) of gestation (the time when birthweight is normally 500 g) and ends seven completed days after live birth" [26]. Although the ICD no longer uses the term stillbirth, the term still appears in the legislation of individual countries, such as the countries of the UK.

The relevance of the upper cutoff point for the perinatal period has often been questioned in recent years. Increasingly, the use of intensive care is enabling very immature babies to survive, but there is also a tendency for those that die to do so later after birth. One response to this is to redefine perinatal deaths as the sum of all stillbirths and neonatal deaths, as is done in Australia. Another, which takes into account the view that there are increasing differences between stillbirths and neonatal deaths, is to tabulate stillbirths, neonatal and postneonatal deaths separately and drop the use of the perinatal mortality rate.

The ninth revision of the ICD recommended using a special form of certificate for perinatal deaths, with the cause section subdivided into "main and other diseases or conditions in the fetus or infant," "main and other maternal conditions affecting the fetus or infant" and "other relevant circumstances" [25]. It did not indicate how these data should be analyzed. In response to this problem, the Office of Population Censuses and Surveys, now known as the Office for National Statistics, has devised a hierarchical classification to group causes of stillbirth and neonatal death from the forms of certificate it introduced in 1986 [1, 2]. This classification uses categories first proposed by Jonathan Wigglesworth for use with information derived from case notes [20] and also builds on the extensive research done over many years in Aberdeen, Scotland.

Sources of Data on Infant and Perinatal Mortality

By the end of the twentieth century, most developed countries had well-established and complete systems for the civil registration of live births, stillbirths and deaths. These are used to derive stillbirth and infant mortality statistics published by individual countries and international organizations, notably the World Health Organization. In contrast, less-developed countries tend either to have registrations which are incomplete, or to have no registration system at all. Methods have been developed to estimate stillbirth and infant mortality rates for these countries by asking women about previous births and their outcome in population surveys or when they have a subsequent baby [21].

Infant mortality rates are published annually by the United Nations Children's Fund (UNICEF) [22]. These showed that by 1997, infant mortality rates for most developed countries were below 10 per thousand live births. Meanwhile, a minority of less-developed countries still had infant rates as high as 100 per thousand live births, with a few having rates above 160 per thousand live births.

References

[1]   Alberman, A., Botting, B., Blatchley, N. & Twidell, A. (1994). A new hierarchical classification of causes of infant deaths in England and Wales, *Archives of Disease in Childhood* **70**, 403–409.

[2]   Alberman, A., Blatchley, N., Botting, B., Schuman, J. & Dunn A. (1997). Medical causes on stillbirth certificates in England and Wales; distribution and results of hierarchical classifications tested for the Office for National Statistics, *British Journal of Obstetrics and Gynaecology* **104**, 1043–1049.

[3]   Armstrong, D. (1986). The invention of infant mortality, *Sociology of Health and Illness* **8**, 211–232.

[4]   Dudfield, R. (1912). Still-births in relation to infant mortality, *Journal of the Royal Statistical Society* **76**, 1–26.

[5]   Farr, W. (1877). Letter to the Registrar General, in *Thirty-eighth Annual Report of the Registrar General of Births, Deaths and Marriages in England*. Abstracts of 1875. Cd 1786. HMSO, London.

[6]   General Register Office (1929). *The Registrar General's Statistical Review of England and Wales for the Year 1927*. HMSO, London.

[7]   General Register Office (1954). *The Registrar General's Statistical Review of England and Wales for the Year 1951*. HMSO, London.

[8]   Gourbin, C. & Masuy-Stroobant, G. (1995). Registration of vital data: are live and stillbirths comparable all over Europe?, *Bulletin of the World Health Organization* **73**, 449–460.

[9]   Holt, L.E. (1913). Infant mortality, ancient and modern. An historical sketch, *Archives of Pediatrics* **30**, 885–915.

[10]   House of Commons(1893). *Still-births in England and Other Countries*. Return to House of Commons. No 279. HMSO, London.

[11]   Macfarlane, A.J. & Mugford, M. (1999). *Birth Counts: Statistics of Pregnancy and Childbirth*, 2nd Ed. The Stationery Office, London.

[12]   McKinlay, P.L. (1929). Some statistical aspects of infant mortality, *Journal of Hygiene* **28**, 394–417.

[13]   Mugford, M. (1983). A comparison of reported differences of vital events and statistics, *WHO Statistics Quarterly* **26**, 201–212.

[14]   Newsholme, A. (1910). *Report by the Medical Officer on Infant and Child Mortality*, Supplement to the Thirty-Ninth Annual Report of the Local Government Board for 1909–10. Cd 5263. HMSO, London.

[15]   Pearson, K. (1912). The intensity of natural selection in man, *Proceedings of the Royal Society of London, Series B* **85**, 469–476.

[16]   Peller, S. (1948). Mortality past and future, *Population Studies* **1**, 405–456.

[17]   Royal Statistical Society (1912). Report of Special Committee on Infantile Mortality, *Journal of the Royal Statistical Society* **76**, 27–87.

[18]   Simon, J. (1858). Introductory report, in *Papers Relating to the Sanitary State of the People of England*. HMSO, London.

[19]   Stouman, K. (1934). The perilous threshold of life. League of Nations, *Quarterly Bulletin of the Health Organisation* **3**, 531–612.

[20]   Wigglesworth, J.S. (1980). Monitoring perinatal mortality – a patho-physiological approach, *Lancet* **ii**, 684–686.

[21]   United Nations (1983). *Indirect Techniques for Demographic Estimation. Manual X*. United Nations, New York.

[22]   United Nations Children's Fund (1999). *The State of the World's Children, 1999*. Oxford University Press, Oxford.

[23]   Woodbury, R.M. (1925). *Causal Factors in Infant Mortality. A Statistical Study Based on Investigation in Eight Cities*, Children's Bureau Publication No 25. Government Printing Office, Washington.

[24]   World Health Organization (1957). *Manual of the International Statistical Classification of Diseases, Injuries and Causes of Death*, 7th Rev., Vol. 1. WHO, Geneva.

[25]   World Health Organization (1977). *Manual of the International Statistical Classification of Diseases, Injuries and Causes of Death*, 9th Rev., Vol. 1. WHO, Geneva.

[26]   World Health Organization (1992). *International Classification of Diseases and Related Health Problems*, 10th Rev., Vol. 1. WHO, Geneva.

(*See also* **Cause of Death, Underlying and Multiple**; **Death Certification**; **Vital Statistics, Overview**)

ALISON J. MACFARLANE

Infectious Disease Models

There are two major roles for stochastic infectious disease models. Their study provides insights into the spread of disease in a community, and they are an essential component in the analysis of data from empirical studies of infectious disease (*see* **Epidemic Models, Stochastic**).

The Epidemic Threshold Theorem

A major insight provided by epidemic models is that major epidemics can be prevented in a large community by immunizing only a fraction of the individuals. This property is sometimes referred to

as herd immunity, and is quantified by the **epidemic threshold** theorem. Deterministic models for infectious diseases (*see* **Epidemic Models, Deterministic**) indicate this result, but these models assume that both the group of susceptible individuals and the group of infective individuals are large throughout the epidemic. The stochastic version of the threshold theorem also requires a large susceptible group, but the infection process may start with only one infective individual. The stochastic threshold theorem is also richer in that it quantifies the probability of a major epidemic when a small number of infective individuals enter a large community that is currently free from the disease.

In the overly simple setting of a large community of homogeneous individuals, who mix uniformly, the threshold theorem indicates that the probability of a major epidemic is zero when the proportion of individuals who are susceptible to infection is less than $1/\theta$. The parameter θ, known as the basic reproduction number, is the mean number of individuals infected by the direct contacts of an infective entering the community when all other individuals are susceptible.

The epidemic threshold theorem holds under quite general conditions, but the bound $1/\theta$ then depends on the community structure and the heterogeneity among individuals (see [7] and [8]).

Data on Outbreaks in Households

Infectious disease data have three features that distinguish them from other data. There is usually some knowledge about the mechanism that generates the data, the data are dependent, and the infection process is only partially observable. A consequence of these features is that the analysis of data is usually most effective when it is based on a model that describes aspects of the infection process. The level of detail that should be incorporated into the model depends on the objective of the study.

Disease transmission and the natural history of diseases evolve in continuous time, but discrete time models are often appropriate for data analysis. It may be that events are only recorded to the nearest day, say, or only the eventual outcomes of outbreaks are observed. Data on the eventual number of cases in households are often collected, because households are a manageable unit size and data on eventual infection can be verified by laboratory tests, which makes them relatively reliable.

Chain Binomial Models

In a household having initially s susceptible individuals, there will be $1, 2, \ldots,$ or s eventual cases. The probability of a specified number of eventual cases in an infected household is computed in terms of disease transmission probabilities by considering the likelihood of the various chains of infection. To illustrate, suppose that one of a total of five susceptible individuals of a household is infected and starts an outbreak in the household. Assume that the outbreak evolves without further infection from outside. Four eventual cases in the household could result via a number of different chains of infection. One such chain is $1 \rightarrow 2 \rightarrow 1 \rightarrow 0$, which means that the single initial infective infected exactly two household members, who in turn infected exactly one member, and the last remaining susceptible member escaped infection throughout.

A simple chain binomial model would compute the probability for this chain, given one introductory case, as

$$\binom{4}{2} p_1^2 q_1^2 \binom{2}{1} p_2 q_2 \binom{1}{0} p_1^0 q_1 = 12 p_1^2 q_1^3 p_2 q_2,$$

where q_i is the probability that a susceptible escapes infection when exposed to i infectives for the duration of their infectious periods and $p_i = 1 - q_i$. The probability that the number of eventual cases in a household is x is the sum of chain probabilities over all chains with x eventual cases.

The expectation-maximization (EM) algorithm is a convenient tool for finding maximum likelihood estimates when fitting chain binomial models to size of household outbreak data. This is pointed out with reference to partner studies for human immunodeficiency virus (HIV) infection in [11] and is discussed more fully in the review paper [6].

Models that capture the infection mechanism of the data generally contain parameters with clear interpretations and are well suited for testing epidemiologically important hypotheses. For example, with a chain binomial model for the size of household outbreaks, we can test the Reed–Frost hypothesis $q_2 = q_1^2$, or the Greenwood hypothesis $q_2 = q_1$.

The Reed–Frost assumption is appropriate for diseases that spread primarily by direct person-to-person contact.

Many methods of analysis of household data assume that each household outbreak evolves essentially independently after the initial infection of the household. This assumption is often of concern. Longini & Koopman [10] propose an analysis based on a pragmatic chain binomial model that also allows infection from outside the household.

Epidemic Chain Models with Random Effects

It is instructive to think about disease transmission in terms of a continuous infectivity function $\lambda(t)$ that indicates how infectious an infective is t time units after being infected. The infectivity function reflects both the level of infectious agent emitted by the infective and his or her rate of making contacts with others. Often, the infectivity function is zero for a period immediately after infection, because the infectious organism is developing within the body and no infectious agent is emitted. When disease transmission is person-to-person, the probability that a given susceptible individual escapes infection when exposed to a given infective is $q_1 = \exp[-\int_0^T \lambda(t)\,dt]$, where T is the duration of time from infection until the end of the infectious period.

Epidemic chain binomial models assume that infectives are homogeneous, in the sense that they all have the same infectivity function. When infectives have different infectivity functions, we still use chain binomial models if the infectives can be partitioned into homogeneous groups. Otherwise, we proceed by considering the q_1 for each infective to be a realization from a probability distribution. In these random effects models, see [4, Chapter 3], the probabilities of the epidemic chains are expressed in terms of the moments of q_1. This allows for heterogeneity in the infectivity of infected individuals. Heterogeneity in susceptibility or among households can be allowed for in a similar way. An application of random effects models to data on *Shigella sonnei* in households is given by Baker & Stevens [3].

A comprehensive analysis of infectious disease data on household outbreaks, allowing infection from outside the household, variation in the duration of the infectious period, and covariates, is described by Addy et al. [1].

Continuous Time Data for Households

Sometimes, when daily data are available on symptoms shown by infected individuals, the analysis is based on a continuous time model. The standard model used is a compartmental model for the irreversible compartments Susceptible → Exposed → Infective → Removed, referred to as the SEIR model. An individual in the exposed category is infected, but not yet infectious, and said to be in the **latent period**. The final category is called removed, because these individuals play no further part in the infection process. These individuals may simply have recovered and have acquired immunity from further infection for the duration of the epidemic. It is of interest to estimate characteristics, such as the mean and variance, of the latent and infectious periods. This can be done by assuming a parametric model for the distribution of the latent and infectious periods, as described in [2, Chapter 15] and [4, Chapter 4]. It is also of interest to make inferences about the functional form of the infectivity function, which is considered in the context of transmission of HIV by Shiboski & Jewell [12] on the basis of data on partners of individuals infected with HIV.

Data on an Epidemic in a Community

Regression Analysis

When data are available on the days on which individuals show symptoms of disease, and these can be used to deduce the date of infection, with reasonable accuracy, then a comprehensive regression analysis is possible. The response variable is the indicator of infection for each susceptible individual on each day. The **Mantel–Haenszel** test statistic has been suggested as a way of reducing the number of covariates, see [4, Chapter 5]; however, a **logistic regression** model is also convenient for determining which covariates are needed in the model. When a final set of covariates is arrived at it is useful to fit a loglinear regression model in these covariates to the binary data. The preference for the loglinear model stems from the more direct epidemiologic interpretation of its parameters in the infectious disease context. More specifically, if Y is the indicator of escaping infection for a given susceptible on a given day, then fitting the model $Y \simeq \text{binomial}[1, \exp(-\beta'\mathbf{x})]$ is useful, because

with this model $\beta'\mathbf{x}$ can be interpreted as the force of infection acting on the susceptible on that day. The covariate $\mathbf{x}$ might include the number of infectives in the community and the number of infectives in the susceptible's household, for example. An illustration of such a regression analysis is given in [4, Chapter 6].

Martingale Methods

The fact that the infection process is observed only partially causes the likelihood function based on continuous time data to be very complicated. This has encouraged the development of pragmatic methods based on simplifying assumptions and approximations. In contrast, methods of analysis derived from martingales for counting processes have proved successful for developing simple methods of statistical inference for some crucial parameters, such as the basic reproduction number, for quite general models. Tutorial accounts of these methods are given in [5] and [4, Chapter 7].

Vaccine Efficacy

A major motivation for the study of infectious diseases is to gain insight into ways in which they can be controlled and to determine requirements for their control. The most successful method of intervention continues to be vaccination. The epidemic threshold theorem plays a key role here, but it can only be applied if parameter estimates are available. A crucial parameter is the vaccine efficacy. Traditionally, vaccine efficacy has been estimated by $1 - (AR_V/AR_U)$, where AR_V is the attack rate among vaccinated individuals and AR_U is the attack rate among unvaccinated individuals. The attack rate is the proportion of individuals infected in the specified risk group over a nominated period of time. As a measure of the protective effect that the vaccine provides, this concept of vaccine efficacy suffers from depending on both the community from which the data come and on the time period over which the data are collected. Recently, there has been a more careful study of the interpretation and estimation of vaccine efficacy, see [9]. Typically, as a concept of protection against infection, vaccine efficacy might be interpreted as α, where the force of infection acting on vaccinated individuals is

$\alpha g(t)$ at chronological time t when the force of infection exerted on an unvaccinated susceptible is $g(t)$. Depending on the vaccine, α may be a constant in [0, 1] or a separate realization on a random variable for each vaccinated individual.

The HIV/AIDS Epidemic

The appearance of acquired immune deficiency syndrome (AIDS) stimulated new interest in the problems of modeling and data analysis for infectious disease studies. A distinguishing feature of infection with HIV is the very long time between infection and diagnosis with AIDS. This has made it feasible, and of interest, to assess the size of the epidemic, forecast its progress, and study characteristics of disease progression during the course of the epidemic.

References

[1] Addy, C.L., Longini, I.M. & Haber, M. (1991). A generalized stochastic model for the analysis of infectious disease final size data, *Biometrics* **47**, 961–974.
[2] Bailey, N.T.J. (1975). *The Mathematical Theory of Infectious Diseases and its Applications*. Griffin, London.
[3] Baker, R.D. & Stevens, R.H. (1995). A random effects model for analysis of infectious disease final-state data, *Biometrics* **51**, 956–968.
[4] Becker, N.G. (1989). *Analysis of Infectious Disease Data*. Chapman & Hall, London.
[5] Becker, N.G. (1993). Martingale methods for the analysis of epidemic data, *Statistical Methods in Medical Research* **2**, 93–112.
[6] Becker, N.G. (1997). Uses of the EM algorithm in the analysis of data on HIV/AIDS and other infectious diseases, *Statistical Methods in Medical Research* **6**, to appear.
[7] Becker, N.G. & Dietz, K. (1995). The effect of household distribution on transmission and control of highly infectious diseases, *Mathematical Biosciences* **127**, 207–219.
[8] Becker, N.G. & Hall, R. (1996). Immunization levels for preventing epidemics in a community of households made up of individuals of different types, *Mathematical Biosciences* **132**, 205–216.
[9] Halloran, M.E., Haber, M. & Longini, I.M. (1992). Interpretation and estimation of vaccine efficacy under heterogeneity, *American Journal of Epidemiology* **136**, 328–343.
[10] Longini, I.M. & Koopman, J.S. (1982). Household and community transmission parameters from final distributions of infections in households, *Biometrics* **38**, 115–126.
[11] Madger, L. & Brookmeyer, R. (1993). Analysis of infectious disease data from partner studies with unknown source of infection, *Biometrics* **49**, 1110–1116.
[12] Shiboski, S.C. & Jewell, N.P. (1992). Statistical analysis of the time dependence of HIV infectivity based on partner study data, *Journal of the American Statistical Association* **87**, 360–372.

(*See also* **Communicable Diseases; Incubation Period of Infectious Diseases**)

Niels G. Becker

Infectious Diseases *see* Communicable Diseases

Information Bias *see* Bias in Case–Control Studies; Bias in Observational Studies

Initiation of Disease *see* Incidence–Prevalence Relationships

Instantaneous Incidence Rate *see* Hazard Rate

Instrumental Data *see* Measurement Error in Epidemiologic Studies

Interaction

Interaction is most often considered in the context of regression models, including the special case of models underlying the analysis of variance (ANOVA). In these models, the response variable is linked in some manner to a linear predictor of the form

$$\alpha + \beta_1 X_1 + \beta_2 X_2 + \cdots + \beta_k X_k,$$

where the X_is represent explanatory variables, and α and the β_is represent parameters to be estimated. Here, for exposition purposes, the X_is will be regarded as representing separate factors of interest, or perhaps functions of a measurement or coding of a single factor. In this case, the linear predictor reflects an additive relationship such that a change in X_i induces the same change in the linear predictor whatever the values of the other explanatory variables.

In this framework, an interaction term is defined by the product of two or more X_is. Consider the special case of two explanatory variables. Then the linear predictor can be expanded and be represented by

$$\nu(X_1, X_2) = \alpha + \beta_1 X_1 + \beta_2 X_2 + \beta_{12} X_1 X_2.$$

The coefficient β_{12} then represents a departure from an **additive model** for the simultaneous effect of X_1 and X_2 on the response. A test of the hypothesis $\beta_{12} = 0$ is used to examine whether there is evidence for such a departure. Technically, such a test is undertaken as a standard test for a nonzero regression coefficient in the regression model being considered.

If X_1 is continuous, then plots of ν against X_1, with X_2 fixed, provide an illustration of interaction effects. In the absence of interaction, the curves are parallel for different values of X_2. If X_2 is also continuous, then parallel curves also arise when ν is plotted against X_2 with X_1 fixed. The nature of the variables may determine the most natural means of presentation. For example, if X_1 represents an experimental treatment level and X_2 a covariate that specifies some intrinsic characteristic of a subject, then it is natural to plot ν against X_1 with X_2 fixed. If X_1 and X_2 are *categorical*, then interaction effects are often displayed by the presentation of values of ν for different values of X_1 and X_2 in a two-way table.

The absence of interaction, when there is particular interest in the effect of both X_1 and X_2 on the response variable, indicates that the separate effects of the two variables are additive. If interest primarily focuses only on X_1, and X_2 is regarded as a covariate, then the lack of interaction indicates that the effect of X_1 is independent of X_2. Particularly in analysis of variance procedures, the interaction of a treatment variable X_1, with a covariate X_2 which varies in a haphazard or largely uncharacterizable way, may be regarded as random variation that may be used in the estimation of the error of treatment contrasts.

When the term $\beta_{12} X_1 X_2$ is referred to as an interaction term, terms of the form $\beta_i X_i$ are often referred to as main-effect terms. This derives predominantly from the ANOVA literature, and is particularly relevant to the orthogonal effects that derive from the coding of explanatory variables commonly used there. More generally, the interpretation of main-effect terms may depend very critically on the particular representation of the explanatory variables used to define X_i, particularly in the presence of interaction terms.

A distinction is sometimes made between qualitative and quantitative interactions. A qualitative interaction is one in which the direction of the effect of X_1, say, differs depending on the value of X_2. A quantitative interaction would reflect changes in the magnitude of the X_1 effect with X_2, which do not induce a change in the direction of the effect.

Another distinction is between synergistic (*see* **Synergy of Exposure Effects**) and antagonistic interactions. Assume that a change in X_1 induces a change δ_1 in the linear predictor through the term $\beta_1 X_1$, and a change in X_2 similarly induces a change δ_2. If δ_1 and δ_2 have the same sign, say "+", then a synergistic interaction is one which causes the change in the linear predictor due to changes in both X_1 and X_2 to be greater than $\delta_1 + \delta_2$. In contrast, an antagonistic interaction will result in a change less than the sum of the individual effects.

Interactions are always defined in terms of a specific model. Another model which is defined with a transformation of the response variable or a different relationship between the response variable and the linear predictor will not necessarily manifest the same interactions. Some formal attention has been paid to defining "removable interactions", but it is probably best to consider alternative models for this purpose on a case by case basis.

For models with more than two factors, products of all pairs of variables can be considered, and would be termed second-order or two-way interactions. In the obvious way, interactions of order m can be defined by introducing a product of *m* variables. When factors are defined with a set of binary dummy variables, interactions between factors involve products of these dummy variables, and the set of cross products corresponding to a pair of factors can be regarded as a single interaction term with degrees of freedom corresponding to the number of nonlinearly dependent cross products that can be defined. For factors with I and J levels, the degrees of freedom would be $(I-1)(J-1)$.

It has been argued that any model with an interaction term must have all main effects corresponding to terms in the interaction in the model. Such an approach produces what are called hierarchical models. While there are examples in which this requirement is viewed as too strong, it is in almost all situations sensible formally to test for nonzero interaction effects in the presence of the main effects.

A comprehensive review of interaction has been given by Cox [1]. In epidemiology, interaction is closely linked with the term **effect modification**.

Reference

[1]   Cox, D.R. (1984). Interaction, *International Statistical Review* **52**, 1–31.

V.T. FAREWELL

Internal Control Group *see* Biased Sampling of Cohorts in Epidemiology

Internal Validation Sample *see* Misclassification Error

Internal Validity *see* Validity and Generalizability in Epidemiologic Studies

International Classification of Diseases (ICD)

The ICD is a classification system designed to group together similar diseases, injuries, and related health problems to facilitate statistical analysis of these conditions. The classification is designed to have a finite number of categories encompassing the entire range of morbid conditions. A specific disease or condition is given its own separate category title in the classification only when separate identification is warranted because of its frequency of occurrence or importance as a medical or public health concern. However, many category titles in the classification contain groups of separate but usually related morbid conditions. There is a unique place for inclusion into one of the categories for every disease or morbid condition; therefore, a number of residual categories are reserved throughout the classification for those conditions which do not belong under one of the more specific titles. The ICD is a statistical classification, not a nomenclature or extensive list of approved names for morbid conditions; however, the concepts of classification and nomenclature are closely related. Some classifications are so detailed (e.g. in zoology and botany) that they in fact become nomenclatures, but these very detailed classifications often lose their value for statistical purposes.

History and Development of the International Classification of Diseases

Interest in classifying diseases and studying disease patterns is usually traced back to the work of John Graunt and his tabulations of causes of death based on the London Bills of Mortality in the seventeenth century. During the eighteenth and early nineteenth centuries, several classifications of diseases were prepared. The first to approach classification of diseases systematically was François Bossier de Lacroix (1706–1777), writing under the name Sauvages, in his treatise, *Nosologia Methodica*. During the same period, the naturalist and physician Carolus Linnaeus (1707–1778) prepared, in addition to his seminal classification of botany, a treatise entitled *Genera Morborum*. By the beginning of the nineteenth century, the disease classification in general use was *Synopsis Nosologiae Methodicae*, prepared by William Cullen (1710–1790) and published in 1785 [1].

When the General Register Office of England and Wales was established in 1837, William Farr (1807–1883) was named as its first medical statistician. Farr found the Cullen classification, still in use, to be outdated and not sufficiently useful for statistical summarization. In his annual "Letters", published in the Annual Reports of the Registrar General, Farr urged the adoption of a new, uniform, statistical classification of diseases. He noted that many diseases were denoted by more than one term, some terms were used to describe more than one disease, vague terms were used, and complications were recorded instead of primary diseases [2].

The importance of a uniform statistical classification was recognized at the first International Statistical Congress meeting in Brussels in 1853. The Congress asked Farr and Marc d'Espine of Geneva to prepare an internationally acceptable uniform classification of causes of death. At the next meeting of the Congress in 1855 in Paris, Farr and d'Espine each submitted his own classification and the Congress adopted a compromise list of 139 rubrics; the compromise list reflected Farr's arrangement into five groups: epidemic diseases, constitutional (general) diseases, local diseases arranged according to anatomical site, developmental diseases, and diseases directly resulting from violence. Over the next 30 years, this classification was revised four times but it maintained the general structure proposed by Farr.

In 1891, the International Statistical Institute, successor to the International Statistical Congress, charged a committee to prepare a new classification of causes of death. The committee, chaired by Jacques Bertillon (1851–1922), submitted its classification to the Institute in 1893, and it was adopted. This Bertillon Classification, as it was called, consisted of 161 rubrics as well as an abridged classification of 44 titles and another of 99 titles. These were based on Farr's principle of distinguishing between general diseases and those localized to a particular organ or anatomical site. The Bertillon Classification received general approval and was put into use by several countries and a number of cities. The 1899 meeting of the Institute passed a resolution acknowledging the use of this "system of cause of death nomenclature" in all the statistical offices in North America, and some in South America and Europe.

The resolution further "insists vigorously that this system of nomenclature be adopted in principle and without revision, by all the statistical institutions of Europe" and "approves…the system of decennial revision proposed by the American Public Health Association …".

The French Government, as a response to the International Statistical Institute's 1899 resolution, convened in Paris, in 1900, the first International Conference for the Revision of the Bertillon or International List of Causes of Death. This conference adopted a classification consisting of 179 groups and an abridged list of 35 groups, and it reaffirmed the desirability of decennial revisions. Accordingly, the International List of Causes of Death, and its successor classifications, has been revised approximately every 10 years thereafter.

Bertillon continued his leadership in classification matters, and the revisions of 1900, 1910, and 1920 were carried out under his guidance. During the decade following his death in 1922, there was an increasing interest in expanding the classification to accommodate morbidity and other **vital statistics** interests. At the same time, there was recognition of the need to involve other international agencies, particularly the Health Organization of the League of Nations, in future revision activity. To coordinate efforts, an international commission, known as the Mixed Commission, was created with equal representation from the International Statistical Institute and the Health Organization of the League of Nations. This Commission drafted the proposals for the fourth (1929) and fifth (1938) revisions of the International List of Causes of Death.

In 1946, the newly established World Health Organization (WHO) was given the responsibility for the next (sixth) revision of the International List of Causes of Death and to develop an International List of Causes of Morbidity. In 1948, the International Conference for the Sixth Revision of the International Lists of Diseases and Causes of Death met in Paris. The Conference secretariat was the joint responsibility of competent French authorities and the WHO. The Sixth Decennial Revision Conference introduced a new era in international vital and health statistics. In addition to recommending a comprehensive list of conditions for both morbidity and mortality, the *Manual of the International Statistical Classification of Diseases, Injuries, and Causes of Death*, the Conference agreed on rules for selecting the underlying **cause of death**, a Medical Certificate of Cause of Death form (*see* **Death Certification**), and special lists and guidelines for tabulation. These recommendations were endorsed by the first World Health Assembly in 1948, resulting in WHO Nomenclature Regulations which member countries have agreed to follow.

The International Conference for the Seventh Revision of the International Classification of Diseases was held under WHO auspices in 1955; the Eighth Revision Conference took place in 1965. The seventh revision was limited to a few essential changes and amendments or corrections. The eighth revision, while more extensive than the seventh, still maintained the basic structure of the classification and the general concept of classifying diseases according to etiology rather than manifestation.

The International Conference for the Ninth Revision of the International Classification of Diseases, again convened by WHO, took place in 1975. During the period when the seventh and eighth revisions were in force, there was a growing use of the International Classification of Diseases for indexing hospital records and for other morbidity applications. These expanding uses were recognized in the ninth revision, which added considerable detail and specificity to the classification. Also introduced was an optional method of classifying selected conditions according to their manifestation in a particular organ or site as well as by the underlying general disease. In addition, based on recommendations of the Ninth Revision Conference, the World Health Assembly approved the publication by WHO of two supplementary classifications on a trial basis: one for Impairments, Disabilities, and Handicaps [4] and one for Procedures in Medicine [3]. These were to be adjuncts to the International Classification of Diseases, not integral parts of the basic classification.

Planning for the preparation of the tenth revision began even before the publication of the ninth revision. Early on, it was apparent that the expanded uses of the classification and the resultant complexities and additional detail required more than the usual 10-year cycle for this revision. The longer time period would not only allow broad solicitation of input from users and producers of the data but would also permit trials of some of the major changes being proposed. Therefore, WHO, with the concurrence of member states, postponed the Tenth Revision Conference from 1985 to 1989, with the planned implementation of the tenth revision consequently also delayed.

Characteristics of the Tenth Revision

The formal title of the tenth revision of the ICD (usually refered to as ICD-10) is *International Statistical Classification of Diseases and Related Health Problems, Tenth Revision* [6]. It comprises three volumes: Vol. 1 contains the main classifications; Vol. 2 contains guidance and rules for use of the ICD; and Vol. 3 is the alphabetic index.

ICD-10 is a variable-axis classification evolved from the original principles of organization proposed by Farr. It is designed as a three-character code with fourth-character subdivisions where appropriate. A letter is used in the first position and a numerical digit in the second, third, and fourth positions. The fourth character is preceded by a decimal point. Therefore, individual alphanumeric codes range from A*nn.n* to Z*nn.n*, where *n* represents any of the ten digits from 0 to 9. The letter U is not used. The alphanumeric characteristic of ICD-10 codes is an innovation designed to permit more flexibility in maintaining a hierarchical sequence of diseases while adding more detail to the classification; previous revision code numbers were completely numeric. Vol. 1 contains the list of three-character categories and the tabular list of inclusions and four-character subdivisions. The "core" classification is the list of three-character categories representing the level of reporting required for the WHO mortality database and for routine international comparisons. Many countries use the ICD only at this level of detail; further subdivision of disease categories may not be possible given the quality of the original diagnostic data. Both the core classification and the fully detailed tabular list with its fourth-character detail are arranged into 21 main chapters, and chapters into blocks of related conditions headed by an appropriate block title. In the tabular list, but not in the list of three-character categories, inclusion terms are provided under each code number as examples or guides to the intended content of the category. However, the inclusion terms so listed are not intended to be exhaustive for any given category, and the Alphabetic Index (Vol. 3) serves as a much more detailed guide to the correct placement of conditions into ICD categories.

Vol. 1 also contains a separate classification of morphology of neoplasms which may be used in addition to the main ICD codes which usually classify neoplasms only by behavior and site. These morphology codes are the same as those appearing in the adaptation of the ICD called the *International Classification of Diseases for Oncology* (ICD-O) [5]. In addition, Vol. 1 contains key definitions adopted by the World Health Assembly to facilitate international comparisons of data, and special tabulation lists recommended for the uniform statistical summarization and presentation of both morbidity and mortality data based on the ICD.

ICD-10 came into force on January 1, 1993; however, the actual implementation of this revision of the classification in countries around the world did not begin in earnest until 1995 and the next several years thereafter.

References

[1]   Knibbs, G.H. (1929). The International Classification of Disease and Causes of Death and its Revision, *Medical Journal of Australia* **1**, 2–12.

[2]   Registrar General of England and Wales (1839). *First Annual Report*. Registrar General of England and Wales, London.

[3]   World Health Organization (1978). *International Classification of Procedures in Medicine*, Vols 1 and 2. World Health Organization, Geneva.

[4]   World Health Organization (1980). *International Classification of Impairments, Disabilities and Handicaps. A Manual of Classification Relating to the Consequences of Disease*. World Health Organization, Geneva.

[5]   World Health Organization (1990). *International Classification of Diseases for Oncology*, 2nd Ed. World Health Organization, Geneva.

[6]   World Health Organization (1992). *International Statistical Classification of Diseases and Related Health Problems*, 10th Rev., 3 Vols. World Health Organization, Geneva.

(*See also* **Cause of Death, Automatic Coding**; **Mortality, International Comparisons**)

ROBERT A. ISRAEL

Interviewer Bias

Interviewer bias is a type of information **bias** (*see* **Bias in Observational Studies**; **Bias, Overview**) that arises when an interviewer consciously or unconsciously elicits inaccurate information from study subjects. Interviewer bias can result in **differential error**, which can seriously distort disease–exposure associations, if the interviewer is aware of the disease status and exposure hypothesis in a **case–control study**, or if the interviewer is aware of the exposure status and outcome hypothesis in a **cohort study**. In the former case, the interviewer may probe more deeply for evidence of exposure among cases than among **controls**. In the latter case, the interviewer may try to elicit evidence of health effects more assiduously in exposed than in unexposed cohort members. Methods used to minimize interviewer bias include providing structured questionnaires, training interviewers to follow a fixed pattern of questioning, and, where possible, keeping interviewers unaware of the disease status and exposure hypotheses of greatest interest in case–control studies, and unaware of exposure status and health outcome hypotheses of greatest interest in cohort studies.

(*See also* **Bias in Case–Control Studies**; **Bias in Cohort Studies**).

M.H. GAIL

Inter-Rater Reliability *see* Agreement, Measurement of

Intracluster Correlation *see* Sample Surveys

Isodemographic Base Map *see* Mapping Disease Patterns

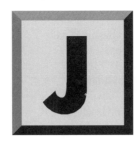

Jaccard Coefficient of Numerical Taxonomy *see* Agreement, Measurement of

Job-Exposure Matrices

Epidemiologic investigation of occupational hazards requires information on illness among workers and on their occupations or occupational exposures. Two families of epidemiologic investigations can be distinguished: industry-based studies and community-based studies. Each has unique advantages and disadvantages. Historically, community-based studies were based on analyses of job titles. With growing realization that there can be substantial variation in exposure profiles among workers who share the same job title, and that workers in different occupations can have common exposures, increasing attention has been paid to ascertaining subjects' occupational exposures (*see* **Occupational Epidemiology**; **Occupational Health and Medicine**; **Occupational Mortality**).

Since taking measurements in subjects' current workplaces is usually neither feasible nor useful for diseases of long latency, other approaches have been developed to ascertain subjects' past occupational exposures. If subjects can be interviewed, they can be asked about their exposure to various chemicals, but information thereby obtained is not sufficiently valid. Another approach is to obtain information about the jobs that subjects did and then have experts

in industrial hygiene estimate the chemicals that may have been present in such workplaces. If the information collected about subjects' jobs is reasonably detailed, and the experts knowledgeable, then this can lead to quite valid exposure estimates. However, it is an expensive labor-intensive enterprise.

The job-exposure matrix (JEM) approach was developed to provide a relatively inexpensive way of inferring exposures when the investigator has information on subjects' job histories. A JEM is simply a correspondence system for translating any occupation code into a list of exposures. The JEM provides the means for bringing together, for the purpose of statistical analysis, groups of subjects who share common exposures, irrespective of their occupations. A JEM consists of two primary axes, an exhaustive and mutually exclusive classification of occupations, and a list of substances. The occupation axis can be further subdivided by industries, by time periods, and conceivably by geographic areas. In the simplest form, the entry in the matrix could be a binary indicator of whether a worker in occupation i should be considered exposed to substance j. Applying each column in turn to a set of occupation histories allows the investigator to infer the exposure status of each study subject to each substance in the JEM. A more refined JEM could contain quantitative indicators of the probability of exposure to the substance in the job and estimates of the degree of exposure.

If the number of JEM substances is lengthy and the matrix entries are valid, this could generate useful data. While a handful of community-based JEMs have been developed in a few countries [1], they have not found wide applicability. The main limiting factor is the lack of valid and generalizable JEMs which are sufficiently broad in scope as to satisfy a wide range of research needs [3] (*see* **Validity and Generalizability in Epidemiologic Studies**). By contrast, a JEM can also be developed in the context of a **cohort study** and can be very useful if based on company records or expertise [2]. Such a JEM would not normally be applicable outside the cohort for which it was developed.

References

[1]   Coughlin, S.S. & Chiazze, L. (1990). Job-exposure matrices in epidemiologic research and medical surveillance, *State of the Art Reviews in Occupational Medicine* **5**, 633–646.
[2]   Goldberg, M., Kromhout, H., Guenel, P., Fletcher, A.C., Gerin, M., Glass, D.C., Heedrok, D., Kauppinen, T. & Ponti, A. (1993). Job-exposure matrices in industry, *International Journal of Epidemiology* **22**, Supplement 2, S10–S15.
[3]   Siemiatycki, J. (1996). Exposure assessment in community-based studies of occupational cancer, *Occupational Hygiene* **3**, 41–58.

JACK SIEMIATYCKI

Job-Exposure Matrix *see* Cohort Study, Historical

Join-Count Statistics *see* Clustering

Joint Action *see* Synergy of Exposure Effects

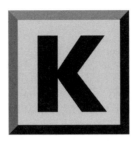

Kappa

In medical research it is frequently of interest to examine the extent to which results of a classification procedure concur in successive applications. For example, two psychiatrists may separately examine each member of a group of patients and categorize each one as psychotic, neurotic, suffering from a personality disorder, or healthy. Given the resulting data, questions may then be posed regarding the diagnoses of the two psychiatrists and their relationship to one another. The psychiatrists would typically be said to exhibit a high degree of agreement if a high percentage of their diagnoses concurred, and poor agreement if they often made different diagnoses. In general, this latter outcome could arise if the categories were ill-defined, the criteria for assessment were different for the two psychiatrists, or their ability to examine these criteria differed sufficiently, possibly as a result of different training or experience. Poor empirical agreement might therefore lead to a review of the category definitions and diagnostic criteria, or possibly retraining with a view to improving agreement and hence consistency of diagnoses and treatment. In another context, one might have data from successive applications of a test for dysplasia or cancer from cervical smears. If the test indicates normal, mild, moderate, or severe dysplasia, or cancer, and the test is applied at two time points in close proximity, ideally the results would be the same. Variation in the method and location of sampling as well as variation in laboratory procedures may, however, lead to different outcomes. In this context, one would say that

there is empirical evidence that the test is reliable if the majority of the subjects are classified in the same way for both applications of the test. Unreliable tests would result from the sources of variation mentioned earlier. Again, empirical evidence of an unreliable test may lead to refinements of the testing procedure.

The Kappa Index of Reliability for a Binary Test

For convenience, consider a diagnostic testing procedure generating a binary response variable T indicating the presence $(T = 1)$ or absence $(T = 2)$ of a particular condition. Suppose this test is applied twice in succession to each subject in a sample of size n. Let T_k denote the outcome for the kth application with the resulting data summarized in the two-by-two table (Table 1). where x_{ij} denotes the frequency at which $T_1 = i$ and $T_2 = j$, $x_{i.} = \sum_{j=1}^{2} x_{ij}$, and $x_{.j} = \sum_{i=1}^{2} x_{ij}$, $i = 1, 2$, $j = 1, 2$. Assuming that test results on different subjects are independent, conditioning on n leads to a multinomial distribution for the outcome of a particular table with

$$ f(\mathbf{x}; \mathbf{p}) = \binom{n}{x_{11} \ x_{12} \ x_{21} \ x_{22}} \prod_{i=1}^{2} \prod_{j=1}^{2} p_{ij}^{x_{ij}}, $$

$\mathbf{x} = (x_{11}, x_{12}, x_{21}, x_{22})'$, $\mathbf{p} = (p_{11}, p_{12}, p_{21}, p_{22})'$, and $p_{22} = 1 - p_{11} - p_{12} - p_{21}$. Let $p_{i.} = \sum_{j=1}^{2} p_{ij}$ and $p_{.j} = \sum_{i=1}^{2} p_{ij}$. Knowledge of $\mathbf{p}$ would correspond to a complete understanding of the

Table 1

	$T_2 = 1$	$T_2 = 2$	Total
$T_1 = 1$	x_{11}	x_{12}	$x_{1\cdot}$
$T_1 = 2$	x_{21}	x_{22}	$x_{2\cdot}$
Total	$x_{\cdot 1}$	$x_{\cdot 2}$	$x_{\cdot\cdot} = n$

reliability of the test. Since knowledge of $\mathbf{p}$ is generally unattainable and estimation of $\mathbf{p}$ does not constitute a sufficient data reduction, indices of reliability/agreement typically focus on estimating one-dimensional functions of $\mathbf{p}$ (*see* **Agreement, Measurement of**).

A natural choice is $p_0 = \sum_{i=1}^{2} p_{ii}$, the probability of raw agreement, which is estimated as $\hat{p}_0 = \sum_{i=1}^{2} x_{ii}/n$. If $p_0 = 1$, then the test is completely reliable since the probability of observing discordant test results is zero. Similarly, if $\hat{p}_0$ is close to unity, then it suggests that the outcomes of the two applications concurred for the vast majority of the subjects. However, several authors have expressed reluctance to base inferences regarding reliability on the observed level of raw agreement (see [3] and references cited therein). The purported limitations of $\hat{p}_0$ as a measure of reliability stem from the fact that p_0 reflects both "chance" agreement and agreement over and above that which would be expected by chance. The agreement expected by chance, which we denote by p_e, is computed on the basis of the marginal distribution, defined by $p_{1\cdot}$ and $p_{\cdot 1}$, and under the assumption that the outcomes of the two tests are independent conditional on the true status. Specifically, $p_e = \sum_{i=1}^{2} p_{i\cdot}\cdot p_{\cdot i}$ is estimated by $\hat{p}_e = \sum_{i=1}^{2} x_{i\cdot}x_{\cdot 1}/n^2$. To address concerns regarding the impact of nonnegligible chance agreement, Cohen [3] defined the index kappa which takes the form

$$\kappa = \frac{p_0 - p_e}{1 - p_e},$$

and indicated that it can be interpreted as reflecting "the proportion of agreement *after* chance agreement is removed from consideration". This can be seen by noting that $p_0 - p_e$ is the difference in the proportion of raw agreement and the agreement expected by chance, this being the agreement arising due to factors not driven by chance. If $p_0 - p_e > 0$, then there is agreement arising from nonchance factors; if $p_0 - p_e = 0$, then there is no additional agreement over

that which one would expect based on chance; and if $p_0 - p_e < 0$, then there is less agreement than one would expect by chance. Furthermore, $1 - p_e$ is interpreted by Cohen [3] as the proportion "of the units for which the hypothesis of no association would predict disagreement between the judges". Alternatively, this can be thought of as the maximum possible agreement beyond that expected by chance. An estimate of κ, denoted $\hat{\kappa}$, is referred to as the kappa statistic and may be obtained by replacing p_0 and p_e with their corresponding point estimates, giving

$$\hat{\kappa} = \frac{\hat{p}_0 - \hat{p}_e}{1 - \hat{p}_e}. \tag{1}$$

The Kappa Index of Reliability for Multiple Categories

When the classification procedure of interest has multiple nominal categories, assessment of agreement becomes somewhat more involved. Consider a diagnostic test with R possible outcomes and let T_k denote the outcome of the kth application of the test, $k = 1, 2$. Then T_k takes values on $\{1, 2, 3, \ldots, R\}$ and interest lies in assessing the extent to which these outcomes agree for $k = 1$ and $k = 2$. An $R \times R$ contingency table may then be constructed (see Table 2), where again x_{ij} denotes the frequency with which the first application of the test led to outcome i and the second led to outcome j, $i = 1, 2, \ldots, R$, $j = 1, 2, \ldots, R$. A category-specific measure of agreement may be of interest to examine the extent to which the two applications tend to lead to consistent conclusions with respect to outcome r, say. In this problem there is an implicit assumption that the particular nature of any disagreements are not of interest.

Table 2

	$T_2 = 1$	$T_2 = 2$	$T_2 = 3$	$\cdots$	$T_2 = R$	Total
$T_1 = 1$	x_{11}	x_{12}	x_{13}	$\cdots$	x_{1R}	$x_{1\cdot}$
$T_1 = 2$	x_{21}	x_{22}	x_{23}	$\cdots$	x_{2R}	$x_{2\cdot}$
$T_1 = 3$	x_{31}	x_{32}	x_{33}	$\cdots$	x_{3R}	$x_{3\cdot}$
$\vdots$	$\vdots$	$\vdots$	$\vdots$	$\cdots$	$\vdots$	$\vdots$
$T_1 = R$	x_{R1}	x_{R2}	x_{R3}	$\cdots$	x_{RR}	$x_{R\cdot}$
Total	$x_{\cdot 1}$	$x_{\cdot 2}$	$x_{\cdot 3}$	$\cdots$	$x_{\cdot R}$	$x_{\cdot\cdot} = n$

One can then collapse the $R \times R$ table to a 2×2 table constructed by cross-classifying subjects with binary indicators such that $T_k = 1$ if outcome r was selected at the kth application, $T_k = 2$ otherwise, $k = 1, 2$. A category-specific kappa statistic can then be constructed in the fashion indicated earlier. This can be repeated for each of the R categories giving R such statistics.

In addition to these category-specific measures, however, an overall summary index of agreement is often of interest. The kappa statistic in (1) is immediately generalized for the $R \times R$ ($R > 2$) table as follows. Let p_{ij} denote the probability of $T_1 = i$ and $T_2 = j$, one of the R^2 multinomial probabilities, $p_{i\cdot} = \sum_{j=1}^{R} p_{ij}$, and $p_{\cdot j} = \sum_{i=1}^{R} p_{ij}$, $i = 1, 2, \ldots, R$, $j = 1, 2, \ldots, R$. Then, as before, $\hat{p}_{ij} = x_{ij}/n$, $\hat{p}_{i\cdot} = x_{i\cdot}/n$, $\hat{p}_{\cdot j} = x_{\cdot j}/n$, $\hat{p}_0 = \sum_{i=1}^{R} \hat{p}_{ii}$, $\hat{p}_e = \sum_{i=1}^{R} \hat{p}_{i\cdot} \hat{p}_{\cdot i}$, and the overall kappa statistic takes the same form as in (1). This overall kappa statistic can equivalently be written as a weighted average of category-specific kappa statistics [6].

The kappa statistic has several properties that are widely considered to be attractive for measures of agreement. First, when the level of observed agreement, reflected by $\hat{p}_0$, is equal to the level of agreement expected by chance ($\hat{p}_e$), $\hat{\kappa} = 0$. Secondly, $\hat{\kappa}$ takes on its maximum value of 1 if and only if there is perfect agreement (i.e. $\hat{p}_0 = 1$ arising from a diagonal table). Thirdly, the kappa statistic is never less than -1. The latter two features require further elaboration, however, as the actual upper and lower limits on $\hat{\kappa}$ are functions of the marginal frequencies. In particular, $\hat{\kappa}$ takes on the value 1 only when the marginal frequencies are exactly equal and all off-diagonal cells are zero. Values less than 1 occur when the marginal frequencies are the same but there are different category assignments in the table or, more generally, when the marginal frequencies differ (when the marginal frequencies differ there are necessarily nonzero diagonal cells and hence some disagreements). It is natural then to expect the kappa statistic for such a table to be less than unity. Cohen [3] shows that the maximum possible value of $\hat{\kappa}$ takes the form

$$\hat{\kappa}_M = \frac{x_{\cdot\cdot} \sum_{i=1}^{R} \min(x_{i\cdot}, x_{\cdot i}) - \sum_{i=1}^{R} x_{i\cdot} x_{\cdot i}}{x_{\cdot\cdot}^2 - \sum_{i=1}^{R} x_{i\cdot} x_{\cdot i}}, \quad (2)$$

and argues that this is intuitively reasonable since differences in the marginal frequencies necessarily lead to a reduction in the level of agreement and hence $\hat{\kappa}$. Cohen then suggests that if one is interested in assessing the proportion of the agreement permitted by the margins (correcting for chance), then one computes $\hat{\kappa}/\hat{\kappa}_M$. We return to the topic of marginal frequencies and their influence on the properties of κ later in the article.

If the marginal frequencies for the two tests are uncorrelated (as measured by the product–moment correlation of the margins [3]), then the lower bound for $\hat{\kappa}$ is $\hat{\kappa}_L = -(R-1)^{-1}$. When the marginal frequencies are negatively correlated, $\hat{\kappa}_L > -(R-1)^{-1}$. However, when the marginal frequencies are positively correlated, $\hat{\kappa}_L < -(R-1)^{-1}$. It is only as the number of categories reduces to two, the correlation of the marginal frequencies approaches 1, and the variances of the marginal frequencies increase, that $\hat{\kappa}_L$ approaches -1 [3].

Having computed a kappa statistic for a given contingency table it is natural to want to characterize the level of agreement in descriptive terms. Landis & Koch [11] provide ranges that suggest, beyond what one would expect by chance, $0.75 < \hat{\kappa}$ typically represents excellent agreement, $0.40 < \hat{\kappa} < 0.75$ fair to good agreement, and $\hat{\kappa} < 0.40$ poor agreement. While there is some appeal to this convenient framework for the interpretation of $\hat{\kappa}$, caution is warranted.

Frequently, it will be of interest to construct confidence intervals for the index kappa. Fleiss et al. [8] derive an approximate large sample estimate for the variance of $\hat{\kappa}$, $\widehat{\text{var}}(\hat{\kappa})$, as

$$\left(\sum_{i=1}^{R} \hat{p}_{ii}[1 - (\hat{p}_{i\cdot} + \hat{p}_{\cdot i})(1 - \hat{\kappa})]^2 \right.$$
$$+ (1 - \hat{\kappa})^2 \sum_{i} \sum_{j \neq i} \hat{p}_{ij}(\hat{p}_{\cdot i} + \hat{p}_{j\cdot})^2$$
$$\left. - [\hat{\kappa} - \hat{p}_e(1 - \hat{\kappa})]^2 \right) \Big/ [x_{\cdot\cdot}(1 - \hat{p}_e)^2], \quad (3)$$

and Fleiss [6] recommends carrying out tests and constructing confidence intervals by assuming approximate normality of $(\hat{\kappa} - \kappa)/[\widehat{\text{var}}(\hat{\kappa})]^{1/2}$ and proceeding in the standard fashion. For tests regarding the null hypothesis $H_0 : \kappa = 0$, an alternate variance estimate may be derived from (3) by substituting 0 for $\hat{\kappa}$, and

$\hat{p}_{i\cdot}\hat{p}_{\cdot j}$ for $\hat{p}_{ij}$, giving

$$\widehat{\mathrm{var}}_0(\hat{\kappa})$$

$$= \left(\sum_{k=1}^{R} \hat{p}_{i\cdot}\hat{p}_{\cdot i}[1-(\hat{p}_{i\cdot}+\hat{p}_{\cdot i})]^2 + \sum_{i\neq j} \hat{p}_{i\cdot}\hat{p}_{\cdot j} \right.$$

$$\left. \times (\hat{p}_{\cdot i}+\hat{p}_{j\cdot})^2 - p_e^2 \right) \Big/ [x_{\cdot\cdot}(1-\hat{p}_e)^2], \quad (4)$$

with tests carried out as described above.

The Weighted Kappa Index

The discussion thus far has focused on situations in which the test serves as a nominal classification procedure (e.g. as in the psychiatric diagnosis example at the beginning of the article). In such settings, since there is no natural ordering to the outcomes, any disagreements are often considered to be equally serious and the methods previously described are directly applicable. In some circumstances with nominal scales, however, certain types of disagreements are more serious then others and it is desirable to take this into account. Furthermore, when the outcome is ordinal (as in the cervical cancer screening example), it is often of interest to adopt a measure of agreement that treats disagreements in adjacent categories as less serious than disagreements in more disparate categories. For the test based on cervical smears designed to classify the condition of the cervix as healthy, mildly, moderately, or severely dysplastic, or cancerous, if on one occasion the test suggested mild dysplasia and on another moderate, this type of disagreement would be considered less serious than if a cervix previously diagnosed as cancerous was subsequently classified as mildly dysplastic. In general, the seriousness reflects clinical implications for treatment and the consequences of wrong decisions.

Weighted versions of the kappa statistic were derived by Cohen [4] to take into account the additional structure arising from ordinal measures or from nominal scales in which certain types of disagreement are of more importance than others. In particular, the objective of adopting a weighted kappa statistic is to allow "different kinds of disagreement" to be differentially weighted in the construction of the overall index. We begin by assigning a weight to each of the R^2 cells; let w_{ij} denote the weight for cell (i, j). These weights may be determined quite arbitrarily but

it is natural to restrict $0 \leq w_{ij} \leq 1$, set w_{ii} to unity to give exact agreement maximum weight, and set $0 \leq w_{ij} < 1$ for $i \neq j$, so that all disagreements are given less weight than exact agreement. The selection of the weights plays a key role in the interpretation of the weighted kappa statistic and also impacts the corresponding variance estimates, prompting Cohen [4] to suggest these be specified prior to the collection of the data.

Perhaps the two most common sets of weights are the quadratic weights, with $w_{ij} = 1 - (i-j)^2/(R-1)^2$, and the so-called Cicchetti weights, with $w_{ij} = 1 - |i-j|/(R-1)$ [1, 2]. The quadratic weights tend to weight disagreements just off the main diagonal more highly than Cicchetti weights, and the relative weighting of disagreements farther from the main diagonal is also higher with the quadratic weights. Clearly, these two weighting schemes share the minimal requirements cited above. The weighted kappa statistic then takes the form

$$\hat{\kappa}^{(w)} = \frac{\hat{p}_0^{(w)} - \hat{p}_e^{(w)}}{1 - \hat{p}_e^{(w)}}, \quad (5)$$

where $\hat{p}_0^{(w)} = \sum_{i=1}^{R}\sum_{j=1}^{R} w_{ij}\hat{p}_{ij}$ and $\hat{p}_e^{(w)} = \sum_{i=1}^{R}\sum_{j=1}^{R} w_{ij}\hat{p}_{i\cdot}\hat{p}_{\cdot j}$. If $\bar{w}_{i\cdot} = \sum_{j=1}^{R}\hat{p}_{\cdot j}w_{ij}$ and $\bar{w}_{\cdot j} = \sum_{i=1}^{R}\hat{p}_{i\cdot}w_{ij}$, then the large-sample variance of $\hat{\kappa}^{(w)}$ is estimated by

$$\widehat{\mathrm{var}}(\hat{\kappa}^{(w)})$$

$$= \left(\sum_{i=1}^{R}\sum_{j=1}^{R} \hat{p}_{ij}[w_{ij}-(\bar{w}_{i\cdot}+\bar{w}_{\cdot j})(1-\hat{\kappa}^{(w)})]^2 \right.$$

$$\left. - [\hat{\kappa}^{(w)}-\hat{p}_e^{(w)}(1-\hat{\kappa}^{(w)})]^2 \right) \Big/ [x_{\cdot\cdot}^2(1-\hat{p}_e^{(w)})^2]$$

$$(6)$$

and, as before, tests and confidence intervals may be carried out and derived in the standard fashion assuming asymptotic normality of the quantity $(\hat{\kappa}^{(w)}-\kappa^{(w)})/[\widehat{\mathrm{var}}(\hat{\kappa}^{(w)})]^{1/2}$. As in the unweighted case, a variance estimate appropriate for testing $H_0: \kappa^{(w)} = 0$ may be derived by substituting $\hat{p}_{i\cdot}\hat{p}_{\cdot j}$ for $\hat{p}_{ij}$, and 0 for $\hat{\kappa}^{(w)}$ in (6).

We note in passing that the weighted kappa with quadratic weights has been shown to bear connections to the intraclass correlation coefficient. Suppose that with an ordinal outcome the categories are assigned the integers 1 through R from the "lowest" to "highest" categories, respectively, and assignment to these categories is taken to correspond to a realization of the appropriate integer value. Fleiss & Cohen [7] show that the intraclass correlation coefficient computed by treating these integer responses as coming from a Gaussian general linear model for a two-way analysis of variance, is asymptotically equivalent to the weighted kappa statistic with quadratic weights.

The Kappa Index for Multiple Observers

Thus far we have restricted consideration to the case of two applications of the classification procedure (e.g. two successive applications of a diagnostic test, two physicians carrying out successive diagnoses, etc.). In many situations, however, there are multiple (> 2) applications and interest lies in measuring agreement on the basis of several applications. Fleiss [5] considered the particular problem in which a group of subjects was examined and classified by a fixed number of observers, but where it was not necessarily the same set of observers carrying out the assessments for each patient. Moreover, Fleiss [5] assumed that it was not possible to identify which observers were involved in examining the patients.

For this problem, we require some new notation. Let M denote the number of subjects, N denote the number of observers per subject, and R denote the number of categories as before. Therefore, NM classifications are to be made. Let n_{ij} denote the number of times the ith subject was assigned to the jth category. A measure of overall raw agreement for the assignments on the ith subject is given by

$$\hat{q}_i = \frac{\sum_{j=1}^{R} n_{ij}(n_{ij} - 1)}{N(N-1)}, \qquad (7)$$

which can be interpreted as follows. With N observers per subjects there are $\binom{N}{2}$ possible pairs of assignments. There are $\binom{n_{ij}}{2}$ which agree on category j and hence a total number of $\sum_{j=1}^{R} \binom{n_{ij}}{2}$ pairs of assignments which concur altogether for the ith subject. Thus, (7) simply represents the proportion of all paired assignments on the ith subject for which there was agreement on the category. The overall measure of raw observed agreement over all subjects

is then given by $\hat{q}_0 = M^{-1} \sum_{i=1}^{M} \hat{q}_i$, which equals

$$\hat{q}_0 = \frac{\sum_{i=1}^{M} \sum_{j=1}^{R} n_{ij}^2}{MN(N-1)} - \frac{1}{N-1}. \qquad (8)$$

As before, however, some agreement would be expected among the observers simply by chance and the kappa statistic in this setting corrects for this. The expected level of agreement is computed by noting that

$$\hat{p}_j = \frac{\sum_{i=1}^{M} n_{ij}}{MN}$$

is the sample proportion of all assignments made to category j, with $\sum_{j=1}^{R} \hat{p}_j = 1$. So if pairs of observers were simply assigning subjects to categories at random and independently one can estimate that they would be expected to agree according to

$$\hat{p}_e = \sum_{j=1}^{R} \hat{p}_j^2, \qquad (9)$$

then the kappa statistic is computed by correcting for chance in the usual way as

$$\hat{\kappa} = \frac{\hat{q}_0 - \hat{p}_e}{1 - \hat{p}_e}. \qquad (10)$$

The sample variance for (10) is derived by Fleiss et al. [9] to be

$$\widehat{\mathrm{var}}(\hat{\kappa})$$

$$= 2 \left[\left(\sum_{j=1}^{R} p_j(1 - p_j) \right)^2 - \sum_{j=1}^{R} p_j(1 - p_j) \right.$$

$$\left. (1 - 2p_j) \right] \bigg/ MN(N-1) \left(\sum_{j=1}^{R} p_j(1 - p_j) \right)^2$$
$$\qquad (11)$$

and is typically used for tests or interval estimation in the standard fashion.

When the same set of raters assesses all subjects and individual raters scores are known, it is not possible to use the results of Fleiss [5] without ignoring the rater-specific assignments. For this context, Schouten [13] proposed the use of indices based on weighted sums of pairwise measures of observed and expected levels of agreement. In particular, for a given pair of raters and a given pair of categories, observed and expected measures of agreement may be computed as earlier. Then, for each pair of raters, a measure of overall observed agreement may be obtained by taking a weighted average of such measures over all pairwise combinations of categories. Given a corresponding measure of expected agreement, an overall kappa statistic can be computed in the usual fashion. Schouten [13] then described how to obtain kappa statistics reflecting agreement over all observers, agreement between a particular observer and the remaining observers, and agreement within and between subgroups of observers.

General Remarks

MaClure & Willett [12] provide a comprehensive review and effectively highlight a number of limitations of the kappa statistics. In particular, they stress that for ordinal data derived from categorizing underlying continuous responses, the kappa statistic depends heavily on the often arbitrary category definitions, raising questions about interpretability. They also suggest that the use of weights, while attractive in allowing for varying degrees of disagreement, introduces another component of subjectivity into the computation of kappa statistics. Perhaps the issue of greatest debate is the so-called prevalence, or base-rate, problem of kappa statistics. Several other authors have examined critically the properties and interpretation of kappa statistics [10, 14, 15], and the debate of the merits and demerits continues unabated. Despite the apparent limitations, the kappa statistic enjoys widespread use in the medical literature and has been the focus of considerable statistical research.

References

[1]   Cicchetti, D.V. (1972). A new measure of agreement between rank ordered variables, *Proceedings of the American Psychological Association* **7**, 17–18.

[2]   Cicchetti, D.V. & Allison T. (1973). Assessing the reliability of scoring EEG sleep records: an improved method, *Proceedings and Journal of the Electro-physiological Technologists' Association* **20**, 92–102.

[3]   Cohen, J. (1960). A coefficient of agreement for nominal scales, *Educational and Psychological Measurement* **20**, 37–46.

[4]   Cohen, J. (1968). Weighted kappa: nominal scale agreement with provision for scaled disagreement or partial credit, *Psychological Bulletin* **70**, 213–220.

[5]   Fleiss, J.L. (1971). Measuring nominal scale agreement among many raters, *Psychological Bulletin* **76**, 378–382.

[6]   Fleiss, J.L. (1981). *Statistical Methods for Rates and Proportions*, 2nd Ed. Wiley, New York.

[7]   Fleiss, J.L. & Cohen, J. (1973). The equivalence of weighted kappa and the intraclass correlation coefficient as measures of reliability, *Educational and Psychological Measurement* **33**, 613–619.

[8]   Fleiss, J.L., Cohen, J. & Everitt, B.S. (1969). Large sample standard errors of kappa and weighted kappa, *Psychological Bulletin* **72**, 323–327.

[9]   Fleiss, J.L., Nee, J.C.M. & Landis, J.R. (1979). Large sample variance of kappa in the case of different sets of raters, *Psychological Bulletin* **86**, 974–977.

[10]   Kraemer, H.C. & Bloch, D.A. (1988). Kappa coefficients in epidemiology: an appraisal of a reappraisal, *Journal of Clinical Epidemiology* **41**, 959–968.

[11]   Landis, J.R. & Koch, G.G. (1977). The measurement of observer agreement for categorical data, *Biometrics* **33**, 159–174.

[12]   MaClure, M. & Willett, W.C. (1987). Misinterpretation and misuse of the kappa statistic, *American Journal of Epidemiology* **126**, 161–169.

[13]   Schouten, H.J.A. (1982). Measuring pairwise interobserver agreement when all subjects are judged by the same observers, *Statistica Neerlandica* **36**, 45–61.

[14]   Thompson, W.D. & Walter S.D. (1988). A reappraisal of the kappa coefficient, *Journal of Clinical Epidemiology* **41**, 949–958.

[15]   Thompson, W.D. & Walter S.D. (1988). Kappa and the concept of independent errors, *Journal of Clinical Epidemiology* **41**, 969–970.

(*See also* **Agreement, Measurement of**)

RICHARD J. COOK

Kermack–McKendrick Threshold Theorem *see* Epidemic Thresholds

Knox's Test *see* Clustering

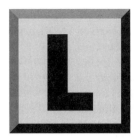

Lagged Cumulative Exposure *see*
Occupational Health and Medicine

Latent Failure Times Model *see*
Competing Risks

Latent Period

Latency or *latent period* is defined as the time interval between the initiation time, say t_0, of a disease process and the time, say t_1, of the first occurrence of a specifically defined manifestation of the disease. For infectious diseases (*see* **Communicable Diseases**), t_0 is the time of infection by the infectious agent and the manifestation may either be a specific serologic marker, or a laboratory abnormality, or a symptom [31]. If the manifestation is the occurrence of a symptom, then the latent period is the same as the **incubation period**, which is the term usually used by statisticians for infectious diseases (e.g. Alcabes [1]). In the case of cancer epidemiology, t_0 is the time of initial exposure to a carcinogen (cancer initiation) and t_1 the time of the first clinical occurrence of the disease [3, 14]. For example, the initial exposure may be the time of exposure to radiation or the time of exposure to a chemical carcinogen, and the first clinical occurrence may be detected by a biological marker

for cancer or by clinical evidence of a tumor [15]. For A-bomb survivors such as those from Hiroshima or Nagasaki, Japan, t_0 is thus the actual time of explosion of the bomb whereas t_1 is the time the disease first appears.

Other Definitions

For infectious diseases, Bailey [5] and Anderson & May [2] have used "the time to first become infectious" as the specified manifestation so that they define the latent period of the disease as the time interval from the point of infection to the beginning of the state of infectiousness of the infected host. This latter definition is not necessarily synchronous with the incubation period except in cases (e.g. yellow fever) in which both the average intervals from the point of infection to the infectiousness of the host and from the point of infection to the onset of a symptom are very short. For many infectious diseases caused by parasites, a distinction can usually be made between infection according to some laboratory criteria and symptoms of illness [2]. For infectious diseases caused by viruses and bacteria, however, such a distinction may be difficult; furthermore, for some viral diseases such as smallpox and yellow fever, an infected individual may be immune to the disease so that illness may never occur in some individuals [2, 30].

For exposure to a carcinogen, distinctions have been made between the biologic latent period and the epidemiologic latent period. For exposure to radiation, such as in A-bomb survivors, the biologic latent period is defined in [41] as the interval during which an elevation of the risk of the disease occurs between the exposed and nonexposed individuals (see Example 3 in the next section for illustration), whereas the epidemiologic latent period is defined in [41] as the interval between the first exposure and the time of death from the cause of interest. For exposure to a chemical carcinogen, the beginning of the biologic latent period is the time that a deoxyribonucleic acid (DNA) adduct of the carcinogen first appears because carcinogenesis starts with the interaction between the DNA adduct of the carcinogen and the genome of the host [18, 39]. The endpoint of the biologic latent period is the time of first occurrence of a cancer tumor cell; see [36]. For the epidemiologic latent period, the initial time is the time of first exposure to the carcinogen, whereas the endpoint is the time of first appearance of a detectable cancer tumor. It is shown in [18] that it is not the exposed dose but the dose of the DNA adduct of the agents that gives a linear **dose–response** curve for small doses; furthermore, detectable cancer tumors arise by clonal expansion from cancer tumor cells [47]. Thus, in most cases there are significant differences between the biologic latent period and the epidemiologic latent period.

Some Examples

The latent period of a disease may be very short and fairly constant. In some chronic infectious diseases, and in cancer, the latent period may be very long and varies greatly among individuals, in which case one should treat it as a random variable and work with the probability distribution of this variable.

Example 1. Yellow Fever

Yellow fever is an infectious disease caused by a yellow fever virus which is the prototype of the flavivirus genus (family Flaviviridae). It is an acute, mosquito-borne viral infection that occurs in epidemic and endemic form in tropical America and Africa. Clinical symptoms of this disease include fever, headache, malaise, and lassitude which persist for 2 to 4 days and occur in 10%–20% of the infected individuals. For this disease, the incubation period is very short (3 to 6 days) and can be considered as fairly constant [30].

Example 2. Malaria

Malaria is an infectious disease caused by parasites called Plasmodia. This disease occurs mainly in tropical areas and is transmitted to humans by the bite of malaria-infected female Anopheles mosquitoes. The four major *Plasmodium* species are *P. falciparum* (Africa, Asia, Oceania, Central America, and South America), *P. vivax* (Asia, Oceania, Central America, and South America), *P. ovale* (Africa and Oceania), and *P. malariae* (Africa and South America). The incubation periods for these four *Plasmodium* species are 8–27 days (average 12 days), 8–27 days (average 14 days), 9–17 days (average 15 days), and 16–28 days, respectively [33]. For this disease the human host becomes infectious with the accumulation of gametocytes in the blood. Hence the interval from infection to infectiousness is the time from initial infection to the first appearance of gametocytes in the blood. (This is the definition of latent period used by Anderson & May [2].) For the above four species, this period is given by 9–10 days, 9–10 days, 10–14 days, and 15–16 days, respectively [2].

Example 3. Leukemia in A-Bomb Survivors

Land & Norman [24] have studied the biologic latent periods of radiogenic cancers occurring among Japanese A-bomb survivors in Hiroshima and Nagasaki, Japan. The leukemias (acute leukemia and chronic granulocytic leukemia) are particularly interesting since the cumulative distributions of those who have been exposed to an A-bomb with kerma doses of 100 rads or more lie on the far left of those who have not been exposed to an A-bomb or those who have been exposed to an A-bomb but with the kerma doses of 0–9 rads. The magnitude of the elevation of the cumulative probability of leukemia over the biologic latent period depends on the age of the survivor at the time of exposure, with the age group 10–19 years at exposure having the largest elevation followed by the age groups 20–34 and 35–49 years at exposure. The biologic latent periods for leukemia are intervals from five years since exposure (time of explosion of the bomb) to an endpoint, say t_1, which is less than 29 years since exposure and which depends on the age of the survivor at the time of exposure. For the age groups 10–19 and 20–34 years at exposure, t_1 is

29 years since exposure, but for age groups 0–9 and 35–49 years at exposure, t_1 is approximately 25 years since exposure.

Example 4. Incubation Period of Acquired Immune Deficiency Syndrome (AIDS)

The infectious chronic disease AIDS is caused by a retrovirus called the human immunodeficiency virus (HIV). This is an endemic fatal infectious disease without cure at the present time. (For a summary of basic facts about AIDS, see [34].) Following infection by HIV, it usually takes several months to develop HIV antibodies in the blood. (For the time interval from infection to the development of antibodies, the estimate by Horsburgh et al. [20] is 3.5 months.) According to the 1993 surveillance definition of AIDS used by the US Centers for Disease Control (CDC), the incubation period is the time interval between infection by HIV and the first time that the total CD4 T-cell counts falls below $200/mm^3$ or the first time that the absolute percentage of CD4 T-cells falls below 14% or the first time that one of the 25 symptoms listed in [12] appears. This period is usually several years and depends on age [35], treatment with antiviral drugs [29], the presence of mutations of the gene CCR5 [16] (long or short AIDS survivors), and possibly other covariates. For untreated subjects aged 20–50 years at infection, the average incubation period is about 10 years. Note, however, that the AIDS definition used by CDC has been broadened three times, first in June 1985, next in July 1987, and then in December 1992. Hence, the incubation times measured before 1993 tend to be longer than the incubation times based on the 1993 AIDS definition.

The Latent Period of Infectious Diseases

For some infectious diseases such as yellow fever and malaria, the incubation period is relatively short and can be regarded as approximately constant. However, for some chronic infectious diseases such as AIDS, the incubation period is long and variable. In this latter case it makes more sense to treat the incubation period as a random variable, rather than as a fixed constant "latency", and to describe the process in terms of the probability distribution of incubation times. For example, the probability distribution of the incubation period of AIDS has been studied extensively, as summarized in Brookmeyer & Gail [9], Becker & Motika [6], and Tan et al. [40]. This probability distribution has been estimated by both parametric and nonparametric methods. However, all the estimates in the literature are based on the 1987 definition of AIDS: estimates of the HIV incubation period based on data and the 1993 AIDS definition have yet to be published.

The Latent Period of Cancer

Some researchers have used the concept of latency and average latent period to describe the interval between exposure to the A-bomb and the subsequent cancer onset in Hiroshima and Nagasaki, Japan [24, 7]. For example, leukemias tend to arise about five years following exposure to nuclear radiation [7]. However, Brookmeyer [8] pointed out that such estimates might be misleading because of censoring and competing causes (*see* **Competing Risks**) of death.

Many investigators prefer to consider the distribution of time to cancer onset, especially investigators who study cancer onset in animals exposed to low doses of a carcinogen [15]. In such cases the latent period is usually very long, and the expected time-to-tumor may exceed vastly the normal life span of the animal. In such circumstances, information on the mean latent period is not sufficient to determine the probability of developing a tumor before dying of some other causes. Moreover, different distributions may have the same mean time to tumor in the high dose range but give vastly different risk estimates when extrapolated to low doses [17, 45]. Thus, some scientists have avoided the use of mean latency for risk assessment based on low dose extrapolation [15]; rather, they describe carcinogens as altering the probability distribution of time to detectable cancer. This probability distribution depends on the mechanism of carcinogenesis and is influenced by many factors. In particular, the incidence of cancer is altered by changing the dose of the carcinogen to which the individual is exposed.

Armitage & Doll [4] developed the first stochastic model of carcinogenesis for the time-to-tumor distribution. This model is referred to as the multistage model (*see* **Multistage Carcinogenesis Models**) as described in reviews by Whittemore & Keller [44] and Kalbfleish et al. [21]. The

Armitage–Doll multistage model assumes that a tumor develops from a normal stem cell by k ($k \geq 2$) consecutive and irreversible genetic changes. These assumptions and the assumptions of low transition rates imply a Weibull model for the cancer **incidence rate**, $\lambda(t)$, and the following dose–response relationship between cancer incidence rate and the dose, d, of carcinogen:

$$\lambda(t) \propto \eta(d) \times t^{k-1}, \tag{1}$$

where $\eta(d)$ is a function of the dose d and is independent of time t.

The Armitage–Doll multistage model has been widely used by statisticians to assess how exposure to carcinogens alters the cancer incidence rates and the distributions of time-to-tumor. Breslow & Day [7] and others [13, 10] applied this model to study the effects of cigarette smoking on lung cancer risk, of asbestos exposure on risk of lung cancer and mesothelioma, and of radiation exposure on risks of leukemia, breast cancer, and bone cancer. While it is widely accepted that cancer results from a multistage process, recent results from molecular biology and molecular genetics have raised questions about some details of the assumptions in the Armitage–Doll multistage model (see [36] and [19]).

For risk assessment of carcinogens by low dose extrapolation, it has been documented that the same observable data can be fitted equally well by different models that yield very different estimates of risk at low doses [43]. Such extrapolation should be based on biologically plausible models, preferably models suggested by data. Thorslund et al. [42] and Moolgavkar et al. [32] proposed the Moolgavkar–Venzon–Knudson (MVK) two-stage model (see [36]) for risk assessment. In this model, the first stage is a Poisson process describing how normal stem cells are changed into initiated cells by mutation (initiation); in the second stage the model incorporates stochastic birth and death for proliferation of initiated cells (promotion), that change into malignant tumor cells by another mutation. Dose–response curves based on the MVK two-stage model have been developed by Chen & Moini [11], and by Krewski & Murdoch [23]. They have used these dose–response curves to assess how a carcinogen alters cancer incidence through its effects on initiating mutations or on the rate of proliferation of initiated cells. If the carcinogen is a pure initiator, then the dose–response curve for cancer incidence can be factorized as a product of a function of dose and a function of time and age; in these cases, the pattern of dose–response curves of the MVK model is quite similar to that of the Armitage–Doll multistage model. However, if the carcinogen is a promoter or a complete carcinogen, then the dose–response curves of the MVK model cannot be factorized, and they differ qualitatively from the Armitage–Doll model.

The MVK two-stage model, and extensions of it, together with many other biologically supported models have been analyzed in Tan [36] and in Yakovlev & Tsodikov [46]. Some extensions and modifications have recently been developed by Little and his colleagues [25]–[28]. (Little [25, 26] has called the multievent model in Tan [36] the generalized MVK model.) To extend the model to complex situations and to bring together information from various sources, Tan & Chen [37] and Tan et al. [38] have recently developed Kalman filter models for many models of carcinogenesis. By merging initiation and promotion, alternate modeling approaches have been proposed by Klebanov et al. [22] for radiation carcinogenesis.

References

[1] Alcabes, P. (1993). The incubation period of human immunodeficiency virus, *Epidemiologic Reviews* **15**, 303–318.

[2] Anderson, R.M. & May, R.M. (1992). *Infectious Diseases of Humans: Dynamics and Control*. Oxford University Press, Oxford.

[3] Armitage, P. & Doll, R. (1961). Stochastic models for carcinogenesis, in *Proceedings of the Fourth Berkeley Symposium on Mathematical Statistics and Probability: Biology and Problems of Health*. University of California Press, Berkeley, pp. 19–38.

[4] Armitage, P. & Doll, R. (1954). The age distribution of cancer and a multi-stage theory of carcinogenesis, *British Journal of Cancer* **8**, 1–12.

[5] Bailey, N.T.J. (1975). *The Mathematical Theory of Infectious Diseases and Its Applications*. Griffin, London.

[6] Becker, N.G. & Motika, M. (1993). Smoothed nonparametric back-projection of AIDS incidence data with adjustment for therapy, *Mathematical Biosciences* **118**, 1–23.

[7] Breslow, N.E. & Day, N.E. (1987). *Statistical Methods in Cancer Research*, Vol. II: *The Design and Analysis of Cohort Studies*. International Agency for Research on Cancer, Lyon.

[8] Brookmeyer, R. (1988). Time and latency considerations in the quantitative assessment of risk, in *Epidemiology and Health Risk Assessment*, L. Gordis, ed. Oxford University Press, Oxford, pp. 178–188.

[9] Brookmeyer, R. & Gail, M.H. (1994). *AIDS Epidemiology: A Quantitative Approach*. Oxford University Press, Oxford.

[10] Brown, C.C. & Chu, K.C. (1983). Implications of multistage theory of carcinogenesis applied to occupational arsenic exposure, *Journal of the National Cancer Institute* **70**, 455–463.

[11] Chen, C.W. & Moini, A. (1990). Cancer dose–response models incorporating clonal expansion, in *Scientific Issues in Quantitative Cancer Risk Assessment*, S.H. Moolgavkar, ed. Birkhauser, Boston, pp. 153–175.

[12] CDC (1992). Revised classification system for HIV infection and expanded surveillance case definition for AIDS among adolescents and adults, *Morbidity and Mortality Weekly Report* **41** (RR-17), 1–19.

[13] Day, N.E. & Brown, C.C. (1980). Multistage models and primary prevention of cancer, *Journal of the National Cancer Institute* **64**, 977–989.

[14] Druckrey, H. (1967). Quantitative aspects of carcinogenesis, in *Potential Carcinogenic Hazards from Drugs*, R. Truhaut, ed. UICC Monograph Series, Vol. 7, Springer-Verlag, New York, pp. 60–78.

[15] Guess, H.A. & Hoel, D.G. (1977). The effect of dose on cancer latency period, *Journal of Environmental Pathology and Toxicology* **1**, 279–286.

[16] Hill, C.M. & Littman, D.R. (1996). Natural resistance to HIV, *Nature* **382**, 668–669.

[17] Hoel, D.G., Gaylor, D.W., Kirschstein, R.L. & Saffiotti, U. (1975). Estimation of risks of irreversible delayed toxicity, *Journal of Toxicology and Environmental Health* **1**, 133–151.

[18] Hoel, D.G., Kaplan, N.L. & Anderson, N.W. (1983). Implication of nonlinear kinetics on risk estimation in carcinogenesis, *Science* **210**, 1032–1037.

[19] Hopkin, K. (1996). Tumor evolution: survival of the fittest cells, *Journal of NIH Research* **8**, 37–41.

[20] Horsburgh, C.R. Jr, Qu, C.Y. & Jason, I.M. (1989). Duration of human immunodeficiency virus infection before detection of antibody, *Lancet* **2**, 637–640.

[21] Kalbfleisch, J.D., Krewski, D.R. & Van Ryzin, J. (1983). Dose–response models for time-to-response toxicity data, *Canadian Journal of Statistics* **11**, 25–50.

[22] Klebanov, L.B. Rachev, S.T. & Yakovlev, A.Y. (1993). A stochastic model of radiation carcinogenesis: latent time distributions and their properties, *Mathematical Biosciences* **113**, 51–75.

[23] Krewski, D.R. & Murdoch, D.J. (1990). Cancer modeling with intermittent exposure, in *Scientific Issues in Quantitative Cancer Risk Assessment*, S.H. Moolgavkar ed. Birkhauser, Boston, pp. 196–214.

[24] Land, C.E. & Norman, J.E. (1978). Latent periods of radiogenic cancers occurring among Japanese A-bomb survivors, in *Late Biological Effects of Ionizing Radiation*, Vol. 1. International Atomic Energy Agency, Vienna.

[25] Little, M.P. (1995). Are two mutations sufficient to cause cancer? Some generalizations of the two-mutation model of carcinogenesis of Moolgavkar, Venzon and Knudson, and of the multistage model of Armitage and Doll, *Biometrics* **51**, 1278–1291.

[26] Little, M.P. (1996). Generalizations of the two-mutation and classical multi-stage models of carcinogenesis fitted to the Japanese atomic bomb survivor data, *Journal of Radiology Protection* **16**, 7–24.

[27] Little, M.P., Muirhead, C.R., Boice, J.D. & Kleinerman, R.A. (1995). Using multistage models to describe radiation-induced leukaemia, *Journal of Radiology Protection* **15**, 315–334.

[28] Little, M.P., Muirhead, C.R. & Stiller, C.A. (1996). Modeling lymphocytic leukaemia incidence in England and Wales using generalizations of the two-mutation model of carcinogenesis of Moolgavkar, Venzon and Knudson, *Statistics in Medicine* **15**, 1003–1022.

[29] Longini, I.R. Jr, Clark, W.S. & Karon, J. (1993). The effect of routine use of therapy in showing the clinical course of human immunodeficiency virus (HIV) infection in population-based cohort, *American Journal of Epidemiology* **137**, 1229–1240.

[30] Monath, T.P. (1994). Yellow fever, in *Infectious Disease: A Treatise of Infectious Diseases*, 5th Ed. P.D. Hoeprich, M.C. Jordan & A.R. Ronald, eds. Lippincott, Philadelphia, pp. 826–828.

[31] Mosley, J.W. (1994). Epidemiology, in *Infectious Disease: A Treatise of Infectious Diseases*, 5th Ed. P.D. Hoeprich, M.C. Jordan & A.R. Ronald, eds. Lippincott, Philadelphia, pp. 20–31.

[32] Moolgavkar, S.H. Cross, F.T. & Luebeck, E.G. (1990). A two-mutation model for radon-induced lung tumors in rats, *Radiation Research* **121**, 28–37.

[33] Redd, S.C. & Campbell, C.C. (1994). Malaria, in *Infectious Disease: A Treatise of Infectious Diseases*, 5th Ed. P.D. Hoeprich, M.C. Jordan & A.R. Ronald, eds. Lippincott, Philadelphia, pp. 1335–1344.

[34] Rhame, F.S. (1994). Acquired immunodeficiency syndrome, in *Infectious Disease: A Treatise of Infectious Diseases*, 5th Ed. P.D. Hoeprich, M.C. Jordan & A.R. Ronald, eds. Lippincott, Philadelphia, pp. 628–652.

[35] Rosenberg, P.S. (1995). Scope of the AIDS epidemic in the United States, *Science* **270**, 1372–1375.

[36] Tan, W.Y. (1991). *Stochastic Models of Carcinogenesis*. Marcel Dekker, New York.

[37] Tan, W.Y. & Chen, C.W. (1998). Stochastic modeling of carcinogenesis: some new insights, *Mathematical and Computer Modeling* **28**, 49–71.

[38] Tan, W.Y., Chen, C.W. & Wang, W. (1998). Some state space models of carcinogenesis, in *Proceedings of 1999 Medical Science Simulation*. J.G. Anderson & M. Katzper, eds. Society for Computer Simulation. San Diego, pp. 183–189.

[39] Tan, W.Y. & Singh, K.P. (1987). Assessing the effects of metabolism of environmental agents on cancer tumor development by a two-stage model of carcinogenesis, *Environmental Health Perspective* **74**, 203–210.

[40] Tan, W.Y. Tang, S.C. & Lee, S.R. (1996). Characterization of the HIV incubations and some comparative studies, *Statistics in Medicine* **15**, 197–220.

[41] Thomas, D.C. & McNeill, K.G. (1982). Risk estimates for the health effects of alpha radiation, in *Appendix M, Research Report*. Atomic Energy Control Board, Ottawa.

[42] Thorslund, T.W., Brown, C.C. & Charnley, C. (1987). Biologically motivated cancer risk models, *Risk Analysis* **7**, 109–119.

[43] Van Ryzin, J. (1980). Quantitative risk assessment, *Occupational Medicine* **22**, 321–326.

[44] Whittemore, A.S. & Keller, J.B. (1978). Quantitative theories of carcinogenesis, *SIAM Review* **20**, 1–30.

[45] Whittemore, A. & Altshuler, B. (1976). Lung cancer incidence in cigarette smokers: further analysis of Doll and Hill's data for British physicians, *Biometrics* **32**, 805–816.

[46] Yakovlev, A.Y. & Tsodikov, A.D. (1996). *Stochastic Models of Tumor Latency and Their Biostatistical Applications*. World Scientific, Singapore.

[47] Yang, G.L. & Chen, C.W. (1991). A stochastic two-stage carcinogenesis model: a new approach to computing the probability of observing tumor in animal bioassays, *Mathematical Biosciences* **104**, 247–258.

WAI-YUAN TAN & CHAO W. CHEN

Latent Predictor *see* Measurement Error in Epidemiologic Studies

Length Bias

The length-biased distribution is a probability distribution resulting from a biased sampling scheme in which the probability of observing a positive-valued random variable is proportional to the value of the variable.

Length Bias in Renewal Theory

The presence of length bias is a natural phenomenon in renewal theory. Consider a sequence of random variables

$$X_1, \quad X_1 + X_2, \quad X_1 + X_2 + X_3, \ldots,$$

where the Xs are positive-valued, nondegenerate, independent and identically distributed (iid) random variables. Suppose the process starts from time 0 and is observed at the time τ_0, where τ_0 is a positive constant. Let α be the index so that

$$\sum_{i=1}^{\alpha-1} X_i < \tau_0 \leq \sum_{i=1}^{\alpha} X_i.$$

Let Y, T, and R respectively denote the length of the interval containing τ_0, the backward recurrence time, and the forward recurrence time, or equivalently,

$$Y = X_\alpha, \qquad T = \tau_0 - \left\{ \sum_{i=1}^{\alpha-1} X_i \right\},$$

$$R = \left\{ \sum_{i=1}^{\alpha} X_i \right\} - \tau_0.$$

Let f, S, and μ represent the density function, survivorship function, and mean of X_1, respectively. When τ_0 is sufficiently large so that an *equilibrium condition* is reached [3], the joint density of (T, R) can then be derived as

$$p_{T,R}(t, r) = f(t + r)I(t \geq 0, r \geq 0)/\mu. \qquad (1)$$

The marginal density functions of Y, T, and R can be derived, based on (1), as

$$p_Y(y) = yf(y)I(y \geq 0)/\mu, \qquad (2)$$

$$p_T(t) = S(t)I(t \geq 0)/\mu, \qquad (3)$$

$$p_R(r) = S(r)I(r \geq 0)/\mu. \qquad (4)$$

The distribution of (2) is generally referred to as the *length-biased distribution*.

Although the length-biased distribution in renewal theory is usually derived under the iid assumption on the Xs, as a general result the independence assumption can be removed and the density formulas (1)–(4) still remain valid [6].

Statistical Methods

Length-biased sampling is recognized in many research fields including epidemiology, ecology, and reliability. A number of methods for length-biased data have been developed in the statistical literature. Cox [4] proposed estimating the survivorship function by a weighted empirical distribution function, with weight inversely proportional to y_i:

$$\hat{S}_n(y) = n^{-1}\hat{\mu}\sum_{i=1}^{n}\left[y_i^{-1}I(y_i > y)\right],$$

where $\hat{\mu} = \{n^{-1}\sum_j y_j^{-1}\}^{-1}$ serves as an appropriate estimate of μ, since $n^{-1}\sum_j y_j^{-1}$ estimates μ^{-1}. The estimator $\hat{S}_n$ can be proven to be the nonparametric maximum likelihood estimator of S, a special case under Vardi's **selection bias** models [12, 13]. Following the same weighting procedure, a kernel estimator of the density function f was proposed in [7] as

$$\hat{f}_n(y) = n^{-1}\hat{\mu}\sum_{i=1}^{n}\left[y_i^{-1}K_h(y - y_i)\right],$$

where $K_h(x) = h^{-1}K(h^{-1}x), h > 0$, with K a kernel function. Alternatively, one could first estimate the length-biased density, (2), by an ordinary kernel estimator and then use the relationship of (2) and f to obtain an estimator of f [2]. Under the proportional hazards model [5], a risk set sampling technique was developed in [17] for estimating regression parameters. For $y_j \geq y_i$, let $\Delta_j(y_i)$ be a binary variable which equals 1 with probability y_i/y_j, and 0 with probability $1 - (y_i/y_j)$. The indicators $\Delta_j(y_i)$ are used to identify bias-adjusted risk sets and to construct pseudo-likelihood equations. Regression parameter estimates are then derived by solving the score equations.

Length Bias in Prevalent Cohorts

Length-biased sampling could arise in many epidemiologic studies when survival data are collected from a disease population (*see* **Prevalent Case**). As an illustration, suppose a random sample of women with breast cancer (BC) are recruited for observation of survival. Assume (i) the rate of occurrence of BC remains constant over time, and (ii) the density function of the time from BC to death, f, is independent of the calendar time when BC occurred. Conditions (i) and (ii) together are referred to as the *equilibrium condition*. Denote by τ_i the calendar time when woman i with BC is recruited, t_i the time from the

initial diagnosis of BC to τ_i, and y_i the time from the initial diagnosis of BC to death. Under the equilibrium condition, the joint density of (t_i, y_i) is an equivalent of (1), namely

$$p_{T,Y}(t, y) = f(y)I(0 \leq t \leq y)/\mu, \qquad (5)$$

and the distribution of y_i is length-biased with density (2). Suppose a sample of iid $(t_1, y_1), \ldots, (t_n, y_n)$ is observed. By the factorization theorem

$$\begin{aligned}p_{T,Y}(t, y) &= p_Y(y)p_{T|Y}(t|y)\\ &= \{yf(y)I(y \geq 0)\}\{I(0 \leq t \leq y)/y\},\end{aligned}$$

the observed failure times $\{y_i\}$ serve as sufficient statistics for parameters of f. In this case, the variables $\{t_i\}$ do not contain additional information for f.

The preceding length-biased sample can be described more generally as disease prevalent data. Suppose there are two chronologically ordered and nonrecurrent events, termed the initiating and terminating events. Replacing the events of BC and death by the initiating and terminating events, the sample $\{y_i\}$ is length-biased when study individuals are recruited from those who have experienced the initiating event but have not experienced the terminating event [16]. Samples of this type could also be collected in a **screening** program for chronic diseases. It was indicated by Zelen & Feinleib [20] that the screen does not detect people at random, but detects people with longer preclinical sojourn times.

Although statistical methods can be formulated on the basis of length-biased observations as discussed earlier, the analysis could be further complicated by the presence of right censoring. We next make connection between length-biased sampling and left truncation in this context.

Length Bias and Left Truncation

Using formula (5), the density function of y_i given t_i can be derived as $f(y)I(y > t)/S(t)$, a truncated density function. The observed t_i in left truncation models [8, 10, 11, 15, 16, 19] is usually termed the *truncation time* and has density function $S(t)I(t > 0)/\mu$. Given the observations $(t_1, y_1), \ldots, (t_n, y_n)$, the full density can be expressed as the product of the marginal density of the t_i,

$$\prod_{i=1}^{n} [S(t_i)/\mu] ,$$

and the conditional density of y_i given the t_i,

$$\prod_{i=1}^{n} [f(y_i)/S(t_i)] . \qquad (6)$$

In length-biased models the truncation times in general do not serve as ancillary statistics for parameters of f, and thus the conditional likelihood (6) is used subject to loss of information. On the other hand, the conditional likelihood approach allows for broader applications because the construction of (6) requires the validity of Assumption (ii) but not (i).

Suppose now the observation of the terminating event is subject to right-censoring. Assume the following independent censoring condition: conditional on the observed t_i, the time from τ_i to the terminating event, r_i, is independent of the time from τ_i to censoring, d_i. This independent censoring condition does not, however, imply independence between the length-biased time, $y_i(= t_i + r_i)$, and the censoring time, $c_i(= t_i + d_i)$ [14, 16]. Let $w_i = \min\{y_i, c_i\}$ be the time from the initiating event to the end of observation, and $\delta_i = I(w_i = y_i)$ the censoring indicator. Conditional on t_i, under the independent censoring condition the density of (w_i, δ_i) is proportional to $f(w_i)^{\delta_i} S(w_i)^{1-\delta_i}/S(t_i)$. Given a sample of iid observations $(t_1, w_1, \delta_1), \ldots, (t_n, w_n, \delta_n)$, statistical approaches based on the conditional likelihood,

$$\prod_{i=1}^{n} \left[f(w_i)^{\delta_i} S(w_i)^{1-\delta_i}/S(t_i) \right],$$

are considered as methods for left-truncated and right-censored data. These approaches replace the usual risk sets $R(w) = \{w_i : w_i \geq w\}$ by $R^*(w) = \{w_i : t_i \leq w \leq w_i\}$ and result in an interesting contrast with the familiar techniques used in survival analysis [11, 15, 16, 19]. These methods can be alternately derived using counting process techniques with left-filtering [1, 8, 10]. The connection between renewal processes and left truncation can also be made by various approaches [9, 18]. While the methods provide "simple solutions" for analyzing censored length-biased data, these conditional approaches, similar to the left-truncation case, are used subject to loss

of efficiency because marginal information from the truncation times is not used in the construction of the methods. Furthermore, the applicability of these methods requires that the truncation time, t_i, be observable, and such a requirement might not be met in some applications.

Length Bias and Cross-Sectional Sampling

In the example of prevalent cohorts, the initiating and terminating events are required to be nonrecurrent. Nevertheless, the problem of length bias could also be encountered in studies that adopt **cross-sectional** sampling techniques to collect failure times from univariate or bivariate recurrent event processes. In these studies the outcome variable of interest is the length between two successive events. The crucial condition assumed, for the validity of length-biased distribution, is the equilibrium condition for the recurrent events. With cross-sectional samplings, the intervals which contain the sampling times are observed and form the length-biased sample. Examples include cross-sectional samples of (i) fibre length [4], where the recurrent events are of the same type and the location of an event is specified as the left end of a fibre, and (ii) length of stay in a hospital, in which the bivariate recurrent events are admission to and discharge from a hospital.

References

[1]   Andersen, P.K., Borgan, O., Gill, R.D. & Keiding, N. (1992). *Statistical Models Based on Counting Processes.* Springer-Verlag, New York.

[2]   Bhattacharyya, B.B., Franklin, L.A. & Richardson, G.D. (1988). A comparison of nonparametric unweighted and length-biased density estimation of fibres, *Communications in Statistics – Theory and Methods,* **17**, 3629–3644.

[3]   Cox, D.R. (1962). *Renewal Theory.* Methuen, London.

[4]   Cox, D.R. (1969). Some sampling problems in technology, in *New Development in Survey Sampling,* N.L. Johnson & H. Smith, Jr, eds. Wiley–Interscience, New York, pp. 506–527.

[5]   Cox, D.R. (1972). Regression models and life tables (with discussion), *Journal of the Royal Statistical Society, Series B* **34**, 187–220.

[6]   Cox, D.R. & Isham, V. (1980). *Point Processes.* Chapman & Hall, London.

[7]   Jones, M.C. (1991). Kernel density estimation for length biased data, *Biometrika* **78**, 511–519.

[8]   Keiding, N. (1992). Independent delayed entry, in *Survival Analysis: State of the Art*, J.P. Klein & P.K. Goel, eds. Kluwer, Dordrecht, pp. 309–326.

[9]   Keiding, N. & Gill, R.D. (1988). Random truncation models and Markov processes. *Technical Report*. Centre for Mathematics and Computer Science, Amsterdam, The Netherlands.

[10]   Keiding, N. & Gill, R.D. (1990). Random truncation models and Markov processes, *Annals of Statistics* **18**, 582–602.

[11]   Lai, T.-L. & Ying, Z. (1991). Rank regression methods for left-truncated and right-censored data, *Annals of Statistics* **19**, 417–442.

[12]   Vardi, Y. (1982). Nonparametric estimation in the presence of length bias, *Annals of Statistics* **10**, 616–620.

[13]   Vardi, Y. (1985). Empirical distributions in selection bias models, *Annals of Statistics* **13**, 178–203.

[14]   Vardi, Y. (1989). Multiplicative censoring, renewal processes, deconvolution and decreasing density: nonparametric estimation, *Biometrika* **76**, 751–761.

[15]   Wang, M.-C., Jewell, N.P. & Tsai W.-Y. (1986). Asymptotic properties of the product-limit estimate under random truncation, *Annals of Statistics* **14**, 1597–1605.

[16]   Wang, M.-C. (1991). Nonparametric estimation from cross-sectional survival data, *Journal of the American Statistical Association* **86** 130–143.

[17]   Wang, M.-C. (1996). Hazards regression analysis for length-biased data, *Biometrika* **83**, 343–354.

[18]   Winter, B.B. & Foldes, A. (1988). A product-limit estimator for use with length-biased data, *Canadian Journal of Statistics* **16**, 337–355.

[19]   Woodroofe, M. (1985). Asymptotic properties of the product-limit estimate under random truncation, *Annals of Statistics* **13**, 163–177.

[20]   Zelen, M. & Feinlieb, M. (1969). On the theory of screening for chronic diseases, *Biometrika* **56**, 601–614.

(*See also* **Biased Sampling of Cohorts in Epidemiology**)

MEI-CHENG WANG

Lexis Diagram

A Lexis diagram is a (time, age) coordinate system, representing individual lives by line segments of unit slope, joining (time, age) of birth and death [13] (see Table 1 and Figure 1). The Lexis diagram is an important descriptive tool in epidemiology and **demography**. However, it also has several applications in **survival analysis** and analytical epidemiology as a tool for several classes of statistical models,

as surveyed by Keiding [8]. These uses of the Lexis diagram are less common and it is the aim of this article to indicate some recent developments.

Lexis [13] in his Figure 1, reproduced here as Figure 2, originally considered a diagram of (calendar time at birth, age) in which life lines will be vertical rather than having unit slope. In his

Table 1   Five lives illustrated in Figure 1

Born	Died	Age at death
1918	1966	48
1926	1944	18
1934	1992	58
1944	1978	34
1954	1968	14

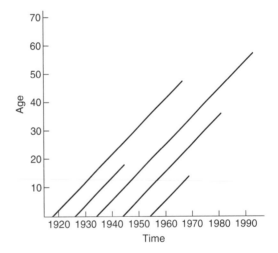

Figure 1   A Lexis diagram representing the five lives of Table 1

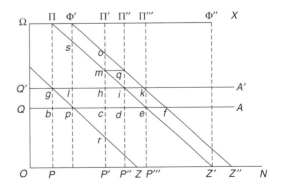

Figure 2   Lexis's diagram [13, Figure 1]

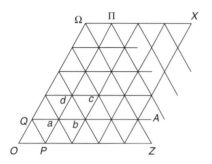

Figure 3 Lexis's equilateral diagram [13, Figure 2]

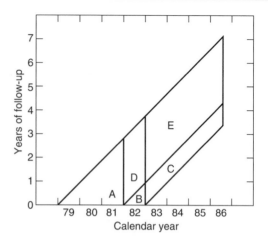

Figure 4 Lexis diagram of the Danish Breast Cancer Cooperative Group (DBCG) DBCG-77 clinical trials on adjuvant treatment of breast cancer. The traditional independent data set for verifying an unexpected finding in A would be based on B and C. However, much more information is obtained by including also D and E, and in fact B and D already would have yielded the independent confirmation not achieved by B and C. Reproduced from Keiding et al. [11] by permission of John Wiley & Sons Ltd

Figure 2, reproduced here as Figure 3, he also mentioned an equilateral diagram in which the time units in the calendar time, age, and cohort (i.e. time of birth) directions are of the same length. Lexis further discussed a three-dimensional extension allowing for an intermediate (irreversible) life event, in Lexis's case exemplified by marriage. This corresponds to the three-state model basic to the modern statistical description of **incidence** and **prevalence** (cf. [9]).

Despite its long history, the Lexis diagram is still being rediscovered among statisticians, cf. Goldman [6] for the standard Lexis diagram and Weinkam & Sterling [18] for the equilateral Lexis diagram.

Applications of the Lexis Diagram in Survival Analysis and Analytical Epidemiology

Clinical Trials with Staggered Entry

In many clinical trials patients arrive sequentially in calendar time but the substantive interest is on survival time since entry. The resulting interplay between the two time scales (calendar time and duration) has generated considerable complications in the development of a satisfactory statistical theory, particularly if comparisons between treatments are intended along the way at certain fixed time points (interim analysis) or sequentially.

As mentioned by Keiding et al. [11], it is sometimes feasible to exploit the remaining life times of individuals (counted with delayed entry) from an interim analysis to supplement new individuals in a confirmatory analysis. This idea is explained in the Lexis diagram of Figure 4.

Disease Incidence Studies

Lexis diagram representations of classical (often historically) prospective studies (*see* **Cohort Study**; **Cohort Study, Historical**) of (calendar time, age)-specific disease incidence are common, and we return to some of the statistical issues below. More intricate sampling plans may also take advantage of this representation, such as the **retrospective** incidence study of a **cross-sectional** sample of prevalent diabetics by Keiding et al. [12], where each incident and surviving case needed to be weighted (in a Horvitz–Thompson fashion) by its inverse survival probability from disease onset to the sampling date.

Prevalent Cohort Studies

A prevalent cohort study is based on a cross-sectional sample of diseased patients, with or without retrospective information on disease onset. Patients are followed until death or a fixed later calendar time, whichever comes first, (see Figure 5, and also [7] for additional examples and the link to the Arjas–Haara theory of innovative and noninnovative marks in the marked point process that accounts

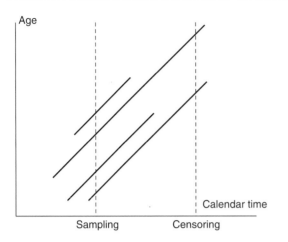

Age

Calendar time

Sampling   Censoring

Figure 5 Lexis diagram of a prevalen cohort study. Four patients are sampled and their disease onset is known. During the follow-up period two of them die; the other two are still alive at the end of follow-up, where they are censored

for the partial observation). The article **Biased Sampling of Cohorts in Epidemiology** provides surveys of design and analysis problems for such studies.

Statistical Inference in the Lexis Diagram

Piecewise Constant Intensity Models

Many disease incidence and mortality studies (perhaps particularly in cancer) have taken piecewise constant intensity models as method of choice (see Clayton & Schifflers [4, 5] for a definitive survey). As is also well known in sociology, there is an inherent unidentifiability of the linear component in a model allowing for dependence on both **age, period and cohort**, although Nakamura [15] showed that a Bayesian framework allowed roughness penalties in the three directions to decide the matter.

Point Processes, Continuous Time

Brillinger [3] initiated an exact use of point processes as a basis for statistical models for incidence and mortality in the Lexis diagram, generalized to morbidity (incidence) and prevalence by Keiding [9, 10] (see also [17]). Without parametric assumptions, statistical analysis requires smoothing formally studied by McKeague & Utikal [14] and embedded in an empirical Bayes interpretation of penalized likelihood by

Berzuini et al. [2], Berzuini & Clayton [1] and Ogata et al. [16], who reanalyzed the retrospective diabetes incidence study by Keiding et al. [12] quoted above.

References

[1] Berzuini, C. & Clayton, D. (1994). Bayesian analysis of survival on multiple time scales, *Statistics in Medicine* **13**, 823–838.

[2] Berzuini, C., Clayton, D. & Bernardinelli, L. (1993). Bayesian inference on the Lexis diagram, *Bulletin of the International Statistics Institute* **55**, 149–165; with discussion **55**, 42–43.

[3] Brillinger, D.R. (1986). The natural variability of vital rates and associated statistics (with discussion), *Biometrics* **42**, 693–734.

[4] Clayton, D. & Schifflers, E. (1987). Models for temporal variation in cancer rates. I: age-period and age-cohort models, *Statistics in Medicine* **6**, 449–467.

[5] Clayton, D. & Schifflers, E. (1987). Models for temporal variation in cancer rates. II: age–period–cohort models, *Statistics in Medicine* **6**, 469–481.

[6] Goldman, A.I. (1992). Eventcharts: Visualizing survival and other timed-events data, *American Statistician* **46**, 13–18.

[7] Keiding, N. (1989). Discussion of E. Arjas: Survival models and martingale dynamics, *Scandinavian Journal of Statistics* **16**, 209–213.

[8] Keiding, N. (1990). Statistical inference in the Lexis diagram, *Philosophical Transaction of the Royal Society of London, Series A* **332**, 487–509.

[9] Keiding, N. (1991). Age-specific incidence and prevalence: a statistical perspective (with discussion), *Journal of the Royal Statistical Society, Series A* **154**, 371–412.

[10] Keiding, N. (1992). Independent delayed entry (with discussion), *Survival Analysis: State of the Art*, J.P. Klein & P.K. Goel, eds. Kluwer, Dordrecht, pp. 309–326.

[11] Keiding, N., Bayer, T. & Watt-Boolsen, S. (1987). Confirmatory analysis of survival data using left truncation of the life times of primary survivors, *Statistics in Medicine* **6**, 939–944.

[12] Keiding, N., Holst, C. & Green, A. (1989). Retrospective estimation of diabetes incidence from information in a prevalent population and historical mortality, *American Journal of Epidemiology* **130**, 588–600.

[13] Lexis, W. (1875). *Einleitung in die Theorie der Bevölkerungsstatistik*. Trübner, Strassburg.

[14] McKeague, I.W. & Utikal, K.J. (1990). Inference for a nonlinear counting process regression model, *Annals of Statistics* **18**, 1172–1187.

[15] Nakamura, T. (1986). Bayesian cohort models for general cohort table analyses, *Annals of the Institute of Statistical Mathematics* **38**, 353–370.

[16] Ogata, Y., Katsura, K., Keiding, N., Holst, C. & Green, A. (1996). Age–period–cohort analysis of incidence from incompletely detected retrospective data,

Research Report 96/2. Department of Biostatistics, University of Copenhagen.

[17] Wang, M.-C., Brookmeyer, R. & Jewell, N.P. (1993). Statistical models for prevalent cohort data, *Biometrics* **49**, 1–11.

[18] Weinkam, J.J. & Sterling, T.D. (1991). A graphical approach to the interpretation of age-period-cohort data, *Epidemiology* **2**, 133–137.

NIELS KEIDING

Life Expectancy

Life expectancy is both the most summary and the most significant measure derived from a **life table**. Life expectancy at age **x** is the average number of years a person aged **x** will live if subject to the mortality rates contained in the life table.

In life table notation, life expectancy at age **x**, $\overset{\circ}{e}_x$, is given by

$$\overset{\circ}{e}_x = T_x/l_x,$$

where T_x is the total years lived in the life table population after exact age **x**, and $l_x =$ the number of survivors in the life table population at exact age **x**. The method for calculating these quantities can be found in standard textbooks [3].

Like the life table itself, life expectancy is determined by the force of mortality or mortality hazard function, $\mu(x)$, over the entire age range (*see* **Hazard Rate**). In continuous notation

$$\overset{\circ}{e}(x) = \int_x^\infty l(x)\mathrm{d}x/l(x),$$

and since

$$l(x) = \exp\left[-\int_0^x \mu(u)\mathrm{d}(u)\right],$$

it can be seen that life expectancy at age **x** reflects both the **cumulative hazard** from birth to age **x** (through l_x), and the cumulative hazard from **x** to the oldest age (through T_x, itself an integral of l_x).

In actuarial analysis it is normal to distinguish between the complete (exact) expectation of life and the curtate or whole year expectation, but in **demography** and epidemiology the complete expectation is universally employed.

In most populations $\overset{\circ}{e}(x)$ tends to rise between birth and age 1, and to decline linearly thereafter, although in very low mortality countries the decline is virtually linear throughout the age range.

The most common life expectancy encountered is $\overset{\circ}{e}(0)$, the expectation of life at birth. Because $\overset{\circ}{e}(0)$ incorporates the entire mortality experience of the cohort or life table population, it may be considered as an age standardized (*see* **Standardization Methods**) measure of mortality, where the standard age distribution is derived from the age pattern of mortality itself.

Life expectancy at birth has increased substantially with modernization, rising from a preindustrial level of perhaps 40 years to current levels of over 80 in countries like Japan. Because of its cumulative impact throughout the age range, improved survival in infancy has made the greatest contribution to this increase.

In recent years there have been unexpected gains in expectation of life at older ages in some very low mortality countries, leading to predictions that expectation of life could rise to 100 years, with significant effects on social security and pension systems. However, 85 seems a more likely upper limit [2].

Traditionally, life table theory has not had a strong statistical component: the focus has primarily been on the average expectation of life, rather than on its distribution. However, Chiang [1] has addressed the sampling theory of the life table, and more recently the homogeneity/heterogeneity of life expectancy has received renewed attention, particularly in the context of expectation of life at advanced ages.

Life expectancy is also used as a powerful tool in association with multistate or multilevel life tables. Expectations of working life, of a healthy life, or of a life free of disability are examples of this. Unlike death, individuals may move in and out of these states, requiring modifications to the logic of the life table to incorporate nonabsorbing states.

References

[1] Chiang, C.L. (1984). *The Life Table and Its Applications.* Krieger, Malabar.

[2] Olshansky, S.J. & Carnes, B.A. (1994). Demographic perspectives on human senescence, *Population and Development Review* **20**, 57–80.

[3] Shryock, H.S. & Siegel, J.S. (1973). *The Methods and Materials of Demography.* US Department of Commerce, Bureau of the Census, Washington.

L. SMITH

Life Table

A life table is a tabular representation of central features of the distribution of a positive random variable, say T, with an absolutely continuous distribution. It may represent the lifetime of an individual, the failure time of a physical component, the remission time of an illness, or some other duration variable. In general, T is the time of occurrence of some event that ends individual survival in a given status. Let its cumulative distribution function (cdf) be $F(t) = \Pr(T \le t)$ and let the corresponding survival function be $S(t) = 1 - F(t)$, where $F(0) = 0$. If $F(\cdot)$ has the probability density function (pdf) $f(\cdot)$, then the risk of event occurrence is measured by the **hazard** $\mu(t) = f(t)/S(t)$, for t where $S(t) > 0$. Because of its sensitivity to changes over time and to risk differentials between population subgroups, $\mu(t)$ is a centerpiece of interest in empirical investigations.

In applications to human mortality, which is where life tables originated, the time variable normally is a person's attained age and is denoted x. The function $\mu(x)$ is then called the *force of mortality* or *death intensity* (*see* **Hazard Rate**). The life-table function $l_x = 100\,000\ S(x)$ is called the *decrement function* and is tabulated for integer x in *complete life tables*; in *abridged life tables* it is tabulated for sparser values of x, most often for five-year intervals of age. The *radix* l_0 is selected to minimize the need for decimals in the l_x table; a value different from $100\,000$ is sometimes chosen. Other life-table functions are the expected number of deaths $d_x = l_x - l_{x+1}$ at age x (i.e. between age x and age $x + 1$), the single-year death probability $q_x = \Pr(T \le x + 1 | T > x) = d_x/l_x$, and the corresponding survival probability $p_x = 1 - q_x$. Simple integration gives

$$q_x = 1 - \exp\left[-\int_x^{x+1} \mu(s)\mathrm{d}s\right]. \qquad (1)$$

Life-table construction consists in the estimation and tabulation of functions of this nature from empirical data. If ungrouped individual-level data are available, then the Kaplan–Meier estimator can be used to estimate l_x for all relevant x and estimators of the other life-table functions can then be computed subsequently. Alternatively, a segment of the Nelson–Aalen estimator can be used to estimate $\int_x^{x+1} \mu(s)\mathrm{d}s$; (1) can then be used to estimate q_x

for each x, and the rest of the computations follow suit. From any given schedule of death probabilities $q_0, q_1, q_2, \ldots$, the l_x table is easily computed sequentially by the relation $l_{x+1} = l_x(1 - q_x)$ for $x = 0, 1, 2, \ldots$. Much of the effort in life-table construction therefore is concentrated on providing such a schedule $\{q_x\}$.

More conventional methods of life-table construction use grouped survival times. Suppose for simplicity that the range of the lifetime T is subdivided into intervals of unit length and that the number of failures observed during interval x is D_x. Let the corresponding total person-time recorded under risk of failure in the same interval be R_x. Then, if $\mu(t)$ is constant over interval x (the assumption of *piecewise constancy*), then the *death rate* $\hat{\mu}_x = D_x/R_x$ is the maximum likelihood estimator of this constant. Relation (1) can again be used to provide an estimator

$$\hat{q}_x = 1 - \exp(-\hat{\mu}_x), \qquad (2)$$

and the crucial first step in the life-table computation has been achieved. Instead of (2), $\hat{\mu}_x/\left(1 + \frac{1}{2}\hat{\mu}_x\right)$ is often used to estimate q_x. This solution is of older vintage and may be regarded as an approximation to (2).

Two kinds of problems may arise: (i) the exact value of R_x may not be known, and (ii) the constancy assumption for the hazard may be violated.

When the exact risk time R_x is not known, some approximation is often used. An Anglo-Saxon tradition is to use the mid-year population in the age interval. Alternatively, suppose that the number N_x of survivors to exact age x and the number W_x of withdrawals (losses to follow-up) in the age interval are known. What has become known as the actuarial method then consists in approximating R_x by $N_x - \frac{1}{2}(D_x + W_x)$. If there are no withdrawals and N_x is known, then D_x/N_x is the maximum likelihood estimator of q_x, and this provides a suitable starting point for the life-table computations.

For the case where only grouped data are available and the piecewise-constancy assumption for the intensity function is implausible, various methods have been developed to improve on (2). For an overview, see Keyfitz [12]. Even if single-year age groups are used, mortality drops too fast in the first year of life to merit an assumption of constancy over this interval. Demographers often use $\hat{\mu}_0/[1 + (1 - a_0)\hat{\mu}_0]$ to estimate q_0, where a_0 is some small figure, say between 0.1 and 0.15 [2]. If it is possible to partition the first year of life into subintervals in each of which mortality *can* be taken as constant, then it is statistically more efficient essentially to build up a life table for this year. This leads to an estimate like $\hat{q}_0 = 1 - \exp(-\sum_i \hat{\mu}_i)$, where the sum is taken over the first-year intervals. See Dublin et al. [5, p. 24] for an example.

The force of mortality is sometimes represented by a function $h(x; \boldsymbol{\theta})$, where $\boldsymbol{\theta}$ is a vector of parameters. Actuaries most often use the classical Gompertz–Makeham function $h(x; a, b, c) = a + bc^x$ for the force of mortality in their life tables. When individual-level data are available, it would be statistically most efficient to estimate the parameters by the maximum likelihood method, but most often they are estimated by fitting $h(\cdot; \boldsymbol{\theta})$ to a schedule of death rates $\{\hat{\mu}_x\}$, perhaps by least squares, minimum chi-square, or some method of moments. This approach is called *analytic graduation*; for its statistical theory, see [11]. One of many alternatives to modeling the force of mortality is to let [10]

$$q_x/p_x = A^{(x+B)^C} + D\exp[-E(\ln x - \ln F)^2] + GH^x.$$

So far we have tacitly assumed that the data come from a group of independent individuals who have all been observed in parallel and whose lifetimes have the same cdf. Staggered (delayed) entries into the study population and voluntary exits (withdrawals) from it are permitted provided they contain no information about the risk in question, be it death, recurrence of a disease, or something else. Nevertheless, the basic idea is that of a connected cohort of individuals that is followed from some significant starting point (like birth or the onset of some disease) and which is diminished over time due to *decrements (attrition)* caused by the risk's operation. In demography, this corresponds to following a **birth cohort** through life or a marriage cohort while their marriages last, and the ensuing tables are called *cohort life tables*.

Because such tables can only be terminated at the end of a cohort's life, it is more common to compute age-specific attrition rates $\hat{\mu}_x$ from data collected for the members of a population during a limited period and to use the mechanics of life-table construction to produce a *period life table* for the population from such rates. If mortality patterns are tied to cohorts, then individuals who live at widely differing ages in the period of observation cannot be expected to have the same risk structure, and the period table is said to reflect the patterns of a *synthetic* (fictitious) cohort exposed to the risk of the period at the various ages.

Multiple-Decrement Tables

When two or more mutually exclusive risks operate on the study population (*see* **Competing Risks**), one may correspondingly compute a *multiple-decrement table* to reflect this. For instance, a period of sickness can end in death or, alternatively, in recovery. Suppose that an integer random variable K represents the *cause of decrement* and define $F_k(t) = \Pr(T \leq t, K = k)$, $f_k(t) = dF_k(t)/dt$, and $\mu_k(t) = f_k(t)/S(t)$, assuming that all $F_k(\cdot)$ are absolutely continuous. Then $\mu_k(\cdot)$ is the cause-specific hazard (intensity) for risk cause k and $\mu(t) = \sum_k \mu_k(t)$ is the total risk of decrement at time t. For the multiple-decrement table, we define the decrement probability

$$q_x^{(k)} = \Pr(T \leq x + 1, K = k | T > x)$$

$$= \int_0^1 \exp\left[-\int_0^t \mu(x+s)ds\right]\mu_k(x+t)dt. \quad (3)$$

For given risk intensities, $q_x^{(k)}$ can be computed by numerical integration in (3). The expected number of decrements at age x as a result of cause k is $d_x^{(k)} = l_x q_x^{(k)}$. When estimates are available for the cause-specific risk intensities, one or two columns can therefore be added to the life table for each cause to include estimates of $d_x^{(k)}$ and possibly $q_x^{(k)}$.

Several further life-table functions can be defined by formal reduction or elimination of one or more of the intensity functions in formulas like those above. In this manner, a *single-decrement life table* can be computed for each cause k, depicting what the normal life table would look like *if* cause k were the only one that operated in the study population and *if* it did so with the risk function estimated from the data. The purpose is to see the effect of the risk cause in question without interference from other causes. Some demographers call this abstraction the risk's *pure* effect. No assumption is made that in practice the total attrition risk can actually be reduced to the level of the one which is in focus or that this cause operates independently of other causes. For instance, a single-decrement life table of recovery from an illness reflects the pure timing effect of the duration structure of the intensity of recovery even though the elimination of mortality is unattainable.

A single-decrement life table is at an extreme end of a class of tables produced by deleting one (or more) of the cause intensities in formulas like those above. To obtain a *cause-deleted life table*, where only cause k has been eliminated, one may introduce $\mu_{-k}(t) = \mu(t) - \mu_k(t)$,

$$q_x^{(-k)} = \int_0^1 \exp\left[-\int_0^t \mu_{-k}(x+s)ds\right]\mu_{-k}(x+t)dt$$

$$= 1 - \exp\left[\int_x^{x+1}\mu_{-k}(s)ds\right], \qquad (4)$$

and so on, and a "normal" life table may be computed with $\mu(t)$ replaced by $\mu_{-k}(t)$ everywhere. A corresponding cause-deleted multiple-decrement life table may be based on reduced cause-specific decrement probabilities like

$$\int_0^1 \exp\left[-\int_0^t \mu_{-k}(x+s)ds\right]\mu_j(x+t)dt,$$
$$\text{for } j \neq k.$$

Such a table would show what a normal table would look like *if* it were possible to eliminate cause k without changing the risk of any other cause. Again no assumption needs to be made about the feasibility of such elimination in real life nor about cause independence. The computations are based on a pure abstraction. The interpretation for real-life applications must be based on substantive considerations and is a different matter.

Life Expectancy

An individual's **life expectancy** (at birth) is the expected value

$$\overset{\circ}{e}_0 = \mathrm{E}(T) = \int_0^\infty [1 - F(x)]dx = \int_0^\infty l_x/l_0 dx$$

of his or her lifetime T, computed for the probability distribution $F(\cdot)$ operating at the time of birth. When the individual has survived to (exact) age x, his or her remaining lifetime, $U = T - x$, is positive and has the survival function $S_x(u) = S(x+u)/S(x) = l_{x+u}/l_x$, and the *residual life expectancy* is

$$\overset{\circ}{e}_x = \mathrm{E}(T-x|T>x) = \int_0^\infty S_x(u)du = \int_0^\infty \frac{l_{x+u}}{l_x}du.$$

If $L_x = \int_0^1 l_{x+t}dt$, we get $L_x \cong \frac{1}{2}(l_x + l_{x+1})$ by the trapezoidal rule of numerical integration, and

$$\overset{\circ}{e}_x = \sum_{t=0}^\infty L_{x+t} \cong \sum_{t=0}^\infty \frac{l_{x+t}}{l_x} - \frac{1}{2}, \qquad (5)$$

which is normally used to compute values for $\overset{\circ}{e}_x$.

Equivalent names for the life expectancies are *mean survival time* for $\overset{\circ}{e}_0$ and *mean residual survival time at age x* for $\overset{\circ}{e}_x$. The *median length of life* is the median in the distribution of T; it used to be called the *probable length of life*. Correspondingly, the *median residual length of life* at age x used to be called the *probable residual length of life*. If we denote the latter by ξ_x, then it is defined by the relation $l_{x+\xi_x} = \frac{1}{2}l_x$.

The above functions can be computed for cohort life tables and for period life tables. Figure 1 shows plots of the function $\overset{\circ}{e}_x$ according to the mortality experience for Swedish women in 1891–1900 and 1990–1994. The life expectancy at birth has increased from 53.6 years in the older table to 80.8 some one hundred years later. Note that in the older table $\overset{\circ}{e}_x$ increases with x up to age 2 and remains above $\overset{\circ}{e}_0$ up through age 11. When mortality is high at very young ages, surviving the first part of life *increases* your expected remaining lifetime. As a consequence of mortality improvements for very young children, these features have disappeared in

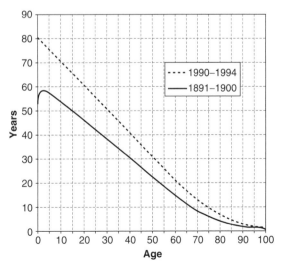

Figure 1 Residual life expectancy for Swedish women, 1891–1900 and 1990–1994

the younger table. Note that the expected *total* lifetime, $x + \overset{\circ}{e}_x$, always increases with x throughout the human lifespan. (One can show that the derivative of this function is always positive.) The longer you have lived already, the longer you can expect the total length of your life to be.

In a multiple-decrement situation, formula (5) can be used to compute a residual life expectancy $\overset{\circ}{e}_x^{(-k)}$ from the decrement series of the cause-deleted life table for risk k. The difference $\overset{\circ}{e}_x^{(-k)} - \overset{\circ}{e}_x$ is the gain one would get in residual life expectancy at age x *if* it were possible to eliminate risk cause k without changing the risk intensity of any other cause of decrement. Dublin et al. [5, p. 96] note that according to the cause-specific mortality of the US in 1939–1941 the gain would be 9.01 years for white men and 8.80 years for white women at age 0 if one could eliminate the risk of death due to cardiovascular–renal diseases at all ages (and change no other cause-specific mortality risks). The gains from eliminating the risk of death in cancer alone were much less (1.39 years for men and 2.05 years for women).

History and Literature

The first step toward the development of the life table was taken when Graunt [9] published his famous *Bills of Mortality*. There were subsequent contributions by Halley, Huygens, Leibniz, Euler, and others. Deparcieux [4] clarified the definition of the life expectancy and identified the need for separate tables for men and women. Wargentin [17] was the first to publish real age-specific death rates, and the first to do so for a whole country. Price [14] included most of the columns now associated with the life table, and the tables by Duvillard [7] contained them all. The basic notions of cause-eliminated life tables go back to Bernoulli [1]. Cournot [3] developed the essentials of their mathematics. See Dupâquier [6] and Seal [15] for historical overviews. Smith & Keyfitz [16] have collected extracts from many original texts.

Life-table techniques are described in most introductory textbooks on the methods of actuarial statistics, biostatistics, demography, or epidemiology. See for example, Chiang [2], Elandt-Johnson & Johnson [8], or Manton & Stallard [13].

References

[1]   Bernoulli, D. (1766). Essai d'une nouvelle analyse de la mortalité causée par la petite vérole, et des avantages de l'inoculation pour la prévenir. *Histoire de l'Académie Royale des Sciences, Mémoires, Année 1760*, pp. 1–45.

[2]   Chiang, C.L. (1984). *The Life Table and its Applications*. Krieger, Malabar.

[3]   Cournot, A. (1843). *Exposition de la théorie des chances et des probabilités*. Hachette, Paris.

[4]   Deparcieux, A. (1746). *Essai sur les probabilités de la durée de la vie humaine*. Guérin Frères, Paris.

[5]   Dublin, L.I., Lotka, A.J. & Spiegelman, M. (1947). *Length of Life*. Ronald Press, New York.

[6]   Dupâquier, J. (1996). *L'invention de la table de mortalité*. Presses Universitaires de France, Paris.

[7]   Duvillard, E. (1806). *Analyse des tableaux de l'influence de la petite vérole, et de celle qu'un préservatif tel que la vaccine peut avoir sur la population et la longévité*. Paris.

[8]   Elandt-Johnson, R.C. & Johnson, N.L. (1980). *Survival Models and Data Analysis*. Wiley, New York.

[9]   Graunt, J. (1662). *Natural and Political Observations Made Upon the Bills of Mortality*. London.

[10] Heligman, L. & Pollard, J. (1980). The age pattern of mortality, *Journal of the Institute of Actuaries* **107**, 49–75.

[11] Hoem, J.M. (1972). Analytic graduation, in *Proceedings of the Sixth Berkeley Symposium on Mathematical Statistics and Probability 1970*, Vol. 1, L.M. Le Cam, J. Neyman & E.L. Scott, eds. University of California Press, Berkeley, pp. 569–600.

[12] Keyfitz, N. (1982). Keyfitz method of life-table construction, in *Encyclopedia of Statistical Sciences*, Vol. 4, S. Kotz & N.L. Johnson, eds. Wiley, New York, pp. 371–372.

[13] Manton, K.G. & Stallard, E. (1984). *Recent Trends in Mortality Analysis*. Academic Press, New York.

[14] Price, R. (1783). *Observations of Reversionary Payments: On Schemes for Providing Annuities for Widows, and for Persons in Old Age; and on the National Debt*. Cadell & Davies, London.

[15] Seal, H. (1977). Studies in the history of probability and statistics, XXV: multiple decrements or competing risks, *Biometrika* **64**, 429–439.

[16] Smith, D. & Keyfitz, N. (1977). *Mathematical Demography: Selected Papers*. Springer-Verlag, Heidelberg.

[17] Wargentin, P. (1766). *Mortaliteten i Sverige, i anledning af Tabell-Verket*. Kongl. Vetenskaps-Academiens Handlingar, Stockholm.

(*See also* **Demography**; **Vital Statistics, Overview**)

JAN M. HOEM

List-Assisted Method *see* Random Digit Dialing Sampling for Case–Control Studies

Little's Equation in Queuing Theory *see* Incidence–Prevalence Relationships

Logistic Regression

The goal of a logistic regression analysis is to find the best fitting and most parsimonious, yet biologically reasonable, model to describe the relationship between an outcome (dependent or response variable) and a set of independent (predictor or explanatory) variables. What distinguishes the logistic regression model from the linear regression model is that the outcome variable in logistic regression is categorical and most usually *binary* or *dichotomous*.

In any regression problem the key quantity is the mean value of the outcome variable, given the value of the independent variable. This quantity is called the *conditional mean* and will be expressed as $E(Y|x)$, where Y denotes the outcome variable and x denotes a value of the independent variable. In linear regression we assume that this mean may be expressed as an equation linear in x (or some transformation of x or Y), such as

$$E(Y|x) = \beta_0 + \beta_1 x.$$

This expression implies that it is possible for $E(Y|x)$ to take on any value as x ranges between $-\infty$ and $+\infty$.

Many distribution functions have been proposed for use in the analysis of a dichotomous outcome variable. Cox & Snell [2] discuss some of these. There are two primary reasons for choosing the logistic distribution. These are: (i) from a mathematical point of view it is an extremely flexible and easily used function, and (ii) it lends itself to a biologically meaningful interpretation.

To simplify notation, let $\pi(x) = E(Y|x)$ represent the conditional mean of Y given x. The logistic regression model can be expressed as

$$\pi(x) = \frac{\exp(\beta_0 + \beta_1 x)}{1 + \exp(\beta_0 + \beta_1 x)}. \tag{1}$$

The *logit transformation*, defined in terms of $\pi(x)$, is as follows:

$$g(x) = \ln\left[\frac{\pi(x)}{1 - \pi(x)}\right] = \beta_0 + \beta_1 x. \tag{2}$$

The importance of this transformation is that $g(x)$ has many of the desirable properties of a linear regression model. The logit, $g(x)$, is linear in its parameters, may be continuous, and may range from $-\infty$ to $+\infty$ depending on the range of x.

The second important difference between the linear and logistic regression models concerns the conditional distribution of the outcome variable. In the linear regression model we assume that an observation of the outcome variable may be expressed as $y = E(Y|x) + \varepsilon$. The quantity ε is called the *error* and expresses an observation's deviation from the conditional mean. The most common assumption is that ε follows a normal distribution with mean zero and some variance that is constant across levels of the independent variable. It follows that the conditional distribution of the outcome variable given x is normal with mean $E(Y|x)$, and a variance that is constant. This is not the case with a dichotomous outcome variable. In this situation we may express the value of the outcome variable given x as $y = \pi(x) + \varepsilon$. Here the quantity ε may assume one of two possible values. If $y = 1$, then $\varepsilon = 1 - \pi(x)$ with probability $\pi(x)$, and if $y = 0$, then $\varepsilon = -\pi(x)$ with probability $1 - \pi(x)$. Thus, ε has a distribution with mean zero and variance equal to $\pi(x)[1 - \pi(x)]$. That is, the conditional distribution of the outcome variable follows a binomial distribution with probability given by the conditional mean, $\pi(x)$.

Fitting the Logistic Regression Model

Suppose we have a sample of n independent observations of the pair $(x_i, y_i), i = 1, 2, \ldots, n$, where y_i denotes the value of a dichotomous outcome variable and x_i is the value of the independent variable for the ith subject. Furthermore, assume that the outcome variable has been coded as 0 or 1 representing the absence or presence of the characteristic, respectively. To fit the logistic regression model (1) to a set of data requires that we estimate the values of β_0 and β_1, the unknown parameters.

In linear regression the method used most often to estimate unknown parameters is least squares. In that method we choose those values of β_0 and β_1 that minimize the sum of squared deviations of the observed values of Y from the predicted values based upon the model. Under the usual assumptions for linear regression the least squares method yields estimators with a number of desirable statistical properties. Unfortunately, when the least squares method is applied to a model with a dichotomous outcome the estimators no longer have these same properties.

The general method of estimation that leads to the least squares function under the linear regression model (when the error terms are normally distributed) is maximum likelihood. This is the method used to estimate the logistic regression parameters. In a very general sense the maximum likelihood method yields values for the unknown parameters that maximize the probability of obtaining the observed set of data. To apply this method we must first construct a function called the *likelihood function*. This function expresses the probability of the observed data as a function of the unknown parameters. The *maximum likelihood estimators* of these parameters are chosen to be those values that maximize this function. Thus, the resulting estimators are those that agree most closely with the observed data.

If Y is coded as 0 or 1, then the expression for $\pi(x)$ given in (1) provides (for an arbitrary value of $\beta' = (\beta_0, \beta_1)$, the vector of parameters) the conditional probability that Y is equal to 1 given x. This will be denoted $\Pr(Y = 1|x)$. It follows that the quantity $1 - \pi(x)$ gives the conditional probability that Y is equal to zero given x, $\Pr(Y = 0|x)$. Thus, for those pairs (x_i, y_i), where $y_i = 1$, the contribution to the likelihood function is $\pi(x_i)$, and for those pairs where $y_i = 0$, the contribution to the likelihood function is $1 - \pi(x_i)$, where the quantity $\pi(x_i)$ denotes the value of $\pi(x)$ computed at x_i. A convenient way to express the contribution to the likelihood function for the pair (x_i, y_i) is through the term

$$\xi(x_i) = \pi(x_i)^{y_i}[1 - \pi(x_i)]^{1-y_i}. \tag{3}$$

Since the observations are assumed to be independent, the likelihood function is obtained as the product of the terms given in (3) as follows:

$$l(\beta) = \prod_{i=1}^{n} \xi(x_i). \tag{4}$$

The principle of maximum likelihood states that we use as our estimate of β the value that maximizes the expression in (4). However, it is easier mathematically to work with the log of (4). This expression, the *log likelihood*, is defined as

$$L(\beta) = \ln[l(\beta)]$$
$$= \sum\{y_i \ln[\pi(x_i)] + (1 - y_i)\ln[1 - \pi(x_i)]\}. \tag{5}$$

To find the value of β that maximizes $L(\beta)$ we differentiate $L(\beta)$ with respect to β_0 and β_1 and set the resulting expressions equal to zero. These equations are as follows:

$$\sum_{i=1}^{n}[y_i - \pi(x_i)] = 0 \tag{6}$$

and

$$\sum_{i=1}^{n} x_i[y_i - \pi(x_i)] = 0, \tag{7}$$

and are called the *likelihood equations*.

In linear regression, the likelihood equations, obtained by differentiating the sum of squared deviations function with respect to β, are linear in the unknown parameters, and thus are easily solved. For logistic regression the expressions in (6) and (7) are nonlinear in β_0 and β_1, and thus require special methods for their solution. These methods are iterative in nature and have been programmed into available logistic regression software. McCullagh & Nelder [6] discuss the iterative methods used by most programs. In particular, they show that the solution to (6) and (7) may be obtained using a generalized weighted least squares procedure.

The value of β given by the solution to (6) and (7) is called the maximum likelihood estimate, denoted as $\hat{\beta}$. Similarly, $\hat{\pi}(x_i)$ is the maximum likelihood estimate of $\pi(x_i)$. This quantity provides an estimate of the conditional probability that Y is equal to 1, given that x is equal to x_i. As such, it represents the fitted or predicted value for the logistic regression model. An interesting consequence of (6) is that

$$\sum_{i=1}^{n} y_i = \sum_{i=1}^{n} \hat{\pi}(x_i).$$

That is, the sum of the observed values of y is equal to the sum of the predicted (expected) values.

After estimating the coefficients, it is standard practice to assess the significance of the variables in the model. This usually involves testing a statistical hypothesis to determine whether the independent variables in the model are "significantly" related to the outcome variable. One approach to testing for the significance of the coefficient of a variable in any model relates to the following question. *Does the model that includes the variable in question tell us more about the outcome (or response) variable than does a model that does not include that variable?* This question is answered by comparing the observed values of the response variable with those predicted by each of two models; the first with and the second without the variable in question. The mathematical function used to compare the observed and predicted values depends on the particular problem. If the predicted values with the variable in the model are better, or more accurate in some sense, than when the variable is not in the model, then we feel that the variable in question is "significant". It is important to note that we are not considering the question of whether the predicted values are an accurate representation of the observed values in an absolute sense (this would be called *goodness of fit*). Instead, our question is posed in a relative sense.

For the purposes of assessing the significance of an independent variable we compute the value of the following statistic:

$$G = -2 \ln \left(\frac{\text{likelihood without the variable}}{\text{likelihood with the variable}} \right). \quad (8)$$

Under the hypothesis that β_1 is equal to zero, the statistic G will follow a chi-square distribution with one degree of freedom. The calculation of the log likelihood and this generalized likelihood ratio test are standard features of any good logistic regression package. This makes it possible to check for the significance of the addition of new terms to the model as a matter of routine. In the simple case of a single independent variable, we can first fit a model containing only the constant term. We can then fit a model containing the independent variable along with

the constant. This gives rise to a new log likelihood. The likelihood ratio test is obtained by multiplying the difference between the log likelihoods of the two models by -2.

Another test that is often carried out is the Wald test, which is obtained by comparing the maximum likelihood estimate of the slope parameter, $\hat{\beta}_1$, with an estimate of its standard error. The resulting ratio

$$W = \frac{\hat{\beta}_1}{\widehat{se}(\hat{\beta}_1)},$$

under the hypothesis that $\beta_1 = 0$, follows a standard normal distribution. Standard errors of the estimated parameters are routinely printed out by computer software. Hauck & Donner [3] examined the performance of the Wald test and found that it behaved in an aberrant manner, often failing to reject when the coefficient was significant. They recommended that the likelihood ratio test be used. Jennings [5] has also looked at the adequacy of inferences in logistic regression based on Wald statistics. His conclusions are similar to those of Hauck & Donner.

Both the likelihood ratio test, G, and the Wald test, W, require the computation of the maximum likelihood estimate for β_1. For a single variable this is not a difficult or costly computational task. However, for large data sets with many variables, the iterative computation needed to obtain the maximum likelihood estimates can be considerable.

The logistic regression model may be used with matched study designs. Fitting **conditional logistic regression** models requires modifications, which are not discussed here. The reader interested in the conditional logistic regression model may find details in [4, Chapter 7].

The Multiple Logistic Regression Model

Consider a collection of p independent variables which will be denoted by the vector $\mathbf{x}' = (x_1, x_2, \ldots, x_p)$. Assume for the moment that each of these variables is at least interval scaled. Let the conditional probability that the outcome is present be denoted by $\Pr(Y = 1|\mathbf{x}) = \pi(\mathbf{x})$. Then the logit of the multiple logistic regression model is given by

$$g(\mathbf{x}) = \beta_0 + \beta_1 x_1 + \beta_2 x_2 + \cdots + \beta_p x_p, \quad (9)$$

in which case

$$\pi(x) = \frac{\exp[g(\mathbf{x})]}{1 + \exp[g(\mathbf{x})]}. \tag{10}$$

If some of the independent variables are discrete, nominal scaled variables such as race, sex, treatment group, and so forth, then it is inappropriate to include them in the model as if they were interval scaled. In this situation a collection of *design variables* should be used. Most logistic regression software will generate the design variables, and some programs have a choice of several different methods.

In general, if a nominal scaled variable has k possible values, then $k - 1$ design variables will be needed. Suppose, for example, that the jth independent variable, x_j has k_j levels. The $k_j - 1$ design variables will be denoted as D_{ju} and the coefficients for these design variables will be denoted as $\beta_{ju}, u = 1, 2, \ldots, k_j - 1$. Thus, the logit for a model with p variables and the jth variable being discrete is

$$g(\mathbf{x}) = \beta_0 + \beta_1 x_1 + \cdots + \sum_{u=1}^{k_j-1} \beta_{ju} D_{ju} + \beta_p x_p.$$

Fitting the Multiple Logistic Regression Model

Assume that we have a sample of n independent observations of the pair $(\mathbf{x}_i, y_i), i = 1, 2, \ldots, n$. As in the univariate case, fitting the model requires that we obtain estimates of the vector $\boldsymbol{\beta}' = (\beta_0, \beta_1, \ldots, \beta_p)$. The method of estimation used in the multivariate case is the same as in the univariate situation, i.e. maximum likelihood. The likelihood

function is nearly identical to that given in (4), with the only change being that $\pi(\mathbf{x})$ is now defined as in (10). There are $p + 1$ likelihood equations which are obtained by differentiating the log likelihood function with respect to the $p + 1$ coefficients. The likelihood equations that result may be expressed as follows:

$$\sum_{i=1}^{n} [y_i - \pi(\mathbf{x}_i)] = 0$$

and

$$\sum_{i=1}^{n} x_{ij} [y_i - \pi(\mathbf{x}_i)] = 0,$$

for $j = 1, 2, \ldots, p$.

As in the univariate model, the solution of the likelihood equations requires special purpose software which may be found in many packaged programs. Let $\hat{\beta}$ denote the solution to these equations. Thus, the fitted values for the multiple logistic regression model are $\hat{\pi}(\mathbf{x}_i)$, the value of the expression in (13) computed using $\hat{\beta}$ and $\mathbf{x}_i$.

Before proceeding further we present an example that illustrates the formulation of a multiple logistic regression model and the estimation of its coefficients.

Example

To provide an example of fitting a multiple logistic regression model, consider the data for the low birth weight study described in Appendix 1 of Hosmer & Lemeshow [4]. The code sheet for the data set is given in Table 1.

Table 1 Code sheet for the variables in the low birth weight data set

Variable	Abbreviation
Identification code	ID
Low birth weight (0 = birth weight $\geq$2500 g, 1 = birth weight <2500 g)	LOW
Age of the mother in years	AGE
Weight in pounds at the last menstrual period	LWT
Race (1 = white, 2 = black, 3 = other)	RACE
Smoking status during pregnancy (1 = yes, 0 = no)	SMOKE
History of premature labor (0 = none, 1 = one, etc.)	PTL
History of hypertension (1 = yes, 0 = no)	HT
Presence of uterine irritability (1 = yes, 0 = no)	UI
Number of physician visits first trimester visits during the first trimester (0 = none, 1 = one, 2 = two, etc.)	FTV
Birth weight (g)	BWT

Table 2 Coding of design variables for RACE

	Design variable	
RACE	RACE 1	RACE 2
White	0	0
Black	1	0
Other	0	1

The goal of this study was to identify risk factors associated with giving birth to a low birth weight baby (weighing less than 2500 g). In this study data were collected on 189 women; $n_1 = 59$ of them delivered low birth weight babies and $n_0 = 130$ delivered normal birth weight babies. In this example the variable race has been recoded using the two design variables shown in Table 2. FTV was recoded to $0 = $ some, $1 = $ none, and PTL was recoded to $0 = $ none, $1 = $ one or more. The two newly coded variables are called FTV01 and PTL01.

The results of fitting the logistic regression model to these data are given in Table 3.

In Table 3 the estimated coefficients for the two design variables for race are indicated in the lines denoted by "RACE 1" and "RACE 2". The estimated logit is given by

$$\hat{g}(\mathbf{x}) = 0.545 - 0.035 \times \text{AGE} - 0.015 \times \text{LWT}$$
$$+ 0.815 \times \text{SMOKE} + 1.824 \times \text{HT} + 0.702$$
$$\times \text{UI} + 1.202 \times \text{RACE 1} + 0.773 \times \text{RACE 2}$$
$$+ 0.121 \times \text{FTV01} + 1.237 \times \text{PTL01}.$$

The fitted values are obtained using the estimated logit, $\hat{g}(\mathbf{x})$, as in (10).

Testing for the Significance of the Model

Once we have fit a particular multiple (multivariate) logistic regression model, we begin the process of assessment of the model. The first step in this process is usually to assess the significance of the variables in the model. The likelihood ratio test for overall significance of the p coefficients for the independent variables in the model is performed based on the statistic G given in (8). The only difference is that the fitted values, $\hat{\pi}$, under the model are based on the vector containing $p + 1$ parameters, $\hat{\boldsymbol{\beta}}$. Under the null hypothesis that the p "slope" coefficients for the covariates in the model are equal to zero, the distribution of G is chi-square with p degrees of freedom.

As an example, consider the fitted model whose estimated coefficients are given in Table 3. For that model the value of the log likelihood is $L = -98.36$. A second model, fit with the constant term only, yields $L = -117.336$. Hence $G = -2[(-117.34) - (-98.36)] = 37.94$ and the P value for the test is $\Pr[\chi^2(9) > 37.94] < 0.0001$ (see Table 3). Rejection of the null hypothesis (that all of the coefficients are simultaneously equal to zero) has an interpretation analogous to that in multiple linear regression; we may conclude that at least one, and perhaps all p coefficients are different from zero.

Table 3 Estimated coefficients for a multiple logistic regression model using all variables from the low birth weight data set

Logit estimates Number of obs. = 189 $\chi^2(9) = 37.94$ Prob $> \chi^2 = 0.0000$

Log likelihood $= -98.36$

Variable	Coeff.	Std. error	z	$\Pr > |z|$	[95% conf. interval]	
AGE	−0.035	0.039	−0.920	0.357	−0.111	0.040
LWT	−0.015	0.007	−2.114	0.035	−0.029	−0.001
SMOKE	0.815	0.420	1.939	0.053	−0.009	1.639
HT	1.824	0.705	2.586	0.010	0.441	3.206
UI	0.702	0.465	1.511	0.131	−0.208	1.613
RACE 1	1.202	0.534	2.253	0.024	0.156	2.248
RACE 2	0.773	0.460	1.681	0.093	−0.128	1.674
FTV01	0.121	0.376	0.323	0.746	−0.615	0.858
PTL01	1.237	0.466	2.654	0.008	0.323	2.148
cons	0.545	1.266	0.430	0.667	−1.937	3.027

Before concluding that any or all of the coefficients are nonzero, we may wish to look at the univariate Wald test statistics, $W_j = \hat{\beta}_j / \widehat{se}(\hat{\beta}_j)$. These are given in the fourth column (labeled z) in Table 3. Under the hypothesis that an individual coefficient is zero, these statistics will follow the standard normal distribution. Thus, the value of these statistics may give us an indication of which of the variables in the model may or may not be significant. If we use a critical value of 2, which leads to an approximate level of significance (two-tailed) of 0.05, then we would conclude that the variables LWT, SMOKE, HT, PTL01 and possibly RACE are significant, while AGE, UI, and FTV01 are not significant.

Considering that the overall goal is to obtain the best fitting model while minimizing the number of parameters, the next logical step is to fit a reduced model, containing only those variables thought to be significant, and compare it with the full model containing all the variables. The results of fitting the reduced model are given in Table 4.

The difference between the two models is the exclusion of the variables AGE, UI, and FTV01 from the full model. The likelihood ratio test comparing these two models is obtained using the definition of G given in (8). It has a distribution that is chi-square with three degrees of freedom under the hypothesis that the coefficients for the variables excluded are equal to zero. The value of the test statistic comparing the models in Tables 3 and 4 is $G = -2[(-100.24) - (-98.36)] = 3.76$ which, with three degrees of freedom, has a P value of $P[\chi^2(3) > 3.76] = 0.2886$. Since the P value is large, exceeding 0.05, we conclude that the reduced model is as good as the full model. Thus there is no advantage to including AGE, UI, and FTV01 in the model. However, we must not base our models entirely on tests of statistical significance. Numerous other considerations should influence our decision to include or exclude variables from a model.

Interpretation of the Coefficients of the Logistic Regression Model

After fitting a model the emphasis shifts from the computation and assessment of significance of estimated coefficients to interpretation of their values. The interpretation of any fitted model requires that we can draw practical inferences from the estimated coefficients in the model. The question addressed is: *What do the estimated coefficients in the model tell us about the research questions that motivated the study?* For most models this involves the estimated coefficients for the independent variables in the model. The estimated coefficients for the independent variables represent the slope or rate of change of a function of the dependent variable per unit of change in the independent variable. Thus, interpretation involves two issues: (i) determining the functional relationship between the dependent variable and the independent variable, and (ii) appropriately defining the unit of change for the independent variable.

For a linear regression model we recall that the slope coefficient, β_1, is equal to the difference between the value of the dependent variable at $x + 1$ and the value of the dependent variable at x, for any value of x. In the logistic regression model $\beta_1 = g(x + 1) - g(x)$. That is, the slope coefficient

Table 4 Estimated coefficients for a multiple logistic regression model using the variables LWT, SMOKE, HT, PTL01 and RACE from the low birth weight data set

Logit estimates   Number of obs. = 189

$\chi^2(6) = 34.19$

Prob $> \chi^2 = 0.0000$

Log likelihood = 100.24

Variable	Coeff.	Std. error	z	Pr $> |z|$	[95% conf. interval]	
LWT	−0.017	0.007	−2.407	0.016	−0.030	−0.003
SMOKE	0.876	0.401	2.186	0.029	0.091	1.661
HT	1.767	0.708	2.495	0.013	0.379	3.156
RACE 1	1.264	0.529	2.387	0.017	0.226	2.301
RACE 2	0.864	0.435	1.986	0.047	0.011	1.717
PTL01	1.231	0.446	2.759	0.006	0.357	2.106
cons	0.095	0.957	0.099	0.921	−1.781	1.970

represents the change in the logit for a change of one unit in the independent variable x. Proper interpretation of the coefficient in a logistic regression model depends on being able to place meaning on the difference between two logits. Consider the interpretation of the coefficients for a univariate logistic regression model for each of the possible measurement scales of the independent variable.

Dichotomous Independent Variable

Assume that x is coded as either 0 or 1. Under this model there are two values of $\pi(x)$ and equivalently two values of $1 - \pi(x)$. These values may be conveniently displayed in a 2×2 table, as shown in Table 5.

The **odds** of the outcome being present among individuals with $x = 1$ is defined as $\pi(1)/[1 - \pi(1)]$. Similarly, the odds of the outcome being present among individuals with $x = 0$ is defined as $\pi(0)/[1 - \pi(0)]$. The **odds ratio**, denoted by ψ, is defined as the ratio of the odds for $x = 1$ to the odds for $x = 0$, and is given by

$$\psi = \frac{\pi(1)/[1 - \pi(1)]}{\pi(0)/[1 - \pi(0)]}. \tag{11}$$

The log of the odds ratio, termed log odds ratio, or *log odds*, is

$$\ln(\psi) = \ln\left\{\frac{\pi(1)/[1 - \pi(1)]}{\pi(0)/[1 - \pi(0)]}\right\} = g(1) - g(0),$$

which is the *logit difference*, where the log of the odds is called the logit and, in this example, these are

$$g(1) = \ln\{\pi(1)/[1 - \pi(1)]\}$$

and

$$g(0) = \ln\{\pi(0)/[1 - \pi(0)]\}.$$

Using the expressions for the logistic regression model shown in Table 5 the odds ratio is

$$\psi = \frac{\left(\dfrac{\exp(\beta_0 + \beta_1)}{1 + \exp(\beta_0 + \beta_1)}\right)\left(\dfrac{1}{1 + \exp(\beta_0)}\right)}{\left(\dfrac{\exp(\beta_0)}{1 + \exp(\beta_0)}\right)\left(\dfrac{1}{1 + \exp(\beta_0 + \beta_1)}\right)}$$

$$= \frac{\exp(\beta_0 + \beta_1)}{\exp(\beta_0)} = \exp(\beta_1).$$

Hence, for logistic regression with a dichotomous independent variable

$$\psi = \exp(\beta_1), \tag{12}$$

and the logit difference, or log odds, is

$$\ln(\psi) = \ln[\exp(\beta_1)] = \beta_1.$$

This fact concerning the interpretability of the coefficients is the fundamental reason why logistic regression has proven such a powerful analytic tool for epidemiologic research. A confidence interval (CI) estimate for the odds ratio is obtained by first calculating the endpoints of a confidence interval for the coefficient β_1, and then exponentiating these values. In general, the endpoints are given by

$$\exp\left[\hat{\beta}_1 \pm z_{1-\alpha/2} \times \widehat{se}(\hat{\beta}_1)\right].$$

Because of the importance of the odds ratio as a measure of association, point and interval estimates are often found in additional columns in tables presenting the results of a logistic regression analysis.

Table 5 Values of the logistic regression model when the independent variable is dichotomous

		Independent variable X	
		$x = 1$	$x = 0$
Outcome variable Y	$y = 1$	$\pi(1) = \dfrac{\exp(\beta_0 + \beta_1)}{1 + \exp(\beta_0 + \beta_1)}$	$\pi(0) = \dfrac{\exp \beta_0}{1 + \exp \beta_0}$
	$y = 0$	$1 - \pi(1) = \dfrac{1}{1 + \exp(\beta_0 + \beta_1)}$	$1 - \pi(0) = \dfrac{1}{1 + \exp \beta_0}$
	Total	1.0	1.0

Table 6 Cross-classification of hypothetical data on RACE and CHD status for 100 subjects

CHD status	White	Black	Hispanic	Other	Total
Present	5	20	15	10	50
Absent	20	10	10	10	50
Total	25	30	25	20	100
Odds ratio ($\hat{\psi}$)	1.0	8.0	6.0	4.0	
95% CI		(2.3, 27.6)	(1.7, 21.3)	(1.1, 14.9)	
$\ln(\hat{\psi})$	0.0	2.08	1.79	1.39	

In the previous discussion we noted that the estimate of the odds ratio was $\hat{\psi} = \exp(\hat{\beta}_1)$. This is correct when the independent variable has been coded as 0 or 1. This type of coding is called "reference cell" coding. Other coding could be used. For example, the variable may be coded as -1 or $+1$. This type of coding is termed "deviation from means" coding. Evaluation of the logit difference shows that the odds ratio is calculated as $\hat{\psi} = \exp(2\hat{\beta}_1)$ and if an investigator were simply to exponentiate the coefficient from the computer output of a logistic regression analysis, the wrong estimate of the odds ratio would be obtained. Close attention should be paid to the method used to code design variables.

The method of coding also influences the calculation of the endpoints of the confidence interval. With deviation from means coding, the estimated standard error needed for confidence interval estimation is $\hat{se}(2\hat{\beta}_1)$, which is $2 \times \hat{se}(\hat{\beta}_1)$. Thus the endpoints of the confidence interval are

$$\exp\left[2\hat{\beta}_1 + z_{1-\alpha/2} \times 2 \times \hat{se}(\hat{\beta}_1)\right].$$

In summary, for a dichotomous variable the parameter of interest is the odds ratio. An estimate of this parameter may be obtained from the estimated logistic regression coefficient, regardless of how the variable is coded or scaled. This relationship between the logistic regression coefficient and the odds ratio provides the foundation for our interpretation of all logistic regression results.

Polytomous Independent Variable

Suppose that instead of two categories the independent variable has $k > 2$ distinct values. For example, we may have variables that denote the county of residence within a state, the clinic used for primary health care within a city, or race. Each of these variables has a fixed number of discrete outcomes and the scale of measurement is nominal.

Suppose that in a study of coronary heart disease (CHD) the variable RACE is coded at four levels, and that the cross-classification of RACE by CHD status yields the data presented in Table 6. These data are hypothetical and have been formulated for ease of computation. The extension to a situation where the variable has more than four levels is not conceptually different, so all the examples in this section use $k = 4$.

At the bottom of Table 6 the odds ratio is given for each race, using white as the reference group. For example, for hispanic the estimated odds ratio is $(15 \times 20)/(5 \times 10) = 6.0$. The log of the odds ratios are given in the last row of Table 6. This display is typical of what is found in the literature when there is a perceived referent group to which the other groups are to be compared. These same estimates of the odds ratio may be obtained from a logistic regression program with an appropriate choice of design variables. The method for specifying the design variables involves setting all of them equal to zero for the reference group, and then setting a single design variable equal to one for each of the other groups. This is illustrated in Table 7.

Use of any logistic regression program with design variables coded as shown in Table 7 yields the

Table 7 Specification of the design variables for RACE using white as the reference group

| RACE (code) | Design variables | | |
	D_1	D_2	D_3
White (1)	0	0	0
Black (2)	1	0	0
Hispanic (3)	0	1	0
Other (4)	0	0	1

Table 8 Results of fitting the logistic regression model to the data in Table 6 using the design variables in Table 7

Variable	Coeff.	Std. error	z	$P > |z|$	[95% conf. interval]	
RACE 1	2.079	0.632	3.288	0.001	0.840	3.319
RACE 2	1.792	0.645	2.776	0.006	0.527	3.057
RACE 3	1.386	0.671	2.067	0.039	0.072	2.701
cons	−1.386	0.500	−2.773	0.006	−2.367	−0.406

Variable	Odds ratio	[95% conf. interval]	
RACE 1	8	2.32	27.63
RACE 2	6	1.69	21.26
RACE 3	4	1.07	14.90

estimated logistic regression coefficients given in Table 8.

A comparison of the estimated coefficients in Table 8 with the log odds in Table 6 shows that $\ln[\hat{\psi}(\text{black, white})] = \hat{\beta}_{11} = 2.079$, $\ln[\hat{\psi}(\text{hispanic, white})] = \hat{\beta}_{12} = 1.792$, and $\ln[\hat{\psi}(\text{other, white})] = \hat{\beta}_{13} = 1.386$.

In the univariate case the estimates of the standard errors found in the logistic regression output are identical to the estimates obtained using the cell frequencies from the contingency table. For example, the estimated standard error of the estimated coefficient for design variable (1), $\hat{\beta}_{11}$, is $0.6325 = (1/5 + 1/20 + 1/20 + 1/10)^{1/2}$. A derivation of this result appears in Bishop et al. [1].

Confidence limits for odds ratios may be obtained as follows:

$$\hat{\beta}_{ij} \pm z_{1-\alpha/2} \times \widehat{se}(\hat{\beta}_{ij}).$$

The corresponding limits for the odds ratio are obtained by exponentiating these limits as follows:

$$\exp[\hat{\beta}_{ij} \pm z_{1-\alpha/2} \times \widehat{se}(\hat{\beta}_{ij})].$$

Continuous Independent Variable

When a logistic regression model contains a continuous independent variable, interpretation of the estimated coefficient depends on how it is entered into the model and the particular units of the variable. For purposes of developing the method to interpret the coefficient for a continuous variable, we assume that the logit is linear in the variable.

Under the assumption that the logit is linear in the continuous covariate, x, the equation for the logit is $g(x) = \beta_0 + \beta_1 x$. It follows that the slope coefficient, β_1, gives the change in the log odds for an increase of "1" unit in x, i.e. $\beta_1 = g(x + 1) - g(x)$ for any value of x. Most often the value of "1" will not be biologically very interesting. For example, an increase of 1 year in age or of 1 mmHg in systolic blood pressure may be too small to be considered important. A change of 10 years or 10 mmHg might be considered more useful. However, if the range of x is from zero to one, as might be the case for some created index, then a change of 1 is too large and a change of 0.01 may be more realistic. Hence, to provide a useful interpretation for continuous scaled covariates we need to develop a method for point and interval estimation for an arbitrary change of c units in the covariate.

The log odds for a change of c units in x is obtained from the logit difference $g(x + c) - g(x) = c\beta_1$ and the associated odds ratio is obtained by exponentiating this logit difference, $\psi(c) = \psi(x + c, x) = \exp(c\beta_1)$. An estimate may be obtained by replacing β_1 with its maximum likelihood estimate, $\hat{\beta}_1$. An estimate of the standard error needed for confidence interval estimation is obtained by multiplying the estimated standard error of $\hat{\beta}_1$ by c. Hence the endpoints of the $100(1 - \alpha)\%$ CI estimate of $\psi(c)$ are

$$\exp[c\hat{\beta}_1 \pm z_{1-\alpha/2}c\widehat{se}(\hat{\beta}_1)].$$

Since both the point estimate and endpoints of the confidence interval depend on the choice of c, the particular value of c should be clearly specified in all tables and calculations.

Multivariate Case

Often logistic regression analysis is used to *adjust statistically* the estimated effects of each variable in the model for differences in the distributions of and associations among the other independent variables. Applying this concept to a multiple logistic regression model, we may surmise that each estimated coefficient provides an estimate of the log odds adjusting for all other variables included in the model. The term confounder is used by epidemiologists to describe a covariate that is associated with both the outcome variable of interest and a primary independent variable or risk factor. When both associations are present the relationship between the risk factor and the outcome variable is said to be *confounded* (*see* **Confounding**). The procedure for adjusting for confounding is appropriate when there is no interaction.

If the association between the covariate and an outcome variable is the same within each level of the risk factor, then there is no interaction between the covariate and the risk factor. When interaction is present, the association between the risk factor and the outcome variable differs, or depends in some way on the level of the covariate. That is, the covariate modifies the effect of the risk factor (*see* **Effect Modification**). Epidemiologists use the term effect modifier to describe a variable that interacts with a risk factor.

The simplest and most commonly used model for including interaction is one in which the logit is also linear in the confounder for the second group, but with a different slope. Alternative models can be formulated which would allow for other than a linear relationship between the logit and the variables in the model within each group. In any model, interaction is incorporated by the inclusion of appropriate higher order terms.

An important step in the process of modeling a set of data is to determine whether or not there is evidence of interaction in the data. Tables 9 and 10 present the results of fitting a series of logistic regression models to two different sets of hypothetical data. The variables in each of the data sets are the same: SEX, AGE, and CHD. In addition to the estimated coefficients, the log likelihood for each model and minus twice the change (deviance) is given. Recall that minus twice the change in the log likelihood may be used to test for the significance of coefficients for variables added to the model. An interaction is added to the model by creating a variable that is equal to the product of the value of the sex and the value of age.

Examining the results in Table 9 we see that the estimated coefficient for the variable SEX changed from 1.535 in model 1 to 0.979 when AGE was added in model 2. Hence, there is clear evidence of a confounding effect owing to age. When the interaction term "SEX × AGE" is added in model 3 we see that the change in the deviance is only 0.52 which, when compared with the chi-square distribution with one degree of freedom, yields a P value of 0.47, which clearly is not significant. Note that the coefficient for sex changed from 0.979 to 0.481. This is not surprising since the inclusion of an interaction term, especially when it involves a continuous variable, will usually produce fairly marked changes in the estimated coefficients of dichotomous variables involved in the interaction. Thus, when an interaction

Table 9 Estimated logistic regression coefficients, log likelihood, and the likelihood ratio test statistic (G) for an example showing evidence of confounding but no interaction

Model	Constant	SEX	AGE	SEX × AGE	Log likelihood	G
1	−1.046	1.535			−61.86	
2	−7.142	0.979	0.167		−49.59	24.54
3	−6.103	0.481	0.139	0.059	−49.33	0.52

Table 10 Estimated logistic regression coefficients, log likelihood, and the likelihood ratio test statistic (G) for an example showing evidence of confounding and interaction

Model	Constant	SEX	AGE	SEX × AGE	Log likelihood	G
1	−0.847	2.505			−52.52	
2	−6.194	1.734	0.147		−46.79	11.46
3	−3.105	0.047	0.629	0.206	−44.76	4.06

term is present in the model we cannot assess confounding via the change in a coefficient. For these data we would prefer to use model 2 which suggests that age is a confounder but not an effect modifier.

The results in Table 10 show evidence of both confounding and interaction due to age. Comparing model 1 with model 2 we see that the coefficient for sex changes from 2.505 to 1.734. When the age by sex interaction is added to the model we see that the deviance is 4.06, which yields a P value of 0.04. Since the deviance is significant, we prefer model 3 over model 2, and should regard age as both a confounder and an effect modifier. The net result is that any estimate of the odds ratio for sex should be made with respect to a specific age.

Hence, we see that determining if a covariate, X, is an effect modifier and/or a confounder involves several issues. Determining effect modification status involves the parametric structure of the logit, while determination of confounder status involves two things. First, the covariate must be associated with the outcome variable. This implies that the logit must have a nonzero slope in the covariate. Secondly, the covariate must be associated with the risk factor. In our example this might be characterized by having a difference in the mean age for males and females. However, the association may be more complex than a simple difference in means. The essence is that we have incomparability in our risk factor groups. This incomparability must be accounted for in the model if we are to obtain a correct, unconfounded estimate of effect for the risk factor.

In practice, the confounder status of a covariate is ascertained by comparing the estimated coefficient for the risk factor variable from models containing and not containing the covariate. Any "biologically important" change in the estimated coefficient for the risk factor would dictate that the covariate is a confounder and should be included in the model, regardless of the statistical significance of the estimated coefficient for the covariate. On the other hand, a covariate is an effect modifier only when the interaction term added to the model is both biologically meaningful and statistically significant. When a covariate is an effect modifier, its status as a confounder is of secondary importance since the estimate of the effect of the risk factor depends on the specific value of the covariate.

The concepts of adjustment, confounding, interaction, and effect modification may be extended to cover the situations involving any number of variables on any measurement scale(s). The principles for identification and inclusion of confounder and interaction variables into the model are the same regardless of the number of variables and their measurement scales.

Much of this article has been abstracted from [4]. Readers wanting more detail on any topic should consult this reference.

References

[1] Bishop, Y.M.M., Fienberg, S.E. & Holland, P. (1975). *Discrete Multivariate Analysis: Theory and Practice.* MIT Press, Boston.
[2] Cox, D.R. & Snell, E.J. (1989). *The Analysis of Binary Data*, 2nd Ed. Chapman & Hall, London.
[3] Hauck, W.W. & Donner, A. (1977). Wald's Test as applied to hypotheses in logit analysis, *Journal of the American Statistical Association* **72**, 851–853.
[4] Hosmer, D. & Lemeshow, S. (1989). *Applied Logistic Regression*. Wiley, New York.
[5] Jennings, D.E. (1986). Judging inference adequacy in logistic regression, *Journal of the American Statistical Association* **81**, 471–476.
[6] McCullagh, P. & Nelder, J.A. (1983). *Generalized Linear Models*. Chapman & Hall, London.

STANLEY LEMESHOW &
DAVID W. HOSMER, JR

Logistic Regression, Conditional

An important extension of the **logistic regression** model is the analysis of data from stratified samples (*see* **Stratification**). Examples of this application include studies where data are collected from several different sites such as schools, hospitals, or clinics as well as analyses where covariates are controlled for by defining *post hoc* stratification variables. The most frequently encountered stratified study design employing the logistic regression model is the matched **case–control study** used in epidemiology (*see* **Matched Analysis**). A discussion of the rationale for these matched studies may be found in epidemiology texts such as Breslow & Day [1], Kleinbaum et al. [5], Schlesselman [8], Kelsey et al. [4], and Rothman [7].

The basic idea is to expand the logistic model by inclusion of stratification variables. Assume the sampled data may be represented as a triple $(y_{kj}, \mathbf{x}_{kj}, \mathbf{z}_k)$, where $j = 1, 2, \ldots, n_k$ represents the particular subject observed within stratum $k = 1, 2, \ldots, K$, $y_{kj} = 0$ or 1 is the observed value of the binary outcome variable for subject j in stratum k, $\mathbf{x}'_{kj} = (x_{kj1}, x_{kj2}, \ldots, x_{kjp})$ is a vector of p nonconstant covariates, and $\mathbf{z}'_k = (z_{k1}, z_{k2}, \ldots, z_{kq})$ is a vector of q covariates defining stratum characteristics. The quantity n_k denotes the number of observations in stratum k. The vector $\mathbf{z}$ may simply contain one variable to indicate the stratum, $z_k = k$, or a set of values of q covariates may be used to define strata. For example, if one defined strata by gender and race coded at three levels, then $\mathbf{z}'_k = (z_{k1}, z_{k2})$ with $z_{k1} = 0$ or 1, $z_{k2} = 1, 2,$ or 3, and $k = 1, 2, \ldots, 6$.

A number of different stratified logistic regression models are possible. The simplest logistic regression model has a logit function with one design variable for the stratum specific effect and constant slope across strata for the covariates, namely

$$g(\mathbf{x}_{kj}, z_k) = \beta_0 + \alpha_k + \boldsymbol{\beta}'\mathbf{x}_{kj}. \tag{1}$$

The logit function is discussed in detail in the article on **Logistic Regression**. It is defined in terms of the model conditional probability as $g(\mathbf{x}_{kj}, z_k) = \ln\{\pi(\mathbf{x}_{kj}, z_k)/[1 - \pi(\mathbf{x}_{kj}, z_k)]\}$ and $\pi(\mathbf{x}_{kj}, z_k) = \Pr(Y_{kj} = 1|\mathbf{x}_{kj}, z_k)$. In the parameterization in (1) one may think of the values of α_k as the coefficients for design variables generated by the K levels of the stratum variable. These design variables may be created using any method but the most frequent choice is either referent cell or deviation from means coding. There are $K - 1$ parameters or degrees of freedom associated with the stratification variable. The model in (1) has a stratum-specific intercept and constant slopes. Thus the effect of the covariates is the same for all strata. The covariate vector, $\mathbf{x}$, may contain both main effects as well as higher-order terms such as interactions and squared terms, but may not contain terms that indicate the stratum.

An extension of the model in (1) is possible when the vector $\mathbf{z}$ contains covariates that measure stratum characteristics, e.g. gender and race as noted above. The vector may also contain continuous covariates. Age is often used as a stratification variable. In this setting one may add interactions to (1), which yield a model with stratum-specific slopes. Suppose strata are defined by gender and $z_k = 0$ or $1(1 = \text{male})$ records

the gender of the subject. The logit for an extended model is

$$g(\mathbf{x}_{kj}, z_k) = \beta_0 + \alpha_k z_k + \boldsymbol{\beta}'\mathbf{x}_{kj} + z_k \times \boldsymbol{\gamma}'\mathbf{x}_{kj}. \tag{2}$$

The model for females is

$$g(\mathbf{x}_{kj}, z_k = 0) = \beta_0 + \boldsymbol{\beta}'\mathbf{x}_{kj},$$

and the model for males is

$$g(\mathbf{x}_{kj}, z_k = 1) = \beta_0 + \alpha_1 + (\boldsymbol{\beta} + \boldsymbol{\gamma})'\mathbf{x}_{kj}.$$

The model in (2) allows for stratum-specific intercepts as well as stratum-specific slopes. Maximum likelihood estimators of the parameters in (1) or (2) are obtained by extending the likelihood function (*see* **Logistic Regression**) to include a product over strata. The likelihood function for the model in (1) is

$$l(\alpha, \beta,) = \prod_{k=1}^{K} \prod_{j=1}^{n_k} \zeta(\mathbf{x}_{kj}, z_k), \tag{3}$$

where $\zeta(\mathbf{x}_{kj}, z_k) = \pi(\mathbf{x}_{kj}, z_k)^{y_{kj}}[1 - \pi(\mathbf{x}_{kj}, z_k)]^{1-y_{kj}}$. Application of the likelihood function in (3) to the model in (2) is accomplished by adding the requisite additional terms to the logit. Estimators of the parameters may be obtained from logistic regression software (*see* **Software, Biostatistical**) by inclusion of the variables recording stratum-specific data into the model.

Thus the model as shown in (1) or (2) does not represent anything particularly new or difficult for the investigator familiar with the logistic regression model. The model-building issues and details are identical to those of the ordinary logistic model, or for that matter any regression model.

Problems begin to arise which require a different approach when the number of strata becomes large and, at the same time, the number of observations within each stratum remains fixed. Application of the logistic regression model to this setting will be described in the remainder of this article.

Logistic Regression with Highly Stratified Data

A convenient setting to illustrate the use of logistic regression with highly stratified data is the matched case–control study design. In this study design subjects are stratified on the basis of covariates believed to be associated with the outcome. Age and gender are examples of commonly used stratification variables. Within each stratum a sample of subjects with the outcome present, called cases ($y = 1$), and a sample of subjects without the outcome, called controls ($y = 0$), is chosen. The number of cases and controls need not be constant across strata, but the most common matched design is one where each stratum includes one case and one control. Study variables are collected on all subjects. We develop the methods for analysis of highly stratified data for the general case. Greater detail is provided for the one-to-one matched design because it can be analyzed using standard logistic regression software.

The methods to be described may be used in settings other than matched case–control studies. For example, suppose that, in a study of student performance, data were collected from 1000 different schools and a fixed number of students was selected from each school. The outcome variable is whether the student "passed" a particular course or standardized test. In this example there are 1000 strata defined by school. The conditional likelihood approach described below is the same for both the case–control study and the general highly stratified design. More stringent sampling assumptions are required in the case–control study, see [3, Chapter 6].

We begin by providing some motivation for the need for special methods for the highly stratified study. We noted in (1) that we could handle the stratified sample by including variables created from the stratification variables in the model. This approach works well when the number of subjects in each stratum is large and strata are few. However, matched studies have few subjects per stratum. For example, in the one-to-one matched design with K case–control pairs we have only two subjects per stratum. A fully stratified analysis of the model in (1) with p covariates would require estimation of $(K + p)$ parameters, the $p + 1$ slope coefficients for the covariates, and the $K - 1$ coefficients for the stratum-specific design variables, using a sample of size $2K$. The optimality properties of the method of maximum likelihood, derived by letting the sample size, K, become large, hold only when the number of parameters remains fixed. In any matched study this is not the case, as the number of parameters increases at the same rate as the sample size. For example, when analyzing a matched one-to-one design via the fully stratified likelihood in (3) using a logistic regression model containing one dichotomous covariate and the $K - 1$ design variables

for strata, it can be shown (see [1, p. 250]) that the bias in the estimate of the coefficient is 100%. If we regard the stratum-specific parameters as (nuisance) parameters whose values are neither of great interest to us nor are essential for the inferences required in the study, and we are willing to forgo their estimation, then we can create a conditional likelihood which will yield maximum likelihood estimators of the slope coefficients in the logistic regression model that are consistent and asymptotically normally distributed. The mathematical details of conditional likelihood analysis may be found in [2]. We summarize its application to the matched design. Liang [6], in related work, considers a general approach to the analysis of highly stratified data.

The Conditional Logistic Regression Model

Suppose that there are K strata with n_{k1} cases (subjects with $y = 1$) and n_{k0} controls (subjects with $y = 0$) in stratum k, $k = 1, 2, \ldots, K$. The conditional likelihood for the kth stratum is obtained as the probability of the observed data conditional on the stratum total sample size (fixed by the sampling design) and the total number of cases, the sufficient statistic for the stratum-specific nuisance parameter. This probability is the ratio of the probability of the observed outcome to the probability for all possible assignments of n_{k1} subjects with $y = 1$ and n_{k0} subjects with $y = 0$ to $n_k = n_{k0} + n_{k1}$ subjects. The number of possible assignments is the n_k choose n_{k1} combinations. Let the subscript j denote any one of these assignments. For any assignment we let subjects 1 to n_{k1} correspond to the subjects with $y = 1$ and subjects $n_{k1} + 1$ to n_k to the subjects with $y = 0$. This will be indexed by i for the observed data and by i_j for the jth possible assignment. The contribution to the conditional likelihood for the kth stratum is

$$l_k(\boldsymbol{\beta})$$
$$= \frac{\prod_{i=1}^{n_{k1}} \Pr(y_{ki} = 1|\mathbf{x}_{ki}) \prod_{i=n_{k1}+1}^{n_k} \Pr(y_{ki} = 0|\mathbf{x}_{ki})}{\sum_j \left[\prod_{i_j=1}^{n_{k1}} \Pr(y_{ki_j} = 1|\mathbf{x}_{ki_j}) \times \prod_{i_j=n_{k1}+1}^{n_k} \Pr(y_{ki_j} = 0|\mathbf{x}_{ki_j}) \right]}, \quad (4)$$

where the summation over j in the denominator is over the n_k choose n_{k1} combinations. The full conditional likelihood is the product of the $l_k(\boldsymbol{\beta})$ over the K strata,

$$l(\boldsymbol{\beta}) = \prod_{k=1}^{K} l_k(\boldsymbol{\beta}). \tag{5}$$

If we substitute the logistic regression model with the logit defined in (1), $\pi(\mathbf{x}_{ki}) = \Pr(y_{ki} = 1 | \mathbf{x}_{ki})$, into (4), then (5) simplifies to

$$l_k(\boldsymbol{\beta}) = \frac{\displaystyle\prod_{i=1}^{n_{k1}} \pi(\mathbf{x}_{ki}) \prod_{i=n_{k1}+1}^{n_k} [1 - \pi(\mathbf{x}_{ki})]}{\displaystyle\sum_j \left\{ \prod_{i_j=1}^{n_{k1}} \pi(\mathbf{x}_{ki_j}) \prod_{i_j=n_{k1}+1}^{n_k} [1 - \pi(\mathbf{x}_{ki_j})] \right\}}. \tag{6}$$

Since the terms of the form $\exp(\beta_0 + \alpha_k)/[1 + \exp(\beta_0 + \alpha_k + \mathbf{x}'_{ki}\boldsymbol{\beta})]$ appear equally in both the numerator and denominator of (6) they cancel out, and (6) simplifies to

$$l_k(\boldsymbol{\beta}) = \frac{\displaystyle\prod_{i=1}^{n_{k1}} \exp(\boldsymbol{\beta}'\mathbf{x}_{ki})}{\displaystyle\sum_j \left(\prod_{i_j=1}^{n_{k1}} \exp(\boldsymbol{\beta}'\mathbf{x}_{ki_j}) \right)}, \tag{7}$$

which depends only on the unknown parameter vector $\boldsymbol{\beta}$. The conditional maximum likelihood estimator for $\boldsymbol{\beta}$ is that value which maximizes (5) when the expression in (7) is used for $l_k(\boldsymbol{\beta})$. Most software packages performing logistic regression have the capability to fit this conditional logistic regression model (*see* **Software, Biostatistical**).

The argument leading to expression (7) is more complicated for a case–control study and requires assumptions about sampling of cases and controls and applications of Bayes' theorem. The details will not be presented here but may be found in [3, Chapters 6 and 7].

One must always keep in mind when using the conditional likelihood in (7) that it was obtained by beginning with the usual logistic regression model. Thus, one still interprets the coefficients as "log-odds ratios". The original logistic regression model (1) or (2) tends to become lost in the arithmetic process of re-expressing the likelihood in (7). This point can be

especially confusing to those analyzing data from a one-to-one matched case–control study.

The one-to-one matched design is probably the most frequent example of the use of a conditional logistic regression model. We show how one may analyze this design using standard logistic regression software, since not all packages have the capability to perform conditional logistic regression. More general software must be used in other matched designs and in the general highly stratified setting.

Logistic Regression Analysis for the One-to-One Matched Study

In the one-to-one matched study there are two subjects within each stratum. To simplify the notation, let $\mathbf{x}_{k1}$ denote the covariate vector for the case and $\mathbf{x}_{k0}$ the covariate vector for the control in the kth stratum. Using this notation, the conditional likelihood, (7), for the kth stratum is

$$l_k(\beta) = \frac{\exp(\boldsymbol{\beta}'\mathbf{x}_{k1})}{\exp(\boldsymbol{\beta}'\mathbf{x}_{k1}) + \exp(\boldsymbol{\beta}'\mathbf{x}_{k0})}. \tag{8}$$

Further simplification is obtained by dividing the numerator and denominator of (8) by $\exp(\boldsymbol{\beta}'\mathbf{x}_{k0})$, yielding

$$l_k(\beta) = \frac{\exp[\boldsymbol{\beta}'(\mathbf{x}_{k1} - \mathbf{x}_{k0})]}{1 + \exp[\boldsymbol{\beta}'(\mathbf{x}_{k1} - \mathbf{x}_{k0})]}. \tag{9}$$

The expression on the right-hand side of (9) is identical to a logistic regression model with the constant term set equal to zero, $\beta_0 = 0$, and covariate vector equal to the value of the case minus the value of the control, $\mathbf{x}_k^* = \mathbf{x}_{k1} - \mathbf{x}_{k0}$. This algebraic simplification allows one to use standard logistic regression software to compute the conditional maximum likelihood estimators of the coefficients and their standard errors. To accomplish this, one performs the following data modifications: define the sample size as the number of case–control pairs, compute the difference vector $\mathbf{x}_k^*$, compute a *pseudo*-response variable equal to 1, $y_k^* = 1$, and exclude the constant term from the model, e.g. force its value to be equal to zero. Thus, from a computational point of view, the one-to-one matched design presents no new challenges.

We have found that in the process of creating the differences and setting the "outcome" equal to

1, one can lose sight of the model. It is important to distinguish between the logistic regression model being fit to the data and the computational manipulations required to fit this model with standard logistic regression software. The process is less confusing if one focuses on the logistic regression model first and then considers the computations needed to obtain the parameter estimates. A few examples should help to illustrate this point.

Suppose we have a dichotomous independent variable coded zero or one. This variable is correctly modeled via a single coefficient in the logit, irrespective of whether we enter the variable via a design variable or treat it as continuous. The difference variable which we obtain by subtracting the value of the case from that of the control may take on one of three possible values: $(-1, 0$ or $1)$. If we had mistakenly thought of the difference variable as being the actual data, then we would have incorrectly modeled the variable by including two design variables in the model. The correct method is to create a difference variable and treat it as if it were continuous.

As a second example, suppose we have a variable such as race, coded at three levels. To model this variable correctly in the one-to-one matched design, we create, for each case and control in a pair, the values of the two design variables representing race. We compute the difference between these two design variables for the case and control and model each of these differences as if it were continuous. The same process is followed for any categorical scaled covariate. Note that the computer software may not recognize the differences in design variables as being created from the same variable, so one has to be sure that all design variables are included in the model. Another point to keep in mind is that differences between variables used to form strata are equal to zero for all strata and thus will not be useful as main effects. However, one may include interaction terms between stratification variables and other covariates, because differences in these interaction variables will likely not be zero.

In summary, the conceptual process for modeling matched or highly stratified data is identical to that of the usual logistic regression model. If one develops the modeling strategy for highly stratified data as if one had unstratified data, and then uses the conditional likelihood, then one will always be proceeding correctly.

Examples of the Use of the Conditional Logistic Regression Model

For illustrative purposes we use a small one-to-one matched data set obtained from a study of factors associated with the birth of a low birthweight baby (less than 2500 g). These data are in [3, Appendix 3]. These data, as well as the other data sets used in [3], may be obtained in the logistic regression menu at internet address http://www-unix.oit.umass.edu/~statdata. A one-to-one matched data set was obtained from an unmatched study of 189 births of which 59 were low weight. The matched data were obtained by randomly selecting, for each woman who gave birth to a low birthweight baby, a mother of the same age who did not give birth to a low birthweight baby. For three of the young mothers (age less than 17) it was not possible to identify a match since there were no mothers of normal weight babies of that age. The data consist of 56 age-matched case–control pairs. Variables selected for use in this example are a prior pre-term delivery (PTD, $1 =$ yes, $0 =$ no), smoking status (during pregnancy) of the mother (SMOKE, $1 =$ yes, $0 =$ no), history of hypertension (HT, $1 =$ yes, $0 =$ no), presence of uterine irritability (UI, $1 =$ yes, $0 =$ no), and the weight of the mother at the last menstrual period (LWT, pounds).

In ordinary logistic regression the coefficient for a model containing only one dichotomous variable is equal to the log of the cross-product ratio (odds ratio) from the two-by-two table of outcome by the dichotomous variable. The same result is true when the conditional logistic model is used with a one-to-one matched study and the model contains a single dichotomous variable. The estimator of the odds ratio in a one-to-one matched study is the ratio of the frequencies of the discordant pairs. These are the frequencies in the off main diagonal cells of a 2×2 table cross-classifying the dichotomous variable for the case by the control. For example, consider the smoking status of the mother. The 2×2 table is shown in Table 1 and the results from fitting the conditional logistic regression model containing this variable are shown in Table 2. The odds ratio computed from Table 1 is $\hat{\psi} = 22/8 = 2.75$ and its log is $\ln \hat{\psi} = 1.012$. The results presented in Table 2 show that the coefficient for smoke is identically equal to the log of the odds ratio from Table 1. A confidence interval (CI) for the odds

Table 1 Cross-classification of the smoking status of the case by the control

Case	Control		Total
	No	Yes	
No	18	8	26
Yes	22	8	30
Total	40	16	56

Table 2 Results from fitting a conditional logistic regression model containing the dichotomous variable, smoking status of the mother

Variable	Coeff.	Std. error	z	P	95% CI
SMOKE	1.012	0.413	2.45	0.014	(0.202, 1.821)

ratio may be obtained by exponentiating the end points of the CI for the coefficient shown in Table 2. The resulting interval is (1.22, 6.18) indicating that, in these data, smoking during pregnancy is a risk factor for giving birth to a low birthweight baby. The significance of the coefficient may be tested using the Wald statistic, labeled as z in Table 2, and whose two-tailed P value is 0.014. The appropriateness of both the CI and test depend on an assumption that the sample size, 56 in this case, is large enough to employ the large-sample distributional properties (normality) of maximum likelihood estimators.

If one did not have available software specifically to perform conditional logistic regression, then the previously described method of creating difference variables could be used before beginning full-scale modeling of the data. This technique is not as important as it once was as most of the commonly available packages either have specific conditional logistic regression routines, or methods for adapting other routines are explained in their manuals. Again we wish to reinforce the point that the method of creating difference variables will only work for the one-to-one matched study. Any other design must be modeled through specific conditional logistic regression software.

We present in Table 3 the results of fitting a more complex model. The purpose of this model is to illustrate the use and interpretation of results from a multivariable conditional logistic regression model. See [3, Chapter 7] for a discussion of the issues involved in

Table 3 Results from fitting a conditional logistic regression model containing prior PTD, SMOKE, HT, UI, and LWT to 56 matched pairs

Variable	Coeff.	Std. error	z	P	95% CI
PTD	1.671	0.747	2.24	0.025	(0.207, 3.135)
SMOKE	1.480	0.562	2.63	0.009	(0.378, 2.582)
HT	2.330	1.003	2.32	0.020	(0.364, 4.296)
UI	1.345	0.694	1.94	0.052	(−0.015, 2.705)
LWT	−0.015	0.008	−1.88	0.060	(−0.031, 0.001)

Table 4 Estimated odds ratios and 95% CIs for prior PTDs, SMOKE, HT, UI, and LWT (10 lb increase)

Variable	Odds ratio	95% CI
PTD	5.32	(1.23, 22.99)
SMOKE	4.39	(1.46, 13.22)
HT	10.28	(1.44, 73.41)
UI	3.84	(0.99, 14.95)
LWT	0.86	(0.73, 1.01)

developing a model within the context of the current example and conditional logistic regression.

We obtain estimates of the odds ratios and their CIs by exponentiating the estimated coefficients and end points of their CIs in Table 3. These are shown in Table 4. The odds ratio and CI presented for the LWT is for a 10 pound increase in weight. The results for LWT are obtained from Table 3 by multiplying the coefficient and end points of the CI by 10 before exponentiating. This is done since LWT is measured in pounds, and an odds ratio for a one pound weight difference is likely not to be clinically meaningful.

The odds ratios in Table 4 suggest an important increase in risk of delivering of a low birthweight baby for prior PTD, SMOKE, HT, UI. The odds ratio for the LWT suggests an approximate 14% decrease in risk per 10 pound increase in weight. This interpretation assumes that the logit is linear in LWT. One should always check the scale of all continuous variables in any regression model. We did this using a method based on design variables for the quartiles of LWT (see [3, p. 194]), which supported the linearity assumption for LWT.

The CI estimates in Table 4 are quite wide for the dichotomous variables. This instability is due to the fact that the variance estimator is inversely related to the number of discordant pairs. The analysis presented in Tables 2 and 3 is based on 56 pairs and the numbers of discordant pairs are 19, 30, 10, and

16, respectively, for the dichotomous variables. The widths of the CIs in Table 4 are a result of the relatively few discordant pairs. This points out an important consideration that must be kept in mind at the design stage of a study. The gain in precision obtained from matching and using conditional logistic regression may be offset by a loss owing to few discordant pairs for dichotomous covariates. In general, the variance estimator of the slope coefficient is a function of how different the subjects with $y = 1$ are from those with $y = 0$ within each stratum.

Likelihood ratio tests may be used for model testing and refinement in a manner similar to that discussed in the article on logistic regression. In the case of conditional logistic regression the likelihood for model zero, "the no data model", is obtained by setting the coefficient vector equal to zero in (7). This model is essentially a coin toss with stratum specific probability $\Pr(Y_{kj} = 1) = n_{k1}/n_k$.

Application of the conditional logistic regression model to other, more complicated, matched or highly stratified designs is, for all intents and purposes, identical to the one-to-one matched study discussed. The essential point to keep in mind is that one uses and interprets the estimated coefficients in a manner identical to ordinary logistic regression. Although not illustrated in the example, because of relatively few matched pairs, one may use matching or stratification variables to form interactions with variables in the model but one may not include them as main effect terms. Much of the content of this article is based on [3].

References

[1] Breslow, N.E. & Day, N.E. (1980). *Statistical Methods in Cancer Research*. Vol. 1. *The Analysis of Case–Control Studies*. Oxford University Press, New York.
[2] Cox, D.R. & Hinkley, D.V. (1974). *Theoretical Statistics*. Chapman & Hall, New York.
[3] Hosmer, D.W. & Lemeshow, S. (1989). *Applied Logistic Regression*. Wiley, New York.
[4] Kelsey, J.L., Thompson, W.D. & Evans, A.S. (1986). *Methods in Observational Epidemiology*. Oxford University Press, New York.
[5] Kleinbaum, D.G., Kupper, L.L. & Morgenstern, H. (1982). *Epidemiologic Research: Principles and Quantitative Methods*. Van Nostrand Reinhold, New York.
[6] Liang, K.Y. (1987). Extended Mantel–Haenszel estimating procedure for multivariate logistic regressions, *Biometrics* **43**, 289–300.
[7] Rothman, K.J. (1986). *Modern Epidemiology*. Little, Brown & Company, Boston.
[8] Schlesselman, J.J. (1982). *Case–Control Studies*. Oxford University Press, New York.

DAVID W. HOSMER & STANLEY LEMESHOW

Logit *see* Logistic Regression

Loss-to-Follow-Up Bias *see* Bias from Loss to Follow-Up

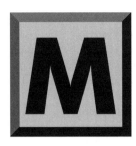

Malaria *see* Epidemic Models, Deterministic

Manski−Lerman Sampling *see* Case−Control Study, Two-Phase

Mantel−Haenszel Methods

Biomedical, clinical, patient-oriented, and public health research investigations frequently focus on the relationship between a primary factor, such as an exposure, a new therapy, or an intervention, and a response variable such as disease classification, functional status, or degree of improvement. When both of these variables are reported on categorical data scales, the resulting data typically are summarized as observed frequencies in a two-way contingency table. However, this *factor−response* relationship may be influenced by other *covariables* or covariates, such as clinical centers or baseline characteristics. Consequently, appropriate adjustments for these covariables must be incorporated into the data analysis.

The historical review of Mantel−Haenszel methods outlined in this article is drawn heavily from the extensive review article by Kuritz et al. [34].

In a classic paper, Cochran [13] proposed a test for several two-by-two tables based on binomial model assumptions. Five years later, Mantel & Haenszel (MH) [46] approached this same problem using a hypergeometric probability model, which permits either exact tests or requires only the overall sample size to be large for asymptotic results to hold. The resulting test statistics from these two procedures are nearly identical, except for applications in which the within-table sample sizes are sparse. In particular, the MH test statistic is entirely appropriate for within-table sample sizes as small as two, provided that there are enough tables. Birch [5] demonstrated that when within-table **odds ratios** are homogeneous, the MH test statistic is the uniformly most powerful unbiased (UMPU) test. Also, it is asymptotically equivalent to specific likelihood ratio (LR) tests from unconditional **logistic regression** when within-table sample sizes are large, and to specific LR tests from **conditional logistic regression** when within-table sample sizes are small [9].

MH procedures are most useful to test H_0: "no partial association" against alternatives encompassing an average effect of the *factor* on the *response* across strata based on the set of *covariables*. In many situations, the sample sizes for some tables may be sparse, the magnitude of the partial association may vary across tables, and the association may be small within subtables. However, if the association is slight, but consistent across the tables, MH procedures will be effective in detecting that association.

Perhaps the most important distinguishing feature of the MH procedures are their connections to randomization model considerations. Quite frequently, health research data are collected under observational study designs such as **case–control studies**, or convenience sampling for a randomized, multicenter efficacy trial. For such situations, MH procedures provide a randomization, design-based approach to hypothesis testing. These methods require no assumptions other than the randomization of subjects to factor levels, either explicitly as in randomized controlled clinical trials, or implicitly by hypothesis or from conditional distribution arguments for observational data from restrictive populations such as **retrospective studies**, nonrandomized **cohort** studies or case–control studies [30, 35].

In a strict statistical sense, the conclusions from an MH analysis might apply only to the study sample. Consequently, generalizations to a target population require nonstatistical arguments concerning the representativeness of the study subjects to the individuals in the target population. These issues of "extended inference," in contrast to "local inference," are discussed in more detail in Koch et al. [30, 31].

The MH methods for hypothesis testing and estimation of an average odds ratio for a set of 2×2 tables are reviewed in this article, both for factor-response and repeated measures study designs. Extensive details on the variance formulae for this average odds ratio are provided in [34], using a unified set of notation. The applications of these methods for investigating treatment differences and within-treatment change over time are illustrated using data from two different randomized, controlled clinical trials.

For the sake of brevity, the extensions of this MH methodology to a set of $s \times r$ contingency tables are summarized, but are illustrated only once using repeated measures ordinal data. The matrix formulations for these generalized MH methods are outlined in the Appendix.

The extent to which the factor–response partial association varies across tables is of critical concern to the interpretation of final results. For a set of 2×2 tables, methods assessing the variation of stratum-specific odds ratios are reviewed in Gart [24], and a popular method to test for homogeneity of the odds ratios across strata under minimal assumptions is described in Breslow & Day [9]. In settings in which sample sizes are adequate within each table, additive loglinear models can be fitted to the data and interaction evaluated through tests for their goodness of fit [2, 7]. Otherwise, an exact

procedure based on the extended hypergeometric distribution is described in [40] and [50], and has been implemented in the StatXact software of Mehta & Patel [50].

Notation and General Methodology

Let $h = 1, 2, \ldots, t$ index strata and let n_{hij} denote the number of sample subjects jointly classified as belonging to the ith factor level, the jth level of response, and the hth stratum. The resulting $s \times r$ contingency table for the hth stratum can be summarized as in Table 1.

For hypotheses involving the *factor–response* association, h indexes the t levels of stratification determined by the cross-classification of the covariables. However, for repeated measurement designs, the primary hypothesis involves homogeneity of the response distribution across levels of the repeated measurement dimension, so that h indexes the t subjects or unique matched sets.

If the row marginal totals $\{n_{hi.}\}$ and column marginal totals $\{n_{h.j}\}$ in Table 1 are assumed fixed, the overall H_0: "no partial association" can be stated as

H_0: For each of the stratum levels indexed by

$h = 1, 2, \ldots, t,$ the response variable is

distributed at random with respect

to the factor levels   (1)

In other words, from a finite population sampling perspective, H_0 assumes that the observed data in each row of the hth stratum can be regarded as a successive set of simple random samples of sizes $\{n_{hi.}\}$ from a fixed population corresponding to the column marginal totals $\{n_{h.j}\}$.

Table 1 The observed contingency table for stratum h

Factor levels	Response variable categories				Total
	1	2	$\ldots$	r	
1	n_{h11}	n_{h12}	$\ldots$	n_{h1r}	$n_{h1.}$
2	n_{h21}	n_{h22}	$\ldots$	n_{h2r}	$n_{h2.}$
$\vdots$	$\vdots$	$\vdots$		$\vdots$	$\vdots$
s	n_{hs1}	n_{hs2}	$\ldots$	n_{hsr}	$n_{hs.}$
Total	$n_{h.1}$	$n_{h.2}$	$\ldots$	$n_{h.r}$	n_h

Under H_0 in (1), the observed frequencies, $\{n_{hij}\}$, follow the multiple hypergeometric probability model,

$$\Pr(\mathbf{n}_h|H_0) = \frac{\prod\limits_{i=1}^{s} n_{hi.}! \prod\limits_{j=1}^{r} n_{h.j}!}{n_h! \prod\limits_{i=1}^{s} \prod\limits_{j=1}^{r} n_{hij}!}. \qquad (2)$$

The expression in (2) simplifies to the familiar Fisher's exact probability for a single 2×2 table. In general, under H_0 in (1), we can compute expected values for each frequency and the covariance of each frequency with each of the other frequencies in Table 1 as outlined in the Appendix. Using these quantities, we can investigate a series of alternative hypotheses involving "average effects" of the primary factor on the distribution of the response variable, adjusted for the strata effects, depending on the measurement scales of each.

Alternative Hypothesis: General Association

When both row and column variables are measured on nominal scales, H_0 can be rejected in favor of the response variable differing in nonspecific patterns across factor levels, adjusted for the covariates. As noted in the Appendix, the generalized MH chi-square test statistic in (A3), with $(s-1)(r-1)$ degrees of freedom (df) is based on the sums of the differences between the observed and expected frequencies, relative to the sum of the covariance matrices over the t tables.

In unmatched studies, for the special case in which $s = r = 2$, the resulting data can be summarized in a set of t 2×2 tables. Here $Q_{\text{MH}(1)}$ is identical to the test statistic proposed in Birch [5], is identical (except for the lack of a continuity correction) to the statistic recommended in Mantel & Haenszel [46], and differs from the test statistic proposed in Cochran [13] only by a factor of $(n_h - 1)/n_h$ in the variance term for each table.

In repeated measurement or matched design, $Q_{\text{MH}(1)}$ simplifies to a number of familiar test statistics as noted in White et al. [62] and Somes [58]. In particular, if the response variable is dichotomous $r = 2$, $Q_{\text{MH}(1)}$ is equivalent to McNemar's test [48] when $s = 2$ and to Cochran's Q criterion [12] when $s > 2$. Furthermore, for $r > 2$

and $s > 2$, this result is identical to the "Lagrange multiplier" test derived in Birch [6], the test of interchangeability due to Madansky [41], and the extended MH criterion described in Darroch [14], Mantel & Byar [44], and White et al. [62].

Alternative Hypothesis: Mean Responses Differ

If the response variable is ordinal, then the average response for each factor level can be estimated by assigning column scores, say $a_{h1}, a_{h2}, \ldots, a_{hr}$, and forming the mean score,

$$\bar{f}_{hi} = \sum_{j=1}^{r} \frac{a_{hj} n_{hij}}{n_{hi.}}, \qquad (3)$$

for the ith row within the hth stratum. The specific choice of the scores is not discussed here; further details are available in Landis et al. [36], Koch & Edwards [29], and Koch et al. [32].

As summarized in the Appendix, differences of these s mean scores from their corresponding expected values across the subtables, relative to their covariances, can be used to create a test statistic, $Q_{\text{MH}(2)}$ in (A4), that reflects the extent to which the mean scores for certain levels of the factor consistently exceed (or are exceeded by) the mean scores for other levels of the factor. In particular, for $s = 2$ this test is identical to the extended MH test statistic proposed in Mantel [42]. Moreover, if marginal rank or ridit-type scores are obtained from each table, with midranks assigned for ties, $Q_{\text{MH}(2)}$ is equivalent to an extension of the Kruskal–Wallis analysis of variance (ANOVA) test on ranks, conditioning on the levels of the strata; for $s = 2$, this is the van Elteren [61] test, for which additional discussion is given in Lehmann & Dabrerd [38]. More recent evaluation of the MH mean score statistic is found in Davis & Chung [15].

Within repeated measures designs, $Q_{\text{MH}(2)}$ is equivalent to the MH statistic provided in Breslow & Day [9] for matched case–control data with an ordinal risk factor. Where marginal rank scores are assigned within each stratum, $Q_{\text{MH}(2)}$ simplifies to the Friedman [20] chi-square criterion from a two-way rank ANOVA within blocks for subjects. In both designs, $Q_{\text{MH}(2)}$ with df $= (s-1)$ provides increased statistical power to detect departures from homogeneity across factor levels for an ordered response variable, relative to $Q_{\text{MH}(1)}$ with df $= (s-1)(r-1)$, although more complex patterns of association will not necessarily be detected.

Alternative Hypothesis: Linear Trend in Mean Responses

When both rows and columns are measured on an ordinal scale, we can assign row scores, say $c_{h1}, c_{h2}, \ldots, c_{hs}$, to the rows, as well as $a_{h1}, a_{h2}, \ldots, a_{hr}$ assigned to the columns. Then, as outlined in the Appendix, the generalized MH test statistic with df $= 1$ investigates the extent to which there is a consistent positive (or negative) association between the response scores and the factor level scores in the respective strata. Specifically, $Q_{MH(3)}$ in (A5) is directed at the extent to which H_0 is contradicted in favor of a linear progression in the average response across the levels of the factor relative to the assigned scores.

This statistic, $Q_{MH(3)}$, is identical to the correlation statistic proposed by Mantel [42] and Birch [6]. If marginal rank or ridit-type scores are assigned to both the rows and columns of each table, with midranks assigned for ties, this statistic is equivalent to an extension of the Spearman rank correlation test, conditioning on the levels of the covariates. With only one degree of freedom, this statistic has increased power relative to either $Q_{MH(1)}$ or $Q_{MH(2)}$ for linear correlation alternatives relative to the assigned scores.

Factor–Response Designs

The MH methods for the standard *factor–response* designs will be described, first beginning with the familiar 2×2 table layout.

2×2 Tables

In this simplest case, the data can be arranged in a series of t 2×2 tables. All three test statistics outlined in the Appendix are identical, having df $= 1$, and simplify (except for the lack of a continuity correction) to the familiar MH statistic,

$$Q_{MH(1)} = \frac{\left[\sum_{h=1}^{t} n_{h11} - \sum_{h=1}^{t} \frac{n_{h1.} n_{h.1}}{n_h} \right]^2}{\sum_{h=1}^{t} \frac{n_{h1.} n_{h2.} n_{h.1} n_{h.2}}{n_h^2 (n_h - 1)}}. \tag{4}$$

Guidelines concerning sample size requirements in order for the chi-square approximation for $Q_{MH(1)}$ to be appropriate are provided by Mantel & Fleiss [45]; briefly, the sum across the t strata of the observed frequency for each cell of the 2×2 table should have an expected value exceeding 5 and an allowable range of 5 on each side of the expected value. Further sample size discussions are available in Breslow & Day [9], Fleiss [19], and Koch et al. [32].

This MH statistic in (4) can be viewed as a test directed at the alternative hypothesis that a weighted average of the stratum-specific odds ratios, say $\overline{\psi} = \sum_h w_h \psi_h / \sum_h w_h$, differs from 1, the expected value under H_0. Having rejected H_0, the most widely accepted estimator for $\overline{\psi}$ is

$$\hat{\overline{\psi}}_{MH} = \frac{\sum_{h=1}^{t} n_{h11} n_{h22} / n_h}{\sum_{h=1}^{t} n_{h12} n_{h21} / n_h}, \tag{5}$$

as proposed in the original MH paper [46]. In addition, many estimators have been proposed for the common odds ratio, ψ, under the assumption of homogeneity of the stratum-specific odds ratios. Among these are the unconditional maximum likelihood [21, 24], Woolf [63], and the modified Woolf [22, 25] estimator. These estimators require large within-stratum sample sizes, assuming that the number of strata t remains fixed, but the total number of subjects increases without bound. In contrast, the conditional maximum likelihood estimator [5, 23] is appropriate with as few as $n_h = 2$ observations per stratum, provided that t is sufficiently large.

All of these estimators are consistent, asymptotically normal, and (at $\psi = 1$ for $\hat{\overline{\psi}}_{MH}$) asymptotically efficient [8, 60]. Simulation work by McKinlay [47] and Hauck et al. [28] has demonstrated that there is little difference among the estimators in terms of bias and precision for the unmatched design with large numbers of subjects in each stratum. The Woolf and modified Woolf statistics have been shown to have a large bias problem as stratum sample sizes become more moderate. When considering ease of computation together with statistical properties, McKinlay [47] has recommended using the MH estimator in (5).

A number of variance formulas for the average odds ratio in (5) have been proposed over the years, as summarized in Kuritz et al. [34]. Based on theoretical considerations, as well as simulation studies [10, 18, 53], the estimator of choice for computing the asymptotic variance of the MH average odds ratio in (5) is

$$
\mathrm{var}_{\mathrm{RBG}}(\widehat{\psi}_{\mathrm{MH}})
$$

$$
= \frac{(\widehat{\psi}_{\mathrm{MH}}^2) \sum\limits_{h=1}^{t} \left\{ \dfrac{S_h}{n_h} \left[\dfrac{n_{h22}}{\widehat{\psi}_{\mathrm{MH}}} + n_{h12} \right] + \dfrac{R_h}{n_h} \left[\dfrac{n_{h21}}{\widehat{\psi}_{\mathrm{MH}}} + \dfrac{n_{h11}}{\widehat{\psi}_{\mathrm{MH}}^2} \right] \right\}}{\left(\sum\limits_{h=1}^{t} S_h \right)^{-2}}
$$

$$(6)$$

where $R_h = n_{h11} n_{h22}/n_h$, $S_h = n_{h12} n_{h21}/n_h$, and the subscript "RBG" denotes "Robins, Breslow and Greenland". This variance estimator has been selected for the asymptotic method of choice in the StatXact software system [50].

When there is only one stratum ($t = 1$), this RBG variance estimator simplifies to the usual large-sample variance for the odds ratio from a single 2×2 table, as presented in Fleiss [19], which is

$$
\mathrm{var}(\hat{\psi}) = \hat{\psi}^2 \left(\frac{1}{n_{11}} + \frac{1}{n_{12}} + \frac{1}{n_{21}} + \frac{1}{n_{22}} \right). \quad (7)
$$

Unlike the alternative model-based estimates of "partial association", the MH estimate in (5) was intended to be a weighted average of the individual odds ratios [43], where the weights are related to the precision of $\hat{\psi}_h$ [9, 17]. In fact, Mantel & Haenszel [46] indicated their disbelief in the constancy of the underlying odds ratio, stating that the assumption of a constant relative risk is usually untenable. McKinlay [47] interpreted (5) as representing the constant component of an association across strata; whereas Landis et al. [35] and others refer to this quantity as "average partial association". Even though the stratum-specific odds ratios may be heterogeneous, one often is interested in a summary measure [26]. However, most investigators generally agree that a combined odds ratio, which is based on individual odds ratios that differ substantially in direction, some being less than unity and others greater than unity, can be difficult to interpret and perhaps should not be used.

Formal statistical tests for this hypothesis of homogeneous odds ratios across strata can be conducted within the context of fitting an additive logit-linear model with either maximum likelihood or weighted least squares methods, provided that the within-stratum sample sizes are adequate. Details of these methods are provided in Koch et al. [32] and Agresti [2]. Otherwise, under an extension of the hypergeometric probability model in (2), Breslow & Day [9] proposed a test statistic directed at the potential lack of homogeneity of odds ratios,

$$
Q_{\mathrm{BD}} = \sum_{h=1}^{t} \frac{\left[n_{h11} - \mathrm{E}(n_{h11}|\widehat{\psi}_{\mathrm{MH}}) \right]^2}{\mathrm{var}(n_{h11}|\widehat{\psi}_{MH})}, \quad (8)
$$

where $\mathrm{E}(n_{h11}|\widehat{\psi}_{\mathrm{MH}})$ is the expected value of n_{h11} under the hypothesis of homogeneity of odds ratios, $\mathrm{var}(n_{h11}|\widehat{\psi}_{\mathrm{MH}})$ is the variance of n_{h11} under the same hypothesis, and $\widehat{\psi}_{\mathrm{MH}}$ is the estimate of the average odds ratio under this homogeneity hypothesis. Assuming acceptably large sample sizes in each subtable, Q_{BD}, where the subscript BD denotes Breslow & Day, can be compared with the chi-square distribution with df $= t - 1$ for assessing statistical significance. This test statistic and p value is produced within the FREQ procedure in SAS [54]. Further work has recently been done evaluating tests of association and homogeneity, along with estimators of common odds ratios and risk ratios, in sparse data situations [51, 56, 57].

The data in Table 2 were obtained from a randomized, controlled clinical trial conducted at each of eight clinics, as reported in Beitler & Landis [4]. The purpose of the study was to investigate the effect of a topical cream drug therapy in curing nonspecific gynecologic infections. The binary response variable was classified as favorable or unfavorable response to treatment.

The data displayed in Table 2, collapsed over the eight clinics, indicate that 42.3% of women receiving the active drug reported a favorable response, compared with 32.9% of women receiving the control, resulting in an (unadjusted) odds ratio of 1.50, and a relative risk of 1.29. By applying the MH method for 2×2 tables in (4) to a single table, we note that the observed "pivot cell" frequency is $\sum_{h=1}^{t} n_{h11} = 55$, with expected value under H_0 of 48.57, and variance of 15.99, yielding a test statistic of $Q_{\mathrm{MH}(1)} = 2.59$, with $p = 0.11$. Consequently, at the standard 5% level of statistical significance, we would conclude that this drug is not different from the control therapy.

However, the same data from Table 2 are shown again in Table 3, stratified by clinic, sorted by

Table 2   The distribution of favorable response to active drug and control treatments in the multicenter randomized clinical trial: collapsed over clinics

| Clinic no. | Treatment | Response | | Total | Proportion favorable | Risk estimates | |
		Favorable	Unfavorable			Relative risk	Odds ratio
Collapsed	Drug	55	75	130	0.423	1.29	1.50
	Control	47	96	143	0.329		
	Subtotal	102	171	273	0.374		

Source: Beitler & Landis [4].

Table 3   The distribution of favorable response to active drug and control treatments in the multicenter randomized clinical trial

| Clinic no. | Treatment | Response | | Total | Proportion favorable | Risk estimates | |
		Favorable	Unfavorable			Relative risk	Odds ratio
1	Drug	11	25	36	0.306	1.13	1.19
	Control	10	27	37	0.270		
	Subtotal	21	52	73	0.288		
2	Drug	16	4	20	0.800	1.16	1.82
	Control	22	10	32	0.688		
	Subtotal	38	14	52	0.731		
3	Drug	14	5	19	0.737	2.00	4.80
	Control	7	12	19	0.368		
	Subtotal	21	17	38	0.553		
4	Drug	2	14	16	0.125	2.13	2.29
	Control	1	16	17	0.059		
	Subtotal	3	30	33	0.091		
5	Drug	6	11	17	0.353	9.29	14.13
	Control	0	12	12	0.000		
	Subtotal	6	23	29	0.207		
6	Drug	1	10	11	0.091	2.74	3.00
	Control	0	10	10	0.000		
	Subtotal	1	20	21	0.048		
7	Drug	1	4	5	0.200	1.80	2.00
	Control	1	8	9	0.111		
	Subtotal	2	12	14	0.143		
8	Drug	4	2	6	0.667	0.78	0.33
	Control	6	1	7	0.857		
	Subtotal	10	3	13	0.769		

Source: Beitler & Landis [4].

largest sample size ($n_1 = 73$) to smallest sample size ($n_8 = 13$).

Now the MH test in (4), with df $= 1$, for the statistical significance of the treatment effect is $Q_{MH(1)} = 6.38$, with $p = 0.01$. Thus, in contrast to the test on the data collapsed over the eight clinics ($p = 0.11$), we reject the null hypothesis of "no partial association", in favor of the alternative hypothesis suggesting that the treatments (drug vs. control) on average are not homogeneous across the eight clinics.

Note that although seven of the eight odds ratios from the eight clinics indicate that drug therapy constitutes a more effective treatment for curing nonspecific gynecologic infections than the control treatment, they differ in magnitude from a low of 1.2 (stratum 1) to a high of 14.1 (stratum 5). Also note that these individual table estimates of the odds ratio for strata 5 and 6 were obtained after adding 0.5 to each cell of the 2×2 table due to the observed zero frequency [19]. The only stratum showing an inverse relationship was clinic 8. Using the Breslow–Day test in (8) for homogeneity of odds ratios, we obtain $Q_{BD} = 7.80$ with df = 7, ($p = 0.33$). Thus, despite this wide range in the magnitude of the stratum-specific odds ratios, these data do not provide sufficient evidence to reject the hypothesis of homogeneous odds ratios.

The MH average odds ratio in (5), adjusting for these strata effects, is $\widehat{\psi}_{MH} = 2.14$, somewhat larger than the unadjusted estimate of 1.50. Furthermore, the 95% confidence interval (CI) for the MH average odds ratio, using the RBG variance in (6), is (1.197, 3.807). This CI, by not containing 1.0, suggests that after adjustments for the variability in the response by clinic, the drug is significantly associated with a favorable response.

General $s \times r$ Tables

In general, there are s levels of the row factor and r levels of the response variable, giving rise to t $s \times r$ contingency tables, as in Table 1. For these settings, the generalized MH methods outlined in the Appendix are illustrated in Kuritz et al. [34] and Landis et al. [35, 37]. For purposes of brevity in this article, we will defer the application of these generalized MH hypothesis testing methods until Example 3 in the subsequent section.

Estimation of treatment effects is much more complex for the general $s \times r$ table situation, particularly if one or both of the dimensions of the tables are not ordinally scaled. Investigators have been developing some extensions of the MH estimating procedure, including variance and covariance estimators and in sparse data situations [15, 16, 27, 39, 49, 55], although none appears to be fully generalizable to a series of $s \times r$ tables. Ordinal models provide summary measures [1, 11], but the sample size requirements and structural model assumptions,

such as proportional odds, are much more restrictive than required for the MH methods to be applied.

Repeated Measures Designs

The use of MH methods for the analysis of categorical data obtained from repeated measures designs was described in the early papers by Mantel & Haenszel [46], and by Birch [5, 6] and Gart [24]. Breslow & Day [9] illustrated the use of these methods for matched case–control data, including the incorporation of scores for an ordinal risk factor. Otherwise, Agresti [2], Darroch [14], Kuritz et al. [34], Landis et al. [37], Mantel & Byar [44], White et al. [62] and others [3, 33, 52] described the use of these methods for a variety of repeated measures and longitudinal designs.

The hypotheses within these designs involve the extent to which the response variable varies across the repeated measures factor (within-subject conditions, case–control status), on average, across the strata (subjects, matched sets). For example, all the matched analyses illustrated in Breslow & Day [9] can be formulated within this framework utilizing the MH methods.

2×2 Tables

Researchers are frequently interested in comparing the prevalence of a condition under two different circumstances or time periods for the same set of subjects, or in comparing the risk factor prevalence in a matched-pair set of subjects. In such applications, a 2×2 table is constructed, in which the row and column dimensions correspond to the level of the condition or risk factor for each dimension of the repeated measure. To illustrate these methods, consider the data in Table 4, summarizing the binary level of obstetrical post-partum pain [Some/More (2–4) vs. None/Little (0–1)] at 4 hours and subsequently at 8 hours after delivery, for each mother from the subgroup of 185 women receiving a combination drug labeled (A and B). More extensive descriptions and analyses of these data are provided in Koch et al. [32] and Kuritz et al. [34].

We can utilize the same MH test statistic in (4) to test the null hypothesis that the prevalence of pain (Some/More) is the same at 4 and 8 hours after delivery. In order to implement this test, with

Table 4 The general layout for the cross-classification of two binary repeated measures using post-partum pain[a] at 4 and 8 hours after delivery for all patients assigned to the combination drugs A and B

Treatment subgroup	Initial pain	Pain at 4 hours	Pain at 8 hours		Totals
			Some/More	None/Little	
A and B	Combined	Some/More	19 (a)	31 (b)	50
		None/Little	6 (c)	129 (d)	135
		Total	25	160	185
			$(a+c)$	$(b+d)$	

[a]Pain level reported as $0 = $ None, $1 = $ Little, $2 = $ Some, $3 = $ Lots, $4 = $ Terrible, at each hour of follow-up; Some/More pain obtained by combining levels 2–4.
Source: Kuritz et al. [34].

appropriate adjustments for the paired data structure within subjects, the data for each woman must be summarized in a 2×2 frequency table with entries of 1s and 0s, as displayed in Table 5. Note that the frequency of women reporting Some/More pain at both 4 and 8 hours ($a = 19$) in Table 4 gives rise to 19 2×2 tables of profile type 1 in Table 5. In total, there are $n = 185$ subtables in Table 5, although those of profile type 1 ($a = 19$) and type 4 ($d = 129$) do not contribute to the test statistic in (4), due to the equality of observed and expected frequencies and a variance term of zero in the denominator.

In summarizing these data in Tables 4 and 5, it should also be noted that this layout is identical to the format used to summarize the frequencies for case–control data from epidemiologic investigations involving matched pairs, where the rows in Table 4 represent the exposure categories for the cases, and the columns represent the exposure categories for the controls.

In this context, the randomization model test statistic in (4) simplifies to $Q_{\text{MH}(1)} = (b - c)^2/(b + c)$, which is identical to the McNemar [48] statistic for repeated measures data from 2×2 tables. This test statistic asymptotically follows the chi-square distribution with df $= 1$. Note, however, that it is completely determined by the off-diagonal cells "b" and "c", and thus the asymptotics for this statistic are linked directly to the number of discordant pairs of observations, $b + c$, rather than the total sample size n. When $b + c$ does not exceed 20, it is preferable to perform an exact conditional test based on the binomial distribution, as implemented within StatXact [40, 50].

The usual MH average odds ratio as defined in (5) simplifies to $\widehat{\psi}_{\text{MH}} = b/c$, using the notation for 2×2

Table 5 The binary level of post-partum pain[a] at 4 and 8 hours after delivery by individual patient profiles for a representative subgroup in the multicenter randomized clinical trial

Profile type	No. of tables (patients)	No. of hours	Level of post-partum pain		Total
			Some/More (2–4)	None/Little (0–1)	
1	$a = 19$	4	1	0	1
		8	1	0	1
		Subtotal	2	0	2
2	$b = 31$	4	1	0	1
		8	0	1	1
		Subtotal	1	1	2
3	$c = 6$	4	0	1	1
		8	1	0	1
		Subtotal	1	1	2
4	$d = 129$	4	0	1	1
		8	0	1	1
		Subtotal	0	2	2

[a]Pain level reported as $0 = $ None, $1 = $ Little, $2 = $ Some, $3 = $ Lots, and $4 = $ Terrible, at each hour of follow-up; Some/More pain obtained by combining levels 2–4.
Source: Kuritz et al. [34].

tables from repeated measures designs as in Table 4. Furthermore, the preferred CI approach for this estimator is to use either the RBG variance in (6) or the exact procedure based on the binomial distribution, which applies to b given $b + c$. Both the RBG and the exact procedure are computed easily within the StatXact [50] package.

These odds ratio and CI procedures are illustrated for nine subsets of the post-partum data from the multicenter study described in Kuritz et al. [34].

Table 6 A cross-classification of two binary repeated measures using post-partum pain[a] at 4 and 8 hours after delivery: patients stratified by treatment and initial pain

Treatment subgroup	Initial pain	Response profile at hours 4 and 8				Total	MH average odds ratio	RBG 95% CIs
		SS (a)	SN (b)	NS (c)	NN (d)			
Placebo	Some	17	16	7	40	80	2.29	(0.94, 5.56)
	Lots	41	11	8	30	90	1.38	(0.55, 3.42)
	Combined	58	27	15	70	170	1.80	(0.96, 3.38)
A only	Some	11	15	6	46	78	2.50	(0.97, 6.44)
	Lots	31	20	6	41	98	3.33	(1.34, 8.30)
	Combined	42	35	12	87	176	2.92	(1.51, 5.62)
A and B	Some	5	12	4	64	85	3.00	(0.97, 9.30)
	Lots	14	19	2	65	100	9.50	(2.21, 40.79)
	Combined	19	31	6	129	185	5.17	(2.16, 12.38)

[a]Pain level reported as 0 = None, 1 = Little, 2 = Some, 3 = Lots, and 4 = Terrible, at each hour of follow-up; Some/More pain obtained by combining levels 2–4.
Source: Kuritz et al. [34].

In particular, for each combination of treatment (Placebo, A only, and A and B) subgroup and initial pain status (Some, Lots, and Combined), these MH average odds ratios, and their RBG 95% CIs were computed and are presented in Table 6. Note that the MH odds ratios for women reporting "Some" initial pain are similar across treatments, ranging from 2.3 for those receiving Placebo to 3.0 for those receiving both A and B. However, due to the small sample sizes of $b + c$, the RBG 95% CIs around each of these odds ratios barely include 1, suggesting only slight evidence that the level of pain at 8 hours differs from that at 4 hours.

In contrast, among women who reported "Lots" of initial pain, the MH average odds ratio ranged from ($\widehat{\psi}_{MH} = 1.38$) in the Placebo subgroup, to ($\widehat{\psi}_{MH} = 9.50$) among women randomized to the A and B combination drug. Furthermore, the RBG 95% CIs suggest that the levels of pain at 4 and 8 hours are different (improved at 8 hours) for those on Drug A only (1.34, 8.30), and particularly so for those receiving the combination A and B drugs (2.21, 40.79).

When initial pain status (Some or Lots) is ignored, by combining the strata within treatment, the odds ratios again demonstrate a clear gradient across treatment subgroups, with the least evidence for a difference in level of pain at 4 and 8 hours among women receiving Placebo ($\widehat{\psi}_{MH} = 1.80$) and the strongest evidence for such a difference among

women receiving both A and B ($\widehat{\psi}_{MH} = 5.17$). For each treatment subgroup, these measures of association are somewhat smaller for the combined group of women than for the subset with "Lots" of initial pain.

General $d \times L$ Tables

In the most general case, a repeated measures design involves d measurement conditions (within-subject treatments, time points, and matched-set members) and L levels of the response variable. To illustrate this situation, consider the data displayed in Table 7 from a pediatric cardiology study conducted at the C.S. Mott Children's Hospital, Ann Arbor, Michigan. As described further in Landis et al. [37], each of 14 puppies was administered each of five variable pulse duration treatments, delivered at a separate site in the esophagus for 30 minutes. The purpose of the study was to investigate the effect of variable pulse duration on the development of acute electrical injury during transesophageal atrial pacing.

Each of the five treatments, distinguished by pulse durations of either 2, 4, 6, 8, or 10 ms, was applied at a separate site of the esophagus. At the conclusion of the experiment, the electrical injury lesion at each site was classified according to the depth of injury by histologic examination using an ordinal staging scale from 0 (no lesion) to 5 (acute inflammation of the fascia). These lesion severity data are displayed

Table 7 Lesion severity[a] of acute electrical injury by variable pulse duration for each of 14 puppies

Puppy no.	Pulse duration (ms)					Mean response
	2	4	6	8	10	
6	0	0	5	0	3	1.60
7	0	3	3	4	5	3.00
8	0	3	4	3	2	2.40
9	2	2	3	0	4	2.20
10	0	0	4	4	3	2.20
12	0	0	0	4	4	1.60
13	0	4	4	4	0	2.40
15	0	4	0	0	0	0.80
16	0	3	0	1	1	1.00
17	–	–	0	1	0	0.33
19	0	0	1	1	0	0.40
20	–	0	0	2	2	1.00
21	0	0	2	3	3	1.60
22	–	0	0	3	0	0.75

[a]Lesion severity graded as 0 = no lesion to 5 = acute inflammation of extraesophageal fascia: – denotes missing data.
Source: data provided by Dr C.L. Webb, and C.S. Mott, Children's Hospital, Ann Arbor.

in Table 7, showing the response at each pulse duration, together with the mean response across pulse durations, for each puppy.

The primary hypothesis under investigation in this experiment is whether the mean lesion severity differs by pulse duration (mean responses differ), and in particular, whether mean lesion severity increases with increasing pulse duration (linear trend in mean responses). By collapsing these responses over individual puppies, the overall response profiles of lesion severity for each condition (pulse duration) are displayed in Table 8. In particular, note that the mean lesion severity increases from 0.18 (due to 10 of 11 puppies having a response of "0") at 2 ms to 1.93 at 10 ms.

To incorporate the appropriate adjustments for the repeated measures (within puppy) across measurement conditions (pulse duration levels), the data for each puppy must be structured in a separate table which displays the response of the puppy at each of the measurement conditions. Let $h = 1, \ldots, N$ index subjects, $k = 1, \ldots, L$ index the response categories, and $g = 1, \ldots, d$ index the measurement conditions. Then, in the cells of each table, $y_{hgk} = 1$ if the hth subject is classified into the kth response category at the gth repeated measure, and is equal to 0 otherwise.

This general $d \times L$ table is illustrated using the data for puppy number 7 from Table 7, as displayed in Table 9. In particular, the response pattern for this puppy was no lesion (severity 0) at pulse duration of 2 ms, a lesion severity of 3 measured at both 4 and 6 ms, a lesion of severity 4 at 8 ms, and an acute inflammation of extraesophageal fascia (severity 5) was measured at the pulse duration of 10 ms.

These data in Table 7, restructured according to the format in Table 9, permit investigation of all three alternative hypotheses relative to the null hypothesis of "no partial association". For comparative

Table 9 Distribution of severity of lesion[a] by pulse duration for puppy number 7

Pulse duration (ms)	Severity of lesion						Total
	0	1	2	3	4	5	
2	1	0	0	0	0	0	1
4	0	0	0	1	0	0	1
6	0	0	0	1	0	0	1
8	0	0	0	0	1	0	1
10	0	0	0	0	0	1	1
Total	1	0	0	2	1	1	5

[a]Lesion severity graded as 0 = no lesion to 5 = acute inflammation of extraesophageal fascia.

Table 8 Distribution of severity of lesion[a] by pulse duration: collapsed across 14 puppies

Pulse duration (ms)	Severity of lesion						Total	Mean response
	0	1	2	3	4	5		
2	10	0	1	0	0	0	11	0.18
4	7	0	1	3	2	0	13	1.46
6	6	1	1	2	3	1	14	1.86
8	3	3	1	3	4	0	14	2.14
10	5	1	2	3	2	1	14	1.93
Total	31	5	6	11	11	2	66	1.58

[a]Lesion severity graded as 0 = no lesion to 5 = acute inflammation of extraesophageal fascia.

Table 10 Randomization model test statistics for association between pulse duration and lesion severity under SRS and repeated measurement sample assumptions: 14 puppies

Alternative hypothesis	Equation number in Appendix	df	SRS sample covariance structure		Repeated measures covariance structure	
			Test statistic	Significance level	Test statistic	Significance level
General association	(A3)	20	21.20	0.39	22.85	0.30
Row mean scores differ	(A4)	4	9.88	0.04	12.35	0.02
Nonzero correlation	(A5)	1	6.76	0.01	8.80	<0.01

purposes, we present each of these three test statistics in Table 10, first of all unadjusted for the 14 strata (puppies), assuming simple random sampling (SRS) and labeled "SRS Sample Covariance Structure". Secondly, each of these three alternative hypotheses is investigated within the MH framework adjusted for the 14 strata (puppies) and labeled "Repeated Measures Covariance Structure".

By treating both the factor levels (pulse duration) and response levels (severity of lesion) as nominal scale variables, the randomization model test statistic in (A3) in the Appendix provides a test of the null hypothesis given in (1) relative to the alternative that there is a general, nonspecific association between pulse duration and severity of lesion. As shown in Table 10, the adjusted test statistic is $Q_{MH(1)} = 22.85$, in contrast to the unadjusted SRS test, $Q_{MH(1)} = 21.20$. In this case, this nonspecific test for general association with df = 20 shows only minimal effects due to adjusting for the within-puppy correlation. Furthermore, without incorporating the ordinal nature of both of these variables, there is no evidence of an association between pulse duration and severity of the lesions ($p = 0.30$). However, the sample size is not large enough for $Q_{MH(1)}$ to follow a chi-square distribution with df = 20, or to detect general association departures from H_0.

On the other hand, if we do incorporate the ordinal nature of lesion severity, assigning scores of $0, 1, \ldots, 5$, but still consider pulse duration as a nominal variable, we can compute an observed mean lesion severity score as in (3), which is summarized for the unadjusted data (collapsed over the 14 puppies) in the last column of Table 8. Consequently, the randomization model test statistic in (A4) of the Appendix can be used to test the null hypothesis of "no partial association" in (1) against the more specific alternative hypothesis that the mean scores for the five pulse durations are different, adjusting for the strata.

As displayed in Table 10, the adjusted test statistic is $Q_{MH(2)} = 12.35$, in contrast to the unadjusted test statistic of $Q_{MH(2)} = 9.88$. Since these tests compare the five mean lesion severity scores (in a fashion equivalent to a two-way ANOVA), the degrees of freedom have been reduced from 20 to 4, resulting in increased statistical power to reject H_0. In fact, not only does the significance level for the adjusted statistic decrease from $p = 0.30$ to $p = 0.02$, indicating that the five pulse durations do not give rise to the same mean levels of lesion severity, but the significance level for the unadjusted test (ignoring within-puppy correlation) is only $p = 0.04$, twice as large as for the adjusted test statistic. This increase in power due to adjustments for within-puppy correlation is already noticeable with only 14 puppies, and small $d = 5$ repeated measures within puppy.

Finally, we can investigate the alternative hypothesis of a linear progression in mean lesion severity scores by computing the test statistic in (A5) in the Appendix using equally spaced row scores of 1, 2, 3, 4, and 5 for the pulse duration levels. The resulting adjusted test statistic is $Q_{MH(3)} = 8.80$, in contrast to the unadjusted test statistic, $Q_{MH(3)} = 6.76$. With one degree of freedom, these test statistics for "nonzero correlation" are highly significant ($p < 0.01$). Thus, when incorporating the ordinal nature of both variables, these data provide strong evidence that increasing the pulse duration (from 2 ms to 10 ms) is associated with a linear increase in the mean lesion severity. Not only does this df = 1 test for linear trend in mean severity most closely address the clinical research question, but it is also most justified in terms of sample size adequacy.

References

[1]   Agresti, A. (1980). Generalized odds ratios for ordinal data, *Biometrics* **36**, 59–67.

[2] Agresti, A. (1990). *Categorical Data Analysis*. Wiley, New York.

[3] Arndt, S., Davis, C.S., Miller, D.D. & Andreasen, N.C. (1993). Effect of antipsychotic withdrawal on extrapyramidal symptoms: statistical methods for analyzing single-sample repeated-measures data, *Neuropsychopharmacology* **8**, 67–75.

[4] Beitler, P.J. & Landis, J.R. (1985). A mixed-effects model for categorical data, *Biometrics* **41**, 991–1000.

[5] Birch, M.M. (1964). The detection of partial association, I: the 2 × 2 case, *Journal of the Royal Statistical Society, Series B* **26**, 313–324.

[6] Birch, M.W. (1965). The detection of partial association, II: the general case, *Journal of the Royal Statistical Society, Series B* **27**, 111–124.

[7] Bishop, Y.M.M., Fienberg, S.E. & Holland, P.W. (1975). *Discrete Multivariate Analysis*. MIT Press, Cambridge, Mass.

[8] Breslow, N.E. (1981). Odds ratio estimators when the data are sparse, *Biometrika* **68**, 73–84.

[9] Breslow, N.E. & Day, N.E. (1980). *Statistical Methods in Cancer Research*, Vol. 1, IARC Science Publication No. 32. International Agency for Research on Cancer, Lyon.

[10] Breslow, N.E. & Liang, K.Y. (1982). The variance of the Mantel–Haenszel estimator, *Biometrics* **38**, 943–952.

[11] Clayton, D.G. (1974). Some odds ratio statistics for the analysis of ordered categorical data, *Biometrika* **61**, 525–531.

[12] Cochran, W.G. (1950). The comparison of percentages in matched samples, *Biometrika* **37**, 256–266.

[13] Cochran, W.G. (1954). Some methods for strengthening the χ^2 test, *Biometrics* **10**, 417–457.

[14] Darroch, J.N. (1981). The Mantel–Haenszel test and tests of marginal symmetry: fixed effects and mixed models for a categorical response, *International Statistical Review* **49**, 285–307.

[15] Davis, C.S. & Chung, Y. (1995). Randomization model methods for evaluating treatment efficacy in multicenter clinical trials, *Biometrics* **51**, 1163–1174.

[16] Davis, L.J. (1985). Generalization of the Mantel–Haenszel estimator to nonconstant odds ratios, *Biometrics* **41**, 487–495.

[17] Dayal, H.H. (1978). On the desirability of the Mantel–Haenszel summary measure in case-control studies of multi-factor etiology of disease, *American Journal of Epidemiology* **108**, 506–511.

[18] Flanders, W.D. (1985). A new variance estimator for the Mantel–Haenszel odds ratio, *Biometrics* **41**, 637–642.

[19] Fleiss, J.L. (1981). *Statistical Methods for Rates and Proportions*, 2nd Ed. Wiley, New York.

[20] Friedman, M. (1937). The use of ranks to avoid the assumption of normality implicit in the analysis of variance, *Journal of the American Statistical Association* **32**, 675–701.

[21] Gart, J.J. (1962). On the combination of relative risks, *Biometrics* **18**, 601–610.

[22] Gart, J.J. (1966). Alternative analyses of contingency tables, *Journal of the Royal Statistical Society, Series B* **28**, 164–179.

[23] Gart, J.J. (1970). Point and interval estimation of the common odds ratio in the combination of 2 × 2 tables with fixed marginals, *Biometrics* **57**, 471–475.

[24] Gart, J.J. (1971). The comparison of proportions: a review of significance tests, confidence intervals and adjustment for stratification, *Review of the International Statistical Institute* **39**, 48–61.

[25] Gart, J.J. & Zweifel, J.R. (1967). On the bias of various estimators of the logit and its variance with application to quantal bioassay, *Biometrika* **54**, 181–187.

[26] Greenland, S. (1982). Interpretation and estimation of summary ratios under heterogeneity, *Statistics in Medicine* **1**, 217–227.

[27] Greenland, S. (1989). Generalized Mantel–Haenszel estimators for K 2 × J tables, *Biometrics* **45**, 183–191.

[28] Hauck, W.W., Anderson, S. & Leahy, F.J. (1982). Finite-sample properties of some old and some new estimators of a common odds ratio from multiple 2 × 2 tables, *Journal of the American Statistical Association* **77**, 145–152.

[29] Koch, G.G. & Edwards, S. (1987). Clinical efficacy trials with categorical data, in *Statistical Methods in the Pharmaceutical Industry*, K. Peace, ed. Marcel Dekker, New York, see Chapter 9.

[30] Koch, G.G., Gillings, D.B. & Stokes, M.E. (1980). Biostatistical implications of design, sampling, and measurement to health science data analysis, *Annual Review of Public Health* **1**, 163–225.

[31] Koch, G.G., Amara, I.A., Davis, G.W. & Gillings, D.B. (1982). A review of some statistical methods for covariance analysis of categorical data, *Biometrics* **38**, 563–595.

[32] Koch, G.G., Imrey, P.B., Singer, J.M., Atkinson, S.S. & Stokes, M.E. (1985). *Analysis of Categorical Data*. Presses de l'Université Montreal, Montreal.

[33] Kuritz, S.J. & Landis, J.R. (1988). Attributable risk estimation from matched case–control data, *Biometrics* **44**, 355–367.

[34] Kuritz, S.J., Landis, J.R. & Koch, G.G. (1988). A general overview of Mantel–Haenszel methods: applications and recent developments, *Annual Review of Public Health* **9**, 123–160.

[35] Landis, J.R., Heyman, E.R. & Koch, G.G. (1978). Average partial association in three way contingency tables: a review and discussion of alternative tests, *International Statistical Review* **46**, 237–254.

[36] Landis, J.R., Cooper, M.M., Kennedy, T. & Koch, G.G. (1979). A computer program for testing average partial association in three-way contingency tables (PARCAT), *Computer Programs in Biomedicine* **9**, 223–246.

[37] Landis, J.R., Miller, M.E., Davis, C.S. & Koch, G.G. (1988). Some general methods for the analysis of

categorical data in longitudinal studies, *Statistics in Medicine* **7**, 109–137.

[38]   Lehmann, E.L. & Dabrerd, H.J.M. (1975). *Nonparametrics: Statistical Methods Based on Ranks.* Holden–Day, San Francisco.

[39]   Liang, K.Y. (1987). Extended Mantel–Haenszel estimating procedure for multivariate logistic regression models, *Biometrics* **43**, 289–299.

[40]   Lynch, J.C., Landis, J.R. & Localio, A.R. (1991). StatXact. *American Statistician* **45**, 151–154.

[41]   Madansky, A. (1963). Tests of homogeneity for correlated samples, *Journal of the American Statistical Association* **58**, 97–119.

[42]   Mantel, N. (1963). Chi-square tests with one degree of freedom: extensions of the Mantel–Haenszel procedure, *Journal of the American Statistical Association* **58**, 690–700.

[43]   Mantel, N. (1977). Tests and limits for the common odds ratio of several 2 × 2 contingency tables: methods in analogy with the Mantel–Haenszel procedure, *Journal of Statistical Planning and Inference* **1**, 179–189.

[44]   Mantel, N. & Byar, D.P. (1978). Marginal homogeneity, symmetry and independence, *Communications in Statistics – Theory and Methods A* **7**, 953–976.

[45]   Mantel, N. & Fleiss, J.L. (1980). Minimum expected cell size requirements for the Mantel–Haenszel one degree of freedom chi-square test and a related rapid procedure, *American Journal of Epidemiology* **112**, 129–134.

[46]   Mantel, N. & Haenszel, W. (1959). Statistical aspects of the analysis of data from retrospective studies of disease, *Journal of the National Cancer Institute* **22**, 719–748.

[47]   McKinlay, S.M. (1978). The effect of nonzero second-order interaction on combined estimators of the odds ratio, *Biometrika* **65**, 191–202.

[48]   McNemar, Q. (1947). Note on the sampling error of the difference between correlated proportions or percentages, *Psychometrika* **12**, 153–157.

[49]   Mickey, R.M. & Elashoff, R.M. (1985). A generalization of the Mantel–Haenszel estimator of partial association for 2 × J × K tables, *Biometrics* **41**, 623–635.

[50]   Mehta, C. & Patel, N. (1995). *StatXact.* CYTEL Software Corporation, Cambridge.

[51]   O'Gorman, T.W., Woolson, R.F., Jones, M.P. & Lemke, J.H. (1990). Statistical analysis of *K* 2 × 2 tables: a comparative study of estimators/test statistics for association and homogeneity, *Environmental Health Perspectives* **87**, 103–107.

[52]   Ramakrishnan, V., Goldberg, J., Henderson, W.G., Eisen, S.A., True, W., Lyons, M.J. & Tsuang, M.T. (1992). Elementary methods for the analysis of dichotomous outcomes in unselected samples of twins, *Genetic Epidemiology* **9**, 273–287.

[53]   Robins, J., Breslow, N. & Greenland, S. (1986). Estimators of the Mantel–Haenszel variance consistent in both sparse data and large strata limiting models, *Biometrics* **42**, 311–324.

[54]   SAS Institute Inc. (1989). *SAS/STAT User's Guide, Version 6*, 4th Ed., Vol. 1. SAS Institute Inc., Cary.

[55]   Sato, T. (1991). An estimating equation approach for the analysis of case-control studies with exposure measured at several levels, *Statistics in Medicine* **10**, 1037–1042.

[56]   Sato, T. (1992). Estimation of a common risk ratio in stratified case–cohort studies, *Statistics in Medicine* **11**, 1599–1605.

[57]   Sato, T. (1994). Risk ratio estimation in case–cohort studies, *Environmental Health Perspectives* **102**, Supplement 8, 53–56.

[58]   Somes, G.W. (1986). The generalized Mantel–Haenszel statistic, *American Statistician* **40**, 106–108.

[59]   Stokes, M., Davis, C.S. & Koch, G.G. (1995). *SAS for Categorical Data Analysis.* SAS Institute Inc., Cary.

[60]   Tarone, R.E., Gatt, J.J. & Hauck, W.W. (1983). On the asymptotic inefficiency of certain noniterative estimators of a common relative risk or odds ratio, *Biometrika* **70**, 519–522.

[61]   van Elteren, P.H. (1960). On the combination of independent two-sample tests of Wilcoxon, *Bulletin of the International Statistical Institute* **37**, 351–361.

[62]   White, A.A., Landis, J.R. & Cooper, M.M. (1982). A note on the equivalence of several marginal homogeneity test criteria for categorical data, *International Statistical Review* **50**, 27–34.

[63]   Woolf, B. (1955). On estimating the relation between blood group and disease, *Annals of Human Genetics* **19**, 251–253.

Appendix

Under H_0 in (1), the observed frequencies in Table 1 have expected values,

$$E\{\mathbf{n}_h | H_0\} = n_h[\mathbf{p}_{h.*} \otimes \mathbf{p}_{h*.}] = \mathbf{m}_h, \qquad (A1)$$

where $\mathbf{p}_{h.*}$ contains the marginal column proportions $(n_{h.j}/n_h)$ in the hth stratum, $\mathbf{p}_{h*.}$ contains the marginal row proportions $(n_{hi.}/n_h)$ in the hth stratum, and $\otimes$ denotes left-hand Kronecker product multiplication, where the matrix on the left multiplies each element in the matrix on the right.

Furthermore, the covariance matrix for these observed frequencies under the null hypothesis of randomness in (1) is

$$V\{\mathbf{n}_h | H_0\} = \frac{n_h^2}{n_h - 1}(\mathbf{D}_{\mathbf{p}_{h.*}} - \mathbf{p}_{h.*}\mathbf{p}'_{h.*})$$

$$\otimes (\mathbf{D}_{\mathbf{p}_{h*.}} - \mathbf{p}_{h*.}\mathbf{p}'_{h*.}) = \mathbf{V}_h, \quad (A2)$$

where $\mathbf{D}_{\mathbf{p}_h}$ is a diagonal matrix with elements of the vector $\mathbf{p}_h$ on the main diagonal.

Without loss of generality, let $\mathbf{A}_{1h} = [(\mathbf{I}_{(r-1)}, \mathbf{0}_{(r-1)}) \otimes (\mathbf{I}_{(s-1)}, \mathbf{0}_{(s-1)})]$ be a linear operator matrix, which eliminates the last row and last column frequencies from each stratum. Then the generalized MH test for H_0 against the nonspecific alternative that the distributions of the response variable are not homogeneous across the s factor levels is

$$Q_{\text{MH}(1)} = \left\{ \sum_{h=1}^{t} (\mathbf{n}_h - \mathbf{m}_h)' \mathbf{A}_{1h}' \right\} \left\{ \sum_{h=1}^{t} \mathbf{A}_{1h} \mathbf{V}_h \mathbf{A}_{1h}' \right\}^{-1}$$
$$\times \left\{ \sum_{h=1}^{t} \mathbf{A}_{1h} (\mathbf{n}_h - \mathbf{m}_h) \right\}, \qquad (A3)$$

which follows a chi-square distribution with df $= (s-1)(r-1)$ under H_0 for large $n_{.ij}$.

If the response variable is reported on an ordinal scale, scores can be assigned to the response levels to compute row mean scores. In this case, the alternative hypothesis to "no partial association" is that there are location shifts for these mean scores across factor levels of the row variable. Let $\mathbf{A}_{2h} = \mathbf{a}_h' \otimes [\mathbf{I}_{(s-1)}, \mathbf{0}_{(s-1)}]$ be an $(s-1) \times sr$ matrix with $\mathbf{a}_h' = (a_{h1}, \ldots, a_{hr})$, where a_{hj} is the score chosen to reflect the ordinal nature of the jth level of response for the hth stratum. Then the MH test for equality among the mean responses for the s subpopulations relative to the response variable score vectors $\{\mathbf{a}_h\}$ is

$$Q_{\text{MH}(2)} = \left\{ \sum_{h=1}^{t} (\mathbf{n}_h - \mathbf{m}_h)' \mathbf{A}_{2h}' \right\} \left\{ \sum_{h=1}^{t} \mathbf{A}_{2h} \mathbf{V}_h \mathbf{A}_{2h}' \right\}^{-1}$$
$$\times \left\{ \sum_{h=1}^{t} \mathbf{A}_{2h} (\mathbf{n}_h - \mathbf{m}_h) \right\}, \qquad (A4)$$

which follows a chi-square distribution with df $= (s-1)$ under H_0 for large $n_{.i.}$.

When both the response variable and the row variable are ordinally scaled, scores can be assigned to both the response levels and the factor levels in the hth stratum. In this situation, the test is directed at the extent to which there is a linear trend on the mean scores across the levels of the row variable, or equivalently, a nonzero correlation between the row and column variables. For this case, let $\mathbf{A}_{3h} = [\mathbf{a}_h' \otimes \mathbf{c}_h']$, where the $\{\mathbf{a}_h\}$ are defined as before and the $\{\mathbf{c}_h\} = (c_{h1}, c_{h2}, \ldots, c_{hs})$ specify a set of scores for the ith level of the row variable in the hth stratum.

The resulting test statistic

$$Q_{\text{MH}(3)} = \left\{ \sum_{h=1}^{t} (\mathbf{n}_h - \mathbf{m}_h)' \mathbf{A}_{3h}' \right\} \left\{ \sum_{h=1}^{t} \mathbf{A}_{3h} \mathbf{V}_h \mathbf{A}_{3h}' \right\}^{-1}$$
$$\times \left\{ \sum_{h=1}^{t} \mathbf{A}_{3h} (\mathbf{n}_h - \mathbf{m}_h) \right\}, \qquad (A5)$$

follows a chi-square distribution with df $= 1$ under H_0 for large $N = \sum_{h=1}^{t} n_h$. Further discussion of these three expressions of the MH statistic and their implementation using SAS [54] can be found in Stokes et al. [59].

J. RICHARD LANDIS, TONYA J. SHARP, STEPHEN J. KURITZ & GARY G. KOCH

Mantel's Test for Clustering *see* Clustering

Mapping Disease Patterns

For as long as disease patterns have been mapped there has been skepticism over the value of the pictures which are drawn. For instance, a map of the geography of the 1832 influenza epidemic in Glasgow (Scotland) was produced by the inmates of a lunatic asylum, mainly to occupy their time [1]. Later, in the nineteenth century, the value of mapping disease patterns was recognized as specific epidemiologic breakthroughs were attributed to the insight gained from mapping. Often cited is a map of the distribution of deaths from the 1848 cholera epidemic in London (England) which, so the tale goes, inspired the removal of the handle of the water pump at the center of a cluster of dots on the map, resulting in the curtailing of the epidemic [12].

Maps of diseases are like news pictures of crowd trouble. Viewers should always ask themselves what is not being shown in the map while looking at what is there. In particular, look around the edge of the map. Ask why it ends where it does. For instance, maps of diseases are often centered on the point the

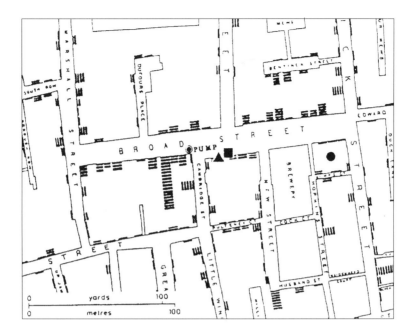

Figure 1 John Snow's map of cholera deaths in Soho, London, 1854 – taken from Cliff & Haggett [1, Figure 1.15D]

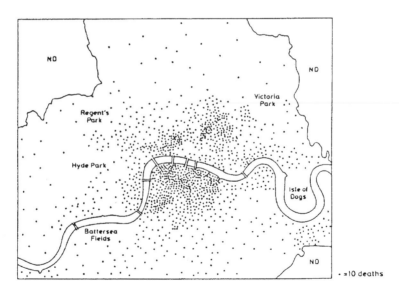

Figure 2 Cholera deaths in London in 1849 – taken from Cliff & Haggett [1, Figure 1.3B]

author thinks is most important. Figure 1 shows the central section of John Snow's map of deaths from cholera in Soho. Note how the eye is drawn to the pump in the center, particularly by the very high number of deaths at the intersection of Cambridge and Broad Streets. Had Snow drawn his map of all of London he would have discovered a greater density of deaths just south of the river Thames, as shown in Figure 2. This concentration would have changed location again had Snow had recourse to an

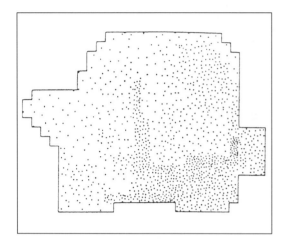

Figure 3 Figure 2 on a population cartogram – taken from Cliff & Haggett [1, Figure 1.18D]

isodemographic base map, as shown in Figure 3. As our picture of a disease pans out, as we include more cases and as we change the way we view the picture, the patterns on our maps show change too.

Disease mapping has been most strongly influenced by the history of diseases. Figure 4 shows the prevalence of 12 major causes of death in England and Wales since the publication of Snow's map of cholera. Infectious diseases now account for a tiny fraction of deaths in developed countries (which can afford most disease mapping

and research). It is causes of death which are not declining, such as suicide, and those which are rising in importance, such as cancers, which increasingly interest researchers. For these causes of illness and death the analysis of point patterns around particular sites is still a major issue, but the patterns are usually far less clearly spatially defined than were outbreaks of cholera. More importantly, it is increasingly being accepted that more abstract factors, such as social inequality, can lie behind particular patterns of disease, and these require more abstract mappings for their study.

There are many different ways of mapping disease but here there is only space to explore one alternative. The alternatives include traditional choropleth mapping, where areas on a map are shaded according to statistics about the population. Most common in epidemiology is the mapping of areas colored by their standardized mortality ratios. Another common form of mapping is to map points or the incidences of disease, and often color is also used here to highlight different types of disease. Various different point symbols can be used in mapping, particularly common is the use of proportional circles which are colored or segmented to highlight different features of a disease. The size of the circles is often made proportional to the population at risk of contracting a disease, at which point this type of cartography begins to merge into isodemographic mapping [4, 5].

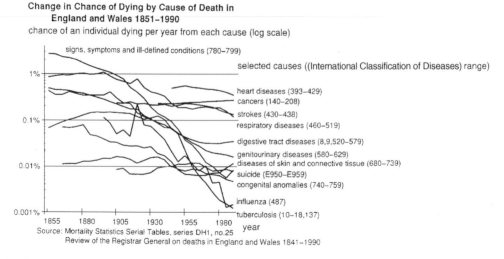

Figure 4 Cause of death 1855–1990 – taken from Dorling [3, Figure 5.21]

Diseases occur across a population as much as across land. That is not to say that geographic distributions are not important, but that we should take account of the distribution of the population at risk to a particular disease, or cause, before mapping its pattern. One way in which this can be done is to use a map projection which draws every area in proportion to the number of people at risk living in that area – hence the term isodemographic ("equal people"). Isodemographic maps, more commonly called cartograms, are used for many purposes, mostly obviously in mapping the geography of elections. However, their most established use has been in disease mapping. Figure 5 shows one of the earliest examples of a cartogram designed for epidemiologic purposes [15, p. 1023]. Figure 5(a) is the conventional map of the counties of Iowa State, and Figure 5(b) is an equal population cartogram upon which colored pins were placed to show the locations of reportable diseases. The square in the middle of the cartogram is Des Moines city in Polk County.

The designer of the Iowa cartogram was a doctor working in the state department of health. Many researchers have been struck by the idea that they could learn more about disease through mapping it in unconventional ways. The first cartogram of London was an "epidemiologic map" produced by a doctor working for the then London County Council Department of Public Health [14]. The cartogram (Figure 6) contained crosses drawn in the borough rectangles to show the incidence of polio during the 1947 epidemic. Because the rectangles were each drawn with the same height, their widths are proportional to population as well as their areas. The borough with the highest rate of polio and hence the tallest column of crosses in the Figure was Shoreditch. Almost exactly 100 years separates the two London epidemics, which were first drawn on a map and cartogram, respectively. Cartograms showing distributions within countries came later.

A claim was made to have produced the first cartograms showing national disease distributions only a decade after the crude cartogram of London was first drawn [6]. The nation was Scotland, and a separate cartogram was constructed by hand for each of eight age–sex groups. Figure 7 shows the cartogram being used to study the 1959–1963 mortality of women in Scotland aged 45–54. The author of this cartogram concluded that a national series of cartograms should

be produced for each age–sex group for use in epidemiologic studies in Britain. This was never done, and it is debatable whether such an exact mapping base is needed in most studies. A single isodemographic base map of the whole population will usually suffice to uncover all but the most subtle of patterns.

A National Atlas of Disease Mortality in the UK was published in 1963 under the auspices of the Royal Geographical Society; the atlas contained no cartograms. However, a revised edition was published a few years later which made copious use of a "demographic base map" [7]. It is interesting to note that, when the revised edition was being prepared, the president of the Society was Dudley Stamp, who believed that "The fundamental tool for the geographical analysis is undoubtedly the map or, perhaps more correctly, the cartogram" [13, p. 135]. In the cartogram which was used in the revised national atlas (Figure 8), squares were used to represent urban areas, while diamonds were used to show statistics for rural districts. No attempt was made to maintain contiguity, but a stylized coastline was placed around the symbols, which were all drawn with their areas in proportion to the populations at risk from the disease being shown on each particular cartogram.

In the *National Atlas of Disease Mortality in the United Kingdom*, Howe used a national cartogram to display the distribution of standardized mortality between 1959 and 1963 from separate as well as all causes of death for both men and women. High rates were seen in northern districts and some Inner London boroughs (including Shoreditch, which is also highlighted on one of the earliest cartograms of London; see above). Extremely high rates in central Scotland were particularly noticeable, as were the low rates in districts which surround London. At the extremes the average man living in Salford was 50% more likely to die each year than his counterpart in Bournemouth [7]. Both these areas are shrunk on a "normal" map. The pattern for women was very similar to that for men although, in general, it was less pronounced. However, women did have the highest mortality rate of any area on the map in rural Dunbartonshire, where they were more than twice as likely to die each year than were women nationally (allowing for local age structure). The cartogram highlights this area, but also puts it in the perspective of the populations at risk from the high mortality rates for women in and around the Glasgow area. Questions for investigation are immediately

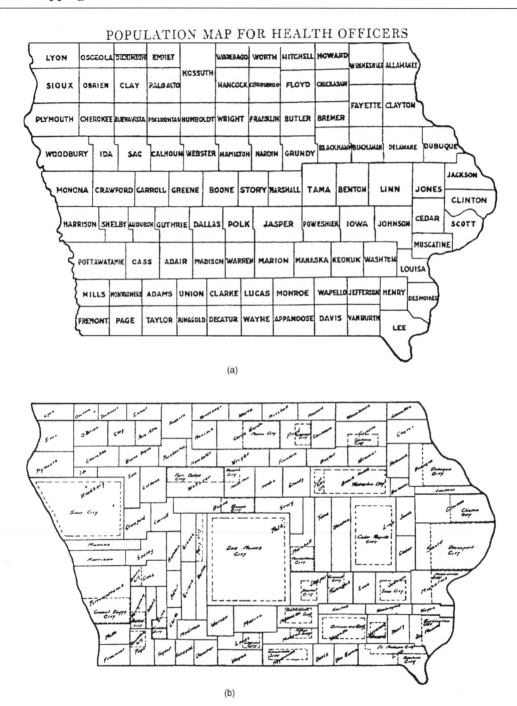

Figure 5   The use of cold vaccine in Iowa County Area, 1926 – taken from Wallace [15, p. 1023]

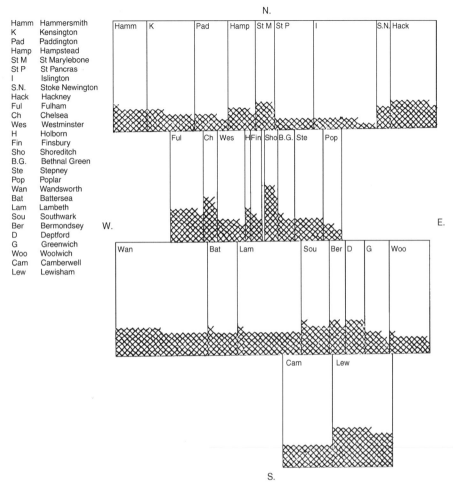

Figure 6 London borough cartogram showing 1947 poliomyelitis notifications – taken from Taylor [14, p. 201]

generated by comparing the maps in Howe's atlases with those produced by Forster for a decade earlier (see Figure 7).

Isodemographic mapping is also used to study the prevalence of disease – individual cases of a disease or death which together might possibly be connected. Figure 9 shows the distribution of cases of Wilm's tumor, a childhood cancer, identified in New York State between 1958 and 1962, drawn upon an equal land area map. Apparent clusters of cases have been marked on the map [8]. In the second diagram in Figure 9, the same cases are drawn upon an equal population cartogram and the apparent clusters can be seen to have been quite evenly dispersed across the population. The same process has been used in

Figure 10 to illustrate how cases of Salmonella food poisoning occurring in Arkansas in 1974 were not unduly clustered in Pulaski county [2].

In recent years researchers have turned their attention to trying to develop cartograms upon which actual, rather than illusory, clusters of disease can be identified (*see* **Clustering**). The major problem with using population cartograms to identify clusters of disease is that the choice of which areas are closest to which on a cartogram can be quite arbitrary. For instance, if the same set of incidences of one particular disease were plotted on three different cartograms, then different parts of the country may appear to have dense clusters of cases depending on which cartogram was chosen. This would be

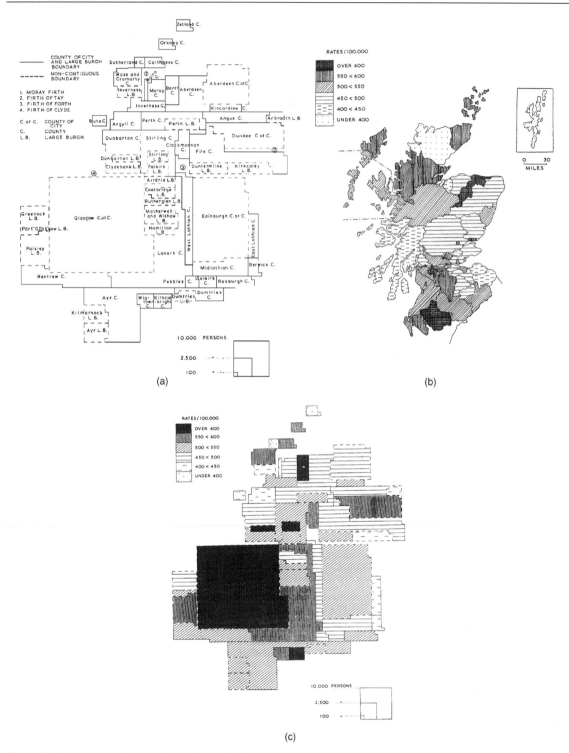

Figure 7   Cartogram and map of Scottish health districts – taken from Forster [6]. (a) Cartogram of females aged 45–54 in 1961 by Scottish health districts; (b) map of 1959–63 mortality rates of females aged 45–54 by district; (c) 1959–63 mortality rates of females aged 45–54 shown in (a)

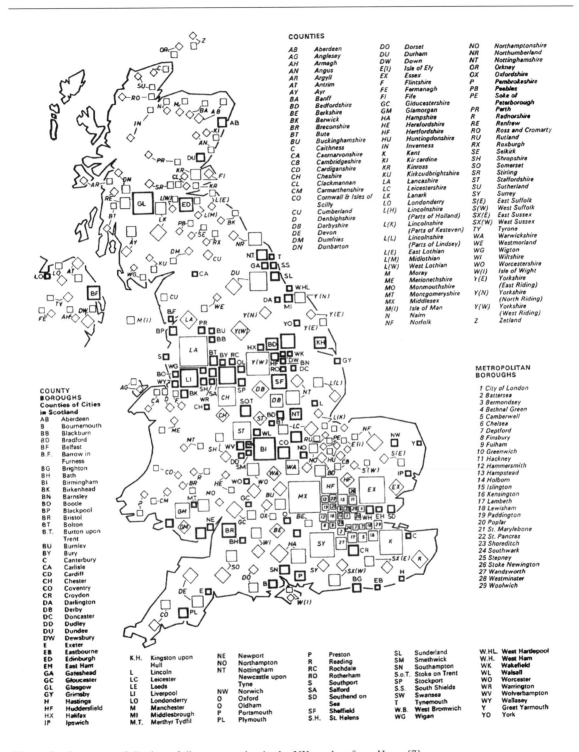

Figure 8 Cartogram of districts of disease mapping in the UK – taken from Howe [7]

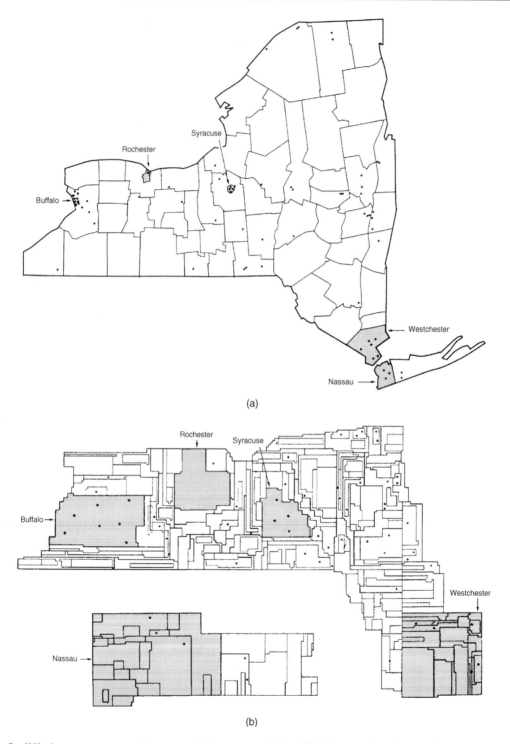

(a)

(b)

Figure 9   Wilm's tumour cases on (a) map and (b) cartogram in New York State – taken from Levison & Haddon [8]

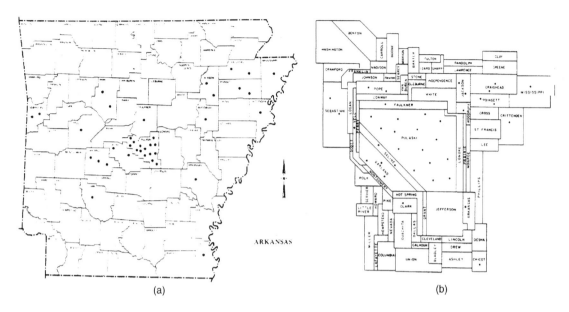

Figure 10   Salmonella Newport cases on (a) map and (b) cartogram in Arkansas State – taken from Dean [2]

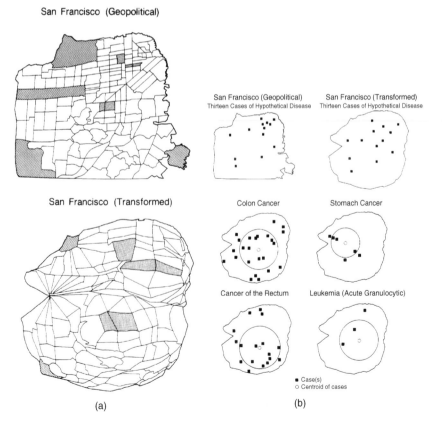

Figure 11   San Francisco map (a) for 1980 census, and cartogram (b) of hypothetical and actual diseases – taken from Selvin et al. [11]

true regardless of whether the clusters were to be identified by eye or by statistical procedures; the different base maps would result in different patterns emerging. The proposition that there is no single "true answer" as to whether a disease is clustered does not go down too well in some circles. Because of this problem a group of researchers at Berkeley developed a computer algorithm for identifying incidences of disease [9]. The algorithm was used to produce the cartogram in Figure 11 of San Francisco county, upon which apparent clusters of disease were shown to be false [11]. However, application of the method to another California county did provide evidence of some clustering of high cancer rates near oil refineries [10].

Mapping of disease patterns is becoming increasingly common due to the proliferation of computer mapping. However, many of these programs were designed to produce general maps of any subject and are often most appropriate to show land use or the distribution of points in physical space. Over most of the course of the last century, doctors, public health officials, and researchers have discovered and rediscovered that traditional maps often do not provide the most appropriate projection to look for patterns of disease. Here, a few alternatives have been shown of just one different form of disease mapping to try to explain why it involves more than just sticking pins in paper.

Acknowledgments

The author is grateful to Robert Israel for commenting on a draft of this article and to the following people for permission to reproduce the copyright material shown here: Peter Haggett (*Atlas of Disease Distributions*) for Figures 1–3; Pam Beckley (Her Majesty's Stationery Office) for Figure 5; Michael Plommer (Office for National Statistics) for Figure 6; Carol Torselli (*British Medical Journal*) for Figure 7; Marian Tebben (*Public Health Reports*) for Figure 9; and Mina Chung (American Public Health Association) for Figure 10.

References

[1]   Cliff, A.D. & Haggett, P. (1988). *Atlas of Disease Distributions. Analytical Approaches to Epidemiological Data*. Blackwell, Oxford.

[2]   Dean, A.G. (1976). Population-based spot maps: an epidemiologic technique, *American Journal of Public Health* **66**, 988–989.

[3]   Dorling, D. (1995). *A New Social Atlas of Britain*. Wiley, Chichester.

[4]   Dorling, D. (1996). *Area Cartograms: Their Use and Creation*, Concepts and Techniques in Modern Geography (CATMOG) no. 59. School of Environmental Sciences, University of East Anglia, Norwich.

[5]   Dorling, D. & Fairbairn, D. (1997). *Mapping: Ways of Representing the World*. Longman, London.

[6]   Forster, F. (1966). Use of a demographic base map for the presentation of areal data in epidemiology, *British Journal of Preventive and Social Medicine* **20**, 165–171.

[7]   Howe, G.M. (1970). *National Atlas of Disease Mortality in the United Kingdom*, Revised and Enlarged Edition. Nelson, London.

[8]   Levison, M.E. & Haddon, W. (1965). The area adjusted map: an epidemiological device, *Public Health Reports* **80**, 55–59.

[9]   Selvin, S., Merrill, D., Sacks, S., Wong, L., Bedell, L. & Schulman, J. (1984). *Transformations of Maps to Investigate Clusters of Disease*. Laboratory Report, LBL-18550, Lawrence, Berkeley.

[10] Selvin, S., Shaw, G., Schulman, J. & Merrill, D. (1987). Spatial distribution of disease: three case studies, *Journal of the National Cancer Institute* **79**, 417–423.

[11] Selvin, S., Merrill, D., Schulman, J., Sacks, S., Bedell, L. & Wong, L. (1988). Transformations of maps to investigate clusters of disease, *Social Science and Medicine* **26**, 215–221.

[12] Snow, J. (1854). *On the Mode of Communication of Cholera*. Churchill Livingstone, London.

[13] Stamp, L.D. (1962). A geographer's postscript, in *Taxonomy and Geography*, D. Nichols, ed. The Systematics Association, London, pp. 153–158.

[14] Taylor, I. (1955). An epidemiology map, *Ministry of Health Monthly Bulletin* **14**, 200–201.

[15] Wallace, J.M. (1926). Population map for health officers, *American Journal of Public Health* **16**, 1023.

(*See also* **Geographic Patterns of Disease**; **Geographical Analysis**)

DANIEL DORLING

Markers *see* Biased Sampling of Cohorts in Epidemiology

Mass Action *see* Epidemic Models, Deterministic

Matched Analysis

On grounds of both validity and efficiency, the appropriate analysis of data involving category matching mandates the use of stratified analysis methods based on the strata used in the matching process [6] (*see* **Stratification**). Two important methods for analyzing category matched (or, more generally, stratified) data are the **Mantel–Haenszel** procedure [9] and **conditional logistic regression** (see [1, Chapter 7], and [5, Chapter 20]).

The Mantel–Haenszel (MH) test statistic [9] is the most widely used and recommended method for testing for overall association in a stratified analysis. And, as we will see, the MH test statistic for stratified data analysis is based on the (central) hypergeometric distribution. For dichotomous disease and exposure variables (the setting for this presentation), the MH testing procedure involves a one degree-of-freedom (continuity-corrected) chi-squared statistic of the general form

$$\chi^2_{\text{MH}} = [|A - \text{E}_0(A)| - 1/2]^2 / \text{var}_0(A), \quad (1)$$

where A is the random variable denoting the total number (over all strata) of diseased subjects in each stratum who are exposed (i.e. the total number of "exposed cases"), $\text{E}_0(A)$ is the expected total number of exposed cases under the null hypothesis of no association between exposure and disease, and $\text{var}_0(A)$ is the variance of the total number of exposed cases under the same null hypothesis.

Suppose that there are G strata defined by the matching process, with the gth stratum having the structure given in Table 1.

Table 1 Data layout for the gth stratum ($g = 1, 2, \ldots, G$)

	E	$\bar{E}$	
D	A_g	B_g	m_{1g}
$\bar{D}$	C_g	D_g	m_{0g}
	n_{1g}	n_{0g}	n_g

The four marginal frequencies n_{1g}, n_{0g}, m_{1g}, and m_{0g} in the gth stratum convey no information about the strength of the association between exposure and disease in that stratum, but rather indicate only the "amount of information" in that stratum. Consequently, the four marginal frequencies within each stratum may be assumed (with no compromise to validity) to be "fixed" for analysis purposes, even though the sampling scheme actually used may not have imposed such constraints on the margins of these G 2×2 tables.

Conditional on these fixed margins for all strata, it is sufficient to focus entirely on the "A_g cell", namely, the number of exposed cases in the gth stratum, $g = 1, 2, \ldots, G$. The test statistic (1) is then a conditional test since properties of the random variable $A = \sum_{g=1}^{G} A_g$ are based on the condition that the four margins in each stratum are fixed. More specifically, assuming fixed margins and no exposure-disease association, A_g is a (central) hypergeometric random variable, so that

$$\text{E}_0(A) = \sum_{g=1}^{G} (n_{1g} m_{1g})/n_g \quad \text{and}$$

$$\text{var}_0(A) = \sum_{g=1}^{G} (n_{1g} n_{0g} m_{1g} m_{0g})/(n_g - 1)n_g^2.$$

Finally, some algebra can be used to write expression (1) in the form

$$\chi^2_{\text{MH}} = \frac{\left[\left|\sum_{g=1}^{G} (A_g D_g - B_g C_g)/n_g\right| - 1/2\right]^2}{\sum_{g=1}^{G} (n_{1g} n_{0g} m_{1g} m_{0g})/(n_g - 1)n_g^2}; \quad (2)$$

under the null hypothesis of no exposure–disease association, it can be shown that the test statistic (2) has, for "large samples", an approximate chi-square distribution with 1 df.

It is very important to stress that the "large samples" assumption for the test statistic (2) pertains to the pooled information over all G strata, rather than to stratum-specific numbers. Consequently, in the use of the MH test statistic (2), it is permissible to have relatively small numbers in each stratum as long as the total number of subjects on the margins over all strata is sufficiently large. Without going into detail, this form of robustness to sparse stratum-specific data accrues due to the assumption of fixed stratum-specific margins, an assumption that maintains validity at only a slight cost in efficiency.

Specific criteria for appropriate sample sizes to maintain the validity of the chi-squared approximation for (2) have been proposed by Mantel & Fleiss [8]. They recommend using (2) provided that the quantities

$$\mathrm{E}_0(A) - \left[\sum_{g=1}^{G} \max(0, m_{1g} - n_{0g})\right] \quad \text{and}$$

$$\left[\sum_{g=1}^{G} \min(n_{1g}, m_{1g})\right] - \mathrm{E}_0(A)$$

both exceed 5 in value.

It is important to mention that the use of the MH test statistic (2) should be avoided when there is evidence of strong **effect modification** in the data, as would be reflected by widely varying stratum-specific estimated **odds ratios** $\widehat{\mathrm{OR}}_g = A_g D_g / B_g C_g, g = 1, 2, \ldots, G$. Because of the structure of the numerator in (2), the value of (2) can be very small (suggesting no exposure–disease association) when, in fact, some stratum-specific estimated odds ratios are significantly greater than 1 and some are significantly less than 1. Indeed, claims of optimal statistical properties for the MH test [11] are valid only in the situation where stratum-specific population odds ratios all have the same value. Tests for lack of uniformity of stratum-specific odds ratios are discussed in Chapter 4 of [1].

Given the assumption of a common population odds ratio for all strata, it makes sense to compute a summary estimator of this common odds ratio; such an estimator is typically a weighted average of the G stratum-specific estimated odds ratios. Mantel & Haenszel [9] proposed several such summary estimators for use in **case–control studies**. The most notable of these is the $\widehat{\mathrm{mOR}}$, which is defined as

$$\widehat{\mathrm{mOR}} = \left[\sum_{g=1}^{G}(A_g D_g)/n_g\right] \Bigg/ \left[\sum_{g=1}^{G}(B_g C_g/n_g)\right]$$

$$= \sum_{g=1}^{G} W_g(\widehat{\mathrm{OR}}_g) \Bigg/ \sum_{g=1}^{G} W_g, \qquad (3)$$

where $W_g = B_g C_g / n_g$. An interesting property of $\widehat{\mathrm{mOR}}$ is that it equals unity only when expression (2) is zero, a property that is not shared by other summary estimators (see [5, Chapter 17]). Another advantage of the $\widehat{\mathrm{mOR}}$ over other summary estimators

is that it can be used without alteration when there are zero frequencies within the body of some of the stratum-specific tables.

For certain types of matched data, expressions (2) and (3) have simple structures. As one example, for a matched pairs case–control study where each stratum (or pair) consists of one case and one control, then expression (2) reduces to $(b-c)^2/(b+c)$ apart from continuity correction, and expression (3) equals b/c, where b is the number of strata where the case is exposed and the control is not, and c is the number of strata where the control is exposed and the case is not. For the special case of R-to-1 matching, see either Chapter 5 in [1] or Chapter 18 in [5]. For confidence interval methods based on (3) in case–control studies with multiple matching, see [3], [12], and [13]. Finally, some generalizations of the MH test have been developed for situations where the exposure variable is nominal with several categories [9] and where the exposure variable is ordinal in nature [2, 7].

A more general and flexible method for the analysis of matched (or, in general, stratified) data is conditional logistic regression (*see* **Logistic Regression, Conditional**). This multivariable modeling procedure is specifically designed to be used when there are small stratum-specific sample sizes. Hence, it is ideally suited for the analysis of matched study designs or to similar situations involving very fine stratification; in fact, its use in these situations is mandatory to avoid **biased** estimates of important odds ratio parameters. In contrast to stratified data analysis methods, conditional logistic regression methods do not require all variables to be categorized; for example, continuous exposure, **confounding**, and effect-modifying variables can be treated as such. In addition, it is theoretically possible to consider simultaneously in one model several exposure variables and to examine potential confounding and effect modification effects due to covariates not involved in the matching process.

Suppose we consider the case–control format, with $\mathbf{x}_{1g}, \mathbf{x}_{2g}, \ldots, \mathbf{x}_{m_g g}$ denoting the observed data vectors for the total of $m_g = (m_{1g} + m_{0g})$ cases and controls in the gth stratum, $g = 1, 2, \ldots, G$. Without loss of generality, we arrange these data vectors so that the first m_{1g} vectors belong to the m_{1g} cases in the gth stratum. For a dichotomous response variable D with $D = 1$ signifying a case and $D = 0$ signifying a control, consider fitting by conditional logistic regression the logistic model

$$\text{logit}[\Pr(D_{lg} = 1)] = \alpha_g + \boldsymbol{\beta}' \mathbf{x}_{lg},$$

$$l = 1, 2, \ldots, m_g \quad \text{and} \quad g = 1, 2, \ldots, G.$$

Then, the contribution from the gth stratum to the full conditional likelihood (CL) has the structure

$$\text{CL}_g = \prod_{l=1}^{m_{1g}} \exp(\boldsymbol{\beta}' \mathbf{x}_{lg}) \Big/ \sum_u \left[\prod_{l=1}^{m_{1g}} \exp(\boldsymbol{\beta}' \mathbf{x}_{ulg}) \right],$$

(4)

where the sum $\sum_u$ in the denominator is over all partitions of the set of integers $\{1, 2, \ldots, m_g\}$ into two subsets, the first of which contains m_{1g} elements; there are $m_g!/m_{1g}!m_{0g}!$ such partitions. Thus, CL_g is the conditional probability that the first m_{1g} of the m_g data vectors $\mathbf{x}_{1g}, \mathbf{x}_{2g}, \ldots, \mathbf{x}_{m_g g}$ go with the cases (as they actually do) considering all possible arrangements of these m_g data vectors; in other words, CL_g is the conditional probability of the observed data. The full CL is then equal to $\text{CL} = \prod_{g=1}^{G} \text{CL}_g$, and standard maximum likelihood methods can be used to estimate and to make inferences about the elements of $\boldsymbol{\beta}$.

It is important to note that the CL based on (4) depends only on $\boldsymbol{\beta}$, the parameter vector of interest. The nuisance parameters $\alpha_1, \alpha_2, \ldots, \alpha_G$ indexing the matching strata have been eliminated via this permutation procedure, thus precluding the need to estimate unnecessarily an often large number of parameters that provide no information about important exposure–disease odds ratio parameters of interest. In addition, precisely the same CL is obtained regardless of whether we consider the data to have arisen from a follow-up study or from a case–control study. Also, CL has precisely the structure of Cox's partial likelihood [4], based on the **proportional hazards model**, for analyzing follow-up study data. However, an important distinction is that each stratum-specific set in the denominator of CL, instead of involving *all* persons in the study who are disease-free at the time each incident case is identified, consists only of the m_{0g} controls specifically associated with (e.g. sampled at the same time as) the m_{1g} cases.

As an illustration of the CL approach for matched data, consider a matched case–control study involving G cases, where the gth case is individually matched to R_g controls on one or more variables. Then, $m_{1g} = 1, m_{0g} = R_g, m_g = (R_g + 1)$, and the

CL takes the specific form

$$\prod_{g=1}^{G} \left[1 + \sum_{l=2}^{R_g+1} \exp[\boldsymbol{\beta}'(\mathbf{x}_{lg} - \mathbf{x}_{1g})] \right]^{-1}.$$

(5)

Given the structure of this expression, if any of the elements of $\mathbf{x}$ are matching variables, taking the same value for each member of a matched set, then their contribution to the likelihood is zero and the corresponding elements of $\boldsymbol{\beta}$ cannot be estimated. However, by incorporating such matching variables in the model as **interaction** terms with exposure factors, one can model the variation in odds ratios across matched sets.

Finally, to appreciate that these CL methods do, in fact, yield recognizable results in well-known special cases, consider the simple matched pairs case–control study considered earlier, where $R_g = 1$ for all g and where there is a single dichotomous exposure variable. With $e^\beta = \text{EOR}$, the exposure odds ratio parameter, it can be shown that (5) is proportional to

$$[\text{EOR}/(1 + \text{EOR})]^b [1/(1 + \text{EOR})]^c.$$

By differentiating the logarithm of the above expression with respect to EOR, equating it to zero, and solving, one finds that the conditional maximum likelihood estimator of EOR is $\widehat{\text{mOR}} = b/c$, the ratio of discordant pairs. In contrast, the unconditional maximum likelihood estimator of EOR is $(b/c)^2$, which dramatically illustrates the potential bias associated with the use of unconditional likelihood methods for finely stratified data. While not as extreme as illustrated here, the bias of unconditional likelihood methods is found in many other sparse data situations [10]. These findings emphasize the need to consider the use of CL methods when fitting logistic models involving many strata and/or other nuisance parameters to data sets of limited size.

References

[1]   Breslow, N.E. & Day, N.E. (1980). *Statistical Methods in Cancer Research*, Vol. 1: *The Analysis of Case–Control Studies*. International Agency for Research on Cancer, Lyon.

[2]   Clayton, D.G. (1974). Some odds ratio statistics for the analysis of ordered categorical data, *Biometrika* **61**, 525–531.

[3]   Connett, J., Ejigou, A., McHugh, R. & Breslow, N.E. (1982). The precision of the Mantel–Haenszel odds

ratio estimator in case–control studies with multiple matching, *American Journal of Epidemiology* **116**, 875–877.

[4]   Cox, D.R. (1975). *The Analysis of Binary Data.* Methuen, London.

[5]   Kleinbaum, D.G., Kupper, L.L. & Morgenstern, H. (1982). *Epidemiologic Research: Principles and Quantitative Methods.* Lifetime Learning Publications, Belmont.

[6]   Kupper, L.L., Karon, J.M., Kleinbaum, D.G., Morgenstern, H. & Lewis, D.K. (1981). Matching in epidemiologic studies: Validity and efficiency considerations, *Biometrics* **37**, 293–302.

[7]   Mantel, N. (1963). Chi-square tests with one degree of freedom: extensions of the Mantel–Haenszel procedure, *Journal of the American Statistical Association* **58**, 690–700.

[8]   Mantel, N. & Fleiss, J.L. (1980). Minimum expected cell size requirements for the Mantel–Haenszel one-degree of freedom chi-square test and a related rapid procedure, *American Journal of Epidemiology* **112**, 129–134.

[9]   Mantel, N. & Haenszel, W. (1959). Statistical aspects of the analysis of data from retrospective studies of disease, *Journal of the National Cancer Institute* **22**, 719–748.

[10] Pike, M.C., Hill, A.P. & Smith, P.G. (1980). Bias and efficiency in logistic analysis of stratified case–control studies, *International Journal of Epidemiology* **9**, 89–95.

[11] Radhakrishna, S. (1965). Combination of results from several 2 × 2 contingency tables, *Biometrics* **21**, 86–98.

[12] Robins, J., Breslow, N. & Greenland, S. (1986). Estimators of the Mantel–Haenszel variance consistent in both sparse data and large-strata limiting models, *Biometrics* **42**, 311–323.

[13] Sato, T. (1990). Confidence limits for the common odds ratio based on the asymptotic distribution of the Mantel–Haenszel estimator, *Biometrics* **46**, 71–80.

(*See also* **Confounder**; **Confounder Summary Score**; **Matching**)

LAWRENCE L. KUPPER

Matching

Before discussing the procedure known as matching, it is necessary to provide some background and motivation for its use. In epidemiologic studies, it is typically the situation that valid estimation of the strength of the relationship between a response variable D of interest (e.g. the presence, $D = 1$, or not, $D = 0$,

of some particular disease) and an independent variable E of interest (e.g. the presence, $E = 1$, or not, $E = 0$, of some exposure) necessitates the consideration of so-called **confounding** factors (*see* **Confounder**). Ignoring or inappropriately accounting for the effects of confounding factors can often lead to invalid (i.e. statistically inconsistent) and inefficient estimation of the true exposure–disease association of interest.

As a simple example, suppose that the dichotomous response (or disease) variable D of interest is the presence or absence of lung cancer and that the dichotomous independent (or exposure) variable E of interest is the presence or absence of a history of occupational exposure to asbestos. Then, a dichotomous variable C such as cigarette smoking status (e.g. evidence, $C = 1$, or not, $C = 0$, of a history of smoking), which is an established risk factor for the development of lung cancer, will be a confounder if, *in the data under consideration*, its distribution among the group of study subjects with a history of occupational exposure to asbestos (the "exposed group") is different from its distribution among the group of study subjects who do not have a history of occupationally related asbestos exposure (the "unexposed group"). If C is, in fact, a confounder in the data under consideration, then appropriate adjustment for C *at the analysis stage* (e.g. by **stratification** methods or, equivalently, by multivariable modeling) would be needed. In our particular example involving the three dichotomous variables D, E, and C, one could fit the **logistic regression** model logit $[\Pr(D = 1)] = \beta_0 + \beta_1 E + \gamma_1 C$ by appropriate likelihood methods to obtain an adjusted (for C) estimated **odds ratio** $\exp(\hat{\beta}_1)$ and to obtain a corresponding interval estimator for the population E–D odds ratio $\exp(\beta_1)$. Here, we are assuming that C is not an **effect modifier** (i.e. there is no **interaction** between E and C), so that it is not necessary to include the product term EC in the above model; we will make this no interaction assumption in our discussion to follow.

However, adjustment for C at the analysis stage can be problematic. For example, if almost all of the study subjects with a history of smoking have lung cancer (i.e. are "cases"), and if a large proportion of the study subjects with no smoking history are "noncases", then such stratum-specific imbalances can lead to poor statistical efficiency in the point and interval estimation of the odds ratio parameter $\exp(\beta_1)$. In more realistic situations where there are typically several confounders to consider simultaneously, distributional imbalances in strata defined by combinations of levels of these confounders can severely compromise the reliability of multivariable modeling analyses.

Design Options: Restriction and Matching

By using appropriate strategies at the *design stage* of a study, it is often possible to avoid many of the confounder-related distributional imbalance problems mentioned earlier. For example, consider a potentially confounding variable such as gender. One way to avoid completely any possible problems associated with an analysis stage adjustment for the variable gender is to decide, at the design stage, to restrict the study so that it involves either only males or only females. This simple study design option is called (*total*) *restriction* because the potential confounder is completely restricted to have exactly the same value for every study subject. Clearly, the disadvantage of (total) restriction is the lack of generalizability of the study results; in our example, by employing (total) restriction with respect to gender, the study conclusions would necessarily only pertain either to males or to females.

Matching, in contrast to total restriction, is a form of *partial restriction* on study subject selection, partial in the sense that only the so-called "referent (or comparison) group", and not the "index group", is chosen subject to certain restrictions. More specifically, for follow-up studies (*see* **Cohort Study**), once the index group of exposed ($E = 1$) subjects is randomly selected from the population of interest, the referent group of unexposed ($E = 0$) subjects is then chosen to be similar to the exposed group with respect to the distributions of one or more potentially confounding factors. For **case–control studies**, once the index group of diseased ($D = 1$) subjects is chosen at random from the population of interest, the referent group of nondiseased ($D = 0$) subjects is picked to be similar to the cases with respect to the distributions of one or more potentially confounding factors. We use the word "similar", rather than "identical", because the index and matched referent groups will generally not have exactly the same confounder distributions after matching; the degree of similarity will depend on the type and the extent of matching employed.

To discuss types of matching schemes, we need to distinguish between matching on continuous variables (e.g. age, weight, cholesterol level) and matching on categorical variables (e.g. gender, race). Matching on a continuous variable (say, X) necessitates the specification of a rule for deciding when an index subject's value (say, X_1) and a referent subject's value (say, X_0) are "close enough" to declare that the two subjects are "matched" on X. In so-called "caliper matching", one specifies a caliper (or tolerance) value C and declares the index and referent subjects to be matched if $|X_1 - X_0| \leq C$.

The smaller is C, the tighter will be the match on X, but, correspondingly, the harder it will be to find index–referent pairs to satisfy such a stringent matching criterion [8, 9].

Since, in standard epidemiologic practice, variables are generally categorized for matching purposes (e.g. note that caliper matching defines categories of width C), we will henceforth focus on so called *category (or frequency) matching*. In particular, index and referent subjects are said to be matched on a categorized potential confounder if they are in the same category of that variable. In the realistic situation where category matching involves several potential confounding variables, index and referent subjects are said to be matched when they are in the same category for each and every one of the categorized matching variables under consideration. For example, suppose that there are three categorized matching variables of interest: age in four categories (30–39, 40–49, 50–59, and 60–69), race (black, white, and other), and gender (male and female). Then, there will be 24 strata defined by the various combinations of these three matching variables, with, for example, one stratum consisting of black females between the ages of 40 and 49.

In general, then, matching can be considered to be pre (or design stage)-stratification, as opposed to post (or analysis stage)-stratification, with the goal of such matching being to form strata that are sufficiently balanced to permit valid, stable, and efficient statistical analyses. Once matching is employed at the design stage, it is mandatory at the analysis stage to take the matching into account via the use of appropriate stratified analysis methods [5]. Such categorical data analysis procedures include the approach of **Mantel & Haenszel** [6] and the use of conditional logistic regression methods [1, 4] (*see* **Logistic Regression, Conditional**; **Matched Analysis**).

Types of Matching Schemes

There are various types of matching schemes that can be used. One of the more popular matching schemes, especially in case–control studies, is known as *pair matching*. Pair matching refers to the special situation when each stratum is assumed, for analysis purposes, to contain exactly one index subject and one referent subject. However, this assumption will generally lead to an inefficient stratified analysis when the pairing is artificial and unnecessary. For example, for a stratum of cases and controls consisting of black females between the ages of 40 and 49, any case in that stratum could theoretically be paired with any control without altering the basic within-stratum structure. Retaining this "random" pairing in the analysis is clearly unwarranted, and such an "overmatched analysis" generally leads to some loss in statistical efficiency [2]. In contrast, the term "**overmatching**" commonly refers to an undesirable design-stage strategy of matching on variables that make the cases and controls too much alike with respect to exposure status. Such variables are generally of two types, namely, so-called "intervening variables" that are intermediate in the causal pathway between exposure and disease and variables that are (at best) very weak risk factors for the disease in question but are nevertheless highly correlated with exposure status [10]. Such overmatching can sometimes lead to a meaningful loss in statistical efficiency, especially in case–control studies (see "Discussion" below).

A generalization of pair matching is a procedure known as R-to-1 matching, where each stratum is considered to contain one index subject and exactly R referent subjects. Miettinen [7] and others have shown that there is little to gain statistically by taking $R > 4$. For example, when comparing R-to-1 matching with pair matching ($R = 1$) in case–control studies, Ury [11] has shown that the Pitman efficiency of the Mantel–Haenszel test for stratified data is $2R/(R + 1)$, so that the Pitman efficiency only increases from 1.600 for $R = 4$ to 1.667 when $R = 5$.

In the most general category matching situation, a particular stratum (say, the gth of G strata) may contain R_g referent subjects and S_g index subjects, giving a *matching ratio* of R_g/S_g (which is not necessarily an integer). If this matching ratio varies with g, then we have a *variable matching ratio plan*. If the matching ratio does not vary over the strata (e.g. as with R-to-1 matching), then we have a *fixed matching ratio*

plan. With either plan, the appropriate data analysis would still appropriately accumulate stratum-specific information; and, in terms of statistical efficiency, a fixed matching ratio plan is usually somewhat better.

Advantages and Disadvantages of Category Matching

Some of the *positive aspects* of category matching in epidemiologic studies are as follows:

1. Category matching a set of referent subjects to a random sample of index subjects can often lead to a more statistically efficient analysis than can be obtained by choosing the same number of referent subjects by random sampling. This efficiency advantage will tend to occur when the matching variables are well-established determinants of the response variable (e.g. are important risk factors for the disease under study) and are expected to be quite differentially distributed between the exposed and unexposed groups in the observed data (i.e. are anticipated to be strong confounders). For more detailed discussion, see Kupper et al. [5] and Karon & Kupper [3].
2. Matching on a variable like neighborhood of residence can lead to efficient adjustment for the potentially confounding effects of a wide range of social and economic factors that would be difficult, if not impossible, to measure and hence to control.
3. Matching can often lead to savings in time and money. For example, when the cases in a case–control study are chosen from records in different hospitals or in different companies within some industry, it is preferable, for reasons of simplicity and convenience in data collection (and also possibly on validity and efficiency grounds), to choose controls for each case from that same set of hospital or company records.
4. Matching in the selection of the referent group with respect to a given set of potential confounders does not preclude controlling for other nonmatched confounders at the analysis stage via multivariable modeling procedures like conditional logistic regression. In this regard, a recommended strategy would be to match only on important risk factors considered a priori to be highly likely to manifest themselves as

strong confounders in the data, and to adjust (if necessary) for other factors at the analysis stage.

Some possible *negative aspects* of category matching in epidemiologic studies are the following:

1. Category matching can be a costly enterprise, both with regard to the *direct* costs of time and labor required to find the appropriate matches and the *indirect* costs (in terms of information loss) owing to the discarding of available referents not able to satisfy possibly stringent matching criteria.
2. When employing category matching, simultaneous recruitment of cases and controls can be problematic since there is no way to know in advance exactly how many controls will be needed to meet sample size requirements in different matching strata defined by the sample of cases. To circumvent this problem, a new "randomized recruitment" method for matching has been developed [12, 13].
3. The referent group chosen by category matching ends up being more like the index group than like the underlying population of referents being sampled. In particular, matching generally precludes the evaluation of the underlying population relationships between the matching variables and exposure status in follow-up studies or between the matching factors and disease status in case–control studies.
4. If the strata defined by the category matching process are wide (so that there is room for the matching factors each to vary sufficiently in value within particular strata), it is possible that stratum-specific residual confounding due to the matching factors can still be present. Appropriate adjustment for such stratum-specific residual confounding at the analysis stage can be accomplished using multivariable modeling procedures.

Discussion

In summary, category matching on potential confounders can be a fruitful design-based strategy in both follow-up and case–control studies when reliable information, based on knowledge of the disease process under study and previous research findings, indicates that such variables are well-established

disease determinants (i.e. are strong risk factors) expected to be quite differentially distributed between exposed and unexposed groups if matching is not employed (e.g. under random sampling of the referent group).

As a word of caution, the use of matching requires more care in case–control studies than in follow-up studies. Since exposure information is collected *after* the occurrence of disease in case–control studies, indiscriminate *overmatching* of controls to cases simultaneously on several factors can lead to a substantial loss in efficiency relative to random sampling of the control group. For example, consider a pair-matched case–control study involving n case–control pairs, where a is the number of pairs where both the case and control are exposed, b is the number of pairs where the case is exposed and the control is not, c is the number of pairs where the control is exposed and the case is not, and d is the number of pairs where neither the case nor the control is exposed. Then, the Mantel–Haenszel test statistic [6] takes the form $(b-c)^2/(b+c)$, and the appropriate odds ratio estimator is b/c (namely, the ratio of discordant pairs). Hence, the effective sample size in such a study is the total number of discordant pairs $(b+c)$, not n. If the matching variables are each correlated with the exposure variable, then overmatching generally increases the number of uninformative pairs in the observed data, namely $(a+d)$, thus leading to a (possibly substantial) loss in efficiency. Thus, in case–control studies especially, the best policy is to consider as candidate matching variables only well-established strong risk factors for the disease in question. As mentioned earlier, matching either on intervening variables or on very weak risk factors highly correlated with exposure status should be avoided.

References

[1] Breslow, N.E. & Day, N.E. (1980). *Statistical Methods in Cancer Research*, Vol. 1: *The Analysis of Case–Control Studies*. International Agency for Research on Cancer, Lyon.
[2] Brookmeyer, R., Liang, K.Y. & Linet, M. (1986). Matched case–control designs and overmatched analyses, *American Journal of Epidemiology* **124**, 693–701.
[3] Karon, J.M. & Kupper, L.L. (1982). In defense of matching, *American Journal of Epidemiology* **116**, 852–866.

[4]   Kleinbaum, D.G., Kupper, L.L. & Morgenstern, H. (1982). *Epidemiologic Research: Principles and Quantitative Methods*. Lifetime Learning Publications, Belmont.

[5]   Kupper, L.L., Karon, J.M., Kleinbaum, D.G., Morgenstern, H. & Lewis, D.K. (1981). Matching in epidemiologic studies: validity and efficiency considerations, *Biometrics* **37**, 293–302.

[6]   Mantel, N. & Haenszel, W. (1959). Statistical aspects of the analysis of data from retrospective studies of disease, *Journal of the National Cancer Institute* **22**, 719–748.

[7]   Miettinen, O.S. (1969). Individual matching with multiple controls in the case of all-or-none responses, *Biometrics* **22**, 339–355.

[8]   Raynor, W.J. & Kupper, L.L. (1981). Category matching of continuous variables in case–control studies, *Biometrics* **37**, 811–817.

[9]   Rubin, D.R. (1973). Matching to remove bias in observational studies, *Biometrics* **29**, 159–183.

[10] Schlesselman, J.J. (1982). *Case–Control Studies: Design, Conduct, Analysis*. Oxford University Press, New York.

[11] Ury, H.K. (1975). Efficiency of case–control studies with multiple controls per case: continuous or dichotomous data, *Biometrics* **31**, 643–649.

[12] Weinberg, C.R. & Wacholder, S. (1990). The design and analysis of case–control studies with biased sampling, *Biometrics* **46**, 963–975.

[13] Weinberg, C.R. & Sandler, D.P. (1991). Randomized recruitment in case–control studies, *American Journal of Epidemiology* **134**, 421–431.

LAWRENCE L. KUPPER

Matching Coefficient of Numerical Taxonomy *see* Agreement, Measurement of

Matlab *see* Software, Biostatistical

Matrix Method to Adjust for Misclassification *see* Misclassification Error

Measurement Error in Epidemiologic Studies

This article is concerned with relating a response or outcome to an exposure and **confounders** in the presence of measurement error in one or more of the variables. We focus almost entirely on measurement error in a continuous or measured variable. When categorical variables (exposed or not exposed, case or control, quintiles of fat) are measured with error, they are said to be misclassified (*see* **Misclassification Error**). There are also many links in this topic with methods for handling missing data and with validation studies (*see* **Missing Data in Epidemiologic Studies**; **Validation Study**). For further details and a general overview of the topic, see [20]; [30] should be consulted for the linear model.

Before describing the problem, it is useful first to consider a number of specific examples that have had an impact on the development of the field:

1. Measurement error has long been a concern in relating error-prone predictors such as systolic blood pressure (SBP) to the development of coronary heart disease (CHD). That SBP is measured with error is well known, and estimates [23] suggest that approximately one-third of its observed variability is due to measurement error. The Framingham Heart Study is perhaps the best known **cohort study** in which the role of measurement error in SBP has been a concern for many years. MacMahon et al. [44] describe the important public health implications of properly accounting for the measurement error inherent in SBP. In an (as yet) unpublished paper, David Yanez, Richard Kronmal & Lynn Shemanski have discovered an example also in the CHD context where the failure to account properly for measurement error leads to misleading conclusions based on falsely detected statistical significance.

2. In measuring nutrient intake, measurement error has been a long-term concern, as has the impact of this error on the ability to detect nutritional factors leading to cancer, especially breast and colon cancer. Typical cohort studies measure diet by means of food frequency questionnaires which, while related to long-term diet, are known to have biases and measurement errors. Other

instruments are in use in this field, including food records (essentially diaries), 24 h recalls and (for a limited number of variables such as total caloric intake) biomarkers. Measurement error in nutrient instruments can be very large, for example because of the daily and seasonal variability of an individual's diet, and the **biases** in and loss of power to detect nutrient–cancer relationships can be profound. There is still considerable controversy in this field (see [37], [54], and [41]). Because of the cost of cohort studies in nutrition, **case–control studies** are of considerable interest. However, nutrient intakes in case–control studies are measured after the development of disease in cases, and this might cause differential measurement error, a topic we discuss in some detail below.

3. There are a number of ongoing prospective and case–control studies of disease and serum hormone levels, and this is an area of considerable potential. Measurement error is a major concern here, due to within-individual variation of hormones, as well as various laboratory errors.

4. In measuring environmental risk factors (*see* **Environmental Epidemiology**), measurement error is a common problem. For example, measuring household lead levels is an error-prone process, not only because of laboratory and device error, but also because lead levels are inhomogeneous in both space and time, while measurement methods tend to be in fixed locations at fixed times. Because lead exposure has many possible media (air, dust, soil) with possibly correlated errors, the effects of measurement error can be large and complex.

Outline

This article consists of a series of major Sections, as follows:

1. We first outline the basic concepts of measurement error modeling, making particular distinction between **differential** and **nondifferential measurement error**. We also describe the ideas of functional and structural modeling, as well as indicating how the measurement error problem can be treated as a **missing data** problem.

2. Following the introductory concepts, we discuss the problem of measurement error as it pertains to the linear regression model. Here we introduce the idea of attenuation of regression coefficients, and the biases in parameter estimates caused by measurement error. We also discuss hypothesis testing. In the simplest cases, measurement error causes an often large decrease in the power to detect significant effects, while, as indicated above, and as exhibited through the analysis of covariance, in an **observational study**, measurement error in a confounder can cause misleading inferences about exposure effects.

3. Having described the effects of measurement error on estimation and hypothesis testing, we turn to correcting for the effects due to measurement error. We first describe the two most common methods, known as regression calibration and simulation extrapolation (SIMEX), and also a group of techniques called corrected score methods. We also describe the use of instrumental variables.

4. Maximum likelihood and Bayesian estimation form an important component of the measurement error problem, and are described in some detail. We define the likelihood function, and show the crucial difference in the likelihood function between the nondifferential and differential measurement error cases; see (13) and (14).

5. While most of the article is based on measurement error in predictors, there is an important literature on response error, which we also review.

6. Case–control studies are important in epidemiology. A distinguishing feature of case–control studies is that the measurement error may be differential. In the differential measurement error case, we indicate that a specific type of data is required, the validation data sets, in which the true predictor can be observed for a subset of the study participants. If the measurement error is nondifferential, then matters are much easier, and the famous result of Prentice & Pyke [55] on the analysis of case–control studies is shown to have an analogue in the measurement error context.

7. There is a significant and developing literature on measurement error in survival analysis, and we indicate two possible approaches to the problem.

Measurement error models have a common structure; we illustrate the terms using a breast cancer and nutrition example:

1. An underlying model for a response in terms of predictors, e.g. linear regression, **logistic regression,** nonlinear regression; see Carrell & Ruppert [14]. This is the model we would fit if all variables were observed without error. In what follows, we call Y the response. For example, in the breast cancer and nutrition example, Y is breast cancer incidence fit to covariables using logistic regression

2. A variable which is measured subject to error. This could be an exposure or a confounder. We call this variable X. It is often called the *error-prone* predictor or the *latent predictor*. In the breast cancer example, X is long-term nutrient intake

3. The observed value of the mismeasured variable. We call this W, e.g. nutrient intake measured from a food frequency questionnaire

4. Those predictors which for all practical purposes are measured without error, which we call Z, e.g. age, body mass index

5. We are interested in relating the response Y to the true predictors (Z, X). One method, often called the *naive* method, simply replaces the error-prone predictor X with its measured version W. This substitution typically leads to biases in parameter estimates and can lead to misleading inferences

6. The goal of measurement error modeling is to obtain nearly unbiased estimates of exposure effects and valid inferences. Attainment of this goal requires careful analysis. Substituting W for X, but making no adjustments in the usual fitting methods for this substitution, leads to estimates that are biased, sometimes seriously. In assessing measurement error, careful attention needs to be given to the type and nature of the error, and the sources of data which allow modeling of this error.

It should be obvious that one should design studies and instruments in such a way as best to lessen or to eliminate measurement error. In this article, we demonstrate some of the impacts of ignoring measurement error, ranging from bias in parameter estimates (Figure 1), to loss of power, requiring therefore much larger sample sizes to detect effects (Figure 2) to cases where the type I errors occur at higher rates than the usual 5% (Figure 3).

Models for Measurement Error

A fundamental prerequisite for analyzing a measurement error problem is specification of a model for the measurement error process. The *classical error model*, in its simplest form, is appropriate when an attempt is made to determine X directly, but one is unable to do so because of various errors in measurement. For example, consider SBP, which is known to have strong daily and seasonal variations. In trying to measure SBP, the various sources of error include simple machine recording error, administration error, time of day, and season of the year. In such a circumstance, it sometimes makes sense to hypothesize an unbiased **additive error model**, which we write as

$$\text{(the classic model)} \quad W = X + U, \quad (1)$$

where U, the error, is assumed to be independent of X. An alternative model, the *controlled variable or Berkson model* [6], is especially applicable to laboratory studies. As an example, consider the herbicide study of Rudemo et al. [61]. In that study, a nominal measured amount W of herbicide was applied to a plant. However, the actual amount X absorbed by the plant differed from W, e.g. because of potential errors in application. In this case,

$$\text{(the Berkson model)} \quad X = W + U, \quad (2)$$

where U, the error, is assumed to be independent of W.

Determining an appropriate error model to use in the data analysis depends upon the circumstances and the available data. For example, in the herbicide study, the measured concentration W is fixed by design and the true concentration X varies due to error, so that model (2) is appropriate. On the other hand, in the measurement of long-term SBP, it is the true long-term blood pressure which is fixed for an individual, and the measured value which is perturbed by error, so model (1) should be used. Estimation and inference procedures have been developed both for error and controlled-variable models.

This hardly exhausts the possible error models. See [20] and [29] for more details and further examples with more complex structure.

Sources of Data

To perform a measurement error analysis, one needs information about the error structure. These data sources can be broken up into two main categories:

1. *internal* subsets of the primary data
2. *external* or independent studies.

Within each of these broad categories, there are three types of data, all of which might be available only in a random subsample of the data set in question:

1. *validation* data, in which X is observable directly
2. *replication* data, in which replicates of W are available
3. *instrumental* data, in which another variable T is observable in addition to W.

An internal validation data set is the ideal, because it can be used with all known analytical techniques, permits direct examination of the error structure and tests of critical error model assumptions, typically leads to much greater precision of estimation and inference, and has strong links to the well-developed theory of missing data analysis (see below). We cannot express too forcefully that, if at all possible, one should obtain an internal validation data set.

With external validation data, one must assume that the error structure in those data also applies to the primary data (see below).

Replication data are used when it is impossible to measure X exactly, as, for example, when X represents long-term systolic average blood pressure or long-term average nutrient intake. Usually, one would make replicate measurements if there were good reason to believe that the replicated mean is a better estimate of X than a single observation, i.e. the classical error model is the target. In the classical error model (1), replication data can be used to estimate the variance of the measurement error, U.

Internal instrumental data sets containing a second measure T are useful for instrumental variable analysis, discussed briefly later in this article.

Transportability of Models and Parameters

In some studies, the measurement error process is not assessed directly, but instead is estimated from external data sets. We say that parameters of a model can be transported from one study to another if the model holds with the same parameter values in both studies. Typically, in applications only a subset of the model parameters need be transportable.

In many instances, approximately the same classical error model holds across different populations. For example, consider SBP at two different clinical centers. Assuming similar levels of training for technicians making the measurements and a similar measurement protocol, it is reasonable to expect that the distribution of the error in the recorded measure is independent of the clinical center one enters, the technician making the measurement, and the value of X being measured. Thus, in classical error models it is often reasonable to assume that the error distribution is the same across different populations, i.e. transportable.

A common mistake is to transport a correction for measurement error from one study to the next. Such transportation is almost never appropriate. For instance, while the properties of errors of measurement may be reasonably transportable, the distribution of the true (or latent) predictor X is rarely transportable, since it depends so heavily on the population being sampled. Problems arise because corrections for measurement error involve not only the measurement error process but also the distribution of X. For example, SBP measurements in the Multiple Risk Factor Intervention Trial (MRFIT) study and the Framingham Heart Study may well have the same measurement error variance, but the distribution of true blood pressure X appears to differ substantially in the two studies, and the "correction for attenuation" described below cannot be transported from Framingham to MRFIT (see [17] for further details).

Is there an "Exact" Predictor?

We have based our discussion on the existence of an exact predictor X and measurement error models that provide information about this predictor. However, in practice, it is often the case that the definition of "exact" needs to be carefully considered prior to discussion of error models. In the measurement error literature the term "gold standard" is often used for the operationally defined exact predictor, though sometimes this term is used for an exact predictor that cannot be operationally defined. Using an operational definition for an "exact" predictor is often reasonable and justifiable on the grounds that it is the best one could ever possibly hope to accomplish. However, such definitions may be controversial. For example, consider the problem of relating breast cancer risk to the dietary intake of fat.

One way to determine whether decreasing one's fat intake lowers the risk of developing breast cancer is to conduct a clinical trial in which members of the treatment group are encouraged to reduce fat intakes. If instead one uses observational prospective data, along with an operational definition of long-term intake, one should be aware that the results of a measurement error analysis could be invalid if true long-term intake and operational long-term intake differ in subtle ways.

Differential and Nondifferential Error

It is important to make a distinction between *differential* and *nondifferential* measurement error. Nondifferential measurement error occurs in a broad sense when one would not even bother with W if X were available, i.e. W has no information about the response other than what is available in X. Nondifferential measurement error typically holds in **cohort studies**, but is often a suspect assumption in **case–control studies**.

Technically, measurement error is nondifferential if the distribution of Y given (X, Z, W) depends only on (X, Z). In this case W is said to be a *surrogate*. Measurement error is *differential* otherwise.

For instance, consider the Framingham example. The predictor of major interest is long-term SBP, X, but we can only observe blood pressure on a single day, W. It seems plausible that a single day's blood pressure contributes essentially no information over and above that given by true long-term blood pressure, and hence that measurement error is nondifferential. The same remarks apply to the nutrition examples: measuring diet on a single day should not contribute information not already available in long-term diet.

Many problems can be analyzed plausibly assuming nondifferential measurement error, especially when the covariate measurements occur at a fixed point in time, and the response is measured at a later time, as is typical in cohort studies.

There are two exceptions that need to be kept in mind. First, in case–control studies, the disease response is obtained first, and then one measures antecedent exposures and other covariates. In nutrition studies, this ordering of measurement may well cause differential measurement error. For instance, here the true predictor would be long-term dietary intake before diagnosis, but the dietary interview data are obtained only after diagnosis. A woman who develops breast cancer may exaggerate her estimated fat intake, thus introducing **recall bias** (*see* **Bias in Case–Control Studies**). In such circumstances, estimated fat intake will be associated with disease status even after conditioning on true long-term diet before diagnosis.

When measurement error is nondifferential, one can estimate parameters in models for responses given true covariates even when the true covariates are not observable. This is not true when measurement error is differential, except for the linear model. With differential error, one must obtain a validation subsample in which both true covariate measurements and surrogate measurements are available. Most of this article focuses on nondifferential measurement error models. Differential models with a **validation study** are typically best analyzed by techniques for handling missing data (*see* **Missing Data in Epidemiologic Studies**; **Missing Data**).

Prediction

Prediction of a response is different from estimation and inference for parameters. If a predictor X is measured with error, and one wants to predict a response *based on the error-prone version W of X*, then, except for an important case discussed below, it makes little sense to worry about measurement error. The reason for this is quite simple. If one has an original set of data (Y, W) then one can fit a convenient model to Y as a function of W. Predicting Y from W is merely a matter of using this model for prediction. There is no need then for measurement error to play a role in the problem.

The one situation requiring that we model the measurement error occurs when we develop a prediction model using data from one population but we wish to predict in another population. A naive prediction model that ignores measurement error may not be transportable. This context often becomes quite complex, requiring a combination of missing data and measurement error techniques, and to the best of our knowledge has not been investigated in detail in the literature, an exception being [31].

Is Bias Always Towards the Null?

It is commonly thought that the effect of measurement error is to bias estimates of exposure effects "towards the null" (*see* **Bias Toward the Null**). Hence, one could ignore measurement error when testing the null hypothesis of no exposure effect, and one could assume that non-null estimates, if anything, underestimate the effect of exposure. This lovely and appealing folklore is sometimes true but, unfortunately, often wrong. We discuss this point in detail below. A numerical example has recently been provided to us by David Yanez, Richard Kronmal & Lynn Shemanski in a heart disease context with seven covariates and a baseline variable. They found that, while an analysis ignoring measurement error showed highly statistically significant effects in all variables, none of the effects was even close to being statistically significant when the analysis took measurement error into account.

Functional and Structural Models

The words *functional* and *structural* have important places in the area of measurement error models. They act as a shorthand terminology for the basic approach one uses to solve the problem. In *functional modeling* nothing is assumed about the Xs; they could be fixed constants (the usual definition) or random variables. In *structural modeling*, X is assumed to be random, and a parametric distribution (usually the normal) is assumed. There has traditionally been considerable concern in the measurement error literature about the robustness of estimation and inferences based upon structural models for unobservable variates. Fuller [30, p. 263] discusses this issue briefly in the classical nonlinear regression problem, and basically concludes that the results of structural modeling "may depend heavily on the (assumed) form of the X distribution". In probit regression, Carroll et al. [23] report that, if one assumes that X is normally distributed, and it really follows a chi-square distribution with one degree of freedom, then the effect on the likelihood estimate is "markedly negative"; see also [63]. Essentially all research workers in the measurement error field come to a common conclusion: likelihood methods can be of considerable value, but the possible nonrobustness of inference due to model misspecification is a vexing and difficult problem.

The issue of model robustness is hardly limited to measurement error modeling. Indeed, it pervades statistics, and has led to the rise of a variety of semiparametric and nonparametric techniques. From this general point of view, *functional modeling* may be

thought of as a group of semiparametric techniques. Functional modeling uses parametric models for the response, but makes no assumptions about the distribution of the unobserved covariate.

There is no agreement in the statistical literature as to whether functional or structural modeling is more appropriate. Many researchers believe that one should make as few model assumptions as possible and favor functional modeling. The argument is that any extra efficiency gained by structural modeling is more than offset by the need to perform careful and often time-consuming sensitivity analyses. Other researchers believe that appropriate statistical analysis requires one to do one's best to model every feature of the data, and thus favor structural modeling.

We take a somewhat more relaxed view of these issues. There are many problems, e.g. linear and logistic regression with additive measurement error, where functional techniques are easily computed and fairly efficient, and we have a strong bias in such circumstances towards functional modeling. In other problems – for example, the segmented regression problem [38] – structural modeling clearly has an important role to play, and should not be neglected.

Measurement Error as a Missing Data Problem

From one perspective, measurement error models are special kinds of missing data problems, because the Xs, being mostly and often entirely unobservable, are obviously missing as well. Readers who are already familiar with linear measurement error models and functional modeling will be struck by the fact that most of the recent missing data literature has pursued likelihood and Bayesian methods, i.e. structural modeling approaches. Readers familiar with missing data analysis will also be interested to know that, in large part, the measurement error model literature has pursued functional modeling approaches. We feel that both functional and structural modeling approaches are useful in the measurement error context, and this article pursues both strategies.

The usual interpretation of the classical missing data problem [42] is that the values of some of the variables of interest may not be observable for all study participants. For example, a variable may be observed for 80% of the study participants, but unobserved for the other 20%. The techniques for analyzing missing data are continually evolving, but it is fair to say that most of the recent advances (multiple imputation, data augmentation, etc.) have been based on likelihood (and Bayesian) methods.

The classical measurement error problem discussed to this point is one in which one set of variables, which we call X, is *never* observable, i.e. always missing. As such, the classical measurement error model is an extreme form of a missing data problem, but with *supplemental information* about X in the form of a surrogate, which we call W. Part of the art in measurement error modeling concerns how the supplemental information is related to the unobservable covariate.

Because there is a formal connection between the two fields, and because missing data analysis has become increasingly parametric, it is important to consider likelihood and Bayesian analysis of measurement error models – topics taken up later in this article.

Linear Regression and the Effects of Measurement Error

A comprehensive account of linear measurement error models can be found in Fuller [30].

Many textbooks contain a brief description of measurement error in linear regression, usually focusing on simple linear regression and arriving at the conclusion that the effect of measurement error is to bias the slope estimate in the direction of 0. Bias of this nature is commonly referred to as *attenuation* or *attenuation to the null*.

In fact, though, even this simple conclusion has to be qualified, because it depends on the relationship between the measurement, W, and the true predictor, X, and possibly other variables in the regression model as well. In particular, the effect of measurement error depends upon the model under consideration and on the joint distribution of the measurement error and the other variables. In multiple linear regression, the effects of measurement error vary, depending on: (i) the regression model, be it additive or multiple regression; (ii) whether or not the predictor measured with error is univariate or multivariate; and (iii) the presence of bias in the measurement. The effects can range from the simple attenuation described above to situations where: (i) real effects are hidden; (ii) observed data exhibit relationships that are not present in the error-free

data; and (iii) even the signs of estimated coefficients are reversed relative to the case with no measurement error.

The key point is that the measurement error distribution determines the effects of measurement error, and thus appropriate methods for correcting for the effects of measurement error depend on the measurement error distribution.

Simple Linear Regression with Additive Error: Regression to the Mean

We start with the simple linear regression model $Y = \beta_0 + \beta_x X + \varepsilon$, where the scalar X has mean μ_x and variance σ_x^2, and the error in the equation ε is independent of X, has mean zero, and variance σ_ε^2. The error model is additive as in (1). In this classical additive measurement error model, it is well known that an ordinary least squares regression ignoring measurement error produces an estimate not of β_x, but instead of $\beta_{x*} = \lambda \beta_x$, where

$$\lambda = \frac{\sigma_x^2}{\sigma_x^2 + \sigma_u^2} < 1. \tag{3}$$

Thus ordinary least squares regression of Y on W produces an estimator that is attenuated to 0. The attenuating factor, λ, is called the *reliability ratio*.

One would expect that, because W is an error-prone predictor, it has a weaker relationship with the response than does X. This can be seen both by the attenuation and also by the fact that the residual variance of this regression is increased, being not σ_ε^2 but instead

$$\text{var}(Y|W) = \text{residual variance of observed data}$$
$$= \sigma_\varepsilon^2 + \lambda \beta_x^2 \sigma_u^2.$$

This facet of the problem is often ignored, but it is important. *Measurement error causes a double-whammy*: not only is the slope attenuated, but the data are more noisy, with an increased error about the line.

To illustrate the attenuation associated with the classical additive measurement error, the results of a small simulation are displayed in Figure 1.

Ten observations were generated with $\sigma_x^2 = \sigma_u^2 = 1$, $(\beta_0, \beta_x) = (0, 1)$, and $\sigma_\varepsilon^2 = 0.25$. The filled circles and steeper line depict the true but unobservable data (Y,X) and the regression line of Y on X. The empty

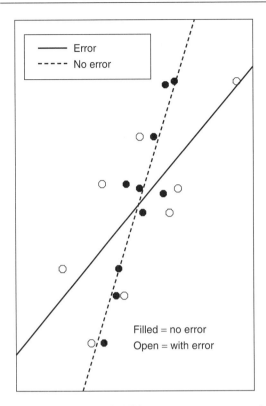

Figure 1 Illustration of additive measurement error model. The filled circles are the true (Y, X) data and the dashed (steeper) line is the least squares fit to these data. The open circles and solid (attenuated) line are the observed (Y, W) data and the associated least squares regression line. For these data $\sigma_x^2 = \delta_u^2 = 1$, $(\beta_0, \beta_x) = (0, 1)$ and $\sigma_\varepsilon^2 = 0.25$

circles and attenuated line depict the observed (Y, W) data and the linear regression of Y on W.

Figure 1 is indicative of a phenomenon called regression to the mean. Intuitively, what this means is that the extremes in the observed (W) data are *too* extreme, and that the true X is closer to the mean of the data. In fact, in normally distributed data, if X has a population mean μ_x, then having observed the fallible instrument, the best prediction of X is $\mu_x(1 - \lambda) + \lambda W$, where $\lambda < 1$ is defined in (3). The net effect is that the best (linear) predictor of X is always closer to the overall mean than any observed W.

The foregoing is one facet of regression to the mean. A more common definition is complementary. In a study participant with an unusually large observed W, if one repeats the measurement and obtains a second (replicated) measure, then this

replicate is generally less (and often much less) than the original extreme value.

For instance, in a study of true long-term fat intake (X) using a 24 h recall instrument (W), if one focuses on the person with the highest reported fat intake, then (i) that person's true fat intake is most likely less than the observed intake, and (ii) if one repeats the 24 h recall instrument, then the new reported fat intake is likely to be less than the original reported fat intake.

The second part of the "double-whammy" is a loss of power. The following example is meant to illustrate this loss of power, and it is easiest to do this illustration in the special case that all variances are known. Suppose that one wants to test the null hypothesis H_0: $\beta_x = 0$ of zero slope against the one-sided alternative H_1: $\beta_x > 0$, using a test with a 5% level (type I error) which has power 80% to detect that the slope $\beta_x = 0.75$. With known variances, in the absence of measurement error, the required sample size is

$$n = \frac{(z_{0.95} + z_{0.80})^2 \sigma_\varepsilon^2}{\sigma_x^2 \beta_x^2},$$

where z_α is the usual α percentile of the normal distribution. With measurement error, the same formula applies, except that, with $\beta_x = 0.75$, one replaces σ_ε^2 by $\sigma_\varepsilon^2 + \lambda \beta_x^2 \sigma_u^2$, σ_x^2 by $\sigma_x^2 + \sigma_u^2$, and β_x by $\lambda \beta_x$. In Figure 2, we plot the sample sizes as a function of the measurement error variance in the case that X has variance $\sigma_x^2 = 1$ and the error about the line has variance $\sigma_\varepsilon^2 = 1$. In the absence of measurement error, approximately 10 observations are required to obtain the desired power. However, if the measurement error variance $\sigma_u^2 = 1$ and thus the reliability = $1/2$, then approximately 30 observations are required. Thus, measurement error causes a loss of power. In planning a study with a large measurement error in a covariate, one will typically require a much larger sample size to meet power goals than if there were no measurement error.

It is a common belief that the effect of measurement error is always to attenuate the slope of the regression line, but in fact attenuation depends critically on the assumed classical additive measurement error model. Very different results are obtained if measurement errors are differential. One example where this problem may arise is in dietary calibration studies. In a typical dietary calibration study,

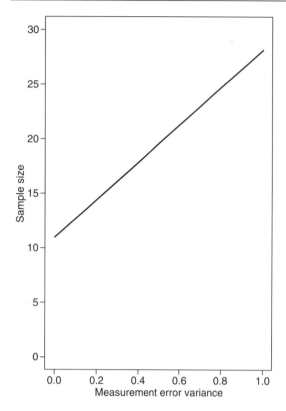

Figure 2 Sample size for 80% power in a one-sided test of level 5% in linear regression, as a function of the measurement error variance. Here the true slope = 0.75, the true variance of X is 1.0, and the true variance about the line is 1.0

one is interested in the relationship between a self-administered food frequency questionnaire (FFQ, the value of Y) and usual (or long-term) dietary intake (the value of X) as measures of, for example, the percentage of calories from fat in a person's diet. FFQs are thought to be biased for usual intake, and in a calibration study researchers will obtain a second measure (the value of W), typically from a food diary, a 24 h recall, or a short-term biomarker. In this context, it is often assumed that the diary, recall, or biomarker is unbiased for usual intake. If, as sometimes occurs, the FFQ and the diary/recall are given very nearly contemporaneously, it is unreasonable to assume that the error in the relationship between the FFQ and usual intake is uncorrelated with the error in the relationship between a diary–recall–biomarker and usual intake. This correlation has been demonstrated [29], and gives rise to differential error. It

can be shown [20] that, if there is significant correlation between the measurement error and the error about the true line, then the regression of Y on W can have a slope biased away from the null. Thus, correction for bias induced by measurement error clearly depends on the nature, as well as the extent, of the measurement error.

Multiple Regression: Single Covariate Measured with Error

In multiple linear regression the effects of measurement error are more complicated, even for the classical additive error model.

We now consider the case where X is scalar, but there are additional covariates Z measured without error. In the linear model the mean is $\beta_0 + \beta_x X + \beta_z Z$. Under the usual conditions of independence of errors, the least squares regression estimator of the coefficient of W consistently estimates $\lambda_1 \beta_x$, where

$$\lambda_1 = \frac{\sigma_{x|z}^2}{\sigma_{w|z}^2} = \frac{\sigma_{x|z}^2}{\sigma_{x|z}^2 + \sigma_u^2}, \qquad (4)$$

and $\sigma_{w|z}^2$ and $\sigma_{x|z}^2$ are the (residual) variances of the regressions of W on Z and X on Z, respectively. Note that λ_1 is equal to the simple linear regression attenuation $\lambda = \sigma_x^2/(\sigma_x^2 + \sigma_u^2)$ only when X and Z are uncorrelated. *The basic point is that the attenuation depends on the relationships among the covariates.*

The problem of measurement-error-induced bias is not restricted to the regression coefficient of X. The coefficient of Z is also biased in general, unless Z is independent of X [19]. In fact, naive ordinary least squares estimates not β_z but rather

$$\beta_{z*} = \beta_z + \beta_x(1 - \lambda_1)\gamma_z, \qquad (5)$$

where γ_z is the coefficient of Z in the regression of X on Z.

This result has important consequences in epidemiology when interest centers on the effects of covariates measured without error. For example, consider the case that Z is a binary exposure variable (exposed or not) which is classified correctly, and X is an important confounder measured with significant error. Then Carroll et al. [19] show that ignoring measurement error produces a consistent estimate of the exposure effect only if the design is balanced, i.e. X has the same mean in both groups and is independent of treatment. With considerable imbalance, the naive analysis may lead to the conclusion that: (i) there is a treatment effect when none actually exists; and (ii) the effects are negative when they are actually positive, and vice versa. In most observational studies the confounder and the exposure are correlated (see [34] and [35]). Errors in measuring the confounders can produce very misleading results.

Multiple Covariates Measured with Error

If multiple covariates are measured with error, then the direction of the bias induced by this error does not follow any simple pattern. One may have attenuation, reverse-attenuation, changes of sign, or an observed positive effect even at a true null model. This is especially the case when the predictors measured with error are correlated or their errors are correlated. In such a problem, there really seems to be no substitute for a careful measurement error analysis.

Correcting for Bias

As we have just seen, the ordinary least squares estimator is typically biased under measurement error, and the direction and magnitude of the bias depends on the regression model and the measurement error distribution. We next describe two commonly used methods for eliminating bias.

In simple linear regression with the classical additive error model, we have seen in (3) that ordinary least squares is an estimate of $\lambda\beta_x$; recall that λ is called the reliability ratio. If the reliability ratio were known, then one could obtain a proper estimate of β_x simply by dividing the ordinary least squares slope by the reliability ratio.

Of course, the reliability ratio is rarely known in practice, and one has to estimate it. If $\hat{\sigma}_u^2$ is an estimate of the measurement error variance (this is discussed below), and if $\hat{\sigma}_w^2$ is the sample variance of the Ws, then a consistent estimate of the reliability ratio is $\hat{\lambda} = (\hat{\sigma}_w^2 - \hat{\sigma}_u^2)/\hat{\sigma}_w^2$. The resulting estimate is $\beta_{x*}/\hat{\lambda}$. In small samples the sampling distribution of this estimate is highly skewed, and in such cases a modified version of the method of moments estimator is recommended [30].

The algorithm described above is called the *method-of-moments* estimator. The terminology is apt, because ordinary least squares and the reliability ratio depend only on moments of the observed data.

The method-of-moments estimator can be constructed for the general linear model, as well as for simple linear regression. Consult the book by Fuller [30], especially Chapter 2.

Another well publicized method for linear regression in the presence of measurement error is *orthogonal regression*. It is fairly rare in epidemiologic situations that the model underlying orthogonal regression holds [15], and we will not discuss the method any further.

Bias vs. Variance

Estimates that do not account for measurement error are typically biased. Unfortunately, correcting for this bias often has a price. In particular, the resulting corrected estimator will be more variable than the biased estimator, and wider confidence intervals result. For example, Rosner et al. [60] describe a problem in logistic regression, where the response is the development of breast cancer, and the predictor measured with error is daily saturated fat intake. Ignoring measurement error, they obtained an estimated **odds ratio** for saturated fat of 0.92, with a 95% confidence interval from 0.80 to 1.05. The corrected estimated odds ratio was 0.83 with a confidence interval from 0.61 to 1.12, which is twice as wide as the previous interval.

Attenuation in General Problems

We have already seen that, with multiple covariates, even in linear regression the effects of measurement error are complex, and not easily described. In this Section, we provide a brief overview of what happens in nonlinear models.

Consider a scalar covariate X measured with error, and suppose that there are no other covariates. In the classical error model for simple linear regression we have seen that the bias caused by measurement error is always in the form of attenuation, so that ordinary least squares preserves the sign of the regression coefficient asymptotically, but is biased towards zero. Attenuation is a consequence then of (i) the simple linear regression model and (ii) the classical additive error model. Without (i) and (ii), the effects of measurement error are more complex; we have already seen that attenuation may not hold if (ii) is violated.

In logistic regression, when X is measured with additive error, attenuation does not always occur, but

Table 1 A hypothetical logistic regression example with nondifferential measurement error. The entries are the expected counts. The true logistic parameters for dummy variables low and high exposure are $\log 2$ and $\log 6$, respectively, while the observed coefficients for the error prone data are $\log 0.46$ and $\log 0.53$, respectively

Disease status	Exposure = none	Exposure = low	Exposure = high
True			
$Y = 1$	4	800	120
$Y = 0$	4	400	20
Observed			
$Y = 1$	52	480	392
$Y = 0$	12	240	172

it is typical and generally much like that of linear regression.

Dosemeci et al. [28] give an example of **misclassification error** that shows that trends are not always preserved under nondifferential measurement error. Suppose that 1348 subjects are exposed at no ($X = 0$), low ($X = 1$), and high ($X = 2$) levels to a harmful substance. Suppose that the chance of an adverse outcome is 1/2, 2/3, and 6/7 for no, low, and high exposures, while the chances of the exposures themselves are 0.0059347, 0.8902077, and 0.1038576, respectively. If true exposure could be ascertained, then the expected outcomes would be as in the section of Table 1 labeled "true". If we were to regress Y on the dummy variables X_1 indicating low exposure ($X_1 = 1$), and X_2 indicating high exposure ($X_2 = 1$), then the true logistic regression parameters for X_1 and X_2 would be $\log 2 = 0.69$ and $\log 6 = 1.79$, respectively, indicating that the two higher exposure levels have response rates higher than the response rate associated with the no-exposure level. The true data clearly indicate a harmful effect due to exposure.

Now suppose, however, that measurement error (in this case misclassification) occurs, so that 40% of those truly at high exposure are misclassified into the no-exposure group, and 40% of those truly at low exposure are misclassified into the high-exposure group. Let W be the resulting variable taking on the three observed levels of exposure, with corresponding dummy variables W_1 and W_2. This is a theoretical example, of course, and one can criticize it for not being particularly realistic, but it is an example of nondifferential measurement error. The observed data we expect to see using the surrogates W_1 and W_2 are also given in Table 1.

The observed logistic regression parameters for W_1 and W_2 are $\log 0.46 = -0.78$ and $\log 0.53 = -0.63$, respectively, indicating that the two higher exposure levels have response rates lower than the response rate associated with the no-exposure level. The observed data suggest a beneficial effect due to exposure, even though the exposure is harmful!

Hypothesis Testing

In this section, we discuss hypothesis tests concerning regression parameters. To keep the exposition simple, we focus on linear regression. However, the results hold in some generality, especially for logistic and **Poisson regression**. We assume nondifferential measurement error and the classical additive error model.

The simplest approach to hypothesis testing calculates the required test statistic from the parameter estimates obtained from a measurement error analysis and their estimated standard errors. Such tests are justified whenever the estimators themselves are justified. However, this approach to testing is only possible when the indicated methods of estimation are possible, and thus requires either knowledge of the measurement error variance, or the presence of validation data, or replicate measurements, or instrumental variables.

There are certain situations in which naive hypothesis tests are justified and thus can be performed without additional data or information of any kind. Here "naive" means that we ignore measurement error and substitute W for X in a test that is valid when X is observed. This Section studies naive tests, describing when they are and are not acceptable.

We use the criterion of asymptotic validity to distinguish between acceptable and nonacceptable tests. We say a test is asymptotically valid if its type I error rate approaches its nominal level as the sample size increases. Asymptotic validity (which we shorten to validity) of a test is a minimal requirement for acceptability.

The main results on the validity of naive tests under nondifferential measurement error are as follows:

1. The naive test of no effects due to X is valid. This means that if one wants to test whether *all* components of X together have no effect, then it is valid to ignore nondifferential measurement

error. Thus, for example, if X is the exposure, then a valid test of the null hypothesis for X is obtained by ignoring measurement error and performing the standard test for the problem at hand.

2. The naive test described above is also fully efficient if X is linearly related to W and Z, but not otherwise [79]. Thus, while in principle one can obtain additional power by a measurement error analysis, many times in practice the naive test of the null hypothesis for X is reasonably efficient.

3. In many problems, more than one covariate is measured with error. For example, suppose that the exposure and one of the confounders are measured with error. Generally, the naive test of the null hypothesis for the exposure is invalid, except under special circumstances, e.g. the exposure and confounder are statistically independent, as are their measurement errors.

4. In general, naive tests for Z are invalid, except possibly if Z is uncorrelated with X. Thus, if X is the exposure and Z is a confounder, then naive tests for significance of the exposure are valid, but they are not valid for testing the significance of the confounder. Somewhat more troubling, though, is the case when X is a confounder related to the exposure Z; here the naive test for the exposure is generally invalid, *even if exposure is measured without error*. We have mentioned this example previously in the case that the exposure is binary (see [19]).

The last point can be demonstrated in the analysis of covariance, in which Z is a binary exposure variable and X is a confounder with strong predictive ability. In the analysis of covariance, the model is

$$Y = \beta_0 + \beta_z Z + \beta_x X + \varepsilon,$$

where ε is the error about the line, with variance σ_ε^2. The binary indicator Z takes on the values ± 1, with 50% of the data being unexposed ($Z = -1$) and 50% of the data being exposed ($Z = 1$). Within the unexposed group, X has mean $-\theta/2$ and variance σ_x^2, while, within the exposed group, X has mean $\theta/2$ and variance σ_x^2. The difference between the means for X in the two groups is θ. In a randomized clinical trial, one would expect that $\theta = 0$, since randomization ensures that the population means of X are

the same in the exposed and unexposed groups. In nonrandomized studies, one would expect that $\theta \neq 0$. Thus, the larger the value of θ, the more unbalanced is the study. In Figure 3, we plot the level (type I error) of the test for the exposure effect which ignores measurement error as a function of the difference in group means θ. This calculation is done for the case that $n = 20$ (10 exposed and 10 unexposed), $\sigma_\varepsilon^2 = 1$, $\sigma_x^2 = 1$, and $\beta_x = 1$, for reliability ratios $\lambda = 1/2$ and $= 2/3$. The graph shows that if the means of the confounders are sufficiently different, then, instead of a type I error of 5%, the test for exposure effect which ignores measurement error in the *confounder* can have type I error rates higher than 10%, even for such small sample sizes.

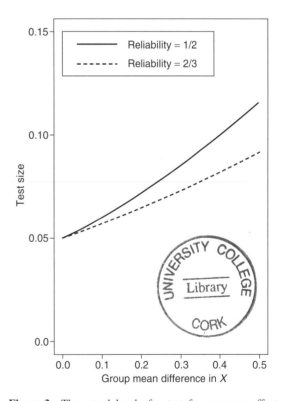

Figure 3 The actual level of a test for exposure effect with a highly predictive covariate measured with error, based on a sample of size $n = 20$. Here the true slope for the covariate $X = 1.0$, the true variance of X is 1.0, the true variance about the line is 1.0, and the reliability is either 2/3 (dashed line) or 1/2 (solid line). The term "Group mean difference in X" is the difference in the mean of X in the exposure group minus the mean of X in the control group

Regression Calibration and SIMEX

We now describe two simple, generally applicable approaches to nondifferential measurement error analysis, regression calibration, and SIMEX.

Regression Calibration

The basis of regression calibration is the replacement of X by the regression of X on (Z,W). After this approximation, one performs a standard analysis. This *regression calibration* algorithm was suggested as a general approach by Carroll & Stefanski [16] and Gleser [33]. Prentice [52] pioneered the idea for the **proportional hazard** model, and a modification of it has been suggested for this topic by Clayton [25]; see below. Armstrong [4] suggests regression calibration for generalized linear models, and Fuller [30, pp. 261–262] briefly mentions the idea. Rosner et al. [59, 60] have developed the idea for **logistic regression** into a workable and popular methodology, complete with a good computer program. Because of the importance of their contribution to epidemiologic applications, regression calibration is often referred to as "Rosner's Method". Other interesting and important applications and methodology related to regression calibration include work by Whittemore [83], Pierce et al. [51], Liu & Liang [43], and Kuha [39]. In some special cases, regression calibration is equivalent to the classical method of moments bias correction.

The main justifications of the regression calibration approximation are that, for some models, e.g. loglinear mean models and linear regression, the regression calibration approximation is often exact except for a change in the intercept parameter. For logistic regression, in many cases the approximation is almost exact.

The Regression Calibration Algorithm.   The regression calibration algorithm is what Pierce et al. [51] call a "replacement method":

1. Using replication, validation or instrumental data, estimate the regression of X on (Z,W) (see below). This is called the *calibration function*.
2. Replace the unobserved X by its estimate from the regression model, and then run a standard analysis to obtain parameter estimates.

3. Adjust the resulting standard errors to account for the estimation at the first step, using either the bootstrap or asymptotic methods [20].

The simplest form of regression calibration is the "correction for attenuation" used in linear regression. It is easiest to describe in the following situation:

1. X is a scalar.
2. The measurement error is additive, with estimated error variance $\hat{\sigma}_u^2$.

For estimating the effect of X, the regression calibration estimator is formed by three steps: (i) form the naive estimator by ignoring measurement error; (ii) let $\hat{\sigma}_{w|z}^2$ be the regression mean square error from a linear regression of W on Z (this is the sample variance of the Ws if there are no other covariates Z); (iii) the regression calibration estimator is defined by multiplying the naive estimator by $\hat{\sigma}_{w|z}^2/(\hat{\sigma}_{w|z}^2 - \hat{\sigma}_u^2)$.

Estimating the Calibration Function Parameters. With *internal validation data*, the simplest approach is to regress X on the other covariates (Z,W) in the validation data. While linear regression will be typical, it is not required.

In some problems, an *unbiased second instrument* T is available for a subset of the study participants. For instance, one might be interested in X = caloric intake over a year, but have available only T = the result of a biomarker experiment using a technique known as doubly labeled water over a 2 week period, which does not equal X because it does not take into account the variability of diet over a year. In this case one uses the regression of T on (Z,W) as the calibration function. This is the method used by Rosner et al. [59] in their analysis of the Nurses' Health Study.

Finally, in the classical additive error model, one often has merely a second measurement (a replicate) for a subset of the study population. One could treat this replicate as an unbiased second instrument and apply the method described in the previous paragraph. If the Ws are not too far from normally distributed, a more efficient method is to use the so-called best linear approximation to the calibration function (see [20, pp. 47–48]). This takes into account that some of the study participants do have a replicated W and hence use the data in a reasonably efficient fashion.

Suppose there are k_i replicate measurements of X_i, and that $\overline{W}_i$ is their mean. Replication enables us to estimate the measurement error covariance matrix σ_u^2 by the usual variance components analysis, as follows:

$$\hat{\sigma}_u^2 = \frac{\displaystyle\sum_{i=1}^{n}\sum_{j=1}^{k_i}(W_{ij} - \overline{W}_{i\cdot})^2}{\displaystyle\sum_{i=1}^{n}(k_i - 1)}. \tag{6}$$

The calibration function is defined as follows. Suppose the observations are $(Z_i, \overline{W}_{i\cdot})$, where $\overline{W}_{i\cdot}$ is the mean of k_i replicates. We use analysis of variance formulas. Let

$$\hat{\mu}_x = \hat{\mu}_w = \sum_{i=1}^{n}k_i\overline{W}_{i\cdot} \Big/ \sum_{i=1}^{n}k_i, \qquad \hat{\mu}_z = \overline{Z}_{\cdot},$$

$$\nu = \sum_{i=1}^{n}k_i - \sum_{i=1}^{n}k_i^2 \Big/ \sum_{i=1}^{n}k_i,$$

$$\hat{\sigma}_z^2 = (n-1)^{-1}\sum_{i=1}^{n}(Z_i - \overline{Z}_{\cdot})^2,$$

$$\hat{\sigma}_{xz} = \sum_{i=1}^{n}k_i(\overline{W}_{i\cdot} - \hat{\mu}_w)(Z_i - \overline{Z}_{\cdot})/\nu,$$

$$\hat{\sigma}_x^2 = \left\{ \left[\sum_{i=1}^{n}k_i(\overline{W}_{i\cdot} - \hat{\mu}_w)^2\right] - (n-1)\hat{\sigma}_u^2 \right\}/\nu.$$

The resulting estimated calibration function which is used to replace $\mathbf{X}$ in the standard analysis is

$$\hat{\mu}_w + (\hat{\sigma}_x^2, \hat{\sigma}_{xz}) \begin{bmatrix} \hat{\sigma}_x^2 + \hat{\sigma}_u^2/k_i & \hat{\sigma}_{xz} \\ \hat{\sigma}_{xz} & \hat{\sigma}_z^2 \end{bmatrix}^{-1} \begin{pmatrix} \overline{W}_{i\cdot} - \hat{\mu}_w \\ Z_i - \overline{Z}_{\cdot} \end{pmatrix}. \tag{7}$$

Expanded Regression Calibration Models.   Rudemo et al. [61], Carroll & Stefanski [16] and Carroll et al. [20] all describe refinements to the regression calibration algorithm. Rudemo et al. [61] describe a bioassay problem with a heteroscedastic Berkson error model. Racine-Poon et al. [56] describe a similar problem.

There is a long history of approximately consistent estimates in nonlinear problems, of which regression calibration and the SIMEX method are the most recent such methods. Readers should also consult

Stefanski & Carroll [70], Stefanski [67], Amemiya & Fuller [3], and Whittemore & Keller [85] for other approaches.

The SIMEX Method

We now describe a method that shares the simplicity of regression calibration and is well suited to problems with additive or multiplicative measurement error. SIMEX is a simulation-based method of estimating and reducing bias due to measurement error. SIMEX estimates are obtained by adding additional measurement error to the data in a resampling-like stage, establishing a trend of measurement error-induced bias vs. the variance of the added measurement error, and extrapolating this trend back to the case of no measurement error. The technique was proposed by Cook & Stefanski [26], and further developed by Carroll et al. [22] and Stefanski & Cook [73]. See also Stefanski [68].

An integral component of SIMEX is a self-contained simulation study resulting in graphical displays that illustrate the effect of measurement error on parameter estimates and the need for bias correction. The graphical displays are especially useful when it is necessary to motivate or explain a measurement error model analysis.

This Section describes the basic idea of SIMEX, focusing on linear regression with additive measurement error. For this simple model the effect of measurement error on the least squares estimator is easily determined mathematically, as we have shown. *The key idea underlying SIMEX is the fact that the effect of measurement error on an estimator can also be determined experimentally via simulation. If we regard measurement error as a factor whose influence on an estimator is to be determined, we are naturally led to consider simulation experiments in which the level of the measurement error, i.e. its variance, is varied intentionally.*

The SIMEX Algorithm

Suppose that, in addition to the original data used to calculate the naive estimate $\hat{\beta}_{x,\text{naive}}$, there are $M-1$ additional data sets available, each with successively larger measurement error variances, say $(1 + \zeta_m)\sigma_u^2$, where $0 = \zeta_1 < \zeta_2 < \ldots < \zeta_M$. Of course, the least squares estimate of slope from the mth data set ignoring measurement error, $\hat{\beta}_{x,m}$, consistently estimates $\beta_x\sigma_x^2/[\sigma_x^2 + (1 + \zeta_m)\sigma_u^2]$.

We can think of this problem as a nonlinear regression model, with dependent variable $\hat{\beta}_{x,m}$ and independent variable ζ_m, having a mean function of the form

$$\mathcal{G}(\zeta) = \frac{\beta_x\sigma_x^2}{\sigma_x^2 + (1 + \zeta)\sigma_u^2}, \zeta \geq 0.$$

The parameter of interest, β_x, is obtained from $\mathcal{G}(\zeta)$ by extrapolation to $\zeta = -1$. We describe the process schematically in Figure 4.

SIMEX imitates the procedure just described. In the *simulation step*, additional independent measurement errors with variance $\zeta_m\sigma_u^2$ are generated and added to the original data, thereby creating data sets with successively larger measurement error variances. For the mth data set, the total measurement error variance is $\sigma_u^2 + \zeta_m\sigma_u^2 = (1 + \zeta_m)\sigma_u^2$. Next, estimates

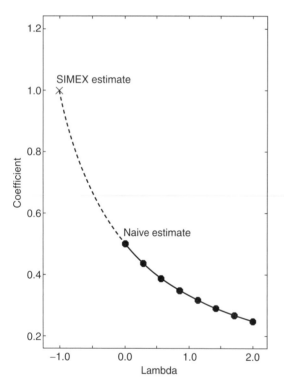

Figure 4 A generic plot of the effect of measurement error of size $(1 + \zeta)\sigma_u^2$ on parameter estimates. The value of ζ is on the x-axis, while the value of the estimated coefficient is on the y-axis. The SIMEX estimate is an extrapolation to $\zeta = -1$. The naive estimate occurs at $\zeta = 0$

are obtained from each of the resulting contaminated data sets. The simulation and reestimation step is repeated a large number of times (to remove simulation variability) and the average value of the estimate for each level of contamination is calculated. These averages are plotted against the ζ values, and regression techniques are used to fit an extrapolant function to the averaged, error-contaminated estimates. Extrapolation back to the ideal case of no measurement error ($\zeta = -1$) yields the SIMEX estimate.

The first part of the algorithm is the simulation step. As described above, this involves using simulation to create additional data sets with increasingly large measurement error $(1 + \zeta)\sigma_u^2$. For any $\zeta \geq 0$, define

$$W_{b,i}(\zeta) = W_i + \zeta^{1/2}U_{b,i},$$

$$i = 1, \ldots, n, b = 1, \ldots, B, \qquad (8)$$

where the computer-generated *pseudo-errors*, $\{U_{b,i}\}_{i=1}^n$, are mutually independent, independent of all the observed data, and identically distributed, normal random variables with mean 0 and variance σ_u^2.

Having generated the new predictors, we compute the resulting naive estimates, component by component. For each ζ, do this B times ($B = 100$ usually works fine) and compute their average, $\hat{\beta}(\zeta)$. It is the points $\{\hat{\beta}(\zeta_m), \zeta_m\}_1^M$ that are plotted as filled circles in Figure 4. This is the simulation component of SIMEX.

The extrapolation step of the proposal entails modeling each of the components of $\hat{\beta}(\zeta)$ as functions of ζ for $\zeta \geq 0$, and extrapolating the fitted models back to $\zeta = -1$. In Figure 4 the extrapolation is indicated by the dashed line and the SIMEX estimate is plotted as a cross. Carroll et al. [20] describe practical modifications of the algorithm, and how to estimate variances of parameters. Inference for SIMEX estimators can also be performed via the bootstrap. Because of the computational burden of the SIMEX estimator, the bootstrap requires considerably more computing time than do other methods. Without efficient implementation of the estimation scheme at each step, the SIMEX bootstrap may take an inconveniently long time to compute. On my computing system for measurement error models the implementation is efficient, and most bootstrap applications take little time.

We have described the SIMEX algorithm in terms of the additive measurement error model. However, SIMEX applies more generally.

For example, consider multiplicative error. Taking logarithms transforms the **multiplicative model** to the **additive model**. SIMEX works naturally here, in that one performs the simulation step (8) on the logarithms of the Ws and not on the Ws themselves.

With replicates, one can also investigate the appropriateness of different transformations. For example, after transformation, the standard deviation of the intraindividual replicates should be uncorrelated with their mean, and one can find the transformation (logarithm, square root, etc.) which makes the two uncorrelated.

Example

To illustrate SIMEX, we use data from the Framingham Heart Study, correcting for bias due to measurement error in SBP measurements. The Framingham study consists of a series of exams taken two years apart. We use Exam #3 as the baseline. There are 1615 men aged 31–65 in this data set, with the outcome, Y, indicating the occurrence of CHD within an 8-year period following Exam #3; there were 128 such cases of CHD. Predictors employed in this example are the patient's age at Exam #2, smoking status at Exam #1, and serum cholesterol at Exams #2 and #3, in addition to SBP at Exam #3, the latter being the average of two measurements taken by different examiners during the same visit. In addition to the measurement error in SBP measurements, there is also measurement error in the cholesterol measurements. However, for this example we ignore the latter source of measurement error and illustrate the methods under the assumption that only SBP is measured with error.

The covariates measured without error, Z, are age, smoking status, and serum cholesterol, with $W = \log(\text{SBP} - 50)$. Implicitly, we are defining X as the long-term average of W. We illustrate the analyses for the case where W is the mean of the two transformed SBPs, and σ_u^2 is estimated using (6). The estimated linear model correction for attenuation, or inverse of the reliability ratio, is 1.16; if only one SBP measurement were used, the correction would be 1.33.

Figure 5 contains plots of the logistic regression coefficients $\hat{\Theta}(\zeta)$ for eight equally spaced values of ζ spanning $[0, 2]$ (solid circles). For this example $B = 2000$. The points plotted at $\zeta = 0$ are the naive estimates $\hat{\Theta}_{\text{naive}}$. The nonlinear least-squares fits of

$\mathcal{G}_{\text{RL}}(\lambda, \Gamma)$ to the components of $\{\hat{\Theta}(\zeta_m), \zeta_m\}_1^8$ (solid curves) are extrapolated to $\zeta = -1$ (dashed curves), resulting in the SIMEX estimators (crosses). The open circles are the SIMEX estimators that result from fitting quadratic extrapolants. To preserve clarity the quadratic extrapolants were not plotted. Note that the quadratic-extrapolant estimates are conservative relative to the rational linear-extrapolant estimates in the sense that they fall between the rational linear-extrapolant estimates and the naive estimates.

We have stated previously that the SIMEX plot displays the effect of measurement error on parameter estimates. This is especially noticeable in Figure 5. In each of the four graphs in Figure 5, the range of the ordinate corresponds to a one-standard-error confidence interval for the naive estimate constructed using the information standard errors. Thus Figure 5 illustrates the effect of measurement error relative to the variability in the naive estimate. It is apparent that the effect of measurement error is of practical importance only on the coefficient of $\log(\text{SBP} - 50)$.

Conditional and Corrected Scores for Functional Modeling

Regression calibration and SIMEX are easily applied general methods for nondifferential error. Although the resulting estimators are consistent in important special cases such as linear regression and loglinear mean models, they are only approximately consistent in general.

For certain generalized linear models and measurement error distributions there are easily applied functional methods that are fully (and not just approximately) consistent, and make no assumptions about the distribution of X.

We focus on the case of additive normally distributed measurement error with measurement error variance σ_u^2. Although the problem has this parametric error assumption, it also has a nonparametric component: no assumptions are made about the true predictors X.

Suppose for the sake of discussion that the measurement error variance σ_u^2 is known. In the functional model, the unobservable Xs are fixed constants, and hence the unknown parameters include the Xs. With additive normally distributed measurement error, one strategy is to maximize the joint density of the observed data with respect to all of the unknown

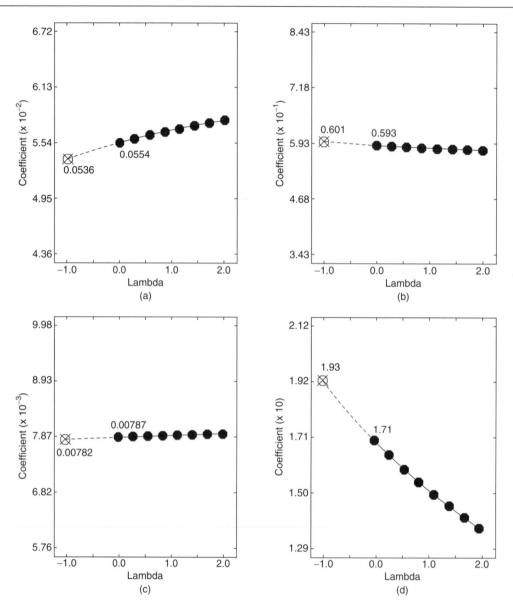

Figure 5 Coefficient extrapolation functions for the Framingham logistic regression modeling. The simulated estimates $\{\hat{\Theta}(\zeta_m), \zeta_m\}_1^8$ are plotted (solid circles) and the fitted rational linear extrapolant (solid line) is extrapolated to $\zeta = -1$ (dashed line), resulting in the SIMEX estimate (cross). Open circles indicate SIMEX estimates obtained with the quadratic extrapolant. (a) Age; (b) Smoking; (c) Cholesterol; (d) log(SBP − 50)

parameters including the Xs. While this works for linear regression [32], it fails for more complex models such as logistic regression. Indeed, the logistic regression functional maximum likelihood estimator is both inconsistent and difficult to compute [70]. An alternative approach is to change to the structural model and apply likelihood techniques (see below).

In this Section, we consider two functional methods, the conditional-score and corrected-score methods. We start with logistic and gamma–loglinear modeling as important examples for which these techniques apply. The conditional methods exploit special structures in important models such as linear, logistic, Poisson loglinear, and gamma-inverse, and then use a traditional statistical device – conditioning on sufficient statistics – to obtain estimators. The corrected-score method effectively estimates the estimator one would use if there were no measurement error.

First consider the multiple linear regression model with mean $\beta_0 + \beta_x X + \beta_z Z$, and write the unknown regression parameter as $\Theta = (\beta_0, \beta_x, \beta_z)$. When the measurement error is additive with nondifferential measurement error variance Σ_{uu}, the usual method-of-moments regression estimator can be derived as the solution to the equation

$$\sum_{i=1}^{n} \psi_* (Y_i, Z_i, W_i, \Theta, \Sigma_{uu}) = 0, \qquad (9)$$

where

$$\psi_* (Y, Z, W, \Theta, \Sigma_{uu}) = (Y - \beta_0 - \beta_x^t X - \beta_z^t Z)$$
$$\times \begin{pmatrix} 1 \\ Z \\ W \end{pmatrix} + \begin{pmatrix} 0 \\ 0 \\ \Sigma_{uu}\beta_x \end{pmatrix}$$

is the *corrected score* for linear regression. If Σ_{uu} is unknown, then one substitutes an estimate of it into (9) and solves for the regression parameters.

The key point to note here is that, in solving (9), we need know nothing about the Xs. This feature is common to all the methods in this Section.

Eq. (9) is an example of an estimating equation approach for estimating a set of unknown parameters. The reader can consult the Appendix of [20] for an overview of estimating equations, although this is unnecessary for the purpose of using the methods. Asymptotic standard errors for the estimators can be derived using either the bootstrap or the sandwich formula.

Logistic regression is best handled using the conditional-score method. For example, consider the usual linear-logistic model, where Y is binary and has success probability following the logistic model $H(\beta_0 + \beta_x X + \beta_z Z)$. The conditional score is

$$\psi_* (Y, Z, W, \Theta, \sigma_u^2)$$
$$= \{Y - H[\beta_0 - \beta_x^t \Delta(\cdot) - 0.5\beta_x^t \sigma_u^2 \beta_x$$
$$- \beta_z^t Z]\} \begin{pmatrix} 1 \\ Z \\ \Delta(\cdot) \end{pmatrix}, \qquad (10)$$

where $\Delta(\cdot) = \Delta(Y, W, \beta_x, \sigma_u^2) = W + Y\sigma_u^2 \beta_x$. Eq. (10) is substituted into (9), and the resulting equation is solved numerically.

When Y has a gamma distribution with loglinear mean $\exp(\beta_0 + \beta_x X + \beta_z Z)$, it has a variance which is ϕ times the square of the mean. For this important example, the corrected-score estimator is obtained from the corrected score

$$\psi_* (Y, Z, W, \Theta, \sigma_u^2)$$
$$= \begin{pmatrix} 1 \\ Z \\ W \end{pmatrix} - \exp[\Delta(Z, W, \Theta, \sigma_u^2)]$$
$$\times \begin{pmatrix} Y \\ ZY \\ Y(W + 0.5\sigma_u^2 \beta_x) \end{pmatrix}, \qquad (11)$$

where $\Delta(Z, W, \Theta, \sigma_u^2) = -\beta_0 - \beta_x^t W - \beta_z^t Z - 0.5 \beta_x^t \sigma_u^2 \beta_x$.

Unbiased Score Functions via Conditioning

The conditional estimators of Stefanski & Carroll [71] and Nakamura [48] are discussed in detail in Carroll et al. [20, Chapter 6]. They apply to linear, logistic, Poisson loglinear, and gamma inverse regression [the mean is $1/(\beta_0 + \beta_x X + \beta_z Z)$]. Their methods have simple formulas for standard errors, although, of course, as usual, the bootstrap applies.

Exact Corrected Estimating Equations

Suppose that it is possible to find a function of the observed data, say $\psi_*(Y, Z, W, \Theta)$, having the property that

$$E[\psi_*(Y, Z, W, \Theta)|Y, Z, X] = \psi(Y, Z, X, \Theta), \quad (12)$$

for all Y, Z, X, and Θ. Then corrected score function estimators simply replace ψ by ψ_*. Corrected score functions satisfying (12) do not always exist, and finding them when they do is not always easy.

One useful class of models that admits corrected functions contains those models with log likelihoods of the form

$$\log[f(y|z, x, \Theta)] = \sum_{k=0}^{2} [c_k(y, z, \Theta)(\beta_x^t x)^k]$$
$$+ c_3(y, z, \Theta) \exp(\beta_x^t x);$$

see the examples given below. Then, using normal distribution moment generating function identities, the required function is

$$\psi_*(y, z, w, \Theta, \sigma_u^2)$$

$$= \frac{\partial}{\partial \Theta^t} \left[\sum_{k=0}^{2} [c_k(y, z, \Theta)(\beta_x^t w)^k] - c_2(y, z, \Theta) \right.$$

$$\left. \times \beta_x^t \sigma_u^2 \beta_x + c_3(y, z, \Theta) \exp(\beta_x^t w - 0.5 \beta_x^t \sigma_u^2 \beta_x) \right].$$

Regression models in this class include:

1. normal linear with mean $= \eta$, variance $= \phi$, $c_0 = -(y - \beta_0 - \beta_z^t z)^2/(2\phi) - \log(\phi^{1/2})$, $c_1 = (y - \beta_0 - \beta_z^t z)/\phi$, $c_2 = -(2\phi)^{-1}$, $c_3 = 0$
2. Poisson with mean $= \exp(\eta)$, variance $= \exp(\eta)$, $c_0 = y(\beta_0 + \beta_z^t z) - \log y!$, $c_1 = y$, $c_2 = 0$, $c_3 = -\exp(\beta_0 + \beta_z^t z)$
3. gamma with mean $= \exp(\eta)$, variance $= \phi \exp(2\eta)$, $c_0 = -\phi^{-1}(\beta_0 + \beta_z^t z) + (\phi^{-1} - 1) \log y + \phi^{-1} \log(\phi^{-1}) - \log[\Gamma(\phi^{-1})]$, $c_1 = \phi^{-1}$, $c_2 = 0$, $c_3 = -\phi^{-1} y \exp(-\beta_0 - \beta_z^t z)$.

Comparison of Methods

The methods are applicable at the same time only in linear regression (where they are identical) and Poisson regression. For Poisson regression the corrected estimating equations are more convenient because they are explicit, whereas the conditional estimator involves numerical summation. For Poisson regression the conditional-score estimator is more efficient than the corrected-score estimator in some practical cases.

Instrumental Variables

We have assumed that it was possible to estimate the measurement error variance, say with replicate measurements or validation data. However, it is not always possible to obtain replicates or validation data, and thus direct estimation of the measurement error variance is sometimes impossible. In the absence of information about the measurement error variance, estimation of the regression model parameters is still possible provided the data contain an *instrumental variable* T, in addition to the unbiased measurement $W = X + U$.

There are three basic requirements that an instrumental variable must satisfy: (i) it must be correlated with X; (ii) it must be independent of $W - X$; and (iii) it must be a surrogate, i.e. subject to nondifferential measurement error.

One possible source of an instrumental variable is a second measurement of X obtained by an independent method. This second measurement need not be unbiased for X. Thus the assumption that a variable is an instrument is weaker than the assumption that it follows the classical additive error model.

Instrumental variable estimation in linear models is covered in depth by Fuller [30]. The work described here, outside the linear model, is based on that of Carroll & Stefanski [17] and Stefanski & Buzas [69]. Other pertinent references include [1], [2], and [13].

We have found that instrumental variables require a slightly different notation. For example, $\beta_{Y|1ZX}$ is the coefficient of **1**, i.e. the intercept, in the regression of Y on **1**, Z, and X; $\beta_{Y|1ZX}$ is the coefficient of Z in the regression of Y on **1**, Z, and X. This notation allows representation of subsets of coefficient vectors, e.g. $\beta_{Y|1ZX} = (\beta_{Y|1ZX}, \beta_{Y|1ZX})$ and $\beta_{X|1ZT} = (\beta_{X|1ZT}, \beta_{X|1ZT}, \beta_{X|1ZT})$.

Our analysis is based upon regression calibration in generalized linear models, e.g. linear, logistic, and Poisson regression. It might be useful simply to think of this Section as dealing with a class of important models, whose details of fitting are standard in many computer programs.

The approximate models and estimation algorithms are best described in terms of the composite vectors

$$\mathbf{X} = (\mathbf{1}, Z, X), \qquad \mathbf{W} = (\mathbf{1}, Z, W),$$

$$\mathbf{T} = (\mathbf{1}, Z, T).$$

Define $\boldsymbol{\beta}_{Y|\tilde{\mathbf{X}}} = (\beta_{Y|1ZX}, \beta_{Y|1ZX}, \beta_{Y|1ZX})$.

We note here that, in addition to the assumptions stated previously, we will also assume that the regression of X on (Z, T, W) is approximately linear. This restricts the applicability of our methods somewhat, but is sufficiently general to encompass many potential applications.

The simplest instrumental variables estimator starts with a (possibly multivariate) regression of **W** on **T** to obtain $\hat{\beta}_{\mathbf{W}|\mathbf{T}}$. Then Y is regressed on the predicted values $\hat{\beta}_{\mathbf{W}|\mathbf{T}}\mathbf{T}$, which results in an estimator of $\boldsymbol{\beta}_{Y|\mathbf{X}}$.

This estimator is easily computed as it requires only linear regression of the components of **W** on **T**, and then the use of standard regression programs to regress Y on the "predictors" $\hat{\beta}_{W|T}\mathbf{T}$.

Carroll et al. [20] describe somewhat more elaborate methods of instrumental variable estimation, which can be more efficient than this simple method, especially if the number of components of T differs from the number of components of W.

Likelihood and Bayesian Structural Methods

This Section describes the use of likelihood methods in measurement error models. There have been a few examples in the literature based on likelihood. See [23], [63], [64], and [78] for probit regression, [84] for a Poisson model, [27], [62] and [81] in logistic regression, and [38] in a change-point problem. The relatively small literature belies the importance of the topic and the potential for further applications.

There are a number of important differences between likelihood methods and the methods described in previous Sections:

1. The previous methods are based on additive or multiplicative measurement error models, possibly after a transformation. Typically, few, if any, distributional assumptions are required. Likelihood methods require stronger distributional assumptions, but they can be applied to more general problems, including those with discrete covariates subject to **misclassification error**.
2. The likelihood for a fully specified parametric model can be used to obtain likelihood ratio confidence intervals. In methods not based on likelihoods, inference is based on bootstrapping or on normal approximations. In highly nonlinear problems, likelihood-based confidence intervals are generally more reliable than those derived from normal approximations.
3. Likelihood methods are often computationally more demanding, whereas the previous methods require little more than the use of standard statistical packages.
4. Robustness to modeling assumptions is a concern for both approaches, but is generally more difficult to understand with likelihood methods.
5. There is a belief that the simpler methods described previously perform just as well as likelihood methods for many statistical models,

including the most common generalized linear models. There is little documentation as to whether the folklore is realistic. The only evidence that we know of is given for logistic regression by Stefanski & Carroll [72], who contrast the maximum likelihood estimate and a particular functional estimate. They find that the functional estimate is fairly efficient relative to the maximum likelihood estimate unless the measurement error is "large" or the logistic coefficient is "large". One should be aware, however, that their calculations indicate that there are situations where *properly parameterized* maximum likelihood estimates are considerably more efficient than estimates derived from functional modeling.

Likelihood Specification: Differential and Nondifferential Error

We consider here only the simplest problem in which X is not observable for all subjects, but there are sufficient data, either internal or external, to characterize the distribution of W given (X, Z) (with validation data, we are in the realm of missing data). To perform a likelihood analysis, one must specify a parametric model for every component of the data. Likelihood analysis starts with a model for the distribution of the response given the true predictors. The likelihood (density or mass) function of Y given (Z, X) will be called $f_{Y|Z,X}(y|z, x, \mathcal{B})$ here, and interest lies in estimating $\mathcal{B}$. For example, if Y is normally distributed with mean $\beta_0 + \beta_x X + \beta_z Z$ and variance σ^2, then $\mathcal{B} = (\beta_0, \beta_x, \beta_z, \sigma^2)$ and

$$f_{Y|Z,X}(y|z, x, \mathcal{B}) = \sigma^{-1}\phi[(y - \beta_0 + \beta_x x + \beta_z z)/\sigma],$$

where $\phi(v) = (2\pi)^{-1/2}\exp(-0.5v^2)$ is the standard normal density function. If Y follows a logistic regression model with mean $H(\beta_0 + \beta_x X + \beta_z Z)$, then $\mathcal{B} = (\beta_0, \beta_x, \beta_z)$ and

$$f_{Y|Z,X}(y|z, x, \mathcal{B}) = H^y(\beta_0 + \beta_x x + \beta_z z)$$
$$\times [1 - H(\beta_0 + \beta_x x + \beta_z z)]^{1-y}.$$

A likelihood analysis starts with determination of the joint distribution of Y and W given Z, as these are the observed variates. There are three components required:

1. A model relating the response to the "true" covariates, see just above.
2. An error model, here called $f_{W|Z,X}(w|z, x, \tilde{\alpha}_1)$. In many applications, the error model does not depend on Z. For example, in the classical additive measurement error model (1) with normally distributed measurement error, σ_u^2 is the only component of $\tilde{\alpha}_1$, and the error model density is $\sigma_u^{-1}\phi[(w - x)/\sigma_u]$, where $\phi(\cdot)$ is the standard normal density function. In the classical error model with independent replicates, W consists of the k replicates, and $f_{W|Z,X}$ is the k-variate normal density function with mean zero, common variance σ_u^2, and zero correlation. A generalization of this error model that allows for correlations among the replicates has been studied [81]. In some application areas, error model structures are studied independently of their role in measurement error modeling, and one can use this research to estimate error models for the problem at hand.
3. A model for the distribution of the latent variable, here called $f_{X|Z}(x|z, \tilde{\alpha}_2)$. Specifying a model for the distribution of the true covariate X given all the other covariates, Z is more difficult. Difficulties arise because: (i) the distribution is usually not transportable, so that different studies yield very different models; and (ii) X is not observed.

Having hypothesized the various models, the likelihood of the observed data under nondifferential measurement error is

$$f_{Y,W|Z}(y, w|z, \mathcal{B}, \tilde{\alpha}_1, \tilde{\alpha}_2)$$
$$= \int f_{Y|Z,X}(y|z, x, \mathcal{B}) f_{W|Z,X}(w|z, x, \tilde{\alpha}_1)$$
$$\times f_{X|Z}(x|z, \tilde{\alpha}_2) d\mu(x). \qquad (13)$$

The notation $d\mu(x)$ indicates that the integrals are sums if X is discrete and integrals if X is continuous. The likelihood for the problem is just the product over the sample of these terms.

There is a significant difference between the likelihood function in the differential and nondifferential cases. This can be expressed in various ways, but the simplest is as follows. In general, and dropping parameters, the likelihood of the observed data is

$$f_{Y,W|Z}(y, w|z) = \int f_{Y,W,X|Z}(y, w, x|z) d\mu(x).$$

Using standard conditioning arguments, this becomes

$$f_{Y,W|Z}(y, w|z) = \int f_{W|Y,Z,X}(w|y, z, x) f_{Y|Z,X}(y|z, x)$$
$$\times f_{X|Z}(x|z) d\mu(x)$$
$$= \int f_{Y|Z,X}(y|z, x) f_{W|Y,Z,X}(w|y, z, x)$$
$$\times f_{X|Z}(x|z) d\mu(x). \qquad (14)$$

Note that the only difference between (13) and (14) is in the error term. In the former, under nondifferential measurement error, W and Y are independent, so that $f_{W|Y,Z,X}(w|y, z, x) = f_{W|Z,X}(w|z, x)$.

What makes differential error so difficult is that, under differential measurement error, we must ascertain the distribution of W given the other covariates *and the response Y*. This is essentially impossible to do in practice unless one has a subset of the data in which all of (Y, Z, X, W) are observed, i.e. a *validation* data set (*see* **Validation Study**).

Numerical Computation of Likelihoods

Typically one maximizes the logarithm of the overall likelihood in the unknown parameters. There are two ways one can maximize the likelihood function. The most direct is to compute the likelihood function itself, and then use numerical optimization techniques to maximize the likelihood. Below we provide a few details about computing the likelihood function. The second general approach is to view the problem as a missing data problem, and then use missing data techniques (*see* **Missing Data**); see, for example, [42] and [75].

Computing the likelihood analytically is easy if X is discrete, as the conditional expectations are simply sums of terms. Likelihoods in which X has some continuous components can be computed using a number of different approaches. In some problems the log likelihood can be computed or very well approximated analytically. In most problems that we have encountered, X is a scalar or a 2×1 vector. In these cases, standard numerical methods such as Gaussian quadrature can be applied, although they are not always very good. When sufficient computing resources are available, the likelihood can be computed using Monte Carlo techniques.

Bayesian Methods

Bayesian estimation and inference in the measurement error problem is a promising approach under active development. Examples of this approach are given by Schmid & Rosner [65], Richardson & Gilks [57], Stephens & Dellaportas [74], Müller & Roeder [47], Mallick & Gelfand [45], and Kuha [40].

Bayesian analysis of parametric models requires specifying a likelihood (as described above) and a prior distribution for the parameters, the latter representing knowledge about the parameters prior to data collection. The product of the prior and likelihood is the joint density of the data and the parameters. Using Bayes' Theorem, one can in principle obtain the posterior density, i.e. the conditional density of the parameters given the data. The posterior summarizes all of the information about the values of the parameters and is the basis for all Bayesian inference. For example, the mean, median, or mode of the posterior density are all suitable point estimators. A region with probability $1 - \alpha$ under the posterior is called a "credible set," and is a Bayesian analog to a confidence region.

Computing the posterior distribution is often a nontrivial problem, because it usually requires high-dimensional numerical integration. This computational problem is the subject of much recent research, with many major advances. The method currently receiving the most attention in the literature is the Gibbs sampler (see [66] and [24]). Also, see Tanner [75] for a book-length introduction to modern methods for computing posterior distributions.

In the Bayesian approach with Gibbs sampling, the Xs are treated as "missing data" (they just happen to be missing for all study subjects unless there is a validation study!). The approach for the classical additive error model is:

1. Assuming nondifferential error, write the likelihood of Y given (X, Z), the likelihood of W given (X, Z), and the likelihood of X given Z depending on parameters, just as in a regular likelihood problem.
2. If X were observable, then the likelihood would be the product of the three terms given above.
3. Select a starting value for the parameters, e.g. from SIMEX.
4. Use a simulation approach to fill in the "missing" Xs, i.e. from the posterior distribution of X given the observed data and the current values of the

parameters. In this step, it is rare that the posterior distribution is known exactly, and so one has to use a device such as the Metropolis–Hastings algorithm.

5. Now one has complete data, with Xs all filled in, and one uses simulation to draw a sample of parameters from the posterior distribution of the parameters given the observed data and the current Xs.
6. Repeat the process of generating X and the parameters. These multiple samples of parameters are used to evaluate features of the posterior distribution.

While the procedure is easy to write down, the computations may be difficult.

More importantly, though, is the need to consider the distribution of X given Z. As we emphasized above, the simplest structural approach assumes that X is normally distributed, but this is often a strong assumption. The popularity of functional methods lies in the fact that such methods require no distributional assumptions about the Xs. There is considerable current effort being made to circumvent the problem of model robustness by specifying a flexible distribution for X.

Mixture Modeling

When there are no covariates measured without error, the nonlinear measurement error problem can be viewed as a special case of what are called mixture problems (see [77]). The idea is to pretend that X has a distribution, but to estimate this distribution nonparametrically. Applications of nonparametric mixture methods to nonlinear measurement error models have only recently been described by Thomas et al. [76] and Roeder et al. [58].

An alternative formulation is to let X have a flexible distribution, which covers a wide range of possibilities including the normal distribution. The simplest such model is the mixture of normals, which has been applied by Wang et al. [81] and by Küchenhoff & Carroll [38].

Response Error

In preceding Sections we have focused exclusively on problems associated with measurement error in predictor variables. Here we consider problems that arise when a true response is measured with error. For example, in a study of factors affecting dietary intake of fat, e.g. sex, race, age, socioeconomic status, etc., true long-term dietary intake is impossible to determine and instead it is necessary to use error-prone measures of long-term dietary intake. Wittes et al. [86] describe another example in which damage to the heart muscle caused by a myocardial infarction can be assessed accurately, but the procedure is expensive and invasive, and instead it is common practice to use the peak cardiac enzyme level in the bloodstream as a proxy for the true response.

For a binary response (case or control), see **Misclassification Error**.

The exclusive attention paid to predictor measurement error earlier in this article is explained by the fact that predictor measurement error is seldom ignorable, by which is meant that the usual method of analysis is statistically valid, whereas response measurement error is often ignorable when the response is continuous. Here, "ignorable" means that the model holding for the true response holds also for the proxy response with parameters unchanged, except that a measurement error variance component is added to the response variance. For example, in linear regression models with simple types of response measurement error, the response measurement error is **confounded** with equation error and the effect is simply to increase the variability of parameter estimates. Thus, response error is ignorable in these cases, although of course power will be lost. However, in more complicated regression models, certain types of response error are not ignorable and it is important to account for the response error explicitly in the regression analysis.

Although the details differ between methods for predictor error and response error, many of the basic ideas are similar. Throughout this section, the response proxy is denoted by S. We consider only the case of measurement error in the response, and not the more complex problem where both the response and some of the predictors are measured with error.

We first consider the analysis of the observed data when the response is subject to independent additive or multiplicative measurement error. Suppose that the proxy response S is unbiased for the true response. Then, in either case, the proxy response has the same mean (as a function of exposure and confounders) as the true response, although the variance structure differs. In models such as linear regression, or

more generally for quasi-likelihood estimation, this means that the parameter estimates are consistent, but inferences may be affected. For example, in linear regression, additive, unbiased response error does not change the mean and simply increases the variance by a constant, so that there is no effect of measurement error other than loss of power. However, for multiplicative, unbiased response error, while the mean remains unchanged, the variances now are no longer constant, and hence inferences which pretend that the variances are constant would be affected. The usual solution is to use a robust covariance estimator, also known as the sandwich estimator.

If the proxy response S is not unbiased for the true response, then a validation study is required to understand the nature of the bias and to correct for it. In a series of papers, Buonaccorsi [8, 9, 11] and Buonaccorsi & Tosteson [12] discuss the use of adjustments for a biased response. See Carroll et al. [20] for further details.

We call S a *surrogate response* if its distribution depends only on the true response and not otherwise on the covariates, i.e. the information about the surrogate response contained in the true response is the same no matter what the values of the covariates. In symbols, if $f_{S|Y,Z,X}(s|y, z, x, \gamma)$ denotes the density or mass function for S given (Y, Z, X), then $f_{S|Y,Z,X}(s|y, z, x, \gamma) = f_{S|Y}(s|y, \gamma)$. In both the additive and multiplicative error models, S is a surrogate. This definition of a surrogate response is the natural counterpart to a surrogate predictor, because it implies that all the information in the relationship between S and the predictors is explained by the underlying response. See Prentice [53] and Carroll et al. [20] for further details.

In general, i.e. for a possibly nonsurrogate response, the likelihood function for the observed response is

$$f_{S|Z,X}(s|z, x, \mathcal{B}, \gamma)$$

$$= \int f_{Y|Z,X}(y|z, x, \mathcal{B}) f_{S|Y,Z,X}(s|y, z, x, \gamma) \mathrm{d}\mu(y).$$

$$(15)$$

There are a number of implications of this formula:

1. If S is a surrogate, and if there is no relationship between the true response and the predictors, then neither is there one between the observed response and the predictors. Hence, if interest

lies in determining whether *any of the predictors* contains any information about the response, then one can use naive hypothesis tests and ignore response error. The resulting tests have an asymptotically correct level, but a decreased power relative to tests derived from true response data. This property of a surrogate is important in clinical trials; see Prentice [53].

2. If S is *not* a surrogate, then there may be no relationship between the true response and the covariates, but the observed response may be related to the predictors. Hence, naive tests will not be valid in general if S is not a surrogate.

Note that one implication of (15) is that a likelihood analysis with mismeasured responses requires a model for the distribution of response error. Except for additive and multiplicative error, understanding such a model requires a validation study.

Case–Control Studies

A *case–control study* is one in which sampling is conditioned on the disease response; it is useful to think that the response is first observed and only later are the predictors observed. A similar design, *choice-based sampling*, is used in econometrics. We use case–control terminology and concentrate on logistic regression models. A distinguishing feature of case–control studies is that the measurement error may be differential.

Two-phase case–control designs, where X is observed on a subset of the data, have been studied by Breslow & Cain [7], Zhao & Lipsitz [87], Tosteson & Ware [80], and Carroll et al. [18], among others. These designs are significant because the validation, if done on both cases and controls, frees us from the nondifferential error assumption.

We assume that the data follow a logistic model in the underlying source population, although the results apply equally well to the more general models described by Weinberg & Wacholder [82]. For such models, Prentice & Pyke [55] and Weinberg & Wacholder [82] show that when analyzing a classical case–control study one can ignore the case–control sampling scheme entirely, at least for the purpose of estimating **relative risk**. Furthermore, these authors show that, if one *ignores the case–control sampling scheme and runs an ordinary logistic regression*, then the resulting relative risk estimates are consistent and the standard errors are asymptotically correct.

The effect of measurement error in logistic case–control studies is to bias the estimates. Carroll et al. [21] show that, for many problems, one can ignore the case–control study design and proceed to correct for the bias from measurement error as if one were analyzing a random sample from the source population. With nondifferential measurement error, this result applies to the methods we have described previously for prospective studies. Regression calibration needs a slight modification, namely that the regression calibration function should be estimated using the controls only.

Michalek & Tripathi [46], Armstrong et al. [5], and Buonaccorsi [10] consider the normal discriminant model. Satten & Kupper [62] have an interesting example of likelihood analysis for nondifferential error validation studies when the validation sampling is in the controls.

Survival Analysis

One of the earliest applications of the regression calibration method was discussed by Prentice [52] in the context of **survival analysis**. Further results in survival analysis were obtained by Pepe et al. [50], Clayton [25], Nakamura [49], and Hughes [36]. While the details differ in substantive ways, the ideas are the same as put forward in the rest of this article, and here we provide only a very brief overview in the case of covariates which do not depend on time.

Suppose that the instantaneous risk that the time T of an event equals t conditional on no events prior to time t and conditional on the true covariate X is denoted by

$$\psi(t, X) = \psi_0(t)\exp(\beta_x X), \qquad (16)$$

where $\psi_0(t)$ is the baseline **hazard** function. When the baseline hazard is not specified, (16) is commonly called the **proportional hazards** assumption. When X is observable, it is well known that estimation of β_x is possible without specifying the form of the baseline hazard function.

If X is unobservable and instead we observe a surrogate W, then the induced hazard function is

$$\psi^*(t, W, \beta_x) = \psi_0(t)\mathrm{E}[\exp(\beta_x X)|T \geq t, W]. \quad (17)$$

The difficulty is that the expectation in (17) for the observed data depends upon the unknown baseline hazard function ψ_0. Thus, the hazard function does not factor into a product of an arbitrary baseline hazard times a term that depends only on observed data and an unknown parameter, and the technology for proportional hazards regression cannot be applied without modification.

The problem simplifies when the event is rare, so that $T \geq t$ occurs with high probability for all t under consideration. As shown by Prentice [53] and others, under certain circumstances this leads to the regression calibration algorithm. The rare event assumption allows the hazard of the observed data to be approximated by

$$\psi^*(t, W, \beta_x) = \psi_0(t)\mathrm{E}[\exp(\beta_x X)|W]. \qquad (18)$$

The hazard function (18) requires a regression calibration formulation! If one specifies a model for the distribution of X given W, then (18) is in the form of a proportional hazards model (16), but with $\beta_x X$ replaced by $\log\{\mathrm{E}[\exp(\beta_x X)|W]\}$. An important special case leads directly to the standard regression calibration model, namely when X given W is normally distributed.

Clayton [25] proposed a modification of regression calibration which does not require events to be rare. At each time $t_i, i = 1, \ldots, k$, for which an event occurs, define the risk set $R_i \subseteq \{1, \ldots, n\}$ as the case numbers of those members of the study cohort for whom an event has not occurred and who were still under study just prior to t_i. If the Xs were observable, and if X_i is the covariate associated with the ith event, in the absence of ties the usual proportional hazards regression would maximize

$$\prod_{i=1}^{k} \frac{\exp(\beta_x X_i)}{\displaystyle\sum_{j \in R_i} \exp(\beta_x X_j)}.$$

Clayton basically suggests using regression calibration within each risk set. He assumes that the true values X within the ith risk set are normally distributed with mean μ_i and variance σ_x^2, and that within this risk set $W = X + U$, where U is normally distributed with mean zero and variance σ_u^2. Neither σ_x^2 nor σ_u^2 depend upon the risk set in his formulation.

Given an estimate $\hat{\sigma}_u^2$, one applies the usual regression calibration calculations to construct an estimate of $\hat{\sigma}_x^2$.

Clayton modifies regression calibration by using it within each risk set. Within each risk set, he applies the formula (7) for the best unbiased estimate of the Xs. Specifically, in the absence of replication, for any member of the ith risk set, the estimate of the true covariate X from an observed covariate W is

$$\hat{X} = \hat{\mu}_i + \frac{\hat{\sigma}_x^2}{\hat{\sigma}_x^2 + \hat{\sigma}_u^2}(W - \hat{\mu}_i),$$

where $\hat{\mu}_i$ is the sample mean of the Ws in the ith risk set.

As with regression calibration in general, the advantage of Clayton's method is that no new software need be developed, other than to calculate the means within risk sets.

Acknowledgment

This work was supported by a grant from the National Cancer Institute (CA-57030).

References

[1] Amemiya, Y. (1985). Instrumental variable estimator for the nonlinear errors in variables model, *Journal of Econometrics* **28**, 273–289.

[2] Amemiya, Y. (1990). Instrumental variable estimation of the nonlinear measurement error model, in *Statistical Analysis of Measurement Error Models and Application*, P.J. Brown & W.A. Fuller, eds. American Mathematics Society, Providence.

[3] Amemiya, Y. & Fuller, W.A. (1988). Estimation for the nonlinear functional relationship, *Annals of Statistics* **16**, 147–160.

[4] Armstrong, B. (1985). Measurement error in generalized linear models, *Communications in Statistics, Part B – Simulation and Computation* **14**, 529–544.

[5] Armstrong, B.G., Whittemore, A.S. & Howe, G.R. (1989). Analysis of case-control data with covariate measurement error: application to diet and colon cancer, *Statistics in Medicine* **8**, 1151–1163.

[6] Berkson, J. (1950). Are there two regressions?, *Journal of the American Statistical Association* **45**, 164–180.

[7] Breslow, N.E. & Cain, K.C. (1988). Logistic regression for two-stage case-control data, *Biometrika* **75**, 11–20.

[8] Buonaccorsi, J.P. (1988). Errors in variables with systematic biases, *Communications in Statistics – Theory and Methods* **18**, 1001–1021.

[9] Buonaccorsi, J.P. (1990). Double sampling for exact values in some multivariate measurement error problems, *Journal of the American Statistical Association* **85**, 1075–1082.

[10] Buonaccorsi, J.P. (1990). Double sampling for exact values in the normal discriminant model with application to binary regression, *Communications in Statistics – Theory and Methods* **19**, 4569–4586.

[11] Buonaccorsi, J.P. (1991). Measurement error, linear calibration and inferences for means, *Computational Statistics and Data Analysis* **11**, 239–257.

[12] Buonaccorsi, J.P. & Tosterson, T. (1993). Correcting for nonlinear measurement error in the dependent variable in the general linear model, *Communications in Statistics – Theory and Methods* **22**, 2687–2702.

[13] Buzas, J.S. & Stefanski, L.A. (1995). A note on corrected score estimation, *Statistics and Probability Letters* **28**, 1–8.

[14] Carroll, R.J. & Ruppert, D. (1988). *Transformation and Weighting in Regression*. Chapman & Hall, London.

[15] Carroll, R.J. & Ruppert, D. (1996). The use and misuse of orthogonal regression in measurement error models, *American Statistician* **50**, 1–6.

[16] Carroll, R.J. & Stefanski, L.A. (1990). Approximate quasilikelihood estimation in models with surrogate predictors, *Journal of the American Statistical Association* **85**, 652–663.

[17] Carroll, R.J. & Stefanski, L.A. (1994). Measurement error, instrumental variables and corrections for attenuation with applications to meta-analyses, *Statistics in Medicine* **13**, 1265–1282.

[18] Carroll, R.J., Gail, M.H. & Lubin, J.H. (1993). Case-control studies with errors in predictors, *Journal of the American Statistical Association* **88**, 177–191.

[19] Carroll, R.J., Gallo, P.P. & Gleser, L.J. (1985). Comparison of least squares and errors-in-variables regression, with special reference to randomized analysis of covariance, *Journal of the American Statistical Association* **80**, 929–932.

[20] Carroll, R.J., Ruppert, D. & Stefanski, L.A. (1995). *Measurement Error in Nonlinear Models*. Chapman & Hall, London.

[21] Carroll, R.J., Wang, S. & Wang, C.Y. (1995). Asymptotics for prospective analysis of stratified logistic case-control studies, *Journal of the American Statistical Association* **90**, 157–169.

[22] Carroll, R.J., Küchenhoff, H., Lombard, F. & Stefanski, L.A. (1996). Asymptotics for the SIMEX estimator in structural measurement error models, *Journal of the American Statistical Association* **91**, 242–250.

[23] Carroll, R.J., Spiegelman, C., Lan, K.K., Bailey, K.T. & Abbott, R.D. (1984). On errors-in-variables for binary regression models, *Biometrika* **71**, 19–26.

[24] Casella, G. & George, E.I. (1992). Explaining the Gibbs sampler, *American Statistician* **46**, 167–174.

[25] Clayton, D.G. (1991). Models for the analysis of cohort and case-control studies with inaccurately measured exposures, in *Statistical Models for Longitudinal Studies of Health*, J.H. Dwyer, M. Feinleib, P. Lipsert et al., eds. Oxford University Press, New York, pp. 301–331.

[26] Cook, J. & Stefanski, L.A. (1995). A simulation extrapolation method for parametric measurement error models, *Journal of the American Statistical Association* **89**, 1314–1328.

[27] Crouch, E.A. & Spiegelman, D. (1990). The evaluation of integrals of the form $\int_{-\infty}^{\infty} f(t)\exp(-t^2)\mathrm{d}t$: applications to logistic–normal models, *Journal of the American Statistical Association* **85**, 464–467.

[28] Dosemeci, M., Wacholder, S. & Lubin, J.H. (1990). Does non-differential misclassification of exposure always bias a true effect towards the null value?, *American Journal of Epidemiology* **132**, 746–748.

[29] Freedman, L.S., Carroll, R.J. & Wax, Y. (1991). Estimating the relationship between dietary intake obtained from a food frequency questionnaire and true average intake, *American Journal of Epidemiology* **134**, 510–520.

[30] Fuller, W.A. (1987). *Measurement Error Models*. Wiley, New York.

[31] Ganse, R.A., Amemiya, Y. & Fuller, W.A. (1983). Prediction when both variables are subject to error, with application to earthquake magnitude, *Journal of the American Statistical Association* **78**, 761–765.

[32] Gleser, L.J. (1981). Estimation in multivariate errors in variables regression model: large sample results, *Annals of Statistics* **9**, 24–44.

[33] Gleser, L.J. (1990). Improvements of the naive approach to estimation in nonlinear errors-in-variables regression models, in *Statistical Analysis of Measurement Error Models and Application*, P.J. Brown & W.A. Fuller, eds. American Mathematical Society, Providence.

[34] Greenland, S. (1980). The effect of misclassification in the presence of covariates, *American Journal of Epidemiology* **112**, 564–569.

[35] Greenland, S. & Robins, J.M. (1985). Confounding and misclassification, *American Journal of Epidemiology* **122**, 495–506.

[36] Hughes, M.D. (1993). Regression dilution in the proportional hazards model, *Biometrics* **49**, 1056–1066.

[37] Hunter, D.J., Spiegelman, D., Adami, H.-O., Beeson, L., van der Brandt, P.A., Folsom, A.R., Fraser, G.E., Goldbohm, A., Graham, S., Howe, G.R., Kushi, L.H., Marshall, J.R., McDermott, A., Miller, A.B., Speizer, F.E., Wolk, A., Yaun, S.S. & Willett, W. (1996). Cohort studies of fat intake and the risk of breast cancer–a pooled analysis, *New England Journal of Medicine* **334**, 356–361.

[38] Küchenhoff, H. & Carroll, R.J. (1997). Segmented regression with errors in predictors: semiparametric and parametric methods, *Statistics in Medicine* **16**, 169–188.

[39] Kuha, J. (1994). Corrections for exposure measurement error in logistic regression models with an application to nutritional data, *Statistics in Medicine* **13**, 1135–1148.

[40]   Kuha, J. (1997). Estimation by data augmentation in regression models with continuous and discrete covariates measured with error, *Statistics in Medicine* **16**, 189–201.

[41]   Li, L., Freedman, L., Kipnis, V. & Carroll, R.J. (1997). Effects of bias and correlated measurement errors in the validation of food frequency questionnaires. Preprint.

[42]   Little, R.J.A. & Rubin, D.B. (1987). *Statistical Analysis with Missing Data*. Wiley, New York.

[43]   Liu, X. & Liang, K.Y. (1992). Efficacy of repeated measures in regression models with measurement error, *Biometrics* **48**, 645–654.

[44]   MacMahon, S., Peto, R., Cutler, J., Collins, R., Sorlie, P., Neaton, J., Abbott, R., Godwin, J., Dyer, A. & Stamler, J. (1990). Blood pressure, stroke and coronary heart disease: Part 1, prolonged differences in blood pressure: prospective observational studies corrected for the regression dilution bias, *Lancet* **335**, 765–774.

[45]   Mallick, B.K. & Gelfand, A.E. (1996). Semiparametric errors-in-variables models: a Bayesian approach, *Journal of Statistical Planning and Inference* **52**, 307–322.

[46]   Michalek, J.E. & Tripathi, R.C. (1980). The effect of errors in diagnosis and measurement on the probability of an event, *Journal of the American Statistical Association* **75**, 713–721.

[47]   Müller, P. & Roeder, K. (1997). A Bayesian semiparametric model for case-control studies with errors in variables, *Biometrika* **84**, 523–537.

[48]   Nakamura, T. (1990). Corrected score functions for errors-in-variables models: methodology and application to generalized linear models, *Biometrika* **77**, 127–137.

[49]   Nakamura, T. (1992). Proportional hazards models with covariates subject to measurement error, *Biometrics* **48**, 829–838.

[50]   Pepe, M.S., Self, S.G. & Prentice, R.L. (1989). Further results in covariate measurement errors in cohort studies with time to response data, *Statistics in Medicine* **8**, 1167–1178.

[51]   Pierce, D.A., Stram, D.O., Vaeth, M. & Schafer, D. (1992). Some insights into the errors in variables problem provided by consideration of radiation dose–response analyses for the A-bomb survivors, *Journal of the American Statistical Association* **87**, 351–359.

[52]   Prentice, R.L. (1982). Covariate measurement errors and parameter estimation in a failure time regression model, *Biometrika* **69**, 331–342.

[53]   Prentice, R.L. (1989). Surrogate endpoints in clinical trials: definition and operational criteria, *Statistics in Medicine* **8**, 431–440.

[54]   Prentice, R.L. (1996). Dietary fat and breast cancer: measurement error and results from analytic epidemiology, *Journal of the National Cancer Institute* **88**, 1738–1747.

[55]   Prentice, R.L. & Pyke, R. (1979). Logistic disease incidence models and case-control studies, *Biometrika* **66**, 403–411.

[56]   Racine-Poon, A., Weihs, C. & Smith, A.F.M. (1991). Estimation of relative potency with sequential dilution errors in radioimmunoassay, *Biometrics* **47**, 1235–1246.

[57]   Richardson, S. & Gilks, W.R. (1993). A Bayesian approach to measurement error problems in epidemiology using conditional independence models, *American Journal of Epidemiology* **138**, 430–442.

[58]   Roeder, K., Carroll, R.J. & Lindsay, B.G. (1996). A nonparametric mixture approach to case-control studies with errors in covariables, *Journal of the American Statistical Association* **91**, 722–732.

[59]   Rosner, B., Spiegelman, D. & Willett, W.C. (1990). Correction of logistic regression relative risk estimates and confidence intervals for measurement error: the case of multiple covariates measured with error, *American Journal of Epidemiology* **132**, 734–745.

[60]   Rosner, B., Willett, W.C. & Spiegelman, D. (1989). Correction of logistic regression relative risk estimates and confidence intervals for systematic within-person measurement error, *Statistics in Medicine* **8**, 1051–1070.

[61]   Rudemo, M., Ruppert, D. & Streibig, J.C. (1989). Random effect models in nonlinear regression with applications to bioassay, *Biometrics* **45**, 349–362.

[62]   Satten, G.A. & Kupper, L.L. (1993). Inferences about exposure-disease association using probability of exposure information, *Journal of the American Statistical Association* **88**, 200–208.

[63]   Schafer, D. (1987). Covariate measurement error in generalized linear models, *Biometrika* **74**, 385–391.

[64]   Schafer, D. (1993). Likelihood analysis for probit regression with measurement errors, *Biometrika* **80**, 899–904.

[65]   Schmid, C.H. & Rosner, B. (1993). A Bayesian approach to logistic regression models having measurement error following a mixture distribution, *Statistics in Medicine* **12**, 1141–1153.

[66]   Smith, A.F.M. & Gelfand, A.E. (1992). Bayesian statistics without tears: a sampling–resampling perspective, *American Statistician* **46**, 84–88.

[67]   Stefanski, L.A. (1985). The effects of measurement error on parameter estimation, *Biometrika* **72**, 583–592.

[68]   Stefanski, L.A. (1989). Unbiased estimation of a nonlinear function of a normal mean with application to measurement error models, *Communications in Statistics – Theory and Methods* **18**, 4335–4358.

[69]   Stefanski, L.A. & Buzas, J.S. (1995). Instrumental variable estimation in binary regression measurement error models, *Journal of the American Statistical Association* **90**, 541–549.

[70]   Stefanski, L.A. & Carroll, R.J. (1985). Covariate measurement error in logistic regression, *Annals of Statistics* **13**, 1335–1351.

[71]   Stefanski, L.A. & Carroll, R.J. (1987). Conditional scores and optimal scores in generalized linear measurement error models, *Biometrika* **74**, 703–716.

[72]   Stefanski, L.A. & Carroll, R.J. (1990). Structural logistic regression measurement error models, in *Proceedings*

of the Conference on Measurement Error Models, P.J. Brown & W.A. Fuller, eds. Wiley, New York.

[73] Stefanski, L.A. & Cook, J. (1995). Simulation extrapolation: the measurement error jackknife, *Journal of the American Statistical Association* **90**, 1247–1256.

[74] Stephens, D.A. & Dellaportas, P. (1992). Bayesian analysis of generalized linear models with covariate measurement error, in *Bayesian Statistics 4*, J.M. Bernado, J.O. Berger, A.P. Dawid & A.F.M. Smith, eds. Oxford University Press, Oxford, pp. 813–820.

[75] Tanner, M.A. (1993). *Tools for Statistical Inference: Methods for the Exploration of Posterior Distributions and Likelihood Functions*, 2nd Ed. Springer-Verlag, New York.

[76] Thomas, D., Stram, D. & Dwyer, J. (1993). Exposure measurement error: influence on exposure-disease relationships and methods of correction, *Annual Review of Public Health* **14**, 69–93.

[77] Titterington, D.M., Smith, A.F.M. & Makov, U.E. (1985). *Statistical Analysis of Finite Mixture Distributions*. Wiley, New York.

[78] Tosteson, T., Stefanski, L.A. & Schafer D.W. (1989). A measurement error model for binary and ordinal regression, *Statistics in Medicine* **8**, 1139–1147.

[79] Tosteson, T. & Tsiatis, A. (1988). The asymptotic relative efficiency of score tests in a generalized linear model with surrogate covariates, *Biometrika* **75**, 507–514.

[80] Tosteson, T.D. & Ware, J.H. (1990). Designing a logistic regression study using surrogate measures of exposure and outcome, *Biometrika* **77**, 11–20.

[81] Wang, N., Carroll, R.J. & Liang, K.Y. (1996). Quasi-likelihood and variance functions in measurement error models with replicates, *Biometrics* **52**, 401–411.

[82] Weinberg, C.R. & Wacholder, S. (1993). Prospective analysis of case–control data under general multiplicative-intercept models, *Biometrika* **80**, 461–465.

[83] Whittemore, A.S. (1989). Errors in variables regression using Stein estimates, *American Statistician* **43**, 226–228.

[84] Whittemore, A.S. & Gong, G. (1991). Poisson regression with misclassified counts: application to cervical cancer mortality rates, *Applied Statistics* **40**, 81–93.

[85] Whittemore, A.S. & Keller, J.B. (1988). Approximations for regression with covariate measurement error, *Journal of the American Statistical Association* **83**, 1057–1066.

[86] Wittes, J., Lakatos, E. & Probstfield, J. (1989). Surrogate endpoints in clinical trials: cardiovascular trials, *Statistics in Medicine* **8**, 415–425.

[87] Zhao, L.P. & Lipsitz, S. (1992). Designs and analysis of two-stage studies, *Statistics in Medicine* **11**, 769–782.

(*See also* **Agreement, Measurement of**)

RAYMOND J. CARROLL

Meta-Analysis in Epidemiology

Because of the pressure for timely and informed decisions in public health and clinical practice and because of the explosion of information in the scientific literature, research results must be synthesized to answer urgent questions [2, 27, 72]. Principles of evidence-based methods to assess the effectiveness of health care interventions and to set policy are cited increasingly [17]. Approaches to summarizing evidence include narrative reviews, systematic reviews and meta-analysis.

In general, randomized (controlled) clinical trials (RCTs) provide more useful evidence than do cohort studies, and cohort studies often provide better evidence than do case–control studies [135]. Cross-sectional studies and case series provide a weaker basis for etiologic reasoning. Because there are usually too few RCTs available to test clinical hypotheses, and because RCTs are rarely available to test etiologic hypotheses, particularly for chronic conditions, combining data from observational (cohort and case–control) studies is often necessary [9, 35, 129, 159] (*see* **Case–Control Study**; **Cohort Study**).

Scientific Synthesis

In a traditional narrative review of the epidemiologic or medical literature, subject-matter experts review studies, decide which are relevant to the particular topic, and highlight their findings in terms of results and, to a lesser degree, methodology. The limitations of this or any approach to a literature review include: (a) biases in the original studies, reporting and publication policies; (b) absence in reported studies of specific data needed for the review; (c) investigator bias caused by subjective inclusion of studies; (d) uneven quality of the primary data; and (e) biased interpretation of outcome [152]. Such limitations have caused some authors to disregard the results of such reviews as having been prepared "with disregard for scientific principles" and therefore resulting in misleading decisions with serious consequences, often affecting health and quality of life [25, 110].

Systematic review methods have been adopted to address these problems. Systematic rules for conducting a synthesis include an explicit description of methodology so that results can be interpreted in light of biases and limitations [41]. Use of such systematic rules enables the investigator to refine large amounts of information, provide estimates of variables needed for economic and decision analysts, provide an efficient scientific technique, establish generalizability of scientific findings, assess consistency of relationships, explain data inconsistencies, increase statistical power and increase the precision of estimates [14, 25]. The techniques of meta-analysis use all of the steps of a systematic review, but in addition include a statistical combination of the results of previous studies to arrive at conclusions about a body of research (e.g. [147, 152]). Although systematic reviews in general, and meta-analyses specifically, are not immune to the potential pitfalls of a narrative review, the technique reduces the possibility of such errors and explicitly describes potential limitations (e.g. bias) of the results and interpretation [3, 111].

The statistical roots of systematic reviews can be found as early as the beginning of the twentieth century [125]. The term *meta-analysis* was first used in 1976 in the educational literature [68]: "the statistical analysis of a large collection of results from individual literature, for the purpose of integrating the findings". Since the method usually uses as "data" summary statistics derived from published reports of original studies, it is an *analysis of a statistical analysis* (thus, *meta*-analysis). Meta-analysis is most useful when individual study results are inconsistent and primary study sizes are small [97, 102, 126], since combining studies increases power. Meta-analysis is often recommended before undertaking a new study, to learn from earlier studies and to determine whether a new study will add substantially to what is already known about the topic [75, 95, 96].

While systematic reviews of evidence are usually desirable, meta-analysis (the statistical synthesis of results) should not be used indiscriminately [38, 42, 43, 61, 77]. In fact, legal suits have been brought by industry against researchers, charging "negligent misleading" when disparate findings are summarized by a single "class effect" [83]. The method is inappropriate if the number of studies is small or if there are large differences among the studies in study populations, interventions or effect measures [56, 92].

Approaches to summarizing data other than meta-analysis include vote counting and pooling [120, 121]. Vote counting relies only on the statistical significance of results [105], and may tend to indicate the

wrong decision more often as the amount of evidence (number of studies) increases and does not incorporate characteristics of the original studies [81]; thus, we do not discuss that method here. The use of pooling, or combining original data, may be limited by the availability of data from primary authors [143]. When feasible, however, pooling original data offers definite advantages. Measures of exposure and outcome can be standardized, and adjustment for confounders can be done in a consistent manner across studies if the original data are available. Thus, with pooling, preliminary analyses yielding summary estimates of exposure effect for each study may be rendered more homogeneous than would be the case in more conventional meta-analyses. Once these study-specific estimates are obtained, standard meta-analytic techniques may be used to combine them. Lubin et al. [109] used pooling to combine data from cohort studies of underground miners to estimate the effect of radon exposure on risk of developing lung cancer.

Uses of Meta-analysis in Epidemiology

Meta-analyses were first used in clinical studies to combine results from RCTs [19, 27, 117, 131]. For example, a meta-analysis of 33 trials that compared treatment using intravenous streptokinase with a placebo in patients hospitalized for acute myocardial infarction showed a favorable effect of treatment, whereas only six of the 33 primary trials showed a statistically significant effect [100]. Continuously updated reviews, such as those provided by the Cochrane Database of Systematic Reviews [26, 32] facilitate proper conduct of meta-analyses of RCTs.

Meta-analysis is being used increasingly to combine results from observational studies when randomized controlled designs are not available or not feasible [149]. Here, we define an observational study as an etiologic or effectiveness study using an analysis from an existing database, a cross-sectional study, a case series, a case–control design, a design with historical controls or a cohort design [70, 124]. Observational designs lack the experimental element of a random allocation to an intervention and rely on studies of association between changes or differences in one characteristic (e.g. an exposure or intervention), and changes or differences in an outcome of interest. These designs have long been recommended and used in the evaluation of educational programs [40] and of exposures that might cause disease [92]. For example, studies of risk factors generally cannot be randomized, because they relate to inherent human characteristics or practices, or because such a randomization might be unethical [106, 124]. At times, clinical data on treatments may be summarized in order to design a randomized treatment comparison [89, 155]. Observational data may also be needed to assess how well an intervention works in a community as opposed to the special setting of a controlled trial [110].

Meta-analyses of observational studies present particular challenges because of inherent biases and differences in study designs [88]. Nonrandomized comparisons are subject to both selection bias and other types of confounding, and combining several studies all subject to the same bias will only reinforce that bias [141] (*see* **Bias in Case–Control Studies**; **Bias in Cohort Studies**). In addition, observational studies may lack some of the elements of a well-designed clinical trial, such as careful definition of endpoints, interventions and study population [117]. Also, observational studies may have different exposed populations and control groups, may suffer from measurement error of exposures, and may explore only varying outcome measures. Because such factors may influence various studies differently, a single summary measure for exposure effect may be misleading. A more important use of meta-analysis of observational studies may well be as a tool for understanding and quantifying sources of heterogeneity in results across studies [113, 119].

Although meta-analysis of observational studies may not always be appropriate (e.g. [73, 137]) – particularly if the goal is to produce a single summary estimate of an association [101] – the number of published meta-analyses concerning health issues has increased substantially during the past four decades: from 678 before 1992; to 525 from 1992 through 1995; to approximately 400 in 1996 alone. Furthermore, a 1997 study of published meta-analyses documented that 86% of authors were the first or second author of only a single meta-analysis before the one used in the study [138], indicating the broadening use of this method.

Steps in a Meta-analysis

The basic steps in a meta-analysis include: (a) a clear statement of the problem and hypothesis to be tested; (b) a clearly defined statement of inclusion and exclusion criteria for admission of studies; (c) a methodology for locating research studies; (d) the classification and coding of study characteristics to be combined in the meta-analysis and a quantitative measurement of study characteristics and of the effect of the exposure on outcome; (e) an assessment of the quality of the methods used in the studies; (f) a statistical analysis that includes methods for combining study results when appropriate and determining the sources of heterogeneity of the data; and (g) interpretation of results, including an assessment of bias of individual studies, a discussion of heterogeneity, and identification of areas for further research [126, 152].

Statement of the Problem and Hypothesis to be Tested

Problem formulation is critical and includes the explicit definition of both outcomes and potential confounding variables. This step enables the investigator to abstract accurate and consistent data from reports of studies and to choose appropriate statistical models for the analysis. This step is especially critical for meta-analyses of observational studies. For example, suppose the major task is the exploration of evidence for a theory: Does a high level of homocysteine contribute to increased risk for cardiovascular disease [20]? Such a statement of the problem allows exclusion of studies using patients with competing conditions, which may preclude a clear evaluation of outcome.

As for any study, the protocol is the blueprint for the conduct of the meta-analysis. The protocol should contain a clear statement of the problem, objectives, hypotheses to be tested, background and specifications for information retrieval, data collection and analysis.

Establishing Inclusion and Exclusion Criteria

As in any statistical study, sample design is an important determinant of the utility and scientific validity of results. In a meta-analysis, the sampling units are the results of published or unpublished studies. The study inclusion/exclusion criteria provide the "case definition" for results to be used in the synthesis. Objective exclusion criteria should be determined a priori to meet scientific criteria and not as a matter of convenience. For example, a decision to exclude studies published before a specific date should be based on evidence that a technology or therapy changed at that time (and therefore historical results may not be comparable with more recent results), and not on the fact that earlier studies may not be cataloged electronically. "Fugitive literature" refers to studies that may be published in documents that are difficult to locate, because they are not published, are published but not abstracted, or have limited circulation (e.g. dissertations, conference abstracts and proceedings or government reports). If studies in the "fugitive literature" are to be excluded, a rationale should be given. Similarly, a decision to exclude foreign language studies should follow a determination that studies published in a language other than English are different in some substantive way, and not be made merely on the basis of a lack of translation capability [59, 74, 114]. Although some control over heterogeneity of design may be accomplished through the use of exclusion rules, a more informative approach could be to use broad inclusion criteria for studies, and then to perform analyses to determine whether measured design features influence measurements of exposure effect on outcome [10].

Locating Research Studies

The goal of the search process is to (a) identify all relevant primary studies (published and unpublished) for potential inclusion in the meta-analysis; and (b) to determine which studies are to be included. Accurate and thorough specifications of the search strategy will allow for the replication of the meta-analysis and permit others to evaluate the external validity of the findings. The term "search" implies the entire process, which is usually composed of several different methods of searching. A 1996 review of 103 meta-analyses in education documented that search procedures were described inadequately, fewer than half of the meta-analyses reported details of classifying and coding the primary study data and only 22% assessed quality of the primary studies [138].

The literature search should be systematic and comprehensive. The researcher uses several sources of information to locate data for retrieval, including written indices; computerized searches; bibliographies of published papers; and unreferenced and sometimes unpublished data from academic, private and governmental researchers [23, 37]. Complete searches should go beyond computerized indices,

which have been shown to have a sensitivity as low at 50% in some examples [51]. Researchers estimate that 25%–50% of all initiated randomized controlled trials are never published, and excluding data from unpublished studies may result in bias or loss of precision in estimation of effect size [50].

Several computerized databases exist, many operated by the National Library of Medicine and included in the Medical Library Information Retrieval System (MEDLARS). These include AIDSLINE (for AIDS-related citations, 1980 to the present), CANCERLIT (containing cancer literature from journals, government reports and conferences, 1963 to the present), TOXLINE (containing citations on the effects of drugs and other chemicals), and Dissertation Abstracts (containing abstracts of American and Canadian doctoral dissertations, 1861 to the present). Registries of randomized trials [32, 54] provide information prior to publication of RCTs for topics of interest to the collaborators. For other study designs, or for situations in which registries do not exist, contact with experts in the field may yield more complete ascertainment. It is important to identify and remove redundant reports for the same study [90]. When computerized indices are used, the search strategy should be specified completely to allow replication. The description should include keywords used, fields searched (e.g. whether the search was by text word, title or subject), software used for searching (e.g. OVID), and any software-specific functions (e.g. "explosion" of terms).

Classification, Coding and Measurement of Study Characteristics and Measurement of Exposure Effect on Outcome

The classification and coding of study characteristics follows directly from problem formulation [152]. This step can consume the majority of time invested in a meta-analysis – approximately 90% [86, p. 85]. In addition to increasing the time required for a synthesis, adding characteristics of the studies included increases the probability of finding at least one chance association as significant. Thus, many meta-analysts recommend coding a study characteristic only when theoretical justification exists [146]. This recommendation is controversial, however, since additional information about study characteristics can provide documentation for findings, can assist analysis of sources of heterogeneity and can provide areas for additional research. Furthermore, the requirement for formal theoretical justification can restrict creative hypothesis generation.

Blinding (masking) readers to identifying information about papers (e.g. author's affiliation) has been advocated. In a study of blinding, five meta-analyses of RCTs were conducted in parallel by two groups randomly assigned to read papers that either had or had not been masked as to the identity of the authors and institutions producing the original papers, and as to which treatment group was which. Although the unmasked readers assigned higher quality scores on average than the masked readers, masking made little difference in the summary odds ratios [6, 16]. We are unaware of any published studies of the effects of blinding on meta-analyses of observational data.

Assessment of Quality of Included Studies

The use of quality scoring in meta-analysis is controversial [56, 60]. One potential use of quality scores is to assign greater weight to some studies than others when combining results. A second use is for grouping studies according to quality to determine whether estimates of exposure effect depend on study quality [66, 77]. Quality scores constructed in an *ad hoc* fashion, however, may lack demonstrated validity. Furthermore, examples indicate that estimates of exposure effect are not always associated with quality [73]. Nevertheless, some *particular* aspects of study quality, such as adherence to the randomization scheme in RCTs, have been shown to be associated with effect size [12, 116, 136].

Statistical Methods for Combining Study Results and Analyzing Heterogeneity

Statistical issues related to combining data from multiple sources in meta-analysis are the subject of ongoing research [60, 104]. The most important statistical issues concern which studies should be combined. When feasible, meta-analysis should be restricted to RCTs, the study design that provides most useful evidence. When too few RCTs are available, combining data from observational (cohort and case–control) studies is necessary.

Beyond the determination of studies to be combined, a central question is whether variations in research studies (methodologic or contextual) are related to variations in effect size. This question can

be approached by the use of *fixed-* or *random-effects models*. The simplest fixed-effects models assume that the exposure effect is constant across studies and that variation from one study to the next is due solely to within-study random variation. More elaborate fixed-effects models may allow the outcome to depend on several fixed effects, corresponding to several variables that characterize the studies [80]. Random-effects models allow the intrinsic exposure effect to vary from study to study so that variation in the estimated exposure effects reflects both sampling error within studies and effect variation across studies [82]. Random-effects models assume that the studies included are selected randomly from a population of studies with varying exposure effects and are used to accommodate unexplained heterogeneity of exposure effects [87]. Random-effects models increase the estimated variance around estimates of associations and produce different point estimates than fixed-effects models. It should be emphasized, however, that using random-effects models to account for unexplained heterogeneity should not substitute for a thorough exploratory (fixed-effects) analysis of how study design and population characteristics affect estimates of exposure effects. If random-effects models are used, then the rationale for model selection should be given, and estimates of among-study variation should be reported [52].

Epidemiologic studies undertaken to establish causal explanations of disease–exposure association frequently estimate risks at different levels of exposure [84]. Such dose–response studies yield study-specific slopes that may be combined using meta-analytic techniques [139, 154]. One meta-analytic method for estimating a combined dose–response effect from case–control and cohort studies incorporates the same dose–response model in each component of the likelihood, which is the product of the study-specific likelihoods [15]. Brumback [22] used the estimation–minimization (EM) algorithm (termed the "method of weights") to maximize this likelihood; the calculations use standard weighted regression software.

Regardless of the statistical measure used to combine data, a meta-analysis to combine results across studies should include: (a) presenting the study-specific exposure estimates with estimates of study-specific random error; (b) presenting summary estimates of exposure effect across studies, with estimates of variability; (c) testing for heterogeneity of exposure effects across studies, and, if present, investigating possible causes of heterogeneity; and (d) providing quantitative support for interpreting the results.

Interpretation of Results

The interpretation should focus on a discussion of the strengths and weaknesses of the evidence, including possible biases, and on the justification for combining estimates in the presence of potential heterogeneity of study results. Bias has been defined as any systematic error that leads to the distortion of accurate results (e.g. [126]). In the original studies, bias can result from flaws in the study design that tend to distort the magnitude or direction of associations in the data. In meta-analyses, additional bias can result from the way in which studies are selected for inclusion and from the way in which data are gathered and analyzed (*see also* **Bias, Overview**).

Assessment of Bias in Individual Studies   One approach to assessing the research quality of observational studies is based on "threats to validity" [40]. Thirty-three independent threats to validity are categorized into four groups – internal, external, statistical conclusion and construct validity. Internal validity is "the truthfulness with which statements can be made about whether there is a causal relationship from one variable to another in the form in which the variables were manipulated or measured" [40, p. 38]. External validity reflects the extent to which the relation can be generalized across other populations. Statistical conclusion validity refers to the quality of the statistical analysis and inference. Construct validity concerns threats that may confound cause and effect measurement

In general, quality assessment indicates that not all studies retrieved should be included in the meta-analysis. Construct and external validity can be used to determine whether a study addresses the hypothesis of interest, participants, time period and location; i.e. the relevance of the study to the meta-analysis [133]. Construct validity can also be used in meta-analyses assessing theories [108]. Studies with fewest threats to internal validity should be considered highest quality [161]. Improper statistical techniques may also render a study unacceptable for inclusion (e.g. inappropriate statistical tests, incorrect grouping of values, inappropriate conclusions or the absence of

information needed to calculate effect estimates or variability).

Publication bias   Publication bias, i.e. the selective publication of studies on the basis of the magnitude and direction of their findings, represents a particular threat to the validity of any meta-analysis [50, 55, 130]. Statistical methods assist in the assessment of publication bias and in correcting for this problem [4, 5, 45]. Methods for detecting publication bias include correlating the observed exposure effect size with design features of the studies that might be "risk factors" for publication bias (such as sample size, presence or absence of randomization and prospective vs. retrospective design) [11, 49, 69, 79]. For example, for a meta-analysis using a mixture of randomized and nonrandomized studies, if randomization status appears to be associated with size of risk estimates, then one might eliminate (or analyze separately) the nonrandomized studies [132].

The effect of sample size on publication bias can be assessed graphically by a "funnel plot" of sample size vs. effect size [104]. In the absence of publication bias caused by sample size, the plot should appear as an inverted funnel; that is, large variability will be shown with small studies and decreasing spread as the sample size increases, with constant mean effect size regardless of sample size. If this shape is not apparent, then publication bias should be suspected. For example, if large studies are clustered around the null value with smaller studies skewed around a positive effect, then one suspects that some small negative studies were not included, revealing publication bias [93].

Formal statistical significance tests can be used to determine whether estimates of intervention effects are correlated with sample size [7]. A rank correlation based on Kendall's tau [1] requires no underlying assumptions, but may lack power. Alternatively, a test based on Spearman's rho is more tractable computationally [36].

Statistical methods for correcting for publication bias include sampling methods and analytic methods. Sampling methods are based on the following logic: if publication bias is caused by preferential publication based on study results, then this problem can be prevented by restricting the search to a sampling frame that cannot be influenced by study results, such as registries of prospective trials [54]. There are few registries of observational studies [30]. Attempting to locate all relevant observational studies through contact with experts and use of sources of unpublished reports to supplement standard computerized searches remains an option [44].

Analytic methods for addressing publication bias include the "file drawer" method [130], which addresses the question: If a combined estimate indicates a statistically significant exposure effect, then how many studies with null results must exist somewhere (the file drawer) to overturn the results? Hedges & Olkin [82] answer a similar question for methods that combine evidence from the individual studies' significance levels, rather than methods that obtain a combined estimate of exposure effect. Some methods to correct for publication bias are based on the assumption that a study is included in the meta-analysis with probability proportional to the estimated effect size [29, 123].

Heterogeneity   Heterogeneity of populations (e.g. study subjects), study designs (e.g. case–control vs. cohort studies), methods for measuring exposure and outcomes, analytical approaches to confounding and other issues must be recognized, reported, and, when possible, addressed in the analysis of the data by exploring associations between variation in study design and analysis and variation in estimated exposure effects [10]. In cases where heterogeneity of exposure effects is large, a single summary measure of exposure effect may be inappropriate. Analyses that stratify by study feature or regression analysis with design features as predictors can be useful in assessing whether these features influence estimates of exposure effect. Studies should never be discarded solely on the basis of having results that disagree with those of the majority of other studies [34], but rather should be examined for underlying characteristics of design or analysis that may have led to the discrepant results.

Statistical tests for heterogeneity include DerSimonian & Laird's Q-test [31, 46], an approach based on weighted least squares [107], an application of the likelihood ratio test [148], and methods based on a bootstrap approach [151]. The power of these tests to detect heterogeneity is often small, however, because the number of studies (the effective sample size) is typically less than 30 [75]. Empirical evaluation shows that the DerSimonian and Laird Q-statistic is preferable from the point of view of

validity, power and computational ease [151]. Graphical displays, stratification and regression analysis are useful methods to address criticisms of summarization in the presence of heterogeneity [73]. For the specific case of combining comparative trials with uncontrolled historical studies, Begg & Pilote have proposed a method using a random effects approach [8]. Investigating heterogeneity was a key feature of a meta-analysis of asbestos exposure and risk of gastrointestinal cancer [67]. This example shows that sources of bias and heterogeneity can be hypothesized before analysis and subsequently confirmed by the analysis.

Finally, sensitivity analysis can permit exploration of sources of heterogeneity and can suggest future research directions. Sensitivity analysis can be used in each step of a meta-analysis. During the search and citation retrieval step, use of more than one investigator is helpful when the research question spans disciplines and requires different subject-matter expertise. Exploratory data analysis [71] can be used to investigate features of articles retrieved in the search and reveal factors that may have impact on the choice of more formal statistical procedures. Combining P-values and regression analysis [82, Chapter 12] aids in sensitivity analysis.

Schlesselman [134] used the possible association between endometrial cancer and oral contraceptives to comment on issues related to potential bias in the studies of this association. His meta-analysis combined both cohort and case–control studies and used a sensitivity analysis to illustrate the effect of omitting specific studies. He addressed possible bias caused by restriction to English language articles by performing analyses limited to such studies.

In summary, interpretation should include assessing the internal validity of component studies; namely, whether they were well-designed, executed and analyzed. Discussion of whether the studies included are appropriate for answering the meta-analytic question should include efforts taken to avoid publication bias. For example, do funnel plots support the contention that publication bias has been minimized? If not, how much bias can be anticipated? To what extent should heterogeneity of effect estimates be related either to systematic features of various studies (such as sample size, type of study or study quality) or to nonidentifiable random variation? In view of any heterogeneity of results, is it reasonable to summarize the results in a single measure of exposure effect (with an estimated confidence interval), or rather to state that a single summary is not appropriate and that further research is needed to define the sources of variation and extent of the association?

A Case Study

A 1991 study of the effects of duration of estrogen use on breast cancer risk [145] illustrates many of the decisions made in performing a meta-analysis in epidemiology. Published reports agreed on the risk associated with ever-use of estrogen replacement therapy, but little evidence was shown for increases in risk due to short-term use (less than five years), and there was less agreement on the effect of long-term use. The authors located case–control and cohort studies; among the case–control studies, designs were heterogeneous in choice of controls (e.g. hospital or community). Heterogeneity testing was used to determine criteria for subgroup analysis. Estimated dose–response slopes from primary studies were used for the meta-analysis to account for inter-study variability. Fixed- and random-effects models were computed, and assumptions such as equal baseline risk were evaluated by sensitivity testing. Because tests of homogeneity were significant, the authors analyzed data from studies that used community controls separately from those that used hospital controls [144].

Increased risk of breast cancer with duration of estrogen use was found among studies with community controls (risk of breast cancer after 10 years of estrogen use increased by at least 15%); studies with hospital controls showed a similar increase when a single outlier study conducted in Europe was excluded. Differences in results of fixed- and random-effects models may have been due to this source of variation. Other sources of heterogeneity explored included study design, location of study population (US vs. Europe) indicating differences in estrogen preparation; the two European studies using hospital controls showed an increased risk, while studies in the US showed a small decrease in risk with duration of estrogen use.

This example indicates the role of heterogeneity of study design in the interpretation of results of a meta-analysis. In this case, many health conditions are associated with estrogen use and a woman's decision to use estrogen. Thus, the choice of controls may have been a critical determinant of heterogeneity.

For example, greater use of estrogen among women who receive acute care in hospitals might explain the apparent decrease in breast cancer risk shown by studies that used hospital controls.

Discussion

Taking stock of what is known in epidemiology involves reviewing the existing literature, summarizing it in appropriate ways, exploring the implications of heterogeneity of study designs, and determining how heterogeneity of design might relate to heterogeneity of study results. Meta-analysis provides a systematic way of performing this research synthesis, while indicating when more research is necessary and is a widely used and increasingly popular technique. Nevertheless, some criticisms and caveats are important for using the results of meta-analyses of observational studies [53, 64, 65, 140].

Criticisms of Meta-Analysis in Epidemiology

The use of meta-analysis in epidemiology is not universally accepted due to several limitations [156]. First, bias can occur in the original studies (resulting from flaws in the study design that tend to distort the magnitude or direction of associations in the data), or from the way in which studies are selected for inclusion [18, 62]. Methods have been developed to aid in the detection of publication bias, a particular threat to the validity of meta-analysis of observational studies [55, 130]. In addition, funding source can be an important source of bias affecting results [94].

Secondly, when combining observational studies, heterogeneity of populations (e.g. US vs. international), design (e.g. case–control vs. cohort studies), and outcome (e.g. different studies yielding different relative risks that cannot be accounted for by sampling variation) is expected [10, 153]. In cases where heterogeneity of outcomes is particularly problematic, a single summary measure may be inappropriate. Analyses that stratify by study feature or regression analysis with design features as predictors can be useful in assessing whether study outcomes indeed vary systematically with these features [34, 150].

Thirdly, the use of quality scoring in meta-analysis is controversial [60] because scores constructed in an *ad hoc* fashion may lack demonstrated validity, and results may not be associated with quality [21].

Fourthly, a statistical summary of evidence may be misused to obscure important variations in exposure effects [56]. Meta-analyses have been criticized because of discrepancies between their results and those from large randomized trials [24, 28, 47, 91, 103, 128].

Extensions and Related Areas

Cumulative Meta-Analysis   The concept of the cumulative meta-analysis was introduced in 1993 [27]. In a cumulative meta-analysis, studies are combined and data synthesized on an ongoing basis. As soon as a study relevant to the particular topic is published, its results are entered into the meta-analysis and estimates of effect or relative risk are then updated. Adaptation of methods from interim analyses of clinical trials has been used in this situation [57, 127, 158]. This updating enables the most current estimation of the effect of a particular intervention or particular risk factor. Retrospective analysis of clinical trials for myocardial infarction indicates that a cumulative meta-analysis of the effects of thrombolytic therapy and lidocaine on cardiovascular mortality could have changed clinical practice as much as 10–15 years earlier had such analyses been conducted, published and disseminated adequately [100]. Alternatively, one may perform the cumulative analysis by adding sequentially studies with increasing quality score or increasing study size to investigate the effects of these factors. Attention should be paid to the results of repeated testing by adjusting significance levels.

Cochrane Collaboration, investigators of a particular subject-matter area, aggregate data on an ongoing basis, conduct cumulative meta-analyses and make the results available to clinical researchers and others interested in clinical and public health policy [18, 33, 160].

Statistical Software   Egger et al. [58] attribute part of the growth in the number of meta-analyses to the recent appearance of software packages that implement the methods. Available packages vary in their provision of tutorials, graphical features and flexibility of modeling. Almost all packages include the capability for fixed- and random-effects modeling, tests of homogeneity and ability to handle multiple types of response. Some, such as RevMan© produced by the Cochrane Collaboration, are available via the Internet. For many applications (e.g. dose–response

analyses, or meta-regressions), one must still use preliminary programs to estimate inputs, such as slopes, for use in meta-analytic programs.

Conclusions: The Role of Meta-Analysis in Epidemiology

Regardless of the problems and technical solutions, an analytic synthesis of evidence is critical for policy in epidemiology and public health [157]. When policy-makers attempted to study the effect of passive smoking in public places (inhalation of others' smoke), tobacco-industry lobbyists presented competent studies showing little evidence of harm, and anti-smoking activists presented studies that showed passive smoking to be a cause of lung cancer [85].

The systematic evaluation of any health topic is essential to excellent clinical or public health practice [98]. The results of such evaluations also help define priorities in research. The conduct of meta-analyses, therefore, warrants rigorous implementation. The introduction of systematic reviews and meta-analyses has fostered controversy [48], but it has also initiated a critical examination of the process of research synthesis. This process must continue with careful consideration given to both epidemiologic and statistical issues and appropriate examination of the impact on health and quality of life. In addition to the specific methodologic issues mentioned above, more effort must continue in the design and implementation of primary studies and the reporting of such studies, including methods as well as results [6, 42, 99, 115, 122, 142]. Efforts such as the Cochrane Collaboration have demonstrated the value of careful collection and storage of information in readily accessible computer data banks. The development of computer software both for data manipulation and transport, as well as statistical analysis, will continue to reap rewards for researchers and practitioners. Improved accessibility of the results of meta-analyses is another potential benefit of the computerization of data. At the same time, researchers and practitioners must be trained to understand the benefits and limitations of alternative methods of data synthesis, as should those who make public policy decisions and influence medical care and public health practice. Statisticians have a critical role in developing methods for special problems and assisting in the design, execution and analysis of these studies.

References

[1] Armitage, P. & Berry, G. (1987). *Statistical Methods in Medical Research*, 2nd Ed. Blackwell, Oxford.

[2] Badgett, R.G., O'Keefe, M. & Henderson, M.C. (1997). Using systematic reviews in clinical education, *Annals of Internal Medicine* **126**, 886–891.

[3] Bailar, J.C. (1997). The promise and problems of meta-analysis, *New England Journal of Medicine* **337**, 559–560.

[4] Begg, C. (1994). Publication bias, in *The Handbook of Research Synthesis*, H. Cooper & L.V. Hedges, eds. Russel Sage Foundation, New York, pp. 399–409.

[5] Begg, C.B. & Berlin, J.A. (1989). Publication bias and dissemination of clinical research, *Journal of the National Cancer Institute* **81**, 107–115.

[6] Begg, C.B., Cho, M., Eastwood, S., Horton, R., Moher, D., Olkin, I., Pitkin, R., Rennie, D., Schulz, K.F., Simel, D. & Stroup, D.F. (1996). Improving the quality of reporting of randomized controlled trials: the CONSORT statement, *Journal of the American Medical Association* **276**, 637–639.

[7] Begg, C.B. & Mazumdar, M. (1994). Operating characteristics of a rank correlation test for publication bias, *Biometrics*, 1088–1101.

[8] Begg, C.B. & Pilote, L. (1991). A model for incorporating historical controls into a meta-analysis, *Biometrics* **47**, 899–906.

[9] Beral, V. (1995). The practice of meta-analysis: discussion. Meta-analysis of observational studies: a case study of work in progress, *Journal of Clinical Epidemiology* **48**, 165–166.

[10] Berlin, J.A. (1995). Invited commentary: benefits of heterogeneity in meta-analysis of data from epidemiologic studies, *American Journal of Epidemiology* **142**, 383–387.

[11] Berlin, J.A., Begg, C.B. & Louis, T.N. (1989). An assessment of publication bias using a sample of published clinical trials, *Journal of the American Statistical Association* **84**, 381–392.

[12] Berlin, J.A. & Colditz, G.A. (1999). The role of meta-analysis in the regulatory process for foods, drugs, and devices, *Journal of the American Medical Association* **281**, 830–834.

[13] Berlin, J.A., Laird, N.M., Sacks, H.S. & Chalmers, T.C. (1989). A comparison of statistical methods for combining event rates from clinical trails, *Statistics in Medicine* **8**, 141–151.

[14] Berlin, J.A., Longnecker M.P. & Greenland S. (1993). Meta-analysis of epidemiologic dose–response data, *Epidemiology* **4**, 218–228.

[15] Berlin, J.A., Miles, C.G. & Cirigliano, M.D. (1997). Does blinding of readers affect the results of meta-analyses? Results of a randomized trial, *Journal of Current Clinical Trials*, doc no. 205, online.

[16] Berlin, J.A. & University of Pennsylvania Meta-analysis Blinding Study Group (1997). Does blinding of readers affect the results of meta-analyses? *Lancet* **350**, 185–186.

[17] Bero, L.A. & Jadad, A.R. (1997). How consumers and policymakers can use systematic reviews for decision making, *Annals of Internal Medicine* **127**, 37–42.

[18] Blettner, M., Sauerbrei, W., Schlehofer, B., Scheuchenpflub, T. & Friedenreich, C. (1999). Traditional reviews, meta-analyses and pooled analyses in epidemiology, *International Journal of Epidemiology* **28**, 1–9.

[19] Boissel, J.P., Blanchard, J., Panak, E., Peyrieux, J.C. & Sacks, H. (1989). Considerations for the meta-analysis of randomized clinical trials, *Controlled Clinical Trials* **10**, 254–281.

[20] Boushey, C.J., Beresford, S.A., Omenn, G.S. & Motulsky, A.G. (1995). A quantitative assessment of plasma homocysteine as a risk factor for vascular disease: probable benefits of increasing folic acid intakes, *Journal of the American Medical Association* **274**, 1049–1057.

[21] Breslow, R.A., Ross, S.A. & Weed, D.L. (1998). Quality of reviews in epidemiology, *American Journal of Public Health* **88**, 475–477.

[22] Brumback, B.A., Holmes, L.B. & Ryan, L.M. (1999). Adverse effects of chorionic villus sampling: a meta-analysis, *Statistics in Medicine* **18**, 2163–2175.

[23] Byars, D.P. (1988). The use of data bases and historical controls in treatment comparison, in *On Combining Information: Historical Controls, Overviews, and Comprehensive Cohort Studies. Recent Results in Cancer Research*, Vol. 111, Springer-Verlag, New York.

[24] Cappelleri, J., Ioannidis, J., Schmid, C., de Ferranti, S., Aubert, M., Chalmers, T.C. & Lau, J. (1996). Large trials vs. meta-analysis of smaller trials, *Journal of the American Medical Association* **276**, 1332–1338.

[25] Chalmers, I. & Altman, D.G., eds. (1995). *Systematic Reviews*. British Medical Journal Publishing Groups, London.

[26] Chalmers, I., Dickerson, K. & Chalmers, T.C. (1992). Getting to grips with Archie Cochrane's agenda, *British Medical Journal* **304**, 768–786.

[27] Chalmers, T.C. & Lau, J. (1993). Meta-analytic stimulus for changes in clinical trials, *Statistical Methods in Medical Research* **2**, 161–172.

[28] Chalmers, T.C., Levin, H., Sacks, H.S., Reitman, D., Berrier, J. & Nagalingam, R. (1987). Meta-analysis of clinical trials as a scientific discipline I: Control of bias and comparison with large co-operative trials, *Statistics in Medicine* **6**, 315–325.

[29] Chalmers, T.C., Smith, H., Jr, Blackburn, B., Silverman, B., Schroeder, B., Reitman, D. & Ambroz, A. (1981). A method for assessing the quality of a randomized control trial, *Controlled Clinical Trials* **2**, 31–49.

[30] Chollar, S. (1998). A registry for clinical trials, *Annals of Internal Medicine* **128**, 701–702.

[31] Cochran, W.G. (1954). The combination of estimates from different experiments, *Biometrics* **10**, 101–129.

[32] Cochrane Collaboration. Handbook. INTERNET: http://www.cochrane.co.uk.

[33] Colditz, G.A., Brewer, T.F., Berkey, C.S., Wilson, M.E., Burdick, E., Fineberg, H.V. & Mosteller, F. (1994). Efficacy of BCG vaccine in the prevention of tuberculosis: meta analysis of the published literature, *Journal of the American Medical Association* **271**, 696–702.

[34] Colditz, G.A., Burdick, E. & Mosteller, F. (1995). Heterogeneity in meta-analysis of data from epidemiologic studies: a commentary, *American Journal of Epidemiology* **142**, 371–382.

[35] Cole, M.G. & Bellavance, F. (1997). Depression in elderly medical inpatients: a meta-analysis of outcomes, *Canadian Medical Association Journal* **157**, 1055–1060.

[36] Colton, T. (1974). *Statistics in Medicine*. Little, Brown, Boston, Mass.

[37] Cook, D.J., Guyatt, G.H., Ryan, G., Clifton, J., Buckingham, L., Willan, A., McIlroy, W. & Oxman, A.D. (1993). Should unpublished data be included in meta-analyses? Current conflicts and controversies, *Journal of the American Medical Association* **21**, 2749–2753.

[38] Cook, D.J. & Mulrow, C.D. (1997). Systematic reviews: synthesis of best evidence for clinical decisions, *Annals of Internal Medicine* **126**, 376–380.

[39] Cook, D.J., Sackett, D.L. & Spitzer, W. (1995). Methodologic guidelines for systematic reviews of randomized control trials in health care from the Potsdam consultation on meta-analysis, *Journal of Clinical Epidemiology* **48**, 167–171.

[40] Cook, T.D. & Campbell, D.T. (1979). *Quasi-Experimentation: Design and Analysis Issues for Field Settings*. Houghton-Mifflin, Boston, Mass.

[41] Cook, T.D., Cooper, H., Cordray, D.S., Hartmann, H., Hedges, L.V., Light, R.J., Louis, T.A. & Mosteller, F. (1992). *Meta-Analysis for Explanation: A Casebook*. Russel Sage Foundation, New York.

[42] Cook, T.D. & Leviton, L.C. (1980). Reviewing the literature: a comparison of traditional methods with meta-analysis, *Journal of Personality* **48**, 449–472.

[43] Cooper, H. & Hedges, L.V., eds (1994). *The Handbook of Research Synthesis*. Russell Sage Foundation, New York.

[44] Counsell, C. (1997). Formulating questions and locating primary studies for inclusion in systematic reviews, *Annals of Internal Medicine* **127**, 380–387.

[45] Dear, K.B. & Begg, C.B. (1992). An approach to assessing publication bias prior to performing a meta analysis, *Statistical Science* **7**, 237–245.

[46] DerSimonian, R. & Laird, N. (1986). Meta-analysis in clinical trials, *Controlled Clinical Trials* **7**, 177–188.

[47] DerSimonian, R. & Levine, R.J. (1986). Resolving discrepancies between meta-analysis and a subsequent large controlled trial, *Journal of the American Medical Association* **282**, 664–670.

[48] Dickersin, K. & Berlin J.A. (1992). Meta-analysis: state of the science, *Epidemiologic Reviews* **14**, 54–76.

[49] Dickersin, K., Chan, S., Chalmers, T.C., Sacks, H.S. & Smith, H., Jr (1987). Publication bias and clinical trials, *Controlled Clinical Trials* **8**, 343–353.

[50] Dickersin, K. & Min, Y.I. (1993). NIH clinical trials and publication bias, *Online Journal of Current Clinical Trials*, doc. no.50, online

[51] Dickersin, K., Scherer, R. & Lefebre, C. (1995). Identifying relevant studies for systematic reviews, in *Systematic Reviews*, I. Chalmers & D.G. Altman, eds. British Medical Journal Publishing Group, London.

[52] DuMouchel, W. (1994). *Hierarchical Bayes Linear Models for Meta-analysis*. National Institute of Statistical Sciences, Research Triangle Park, North Carolina.

[53] Dyer, A.R. (1986). A method for combining results from several prospective epidemiologic studies, *Statistics in Medicine* **5**, 303–317.

[54] Easterbrook, P.J. (1992). Directory of registries of clinical trials, *Statistics in Medicine* **11**, 345–423.

[55] Easterbrook, P.J., Berlin, J.A., Gopalan, R. & Matthews, D.R. (1991). Publication bias in clinical research, *Lancet* **337**, 867–872.

[56] Egger, M., Scheider, M. & Davey-Smith, G. (1998). Meta-analysis: spurious precision? Meta-analysis of observational studies, *British Medical Journal* **316**, 140–144.

[57] Egger, M., Smith G.D. & Sterne, J.A. (1998). Meta-analysis: is moving the goal post the answer? *Lancet* **351**, 1517.

[58] Egger, M. & Sterne, J.A. (1998). Software for meta-analysis, *British Medical Journal* **316**, online.

[59] Egger, M., Zellweger-Zähner, T., Schneider, M., Junker, C., Lengeler, C. & Antes, G. (1997). Language bias in randomised controlled trials published in English and German, *Lancet* **350**, 326–329.

[60] Emerson, J.D., Burdick, E., Hoaglin, D.C., Mosteller, F. & Chalmers, T.C. (1990). An empirical study of the possible relation of treatment differences to quality scores in controlled randomized clinical trials, *Controlled Clinical Trials* **11**, 339–352.

[61] Eysenck, H.J. (1984). Meta-analysis: an abuse of research integration, *Journal of Special Education* **18**, 41–59.

[62] Felson, D.T. (1992). Bias in meta-analytic research, *Journal of Clinical Epidemiology* **45**, 885–892.

[63] Fleiss, J.L. (1993). The statistical basis of meta-analysis, *Statistical Methods of Medical Research* **2**, 121–145.

[64] Fleiss, J.L. & Gross, A.J. (1999). Meta-analysis in epidemiology, with special reference to studies of the association between exposure to environmental tobacco smoke and lung cancer: a critique, *Journal of Clinical Epidemiology* **44**, 127–139.

[65] Friedenreich, C. (1993). Methods for pooled analyses of epidemiologic studies, *Epidemiology* **4**, 295–302.

[66] Friedenreich, C. (1994). Influence of methodologic factors in a pooled analysis of 13 case–control studies of colorectal cancer and dietary fiber, *Epidemiology* **5**, 66–67.

[67] Frumkin, H. & Berlin, J. (1988). Asbestos exposure and gastrointestinal malignancy review and meta-analysis [published erratum appears in *American Journal of*

Industrial Medicine 1988, 14(4), 493], *American Journal of Industrial Medicine* **14**, 79–95.

[68] Glass, G.V. (1976). Primary, secondary, and meta-analysis of research, *Educational Researcher* **5**, 3–8.

[69] Gleser, L.J. & Olkin, I. (1996). Models for estimating the number of unpublished studies, *Statistics in Medicine* **15**, 2493–2507.

[70] Green, S.B. & Byars, D.P. (1984). Using observational data from registries to compare treatments: the fallacy of omnimetrics, *Statistics in Medicine* **3**, 361–370.

[71] Greenhouse, J.B. & Iyengar, S. (1994). Sensitivity analysis and diagnostics, in *The Handbook of Research Synthesis*, H. Cooper & L.V. Hedges, eds. Russell Sage Foundation, New York, pp. 383–398.

[72] Greenland, S. (1987). Quantitative methods in the review of epidemiologic literature, *Epidemiological Reviews* **9**, 1–30.

[73] Greenland, S. (1994). Invited commentary: a critical look at some popular meta-analytic methods (Comment in *Am J Epidemiol*, 1994, 1 Aug, **140**(3), 297–299; discussion 300–301, *Am J Epidemiol*, 1995, 1 Nov, **142**(9), 1007–1009), *American Journal of Epidemiology* **140**, 290–296.

[74] Gregoire, G., Derderian, F. & LeLorier, J. (1995). Selecting the language of the publications included in a meta-analysis: is there a Tower of Babel bias?, *Journal of Clinical Epidemiology* **48**, 159–163.

[75] Harwell, M. (1997). An empirical study of Hedges' homogeneity test, *Psychological Methods* **2**, 219–231.

[76] Hasselblad, V. (1995). Meta-analysis of environmental health data, *Science of the Total Environment* **160–161**, 545–558.

[77] Hasselblad, V., Eddy, D.M. & Kotchmar, D.J. (1992). Synthesis of environmental evidence: nitrogen dioxide epidemiology studies, *Journal of the Air and Waste Management Association* **42**, 662–671.

[78] Hassleblad, V., Mosteller, F., Littenberg, B., Chalmers, T.C., Hunink, M.G., Turner, J.A., Morton, S.C., Diehr, P., Wong, J.B. & Powe, N.R. (1995). A survey of current problems in meta-analysis. Discussion from the Agency for Health Care Policy and Research inter-PORT Work Group on Literature Review/Meta-Analysis, *Medical Care* **33**, 202–220.

[79] Hedges, L.V. (1992). Modeling publication selection effects in meta analysis, *Statistical Science* **2**, 246–255.

[80] Hedges, L.V. (1994). Fixed effect models, in *The Handbook of Research Synthesis*, H. Cooper & L.V. Hedges, eds. Russell Sage Foundation, New York.

[81] Hedges, L.V. & Olkin, I. (1980). Vote-counting methods in research synthesis, *Psychological Bulletin* **88**, 359–369.

[82] Hedges, L.V. & Olkin, I. (1985). *Statistical Methods for Meta-Analysis*. Academic Press, Boston, Mass.

[83] Hemminki, E., Hailey, D. & Koivusalo, M. (1999). The courts – a challenge to health technology assessment, *Science* **285**, 203–204.

[84] Hill, A.B. (1965). The environment and disease: association or causation? *Proceedings of the Royal Society of Medicine* **58**, 295–300.

[85] Hunt, M. (1997). *How Science Takes Stock: The Story of Meta-Analysis*. Russell Sage Foundation, New York.

[86] Hunter, J.D. & Schmidt, F.L. (1995). *Methods of Meta-Analysis*. Sage Publications, London.

[87] Hunter, J.E. & Schmidt, F.L. (1994). Correcting for sources of artifactual variation across studies, in *The Handbook of Research Synthesis*, H. Cooper & L.V. Hedges, eds. The Russell Sage Foundation, New York.

[88] Huston, P. (1996). Cochrane Collaboration helping unravel tangled web woven by international research, *Canadian Medical Association Journal* **154**, 1389–1392.

[89] Huston, P. (1996). Health services research: reporting on studies using secondary data sources, *Canadian Medical Association Journal* **155**, 1697–1702.

[90] Huston, P. & Moher, D. (1996). Redundancy, disaggregation, and the integrity of medical research, *Lancet* **347**, 1024–1026.

[91] Ioannidis, J.P., Cappelleri, J.C. & Lau, J. (1998). Issues in the comparison of meta-analysis and large trials, *Journal of the American Medical Association* **279**, 1089–1093.

[92] Ioannidis, J.P. & Lau, J. (1999). Pooling research results: benefits and limitations of meta-analysis, *Journal of Quality Improvement* **25**, 462–469.

[93] Iyengar, S. & Greenhouse, J.B. (1988). Selection models and the file drawer problem, *Statistical Sciences* **3**, 109–135.

[94] Jadad, A.R., Sullivan, C., Luo, D., Allen, I.E., Ross, S.D. & Sheinhait, I.A. (1999). Patients' preferences during the treatment of obstructive airway disease: a systematic review of studies comparing Turbuhaler with pressurized metered dose inhalers, *Annals of Allergy, Asthma, and Immunology*, in press.

[95] Kheifets, L.I., Afifi, A.A., Buffler, P.A., Zhang, Z.W. & Matkin, C.C. (1997). Occupational electric and magnetic field exposure and leukemia. A meta-analysis, *Journal of Occupational and Environmental Medicine* **39**, 1074–1091.

[96] Kleijinen, J., ter Riet, G. & Knipschild, P. (1990). Vitamin B-6 in the treatment of the premenstrual syndrome – a review, *British Journal of Obstetrics and Gynecology* **97**, 847–852.

[97] Krutan, B.M., Taylor, M.L. & Freeman, E. (1990). Vitamin B-6 in the treatment of the premenstrual syndrome, *Journal of the American Dietary Association* **90**, 859–861.

[98] L'Abbe, K.A., Detsky, A.S. & O'Rourke, K. (1987). Meta-analysis in clinical research, *Annals of Internal Medicine* **107**, 224–233.

[99] Lang, T.A. & Secic, M. (1997). *How to Report Statistics in Medicine*. American College of Physicians, New York.

[100] Lau, J., Antman, E.M., Jimenez-Silva, J., Kupelnick, B., Mosteller, F. & Chalmers, T. C. (1992). Cumulative

meta-analysis of therapeutic trials for myocardial infarction, *New England Journal of Medicine* **327**, 248–254.

[101] Lau, J., Ioannidis, J.P. & Schmid, C.H. (1998). Summing up evidence: one answer is not always enough, *Lancet* **351**, 123–127.

[102] Law, M.R., Morris, J.K. & Wald, N.J. (1997). Environmental tobacco smoke exposure and ischaemic heart disease: an evaluation of the evidence, *British Medical Journal* **315**, 973–980.

[103] LeLorier, J., Grégoire, G., Benhaddad, A., Lapierre, J. & Derderian, F. (1997). Discrepancies between meta-analyses and subsequent large randomized, controlled trials, *New England Journal of Medicine* **337**, 536–542.

[104] Light, R.J. & Pillemer, D.B. (1984). *Summing Up: The Science of Reviewing Research*. Harvard University Press, Boston, Mass.

[105] Light, R.J. & Smith, P.B. (1971). Accumulating evidence; procedures for resolving contradictions among different research studies, *Harvard Educational Review* **41**, 429–471.

[106] Lipsett, M. & Campleman, S. (1999). Occupational exposure to diesel exhaust and lung cancer: a meta-analysis, *American Journal of Public Health* **89**, 1009–1017.

[107] Lipsitz, S.R., Dear, K.B., Laird, N.M. & Molenberghs, G. (1998). Tests for homogeneity of the risk difference when data are sparse, *Biometrics* **54**, 148–160.

[108] Lohrer, B.T., Noe, R.A., Moeller, N.L. & Fitzgerald, M.P. (1985). A meta-analysis of the relation of job characteristics to job satisfaction, *Journal of Applied Psychology* **79**, 280–289.

[109] Lubin, J.H., Boice, J.D., Jr, Edling, C., Hornung, R.W., Howe, G., Kunz, E., Kusiak, R.A., Morrison, H.I., Radford, E.P. & Samet, J.M. (1995). Lung cancer in radon-exposed miners and estimation of risk from indoor exposure, *Journal of the National Cancer Institute* **87**, 817–827.

[110] Mann, C.C. (1994). Can meta-analysis make policy?, *Science* **266**, 960–962.

[111] Meinert, C.L. (1989). Meta-analysis: science or religion?, *Controlled Clinical Trials* **10**, 257S–263S.

[112] Miller, N. & Pollock, V.E. (1994). Meta-analytic synthesis for theory development, in *The Handbook of Research Synthesis*, H. Cooper & L.V. Hedges, eds. The Russell Sage Foundation, New York.

[113] Miller, W.C., Koceja, D.M. & Hamilton, E.J. (1997). A meta-analysis of the past 25 years of weight loss research using diet, exercise or diet plus exercise intervention, *International Journal of Obesity and Related Metabolic Disorders* **21**, 941–947.

[114] Moher, D., Fortin, P., Jadad, A.R., Juni, P., Klassen, T., Le Lorier, J., Liberati, A., Linde, K. & Penna, A. (1996). Completeness of reporting of trials published in languages other than English: implication for conduct and reporting of systematic reviews, *Lancet* **347**, 363–366.

[115] Moher, D. & Olkin, I. (1995). Meta-analysis of randomized controlled trials. A concern for standards, *Journal of the American Medical Association* **274**, 1942–1948.

[116] Moher, D., Pham, B., Jones, A., Cook, D.J., Jadad, A.R., Moher, M., Tugwell, P. & Klassen, T.P. (1998). Does quality of reports of randomised trials affect estimates of intervention efficacy reported in meta-analysis?, *Lancet* **352**, 609–613.

[117] Mosteller, F. & Chalmers, T.C. (1992). Some progress and problems in meta-analysis of clinical trials, *Statistical Science* **7**, 227–236.

[118] Mosteller, F. & Colditz, G.A. (1996). Understanding research synthesis (meta-analysis), *Annals of Review of Public Health* **17**, 1–23.

[119] Naylor, C.D. (1997). Meta-analysis and the meta-epidemiology of clinical research, *British Medical Journal* **315**, 617–619.

[120] Ohlsson, A. (1994). Systematic reviews – theory and practice, *Scandinavian Journal of Clinical Laboratory Investigations* **219**, 25–32.

[121] Olkin, I. (1996). Meta-analysis: current issues in research synthesis, *Statistics in Medicine* **15**, 1253–1257.

[122] Olson, C.M. (1994). Understanding and evaluating a meta-analysis, *Academic Emergency Medicine* **1**, 392–398.

[123] Patil, G.P. & Rao, C.R. (1977). The weighted distributions: a survey of their applications, in *Applications of Statistics*, P.R. Krishiaiah, ed. North-Holland, Amsterdam.

[124] Peipert, J.F. & Phipps, M.G. (1998). Observational studies, *Clinical Obstetrics and Gynecology* **41**, 235–244.

[125] Person, K. (1904). Report on certain enteric fever inoculations, *British Medical Journal* **2**, 1243–1246.

[126] Petitti, D. (1994). *Meta-Analysis, Decision Analysis, and Cost Effectiveness Analysis: Methods for Quantitative Synthesis in Medicine*. Oxford University Press, New York.

[127] Pogue, J.M. & Yusuf, S. (1997). Cumulating evidence from randomized trials: utilizing sequential monitoring boundaries for cumulative meta-analysis, *Controlled Clinical Trials* **18**, 580–593.

[128] Pogue, J.M. & Yusuf, S. (1998). Overcoming the limitations of current meta-analysis of randomized controlled trials, *Lancet* **351**, 47–52.

[129] Realini, J.P. & Goldzieher, J.W. (1985). Oral contraceptives and cardiovascular disease: a critique of the epidemiologic studies, *American Journal of Obstetrics and Gynecology* **152**, 729–798.

[130] Rosenthal, R. (1979). The "file drawer problem" and tolerance for null results, *Psychological Bulletin* **86**, 638–641.

[131] Sacks, H.S., Berrier, J., Reitman, D., Ancona-Berk, V.A. & Chalmers, T.C. (1983). Meta-analyses of randomized controlled trials, *New England Journal of Medicine* **316**, 450–455.

[132] Sacks, H.S., Chalmers, T.C. & Smith, H. (1983). Sensitivity and specificity of clinical trials: randomized

versus historical controls, *Archives of Internal Medicine* **143**, 753–755.

[133] Sacks, H.S., Reitman, D., Pagano, D. & Kupelnick, B. (1996). Meta-analysis: an update, *Mount Sinai Journal of Medicine* **63**, 216–224.

[134] Schlesselman, J.J. (1997). Risk of endometrial cancer in relation to use of combined oral contraceptives. A practitioner's guide to meta-analysis, *Human Reproduction* **12**, 1851–1863.

[135] Schulz, K.F. (1998). Randomized controlled trials, *Clinical Obstetrics and Gynecology* **41**, 245–256.

[136] Schulz, K.F., Chalmers, I., Hayes, R.J. & Altman, D.G. (1995). Empirical evidence of bias. Dimensions of methodological quality associated with estimates of treatment effects in controlled trials, *Journal of the American Medical Association* **273**, 408–412.

[137] Shapiro, S. (1994). Meta-analysis/Shmeta-analysis, *American Journal of Epidemiology* **140**, 771–778.

[138] Sipe, T.A. & Curlette, W.L. (1997). A meta-synthesis of factors related to educational achievement: a methodological approach to summarizing and synthesizing meta-analyses, *International Journal of Educational Research* **25**, 583–698.

[139] Smith, S.J., Caudill, S.P., Steinberg, K. & Thacker, S.B. (1995). On combining dose–response data from epidemiologic studies by meta-analysis, *Statistics in Medicine* **14**, 531–544.

[140] Spector, T.D. & Thompson, S.G. (1991). The potential and limitations of meta-analysis, *Journal of Epidemiology and Community Health* **45**, 89–92.

[141] Spitzer, W.O. (1995). The challenge of meta-analysis, *Journal of Clinical Epidemiology* **48**, 1–4.

[142] Standards of Reporting Trials Group (1994). A proposal for structured reporting of randomized controlled trials, *Journal of the American Medical Association* **272**, 1926–1931.

[143] Steinberg, K.K., Smith, S.F., Lee, N., Stroup, D.F., Olkin, I. & Williamson, G.D. (1997). A comparison of meta analysis to pooled analysis: an application to ovarian cancer, *American Journal of Epidemiology* **145**, 1917–1925.

[144] Steinberg, K.K., Smith, S.J., Thacker, S.B. & Stroup, D.F. (1994). Breast cancer risk and duration of estrogen use: the role of study design in meta-analysis, *Epidemiology* **5**, 415–421.

[145] Steinberg, K.K., Thacker, S.B., Smith, S.J., Stroup, D.F., Zack, M.M., Flanders, W.D. & Berkelman, R.L. (1991). A meta-analysis of the effect of estrogen replacement therapy on the risk of breast cancer, *Journal of the American Medical Association* **265**, 1985–1990.

[146] Stock, W.A. (1995). Systematic coding for research synthesis, in *The Handbook of Research Synthesis*, H. Cooper & L.V. Hedges, eds. The Russell Sage Foundation, New York.

[147] Stoto, M. (1995). Research synthesis for public health policy: experience of the Institute of Medicine, in *Evaluation for the 21st Century: A Handbook*, W. Shadish & E. Chelimsley, eds. Sage Publications, New York.

[148] Stram, D.O. & Lee, J.W. (1994). Variance components testing in the longitudinal mixed effects model, *Biometrics* **50**, 1171–1177.

[149] Stroup, D.F., Thacker, S.B., Olson, C.M. & Glass, R.M. (1997). Characteristics of meta-analyses submitted to a medical journal. Presented at the International Congress on Biomedical Peer Review and Global Communications, Prague.

[150] Sutton, A.J., Jones, D.R., Abrams, K.R., Sheldon, T.A. & Song, F. (1999). Systematic reviews and meta-analysis: a structured review of the methodological literature, *Journal of Health Services Research and Policy* **4**, 49–55.

[151] Takkouche, B., Cadarso-Suárez, C. & Spiegelman, D. (1999). Evaluation of old and new tests of heterogeneity in epidemiologic meta-analysis, *American Journal of Epidemiology* **150**, 206–215.

[152] Thacker, S.B. (1988). Meta-analysis: a quantitative approach to research integration, *Journal of the American Medical Association* **259**, 1685–1689.

[153] Thompson, S.G. (1994). Why sources of heterogeneity in meta-analysis should be investigated, *British Medical Journal* **309**, 1351–1355.

[154] Vanhonacker, W.R. (1996). Meta-analysis and response surface extrapolation: a least squares approach, *American Statistician* **50**, 294–299.

[155] Vickers, A., Cassileth, B., Ernst, E., Fisher, P., Goldman, P., Jonas, W., Kang, S.K., Lewith, G., Schulz, K. & Silagy, C. (1997). How should we research unconventional therapies? A panel report from the Conference on Complementary and Alternative Medicine Research Methodology, National Institutes of Health, *International Journal of Technology Assessment in Health Care* **13**, 111–121.

[156] Wachter, K.W. (1998). Disturbed by meta-analysis? *Science* **241**, 1407–1408.

[157] Wachter, K.W. & Straf, M. (1990). *The Future of Meta-analysis*. Russell Sage Foundation, New York.

[158] Ware, J.H., Muller, J.E. & Braunwald, E. (1985). The futility index: an approach to the cost-effective termination of randomized clinical trials, *American Journal of Medicine* **78**, 635–643.

[159] Wells, A.J. (1998). Heart disease from passive smoking in the workplace, *Journal of the American College of Cardiology* **31**, 1–9.

[160] Wilson, M.E., Fineberg, H.V. & Colditz, G.A. (1995). Geographic latitude and the efficacy of bacillus Calmette–Guerin vaccine, *Clinical Infectious Diseases* **20**, 982–991.

[161] Wortman, P.M. (1994). Judging research quality, in *The Handbook of Research Synthesis*, H. Cooper & L.V. Hedges, eds. Russell Sage Foundation, New York.

DONNA F. STROUP & STEPHEN B. THACKER

Midpoint Imputation *see* Incubation Period of Infectious Diseases

Migrant Studies

Studies on migrant populations are based on the assumption that migrants carry a risk that to some extent reflects that of their country of origin rather than the host country. Migrant studies are, therefore, a category of **ecologic studies** in which geographic differences in **risk** are replaced by risk differences among population groups (immigrants vs. host population and vs. population of origin).

Migration can be studied for three main reasons:

1. The study of migrant populations can be used for generating (as opposed to "testing") or confirming hypotheses derived from etiologic studies of environmental risk factors associated with disease occurrence.
2. The study of the health status of minorities who have emigrated from abroad has recently acquired public health significance, because of the effect of migration from the underdeveloped to the developed world on the occurrence of acute and socially relevant diseases in the host country.
3. Migrant status may be used in **case–control** and **cohort** studies as a variable representing possible **confounding** exposures.

Definition of Migrant Status

There are several ways of defining a subject as a migrant.

Place of birth Subjects born abroad are considered to be immigrants. This definition is the most widely used in epidemiologic studies. For diseased subjects, the information is either obtained from **death certificates**, which report the country of birth, or from **disease registries**, such as cancer registries. Furthermore, place of birth is usually enumerated in population censuses, but sometimes only for a subset of the population.

Citizenship Subjects with foreign citizenship are considered to be immigrants. The original citizenship may be retained by residents of foreign countries

Table 1 Number of Italian migrants in the US in the decade 1970–1980

Italian-born	831 000
Italian citizens	230 000
First- and second-generation immigrants	5 000 000
Italian origin	8 800 000
Italian origin identified as one of the subject's roots	12 180 000

Source: [4]. Reproduced with permission of the International Agency for Research against Cancer (IARC).

or obtained by the spouse of a migrant. The foreign offices of some countries provide periodic information on these persons.

Ethnic origin Subjects may be considered as migrants if both parents were born abroad or if they answer positively to the question: "Are you a migrant?"

Each of the above-mentioned definitions identifies a population group of different size. For example, Table 1 shows the number of Italian migrants in the US in the decade 1970–1980 according to each definition [9].

Sources of Information for Migrant Studies

Information on Diseased Subjects

First-Generation Migrants. In the majority of migrant studies, information on diseased subjects is derived from routine **surveillance** systems. These are mortality statistics, when the content of the death certificates allows it, or cancer registries statistics, when the interest is focused on cancer risk. Other pathology reporting systems have begun to include information on migrant status in order to evaluate the effect of migration on the epidemiology of some diseases of emerging interest, such as tuberculosis and acquired immune deficiency syndrome (AIDS).

If information on the date of migration is recorded individually, the duration of stay and the age at migration to the host country can also be computed [4, 39]. This information is, however, seldom routinely available. In the US, the Social Security Number (SSN), which is assigned sequentially to all residents, has been used as a proxy of age at migration. If the SSN is assigned to a migrant after the usual age of entry to work, it is considered most likely that he/she migrated as an adult (late migrant). In contrast, those whose SSN was assigned at the usual age of initial employment are considered to have migrated in childhood (early migrant). Unfortunately, such information can be used only for cases and not for the general population, thus limiting the choice of study design [26].

Second-Generation Migrants.   Parents' birthplace is routinely recorded on death certificates in some countries and by some cancer registries, allowing for the identification of second-generation migrants [10, 17, 33, 38]. Alternatively, studies on second-generation migrants may be based on information on both ethnicity and birthplace. Members of ethnic groups born locally are considered to be second-generation migrants, while those born abroad are first-generation migrants [42].

If second-generation migrants can be identified, the modification of risk between first-generation migrants and their descendants can be estimated. Moreover, disease risk can be studied in individuals of mixed parentage, in whom the genetic susceptibly may be intermediate between those of the two populations; furthermore, environmental exposures, such as lifestyle habits, may be influenced to different extents by the origin of the father and the mother [10, 17, 33, 38].

Information on the Population

First-Generation Migrants.   To estimate incidence or mortality rates by migrant status, information is required on the population at risk of developing the disease under study. This may be provided by censuses, as long as the definition of migrant status in the denominator is the same as that in the numerator.

The use of censuses as a source of information for the denominator tends to limit the number of variables that can be considered in the study, as time since migration, age at migration, and other variables for diseased or deceased subjects, are seldom available for the population at risk.

Second-Generation Migrants.   Only some population censuses include the country of birth of the parents of the enumerated subjects [38]. When available, this allows estimation of disease and death rates for second-generations migrants.

Use of Census Information for Longitudinal Migrant Studies

The identification of a cohort of migrants (first- or second-generation) through censuses may allow follow-up and cross-linking with routine information on diseases and deaths [16] (*see* **Record Linkage**). The number of persons "lost to follow-up" in these cohorts, however, tends to be high, because of the tendency of people who migrate once to move again, often back to the country of origin.

Information on Other Variables: Socioeconomic Level and Lifestyle

In some countries, routine sources of numerators and denominators provide some information on socioeconomic level, usually approximated by occupation, educational level, or a combination of the two [6].

Surveys of the frequency of exposure to disease determinants (tobacco, alcohol, dietary habits) at a population level seldom include information on migrant status [24, 27]. When this is not available, exposure **prevalence** derived from population-based surveys in the country of origin, and in the host country, may be used to interpret differences in the disease risk of migrants [30].

Information on the prevalence of lifestyle habits of migrants may be derived from **control** groups in case–control studies in which migrant status is considered [41, 46].

Exposure to lifestyle, environmental, and other risk factors in migrants, and in control groups, has been determined directly in only a few studies. It can be done through the use of questionnaires in cohort or case–control studies and makes it possible to disentangle the roles of different exposures in determining the risk pattern related to migrant status. The exposures of interest tend to vary widely among first- and second-generation migrants and in relation to duration of stay, providing greater power to detect associations and therefore smaller study size in comparison with populations in which the level of exposure is more homogeneous. Furthermore, direct measurement of exposure makes it possible to study the relationship between time variables, such as age and time at migration, and lifestyle changes. Most studies [43] have addressed the role of diet in determining the risk for cancers at various sites. In some cases, blood samples were obtained so that internal doses of nutrients and micronutrients could be measured in a prospective **cohort** design [32].

Sources of Bias in Migrant Studies

If a different definition of migrant status is used for the denominator than for the numerator in computing mortality or morbidity rates, erroneous estimates of the rates in an unpredictable direction may result.

Because of the infrequency of censuses (commonly at 10-year intervals), censuses must often be interpolated to estimate appropriate denominators for migrants. This may introduce an additional source of **bias**, due to an underestimate of the denominator, when active migration is still occurring during the period of interpolation.

The accuracy of diagnostic information and of the coding of diseases changes geographically. This may lead to artifactual differences when the rates in one country (local-born and migrants) are compared with those in another (country of origin), due to information bias on disease status. If diagnostic procedures and coding practices are not selective by migrant status, this source of bias does not affect comparisons between migrants and locally born people within the host country. It can be hypothesized, however, that the access to certain diagnostic procedures may be different for migrants within the same country, especially for those of low socioeconomic status, owing to communication problems or legal status. This will introduce bias in disease status, partially hampering comparisons of rates with those of locally born persons.

Furthermore, a possible selection of subjects who migrate, in contrast to the population of the country of origin, must be considered.

First, migration may be selective by subarea within the country of origin [9]. If there are different patterns of risk in the population of origin by subarea, any comparison between migrants and the population of country of origin as a whole will be incorrect. If information on the subarea of origin is available, however, a specific comparison with the subarea may be accomplished.

Secondly, subjects who decide to migrate may have a different disease occurrence pattern from that of the population as a whole, as health status is related to the opportunity to migrate. This **selection bias** usually leads in the direction of a lower disease risk among migrants (healthy migrant effect) [28]; however, it may be associated with a higher disease risk if diseased subjects tend to join a family that has previously migrated, or tend to migrate to another country for retirement or care (unhealthy migrant effect). To evaluate the relevance of this selection bias, the disease experience in the first period after migration is sometimes considered separately, when information on the date of migration is available [39] (*see* **Bias, Overview**).

Finally, if migrants are reluctant to use unfamiliar medical services or unable to afford to do so, they may "go back home" when severely ill, thus disappearing from the numerator while still contributing to the denominator [31]. This will lead to an underestimate of mortality and incidence rates.

Statistical Methods

All classical **descriptive epidemiological** methods can be used in migrant studies.

Variables Under Study

Migrant status is the exposure variable for which disease risk is estimated: the reference category is represented by nonmigrants in the host country or by subjects resident in the country or origin. Time variables, when available, can be investigated.

Age.   The first time variable to be considered is age, because changes in risk result from aging and because of the peculiar age structure of migrant populations, which tend to an overrepresentation of young adults, especially in recently migrated groups. Age is, therefore, associated with both disease and migrant status (*see* **Confounding**).

Calendar Time.   Disease rates are likely to change over calendar time. If this happens differentially in the country of origin, in the host country, and in the migrant population, any comparison should take into account the effect of such changes.

Duration of Stay and Age at Migration.   Duration of stay is an index of duration of exposure to determinants of the disease under study during the stay in the host country, and therefore represents a proxy of cumulative exposure levels. If differences in disease risk between migrants and locally born people, and between migrants and the population of origin, are related to differential exposure levels, these should be found to be associated with the duration of stay. Furthermore the speed with which the disease pattern in migrants changes by duration of stay can be interpreted in terms of duration of exposure (or nonexposure) to etiologic agents in the host country.

Age at migration is strictly related to duration of stay, as subjects migrating at younger ages tend to stay longer. In terms of the natural history of the disease, this variable is potentially informative for latency, estimated as the interval between the beginning of exposure and disease occurrence (*see* **Latent Period**). For example, the finding that subjects migrating from a high-risk to a low-risk country at a young age retain a life-long higher risk than that in the host country, and than that of people who migrated during adulthood, indicates that exposure during childhood is relevant for the disease. In cancer studies, and in general for diseases with a multistep etiologic process, it suggests that the determinants involved in migration act as initiators of the disease.

Ideally, one would examine simultaneously the effect of age on arrival and duration of stay in the host country, controlling for the other relevant temporal variables (age and period of occurrence of the disease). This is not feasible, however, as age, duration of stay, and age on arrival are not independent: the definition of two of them implies knowledge of the third. The situation is similar to that of the **age–period–cohort** problem framework. To overcome this difficulty, separate analyses sequentially ignoring one of the two variables (duration of stay or age on arrival) are performed in migrant studies [4].

Other Variables.   Information on other variables related to both disease and exposure may be considered when available. As mentioned above, this is possible in case–control and cohort studies in which individual questionnaires are used. Additional variables can be derived from routine surveys, such as on occupation and education, as a proxy for socio-economic status, and on place of residence in the host country as a proxy for access to diagnostic procedures and care.

Statistical Analysis

The statistical analysis of migrant studies depends upon the data sources available.

Denominator-Based Analysis.
Age-Standardized Rates.   If the information on the denominator is reliable, incidence or mortality rates for migrants can be calculated and compared with those of residents of the host country and/or the country of origin. Direct standardization is used to adjust for age distribution [35]. Standardized rate ratios (SRRs) are generally computed, since interest is focused on the magnitude of the difference between the two rates (migrants vs. locally born and/or migrants vs. country of origin) [3]. The choice of a common standard population (e.g. locally born in the host country) allows the use of rate ratios.

Direct standardization, however, is sensitive to small numbers of events in the study population [35]. For migrants, some age-specific rates may be based on very few cases. The result is unstable rates and large confidence intervals around the rate ratios.

To increase the precision of the measure, indirect standardization, from which a smaller standard error is expected, is used for rare diseases and for small migrant groups, with the estimation of Standardized Mortality Ratios (SMRs) or Standardized Incidence Ratios (SIRs). The standard set of rates are the age-specific rates of the host country as a whole or, more properly, of the local-born, from which migrants have been excluded [45]. It must be considered, however, that SMRs and SIRs are internally standardized and not mutually comparable [35] (*see* **Standardization Methods**).

Other Methods of Adjustment.   When variables other than age are considered in a study, the **Mantel–Haenszel** estimator can be used to obtain a summary estimate of risk, adjusted by age and by the other variables. Loglinear models, however, are currently preferred for migrant studies, when several variables are available for analysis and **stratification** would fail because of insufficient numbers.

Recently, loglinear modeling based on the Poisson distribution has been applied to migrant studies in order to control simultaneously for a number of counfounding factors [19]. This application is based on the following two assumptions:

1. The number of cases per cell is assumed to follow a Poisson distribution, with a mean value proportional to the number of **person-years at risk**.
2. The logarithm of the rate is assumed to be a linear function of the combination of classification variables that best describe the disease risk in the migrant population.

The **relative risks** obtained by model fitting are expected to show a greater numerical stability in comparison with those computed by traditional standardization methods.

A comparison of risk estimates with 95% confidence intervals obtained when different methods were applied to a large set of mortality data for Italian migrants to Canada is shown in Table 2 for deaths from selected cancers [21].

Numerator-Based Analysis. When the denominator is not available, or the population at risk cannot be cross-classified by the variables of interest, the analysis is based on diseased/deceased subjects only. The **proportional mortality ratio (PMR)** or proportional incidence ratio (PIR) is the measure often used in such cases [39], and the relative proportion of diseases in the locally born population other than the one of interest is taken as the standard to adjust by age.

A proportional mortality or incidence study can be classified as a variant of a case–control study, where the cases are deaths or incident events classified by migrant status and the controls are other deaths or incident events of a different disease occurring in the same base population. This study design is based on the assumption that the migrant status among the controls has the same distribution as in the base population, i.e. that the overall rate of the disease/s in the controls is not related to migration.

Instead of PMRs or PIRs, a Mantel–Haenszel or, more frequently, a loglinear modeling approach is used in numerator-based studies when variables of interest other than age are considered. The assumptions described for PMR and PIR studies are used. When **logistic regression** models are applied, the cases in the cells are assumed to follow a binomial distribution, and the logit transformation of the disease probability is considered to be a linear function of the classification variables. If the assumption that the disease or death risk in controls is not related to migration is true, the estimates from the logistic model approximate those derived from the Poisson regression. The choice of appropriate controls is therefore crucial in this study design.

A comparison of the results obtained from the same set of cancer deaths among Italian migrants to Australia using Poisson and logistic regression (the latter using three sets of controls) is shown in Table 3 [21]. The risk estimates obtained using noncancer or all other deaths as controls are consistently greater than those obtained using cancer controls or Poisson regression. This result is due to a lower risk of death from all causes and from causes other than cancer in migrants than among locally born persons. The results, therefore, do not confirm the assumption that the disease in controls are unrelated to migration when these two sets of controls are considered.

Table 2 Comparison of age-adjusted estimates of risks and their 95% confidence intervals obtained by different methods, for male Italian migrants relative to locally born, Canada, 1964–1985

Cancer site	SRR[a]	SMR[b]	RR[c]	RR[d]
Esophagus	0.72(0.60–0.87)	0.69(0.56–0.82)	0.69(0.58–0.83)	0.69(0.57–0.83)
Stomach	1.28(1.18–1.39)	1.30(1.20–1.40)	1.30(1.20–1.40)	1.30(1.20–1.40)
Lung	0.76(0.72–0.80)	0.74(0.70–0.78)	0.74(0.70–0.78)	0.74(0.70–0.78)
Melanoma	0.96(0.71–1.29)	0.86(0.63–1.09)	0.86(0.65–1.14)	0.86(0.65–1.14)
Leukemia	1.18(1.05–1.33)	1.18(1.05–1.31)	1.18(1.05–1.32)	1.18(1.05–1.32)

[a]Standardized rate ratio (SRR) (direct standardization).
[b]SMR (indirect standardization).
[c]Relative risk (RR) estimates according to the Mantel–Haenszel procedure.
[d]RR estimates according to the Poisson regression procedure.
Source: [4]. Reproduced with permission of the IARC.

Table 3 Comparison of age-adjusted estimates of risks and their 95% confidence intervals obtained by Poisson regression and logistic regression, with different choices of controls, for male Italian migrants relative to locally born, Australia, 1964–1985

Cancer site	RR (Poisson regression)	RR (Logistic regression) Controls		
		Other-cancer deaths	Noncancer deaths	Noncancer and other-cancer deaths
Stomach	1.45(1.16–1.82)	1.75(1.61–1.91)	2.39(2.20–2.60)	2.23(2.05–2.42)
Lung	0.95(0.85–1.07)	1.19(1.12–1.26)	1.61(1.52–1.70)	1.51(1.44–1.60)
Melanoma	0.27(0.18–0.40)	0.32(0.24–0.42)	0.49(0.37–0.64)	0.44(0.34–0.57)

Source: [4]. Reproduced with permission of the IARC.

Evaluation of Goodness of Fit of Regression Models – the "Overdispersion" Phenomenon. When the analysis is based on modeling, Goodness of fit can be assessed with the log likelihood ratio statistic [19]. Provided that the Poisson or binomial assumptions hold, and the regression model is correctly specified, this statistic is of the same magnitude as the degrees of freedom, or smaller for small cell sample size. However, especially when a large data set is used and the contingency table is not classified by factors that are relevant to the response, the phenomenon of overdispersion may occur, reflected in a log-likelihood ratio greater than predicted.

This case occurs frequently in migrant studies, especially when the comparison is between those born in the host country and the general population in the country of origin, thus involving very large data sets with few explanatory variables available for the analysis. The problem of overdispersion can be addressed in the analysis by using a conservative approach in estimating the confidence intervals of the effect parameters [1].

Contribution of Migrant Studies to Insight into Disease Etiology

Most studies of migrant populations address cancer incidence or mortality (for some relevant references on this issue, see Geddes et al. [11], Steinitz et al. [39], Haenszel [14], Haenszel et al. [15], and Thomas & Karagas [43]). The published studies refer to migration from high- to low-risk countries for some cancer sites (e.g. stomach cancer in migrants from Japan and Italy to the US and Australia) or from low- to high-risk countries (e.g. breast cancer in migrants from Japan and China to the US). The

analysis of temporal variables, such as duration of stay in the host country, and age at migration, and the study of second-generation migrants have provided valuable information on the size and timing of changes in cancer risk in response to changes in the external environment and/or lifestyle [10, 22, 38].

Another result of migrant studies is information on cancer rates in the migrant's country of origin, when these are not currently recorded or reasonably valid. This is of particular value for migrants from the underdeveloped world who have recently migrated to developed countries. Such estimates should, however, be considered with caution because of the possible **selection bias** of migrants (see above).

The relation of risk to the frequency of exposure to dietary factors, as derived from **cross-sectional studies** of migrants, their offspring, host countries, and countries of origin, has been highlighted in some studies [24, 25, 30].

The results of studies in which dietary and other variables were considered have been used to infer possible environmental factors in the geographic differences in cancer rates. Although such studies are not common, they represent a potential field of development in migrant studies.

Other migrant studies, mainly based on mortality data, address cardiovascular disease and stroke [8, 16, 18, 40]. In these studies, temporal variables and measurement of risk are treated by methods similar to those used in cancer studies.

Another developing field of interest is of diseases and accidents that are suspected of being determined by migration itself, or which are prominent in the migrant population, thus affecting the rates in the host country. This is the case of studies on suicide [23], homicide [37], work-related fatalities [7], tuberculosis [5, 29], birth outcomes [2, 13, 36], psychiatric disorders [34], hepatitis [20, 44] and human immunodeficiency virus (HIV)/AIDS [12].

Most of these studies, however, do not involve use of the methods described above, and risk estimates are not provided for the migrant population in comparison with the locally born population or with the country of origin. This may be due to the lack of population-based registries for the diseases under study and to the relatively small groups of subjects involved.

References

[1] Aitkin, M., Anderson, D., Francis, B. & Hinde, J. (1989). *Statistical Modelling in Glim*. Clarendon Press, Oxford.

[2] Alexander, G.R., Mor, J.M., Kogan, M.D., Leland, N.L. & Kieffer, E. (1996). Pregnancy outcomes of US-born and Japanese Americans, *American Journal of Public Health* **86**, 820–824.

[3] Armstrong, B.K., Woodings, T.L., Stenhouse, N.S. & McCall, M.G. (1983). *Mortality from Cancer in Migrants to Australia 1962 to 1971*. NH & MCR Research Unit in Epidemiology and Preventive Medicine, Raine Medical Statistics Unit, Perth, University of Western Australia.

[4] Balzi, D., Khlat, M. & Matos, E. (1993). Australia: mortality data, in *Cancer in Italian Migrant Populations*, M. Geddes, D.M. Parkin, M. Khlat, D. Balzi, & E. Buiatti, eds. IARC Scientific Publications, Lyon, pp. 125–137.

[5] Bhatti, N., Law, M.R., Morris, J.K., Halliday, R. & Moore-Gillon, J. (1995). Increasing incidence of tuberculosis in England and Wales: a study of the likely causes, *British Medical Journal* **310**, 976–979.

[6] Bouchardy, C. (1993). France, in *Cancer in Italian Migrant Populations*, M. Geddes, D.M. Parkin, M. Khlat, D. Balzi, & E. Buiatti, eds. IARC Scientific Publications, Lyon, pp. 149–159.

[7] Corvalan, C.F., Driscoll, T.R. & Harrison, J.E. (1994). Role of migrant factors in work-related fatalities in Australia, *Scandinavian Journal of Work and Environmental Health* **20**, 364–370.

[8] Fang, J., Madhavan, S. & Alderman, M.H. (1999). Cardiovascular mortality in New York City, *Journal of Urban Health* **76**, 51–61.

[9] Geddes, M. (1993). Italian migration: an overview, in *Cancer in Italian Migrant Populations*, M. Geddes, D.M. Parkin, M. Khlat, D. Balzi & E. Buiatti, eds. IARC Scientific Publications, Lyon, pp. 11–19.

[10] Geddes, M., Balzi, D., Buiatti, E., Brancker, A. & Parkin, D.M. (1994). Cancer mortality in Italian migrants to Canada, *Tumori* **80**, 19–23.

[11] Geddes, M., Parkin, D.M., Khlat, M., Balzi, D. & Buiatti, E. (1993). *Cancer in Italian Migrant Populations*. IARC Scientific Publications, Lyon.

[12] Gellert, G.A., Maxwell, R.M., Higgins, K.V., Mai, K.K., Lowery, R. & Doll, L. (1995). HIV/AIDS knowledge and high risk sexual practices among southern California Vietnamese, *Genitourinarian Medicine* **71**, 216–223.

[13] Guendelman, S. & English, P.B. (1995). Effect of United States residence on birth outcomes among Mexicans immigrants: an exploratory study, *American Journal of Public Health* **142**, S30–S38.

[14] Haenszel, W. (1961). Cancer mortality among the foreign-born in the United States, *Journal of the National Cancer Institute* **26**, 37–132.

[15] Haenszel, W., Kurihara, M., Segi, M. & Lee R.K.C. (1972). Stomach cancer among Japanese in Hawaii, *Journal of the National Cancer Institute* **49**, 969–988.

[16] Harding, S. & Balarajan, R. (1996). Pattern of mortality in second generation Irish living in England and Wales: longitudinal study, *British Medical Journal* **312**, 1389–1392.

[17] Iscovich, J. & Parkin, D.M. (1997). Risk of cancer in migrants and their descendants in Israel: I. Leukaemias and lymphomas, *International Journal of Cancer* **70**, 649–653.

[18] Kagan, A., Harris, B.R., Winkelstein, W., Johnson, K.G., Kato, H., Syme, S.L., Rhoods, G.G., Gay, M.L., Nichaman, M.Z., Hamilton, H.B. & Tillotson, J. (1974). Epidemiologic studies of coronary heart disease and stroke in Japanese men living in Japan, Hawaii and California: demographic, physical, dietary and biochemical characteristics, *Journal of Chronic Disease* **27**, 345–364.

[19] Kaldor, J., Khlat, M., Parkin, D.M., Shiboski, S. & Steinitz, R. (1990). Log-linear models for cancer risk among migrants, *International Journal of Epidemiology* **19**, 233–239.

[20] Karetnyi, Y.V., Mendelson, E., Shlyakhov, E., Rubinstein, E., Golubev, N., Levin, R., Sandler, M., Schreiber, M., Rubinstein, U., Shif, I., Handsher, R., Varsano, N. & Modan, B. (1995). Prevalence of antibodies against hepatitis A virus among new immigrants in Israel, *Journal of Medical Virology* **46**, 61–65.

[21] Khlat, M. & Balzi, D. (1993). Statistical methods, in *Cancer in Italian Migrant Populations*, M. Geddes, D.M. Parkin, M. Khlat, D. Balzi & E. Buiatti, eds. IARC Scientific Publications, Lyon, pp. 37–47.

[22] Khlat, M., Vail, A., Parkin, D.M. & Green, A. (1992). Mortality from melanoma in migrants to Australia: variation by age at arrival and duration of stay, *American Journal of Epidemiology* **135**, 1103–1113.

[23] Kliewer, E.V. & Ward, R.H. (1988). Convergence of immigrant suicide rates to those in the destination country, *American Journal of Epidemiology* **127**, 640–648.

[24] Kolonel, L., Hinds, W. & Hankin, J. (1980). Cancer patterns among migrant and native-born Japanese in Hawaii in relation to smoking, drinking and

dietary habits, in *Genetic and Environmental Factors in Experimental and Human Cancer*, H.V. Gelboin, B. MacMahon, T. Matsushima, T. Sugimura, S. Takayama & H. Takabe, eds. Japanese Scientific Societies Press, Tokyo, pp. 327–340.

[25]   Kolonel, L.N., Nomura, A.M.Y., Hirohata, T., Hankin, J.H. & Hinds, M.W. (1981). Association of diet and place of birth with stomach cancer incidence in Hawaii Japanese and Caucasians, *American Journal of Clinical Nutrition* **34**, 2478–2485.

[26]   Mack, T.M., Walker, A., Mack, W. & Bernstein, L. (1985). Cancer in Hispanics in Los Angeles County, *National Cancer Institute Monograph* **69**, 99–104.

[27]   Margetts, B.M., Hopkins, S.M., Binns, C.W., Miller, M.R. & Armstrong, B.K. (1981). Nutrient intakes in Italian migrants and Australians in Perth, *Food and Nutrition* **31**, 7–10.

[28]   Marmot, M.G., Adelstein, A.M. & Bulusu, L. (1984). Immigrant mortality in England and Wales 1970–78: causes of death by country of birth, *Studies on Medical and Population Subjects*. HMSO, London.

[29]   McKenna, M.T., McCray, E. & Onorato, I. (1995). The epidemiology of tuberculosis among foreign-born persons in the United States, 1986 to 1993, *New England Journal of Medicine* **332**, 1071–1076.

[30]   McMichael, A.J., McCall, M.G., Hartshorne, J.M. & Woodings, T.L. (1980). Patterns of gastro-intestinal cancer in European migrants to Australia: the role of dietary change, *International Journal of Cancer* **25**, 431–437.

[31]   Muir, C.S. & Staszewski, J. (1986). Geographical epidemiology and migrant studies, in *Biochemical and Molecular Epidemiology of Cancer*, C. Harris, ed. Liss, New York, pp. 135–148.

[32]   Nomura, A.M., Stemmermann, G.N., Heilbrun, L.K., Salked, R.M. & Vuilleumier, J.P. (1985). Serum vitamin levels and the risk of cancer of specific sites in men of Japanese ancestry in Hawaii, *Cancer Research* **45**, 2369–2372.

[33]   Parkin, D.M. & Iscovich, J. (1997). Risk of cancer in migrants and their descendants in Israel: II. Carcinomas and germ-cell tumours, *International Journal of Cancer* **70**, 654–660.

[34]   Roberts, N. & Cawthorpe, D. (1995). Immigrant child and adolescent psychiatric referrals: a five-year retrospective study of Asian and Caucasian families, *Canadian Journal of Psychiatry* **40**, 252–256.

[35]   Rothman, K.J. (1986). *Modern Epidemiology*, Little, Brown, & Company, Boston.

[36]   Singh, G.K. & Yu, S.M. (1996). Adverse pregnancy outcomes: differences between US and foreign-born women in major US racial and ethnic groups, *American Journal of Public Health* **86**, 837–843.

[37]   Sorenson, S.B. & Shen, H. (1996). Homicide risk among immigrants in California, 1970 through 1992, *American Journal of Public Health* **86**, 97–100.

[38]   Steinitz, R., Iscovich, J.N. & Katz, L. (1990). Cancer incidence in young offspring of Jewish immigrants to Israel: a methodological study, I: Nasopharyngeal

malignancies and Ewing sarcoma, *Cancer Detection and Prevention* **14**, 547–553.

[39]   Steinitz, R., Parkin, D.M., Young, J.L., Bieber, C.A. & Katz, L. (1989). *Cancer Incidence in Jewish Migrants to Israel 1961–1981*. IARC Scientific Publications, Lyon.

[40]   Stenhouse, N.S. & McCall, M.G. (1970). Differential mortality from cardiovascular disease in migrants from England and Wales, Scotland and Italy, and native-born Australians, *Journal of Chronic Diseases* **23**, 423–431.

[41]   Terracini, B., Siemiatycki, J. & Richardson, L. (1990). Cancer incidence and risk factors among Montreal residents of Italian origin, *International Journal of Epidemiology* **19**, 491–497.

[42]   Thomas, D.B. & Karagas, M.R. (1987). Cancer in first and second generation Americans, *Cancer Research* **47**, 5771–5776.

[43]   Thomas, D.B. & Karagas, M.R. (1996). Migrant studies, in *Cancer Epidemiology and Prevention*, D. Schottenfeld & J.F. Fraumeni Jr, eds. Oxford, University Press, Oxford, pp. 236–254.

[44]   Trautwein, C., Kiral, G., Tillmann, H.L., Witteler, H., Michel, G. & Manns, M.P. (1995). Risk factors and prevalence of hepatitis E in German immigrants from the former Soviet Union, *Journal of Medical Virology* **45**, 429–434.

[45]   Wang, Z.J., Ramcharan, S. & Love, E.J. (1989). Cancer mortality of Chinese in Canada, *International Journal of Epidemiology* **18**, 17–21.

[46]   Wu, A.H., Ziegler, R.G., Horn-Ross, P.L., Nomura, A.M., West, D.W., Kolonel, L.N., Rosenthal, J.F., Hoover, R.N. & Pike, M.C. (1996). Tofu and risk of breast cancer in Asian-Americans, *Cancer Epidemiology Biomarkers and Prevention* **5**, 901–906.

E. BUIATTI & D. BALZI

Minitab *see* Software, Biostatistical

Misclassification Error

It was recognized early [3] that misclassification of categorical variables induces problems of analysis and interpretation. In epidemiology there has been continuing interest in assessing effects of misclassification on exposure–disease associations. More recent attention has been paid to methodology for estimating the misclassification structure and adjusting for resulting **biases**. This involves gathering auxiliary data through validation samples (*see* **Validation Study**) and repeated measurements. Although there are immediate parallels between the rationale for handling misclassification and the discussion on measurement errors in continuous exposure variables, the two topics have different historical paths and the statistical techniques differ in technical detail. **Measurement Error in Epidemiologic Studies** deals with the case of continuous covariates. Early reviews on the effects of misclassification include a bibliography by Dalenius [8] and a paper by Chen [4]. Kuha & Skinner [26] offer a more recent account. Here we describe effects caused by misclassification and present some of the methodology for adjustment.

Effects of Misclassification

Univariate Analyses

Let A^* denote the classification variable subject to error and A the true variable that the classification variable is intended to measure. We refer to A^* as a surrogate for A. For each unit (individual) the outcome of A, and A^*, falls into one of m mutually exclusive categories. Independence between units is assumed. We write the misclassification probabilities

$$\Pr(A^* = j | A = k) = \theta_{jk}, \quad j, k = 1, \ldots m.$$

The parameters θ_{jk} governing the misclassification structure may be collected into an $m \times m$ misclassification matrix $\Theta = [\theta_{jk}]$ with nonnegative elements and columns that sum to one. For a binary response, where $m = 2$ and the categories indicate the presence ($A = 2$) or absence ($A = 1$) of disease, the misclassification matrix involves only two parameters

$$\Theta = \begin{pmatrix} \theta_{11} & \theta_{12} \\ \theta_{21} & \theta_{22} \end{pmatrix} = \begin{pmatrix} \beta & 1 - \alpha \\ 1 - \beta & \alpha \end{pmatrix}. \quad (1)$$

The parameter α in (1) is called the **sensitivity** of the measuring instrument and β the **specificity**.

The effect of using the surrogate classification A^* may be summarized by

$$\pi_{A*} = \Theta \pi_A,$$

where $\pi_{A*} = (\pi_{A*}(1), \ldots, \pi_{A*}(m))'$ and $\pi_A = (\pi_A(1), \ldots, \pi_A(m))'$ are the population proportions in the categories of the surrogate variable and the true variable, respectively. Sample proportions of A^* are

thus biased estimates of π_A. The nature of this bias is most easily described in the binary case, where

$$\pi_{A*}(2) = (1 - \beta)\pi_A(1) + \alpha \pi_A(2) \quad (2)$$

(for example [6]). Even when the misclassification matrix differs from the identity matrix it is clear from (2) that the two errors are mutually compensating if $(1 - \beta)\pi_A(1) = (1 - \alpha)\pi_A(2)$. The degree of compensation depends on the true proportions $\pi_A(1)$ and $\pi_A(2)$. An instrument with given misclassification matrix can thus induce different degrees of bias in different populations.

Bivariate Analyses

2 × 2 Tables. In a two-by-two table, let A define the presence or absence of disease and B two exposure groups, e.g. smokers and nonsmokers. We first consider the case where the response variable is subject to misclassification, i.e. A is measured by the surrogate A^*. Let $\pi_{A|B}(j|l)$ denote the proportion of units in the population for which $A = j$ in exposure group $B = l$, and let $\pi_{A*|B}(j|l)$ denote the corresponding proportion for A^*.

When focus is on the difference in the response proportions between the two exposure groups, then an unbiased estimator of the surrogate difference $\pi_{A*|B}(2|2) - \pi_{A*|B}(2|1)$ will in general be biased for the true difference $\pi_{A|B}(2|2) - \pi_{A|B}(2|1)$. The argument simplifies if both exposure groups have the same sensitivity α and specificity β. In this case the misclassification mechanism for A is said to be **nondifferential** with respect to B. It follows from (2) that under nondifferential misclassification

$$\pi_{A*|B}(2|2) - \pi_{A*|B}(2|1)$$
$$= (\alpha + \beta - 1)[\pi_{A|B}(2|2) - \pi_{A|B}(2|1)]. \quad (3)$$

It is reasonable to expect each of the misclassification probabilities $1 - \alpha$ and $1 - \beta$ to be less than 0.5, in which case the factor $(\alpha + \beta - 1)$ in (3) takes values between 0 and 1. The difference measured by the surrogate A^* is thus always smaller than the true difference based on A. The effect of nondifferential misclassification is to *attenuate*, i.e. "to make seem smaller", the difference in subclass proportions. This was noted by Rubin et al. [30] as early as 1956. Nondifferential misclassification similarly attenuates the ratio $\pi_{A|B}(2|2)/\pi_{A|B}(2|1)$ toward the null value of one (see, for example, [7]) (*see* **Bias Toward the Null**).

If, instead, the response variable A is correctly classified while the exposure B is misclassified as B^*, and if the misclassification of B is nondifferential with respect to A, then

$$\pi_{A|B*}(2|2) - \pi_{A|B*}(2|1)$$
$$= \frac{(\alpha_B + \beta_B - 1)\pi_B(2)\pi_B(1)}{\pi_{B*}(2)\pi_{B*}(1)}$$
$$\times [\pi_{A|B}(2|2) - \pi_{A|B}(2|1)], \qquad (4)$$

where $\pi_B = (\pi_B(1), \pi_B(2))'$ and $\pi_{B*} = (\pi_{B*}(1), \pi_{B*}(2))'$ are the population proportions of B and B^* respectively, and α_B and β_B are the sensitivity and specificity of the classification of B. The factor multiplying $\pi_{A|B}(2|2) - \pi_{A|B}(2|1)$ in (4) is again between 0 and 1, when $0 < \alpha_B + \beta_B - 1 \leq 1$, so that the effect is a similar type of attenuation as described above.

If both the response A and the exposure B are subject to misclassification, and if the surrogate pair (A^*, B^*) is jointly determined by the pair (A, B) through the misclassification probabilities $\Pr(A^* = j^*, B^* = k^*|A = j, B = k)$, then misclassification of A and B is said to be *independent* if

$$\Pr(A^* = j^*, B^* = k^*|A = j, B = k)$$
$$= \Pr(A^* = j^*|A = j, B = k)$$
$$\times \Pr(B^* = k^*|A = j, B = k),$$

and it is *nondifferential* if

$$\Pr(A^* = j^*|A = j, B = k) = \Pr(A^* = j^*|A = j)$$

and

$$\Pr(B^* = k^*|A = j, B = k) = \Pr(B^* = k^*|B = k).$$

Under the condition of independent and nondifferential misclassification in A and B, Gullen et al. [20] show that an unbiased estimator of $\pi_{A*|B*}(2|2) - \pi_{A*|B*}(2|1)$ again attenuates the true difference. If on the other hand A, or B, or both, are subject to *differential* misclassification, then the bias inherent in $\pi_{A*|B*}(2|2) - \pi_{A*|B*}(2|1)$ can take any arbitrary form. A clear account of the possible effects of differential misclassification is presented by Goldberg [16] (*see* **Differential Error**).

Note that changes in the categorization of a misclassified variable may turn a nondifferential misclassification into a differential one. Wachholder et al. [34] discuss the situation in which A has three categories and is subject to nondifferential misclassification with respect to B. They show that combining two of the categories of A induces differential misclassification with respect to B. On a similar note, Flegal et al. [13] show that if a nondifferentially mismeasured continuous variable is dichotomized, this may induce differential error.

2 × m   Tables.   When comparing proportions defined by a binary response A in three or more exposure subgroups ($m > 2$) defined by B, the result in (3) holds when the response A is nondifferentially misclassified with respect to B. The ordering of the response proportions over exposure subgroups is thus preserved, but the differences are attenuated.

If, instead, the response A is correctly classified but the exposure B is subject to nondifferential misclassification, then (i) measures of association for response proportions between the two extreme exposure subgroups $B = 1$ and $B = m$ are again attenuated, but (ii) associations between other exposure subgroups may be biased either away from or towards null [2, 15]. Exposure misclassification can even change the ordering of the response proportions in the intermediate subgroups and distort trends. However, if misclassification is confined to adjacent exposure subgroups, then attenuation occurs, but the ordering of the response proportions is retained [28].

Hypothesis Testing for Two-Way Tables.   An important consequence of the attenuation results is that if there is no association between A and B, then there will be no association between the surrogates A^* and B^* under nondifferential misclassification in one variable [29] or under nondifferential and independent misclassification in both variables [1]. The test of no association between A and B based on A^* and B^* will thus have the correct significance level, but the power is in general reduced. Marshall et al. [28] show similar results for a test of no trend in subclass proportions for tables where the outcome A is binary and a polytomous subgroup variable B is nondifferentially misclassified.

Multivariate Analyses

The simplest multivariate case involves a $2 \times 2 \times 2$ table. Let A be a binary response variable and B and C binary variables defining subgroups of the population. In particular, B may refer to an exposure and C to a potential **confounder**.

If C is correctly classified, then we can consider the two-way tables between A and B separately for the two levels of C, and apply the bivariate results of the previous section. If only A is subject to nondifferential misclassification, then the difference in response proportions between the two exposure groups is attenuated by the factor given in (3). If, however, the exposure B is nondifferentially misclassified, we have from (4) that the degree of attenuation depends on the true proportions, in this case on $\pi_{B|C}(2|2)$ for $C = 2$ and on $\pi_{B|C}(2|1)$ for $C = 1$. If there is association between B and C, then the difference in response proportions between the two exposure groups may be attenuated to a different degree in the two categories of C. Nondifferential misclassification in the exposure may thus induce spurious heterogeneity (or mask true heterogeneity) in the exposure–disease association for different levels of the confounder [17].

If C is subject to nondifferential misclassification (with $0 < \alpha_C + \beta_C - 1 \le 1$) with respect to A and B, which are both classified without error, then $\pi_{A|B,C*}(2|k, l)$ lies between the true proportions $\pi_{A|B,C}(2|k, l)$ and $\pi_{A|B}(2|k)$ for any $k, l = 1, 2$ [17, 26]. The proportions $\pi_{A|B}(2|k)$ are obtained by summing the data over the levels of C. This form of bias is known as residual confounding (for example [31]). It occurs because the analysis is restricted to the wrong levels of the confounder C, and thus the heterogeneity in the proportions due to confounding is not fully controlled for. The bias due to residual confounding may be either away from or toward the null value, and it can even induce a exposure–response association with the wrong sign. Both the size and power of a test of no association between A and B adjusted for C are thus incorrect when C is subject to nondifferential misclassification.

The above example of misclassification in a $2 \times 2 \times 2$ table may be extended in various ways. Some of the variables in a three-way table may be polytomous and there may be independent and nondifferential misclassification in more than one variable. In this case the effect of misclassification is a combination of attenuation and residual confounding [14].

Misclassification that is not both independent and nondifferential can produce any kind of biases (some examples are given by Greenland & Robins [19]).

For tables involving more than three variables it is not in general possible to give even qualitative statements about how misclassification distorts the analysis. One exception is a useful result due to Korn [24]: if there is independent and nondifferential misclassification in several variables in a multiway table, and if each of these misclassified variables appears in only one term of a hierarchical loglinear model specifying the association structure of the table, then this association structure is preserved under the misclassification. A test of goodness of fit for this loglinear model will have the correct significance level but reduced power. Korn [25] evaluates the loss of power due to misclassification when using a likelihood ratio test for comparing two nested models where the association structure is preserved.

Auxiliary Data on Misclassification

Adjustment for potential bias due to misclassification requires some information on the misclassification structure. If the structure is known, either through prior information or by assumption, then adjustment is straightforward. In general, however, the misclassification structure is unknown and estimated from a suitable set of *auxiliary data*, which are assumed to have the same misclassification parameters as the *primary data*. We briefly describe the two main types of auxiliary data: *validation samples* and *repeated measurements*.

Validation Samples

Both the true variable A, say, and the surrogate variable A^*, possibly together with other variables, are measured on each unit in a validation sample. This raises two important questions: (i) How does one measure the true value A? (ii) How should the units in the validation sample be selected?

A measurement of A may be possible using an instrument referred to as the gold standard. It may be too expensive, however, to use the gold standard on all units in the primary study, or the gold standard may be available only for a subset of the units. The gold standard is a key concept in validation studies and the assumption that it measures A accurately, or with negligible error, is crucial (cf. [33], for a discussion of bias induced by using an erroneous or "alloyed" gold standard).

Ideally the validation sample should be a subsample of the primary data, obtained by a known randomized double sampling scheme. Simple random sampling from the primary data gives an *internal validation sample*, where the proportions in the categories of A in the validation sample are unbiased estimates of the corresponding population proportions. Both the misclassification probabilities $\Pr(A^*|A)$ and the **predictive values** $\Pr(A|A^*)$ in the population of interest can thus be consistently estimated from internal validation data. There may, however, be practical reasons that prevent such double sampling. If validation data from an earlier study are used, or if the gold standard is available only in a specific subpopulation, or if validation data are collected after the primary data are in hand, then it may be unreasonable to assume that the distribution over the categories of A are the same for units in the validation sample and in the primary study population. We then say that the validation data are *external*, and only the misclassification probabilities are assumed to be transportable between data sets.

Instead of using simple random sampling it may be useful to draw a prespecified proportion of the validation sample units within each category of A^*. This increases the efficiency in estimating the predictive values $\Pr(A|A^*)$, and is thus useful in internal validation studies [21].

Repeated Measurements

Even without a gold standard it may be possible to estimate misclassification parameters from repeated measurements of the surrogate. The measurements may be replicates using the same instrument or they may be obtained using different instruments. The distinction between internal and external data is relevant also for repeated measures, and which of these is in question depends on how the distributions over categories of A are related in the auxiliary and primary data sets.

For models based on repeated surrogate measures to be identifiable, a sufficient number of the measurements should be conditionally independent given the true value A. The required number depends on the model; some simple models are identifiable from just

two measurements, while three measurements are sufficient for most models (see [35] and [27] for general identifiability conditions).

Adjusting for Effects of Misclassification

Misclassification parameters estimated from auxiliary data may be used to estimate parameters of interest adjusting for the biases induced by misclassification. Here we describe three classes of adjustment methods: simple matrix methods and model-based methods using either validation data or repeated measurements.

Matrix Methods

The most straightforward way to adjust for misclassification is via simple **back-calculation**. We refer to this as the *matrix method* of adjustment. The aim is to estimate the vector of cell proportions π_A for variable A. Here A may represent one variable or the cross-classification of several variables. Suppose that a primary data set and a validation data set are available, with n_p and n_v observations, respectively. The validation data provide an estimate, denoted by $\hat{\Theta}(A^*|A)$, for the matrix of misclassification probabilities $\theta_{jk} = \Pr(A^* = j|A = k)$. A matrix estimate of π_A is given by

$$\hat{\pi}_A^m = \{\hat{\Theta}(A^*|A)\}^{-1}\hat{\pi}_{A^*}, \qquad (5)$$

with $\hat{\pi}_{A^*}$ the vector of observed cell proportions for the surrogate A^* in the primary data set. The analysis of interest is performed on the transformed table $\hat{\pi}_A^m$. An estimated variance matrix for $\hat{\pi}_A^m$, or any quantities derived from it, such as **odds ratios**, can be obtained using the delta method [18]. The simple matrix estimator (5) is well known in the epidemiologic literature. It is straightforward to compute, but has the drawbacks that the estimated probabilities are not constrained to lie between 0 and 1, and its small sample properties may be poor due to the matrix inversion.

The estimator (5) can also be motivated as a maximum likelihood estimator (MLE) of π_A under a model where (i) π_A is unrestricted, (ii) the model for the misclassification probabilities is the one under which $\hat{\Theta}(A^*|A)$ was estimated (or taken as known), and (iii) the validation data are external. For most other models the MLE needs to be computed using iterative methods described in the next section. An important exception is a case where the validation data are internal and the model structure is such that there exists a one-to-one transformation from π_A and $\Theta(A^*|A)$ to π_{A^*} and $\Lambda(A|A^*)$, where $\Lambda(A|A^*)$ denotes the $m \times m$ matrix of predictive values $\Pr(A = i|A^* = j)$. The MLE of π_A is then also a closed-form matrix estimate, given by

$$\hat{\pi}_A^c = f_p \hat{\Lambda}(A|A^*)\hat{\pi}_{A^*} + (1 - f_p)\hat{\pi}_A^{(v)} \quad (6)$$

where $f_p = n_p/(n_p + n_v)$, $\hat{\pi}_A^{(v)}$ is the vector of observed cell proportions of A in the validation data set, and $\hat{\Lambda}(A|A^*)$ is the matrix of predictive values estimated from the validation data. Estimates of this type were proposed by Tenenbein [32] for estimating cell probabilities of a single variable when both π_A and the misclassification probabilities are unrestricted. Tenenbein also gave formulas for the variance of $\hat{\pi}_A^c$.

In cases where (6) is the MLE of π_A, the external validation MLE $\hat{\pi}_A^m$ in (5) is also consistent, but not fully efficient. It may even have a higher variance than $\hat{\pi}_A^{(v)}$ alone. Surprisingly, the same is also true for the estimate $\tilde{\pi}_A^c = f_p\{\hat{\Theta}(A^*|A)\}^{-1}\hat{\pi}_{A^*} + (1 - f_p)\hat{\pi}_A^{(v)}$, which appears to be a compromise between (5) and (6). This estimate should not be used, because it is inconsistent when the validation data are external and less efficient than $\hat{\pi}_A^c$ when they are internal. Its variance may even *increase* with increasing n_p [26].

Matrix adjustments for misclassification are most useful in fairly simple problems with a small number of variables and few categories per variable. The estimates imply a model where the cell probabilities of the true variables are unrestricted and the model for the misclassification structure is either saturated or has a special form such as independent and nondifferential misclassification for all variables. In large problems this may lead to sparse tables and imprecise estimates for the many parameters. It is then desirable to consider more parsimonious models, especially when the focus is on inference about the association structure between the true variables. This can be done, at the expense of further model assumptions and some extra computing, by using model-based adjustment procedures described in the next section.

Modeling

Let A denote a set of variables subject to misclassification and A^* the corresponding set of surrogate variables, and let C be variables classified without error. It is also useful to define a sample indicator variable L which identifies the data set to which a unit belongs. L is binary when there is one primary sample and one validation sample, but other study designs can also be incorporated in this framework. The joint distribution of (A, A^*, C, L) may be specified through two submodels (cf. Espeland & Odoroff [12], who consider a slightly different set of models):

1. A model for the true variables (A, C, L). **Interactions** between L and (A, C) indicate differences in the distribution of the true variables between samples such as when a validation sample is external. The model of interest is the model for (A, C) in the primary sample.
2. A model for the misclassification probabilities, specified by interactions within A^* and between (A, C) and A^*. The model is saturated with respect to the true variables (A, C). Because the misclassification probabilities are assumed to be transportable between data sets, there should not be any interaction terms between L and A^*.

Both submodels are usually taken to be hierarchical loglinear models, but the joint model generated by them will not in general be loglinear [12].

The misclassification problem may be treated as one of incomplete contingency tables, collapsed over the margins corresponding to the unobserved variables. Suppose that there is one primary data set and one validation data set. The log likelihood function for the observed variables can be written as

$$L = \sum_{\text{prim}} n_{A^*C} \log \pi_{A^*,C} + \sum_{\text{val}} n_{AA^*C} \log \pi_{A,A^*,C}^{(v)}$$

$$(7)$$

where n_{A^*C} are the observed cell counts for (A^*, C) in the primary data and $\pi_{A^*,C} = \sum_A \pi_{A,A^*,C}$ are the corresponding cell probabilities satisfying the specified model, and n_{AA^*C} and $\pi_{A,A^*,C}^{(v)}$ are the cell counts and probabilities for (A, A^*, C) in the validation data. The models may be fitted by maximizing (7) using iterative techniques, especially the expectation-maximization (EM) algorithm. At the E step of the algorithm, observations from the observed (A^*, C) table in the primary data are allocated values of A to create a notionally complete (A, A^*, C) table. This is used at the M step, together with the validation sample, to fit the required joint model, and the process is iterated until convergence. Different versions of the EM algorithm for misclassification problems have been proposed by Chen et al. [5] and Espeland & Odoroff [12], who also consider the estimation of standard errors for the resulting estimates. The joint likelihood can also be maximized using other algorithms such as direct Newton–Raphson maximization [10, 11].

Methods Using Repeated Measurements

When the misclassification parameters are estimated from repeated measurements, the true values of the misclassified variables are latent variables which are never observed. The misclassification probabilities and models of interest can be estimated from such data subject to appropriate identifiability assumptions. The analysis proceeds by specifying models for the true variables and misclassification as above and obtaining MLEs for their parameters. In some very simple cases, such as when estimating the proportions of a single binary misclassified variable, estimates are available in a closed form [22]. It is then also possible to use external repeated measurements to estimate the misclassification matrix in the matrix estimate (5) [9]. For most models, however, estimates have to be obtained iteratively, using general techniques of latent class modeling (see, for example, [23]). The calculations may again be conveniently carried out using the EM algorithm.

Conclusions

Misclassification induces bias in the estimates of quantities of interest obtained from observed surrogate variables. In some special cases it is possible to characterize qualitatively the nature of the bias, such as when measures of association are attenuated. In many situations, however, biases in any direction are possible. It is then desirable to collect auxiliary data such as validation data or repeated measurements from which the misclassification probabilities can be estimated, and to use these estimates to adjust analyses explicitly for the effects of misclassification. The most straightforward adjustment methods are simple matrix methods, which may, however, be unsatisfactory in larger models. Model-based adjustment methods may then be used for estimation.

References

[1]   Assakul, K. & Proctor, C.H. (1967). Testing independence in two-way contingency tables with data subject to misclassification, *Psychometrika* **32**, 67–76.

[2]   Birkett, N.J. (1992). Effects of nondifferential misclassification on estimates of odds ratios with multiple levels of exposure, *American Journal of Epidemiology* **136**, 356–362.

[3]   Bross, I. (1954). Misclassification in 2 × 2 tables, *Biometrics* **10**, 488–495.

[4]   Chen, T.T. (1989). A review of methods for misclassified categorical data in epidemiology, *Statistics in Medicine* **8**, 1095–1106.

[5]   Chen, T.T., Hochberg, Y. & Tenenbein, A. (1984). Analysis of multivariate categorical data with misclassification errors by triple sampling schemes, *Journal of Statistical Planning and Inference* **9**, 177–184.

[6]   Cochran, W.G. (1968). Errors of measurement in statistics, *Technometrics* **10**, 637–666.

[7]   Copeland, K.T., Checkoway, H., McMichael, A.J. & Holbrook, R. (1977). Bias due to misclassification in the estimation of relative risk, *American Journal of Epidemiology* **105**, 488–495.

[8]   Dalenius, T. (1977). Bibliography of non-sampling errors in surveys, *International Statistical Review* **45**, 71–89, 181–197, 303–317.

[9]   Duffy, S.W., Rohan, T.E. & Day, N.E. (1989). Misclassification in more than one factor in a case–control study: A combination of Mantel–Haenszel and maximum likelihood approaches, *Statistics in Medicine* **8**, 1529–1536.

[10] Ekholm, A. & Palmgren, J. (1987). Correction for misclassification using doubly sampled data, *Journal of Official Statistics* **3**, 419–429.

[11] Espeland, M.A. & Hui, S.L. (1987). A general approach to analyzing epidemiologic data that contain misclassification errors, *Biometrics* **43**, 1001–1012.

[12] Espeland, M.A. & Odoroff, C.L. (1985). Log-linear models for doubly sampled categorical data fitted by the EM algorithm, *Journal of the American Statistical Association* **80**, 663–670.

[13] Flegal, K.M., Keyl, P.M. & Nieto, F.J. (1991). Differential misclassification arising from nondifferential errors in exposure measurement, *American Journal of Epidemiology* **134**, 1233–1244.

[14] Fung, K.Y. & Howe, G.R. (1984). Methodological issues in case–control studies. III: The effect of joint misclassification of risk factors and confounding factors upon estimation and power, *International Journal of Epidemiology* **13**, 366–370.

[15] Gladen, B. & Rogan, W.J. (1979). Misclassification and the design of environmental studies, *American Journal of Epidemiology* **109**, 607–616.

[16] Goldberg, J.D. (1975). The effects of misclassification on the bias in the difference between two proportions and the relative odds in the fourfold table, *Journal of the American Statistical Association* **70**, 561–567.

[17] Greenland, S. (1980). The effect of misclassification in the presence of covariates, *American Journal of Epidemiology* **112**, 564–569.

[18] Greenland, S. (1988). Variance estimation for epidemiologic effect estimates under misclassification, *Statistics in Medicine* **7**, 745–757.

[19] Greenland, S. & Robins, J.M. (1985). Confounding and misclassification, *American Journal of Epidemiology* **122**, 495–506.

[20] Gullen, W.H., Bearman, J.E. & Johnson, E.A. (1968). Effects of misclassification in epidemiologic studies, *Public Health Reports* **83**, 914–918.

[21] Haitovsky, Y. & Rapp, J. (1992). Conditional resampling for misclassified multinomial data with applications to sampling inspection, *Technometrics* **34**, 473–483.

[22] Harper, D. (1964). Misclassification in epidemiological surveys, *American Journal of Public Health* **54**, 1882–1886.

[23] Kaldor, J. & Clayton, D. (1985). Latent class analysis in chronic disease epidemiology, *Statistics in Medicine* **4**, 327–335.

[24] Korn, E.L. (1981). Hierarchical log-linear models not preserved by classification error, *Journal of the American Statistical Association* **76**, 110–113.

[25] Korn, E.L. (1982). The asymptotic efficiency of tests using misclassified data in contingency tables, *Biometrics* **38**, 445–450.

[26] Kuha, J. & Skinner, C. (1997). Categorical data analysis and misclassification, in *Survey Measurement and Process Quality*, L. Lyberg, P. Biemer, M. Collins, E. De Leeuw, C. Dippo, N. Schwarz & D. Trewin, eds. Wiley, New York, pp. 633–670.

[27] Liu, X. & Liang, K.-Y. (1991). Adjustment for nondifferential misclassification error in the generalized linear model, *Statistics in Medicine* **10**, 1197–1211.

[28] Marshall, J.R., Priore, R., Graham, S. & Brasure, J. (1981). On the distortion of risk estimates in multiple exposure level case–control studies, *American Journal of Epidemiology* **113**, 464–473.

[29] Mote, V.L. & Anderson, R.L. (1965). An investigation of the effect of misclassification on the properties of χ^2-tests in the analysis of categorical data, *Biometrika* **52**, 95–109.

[30] Rubin, T., Rosenbaum, A.B. & Cobb, S. (1956). The use of interview data for the detection of association in field studies, *Journal of Chronic Diseases* **4**, 253–266.

[31] Savitz, D.A. & Barón, A.E. (1989). Estimating and correcting for confounder misclassification, *American Journal of Epidemiology* **129**, 1062–1071.

[32] Tenenbein, A. (1972). A double sampling scheme for estimating from misclassified multinomial data with applications to sampling inspection, *Technometrics* **14**, 187–202.

[33] Wachholder, S., Armstrong, B. & Hartge, P. (1993). Validation studies using an alloyed gold standard, *American Journal of Epidemiology* **137**, 1251–1258.

[34] Wachholder, S., Dosemeci, M. & Lubin, J.H. (1991). Blind assignment of exposure does not always prevent differential misclassification, *American Journal of Epidemiology* **134**, 433–437.

[35] Walter, S.D. & Irwig, L.M. (1988). Estimation of test error rates, disease prevalence and relative risk from misclassified data: a review, *Journal of Clinical Epidemiology* **41**, 923–937.

JOUNI KUHA, CHRIS SKINNER &
JUNI PALMGREN

Missing Data

This article concerns the analysis of biostatistical data that are subject to missing values. It builds on earlier research [63, 65–67]. Missing values arise in biostatistics for many reasons. For example:

1. In longitudinal studies, data are missing because of *attrition*, i.e. subjects drop out prior to the end of the study.

2. In **sample surveys**, some individuals provide no information because of noncontact or refusal to respond (*unit* **nonresponse**). Other individuals are contacted and provide some information, but fail to answer some of the questions (*item* nonresponse). For example, the National Health and Nutrition Examination Survey (NHANES) includes data from an individual interview and a health examination. Some survey respondents miss particular variables because they refused to answer sensitive questions, or measurements were not carried out or were incorrectly recorded, for example they lie outside allowable ranges. Other individuals are missing all the recordings from the health examination since they failed to show up, but have information from the individual interview recorded.

3. Information about a variable is partially recorded. A common example in biostatistics is *right censoring*, where times to an event (death, progression

of disease) are being recorded, and for some individuals the event has still not taken place when the study is terminated. The times for these subjects are known to be greater than that corresponding to the latest time of observation, but the actual time is unknown. Another example of partial information is interval censoring, where it is known that the time to an event lies in an interval. For example, in a longitudinal study of a chronic disease, it may be established that some event (such as reinjury of hip after hip replacement surgery) took place some time between two visits to the doctor for checkups. The time to reinjury is then known to lie in an interval determined by the two checkups. If the interval is narrow compared with the distribution of event times themselves, then the simple approach of locating the event at the midpoint of the interval may be a good approximation, but otherwise methods that treat the event time as partially missing data may be important [13, 19, 38].

4. In clinical studies that involve chart review, charts are often incomplete or lacking in sufficient detail to determine particular items. Often indices are constructed by summing values of particular items, and if any of the items that form the index are missing, then some procedure is needed to deal with the missing data.

5. Missing data can arise by design. For example, suppose one objective in a study of obesity is to estimate the distribution of a measure Y_1 of body fat in the population, and correlate it with other factors. Since Y_1 is expensive to measure, it can only be obtained for a limited sample, but a crude proxy measure Y_2, such as body mass index, can be obtained for a much larger sample. A useful design is to measure Y_2 and covariates for a large sample and Y_1, Y_2, and covariates for a smaller subsample. The subsample allows predictions of the missing values of Y_1 to be generated for the larger sample, using one of the methods of analysis described below, yielding more efficient estimates than are possible from the subsample alone.

Unless missing data are deliberately incorporated by design, the most important step in dealing with missing data is to try to avoid it during the data-collection stage. Given that data are likely to be missing after data collection, however, it is also useful to try to collect covariates that are likely to be predictive of the missing values, so that an adequate adjustment can be made. In addition, the process that leads to missing values should be determined during the collection of data if possible. This assists in modeling the missing-data mechanism when an adjustment for the missing values is performed [62].

Three major approaches to the analysis of missing data can be distinguished:

1. discard incomplete cases and analyze the remainder (complete-case analysis);
2. impute or fill in the missing values and then analyze the filled-in data; and
3. analyze the incomplete data by a method that does not require a complete (that is, a rectangular) data set.

With regard to point 3, I focus on powerful likelihood-based methods, specifically maximum likelihood (ML) and Bayesian simulation. The latter is closely related to multiple imputation [96], an extension of single imputation that allows uncertainty in the imputations to be reflected appropriately in the analysis. Approaches to longitudinal data with missing values are considered in the concluding section.

A basic assumption in all our methods is that missingness of a particular value hides a true underlying value that is meaningful for analysis. This may seem obvious but is not always the case. For example, consider a longitudinal analysis of CD4 counts in a clinical trial for acquired immune deficiency syndrome (AIDS) [9]. For subjects who leave the study because they move to a different location, it makes sense to consider the CD4 counts that would have been recorded if they had remained in the study. For subjects who die during the course of the study, it is less clear whether it is reasonable to consider CD4 counts after time of death as missing values. Rather, it may be preferable to treat death as a primary outcome and restrict the analysis of CD4 counts to individuals who are alive. A more complex missing data problem arises when individuals leave the study for unknown reasons, which may include relocation or death.

Pattern and Mechanism of Missing Data

It is useful to distinguish the *pattern* of the missing data and the missing data *mechanism*. The pattern simply defines which values in the data set are observed and which are missing. Specifically, let

$Y = y_{ij}$ denote an $n \times p$ rectangular data set without missing values, with ith row $y_i = y_{i1}, \ldots, y_{ip}$, where y_{ij} is the value of variable Y_j for subject i. With missing data, define the *missing-data indicator matrix* $M = m_{ij}$, such that $m_{ij} = 1$ if y_{ij} is missing and $m_{ij} = 0$ if y_{ij} is present. The matrix M then defines the pattern of missing data.

When a data set contains missing values, it is important that information is coded so that M can be determined, even if it is not specifically created. This is usually done by designating a special missing-value code for missing values (such as 9999) that lies outside the allowable range for the variable. It is important to distinguish between zero values and missing values, since failure to do this creates considerable problems in analysis.

Some methods for handling missing data apply to any pattern of missing data, whereas other methods assume a special pattern. An important example of a special pattern is *univariate* nonresponse, where missingness is confined to a single variable. Another is *monotone* missing data, where the variables can be arranged so that $Y_{j+1}, \ldots, Y_p$ is missing for all cases where Y_j is missing, for all $j = 1, \ldots, p - 1$ (see Figure 1). This pattern arises commonly in longitudinal data subject to attrition.

The missing-data mechanism concerns the reasons why values are missing, and in particular whether these reasons relate to values in the data set. For example, a subject in a longitudinal study may be more likely to avoid a treatment and drop out of a study because (s)he felt the treatment was ineffective, which might be related to a poor value of an outcome measure. Rubin [93] treated M as a random matrix, and characterized the missing-data mechanism by the conditional distribution of M given Y,

say $f(M|Y, \phi)$, where ϕ denotes unknown parameters. If missingness does not depend on the values of the data Y, missing or observed, that is:

$$f(M|Y, \phi) = f(M|\phi), \quad \text{for all } Y, \phi,$$

then the data are called missing completely at random (MCAR) – note that this assumption does not mean that the pattern itself is random, but rather that missingness does not depend on the data values. A MCAR mechanism is plausible in planned missing-data designs as in example 5 above, but is a strong assumption when missing data do not occur by design because missingness usually depends on recorded variables. Let Y_{obs} denote the observed values of Y and Y_{mis} the missing values. A less restrictive assumption is that missingness depends only on values Y_{obs} that are observed, and not on values Y_{mis} that are missing. That is:

$$f(M|Y, \phi) = f(M|Y_{obs}, \phi), \quad \text{for all } Y_{mis}, \phi.$$

The missing data mechanism is then called missing at random (MAR). Murray & Findlay [80] provided an instructive example of MAR for data from a study of hypertensive drugs where the outcome was diastolic blood pressure. By protocol, the subject was no longer included in the study when the diastolic blood pressure got too large. This mechanism is not MCAR, since it depends on the values of blood pressure. But blood pressure at the time of drop-out was observed before the subject dropped out. Hence the mechanism is MAR, because drop-out only depends on the observed part of Y. Many methods for handling missing data assume the mechanism is MCAR or MAR, and yield **biased** estimates when the data are not MAR.

Complete-Case Analysis

A common and simple method is complete-case (CC) analysis, also known as *listwise* deletion, where incomplete cases are discarded and standard analysis methods applied to the complete cases. In many statistical packages (*see* **Software, Biostatistical**) this is the default analysis. Valid (but often suboptimal) inferences are obtained when the missing data are MCAR, since then the complete cases are a random subsample of the original sample with respect to all variables. However, even when MCAR holds,

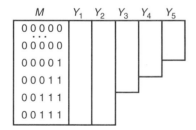

Figure 1 Schematic of a monotone missing data pattern, with rows representing cases, $Y_1, \ldots, Y_5$ repeated measures at five time points, and blocks representing data. M is the missing-data indicator matrix

the rejection of incomplete cases seems an unnecessary waste of information: if the number of variables is large, then even a sparse pattern of missing values can result in a substantial number of incomplete cases. One approach to incorporating the incomplete cases is to drop variables with high levels of nonresponse; Rubin [92] provides systematic methods in the regression context.

Aside from efficiency considerations, a serious problem with dropping incomplete cases is that the complete cases are often a biased sample, i.e., the missing data are not MCAR. The size of the resulting bias depends on the degree of deviation from MCAR, the amount of missing data, and the specifics of the analysis. In particular, the bias in estimating the mean of a variable is easily shown to be the difference in the means for complete and incomplete cases multiplied by the fraction of incomplete cases. Thus, the potential for bias increases with the fraction of missing data (*see* **Bias from Nonresponse**). In sample surveys this motivates strenuous attempts to limit unit nonresponse through multiple follow-ups, and surveys with high rates of unit nonresponse (say 30% or more) are often considered unreliable for making inferences to the whole population. For comparisons of means [69] and more generally regression analysis [59], the bias from CC analysis is often smaller. Specifically, it yields valid inferences in regression provided the model is correctly specified and missingness depends on the predictor variables, observed or missing, but not on the outcome.

When data are MAR but not MCAR, a useful modification of CC analysis is to assign a nonresponse weight to the respondents to remove or reduce nonresponse bias. In probability sampling, a sampling weight inversely proportional to the probability of selection is often used to adjust for differential selection probabilities. If nonresponse is viewed as another stage of probabilistic selection of units, then the product of the probability of selection by design and the probability of response given selection is the probability of being observed, and the inverse of this can be used as a weight in the analysis. Whereas sample design probabilities are known, nonresponse probabilities are unknown and need to be estimated from the data. A standard approach is to form adjustment cells (or subclasses) on the basis of background variables measured for respondents and nonrespondents; for unit nonresponse adjustment these are often based on geographical areas or groupings of similar areas based on aggregate socioeconomic data. All nonrespondents are given zero weight and the nonresponse weight for all respondents in an adjustment cell is then the inverse of the response rate in that cell. If more than one background variable is measured, then adjustment cells can be based on a joint classification, collapsing small cells as necessary. For a health survey application, see Ezzati & Khare [15]. This method removes the component of nonresponse bias attributable to differential nonresponse rates across the adjustment cells, and eliminates bias if within each adjustment cell respondents can be regarded as a random subsample of the original sample within that cell (i.e. the data are MAR given indicators for the adjustment cells).

A useful alternative approach with more extensive background information is *response propensity* **stratification**, where (i) the indicator for unit nonresponse is regressed on the background variables, using the combined data for respondents and nonrespondents and a method such as **logistic regression** appropriate for a binary outcome; (ii) a predicted response probability is computed for each respondent based on the regression in (i); and (iii) adjustment cells are formed on the basis of a categorized version of the predicted response probability. Theory [56, 90] suggests that this is an effective method for removing nonresponse bias attributable to the background variables. For a health survey application, see [30]. Robins et al. [89] and Robins & Rotnitsky [88] apply a similar weighting approach in the more general settings of generalized estimating equations for repeated measures analysis and multivariate regression.

Weighting methods can be useful for removing or reducing nonresponse bias, but they do have serious limitations. First, information in the incomplete cases is still discarded, so the method is inefficient. Weighted estimates can have unacceptably high variance, as when outlying values of a variable are given large weights. Secondly, variance estimation for weighted estimates with estimated weights is problematic. Explicit formulas are available for simple estimators such as means under simple random sampling [82], but methods are not well developed for more complex problems, and often ignore the component of variability from estimating the weight from the data. Bias and variance considerations aside, statisticians rightly resist attempts to analyze data selectively, and hence aim to analyze all the data to the extent possible; alternatives to CC analysis that incorporate the incomplete cases in a satisfactory way are recommended unless the fraction of incomplete cases is very small, say 10% or less.

Available-case (AC) analysis [65, section 3.3] is a straightforward attempt to exploit the incomplete information by using all the cases available to estimate each individual parameter. For example, suppose the objective is to estimate the correlation matrix of a set of continuous variables $Y_1, \ldots, Y_p$. Complete-case analysis uses the set of complete cases to estimate all the correlations; AC analysis uses all the cases with both Y_j and Y_k observed to estimate the correlation of Y_j and Y_k, $1 \le j, k \le p$. Since the sample base of available cases for measuring each correlation includes the set of complete cases, the AC method appears to make better use of available information. The sample base changes from correlation to correlation, however, creating potential problems when the missing data are not MCAR or variables are highly correlated. In the presence of high correlations, there is no guarantee that the AC correlation matrix is even positive definite. Haitovsky's [32] simulations concerning regression with highly-correlated continuous data found AC markedly inferior to CC. However, Kim & Curry [44] found AC superior to CC in simulations based on weakly correlated data. Simulation studies comparing AC regression estimates with ML under normality suggest that ML is superior even when underlying normality assumptions are violated [4, 58, 81]. Although AC estimates are easy to compute standard errors are more complex [109]. The method cannot be generally recommended.

Imputation

Methods that impute, or fill in, the missing values have the advantage that, unlike CC analysis, observed values in the incomplete cases are retained. A common naive approach imputes missing values by their simple unconditional sample means (i.e. marginal means). Wilks [111] and Afifi & Elashoff [1] discussed this method in bivariate settings. Unconditional mean imputation can yield satisfactory point estimates of some parameters such as unconditional means and totals, but it yields inconsistent estimates of other parameters, even if the data are MCAR. In particular, sample variances from the data

filled in by means clearly underestimate actual variances, since the imputed cases contribute zero to the sum of squared deviations from the sample mean. Unconditional mean imputation yields an inconsistent estimate of the covariance matrix and distorted estimates of association [65, Chapter 3]. Inferences (tests and confidence intervals) based on the filled-in data are seriously distorted by bias and overstated precision. Thus, unconditional mean imputation cannot be generally recommended.

An improvement over unconditional mean imputation is *conditional mean* imputation, in which each missing value is replaced by an estimate of its conditional mean given the values of the observed values. For example, in the case of univariate nonresponse with $Y_1, \ldots, Y_{p-1}$ fully observed and Y_p sometimes missing, one approach is to classify cases into cells on the basis of similar values of observed variables, and then to impute missing values of Y_p by the within-cell mean from the complete cases in that cell. A more general approach is regression imputation, in which the regression of Y_p on $Y_1, \ldots, Y_{p-1}$ is estimated from the complete cases, including **interactions** as needed, and the resulting prediction equation is used to impute the estimated conditional mean for each missing value of Y_p. For a general pattern of missing data, the missing values for each case can be imputed from the regression of the missing variables on the observed variables, computed using the set of complete cases. Iterative versions of this method lead (with some important adjustments) to ML estimates under multivariate normality [6, 84].

Although conditional mean imputation incorporates information from the observed variables and yields best predictions of the missing values in the sense of mean square error, imputations should be judged in terms of the quality of inferences about population parameters from the filled-in data. From this perspective, conditional mean imputation leads to distorted estimates of quantities that are not linear in the data, such as percentiles, correlations and other measures of association, and variances and other measures of variability. A solution to this problem is to use random draws rather than best predictions to preserve the distribution of variables in the filled-in data set. An example is *stochastic regression* imputation, in which each missing value is replaced by its regression prediction plus a **random error** with variance equal to the estimated residual variance.

In other approaches, imputations are drawn from the actual values in the data set. A common version of this method in longitudinal studies subject to attrition is to carry the last observation forward in time to fill out the dataset [87]. Clearly, this method is making a very strong assumption about missing data: that the missing values in a case are all identical to the last observed value. Even if we accept the notion that the average level of the variable does not change after drop-out, there is no fluctuation about that average. Little & Su [69] suggested better methods for longitudinal imputation based on simple row and column fits. Another method that imputes respondent values is the *hot deck*, as used by the Census Bureau for imputing income in the Current Population Survey (CPS) [33]. For each nonrespondent on one or more income items, the CPS hot deck finds a matching respondent on the basis of variables that are observed for both; the missing items for the nonrespondent are then replaced by the respondent's values. For matching purposes in the CPS, all variables are categorized, and the number of variables used to define matches is large. When no match can be found for a nonrespondent based on all of the variables, the CPS hot deck searches for a match at a lower level of detail, obtained by omitting some variables and collapsing the categories of others. David et al. [8] compared imputations from the CPS hot deck with imputations using a more parsimonious regression model for income.

A more general approach to hot deck imputation is to define a distance function on the basis of the variables that are observed for both nonrespondents and respondents. The missing values for each nonrespondent are then imputed from a respondent that is close to the nonrespondent in terms of the distance function. One such method is *predictive mean matching* [57, 95]. Consider, for simplicity, univariate nonresponse, and suppose that a model predicting Y_p from the other variables $Y_1, \ldots, Y_{p-1}$ has been estimated using the complete cases. For each nonrespondent, predictive mean matching finds a respondent whose predicted value of Y_p is close to the predicted value of the nonrespondent. The respondent's observed value of Y_p is then imputed to the nonrespondent. Lazzeroni et al. [51] showed in simulations that this method in somewhat robust to misspecification of the model used for matching.

The imputation methods discussed so far assume the missing data are MAR. In contrast, models that are not missing at random (NMAR) assert that even if

a respondent and nonrespondent to Y_p appear identical with respect to observed variables $Y_1, \ldots, Y_{p-1}$, their Y_p values differ systematically. Greenlees et al. [31] and Lillard et al. [54] discussed how imputations for missing CPS data can be based on NMAR models. It is also possible to create an NMAR hot deck procedure; for example, respondents' values that are to be imputed to nonrespondents could be multiplied by an inflation or deflation factor that depends on the variables that are observed. A crucial point about the use of NMAR models is that often there is no direct evidence in the data to address the validity of their underlying assumptions. Thus, whenever NMAR models are being considered it is prudent to consider several NMAR models and explore the sensitivity of analyses to the choice of model [94]. See Little & Wang [70] for an application of this idea to a longitudinal study of treatments of schizophrenia.

A serious defect with imputation is that it seems to be inventing data. More specifically, a single imputed value cannot represent all the uncertainty about which value to impute, so analyses that treat imputed values just like observed values generally underestimate uncertainty, even if nonresponse is modeled correctly and random imputations are created. Large-sample results [97] show that for simple situations with 30% of the data missing, single imputation under the correct model results in nominal 90% confidence intervals having actual coverages below 80%. The inaccuracy of nominal levels is even more extreme in multiparameter testing problems.

A modification of imputation that fixes this problem is multiple imputation (MI) [96, 98]. Instead of imputing a single set of draws for the missing values, a set of M (say $M = 5$) data sets are created, each containing different sets of draws of the missing values from their predictive distribution. We then apply the analysis to each of the M data sets and combine the results in a simple way. In particular for scalar estimands, the MI estimate is the average of the estimates from the M data sets, and the variance of the estimate is the average of the variances from the five data sets plus $1 + 1/M$ times the sample variance of the estimates over the M data sets (the factor $1 + 1/M$ is a small-M correction). The last quantity here estimates the contribution to the variance from imputation uncertainty, missed by single imputation methods. Another benefit of multiple imputation is that the averaging over data sets results in more efficient point estimates than does single random imputation. Often MI is not much more difficult than doing a single imputation – the additional computing from repeating an analysis M times is not a major burden and methods for combining inferences are straightforward. Most of the work is in generating good predictive distributions for the missing values.

ML for Ignorable Models

Complete-case analysis and imputation both result in rectangular data sets for analysis. But there are statistical methods that let us analyze a nonrectangular data set without having to impute the missing values. One such approach is the method of ML with associated large-sample standard errors based on the information matrix.

The ML approach avoids imputation by formulating a statistical model and basing inference on the likelihood function of the incomplete data. Define Y and M as above, and let $X = x_{ij}$ denote an $n \times q$ matrix of fixed covariates, assumed fully observed, with the ith row $x_i = x_{i1}, \ldots, x_{iq}$, where x_{ij} is the value of covariate X_j for subject i. Covariates that are not fully observed should be treated as random variables and modeled with the set of Y_js [64]. The data and missing-data mechanism are modeled in terms of a joint distribution for Y and M given X. *Selection models* specify this distribution as

$$f(Y, M|X, \theta, \Psi) = f(Y|X, \theta)f(M|Y, X, \Psi), \quad (1)$$

where $f(Y|X, \theta)$ is the model in the absence of missing values, $f(M|Y, X, \Psi)$ is the model for the missing-data mechanism, and θ and Ψ are unknown parameters. The likelihood of θ and Ψ given the data Y_{obs}, M, and X is then proportional to the density of Y_{obs} and M given X regarded as a function of the parameters θ and Ψ, and is obtained by integrating out the missing data Y_{mis} from (1), i.e.

$$L(\theta, \Psi|Y_{\mathrm{obs}}, M, X)$$
$$= \mathrm{const} \times \int f(Y, M|X, \theta, \Psi)\mathrm{d}Y_{\mathrm{mis}}. \quad (2)$$

The likelihood of θ *ignoring the missing-data mechanism* is obtained by integrating the missing data from the marginal distribution of Y given X, i.e.

$$L(\theta|Y_{\mathrm{obs}}, X) = \mathrm{const} \times \int f(Y|X, \theta)\mathrm{d}Y_{\mathrm{mis}}. \quad (3)$$

The likelihood (3) is easier to work with than (2) since it is computationally simpler and, more importantly, avoids the need to specify a model for the missing-data mechanism, about which little is known in many situations. Hence it is important to determine when valid likelihood inferences are obtained from (3) instead of the full likelihood (2). Rubin [93] showed that valid inferences about θ are obtained from (3) when the data are MAR, i.e.

$$p(M|X, Y, \Psi) = p(M|X, Y_{\mathrm{obs}}, \Psi),$$
$$\text{for all } Y_{\mathrm{mis}} \text{ and } \Psi.$$

If, in addition, θ and Ψ are distinct in the sense that they have disjoint sample spaces, then likelihood inferences about θ based on (3) are equivalent to inferences based on (2); the missing-data mechanism is then called *ignorable* for likelihood inferences. Large-sample inferences about θ for an ignorable model are based on ML theory, which states that under regularity conditions

$$\theta - \hat{\theta} \sim \mathrm{N}_k(0, C), \quad (4)$$

where $\hat{\theta}$ is the value of θ that maximizes (3), and $\mathrm{N}_k(0, C)$ is the k-variate normal distribution with mean zero and convariance matrix C given by the inverse of an information matrix; for example, $C = I^{-1}(\hat{\theta})$, where I is the observed information matrix $I(\theta) = -\partial^2 \log L(\theta|Y_{\mathrm{obs}}, X)/\partial\theta \partial\theta^{\mathrm{T}}$, or $C = J^{-1}(\hat{\theta})$, where $J(\theta)$ is the expected value of $I(\theta)$. As in [65], (4) is written to be open to a frequentist interpretation if $\hat{\theta}$ is regarded as random and θ fixed, or a Bayesian interpretation if θ is regarded as random and $\hat{\theta}$ fixed. Thus, if the data are MAR, the likelihood approach reduces to developing a suitable model for the data and computing $\hat{\theta}$ and C.

Likelihoods based on incomplete data often have complicated forms and require iterative maximization algorithms. In some situations the method of *factored likelihoods*, first described by Anderson [3], yields explicit ML estimates. The idea is to transform θ to $\phi(\theta) = [\phi_i(\theta), \ldots, \phi_Q(\theta)]$, where the components $\phi_1, \ldots, \phi_Q$ are distinct, and the likelihood of ϕ factors into the product $L(\phi|Y_{\mathrm{obs}}, X) = \prod_{q=1}^{Q} L_q(\phi_q|Y_{\mathrm{obs}}, X)$, where each factor $L_q(\phi_q|Y_{\mathrm{obs}}, X)$ corresponds to a complete-data problem or a simpler incomplete-data problem. The ML estimate $\hat{\phi} = (\hat{\phi}_1, \ldots, \hat{\phi}_Q)$ of ϕ is found by maximizing each factor $L_q(\phi_q|Y_{\mathrm{obs}}, X)$ separately, and the ML estimate of θ is then $\hat{\theta} = \theta(\hat{\phi})$, where $\theta(\phi)$ is the inverse transformation from ϕ to θ. Consider, for example, bivariate normal data:

$$\begin{pmatrix} y_{i1} \\ y_{i2} \end{pmatrix} \sim_{\text{ind}} N_2 \left(\begin{pmatrix} \mu_1 \\ \mu_2 \end{pmatrix}, \begin{pmatrix} \sigma_{11} & \sigma_{12} \\ \sigma_{12} & \sigma_{22} \end{pmatrix} \right),$$

and a monotone pattern with m complete cases $\{(y_{i1}, y_{i2}) : i = 1, \ldots, m\}$ and $n - m$ incomplete cases $\{y_{i1} : i = m + 1, \ldots, n\}$ with Y_2 missing. Let $\theta = (\mu_1, \sigma_{11}, \mu_2, \sigma_{22}, \sigma_{12})$ and $\phi = (\phi_1, \phi_2)$, where $\phi_1 = (\mu_1, \sigma_{11})$, $\phi_2 = (\beta_{20.1}, \beta_{21.1}, \sigma_{22.1})$, and $\beta_{21.1} = \sigma_{12}/\sigma_{11}$, $\beta_{20.1} = \mu_2 - \beta_{21.1}\mu_1$, $\sigma_{22.1} = \sigma_{22} - \sigma_{12}^2/\sigma_{11}$ are, respectively, the slope, intercept, and residual variance of the regression of Y_2 on Y_1. The ignorable model likelihood of ϕ based on Y_{obs} then factorizes into the complete-data likelihood of ϕ_1 based on the n observations $\{y_{i1} : i = 1, \ldots, n\}$ and the complete-data likelihood of ϕ_2 for the regression of Y_2 on Y_1 based on the m complete cases $\{(y_{i1}, y_{i2}) : i = 1, \ldots, m\}$. Explicit expressions for the ML estimates of ϕ and hence θ are readily obtained. In particular:

$$\begin{aligned} \hat{\mu}_2 &= \hat{\beta}_{20.1} + \hat{\beta}_{21.1}\hat{\mu}_1 = \bar{y}_2 - b_{21}\bar{y}_1 + b_{21}\hat{\mu}_1 \\ &= \bar{y}_2 + b_{21}(\hat{\mu}_1 - \bar{y}_1), \end{aligned}$$

where $\bar{y}_1$, $\bar{y}_2$ and b_{21} are the sample means of Y_1 and Y_2 and least squares slope of Y_2 on Y_1 based on the m complete cases and $\hat{\mu}_1$ is the sample mean of Y_1 based on all n cases. This is known as the regression estimate of the mean of Y_2, and is a well-known estimator from double sampling in sample surveys. It is also the average of observed and imputed values from regression imputation, discussed before. For further details on this example, and applications to multivariate normal and multinomial data with a monotone missing data pattern, see [91] or [65, Chapter 6].

The factored likelihood method does not work in the above problem if incomplete cases on Y_2 are also available. Here, and in many other problems, maximization of the likelihood requires numerical methods. Standard optimization methods such as Newton–Raphson or Scoring can be applied; for example, Hartley & Hocking [34] applied a scoring algorithm to multivariate normal data with missing values, and Jennrich & Schluchter [42] applied modified scoring to unbalanced repeated-measures data. Alternatively, the expectation-maximization (EM) algorithm [10] can be applied, a general algorithm for incomplete

data problems that provides an interesting link with imputation methods. The history of EM, which dates back at least to McKendrick [73] for particular problems, is sketched in [65]. For more recent work on extensions, see [77].

For ignorable models, let $L(\theta | Y_{\text{obs}}, Y_{\text{mis}}, X)$ denote the likelihood of θ based on the hypothetical complete data $Y = (Y_{\text{obs}}, Y_{\text{mis}})$ and covariates X. Let $\theta^{(t)}$ denote an estimate of θ at iteration t of EM. Iteration $t + 1$ consists of an E-step and an M-step. The E-step consists of taking the expectation of log $L(\theta | Y_{\text{obs}}, Y_{\text{mis}}, X)$ over the conditional distribution of Y_{mis} given Y_{obs} and X, evaluated at $\theta = \theta^{(t)}$. That is, the expected log likelihood $Q(\theta | \theta^{(t)}) = \int \log L(\theta | Y_{\text{obs}}, Y_{\text{mis}}, X) f(Y_{\text{mis}} | Y_{\text{obs}}, X, \theta^{(t)}) dY_{\text{mis}}$. is formed. When the complete data belong to an exponential family with complete-data sufficient statistics S, the E-step simplifies to computing expected values of these statistics given the observed data and $\theta = \theta^{(t)}$, thus in a sense "imputing" the sufficient statistics [105].

The M-step determines $\theta^{(t+1)}$ to maximize $Q(\theta | \theta^{(1)})$ with respect to θ. In exponential family cases this step is the same as for complete data, except that the complete-data sufficient statistics S are replaced by their estimates from the E-step. Thus, the M-step is often easy or available with existing software, and the programming work is mainly confined to E-step computations. Under very general conditions, each iteration of EM increases the log likelihood, and under more restrictive but still general conditions EM converges to a maximum of the likelihood function [112]. If a unique finite ML estimate of θ exists, then EM will find it.

Little & Rubin [65] provided many applications of EM to particular models, including: (i) multivariate normal data with a general pattern of missing values and the related problem of multivariate linear regression with missing data [6, 84]; (ii) robust inference based on multivariate t models [50, 58]; (iii) loglinear models for multiway contingency tables with missing data [21]; and (iv) the general location model for mixtures of continuous and categorical variables [68, 83], which yields ML algorithms for logistic regression with missing covariates [108]. Schluchter & Jackson [102] provided an EM algorithm for **survival analysis** with missing covariates. An extensive bibliography of the myriad of EM applications is given in [74].

The EM algorithm is reliable, but has a linear convergence rate determined by the fraction of missing information, as defined in [10]. When the fraction of missing information is large, convergence can be painfully slow. Meng & Van Dyk [77] showed how the clear choice of the missing data can be used to speed convergence. There is an extensive literature on extensions and enhancements of EM for cases where the E- or M-step is hard or slow [17, 18, 41, 47, 48, 71, 76, 77]. EM does not involve computation and inversion of an information matrix based on the observed data. This makes the algorithm particularly attractive in problems where the number of parameters is large, as in ML algorithms for biomedical imaging, such as positron emission tomography [17, 18, 49, 103]. This feature of EM has the disadvantage that asymptotic standard errors based on the inverse of the information matrix are not an output. An information matrix can be computed and inverted separately. Alternative approaches to computing standard errors are to use the formulas in [72], to build an information matrix from supplemental EM steps [75], to use bootstrap methods [14, 58], or to switch to a Bayesian simulation method that simulates the posterior distribution of θ (see below).

ML for Nonignorable Models

Ignorable ML is appropriate when the data are MAR. Nonignorable, non-MAR models apply when missingness depends on the missing values. For example, if a subject dropped out of the longitudinal study when his/her blood pressure got too high and we did not observe that blood pressure, or if in an analgesic study measuring pain, the subject dropped out when the pain was high and we did not observe that pain value, missingness depends on the missing value. A correct likelihood analysis must be based on the full likelihood from a model for the joint distribution of Y and M. The standard likelihood asymptotics apply to nonignorable models provided the parameters are identified, and computational tools such as EM also apply to this more general class of models. However, often information to estimate simultaneously the parameters of the missing-data mechanism and the parameters of the complete-data model is limited, and estimates are sensitive to misspecification of the model. Often a sensitivity analysis is needed to see

how much the answers change for various assumptions about the missing-data mechanism.

There are two broad classes of models for the joint distribution of Y and M. *Selection* models model the joint distribution as in (1). *Pattern-mixture* models specify

$$f(Y, M|X, \pi, \phi) = f(Y|X, M, \phi)f(M|X, \pi), \quad (5)$$

where ϕ and π are unknown parameters and now the distribution of Y is conditioned on the missing-data pattern M [29, 60, 65, 94]. Eqs (1) and (5) are simply two different ways of factoring the joint distribution of Y and M. When M is independent of Y the two specifications are equivalent with $\theta = \phi$ and $\psi = \pi$. Otherwise (1) and (5) generally yield different models.

Most of the literature on missing data has concerned selection models of the form (1) for univariate nonresponse. Examples are the probit selection model [2, 36], and the closely related logit model of Greenlees et al. [31], extended to repeated-measures data in [11]. The sensitivity of answers to model misspecification is discussed in [29; 55; 65, Chapter 11; 104] and the discussion in [11]. Nonignorable models for contingency tables are discussed in [5; 16; 65, Chapter 9; 86].

Pattern-mixture models seem more natural when missingness defines a distinct stratum of the population of intrinsic interest, such as individuals reporting "don't know" in an opinion survey. However, pattern-mixture models can also provide inferences for parameters θ of the complete-data distribution by expressing the parameters of interest as functions of the pattern-mixture model parameters ϕ and π. An advantage of the pattern-mixture modeling approach over selection models is that assumptions about the form of the missing-data mechanism are sometimes less specific in their parametric form, since they are incorporated in the model via parameter restrictions. This idea is explained in specific normal models in [61] and [70].

Heitjan & Rubin [40] and Heitjan [39] extended the formation of missing-data problems via the joint distribution of Y and M to more general incomplete data problems involving coarsened data. The idea is to replace the binary missing-data indicators $M = \{m_{ij}\}$ by random coarsening variables $G = \{g_{ij}\}$, which map the y_{ij} values to coarsened versions $z_{ij}(y_{ij})$. Particular values of g_{ij} could map y_{ij} to "completely observed" and "completely missing", as with m_{ij} above, but other values of g_{ij} might map y_{ij} into other sets, for example a finite interval would correspond to interval censoring. The data are then defined as *coarsened completely at random* or *coarsened at random* depending on whether the distribution of G is independent of Y, or depends on Y only through observed data. Full and ignorable likelihoods can be defined for this more general setting. This theory provides a bridge between missing-data theory and theories of censoring in the survival analysis literature. For biomedical applications, see [38].

Bayesian Simulation Methods

Maximum likelihood is most useful when sample sizes are large, since then the log likelihood is nearly quadratic and can be summarized well using the ML estimate θ and its large sample variance–covariance matrix. When sample sizes are small, a useful alternative approach is to add a prior distribution for the parameters and compute the posterior distribution of the parameters of interest. For ignorable models this posterior is

$$p(\theta|Y_{\text{obs}}, M, X) \equiv p(\theta|Y_{\text{obs}}, X) = \text{const}\, p(\theta|X)$$
$$\times f(Y_{\text{obs}}|X, \theta),$$

where $p(\theta|X)$ is the prior and $f(Y_{\text{obs}}|X, \theta)$ is the density of the observed data. Since the posterior distribution rarely has a simple analytic form for incomplete-data problems, simulation methods are often used to generate draws of θ from the posterior distribution $p(\theta|Y_{\text{obs}}, M, X)$. I outline two of these simulation methods for the ignorable case, although the techniques can also be applied to nonignorable models.

For missing data problems where the likelihood can be factored into complete-data components, $L(\phi|Y_{\text{obs}}, X) = \prod_{q=1}^{Q} L_q(\phi_q|Y_{\text{obs}}, X)$ and the parameters $\phi_1, \ldots, \phi_Q$ are also a priori independent, the posteriors of $\phi_1, \ldots, \phi_Q$ are also independent, and draws $\phi^{(d)} = (\phi_1^{(d)}, \ldots, \phi_Q^{(d)})$ can be obtained directly from the complete-data posterior distributions. Draws of θ are then obtained as $\theta^{(d)} = \theta(\phi^{(d)})$, where $\theta(\phi)$ is the inverse transformation from ϕ to θ. This method is analogous to the factored likelihood method for ML estimation described above. For an application to normal data see [65, Chapter 6].

Data augmentation [107] is an iterative method for simulating the posterior distribution of θ that combines features of the EM algorithm and multiple imputation, with M imputations of each missing value at each iteration. It can be thought of as a small-sample refinement of the EM algorithm using simulation, with the imputation step corresponding to the E-step and the posterior step corresponding to the M-step. An important special case of data augmentation arises when M is set equal to one, yielding the following special case of the Gibbs' sampler [22, 25]. Start with an initial draw $\theta^{(0)}$ from an approximation to the posterior distribution of θ. Given a value $\theta^{(t)}$ of θ drawn at iteration t:

1. draw $Y_{\text{mis}}^{(t+1)}$ with density $p(Y_{\text{mis}}|Y_{\text{obs}}, X, \theta^{(t)})$;
2. draw $\theta^{(t+1)}$ with density $p(\theta|Y_{\text{obs}}, Y_{\text{mis}}^{(t+1)}, X)$.

The procedure is motivated by the fact that the distributions in 1 and 2 are often much easier to draw from than the correct posterior distributions, $p(Y_{\text{mis}}|Y_{\text{obs}}, X)$ and $p(\theta|Y_{\text{obs}}, X)$. The iterative procedure can be shown in the limit to yield a draw from the joint posterior distribution of Y_{mis} and θ given Y_{obs} and X. The algorithm was termed *chained data augmentation* in [106]. This algorithm can be run independently K times to generate K iid draws from the approximate joint posterior distribution of θ and Y_{mis}. A number of articles [23, 24, 26, 107] have discussed techniques for monitoring the convergence of the algorithms. Schafer [100] developed algorithms that use iterative Bayesian simulation to multiply impute rectangular data sets with arbitrary patterns of missing values when the missing-data mechanism is ignorable. The methods are applicable when the rows of the complete-data matrix can be modeled as iid observations from the multivariate normal, multinomial loglinear, and general location models.

Methods for Unbalanced Repeated-Measures Data

I conclude by reviewing methods for longitudinal data with unequal numbers of measurements between subjects. For normal outcomes and ignorable missing data, a wide range of problems can be tackled using the random-effects model:

$$(y_i|X_i, \beta_i) \sim_{\text{iid}} N_k(X_{1i}\alpha + X_{2i}\beta_i, \Sigma),$$
$$\beta_i|X_i \sim_{\text{iid}} N_q(0, \Gamma),$$

where $N_p(\alpha, B)$ denotes the p-variate normal distribution with mean α covariance matrix B; X_{1i} is a known $(K \times p)$ design matrix containing fixed within-subject and between-subject covariates, with associated unknown $(p \times 1)$ parameter vector α; β_i is an unknown $(q \times 1)$ random-coefficient vector; and X_{2i} is a known $(K \times q)$ matrix for modeling the random effects. Estimation for this model is discussed in [35, 42, 46], and ML estimation is currently available in SAS PROC MIXED [99], or the Biomedical Data Processing (BMDP) program BMDP5V [12] (*see* **Software, Biostatistical**). For Bayesian inference using the Gibbs' sampler, see [28].

For longitudinal categoric data with unequal numbers of measurements, standard loglinear models are unsatisfactory because of the conditional interpretation of the parameters. ML methods have been proposed on the basis of marginal multinomial models [43, 115]. An alternative approach is to assume categoric outcomes are indicators for underlying continuous outcomes that follow a normal model [27, 37]. Nonlikelihood approaches include the weighted least squares methods [45], and iterative methods based on generalized estimating equations [20, 52, 53, 85, 89]. Another approach is analysis by summary measures, in which we obtain a summary measure for each individual and then analyze it across the subjects.

A variety of nonignorable pattern-mixture and selection models for dropouts in longitudinal data have been proposed, including models for informative dropout where dropout depends on underlying unobserved slopes characterizing a patient's decline [9, 62, 79, 101, 110, 113, 114]. An advantage of pattern-mixture models in this setting is that this part of the model can usually be fit using standard software such as PROC MIXED [99] by simply including the dropout indicator as a covariate in the model for the distribution of the y_is. Nonignorable models for repeated-measures categorical data are considered in [7] and [78].

Acknowledgments

This research was supported by National Science Foundation Grant DMS 9408837. Donald Rubin and Nathaniel Schenker's important influences on this review are gratefully acknowledged.

References

[1] Afifi, A.A. & Elashoff, R.M. (1967). Missing observations in multivariate statistics II: point estimation in simple linear regression, *Journal of the American Statistical Association* **62**, 595–604.

[2] Amemiya, T. (1984). Tobit models: a survey, *Journal of Econometrics* **24**, 3–61.

[3] Anderson, T.W. (1957). Maximum likelihood estimation for the multivariate normal distribution when some observations are missing, *Journal of the American Statistical Association* **52**, 200–203.

[4] Azen, S.P., Van Guilder, M. & Hill, M.A. (1989). Estimation of parameters and missing values under a regression model with non-normally distributed and non-randomly incomplete data, *Statistics in Medicine* **8**, 217–228.

[5] Baker, S.G. & Laird, N.M. (1988). Regression analysis for categorical variables with outcome subject to nonresponse, *Journal of the American Statistical Association* **83**, 62–69.

[6] Beale, E.M.L. & Little, R.J.A. (1975). Missing values in multivariate analysis, *Journal of the Royal Statistical Society, Series B* **37**, 129–145.

[7] Conaway, M.R. (1992). The analysis of repeated categorical measurements subject to nonignorable nonresponse, *Journal of the American Statistical Association* **87**, 817–824.

[8] David, M.H., Little, R.J.A., Samuhel, M.E. & Triest, R.K. (1986). Alternative methods for CPS income imputation, *Journal of the American Statistical Association* **81**, 29–41.

[9] DeGruttola, V. & Tu, X.M. (1994). Modeling progression of CD4-lymphocyte count and its relationship to survival time, *Biometrics* **50**, 1003–1014.

[10] Dempster, A.P., Laird, N.M. & Rubin, D.B. (1977). Maximum likelihood from incomplete data via the EM algorithm (with discussion), *Journal of the Royal Statistical Society, Series B* **39**, 1–38.

[11] Diggle, P. & Kenward, M.G. (1994). Informative dropout in longitudinal data analysis (with discussion), *Applied Statistics* **43**, 49–94.

[12] Dixon, W.J. (1988). *BMDP Statistical Software*. University of California Press, Berkeley.

[13] Dorey, F.J., Little, R.J.A. & Schenker, N. (1993). Multiple imputation for threshold-crossing data with interval censoring, *Statistics in Medicine* **12**, 1589–1603.

[14] Efron, B. (1994). Missing data, imputation and the bootstrap, *Journal of the American Statistical Association* **89**, 463–479.

[15] Ezzati, T. & Khare, M. (1992). Nonresponse adjustments in a National Health Survey, in *American Statistical Association 1992 Proceedings of the Section on Survey Research Methods*. American Statistical Association, Alexandria, pp. 339–344.

[16] Fay, R.E. (1986). Causal models for patterns of nonresponse, *Journal of the American Statistical Association* **81**, 354–365.

[17] Fessler, J.A. & Hero, A.O. (1994). Space-alternating generalized expectation–maximization algorithm, *IEEE Transactions on Signal Processing* **42**, 2664–2677.

[18] Fessler, J.A. & Hero, A.O. (1995). Penalized maximum-likelihood image reconstruction using space-alternating generalized expectation-maximization algorithm, *IEEE Transactions on Image Processing* **4**, 1417–1438.

[19] Finkelstein, D.M. & Wolfe, R.A. (1985). A semiparametric model for regression analysis of interval-censored failure time data, *Biometrics* **41**, 933–945.

[20] Fitzmaurice, G.M., Laird, N.M. & Rotnitzky, A.G. (1993). Regression models for discrete longitudinal responses, *Statistical Science* **8**, 284–309.

[21] Fuchs, C. (1982). Maximum likelihood estimation and model selection in contingency tables with missing data, *Journal of the American Statistical Association* **77**, 270–278.

[22] Gelfand, A.E. & Smith, A.F.M. (1990). Sampling-based approaches to calculating marginal densities, *Journal of the American Statistical Association* **85**, 398–409.

[23] Gelfand, A.E., Hills, S.E., Racine-Poon, A. & Smith, A.F.M. (1990). Illustration of Bayesian inference in normal data models using Gibbs sampling, *Journal of the American Statistical Association* **85**, 972–985.

[24] Gelman, A. & Rubin, D.B. (1992). Honest inferences from iterative simulation (with discussion), *Statistical Science* **4**, 457–511.

[25] Geman, S. & Geman, D. (1984). Stochastic relaxation, Gibbs' distributions and the Bayesian restoration of images, *IEEE Transactions on Pattern Analysis and Machine Intelligence* **6**, 721–741.

[26] Geyer, C.J. (1992). Practical Markov chain Monte Carlo (with discussion), *Statistical Science* **4**, 473–511.

[27] Gibbons, R.D. & Bock, R.D. (1987). Trend in correlated proportions, *Psychometrika* **52**, 113–124.

[28] Gilks, W.R., Wang, C.C., Yvonnet, B. & Coursaget, P. (1993). Random-effects models for longitudinal data using Gibbs' sampling, *Biometrics* **49**, 441–453.

[29] Glynn, R., Laird, N.M. & Rubin, D.B. (1986). Selection modeling versus mixture modeling with non-ignorable nonresponse, in *Drawing Inferences from Self-Selected Samples*, H. Wainer, ed. Springer-Verlag, New York, pp. 119–146.

[30] Goksel, H., Judkins, D.R. & Mosher, W.D. (1991). Nonresponse adjustments for a telephone follow-up to a national in-person survey, in *American Statistical Association 1991 Proceedings of the Section on Survey Reasearch Methods*. American Statistical Association, Alexandria, pp. 581–586.

[31] Greenlees, W.S., Reece, J.S. & Zieschang, K.D. (1982). Imputation of missing values when the probability of nonresponse depends on the variable being imputed, *Journal of the American Statistical Association* **77**, 251–261.

[32] Haitovsky, Y. (1968). Missing data in regression analysis, *Journal of the Royal Statistical Society, Series B* **30**, 67–81.

[33] Hanson, R.H. (1978). The current population survey: design and methodology, *Technical Paper*, No. 40, US Bureau of the Census, Washington.

[34] Hartley, H.O. & Hocking, R.R. (1971). The analysis of incomplete data, *Biometrics* **14**, 174–194.

[35] Harville, D.A. (1977). Maximum likelihood approaches to variance component estimation and to related problems (with discussion), *Journal of the American Statistical Association* **72**, 320–340.

[36] Heckman, J. (1976). The common structure of statistical models of truncation, sample selection and limited dependent variables, and a simple estimator for such models, *Annals of Economic and Social Measurement* **5**, 475–492.

[37] Hedeker, D. (1993). *MIXOR: A Fortran Program for Mixed-Effects Ordinal Probit and Logistic Regression*. Prevention Research Center, University of Illinois at Chicago, Chicago.

[38] Heitjan, D.F. (1993). Ignorability and coarse data: some biomedical examples, *Biometrics* **49**, 1099–1109.

[39] Heitjan, D.F. (1993). Ignorability in general complete-data models, *Biometrika* **81**, 701–708.

[40] Heitjan, D. & Rubin (1991). Ignorability and coarse data, *Annals of Statistics* **19**, 2244–2253.

[41] Jamshidian, M. & Jennrich, R.I. (1993). Conjugate gradient acceleration of the EM algorithm, *Journal of the American Statistical Association* **88**, 221–228.

[42] Jennrich, R.I. & Schluchter, M.D. (1986). Unbalanced repeated-measures models with structured covariance matrices, *Biometrics* **42**, 805–820.

[43] Kenward, M.G., Lesaffre, E. & Molenberghs, G. (1994). An application of maximum likelihood and estimating equations to the analysis of ordinal data from a longitudinal study with cases missing at random, *Biometrics* **50**, 945–953.

[44] Kim, J.O. & Curry, J. (1977). The treatment of missing data in multivariate analysis, *Sociological Methods and Research* **6**, 215–240.

[45] Koch, G.G., Landis, J.R., Freeman, J.L., Freeman, D.H. & Lehnen, R.G. (1977). A general methodology for the analysis of experiments with repeated measurement of categorical data, *Biometrics* **33**, 133–158.

[46] Laird, N.M. & Ware, J.H. (1982). Random-effects models for longitudinal data, *Biometrics* **38**, 963–974.

[47] Lange, K. (1995). A gradient algorithm locally equivalent to the EM algorithm, *Journal of the Royal Statistical Society, Series B* **57**, 425–437.

[48] Lange, K. (1995). A quasi-Newtonian acceleration of the EM algorithm, *Statistica Sinica* **5**, 1–18.

[49] Lange, F. & Carson, R. (1984). EM reconstruction algorithms for emission and transmission tomography, *Journal of Computer-Assisted Tomography* **8**, 306–316.

[50] Lange, K., Little, R.J.A. & Taylor, J. (1989). Robust statistical inference using the *T* distribution, *Journal of the American Statistical Association* **84**, 881–896.

[51] Lazzeroni, L.C., Schenker, N. & Taylor, J.M.G. (1990). Robustness of multiple imputation techniques to model specification, in *American Statistical Association 1990 Proceedings of the Section on Survey Reasearch Methods*. American Statistical Association, Alexandria, pp. 260–265.

[52] Liang, K-Y. & Zeger, S.L. (1986). Longitudinal data analysis using generalized linear models, *Biometrika* **73**, 13–22.

[53] Liang, K-Y., Zeger, S.L. & Qaqish, B. (1992). Multivariate regression analyses for categorical data (with discussion), *Journal of the Royal Statistical Society, Series B* **54**, 3–40.

[54] Lillard, L., Smith, J.P. & Welch, F. (1986). What do we really know about wages: the importance of nonreporting and census imputation, *Journal of Political Economy* **94**, 489–506.

[55] Little, R.J.A. (1985). A note about models for selectivity bias, *Econometrica* **53**, 1469–1474.

[56] Little, R.J.A. (1986). Survey nonresponse adjustments, *International Statistical Review* **54**, 139–157.

[57] Little, R.J.A. (1988). Missing data adjustments in large surveys, *Journal of Business and Economic Statistics* **6**, 287–301.

[58] Little, R.J.A. (1988). Robust estimation of the mean and covariance matrix from data with missing values, *Applied Statistics* **37**, 23–38.

[59] Little, R.J.A. (1992). Regression with incomplete X's; a review, *Journal of the American Statistical Association* **87**, 1227–1237.

[60] Little, R.J.A. (1993). Pattern-mixture models for multivariate incomplete data, *Journal of the American Statistical Association* **88**, 125–134.

[61] Little, R.J.A. (1994). A class of pattern-mixture models for normal missing data, *Biometrika* **81**, 471–483.

[62] Little, R.J.A. (1995). Modeling the drop-out mechanism in longitudinal studies, *Journal of the American Statistical Association* **90**, 1112–1121.

[63] Little, R.J.A. & Rubin, D.B. (1983). Incomplete data, in *Encyclopedia of the Statistical Sciences*, Vol. 4, S. Kotz & N.L. Johnson, eds. Wiley, New York, pp. 46–53.

[64] Little, R.J.A. & Rubin, D.B. (1983). On jointly estimating parameters and missing data by maximizing the complete data likelihood, *American Statistician* **37**, 218–220.

[65] Little, R.J.A. & Rubin, D.B. (1987). *Statistical Analysis with Missing Data*. Wiley, New York.

[66] Little, R.J.A. & Rubin, D.B. (1989). Missing data in social science data sets, *Sociological Methods and Research* **18**, 292–326.

[67] Little, R.J.A. & Schenker, N. (1994). Missing data, in *Handbook for Statistical Modeling in the Social and Behavioral Sciences*, G. Arminger, C.C. Clogg & M.E. Sobel, eds. Plenum Press, New York, pp. 39–75.

[68] Little, R.J.A. & Schluchter, M.D. (1985). Maximum likelihood estimation for mixed continuous and categorical data with missing values, *Biometrika* **72**, 497–512.

[69] Little, R.J.A. & Su, H.L. (1989). Item nonresponse in panel surveys, in *Panel Surveys*, D. Kasprzyk, G. Duncan, G. Kalton & M.P. Singh, eds. Wiley, New York, pp. 400–425.

[70] Little, R.J.A. & Wang, Y.-X. (1996). Pattern-mixture models for multivariate incomplete data with covariates, *Biometrics* **52**, 98–111.

[71] Liu, C. & Rubin, D.B. (1994). The ECME algorithm: a simple extension of EM and ECM with fast monotone convergence, *Biometrika* **81**, 633–648.

[72] Louis, T.A. (1982). Finding the observed information matrix using the EM algorithm, *Journal of the Royal Statistical Society, Series B* **44**, 226–233.

[73] McKendrick, A.G. (1926). Applications of mathematics to medical problems, *Proceedings of the Edinburgh Mathematics Society* **44**, 98–130.

[74] Meng, X.L. & Pedlow, S. (1992). EM: a bibliographic review with missing articles, in *American Statistical Association 1992 Proceedings of the Section on Computing*. American Statistical Association, Alexandria, pp. 24–27.

[75] Meng, X.L. & Rubin, D.B. (1991). Using EM to obtain asymptotic variance–covariance matrices: the SEM algorithm, *Journal of the American Statistical Association* **86**, 899–909.

[76] Meng, X.L. & Rubin, D.B. (1993). Maximum likelihood estimation via the ECM algorithm: a general framework, *Biometrika* **80**, 267–278.

[77] Meng, X.L. & Van Dyk (1997). The EM algorithm – an old folk song sung to a fast new tune (with discussion), *Journal of the Royal Statistical Society, Series B* **59**, 511–567.

[78] Molenberghs, G., Kenward, M.G. & Lesaffre, E. (1997). The analysis of longitudinal ordinal data with informative dropout, *Biometrika* **84**, 33–44.

[79] Mori, M., Woolson, R.F. & Woodsworth, G.G. (1994). Slope estimation in the presence of informative censoring: modeling the number of observations as a geometric random variable, *Biometrics* **50**, 39–50.

[80] Murray, G.D. & Findlay, J.G. (1988). Correcting for the bias caused by drop-outs in hypertension trials, *Statistics in Medicine* **7**, 941–946.

[81] Muthen, B., Kaplan, D. & Hollis, M. (1987). On structural equation modeling with data that are not missing completely at random, *Psychometrika* **52**, 431–462.

[82] Oh, H.L. & Scheuren, F.S. (1983). Weighting adjustments for unit nonresponse, in *Incomplete Data in Sample Surveys*, Vol. 2: *Theory and Bibliographies*, W.G. Madow, I. Olkin & D.B. Rubin, eds. Academic Press, New York, pp. 143–184.

[83] Olkin, I. & Tate, R.F. (1961). Multivariate correlation models with mixed discrete and continuous variables, *Annals of Mathematical Statistics* **32**, 448–465.

[84] Orchard, T. & Woodbury, M.A. (1972). A missing information principle: theory and applications, in *Proceedings of the Sixth Berkeley Symposium on Mathematical Statistics and Probability*, Vol. 1, University of California Press, Berkeley, pp. 697–715.

[85] Park, T. (1993). A comparison of the generalized estimating equation approach with the maximum likelihood approach for repeated measurements, *Statistics in Medicine* **12**, 1723–1732.

[86] Park, T. & Brown, M.B. (1994). Models for categorical data with nonignorable nonresponse, *Journal of the American Statistical Association* **89**, 44–52.

[87]   Pocock, S.J. (1983). *Clinical Trials: A Practical Approach*. Wiley, New York.

[88]   Robins, J. & Rotnitsky, A. (1995). Semiparametric efficiency in multivariate regression models with missing data, *Journal of the American Statistical Association* **90**, 122–129.

[89]   Robins, J., Rotnitsky, A. & Zhao, L.P. (1995). Analysis of semiparametric regression models for repeated outcomes in the presence of missing data, *Journal of the American Statistical Association* **90**, 106–121.

[90]   Rosenbaum, P.R. & Rubin, D.B. (1983). The central role of the propensity score in observational studies for causal effects, *Biometrika* **70**, 41–55.

[91]   Rubin, D.B. (1974). Characterizing the estimation of parameters in incomplete data problems, *Journal of the American Statistical Association* **69**, 467–474.

[92]   Rubin, D.B. (1976). Comparing regressions when some predictor values are missing, *Technometrics* **18**, 201–205.

[93]   Rubin, D.B. (1976). Inference and missing data, *Biometrika* **63**, 581–592.

[94]   Rubin, D.B. (1977). Formalizing subjective notions about the effect of nonrespondents in sample surveys, *Journal of the American Statistical Association* **72**, 538–543.

[95]   Rubin, D.B. (1986). Statistical matching and file concatenation with adjusted weights and multiple imputations, *Journal of Business and Economic Statistics* **4**, 87–94.

[96]   Rubin, D.B. (1987). *Multiple Imputation for Nonresponse in Surveys*. Wiley, New York.

[97]   Rubin, D.B. & Schenker, N. (1986). Multiple imputation for interval estimation from simple random samples with ignorable nonresponse, *Journal of the American Statistical Association* **81**, 366–374.

[98]   Rubin, D.B. & Schenker, N. (1991). Multiple imputation in health-care databases: an overview and some applications, *Statistics in Medicine* **10**, 585–598.

[99]   SAS (1992). The mixed procedure, in *SAS/STAT Software: Changes and Enhancements*, Release 6.07, Technical Report P-229. SAS Institute, Inc., Cary.

[100] Schafer, J.L. (1996). *Analysis of Incomplete Multivariate Data*. Chapman & Hall, London.

[101] Schluchter, M.D. (1992). Methods for the analysis of informatively censored longitudinal data, *Statistics in Medicine* **11**, 1861–1870.

[102] Schluchter, M.D. & Jackson, K.L. (1989). Loglinear analysis of censored survival data with partially observed covariates, *Journal of the American Statistical Association* **84**, 42–52.

[103] Shepp, L.A. & Vardi, Y. (1982). Maximum likelihood reconstruction for emission tomography, *IEEE Transactions on Image Processing* **2**, 113–122.

[104] Stolzenberg, R.M. & Relles, D.A. (1990). Theory testing in a world of constrained research design – the significance of Heckman's censored sampling bias correction for nonexperimental research, *Sociological Methods and Research* **18**, 395–415.

[105] Sundberg, R. (1974). Maximum likelihood theory for incomplete data from an exponential family, *Scandinavian Journal of Statistics* **1**, 49–58.

[106] Tanner, M.A. (1991). *Tools for Statistical Inference: Observed Data and Data Augmentation Methods*. Springer-Verlag, New York.

[107] Tanner, M.A. & Wong, W.H. (1987). The calculation of posterior distributions by data augmentation, *Journal of the American Statistical Association* **82**, 528–550.

[108] Vach, W. (1994). *Logistic Regression with Missing Values in the Covariates*. Springer-Verlag, New York.

[109] Van Praag, B.M.S., Dijkstra, T.K. & Van Velzen, J. (1985). Least-squares theory based on general distributional assumptions with an application to the incomplete observations problem, *Psychometrika* **50**, 25–36.

[110] Wang-Clow, F., Lange, M., Laird, N.M. & Ware, J.H. (1995). Simulation study of estimators for rate of change in longitudinal studies with attrition, *Statistics in Medicine* **14**, 283–297.

[111] Wilks, S.S. (1932). Moments and distribution of estimates of population parameters from fragmentary samples, *Annals of Mathematical Statistics* **3**, 163–195.

[112] Wu, C.F.J. (1983). On the convergence properties of the EM algorithm, *Annals of Statistics* **11**, 95–103.

[113] Wu, M.C. & Bailey, K.R. (1989). Estimation and comparison of changes in the presence of informative right censoring: conditional linear model, *Biometrics* **45**, 939–955.

[114] Wu, M.C. & Carroll, R.J. (1988). Estimation and comparison of changes in the presence of informative right censoring by modeling the censoring process, *Biometrics* **44**, 175–188.

[115] Zhao, L.P. & Prentice, R.L. (1990). Correlated binary regression using a quadratic exponential model, *Biometrika* **77**, 642–648.

(*See also* **Missing Data in Epidemiologic Studies**)

RODERICK J. LITTLE

Missing Data in Epidemiologic Studies

In analytic epidemiologic studies, such as **case–control studies, cohort studies** and related designs, data are usually collected by questionnaire or interview, or are abstracted from existing records, such as hospital records on treatment or diagnosis, personnel employment records on occupational exposures, or death certificates. Except in studies with a two-stage design (see below), complete information is sought for all subjects included in the study.

In case–control studies, one requires data on previous exposures that may have occurred long before the study. Adequate planning and organization are required to try to ensure that data are collected in an identical way for diseased persons (cases) and for healthy subjects (**controls**). Data are also collected on known or suspected **confounding** variables in order to adjust for these variables in the analysis. Preliminary data on matching variables, such as information on sex and age, are needed for matched case–control designs (*see* **Matching**). In cohort studies personal interviews are carried out infrequently, but data are often abstracted from existing files or records. In occupational cohort studies one can use personnel records to obtain data on the occupational history and sometimes on specific exposures; sometimes records from the office of the occupational hygienist or routinely collected data from the medical officer will be useful (*see* **Occupational Epidemiology**). The quality and completeness of such data may differ substantially between companies or even departments of the same company. Data quality may also differ for different job categories and could therefore depend on the exposure of interest. Disease information in cohort studies is sometimes abstracted from hospital records or from cancer registry files (*see* **Disease Registers**). In mortality studies, the date and **cause of death** are abstracted from official death certificates or from other sources. An important issue in planning and organizing cohort studies is to try to guarantee a nonselective retrieval of information for the personal history (occupational history, lifestyle, residential history). It is also important to avoid any selective follow-up to obtain the date of diagnosis or date of death. The diagnosis and/or the causes of death should be assessed in a comparable way for exposed and nonexposed subjects (*see* **Bias in Case–Control Studies**; **Bias in Cohort Studies**).

Sources of Missing Values in Epidemiologic Research

Unplanned Missing Values

Despite well-organized data collection efforts, data may contain errors, the data collection is sometimes incomplete, and missing values occur. Missing data can arise as total **nonresponse** or as item nonresponse. Total nonresponse results from refusal of subjects to participate in the study or from inability to locate the selected subjects. For example, in **population-based case–control studies,** controls may have been selected but are not accessible because they have recently moved. Total nonresponse is a frequent source of **selection bias**. In this article we restrict ourselves to item nonresponse, which refers to the lack of data on one or several items from a study participant but not on all items.

Item nonresponse may arise because a person refuses to answer certain questions. For example, if the question is too sensitive (e.g. alcohol consumption, sexual behavior, income, or health-related questions), a study participant may refuse to answer that item. What is regarded as sensitive may differ from one person to the next, and it may vary with personal behavior and/or depend on the answer to the sensitive question. Older people may be more willing to answer a certain question than younger people. Persons with a very high or very low income may not be willing to report it. Another reason for missing values is that subjects do not know the answer because they are unable to recall certain events. It also happens that a given answer is inconsistent with other answers and can therefore not be used in the analysis, as when a person says on one part of the questionnaire that she never smoked but later reports a consumption of 20 cigarettes daily. Missing values can also occur if the interviewer fails to ask all questions, as may happen if the interview is interrupted. Parts of the questionnaire may not be readable or may be destroyed during the process of editing. If data are abstracted from records, these records may be incomplete, illegible, or simply missing. Operating procedures in some departments of an industrial setting or a hospital may require records to be destroyed. In many situations, records include gaps or insufficient or uninterpretable information, resulting in missing values. Similarly, measures based on chemical or physical procedures may fail to produce a value because required amounts of blood or tissue are not available, or because of a laboratory accident or technical failure. In all these cases the missing values are unplanned, and we usually have limited information on why the data are missing. This lack of information on the mechanism of missingness makes this type of missing value problematic during an analysis.

Planned Missing Values

Because epidemiologic studies may require the collection of data on many variables for many subjects some sampling strategies have been developed that require less data. A two-stage design (*see* **Case–Control Study, Two-Phase**) may be performed in which first-stage data on the disease and crude exposure status are collected for many subjects, but additional information on detailed exposure or on confounding variables is collected only for a subsample in a second stage. The second stage may include equal numbers of crudely exposed and unexposed subjects. In a two-stage design, a large amount of data can be missing, but the missingness is understood and under the control of the investigator. The probability that a value is missing is known or can be calculated easily and can be used for the analysis. Simple and efficient procedures to estimate exposure effects for such designs were proposed by White [62] already in 1982. Closely related ideas of planned missingness are found in **validation studies** in which an easy-to-measure surrogate variable is collected for all subjects, and "gold standard" measurements are made only for a subsample.

Missing Value Mechanisms

Whenever we want to handle a data set with missing values appropriately, the probability law generating the missing values will be of importance. Formally, this law, usually called the missing value mechanism, is the conditional distribution of the missing indicators, given all variables considered. To facilitate the discussion, we introduce some notation and consider here the situation with one exposure and one **confounder** variable, where only the confounder variable may be missing. Hence we consider for each subject four variables: the disease status D, the exposure E, the confounder C, and the response indicator R, such that we actually observe C if and only if $R = 1$. This situation is complex enough to explain most problems and the basic approach to solutions. Some solutions, however, do not generalize to settings with several exposures and/or confounders, especially in the case of arbitrary missing patterns; we will point this out where it is necessary. Also, one can exchange the role of E and C.

Now, the missing value mechanism is given by the conditional probabilities of observing C, i.e. by

$$q(d, e, c) := \Pr(R = 1 | D = d, E = e, C = c).$$

To understand the possible dependencies of the observability of C on D, E and C, we shall discuss some specific situations. In case–control studies, missingness often depends on the disease status, as cases and controls may differ in their behavior and willingness to participate in the investigation and to respond to specific questions. For example, Schlehofer et al. [51] report results of a case–control study on risk factors for brain tumor, including blood group among other factors. For controls, only interview data were available, but for cases hospital records could be used in addition. This results in missing rates of 9% for cases, but of 46% for controls. By contrast, in a prospective cohort study one can usually exclude a dependence of the response probabilities on the disease status, if all covariate data are collected at the start of the study. Retrospective cohort studies (*see* **Cohort Study, Historical**) and most hybrid designs, such as **nested case–control studies**, often exhibit a dependence of missingness probabilities on the disease status.

Also, the exposure variable may have an influence on observability of the confounder. In an investigation of the risk of radiation therapy, a given therapy may be associated with hospital records containing detailed information on potential confounders. In studies of exposure in nuclear plants, higher exposure levels may be associated with frequent medical examinations and increased chance to assess information on confounders.

There exist a variety of settings in which the probability of observing a variable depends on the value of the variable itself. In interviews or studies by questionnaire, heavy drinkers or smokers may refuse to answer questions about such behavior, and very poor or very rich people may refuse to give information on their income. Likewise, long-term unemployed subjects may refuse to give information on their working history. Often the value of a variable may influence the probability of knowing or remembering it. For example, if we ask subjects to recall whether there is any case of a disease among their first and second degree relatives, and if there is no such case, he or she will often answer "I don't know", because he or she does not know all the relatives. But if there is one case, it suffices to know this one to give an answer.

Even "objective" sources like hospital records do not guarantee that there is no dependence on the true value. In looking for exposure to a specific therapy, it is often easy to detect such a treatment if it has been given, but to assert that the treatment has not been given requires a complete search of hospital records over the time period of interest.

In epidemiology we may often have rather complicated missing mechanisms. For example, in case–control studies, cases may refuse more often to admit an unhealthy lifestyle than controls, because they feel guilty. On the other hand, they may remember previous exposures better because they have sought reasons for their illness. Similarly, the willingness to admit to specific sexual behaviors may differ among sex and age groups. As another example, the availability of information on confounder variables may depend both on the disease status and the exposure level. If exposed subjects and cases are willing subjects, only unexposed controls may yield missing values. These possible interactions make handling of incomplete data especially difficult.

So far, we have described possible scenarios. Some of them are more dangerous than others, however, depending on the type of analysis. If one wants to make efficient use of subjects with incomplete confounder information, the missing at random (MAR) assumption is of central importance. In our context, the MAR assumption is

$$q(d, e, c) = q(d, e),$$

namely that the true value of C is conditionally independent of R given D and E. This assumption allows one to estimate the conditional distribution of C, given D, E and $R = 0$ from those subjects with $R = 1$, which is the key to efficient use of all data. Note that the MAR assumption allows a dependence of the occurrence of missing values on D and E. In two-stage designs we can exclude a dependence on C by design, but sampling fractions typically depend on D and E. In the literature on missing values, one sometimes finds the missing completely at random (MCAR) assumption, $q(d, e, c) = q$, but this is seldom realistic in epidemiology.

If one wants to ignore the subjects with incomplete covariate data in the analysis, it is essential to assume that the selection of such subjects introduces no **bias**, which leads to different requirements as discussed later. We should finally mention that in a case–control study the definition of

$q(d, c, e)$ refers to the selected subjects, but it coincides with the values in the total population, provided that selection probabilities really depend only on the case–control status, and not on other information which is a requirement for any well-conducted case–control study.

Fitting Logistic Regression Models with Incomplete Covariate Data

For epidemiologic investigations, **logistic regression** is an important tool to analyze the joint effect of one or several exposure variables on the disease risk adjusted for one or several confounding variables. In the case of one exposure and one confounder variable, the logistic model for risk in the underlying population assumes that the conditional probability of disease given the exposure value e and the confounder value c is given as

$$\Pr(D = 1 | E = e, C = c) = \Lambda(\beta_0 + \beta_E e + \beta_C c)$$
$$=: p_\beta(e, c),$$

with $\Lambda(t) = 1/[1 + \exp(-t)]$. As suggested by this formula, E and C may be binary or continuous variables, extensions to polytomous variables are straightforward, and most statements in this article are valid for any type of covariates.

With complete data we can estimate the parameters β_0, β_E, and β_C by the maximum likelihood principle. There are several proposals of different quality to cope with incomplete data. To understand the behavior of most simple methods for handling incomplete covariate data, we examine the conditional probabilities of the disease status given the actual information we observed. Considering only subjects in the cohort with complete data, we have

$$\Pr(D = 1 | E = e, C = c, R = 1)$$
$$= \Lambda\left(\beta_0 + \log \frac{q(1, e, c)}{q(0, e, c)} + \beta_E e + \beta_C c\right), (1)$$

which can be derived by analogy with the justification of logistic regression models for case-control data, as given by Breslow & Day [5, p. 203]. This result follows by noting that $q(d, e, c)$ are nothing other than the probabilities of selecting these subjects, just as cases and controls have selection probabilities from the base population in a case-control study.

Eq. (1) implies that fitting a logistic regression model to the subjects with complete data only will give valid estimates for β_E and β_C, provided $q(d, e, c)$ can be decomposed into $q(d) \cdot q(e, c)$. For subjects with a missing confounder value we have

$$\Pr(D = 1|E = e, R = 0)$$

$$= \int \Lambda \left(\beta_0 + \log \frac{1 - q(1, e, c)}{1 - q(0, e, c)} + \beta_E e + \beta_C c \right)$$

$$dF(c|E = e, R = 0). \qquad (2)$$

Most simple methods to handle incomplete covariate data try to approximate (1) and (2) by simple logistic models, and the resulting misspecification can cause serious bias. In contrast, methods relying on the likelihood or on appropriately chosen estimating equations have the potential to produce consistent estimates. Hence we now consider the likelihood in the incomplete data case. From the joint distribution of the observed variables, subjects without a missing value contribute

$$q(d, e, c) \times p_\beta(e, c)^d \times [1 - p_\beta(e, c)]^{1-d}$$

$$\times \Pr(C = c|E = e) \times \Pr(E = e),$$

and subjects with a missing value contribute

$$\int [1 - q(d, e, c)] \times p_\beta(e, c)^d \times [1 - p_\beta(e, c)]^{1-d}$$

$$\times \Pr(C = c|E = e) \times \Pr(E = e)dc.$$

If the MAR assumption $q(d, e, c) = q(d, e)$ holds, not only $\Pr(E = e)$ but also the terms involving q can be removed from the likelihood. However, the likelihood still depends on $\Pr(C = c|E = e)$; hence the classical maximum likelihood principle requires specifying the distribution of the covariates, at least in part, which is fundamentally unlike the complete data case. Trying to avoid these difficulties leads to semiparametric approaches. The likelihood presented above is based on a prospective sampling scheme. In the case of complete data, it is well known that such a likelihood also yields valid estimates of β_E and β_C in the analysis of case–control studies [34]. This is also true for incomplete data, as shown by Carroll et al. [9].

In the following we outline the main simple and sophisticated methods for handling incomplete covariate data.

Complete Case Analysis

In a complete case analysis all subjects with a missing value are omitted from the analysis. The validity of this approach is based on the implicit assumption that the regression model for the subjects with complete data is identical to the model for all subjects, i.e. that

$$\Pr(D = 1|E = e, C = c, R = 1)$$

$$= \Pr(D = 1|E = e, C = c)$$

holds. Using (1), this is true, if $q(d, e, c) = q(e, c)$, i.e. if missing probabilities do not depend on the disease status. This is also intuitively clear; if missing probabilities depend only on the covariate values, restriction to subjects without missing values changes only the population, but not the regression model, whereas missing probabilities depending additionally on the outcome introduce some type of **selection bias**. An isolated difference between the missingness probabilities for cases and controls affects the estimation of the intercept but does not affect the estimation of β_E and β_C; in general consistent estimation of the latter is guaranteed if $q(d, e, c) = q(d) \cdot q(e, c)$, which follows directly from (1) [20].

Therefore a complete case analysis has the favorable property that it yields consistent estimates of the regression parameters, even if the MAR assumption is violated. It has the unfavorable property that consistency of parameter estimates depends on the assumption that missingness probabilities do not depend jointly on the disease status and the covariate values. The latter is however often questionable for case–control studies (cf. final section). The bias of the **odds ratio** based on a complete case analysis can be easily computed [57], and it can be shown that realistic differences in the missingness probabilities can lead to substantial bias. For example, if exposed cases are better documented than controls and unexposed cases such that the missingness probability for the exposed cases is 10% and 40% for the other groups, then the odds ratio for exposure is overestimated by a factor of 1.5.

Additional Category or Missing Indicator Method

Epidemiologists often work with categorical variables and sometimes define an additional category for missing observations. Such coding suggests that we analyze the data under the implicit assumption that

$$\Pr(D = 1 | E = e, C = c, R = 1)$$
$$= \Lambda(\beta_0 + \beta_E e + \beta_C c)$$

and

$$\Pr(D = 1 | E = e, R = 0) = \Lambda(\beta_0 + \beta_E e + \beta^*).$$

Equivalently we can impute for the missing values of C the value 0 and add the missing indicator $M = 1 - R$ to the regression model. This "missing indicator method", which is also applied to continuous covariates, results in the same specification and hence the same estimates. The approach is inappropriate, as one cannot expect to achieve good estimates for the adjusted risk β_E if adjustment for the unobserved values of the confounding variable is attempted by introducing the additional parameter β^* in the second equation above. To see this, let us assume that $q(d, e, c) \equiv q$, i.e. MCAR, such that the subjects with and without missing values form two random subsamples. Then in the first equation above β_E corresponds to the adjusted log-odds ratio (OR) of the exposure, whereas in the second line β_E corresponds to the unadjusted log-OR, because $\beta_0 + \beta^*$ can be regarded as one intercept. Consequently, the quantity $\exp(\hat{\beta}_E)$ estimates a quantity between the adjusted and unadjusted OR. Hence the goal of obtaining realistic ORs that describe the effect of exposure adjusted for confounding variables cannot be achieved if missing values in the confounding variables are regarded as an additional category. Moreover, if the missingness probabilities are allowed to depend on the disease status and/or exposure status, then $\exp(\hat{\beta}_E)$ can lead to values outside the range between the adjusted and unadjusted OR. The bias is often accompanied by underestimation of the variability; Greenland & Finkle [21] report the results of a simulation study with two Gaussian covariates, where the missing indicator method results in true coverage probabilities of 55% for nominal 95% confidence intervals.

So far we have considered the effect of coding missing values as an additional category on the estimation of β_E. In the epidemiologic literature the estimate of β^* is often reported, too, and compared with the value of $\hat{\beta}_C$. Often there is an implicit assumption that $\hat{\beta}^*$ has to be between 0 and $\hat{\beta}_C$, or, in the case of several categories, within the range of the effect estimates (including 0 for the baseline category). If

missing probabilities depend only on the exposure, and the degree of correlation between confounder and exposure is small, then this is approximately true, as can be shown using the approximation discussed in the next section. However, if missingness probabilities depend on the disease status, the relative disease frequency among subjects with complete data differs from the relative disease frequency among subjects with incomplete data, and β^* mainly reflects this difference.

Although regarding missing values as an additional category cannot be recommended in general, it can be appropriate in special settings, where missing values characterize a meaningful subset of all individuals. For example, Commenges et al. [11] report a study comparing different procedures to diagnose dementia in a screening setting. They found missing values in those variables corresponding to the results of two tests to be highly predictive, because the missing values reflected a subject's failure to comprehend the test.

Single-Imputation Methods

This class of methods is characterized by imputing for each missing value a single value and analyzing the completed data set. If the confounder C is continuous, the simplest choice is to replace each missing value by the overall mean $\overline{C}$ of the observed values of the confounding variable. Instead of using an estimate for the overall expectation of C, one may use estimates of the conditional expectations: if E is categorical, then we can impute the mean of the observed values of C within each category of E; if E is continuous, then we can compute a regression of the observed values of C on E. If C is binary, then relative frequencies replace the means, and Schemper & Smith [48] proposed the term probability imputation. The imputation of estimates for the conditional expectations yields an approximately valid inference, if missing probabilities do not depend on the disease state and the true, unobserved value, i.e. if $q(d, e, c) = q(e)$. In this situation, we have

by (1) $\Pr(D = 1 | E = e, C = c, R = 1) = p_\beta(e, c)$

and

by (2) $\Pr(D = 1 | E = e, R = 0)$
$$= \int \Lambda(\beta_0 + \beta_E e + \beta_C c) \mathrm{d} F^{C|E=e}(c).$$

If we regard Λ as an approximately linear function, then we have

$$\Pr(D = 1 | E = e, R = 0)$$
$$\approx \Lambda(\beta_0 + \beta_E e + \beta_C \cdot E[C | E = e]).$$

Hence imputing estimates for the conditional expectation results in an approximately correct specification of the conditional disease probabilities, and hence the resulting bias of the parameter estimates is often small. One has to expect, however, that variance estimates tend to be too small, because the imputed values are treated as true ones and no adjustment is made for the additional variability introduced by imputing estimates. Results of simulation studies [47, 48, 55, 60] suggest that both bias and underestimation of the variance are only problematic for extreme parameter constellations with high missingness rates and very influential confounding variables.

The justification so far depends on the assumption that missingness probabilities do not depend on the disease status. This is not necessary, because imputation of conditional expectations can always be regarded as an approximation to simple semi-parametric approaches [60]. However, some care is necessary; if missingness probabilities depend on the disease status, then naive estimates for conditional expectations are wrong; it is necessary to estimate the conditional expectations separately within diseased and undiseased subjects and then to form a weighted average [60]. Moreover, for extreme parameter constellations the bias can be still substantial [55].

Generalizations to several covariates with arbitrary missing patterns are straightforward, as long as there are enough subjects with complete information. But many auxiliary regression models may be required. In general, misspecification of these auxiliary regression models can be a source of additional bias in the parameter estimates, but little is known about this problem.

Modifying the Complete Case Estimates

Under the MAR assumption, the response probabilities $q(d, e)$ can be estimated from the observed data, for example by fitting a logistic regression model with outcome variable R and covariates D and E. The bias of the complete case estimates can be expressed as a function of q, and hence we can correct the bias [55, 57]. Alternatively, one may fit a logistic regression

model with estimated offsets in (1) to the subjects with complete covariate data [4]. If E is categoric and a saturated model is used in estimating q, then both approaches coincide and are identical to maximum likelihood estimates [59]. As simple expressions for the corresponding asymptotic variances can be provided [7], this is a simple method to achieve consistent and efficient estimates in this special setting if the MAR assumption is tenable. Unfortunately there is no simple generalization for arbitrary missingness patterns.

Estimation of the Score Function: Weighting, Filling, and the Mean Score Method

In the complete data case, maximization of the likelihood is equivalent to finding a root of the score function

$$S_n(\beta) = \frac{1}{n} \sum_{i=1}^{n} S_\beta(D_i, E_i, C_i),$$

with

$$S_\beta(d, e, c) = \frac{\partial}{\partial \beta} \{d \log p_\beta(e, c) + (1 - d) \log(1 - p_\beta(e, c))\}.$$

In the incomplete data case the contribution to the score function is unknown for subjects with a missing value. Nevertheless, one can try to estimate $S_n(\beta)$. A first approach is to regard the subjects with complete covariate information as a subsample with selection probabilities $q(d, e, c)$ and to try to estimate the "population average" $ES_\beta(D, E, C)$. The classical Horvitz–Thompson estimator satisfies this task by weighting each contribution of the subsample with $q(d, e, c)^{-1}$. However, $q(d, e, c)$ is unknown, and only under the MAR assumption can we arrive at estimates $\hat{q}(d, e)$ and at a weighted score function

$$\tilde{S}_n(\beta) = \frac{1}{n} \sum_{\substack{i=1 \\ R_i=1}}^{n} S_\beta(D_i, E_i, C_i) / \hat{q}(D_i, E_i).$$

Solving $\tilde{S}_n(\beta) = 0$ results in consistent estimates of β. Solving $\tilde{S}_n(\beta) = 0$ can be done by any software package for logistic regression that allows arbitrary weights (see **Software, Biostatistical**). However, variance estimates obtained this way are invalid, and can be much too small [55, Section 5.11]. If a parametric model $q_\alpha(d, e)$ is used in estimating the response probabilities, explicit estimates of the variance can be provided [35; 55, p. 17], but they cannot be computed with standard software. If E and C are both categorical, then the approach is equivalent to distributing subjects with a missing value to the cells of the contingency table of subjects without a missing value with fractions equal to estimates of the conditional probability for the true value. This intuitive method was called "filling" by Vach & Blettner [57]. The idea to weight contributions to the score function reciprocally to the response probabilities was also used by Flanders & Greenland [16] and Zhao & Lipsitz [63]. However, they consider the analysis of designs for which the response probabilities were known.

An alternative approach to estimating S_β is to replace each unknown contribution $S_\beta(D_i, E_i, C_i)$ for subjects with unknown C_i by an estimate for $E[S_\beta(D_i, E_i, C_i)|D_i, E_i]$, i.e. an estimate for the conditional expectation of the score function given the observed variables. Reilly & Pepe [36] investigate this approach in detail for the special case where E is categorical. In that case, estimates of the conditional expectations are simple averages over the subjects without missing values, and the approach is equivalent to weighting. However, whereas the weighting approach is difficult to generalize to the case of several covariates with arbitrary missingness patterns, this is in principle possible for the individual estimation of the conditional expectations by nonparametric regression.

Finally, estimates based on the weighting or the mean score approach are consistent under the MAR assumption but not always efficient. Especially if missingness rates are large, there can be a substantial loss in comparison to efficient approaches [40; 55, Section 5.2; 63].

Maximum Likelihood Estimation

Application of the maximum likelihood (ML) principle requires a parametric specification $f_\alpha(c|e)$ for the conditional distributions $\Pr(C = c|E = e)$ (cf. above). Then under the MAR assumption the contributions to the likelihood are given by

$$p_\beta(e, c)^d (1 - p_\beta(e, c))^{1-d} f_\alpha(c|e), \quad \text{if } R = 1,$$

$$\int p_\beta(e, c)(1 - p_\beta(e, c))^{1-d} f_\alpha(c|e)\mathrm{d}c, \quad \text{if } R = 0.$$

The integral in the likelihood makes maximization a little bit cumbersome. The expectation-maximization (EM) algorithm [12] is a standard tool to maximize the likelihood in incomplete data problems. However, if C is continuous, even the EM algorithm may require numerical integration. If C is categorical, integration reduces to summation, and both the EM algorithm [25] or a direct maximization using the Newton–Raphson method are feasible. The latter has the advantage of automatically computing the quantities necessary to estimate the variance of the parameter estimates, whereas use of the EM algorithm requires additional effort [32, 54]. The ML principle is also applicable in the general setting with several covariates and arbitrary missingness patterns, as long as we are able to specify a parametric family for the conditional distribution of the covariates affected by missing values given the unaffected covariates.

The ML estimates are consistent and efficient as long as the MAR assumption is valid and the true distribution of the covariates is within the specified family. This specification is a crucial point of the ML approach, because this requirement is not necessary in the complete data case, and our knowledge about the distributions of and dependencies between the covariates is usually limited. Misspecification of the distribution of the covariates, however, can induce a bias in the regression parameter estimates. Thus it becomes necessary to model nuisance features of the problem carefully. If all covariates are categorical, loglinear models provide a simple framework to describe the joint distribution [58], but if continuous covariates are involved, parametric models flexible enough seem to be hard to specify.

If all covariates are categorical, one can also fit a loglinear model to the joint distribution of all variables [17, 61] and use relationships between loglinear and logistic models.

Semiparametric ML Estimation

We have seen in the previous section that ML estimation requires specification of a parametric family for the conditional distribution of C given E. It is an appealing idea to avoid this unpleasant task by replacing $f(c|e)$ by a nonparametric estimate. Pepe & Fleming [33] consider the case of a categorical exposure, such that the empirical distribution within each exposure stratum can be used; Carroll & Wand

[8] consider a continuous exposure and use kernel estimates. Both approaches rely on the assumption that missingness probabilities do not depend on the disease status, but they can be generalized to this setting (Vach & Schumacher [60]). Computations of the resulting estimates of β require special software, as does estimation of the variance. The resulting estimates are not fully efficient in comparison to the estimates of the next section. It is also difficult to generalize these approaches to settings with several covariates and arbitrary missingness patterns, because this requires non-parametric estimation of high-dimensional multivariate conditional distributions.

Semiparametric Efficient Estimation

The last two sections have suggested that the handling of incomplete covariate data is ideally a semiparametric problem; we are interested in the parameters of the regression model describing the conditional distribution of disease status given all exposure and confounding covariates, but the distribution of the covariates, in spite of being essential for the likelihood, should be left unspecified. In recent years there has been substantial progress (for example [3]) in the general field of efficient semiparametric estimation. Robins et al. [40] used this theory to fit generalized linear models with incomplete covariate data. They showed that roughly any consistent estimator for β is asymptotically equivalent to one defined as the solution of an estimating equation $\sum_{i=1}^{n} S_\beta(D_i, E_i, C_i) = 0$, where

$$S_\beta(D, E, C) = R \frac{h(E, C)(D - p_\beta(E, C))}{q(D, E)}$$
$$- \frac{\varphi(D, E)(R - q(D, E))}{q(D, E)}.$$

They were also able to characterize functions h_{opt} and φ_{opt} which lead to a semiparametric efficient estimate, i.e. the asymptotic variance of this estimate is exactly the supremum of the asymptotic variances of all maximum likelihood estimators based on parametric families $f_\alpha(c|e)$ covering the true $f(c|e)$. Of course, this is the best we can expect without imposing parametric assumptions. Unfortunately h_{opt} and φ_{opt} depend on the true values of β and the true distribution of C given E and are moreover not available in closed form.

However, an adaptive procedure is possible which starts with a parametric assumption on the distribution of the covariates, then estimates all parameters, uses an iterative procedure to compute $\hat{h}_{\text{opt}}$ and $\hat{\varphi}_{\text{opt}}$ based on the assumption that the estimates correspond to the true parameters, and finally solves the estimating equations with h and φ replaced by $\hat{h}_{\text{opt}}$ and $\hat{\varphi}_{\text{opt}}$, and q replaced by an appropriate estimate. In contrast to ML estimation, a misspecification of the covariate distribution does not result in inconsistent estimates, and, in spite of the adaptive steps, the estimates are efficient, if the specification of the covariate distribution was correct. Details of this adaptive procedure can be found in Robins et al. [40] and Rotnitzky & Robins [42]. The approach can be also generalized to several covariates with arbitrary missingness patterns; however, here the computation of $\hat{h}_{\text{opt}}$ and $\hat{\varphi}_{\text{opt}}$ is more difficult. One can try to avoid this by considering estimating equations that are intermediate between the efficient ones and simple reweighting [64].

Multiple Imputation

Multiple imputation is a general technique for statistical inference with incomplete data. The basic idea is to create several data sets with different values imputed for the missing values, and to analyze each data set by standard software, such as software for logistic regression. If the imputations are generated in a so-called "proper" manner, the average of the parameter estimates provides a consistent estimate. Furthermore, the average of the variance estimates and the empirical variance of the multiple parameter estimates can be combined to form a total variance estimate; confidence intervals and P values can be computed, too. Rubin & Schenker [46] present an overview of the basic techniques.

It seems reasonable to generate imputations from estimates of the conditional distribution of the unobserved values. However, this is an improper method in the sense that variance estimates tend to be too small, because they do not take into account the variance due to estimating the conditional distribution. Proper methods can be defined by additionally estimating the conditional distribution in each imputation step based on a random sample with replacement of the subjects without missing values [15, 44, 45]. Of course, any attempt to estimate the conditional distribution of the missing values from the observed values depends on the MAR assumption.

With respect to our setting, Reilly & Pepe [36, 37] have considered the special case where E is categoric. Values to be imputed for missing values in C are drawn from the empirical distributions of C within the strata defined by D and E. This hot-deck imputation method is improper, although Reilly & Pepe [37] provided a valid variance estimator. Moreover they showed that hot-deck multiple imputation with infinite imputations is asymptotically equivalent to the mean-score method. In particular, this implies that the hot-deck method has the same deficiencies with respect to efficiency. Greenland & Finkle [21] report results of a simulation study with E and C both continuous and affected by missing values. Imputations were drawn from estimated conditional distributions resulting from fitting bivariate normal distributions within the diseased and undiseased subjects. Although this is an improper method, they observed that confidence intervals keep their nominal level. They also observed a loss of efficiency in comparison to maximum likelihood estimation.

Multiple imputation can be also applied in general settings with arbitrary missingness patterns. The crucial point is the choice of the procedure to estimate the necessary conditional distribution. If we rely on parametric assumptions on the distribution of the covariates, we have the same unpleasant situation as with ML estimation. However, one can alternatively draw imputations from a set of nearest neighbors, i.e. subjects with complete information and similar values with respect to the observed variables. The choice of an appropriate distance measure requires some knowledge about the distribution of the covariates, but not necessarily an explicit model. Heitjan & Little [23] give an illuminating example.

Methods Based on the Retrospective Likelihood

The methods considered so far rely on a prospective sampling scheme implying independence of the disease status among different subjects. In case–control studies this assumption is violated. However, in incomplete data problems the use of the prospective likelihood can also be justified for retrospective data [9]. The resulting estimates are consistent, the estimated standard errors are never too small, and they are correct if we make no assumptions on the distribution of the covariates. Nevertheless, methods based

on the retrospective likelihood are of interest, especially for the analysis of two-stage designs. In such a design, the number of subjects with complete data is fixed in advance, and hence missingness indicators are not independent, which is a further violation of the prospective sampling scheme.

ML estimation with respect to the retrospective likelihood is considered by Scott & Wild [53] and Breslow & Holubkov [6]. Two different pseudo-likelihood approaches, in which some parameters are pre-estimated in a naive manner, are considered by Breslow & Cain [4] and Schill et al. [50]. A weighting approach is due to Flanders & Greenland [16]. Comparisons with respect to the asymptotic relative efficiency and simulation studies [6, 49, 63] often reveal large inefficiencies of the weighting approach and some inefficiencies of the two pseudo-maximum likelihood approaches.

Handling of a Questionable MAR Assumption

All sophisticated, and especially all efficient, approaches to handle incomplete covariate data rely on the MAR assumption. In many applications this assumption is questionable, but one may still want to use methods relying on it. In that case, it is necessary to think about or investigate the possible impact of a violation. One may argue that if there is a pure violation, in the sense that missingness depends only on the true value of the covariate, then the impact must be small, because the association between the covariates and the outcome is not changed. Schemper & Smith [48] provide an informal argument for this conjecture. Investigations for the special case of categorial C and E [59] corroborate the conjecture. These studies further demonstrate that the impact on the exposure effect estimate can be substantial if there are differences in the degree of violation between diseased and undiseased or between exposed and unexposed subjects, which is also intuitively clear, because such differences change the observed association.

If one does not want to rely on such general, theoretical considerations, one may try to investigate the impact of an invalid MAR assumption for a particular data set. This can be easily done within the multiple imputation framework, for example by drawing more larger values for a variable or more values from a specific category (cf. [46]). Vach & Blettner [58] present a framework to specify violations within the framework of ML estimation and perform a sensitivity analysis for two case–control studies. Baker [2] takes an additional step and does not specify, but tries to estimate, the parameters of the non-MAR mechanism. Rotnitzky & Robins [42] consider this step within the framework of semiparametric efficient estimation. However, a (saturated) logistic model and a (saturated) non-MAR model are in general not jointly identifiable; hence any attempt to estimate non-MAR mechanisms relies on restrictions of the two models allowing identifiability. This alone, however, is not enough, as identifiability does not imply reasonable properties of resulting estimates in this setting; Rotnitzky & Robins [42] show in the semiparametric setting that in spite of identifiability there need not exist a $\sqrt{n}$-consistent estimator. Hence, the usefulness of these approaches has to be investigated further before recommendations can be made.

Robins & Gill [39] point out that in settings with arbitrary missingness patterns, the MAR assumption as defined by Rubin [43] allows some configurations of no practical relevance. This fact can be used to change the MAR assumption, allowing some special non-MAR mechanisms to be estimated without problems of identifiability. Robins & Gill [39] and Robins [38] present two examples of this kind.

Handling of Incomplete Data in other Models Used in Analytic Epidemiology

Poisson Regression, Gaussian Regression, and Generalized Linear Models

Nearly everything we have said in the last section with respect to logistic regression is also valid for other regression models where parameters are estimated by maximum likelihood. In particular, the difficulties with maximum likelihood estimation in the incomplete data case are the same, and the semiparametric approaches work in the general setting of generalized linear models. With respect to the simple methods, there are two differences. First, there is no general analogy to the modifications of the complete case estimates. Second, the single imputation methods need more care. We can expect nearly unbiased estimates of the regression parameters after imputation of conditional means, as this implies a roughly correct specification of the conditional expectation of

the outcome variable. Indeed, in the case of Gaussian regression one can prove consistency [19]. However, only in binary regression models does correct specification of the conditional mean imply correct specification of the conditional variance. In general, the conditional variance of the outcome increases if some covariate values are missing; hence, after the imputation of conditional means, a further analysis should be based on a heteroscedastic model. For this reason, weighted least squares estimates are advocated in Gaussian regression after imputation of conditional means. An overview of this and other techniques suitable for Gaussian regression models is given by Little [29]. Some of the proposals depend on the assumption of a multivariate normal distribution of all variables and hence have limited application in epidemiology. The impact of the variance heterogeneity for other types of regression models, especially **Poisson regression**, has not been investigated. Thus we recommend that the single imputation method should be used with caution.

Cox Regression with Incomplete Covariate Data

For the analysis of (censored) survival times the **proportional hazard** model [10] is widely used in epidemiology. Simple methods to handle incomplete covariate data are subject to the same criticism as for logistic regression, with the additional difficulty that, especially in **retrospective studies**, censoring may be associated with missingness in covariates. Even in a complete case analysis, the assumption of noninformative censoring can be violated. With respect to more sophisticated approaches, it is difficult to extend the maximum likelihood approach to survival models (*see* **Survival Analysis, Overview**), as the nuisance parameter involves the baseline hazard, although a semiparametric partial maximum likelihood approach is possible [65]. A weighting approach has been proposed by Pugh et al. [35], and Lin & Ying [27] consider an appropriately modified score function, but their approach requires MCAR. None of these approaches can be easily generalized to situations with general missingness patterns. Robins et al. [40] also point out the difficulty of obtaining a feasible solution from the theory of semiparametric efficient estimation. In the face of this problem, one may be willing to use alternative fully parametric regression models for survival data, such that, especially in the case of categorical covariates, the ML principle can be used. In this spirit, Schluchter & Jackson [52], Baker [1] and Vach [56] suggest approximating the **Cox regression model** by a logistic model for grouped survival data, and Lipsitz & Ibrahim [31] consider Weibull models. The use of single imputation methods has been considered by Schemper & Smith [48].

Analysis of Matched Case–Control Studies

The handling of incomplete covariate data in matched case–control studies has received little attention. Haber & Chen [22] consider the case of a single exposure variable as the only covariate and compare the matched and unmatched odds ratio estimator. They conclude that in the case of missing exposure information for some cases and controls, the advantages of the unmatched estimator increase in comparison to the complete data case. **Conditional logistic regression** (*see* **Matched Analysis**) is a standard tool for the analysis of matched case–control studies. Missing values in the covariates constitute an even greater problem with **conditional logistic regression** than with ordinary logistic regression, as a complete case analysis with one-to-one-matching causes loss of the complete pair if the covariate is missing in either the case or the control. Despite a small simulation study [18], a systematic investigation is still needed. A proposal of Lipsitz et al. [28] for handling incomplete covariate data in conditional logistic regression is unfortunately not directly applicable in matched case–control studies.

Regression Models for Longitudinal and Multivariate Data

Regression models for longitudinal or clustered data (*see* **Clustering**), especially marginal models, are proving useful in epidemiology for the analysis of familial aggregation and of environmental studies (*see* **Environmental Epidemiology**) as well as for studies of biochemical markers. With respect to incomplete covariate data, there is little to add to what we have said previously. However, in these applications outcome variables may also be missing, especially from drop outs in longitudinal studies. We want to restrict ourselves to some basic comments, especially on the differences with the incomplete covariate problem.

First, the MAR assumption is again of central importance. In the case of drop outs, the question is whether we are able to observe the crucial event causing the drop out, or whether the drop out hides this event. Secondly, if the MAR assumption is tenable and if we consider regression models specifying the joint conditional distribution of the outcome variables and allowing the use of the ML principle with complete data case, then the ML principle can also be used in the presence of missing values in the outcome variables and reduces usually to an analysis of all units with measured outcome. Thirdly, the popular marginal models [26] do not belong to this class, and for them the MAR assumption is not sufficient to exclude a bias due to missing values, if only the available units are used; a solution has been provided by Robins et al. [41]. Finally, if the MAR assumption is violated, we have often some rather precise ideas on the drop out mechanism, which may permit adjustment by choosing an appropriate model [13, 14, 24, 30].

Strategies to Cope with Incomplete Data

The best advice is to minimize the possibility for missing values. We should plan appropriate data collection procedures and design interviews and questionnaires so that subjects have little reason to refuse an answer. Adequate planning can also help to avoid differential missingness with respect to disease status or exposure status. The same data collection procedures should be used for cases and controls in case–control studies, and exposed and unexposed subjects should be followed using similar procedures and effort in cohort studies. Usually one knows in advance which variables are most likely to have missing values. Then a fruitful strategy can be to collect data on a surrogate variable that is available on most subjects and to collect the variable of interest with additional effort only in a randomly selected subsample, assuring that the MAR assumption holds. Then it is possible to use statistical methods very similar to the sophisticated methods discussed earlier, except that the surrogate variable is not included in the regression model (*see* **Validation Study**). A general idea is to collect additional data to predict missingness. By incorporating such variables in the analysis, the MAR assumption may become more reliable. Finally, one can try to recontact a representative sample of the nonresponders, and try to collect the missing data. If this succeeds, a valid analysis becomes possible in principle.

If these approaches are infeasible or unsuccessful, then one should at least discuss the possible impact of the missing values on the analysis. The first step is to report the missing rates for all variables, stratified by disease status and exposure levels, and to summarize major associations of missingness with other variables. The second step is to justify the analytical approach. If a complete case analysis is applied in a case–control study, then one should give arguments to exclude an important difference in the missing value mechanism between cases and controls. If one uses methods relying on the MAR assumption, then the latter must be justified or a sensitivity analysis should be conducted.

Conclusions

Missing values are a common problem in the analysis of epidemiologic studies. The problem should be addressed in planning the study so as to minimize their occurrence. Careful planning may also allow one to control or to understand the missingness mechanism and thereby to facilitate valid inference. If one has sufficient insight into the missingness mechanism, then one can take advantage of efficient statistical methods, although there remains a need for more practical experience with these techniques and improved availability of software. Such analytical methods cannot salvage a poorly planned and executed study, however, that has many missing values and offers little insight into the missingness mechanism.

References

[1]   Baker, S.G. (1994). Regression analysis of grouped survival data with incomplete covariates: Nonignorable missing-data and censoring mechanisms, *Biometrics* **50**, 821–826.

[2]   Baker, S.G. (1996). Reader reaction: The analysis of categorical case–control data subject to nonignorable nonresponse, *Biometrics* **52**, 362–369.

[3]   Bickel, P.J., Klaassen, C.A., Ritov, Y. & Wellner, J.A. (1993). *Efficient and Adaptive Estimation for Semiparametric Models*. John Hopkins University Press, Baltimore.

[4]   Breslow, N.E. & Cain, K.C. (1988). Logistic regression for two-stage case–control data, *Biometrika* **75**, 11–20.

[5]   Breslow, N.E. & Day, N.E. (1980). *Statistical Methods in Cancer Research*, Vol. 1: *The Analysis of Case–Control Studies*. IARC Scientific Publications, Lyon, No. 32.

[6]   Breslow, N.E. & Holubkov, R. (1997). Weighted likelihood, pseudolikelihood and maximum likelihood methods for logistic regression two-stage data, *Statistics in Medicine* **16**, 103–116.

[7]   Cain, K.C. & Breslow, N.E. (1988). Logistic regression analysis and efficient design for two-stage studies, *American Journal of Epidemiology* **128**, 1198–1206.

[8]   Carroll, R.J. & Wand, M.P. (1991). Semiparametric estimation in logistic measurement error models, *Journal of the Royal Statistical Society, Series B* **53**, 573–585.

[9]   Carroll, R.J., Wang, S. & Wang, C.Y. (1995). Prospective analysis of logistic case-control studies, *Journal of the American Statistical Association* **90**, 157–169.

[10]   Cox, D.R. (1972). Regression models and life tables (with discussion), *Journal of the Royal Statistical Society, Series B* **34**, 187–220.

[11]   Commenges, D., Gagnon M., Letenneur, L., Dartigues, J.F., Barbarger-Gateau, P. & Salamon R. (1992). Improving screening for dementia in the elderly using mini-mental state examination subscores, Benton's visual retention test, and Isaacs' set test, *Epidemiology* **3**, 185–188.

[12]   Dempster, A.P., Laird, N.M. & Rubin, D.B. (1977). Maximum likelihood estimation from incomplete data via EM algorithm (with discussion), *Journal of the Royal Statistical Society, Series B* **39**, 1–38.

[13]   Diggle, P.J. (1998). Dealing with missing values in longitudinal studies, in *Statistical Analysis of Medical Data–New Developments*, B.S. Everitt & G. Dunn, eds. Arnold, London, pp. 203–228.

[14]   Diggle, P. & Kenward, M.G. (1994). Informative dropout in longitudinal data analysis, *Applied Statistics* **43**, 49–93.

[15]   Efron, B. (1994). Missing data, imputation and the bootstrap (with discussion), *Journal of the American Statistical Association* **89**, 463–479.

[16]   Flanders, W.D. & Greenland, S. (1991). Analytical methods for two-stage case–control studies and other stratified designs, *Statistics in Medicine* **10**, 739–747.

[17]   Fuchs, C. (1982). Maximum likelihood estimation and model selection in contingency tables with missing data, *Journal of the American Statistical Association* **77**, 270–278.

[18]   Gibbons, L.E. & Hosmer, D.W. (1991). Conditional logistic regression with missing data, *Communications in Statistics – Simulation and Computation* **20**, 109–119.

[19]   Gill, R.D. (1986). A note on some methods for regression analysis with incomplete observations, *Sankhyā, Series B* **48**, 19–30.

[20] Glynn, R.J. & Laird, N.M. (1983). Regression estimates and missing data: Complete case analysis. *Unpublished manuscript*, Department of Biostatistics, Harvard University.

[21] Greenland, S. & Finkle, W.D. (1995). A critical look at methods for handling missing covariates in epidemiologic regression analysis, *American Journal of Epidemiology* **142**, 1255–1264.

[22] Haber, M. & Chen, C.C.H. (1991). Estimation of odds ratios from matched case–control studies with incomplete data, *Biometrical Journal* **33**, 673–682.

[23] Heitjan, D.F. & Little, R.J.A. (1991). Multiple imputation for the Fatal Accident Reporting System, *Applied Statistics* **40**, 13–29.

[24] Hogan, J.W. & Laird, N.M. (1997). Model-based approaches to analyzing incomplete longitudinal and failure time data, *Statistics in Medicine* **16**, 259–284.

[25] Ibrahim, J.G. (1990). Incomplete data in generalized linear models, *Journal of the American Statistical Association* **85**, 765–769.

[26] Liang, K.Y. & Zeger, S.L. (1986). Longitudinal data analysis using generalized linear models, *Biometrika* **73**, 13–22.

[27] Lin, D.Y. & Ying, Z. (1993). Cox regression with incomplete covariate measurements, *Journal of the American Statistical Association* **88**, 1341–1349.

[28] Lipsitz, S.R., Parzen, M. & Ewell, M. (1998). Inference using conditional logistic regression with missing covariates, *Biometrics* **54**, 295–303.

[29] Little, R.J.A. (1992). Regression with missing X's: A review, *Journal of the American Statistical Association* **87**, 1227–1237.

[30] Little, R.J.A. (1995). Modeling the drop-out mechanism in repeated-measures studies, *Journal of the American Statistical Association* **90**, 1112–1121.

[31] Lipsitz, S.R. & Ibrahim, J.G. (1996). Using the EM-algorithm for survival data with incomplete categorical covariates, *Lifetime Data Analysis* **2**, 5–14.

[32] Louis, T.A. (1982). Finding the observed information when using the EM algorithm, *Journal of the Royal Statistical Society, Series B* **44**, 226–233.

[33] Pepe, M.S. & Fleming, T.R. (1991). A nonparametric method for dealing with missing covariate data, *Journal of the American Statistical Association* **86**, 108–113.

[34] Prentice, R.L. & Pyke, R. (1979). Logistic disease incidence models and case–control studies, *Biometrika* **66**, 403–412.

[35] Pugh, M., Robins, J., Lipsitz, S. & Harrington, D. (1993). Inference in the Cox Proportional Hazards Model with Missing Covariate Data, *Technical Report 758Z*. Division of Biostatistics, Dana-Farber Cancer Institute, Boston.

[36] Reilly, M. & Pepe, M. (1995). A mean score method for missing and auxiliary covariate data in regression models, *Biometrika* **82**, 299–314.

[37] Reilly, M. & Pepe, M. (1997). The relationship between hot-deck multiple imputation and weighted likelihood, *Statistics in Medicine* **16**, 5–19.

[38] Robins, J.M. (1997). Non-response models for the analysis of non-ignorable missing data, *Statistics in Medicine* **16**, 21–37.

[39] Robins, J.M. & Gill, R. (1997). Non-response models for the analysis of non-monotone ignorable missing data, *Statistics in Medicine* **16**, 39–56.

[40] Robins, J.M., Rotnitzky, A. & Zhao, L.P. (1994). Estimation of regression coefficients when some regressors are not always observed, *Journal of the American Statistical Association* **89**, 846–866.

[41] Robins, J.M., Rotnitzky, A. & Zhao, L.P. (1995). Analysis of semiparametric regression models for repeated outcomes in the presence of missing data, *Journal of the American Statistical Association* **90**, 106–121.

[42] Rotnitzky, A. & Robins, J.M. (1997). Analysis of semiparametric regression models with non-ignorable non-response, *Statistics in Medicine* **16**, 81–102.

[43] Rubin, D.B. (1976). Inference and missing data, *Biometrika* **63**, 581–592.

[44] Rubin, D.B. (1981). The Bayesian bootstrap, *Annals of Statistics* **9**, 130–134.

[45] Rubin, D.B. (1987). *Multiple Imputation for Nonresponse in Surveys*. Wiley, New York.

[46] Rubin, D.B. & Schenker, N. (1991). Multiple imputation in health-care databases: An overview and some applications, *Statistics in Medicine* **10**, 585–598.

[47] Schemper, M. & Heinze, G. (1997). Probability imputation revisited for prognostic factor studies, *Statistics in Medicine* **16**, 73–80.

[48] Schemper, M. & Smith, T.L. (1990). Efficient evaluation of treatment effects in the presence of missing covariate values, *Statistics in Medicine* **9**, 777–784.

[49] Schill, W. & Drescher, K. (1997). Logistic analysis of studies with two-stage sampling: A comparison of four approaches, *Statistics in Medicine* **16**, 117–132.

[50] Schill, W., Jöckel, K.H., Drescher, K. & Timm, J. (1993). Logistic analysis in case–control studies under validation sampling, *Biometrika* **80**, 339–352.

[51] Schlehofer, B., Blettner, M., Becker, N., Martinsohn, C. & Wahrendorf, J. (1992). Medical risk factors and the development of brain tumor, *Cancer* **69**, 2541–2547.

[52] Schluchter, M.D. & Jackson, K.L. (1989). Log-linear analysis of survival data with partially observed covariates, *Journal of the American Statistical Association* **79**, 772–780.

[53] Scott, A.J. & Wild, C.J. (1991). Fitting logistic regression models in stratified case–control studies, *Biometrics* **47**, 497–510.

[54] Tanner, M. (1994). *Tools for Statistical Inference. Methods for the Exploration of Posterior Distributions and Likelihood Functions*. Springer-Verlag, New York.

[55] Vach, W. (1994). *Logistic Regression with Missing Values in the Covariates*, Lecture Notes in Statistics 86. Springer-Verlag, New York.

[56] Vach, W. (1997). Some issues in estimating the effect of prognostic factors from incomplete covariate data, *Statistics in Medicine* **16**, 57–72.

[57] Vach, W. & Blettner, M. (1991). Biased estimation of the odds ratio in case–control studies due to the use of ad-hoc methods of correcting for missing values for confounding variables, *American Journal of Epidemiology* **134**, 895–907.

[58] Vach, W. & Blettner, M. (1995). Logistic regression with incompletely observed categorical covariates – Investigating the sensitivity against violation of the missing at random assumption, *Statistics in Medicine* **14**, 1315–1329.

[59] Vach, W. & Illi, S. (1997). Biased estimation of adjusted odds ratios from incomplete covariate data due to violation of the MAR assumption, *Biometrical Journal* **39**, 13–28.

[60] Vach, W. & Schumacher, M. (1993). Logistic regression with incompletely observed categorical covariates – a comparison of three approaches, *Biometrika* **80**, 353–362.

[61] Williamson, G.D. & Haber, M. (1994). Models for three-dimensional contingency tables with completely and partially cross-classified data, *Biometrics* **50**, 194–203.

[62] White, J.E. (1982). A two-stage design for the study of the relationship between a rare exposure and a rare disease, *American Journal of Epidemiology* **115**, 119–128.

[63] Zhao, L.P. & Lipsitz, S. (1992). Designs and analysis of two-stage designs, *Statistics in Medicine* **11**, 769–782.

[64] Zhao, L.P., Lipsitz, S. & Lew, D. (1996). Regression analysis with missing covariate data using estimating equations, *Biometrics* **52**, 1165–1182.

[65] Zhou, H. & Pepe, M.S. (1995). Auxiliary covariate data in failure time regression, *Biometrika* **82**, 139–149.

(*See also* **Missing Data**)

WERNER VACH & MARIA BLETTNER

Missing Indicator Method for Missing Values *see* Missing Data in Epidemiologic Studies

Mitofsky–Waksberg Design for Telephone Sampling *see* Telephone Sampling

Molecular Epidemiology

Molecular epidemiology (ME) refers to the use of biomarkers in epidemiologic study designs, with emphasis on markers designed to measure exposure, to characterize host susceptibility, and to measure disease. Other terms involving closely related types of studies include biochemical epidemiology [16], pharmacogenetics [5], ecogenetics [10], and transitional studies [4], the last term referring to studies designed to bridge the gap between laboratory investigations and population studies. The first systematic description of the approach was provided by Perera & Weinstein [11]. They defined "molecular cancer epidemiology" as "advanced laboratory methods in combination with analytical epidemiology to identify at the biochemical or molecular level specific exogenous agents and/or host factors that play a role in human cancer causation". Consistent with the broad contribution of molecular biology to a more profound understanding of human disease, laboratory markers have been increasingly integrated into epidemiologic studies.

Objectives

ME can be viewed as a synthesis involving the application of the methods of molecular biology to the study of disease on the population level. The contribution of molecular biology during the last third of the twentieth century has resulted in a redefinition of our basic understanding of human disease. **Population-based studies** have also grown in size and sophistication as the need to understand the cause of disease has been better appreciated, especially in an era where high costs for medical care indicate a need for expanded efforts at disease prevention.

Biological markers used in classical epidemiologic study designs can contribute to understanding **dose–response** relationships by assessing biologically effective dose, making interspecies comparisons, quantifying human interindividual variability, and identifying subsets at altered risk [13, 16]. In addition, biomarkers may provide more sensitive, specific, quantitative, or reproducible indications of study endpoints than traditional approaches, and therefore may in theory improve both study efficiency and validity. Such markers might provide early or specific indications of disease, and thereby identify a cancer at an earlier more treatable stage, or even in time for a preventive intervention. The mechanistic insight gained from biomarkers study may enhance disease understanding in profound ways.

Types of Biomarkers

Biomarkers are used to make three general types of measurements: (i) internal exposure, often measuring a compound of interest bonded to a macromolecule (i.e. hemoglobin or deoxyribonucleic acid (DNA), a critical "target"), but also including substances or their metabolites such as nicotine or its metabolite cotinine as a marker for exposure to tobacco smoke; (ii) host susceptibility factors, typically metabolic traits that are due to hereditary variation; and (iii) early biologic effects, mutations or cytogenetic damage – these are "effect" markers, that is indicators of disease or biological effects of pathologic significance.

Although for discussion purposes these categories are considered distinct, there is overlap. For example, detection of nicotine in the blood might be considered a marker of smoking (exposure), or an indicator of potential pathologic effects (early effect or

disease marker), or might comprise part of a phenotype (e.g. ratio of nicotine to its metabolites) reflecting activity of a metabolizing enzyme (susceptibility factor).

Exposure Markers

The first category, exposure markers, offers the possibility of extending the reach of classic epidemiology beyond traditional questionnaire or external exposure monitoring. The actual dose of a compound of interest in the organism is assessed by the biomarker. Much attention has focused on measurement of adducts to DNA and other macromolecules, as it has been hypothesized that these might reflect both the relevant exposure, metabolic activation (generally considered an obligate step in carcinogenesis), and the actual quantity of compound that has reached a critical cellular target. In light of the target (i.e. DNA) involved, it is plausible that these compounds reflect a biologically relevant measure on the pathway to malignancy. The use of biomarkers is of course not new in the history of epidemiology. Examples include the use of polio antibody patterns to detect immunity. Some of the features of this approach that contrast with conventional epidemiology are indicated in Table 1.

Table 1 Conventional and molecular epidemiology

Feature	Conventional	Molecular
Use of biomarkers	Incidental	Systematic
Size	Varies, but often large	Varies, but typically small
Type of biomarker	Well established measures of exposure or disease	New or investigational markers of exposure, effect, or susceptibility
Cost	Low per subject	High per subject
Goals	Identify relationship between exposure and disease	Clarify mechanism and identify high-risk subgroups
Advantages	Historically the major method used to identify external cancer causes Public health orientation	Enter the "black box", i.e. elucidate mechanism Reduce interindividual variation Identify subsets at risk Potentially refine risk estimates Facile link to animal studies
Disadvantages	For certain cancers no cause is known, in spite of study Variable susceptibility is poorly understood Poor record at identifying reasons for individual susceptibility	Costly and complex Misclassification increased due to laboratory error Biomarker collection compromises validity Little public health benefit has resulted Ethical concerns

"Susceptibility Markers" and Genetic Studies

The second category of markers involves host susceptibility factors, typically but not always genetic (hereditary) traits that control the metabolism of substances involved directly or indirectly with human disease. A susceptibility factor modifies the disease risk conferred by a specific exposure. It is further distinguished from exposure because susceptibility is generally preexisting and nontransitory. An early focus of ME studies was a hypothesized genetic component in cancer. In contrast to earlier studies that searched for an obvious hereditary factor that accounted for the aggregation of specific cancers in families, these studies hypothesized that an influence of certain genes would exist for common apparently sporadic cancers in the general population as well.

Four studies in the 1980s laid the groundwork for the study of genetic susceptibility using epidemiologic study designs. This first generation of studies all involved a determination of a "metabolic phenotype", i.e. a pattern of metabolism of a test substance that would reflect the underlying inherited genetic trait. In 1979, Lower et al. reported a relationship between the acetylation phenotype and incidence of urinary bladder cancer [8]. This early report was an early example of a study involving a relationship between a common genetic factor that controls the metabolism of an environmental contaminant and a disease in a case and control population. The term "molecular epidemiology" appeared in the title. The hypothesis was that "slow acetylators", a group comprising 50% of Western populations, would be less able to acetylate and thereby inactivate carcinogenic aromatic amine carcinogens. The second study examined aryl hydrocarbon hydroxylase (AHH) inducibility in relation to lung cancer [6]. The 20% of the population with the high inducibility phenotype were thought to convert carcinogens in tobacco to their active form at an accelerated rate, accounting for their increased risk of lung cancer. Ayesh et al. studied the relationship of debrisoquine metabolism (*CYP2D6*), to lung cancer [1]. A fourth genetic factor, glutathione *S*-transferase (*GSTM1*) was studied in relation to lung cancer. Subjects without this activity, who were presumably deficient in ability to eliminate carcinogenic epoxides from cigarette smoke, exhibited excess lung cancer risk [14]. All of these studies relied on a laboratory measurement of a phenotype to infer the genetic susceptibility factor. In contrast, more recent studies directly identify the genotype through the study of an individual's DNA. Some of the advantages and disadvantages of the phenotype and genotype approaches are indicated in Table 2. Each of the four genetic traits initially approached with phenotypic measurements is under continued study today.

A major evolution over this period is the superseding of phenotype probe drug approaches by direct genotype assays. The genotype approach has distinct advantages and drawbacks (summarized in Table 2), but generally genotyping is increasingly the study

Table 2   The phenotype and genotype approaches in ME

Consideration	Phenotype	Genotype
Advantage	Approach is historically tested Reflects physiologic, *in vivo* disposition of drug Inducers, inhibitors, substrates all combine to reflect physiology	Identifies heterozygotes Simple, requires only germline DNA sample Unaffected by illness, diet, medications, etc. Can be performed with microquantities Noninvasive samples (i.e. DNA obtained from mouth wash, hair follicles, or standard blood sample)
Disadvantage	Numerous factors may distort measurements, e.g. drug–drug interaction More complex analysis Patient cooperation required Phenotyping protocols difficult to adapt to field study Time-consuming nature of test results in refusal to participate	Functional status of mutations may be unknown Risk of exposure to blood-borne pathogens Ethical questions arise since DNA may be used for other tests Allelic heterogeneity Ethnic differences

approach of choice. Acetylation phenotyping, originally accomplished by administering sulfa drugs or caffeine, is now performed using a direct genotyping approach that detects the major mutations in the *NAT2* gene. The association of slow acetylators (*NAT2*-deficient subjects) with bladder cancer has been repeatedly observed in subjects with occupational exposure to arylamines. The debrisoquine phenotype can likewise be accurately detected by genotyping of the *CYP2D6* gene. The genotype determination is more complex since partially activating and inactivating mutations exist, and many minor variants must be tested. The degree of association of this trait with lung cancer is controversial. It appears most likely that elevated risk for smoking-related cancer in extensive metabolizers is limited to subjects with heavy smoking histories [2]. Investigators have attempted to understand the relationship of AHH activity to polymorphisms of both the *CYP1A1* and *Ah receptor* genes. The precise relationship of the gene polymorphisms to enzyme activity (and presumably to the ability to activate carcinogens in tobacco, thereby accounting for lung cancer risk) is incompletely understood, and may involve other genes such as the Ah receptor. Studies of the phenotype are subject to **bias** (see Table 2) but have often shown an effect, while genotype studies have been negative in Western studies, but positive in Japan. These differences may reflect the fact that both the mutation frequency (i.e. gene frequency) and mutation type (allelic heterogeneity) exhibit ethnic variation. Finally, a summary of the available literature suggests that individuals that lack *GSTM1* activity (i.e. without at least one functional *GSTM1* allele) exhibit consistently increased risk of both lung and bladder cancer (relative risk 1.2–1.6) [3] (*see* **Genetic Epidemiology, Overview**).

Effect Markers

Effect markers comprise the third category. These include nonspecific markers such as mutations in *Salmonella typhimurium* detected in urine or feces, various assays for chromosomal abnormalities (e.g. micronuclei, sister-chromatid exchange), as well as more specific findings, such as the specific chromosome translocations that characterize hematologic malignancies. These markers complement better

known histologic and cytologic markers such as dyplasia or increased mitotic frequency.

Related Approaches

Inborn errors of metabolism were described by Garrod in the early twentieth century and are distinct from the genetic traits of interest to ME in that they invariably produced phenotypic manifestations and clinical consequences. In genetic terms, the associated condition was fully penetrant given the genotype. Most of the genetic traits of interest in ME are not highly penetrant. In pharmacogenetics, an area closely related to ME, the phenotype is detected with laboratory probes and does not always result in clinical sequelae, i.e. the condition is not fully penetrant. Sequelae result after specific exposures, typically to pharmaceutical agents (but also xenobiotics, carcinogens, or endogenous compounds) whose metabolism is dependent upon the enzyme (or receptor, immune factor, or other element) that is subject to pharmacogenetic variability. Chronic conditions are thought to occur with altered frequency based on long-term exposures to specific agents subject to this type of variability.

Criticism

The field has attracted much attention and methodological critique. First, there are those who have questioned whether ME is a true subdiscipline with substantive new content [9]. While no one distinguishing factor can uniquely identify ME studies, the alteration of study design to allow the use of biomarkers is probably characteristic. A second area that has generated negative comment is the small size and inadequate attention to design issues in some studies. The size of certain studies has been constrained by the cost of specific assays. For example, a newly developed or expensive gas chromatography/mass spectroscopy assay could cost over $1000 per sample. Given this limitation it is axiomatic that proper design of a study should be a major concern in order to achieve maximum efficiency. Certain goals of ME such as identifying subsets of the population at elevated risk will necessitate large sample size. Some studies have placed emphasis on the "molecular" aspects but with minimal "epidemiology" or sophistication in the statistical treatment. Both the quality and the co-opting of the "epidemiology" label to cover such studies are unfortunate, but some bad studies do not invalidate the proper use of the approach. Some have also dismissed the "molecular" modifier for epidemiology as unnecessary, stating that it is improper to identify a component of epidemiology based on a measurement technique, compared with recognized fields of epidemiology such as "pediatric", "infectious", "occupational", or "clinical". Such a complaint seems churlish given that the growth of scientific inquiry does not follow a set pattern and nomenclature is anything but consistent.

A more basic issue to emerge is that some goals of ME may not be attainable with the designs being used. For example, some proponents of ME would like to estimate the **absolute risk** of cancer in an individual associated with a specific set of genetic factors. While the general direction of inquiry is laudable, the hospital-based case–control approach (*see* **Case–Control Study, Hospital-Based**) often advocated is incompatible with this goal, and population-based case–control (*see* **Case–Control Study, Population-Based**) or **cohort** designs will be required. In addition, much larger studies (i.e. thousands of subjects rather than hundreds) will be required to detect gene–environment interactions of medical interest. The idea that combinations of factors (i.e. genetic factors plus mutation load) will refine individual risk [15] challenges the traditional public health advocacy of epidemiology and refocuses emphasis on "individual" clinical risk in a way that is disturbing to many [7, 9]. The implicit reductionism of the approach raises worrisome ethical issues. In particular, the improper use of genetic information derived from these studies in an increasing concern.

Two critiques finally emerge as central. The first is that historically, all the major etiologic environmental factors known to cause cancer have been identified not through mechanistic or animal studies, but through **observational studies** in humans. Smoking and lung cancer is a paradigmatic example. Case–control and cohort studies unequivocally demonstrated the association of tobacco use and lung cancer a least a decade before Aurbach's smoking beagles were shown to exhibit characteristic preneoplastic changes in the respiratory tract. Moreover, the history of epidemiology demonstrates that public health and prevention can be accomplished in the absence of detailed mechanistic understanding.

Secondly, it is difficult to demonstrate that specific biomarkers are superior to properly designed traditional questionnaire approaches to exposure assessment. A carefully designed smoking questionnaire will demonstrate a stronger association of tobacco use with lung cancer then either serum cotinine (nicotine metabolite marker of recent smoking) or smoking-related carcinogen adducts of hemoglobin (e.g. 4-aminobiphenyl, a marker of intermediate exposure). It can be argued that these markers relate to recent or intermediate time periods, and the exposure that caused the disease is remote. Nevertheless, without a clear public health benefit, one might ask whether ME studies are worth the cost in time, resources, lost eligible subjects (some will refuse a biospecimen request), and new sources of bias. The roles of questionnaire information and biomarkers are complementary, and there are clearly settings where questionnaire approaches are not suitable. Nevertheless, the tacit assumption that biomarkers are universally superior requires critical scrutiny [12].

Summary

The advances of molecular biology have transformed science in the late twentieth century and may ultimately be more far-reaching than the revolutionary advances of physics in the first half of the century. It is inevitable that this understanding must permeate scientific investigation involving human disease, including the study of disease on the population level. Epidemiology provides the tools for such study, and it is fitting that these tools will be transformed and adapted to optimize the use of biomarkers. The trend towards increasing emphasis on laboratory methods in clinical medicine shows no signs of declining, and such approaches will find application in the studies that define both the diseases and the factors that cause them. Seen in this context, the growth of molecular epidemiology is both natural and inevitable. To achieve the full potential of the ME approach, however, investigators will need to pay close attention to issues of study design and quality control.

References

[1]   Ayesh, R., Idle, J.R., Richie, J.C., Crothers, M.J. & Hetzel, M.R. (1984). Metabolic oxidation phenotypes as markers for susceptibility to lung cancer, *Nature* **312**, 169–170.

[2] Bouchardy, C., Benhamou, S. & Dayer, P. (1996). The effect of tobacco on lung cancer risk, *Cancer Research* **56**, 251–253.

[3] D'Errico, A., Taioli, E., Xiang, C. & Vineis, P. (1996). Genetic metabolic polymorphisms and the risk of cancer: A review of the literature, *Biomarkers* **1**, 174–177.

[4] Hulka, B.S. (1991). Epidemiological studies using biomarkers: issues for epidemiologists, *Cancer Epidemiology Biomarkers and Prevention* **1**, 13–19.

[5] Kalow, W. (1962). *Pharmacogenetics: Heredity and Response to Drugs*. W.B. Saunders, Philadelphia.

[6] Kellerman, G., Shaw, C.R. & Luyten-Kellerman, M. (1973). Aryl hydrocarbon hydroxylase inducibility and bronchogenic carcinoma, *New England Journal of Medicine* **289**, 934–937.

[7] Loomis, D. & Wing, S. (1990). Is molecular epidemiology a Germ Theory for the end of the twentieth century?, *International Journal of Epidemiology* **19**, 1–3.

[8] Lower, G.M., Nilsson, T., Nelson, C.E., Wolf, H., Gamsky, T.E. & Bryan, G.T. (1979). N-Acetyltransferase phenotype and risk in urinary bladder cancer: Approaches in molecular epidemiology. Preliminary results in Sweden and Denmark, *Environmental Health Perspectives* **29**, 71–79.

[9] McMichael, A.J. (1994). Invited commentary – molecular epidemiology: new pathway or new traveling companion?, *American Journal of Epidemiology* **140**, 1–11.

[10] Mulvihill, J.J. (1976). Host factors in human lung tumors, an example of ecogenetics in human oncology, *Journal of the National Cancer Institute* **57**, 3–7.

[11] Perera, F.P. & Weinstein, I.B. (1982). Molecular epidemiology and carcinogen–DNA adduct detection: New approaches to studies of human cancer detection, *Journal of Chronic Diseases* **35**, 581–600.

[12] Rothman, N., Stewart, W.F. & Shulte, P.A. (1995). Incorporating biomarkers into cancer epidemiology: a matrix of biomarker and study design categories, *Cancer Epidemiology Biomarkers and Prevention* **4**, 301–311.

[13] Schulte, P.A. & Mazzuckelli, L.F. (1991). Validation of biological markers for quantitative risk assessment, *Environmental Health Perspectives* **90**, 239–246.

[14] Seidegard, J., Pero, R.W., Miller, D. & Beattie, E.J. (1986). A glutathione transferase in human leukocytes as a marker for susceptibility to lung cancer, *Carcinogenesis* **7**, 751–753.

[15] Shields, P.G. & Harris, C.C. (1991). Molecular epidemiology and the genetics of environmental cancer, *Journal of the American Medical Association* **266**, 681–687.

[16] Vineis, P. & Caporaso, N. (1988). Applications of biochemical epidemiology in the study of human carcinogenesis, *Tumori* **74**, 19–26.

NEIL CAPORASO

Monotonic Agreement *see* Agreement, Measurement of

Morbidity and Mortality, Changing Patterns in the Twentieth Century

The twentieth century has been a period of unprecedented gains in longevity and health status. At the turn of the twentieth century, **life expectancy** at birth in Europe, North America, and Australia and New Zealand was typically around 45–50 years, similar to levels prevailing in Africa today, and not much greater than the levels of 35–40 years which had prevailed in Europe for centuries. As the twentieth century draws to a close, life expectancy in most industrialized countries is of the order of 75–80 years, or even higher for females in some countries. In other words, life expectancy has increased by more than 50% over the last 100 years or so in the industrialized world, but these gains have not been enjoyed equally by all population groups. The twentieth century has seen the emergence of dramatic inequalities in survival, notably between men and women, but also between the better educated and poorer sectors of society.

In this brief review of 100 years of epidemiologic history, trends and differentials in mortality will be presented to the extent that data are available to document them, and the emergence (or decline) of major epidemics and endemic conditions will be discussed. Much of the analysis will be limited to mortality data since this is the most comprehensive, comparable, and unambiguous source of information on health status. With the exception of cancer registries (*see* **Disease Registers**) for some (generally subnational) populations, and **surveillance** sites for vascular events included under the World Health Organization (WHO) Monitoring of Cardiovascular Diseases (MONICA) project, there are no comparable, standardized data on morbidity from which comparative trend analyses can be made. (MONICA is a 10-year (1984–94) epidemiologic surveillance system established in 35 countries, mostly industrialized, to *moni*tor *ca*rdiovascular disease incidence and mortality in defined populations, hence the name.) Equally importantly, there are no comparable data to investigate whether the extra years of life gained, particularly at older ages, have been accompanied by a rise, or fall, in disability. Data sources for assessing disability vary among countries and even within a population over time. Therefore little can be said, with any confidence, about changing patterns of disability, although this information is clearly required to assist policy and program formulation.

Data Sources for Mortality

Vital registration of births and deaths is the most useful source of mortality data for populations where complete recording of events has been achieved (*see* **Vital Statistics, Overview**). Where the death certificate includes diagnosis of the underlying **cause of death**, certified by a registered medical practitioner in accordance with the principles and procedures of the revision of the **International Classification of Diseases (ICD)** currently in force (*see* **Death Certification**), the information can also be used for epidemiologic assessments. Complete (or virtually complete) vital registration exists for industrialized countries, including Eastern Europe and the former USSR. In addition, several countries in developing regions of the world, including Argentina, Chile, Cuba, Mexico, Singapore, Uruguay, and some countries in the Caribbean have virtually complete registration and medical certification of deaths. Of the developing regions, medical certification of deaths is most advanced for Latin America and the Caribbean (43% of deaths), and least advanced in Sub-Saharan Africa (1% of deaths) [2].

Even in the absence of reliable vital registration data, patterns and levels of mortality can still be usefully ascertained through less expensive systems covering a sample of the population. For example, China has established a network of 145 Disease Surveillance Points (DSP) which record over 50 000 deaths annually in a population of 10 million people, representative of mortality conditions throughout China. Causes of death among the rural population in India are assessed via a "verbal autopsy" system operating from 1300 primary health care centers throughout the country. ("Verbal autopsy" is a method for diagnosing the approximate cause of death through a structured interview with relatives of the deceased. The interview is usually administered by a nonmedical person some weeks or months after death. Relatives are asked about a series of symptoms prior to death from which a diagnosis of the cause of death is made, preferably by a qualified physician.) While not as reliable as the DSP system in China, the Indian data are nonetheless useful for delineating broad cause of death patterns throughout the country [2].

Issues of Comparability

The interpretation of analyses of vital registration data on causes of death must be made with caution since the comparability of data is undoubtedly affected by many factors (*see* **Mortality, International Comparisons**). Even among the developed nations, where causes of death over the course of the twentieth century have generally been classified according to standards and principles agreed upon by various international committees (since 1948, under the auspices of WHO), variations in diagnostic practice among countries affect data comparisons. A WHO international comparative study carried out in the 1960s reported significant variations in certification practices among six European countries with major differences in the proportion of deaths which were certified by pathologists [11]. No doubt these differences have diminished in recent decades [3], but the practice of autopsy still varies substantially among industrialized countries, with implications for data comparability [12].

Cultural differences also no doubt are a significant factor in the coding of injuries. Suicides in particular are undoubtedly underreported in some countries owing to the social or religious stigma associated with the act, with the death in such cases usually being coded to accidental injuries [7]. Studies have also revealed "diagnostic preferences" for chronic diseases. For example, in the 1950s and early 1960s, deaths which were coded to chronic respiratory diseases in the UK, Australia, and New Zealand may well have been coded to a cardiovascular disease in the US [6].

The statistical comparability of cause of death data has certainly been affected by the successive revisions of the ICD. The most profound change occurred with the introduction of the Sixth Revision around 1950, in which major alterations to the format of the list of causes were made to accommodate the sweeping changes in the principles of cause of death classification introduced with that revision. The introduction of the Eighth Revision in 1968 substantially affected the time series comparability of certain major causes of death, particularly ischemic heart disease (IHD), with up to 15% more deaths being coded to IHD than to the most comparable cause in the Seventh Revision [10].

The comparability of epidemiologic analyses of mortality data is also very much affected by the extent to which deaths are coded to ill-defined and unspecified diagnoses. This affects both comparisons among countries as well as trends within a country over time. For example, around 1950, approximately 15%–20% of all deaths in Belgium, France, Greece, Poland, and Spain were coded to ill-defined causes, compared with 1%–2% in Australia, Austria, Canada, Denmark, New Zealand, Switzerland, the UK, and the US. Without adjustment for diseases coded to ill-defined conditions, cross-national comparisons might be very misleading [5]. By the early 1990s, ill-defined causes throughout the industrialized world had declined to about 1%–3% of all deaths. For countries where this practice was common four decades ago, time series analyses for specific causes (especially cardiovascular diseases) must be interpreted with great prudence.

Trends in Life Expectancy and Age-Specific Mortality Rates

Life Expectancy

Life expectancy at birth is a convenient summary index of prevailing mortality conditions at each age. The measure is not a linear function of age-specific death rates and hence equal reductions in mortality at different ages will not have an identical impact on life expectancy – a reduction in death rates at younger ages will result in a larger gain in life expectancy at birth than a similar reduction in death rates at older ages. Despite this feature, life expectancy is widely understood and is perhaps still the most commonly used indicator to summarize overall mortality levels in a population.

Table 1 provides an overview of the gains in life expectancy in selected countries over the course of the twentieth century. By far the largest absolute increase has been enjoyed in Japan (34 years for males, 39 years for females), followed by Italy. Much less progress has been registered in Eastern Europe although national trends are not strictly comparable owing to differences in time period, **life table** methodologies, and population coverage around the turn of the century. What the table does suggest, however, is that the pattern of mortality reduction among the industrialized countries is extremely heterogeneous and that, while significant progress has been achieved, there has been more divergence than convergence among the industrialized countries.

Viewing trends in life expectancy over almost a century can conceal significant time trends that have characterized this century of mortality change. Life expectancy at birth has not increased monotonically since the early 1900s. Rather, significant gains were achieved virtually everywhere until the beginning of the 1950s. From the mid-1950s, male life expectancy stagnated, or even declined modestly in some Western European countries, as well as in Australia and North America (see Figure 1). Meanwhile, female life expectancy continued to rise. From the mid-to-late 1960s, male life expectancy began to rise again, quite sharply in some countries. At about the same time, one of the most remarkable reversals in life expectancy began throughout Eastern Europe with male life expectancy declining by up to 4–5 years in most countries, and by even more (7 years) in Russia [9]. Even this general trend has been accompanied by significant national variations with male life expectancy beginning to show signs of a renewed rise in the Czech Republic, Hungary, and Poland, but deteriorating markedly in Russia since 1988, having risen sharply in the former USSR between 1980 and 1987 [9].

Demographers and epidemiologists have been studying these remarkable changes in Eastern Europe for more than two decades. Most would agree that the trends are real and not due to sudden changes in the completeness or accuracy of reporting of deaths following widespread social and political change in the late 1980s. Epidemiologic research suggests that much of the pervasive increase in male mortality in Eastern Europe since the late 1960s is due to tobacco usage [4] or, in the case of the recent dramatic mortality increases in Russia, alcohol abuse [8].

Table 1 Life expectancy at birth, 1900–95, selected countries
(a) Males

Country	Life expectancy at birth in				
	1900–10	1930–40	1950–55[a]	1970–75[a]	1990–95[a]
Japan	42.4	47.9	62.1	70.6	76.4
Sweden	56.6	62.1	70.4	72.1	75.4
Australia	57.6	63.6	69.9	68.4	74.7
Spain		47.2	61.6	70.2	74.6
Netherlands		63.7	70.9	71.1	74.4
Italy	43.0	53.4	64.3	69.2	74.2
Norway	56.4	62.6	70.9	71.4	73.6
UK	45.3		66.7	69.0	73.6
France	43.4	55.2	63.7	68.6	73.0
Denmark		61.4	69.6	70.9	72.5
New Zealand	58.0	63.3	67.5	68.7	72.5
US	45.6	57.6	66.2	67.5	72.5
Poland			58.6	67.0	66.7
Hungary			61.5	66.5	64.5
Russian Federation	30.9	40.4	62.5	63.1	61.7

(b) Females

Country	Life expectancy at birth in				
	1900–10	1930–40	1950–55[a]	1970–75[a]	1990–95[a]
Japan	43.7	50.7	65.9	76.2	82.5
Sweden	59.5	64.2	73.3	77.5	81.1
France	47.0	59.8	69.5	76.3	80.8
Australia	61.4	67.3	72.4	75.2	80.6
Italy	43.7	55.5	67.8	75.2	80.6
Spain		50.8	66.3	75.7	80.5
Netherlands		65.0	73.4	77.0	80.4
Norway	59.3	65.8	74.5	77.6	80.3
US	48.3	61.0	72.0	75.3	79.3
UK	49.3		71.8	75.2	78.7
New Zealand	59.9	66.0	71.8	74.8	78.6
Denmark		63.3	72.4	76.4	78.2
Poland			64.2	74.1	75.7
Hungary			65.8	72.4	73.8
Russian Federation	33.0	46.7	70.5	73.5	73.6

[a]Annual average.

Age-Specific Mortality Change

Given the very close relationship between the age-pattern of mortality and the prevailing cause of death structure – infectious diseases tend to kill many more children than adults, while chronic diseases do the converse – the conquest of the communicable diseases such as tuberculosis, measles, malaria, diarrheal diseases, and acute respiratory infections, which had largely been completed in the industrialized countries by 1950 or thereabouts, has resulted in massive declines in **infant mortality** and child mortality, and a significant reduction of death rates among young adults.

Around 1900, infant mortality rates in Australasia, Europe, or North America typically hovered around 100–150 deaths per 1000 live births, similar to levels currently prevailing in many African countries (see Table 2). Overall child mortality rates (measured as the probability of a newborn infant dying before age

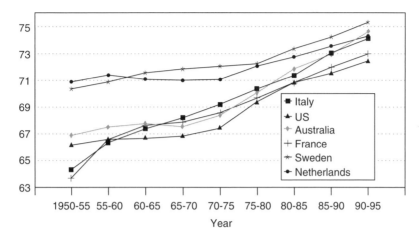

Figure 1 Trends in life expectancy at birth in selected countries, 1950–95, males

Table 2 Infant mortality rate (per 1000 live births)

Country	1900	1930	1950–55	1970–75	1990–95
Japan	168M/147F		51	12	4
Finland			34	12	5
Iceland			21	12	5
Sweden	78M/63F	62M/47F	20	10	5
Belgium			45	19	6
Germany			51	21	6
Switzerland		61M/48F	29	13	6
Australia	74M/59F	45M/36F	24	17	7
Austria			53	24	7
Canada		105M/82F	36	16	7
Denmark		89M/69F	28	12	7
France		80M/63F	45	16	7
Ireland			41	18	7
Luxembourg			44	16	7
Netherland		54M/41F	24	12	7
Spain		150M/130F	62	21	7
UK			29	17	7
Italy	176M/158F	112M/100F	60	26	8
Norway	75M/61F	50M/41F	23	12	8
Czech Republic			43	20	9
Israel			41	23	9
Malta			75	22	9
New Zealand	80M/69F	44M/36F	26	16	9
US	162M/133F	73M/58F	28	18	9
Greece		98M/97F	60	34	10
Portugal		196M/166F	91	45	10
Slovokia			73	24	12
Bulgaria			92	26	14
Hungary			71	34	15
Poland			95	27	15
Yugoslavia			110	47	20
Russian Federation			98	28	21
Romania			101	40	23

5) were of the order of 200 per 1000 live births. In 1995, infant mortality rates in the industrialized countries are typically around 10 or less per 1000 live births, reaching as low as 4–5 per 1000 in Japan and parts of Scandinavia.

Although less dramatic, and with some interruptions for men as noted earlier, adult mortality levels have also declined more or less continuously since the beginning of the twentieth century. This decline has been much more evident for women, although evidence of a stagnation in mortality rates for women in some Eastern European countries first became evident in the early 1970s. Since the late 1970s, several countries, including Australia, the Netherlands, the UK, and the US, have seen further substantial reductions in male (and female) mortality, both in middle and old age. Much of this recent decline in death rates can be attributed to further declines in IHD and stroke mortality, continuing a trend which began in the late 1960s.

From this brief analysis, one may conclude that adult mortality rates tend to be higher in populations with higher overall mortality and tend to decline (more or less monotonically) with declines in general mortality levels. This is perhaps counterintuitive, but is confirmed by recent global mortality analyses which suggest that the risk of adult death throughout the developing world is substantially higher than in Australasia, North America, Japan, and Western Europe [2].

Demographers have developed methods to decompose or disaggregate changes in life expectancy at birth into contributions due to changes in mortality at different ages. These can be either positive contributions (in which case mortality rates in the age group have declined), or negative, whereby life expectancy has increased despite an increase in mortality rates in a given age group. To illustrate the utility of these methods, the age pattern of contributions to life expectancy trends for males in three populations, Australia, England and Wales, and Hungary, are shown in Table 3 for the period 1950–79.

The very substantial contribution (in years) from post-1950 declines in infant and child mortality is evident in all three populations (1.37 years out of a 3.0 year increase in life expectancy in England and Wales, 4.32 years of a 4.9 year increase in Hungary, and 1.48 years out of a 4.2 year gain in Australia) [1]. Since mortality rates at ages 15–34 years were already comparatively low in the early 1950s, further

declines at these ages did not contribute greatly to changes in life expectancy. Reductions in mortality for higher age-groups resulted in similar absolute contributions to increasing life expectancy in both England and Wales, and Hungary, at least until the mid-1960s.

Given the abrupt cessation of overall male mortality decline in Hungary and neighboring countries from the mid-1960s and the rapid increase in male life expectancy in Australia (and other Western countries) since the early 1970s, analyses for these subperiods are also presented in the table.

The complexity of age patterns of mortality change and their influence on overall life expectancy is well illustrated by these two examples which, in many respects, are representative of recent mortality trends in the industrialized countries. In Hungary, male life expectancy remained unchanged between 1960–64 and 1975–78 (but declined subsequently). This was due to rises in mortality (i.e. negative contributions to life expectancy) at all ages 25 years and older, and particularly at ages 45–54 years. Conversely, further declines in infant and child mortality, and, to a much lesser extent, at ages 15–24 years, acted to increase life expectancy but were exactly counteracted by rising death rates at older ages. The pattern of mortality change in Australia over the same period was exactly the reverse. Between 1950–54 and 1970–76, male life expectancy hardly changed at all (up by 1.3 years), almost all of which (0.9 years) was due to declines in infant and child death rates, with only small (positive or negative) contributions from relatively stable adult death rates. During the 1970s, however, male death rates at ages 45 and over declined dramatically in Australia, accounting for 1.9 years of the 2.9 year increase in life expectancy at birth, with much of the remainder (0.6 years) being due to continued declines in infant and child mortality.

Sex Differentials in Mortality

One of the most remarkable features of twentieth century mortality decline in the industrialized countries has been the dramatic widening of male–female differentials in mortality. Around the turn of the century, life expectancy for females was typically 2–3 years higher than for males, and in some countries, such as Ireland and Italy, the gap was less than 1 year.

Table 3 Age components of changing life expectancy at birth, selected nations, 1950–54 to 1979

Country	Life table periods	Sex	Contribution (in years) to change in life expectancy at birth due to mortality trends at ages									Total increase in life expectancy (in years)[a]
			0–14	15–24	25–34	35–44	45–54	55–64	65–74	75+	Interaction	
UK: England and Wales	1950–54 to 1975–78	M	1.37	0.06	0.21	0.20	0.25	0.42	0.24	0.19	0.09	3.0
		F	1.16	0.16	0.29	0.21	0.21	0.35	0.64	0.77	0.20	4.0
		F–M	−0.21	0.10	0.08	−0.01	−0.04	−0.07	0.40	0.58	0.11	1.0
Hungary	1950–54 to 1975–78	M	2.83	0.33	0.29	0.30	0.41	0.27	0.18	0.18	0.16	4.9
		F	2.50	0.37	0.38	0.29	0.33	0.44	0.42	0.30	0.22	5.3
		F–M	−0.33	0.04	0.09	−0.01	−0.08	0.17	0.24	0.12	0.06	0.4
	1960–64 to 1975–78	M	1.49	0.08	−0.02	−0.30	−0.54	−0.27	−0.31	−0.12	0.01	0.0
		F	1.33	0.07	0.07	0.00	−0.06	−0.01	0.17	0.18	0.02	1.8
		F–M	−0.16	−0.01	0.09	0.30	0.48	0.26	0.48	0.30	0.01	1.8
Australia	1950–54 to 1970–74	M	0.87	0.05	0.13	0.10	0.08	0.10	−0.01	−0.01	0.01	1.3
		F	0.79	0.06	0.17	0.20	0.25	0.27	0.41	0.49	0.09	2.7
		F–M	−0.08	0.01	0.04	0.10	0.17	0.17	0.42	0.50	0.08	1.4
	1970–74 to 1979	M	0.61	0.07	0.02	0.19	0.30	0.52	0.55	0.48	0.17	2.9
		F	0.35	0.03	0.07	0.18	0.28	0.39	0.60	0.95	0.18	3.0
		F–M	−0.26	−0.04	0.05	−0.01	−0.02	−0.13	0.05	0.47	0.01	0.1

Source: [1]

[a]The age components and the interaction contribution may not sum exactly to the total due to rounding.

Female mortality rates exceeded those of males in many countries at various ages up to the end of the child-bearing period. Indeed, the contribution of maternal mortality to the sex mortality differential around the turn of the century was sufficiently high to reduce the female advantage in life expectancy over males by 0.3 to 0.5 years [1]. Conversely, accidents and violence were a major cause of male excess mortality, typically accounting for about half of the female advantage in life expectancy at birth.

By far the largest contribution to the increase in male excess mortality by the mid-1960s was the diverging mortality trends for men and women from cardiovascular diseases, at least in Australia and the US. A similar pattern is also evident in the Scandinavian countries (and indeed in most other industrialized nations) after 1950.

The contribution of cancer to widening sex mortality differentials is rather more complex. Prior to about 1930, female mortality from cancer exceeded that for men, largely due to cancers of the genital tract. By the mid-1960s, about half a year had been added to the gap in life expectancy in Australia and Scandinavia due to differential male–female trends from cancer, and almost a full year in the US. Much of this, and subsequent increases after 1960, can be attributed to the massive increase in male lung cancer mortality (see next section). Finally, it is also interesting to observe the growth in the contribution of male excess mortality from motor vehicle accidents. Around 1910, there were too few cars for this to be a significant cause of death. Since then death rates from car crashes rose dramatically, especially for males, so that by 1964, this cause alone contributed about half a year to the gap in life expectancy between the sexes.

Sex differentials in mortality have continued to widen in recent decades with the result that average life expectancy at birth for females is currently typically about 6–7 years higher than for males, and in some countries (e.g. Hungary and France) the gap is closer to 9 years. In others, e.g. Australia and the UK, there is evidence that the sex differential in mortality is no longer increasing. This is due to the very substantial declines in male mortality from lung cancer, IHD, and stroke in these countries, following widespread reductions in smoking by men which began several decades ago.

Cause of Death Trends

The twentieth century has been characterized by a massive decline in **communicable diseases** and maternal and perinatal causes in industrialized countries, and increasingly in many developing countries as well. The extent of this reduction is well illustrated in Figure 2, which shows the **proportionate mortality** for males in selected countries from various broad causes over the last 100 years or so. The pattern for females is broadly similar, with the added feature that maternal deaths have declined from around 2%–5% of female deaths in the early 1900s to less than one-tenth of 1% today. From causing about 30% of deaths around 1900, infectious and parasitic diseases now cause less than 5% of deaths in the industrialized countries, and this figure would be even lower were it not for the acquired immune deficiency syndrome (AIDS) epidemic. Noncommunicable diseases have emerged as the leading causes of death by far as the twentieth century draws to a close, despite the very substantial reductions in vascular disease mortality in some developed countries in recent decades.

The trends in accidents and violence (external causes) are particularly interesting. Although the proportionate contribution of these nonmedical causes to overall mortality has remained relatively constant at around 6%–8%, the composition of causes within the category of accidents and violence has changed dramatically. For example, earlier in the century, industrial accidents were the leading cause of male deaths from external causes, reflecting the risks associated with several occupations commonly practiced at that time (see **Occupational Mortality**). Subsequently, with the modernization of the labor market and legislative reform for occupational safety, these accidents have greatly diminished in frequency. For males, at least, motor vehicle accidents have emerged as the principal cause of death from nonmedical causes, rising from virtually zero around 1900 to account for about 30% of violent deaths among males in many industrialized countries, and an even higher proportion (50% or so) of violent deaths at the young adult ages (15–34 years) (see Figure 3).

An overview of mortality change in the industrialized countries since 1950 is given in Figure 4, which shows the *relative* change (death rate in 1950–54 = 100) in age-standardized death rates from selected

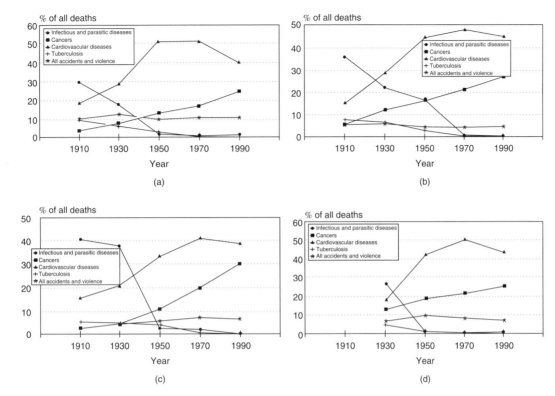

Figure 2 Proportionate mortality (in %) from broad causes, selected countries, males, 1910–90. (a) US, (b) England and Wales, (c) Italy, and (d) Denmark

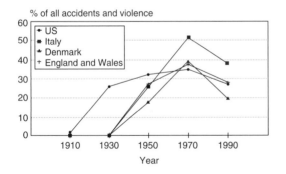

Figure 3 Proportion of all violent deaths due to motor vehicle accidents, selected countries, males, 1910–90

leading causes of death for men and women separately (*see* **Standardization Methods**). The graph shows the average experience of 22 industrialized countries and demonstrates the varied epidemiologic history of the world's richest countries over the last

few decades. The rise (for men) and then steady decline in IHD and stroke mortality is clear, as is the peak in motor vehicle accident mortality in the early 1970s. Since then, death rates from traffic crashes have returned to levels last seen in the 1950s for women, and 25% lower than the 1950–54 level for males. This has occurred despite a dramatic increase in the number of motor cars. This remarkable reversal is due to a number of factors, including improved highway conditions and stricter measures to control drunken driving in these countries.

But perhaps the most dramatic change in mortality since the middle of the century has been the extraordinary growth in lung cancer mortality, for both males and females. Male lung cancer rates have increased, on average, by almost 200% since 1950–54, while for females, the rise, in relative terms at least, has been even greater (more than 300%). Even though the relative increase in lung cancer rates has been

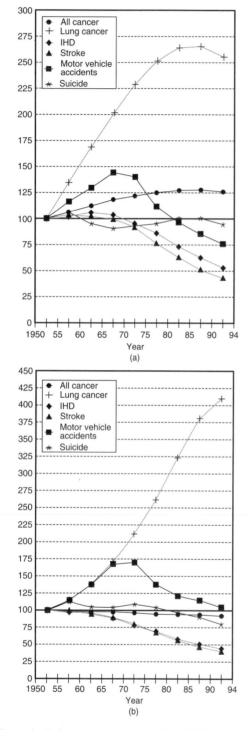

Figure 4 Relative change in mortality (1950–54 = 100) for selected causes of death in 22 industrialized countries, 1950–54 to 1990–94, (a) males, (b) females

higher for females, the absolute level of rates is still much higher in males owing to their longer smoking history. The enormity of the lung cancer epidemic in the industrialized countries during the course of the twentieth century is perhaps best summarized by the trends for the US (see Figure 5).

From a level of around five deaths per 100 000 in 1930, US male lung cancer rates have risen about 15-fold to peak in the early 1990s. Other cancers have remained relatively stable, or, in the case of stomach cancer, declined substantially. For women, the rise in lung cancer only began in the early 1960s, some decades after American women began to smoke in large numbers.

There have been notable successes in reducing lung cancer mortality, particularly in Australia, Finland, the Netherlands, and the UK, where death rates from the disease have been steadily declining and are now at levels 20%–40% below their peaks. Male lung cancer rates in some industrialized countries are still rising, most notably in Japan (an increase of over 1000% since 1950), but also in Greece, Hungary, Portugal, Poland, and Spain. Indeed, lung cancer mortality in Hungary in 1994 reached 122 deaths/100 000 population (age-standardized), exceeding even the highest level reported for UK men (111/100 000) at the height of their epidemic (1974) [12].

Lung cancer death rates for women are rising everywhere except in Australia, New Zealand, and the UK, where death rates appear to have stabilized. The highest mortality rate for women in the mid-1990s is reported for Scottish women (45/100 000), closely followed by Denmark and the US (40/100 000). Indeed, in several populations (see Figure 5), lung cancer now exceeds breast cancer as the leading site for mortality from the disease.

Along with the reversal in lung cancer rates for men in some countries, the other great public health success of the second half of the twentieth century has been the extraordinary decline in IHD mortality and stroke (cerebrovascular disease). Beginning in the mid-to-late 1960s, death rates from these diseases began to decline following a decade or more of rising rates in many countries. Death rates are now less than half their post World War II peak levels and are still declining. Largely as a result of these declines in major vascular diseases, overall mortality levels have fallen by up to 40% in many Western countries.

The other major disease for which significant progress in reducing mortality has been achieved

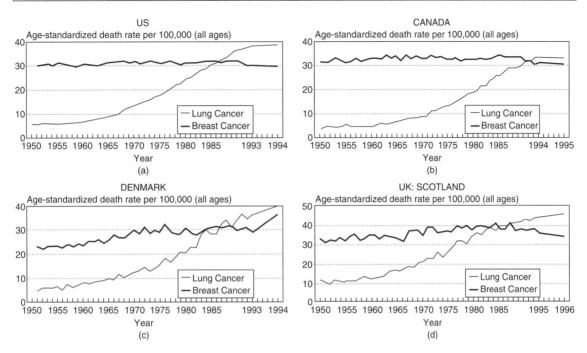

Figure 5 Trends in breast and lung cancer mortality among women, selected countries, 1950–95. (a) US, (b) Canada, (c) Denmark, and (d) UK (Scotland)

is cirrhosis of the liver. In countries such as Australia, France, Germany, Portugal, and Spain, male death rates from the disease rose steadily during the 1950s and 1960s and reached a peak level of 45–55 deaths/100 000 population in the mid-1970s. Since then, death rates have halved in France and Portugal, and have declined by 20%–30% in the other countries where death rates from the disease have been comparatively high. On the contrary, there is limited evidence that mortality has declined among men in Eastern Europe, and indeed it appears to be rising in several of these countries.

Whither the Future: Mortality and Causes of Death in the Twenty-First Century

As the twentieth century draws to a close, it is perhaps important to reflect briefly on major threats to health in the first decades of the twenty-first century. Unquestionably, the two epidemics of greatest public health concern must be use of *tobacco* and human immunodeficiency virus (HIV) infection. Between 1950 and 2000, tobacco will have caused over 60 million deaths in the developed countries

of the world, more than 50 million men and about 10 million women [4]. In 1998, tobacco was estimated to have caused about 8 million deaths globally, about 2 million in the developed countries and about 2 million, but with substantial uncertainty, in less developed countries. In the twentieth century, most of the deaths from tobacco have been in developed populations, but in the twenty-first century the opposite will be true. The annual numbers of deaths are still increasing in developed populations but they are increasing even faster elsewhere. Over the past few decades there has been a massive rise in global cigarette consumption, particularly in developing countries, where 50% of men smoke. On current trends, annual global tobacco deaths are likely to reach 10 million by about 2030. The chief uncertainty is not whether, but when, annual mortality will reach this level. On present smoking patterns, half a billion of the world's current population will eventually be killed by tobacco. These predictions will be substantially wrong only if there are substantial changes in global smoking patterns.

AIDS, caused by HIV, is the only other major cause of death that is rising rapidly. First diagnosed in the early 1980s, the disease is estimated to have caused about 400 000 deaths in 1990, the majority in Sub-Saharan Africa [2]. **Epidemic modeling** of the disease suggests that the peak in global mortality will be attained sometime between 2005 and 2010, when annual deaths are predicted to reach about 1.7 to 1.8 million a year [2]. Beyond then, the epidemic is expected to decline slowly due to the past (and projected) efforts at prevention. As with tobacco, these projections could be gross underestimates if HIV incidence were to increase rapidly in some large population groups. If this were to happen, it would most probably occur in Asia where seroprevalence has been increasing dramatically in some high-risk populations.

The third area for concern is the emergence, or reemergence, of various infectious diseases which, if uncontrolled, could cause a substantial number of deaths in the future. The reemergence of tuberculosis as a significant health issue in the developed countries is an object lesson for the public health profession not to become complacent about past successes in disease control. Equally, the ebola virus as well as significant cholera outbreaks attest to the need for continual vigilance in **surveillance of diseases**. Finally, the very large unfinished agenda of controlling the leading causes of child mortality in developing countries, particularly diarrheal diseases, acute respiratory infections, the vaccine-preventable diseases, and malaria, which each year collectively kill more than 12 million infants and young children [2], must remain a major global public health priority into the next century.

References

[1]   Lopez, A.D. (1983). The sex mortality differential in developed countries, in *Sex Differentials in Mortality: Trends, Determinants and Consequences*, A.D. Lopez & L.T. Ruzicka, eds. Australian National University Press, Canberra, pp. 53–120.

[2]   Murray, C.J.L. & Lopez, A.D. (1996). Estimating causes of death: new methods and global and regional applications in 1990, in *The Global Burden of Disease*, C.J.L. Murray & A.D. Lopez, eds. Harvard University Press on behalf of the World Health Organization and the World Bank, Cambridge, Mass, pp. 117–200.

[3]   Percy, C. & Muir, C. (1989). The international comparability of cancer mortality data: results of an international death certificate study, *American Journal of Epidemiology* **129**, 934–946.

[4]   Peto, R., Lopez, A.D., Boreham, J., Thun, M. & Heath, C. (1994). *Mortality from Smoking in Developed Countries, 1950–2000*. Oxford University Press, Oxford.

[5]   Preston, S.N. (1976). *Mortality Patterns in National Populations*. Academic Press, New York.

[6]   Reid, D.D. & Rose, G.A. (1964). Assessing the comparability of mortality statistics, *British Medical Journal* **2**, 1437–1439.

[7]   Ruzicka, L.T. (1995). Suicide mortality in developed countries, in *Adult Mortality in Developed Countries: From Description to Explanation*, A.D. Lopez, G. Caselli & T. Valkonen, eds. Clarendon Press, Oxford, pp. 83–110.

[8]   Shkolnikov, V. & Nemstov, A. (1997). *The Anti-Alcohol Campaign and Variations in Russian Mortality*. National Academy of Sciences, Washington.

[9]   Shkolnikov, V., Meste, F. & Vallin, J. (1996). Health crisis in Russia II. Changes in causes of death: a comparison with France and England and Wales (1970 to 1993), *Population* **8**, 155–189.

[10]   United States Department of Health, Education and Welfare (1975). *Comparability of Mortality Statistics for the Seventh and Eighth Revisions of the International Classification of Diseases, United States*. Public Health Service, Series 2, No. 66.

[11]   World Health Organization (1967). The accuracy and comparability of death statistics, *World Health Organization Chronicle* **21**, 11–17.

[12]   World Health Organization (1996). *World Health Statistics Annual 1995*. World Health Organization, Geneva.

ALAN D. LOPEZ

Mortality, International Comparisons

The international comparison of mortality or other health-related statistics is probably the most useful, simple, and widely used method to assess the health status of the population of a particular country. In most cases health can be measured only in relative terms, by placing the country on a scale between the best and worst achievements being observed in other countries. Most often, comparisons are made between countries in a specific geographic region or with similar level of socioeconomic development. Such comparisons form an important part of national public health reports or documents on national health policies. Publications and reports of international organizations active in the field of health are usually also largely based on international comparisons of health statistics including mortality data. International mortality comparisons are often the subject of research papers.

To make international comparisons of health data possible, there are several essential and obvious conditions. Data have to be available from a sufficient number of countries and they must be based on the same definitions in order to be comparable. In this respect, mortality statistics are probably the best presently available health data for international comparisons. The World Health Organization (WHO) has been collecting mortality information since the early 1950s, just after the establishment of the Organization. Currently, about 70 countries are regularly reporting detailed data to the WHO on an annual basis. These statistics are based on the concept of the underlying cause of death (*see* **Death Certification**) and are usually coded using the **International Classification of Diseases** (ICD). Generally, these data can be estimated as being of good quality (accuracy) particularly in developed countries with well established and functioning systems of **vital statistics**. However, there are many potential methodologic problems limiting the comparability of mortality data even among developed countries. These problems are mostly related to the coding of the underlying cause of death (*see* **Cause of Death, Underlying and Multiple**). However, the impact of variations in coding procedures on actual cause-specific mortality statistics is very difficult to measure regularly in quantitative terms, as it requires special studies to compare actual methods and practices of coding death certificates between countries. Studies which have been carried out so far have confirmed the perception that in some cases differences in the coding methods and practices may cause significant **bias** in the number of deaths from specific diseases. There are several elements in death registration which may have an influence on the international comparability or may cause an artifact in the trend of particular cause-specific mortality within the country. At least the following could be mentioned:

1. the level of training and corresponding practices in filling in death certificates by health professionals;
2. the form of the certificate itself – for example, the number of lines provided to list underlying and intermediate causes of death;
3. the regulations and administrative structures defining further transfer and processing of death certificates – for example, whether completeness and quality are controlled locally;

4. the coding of the cause of death from the written textual form into the ICD code – for example, whether it is done locally or centrally, manually or automated.

Another factor that is often forgotten, but which may cause significant bias in mortality rates used for international comparisons, is related to the population estimates used as a denominator to calculate mortality rates; for example, the number of deaths per 100 000 population. The total resident population in a given country is counted more or less accurately only during population censuses, which in most countries are carried out once every 10 years. In between census periods, population estimates are calculated on the basis of births, deaths, immigration, emigration, and aging of the population (*see* **Demography**). In practice, these estimates may not be accurate enough. When such estimates are used to calculate mortality rates, these inaccuracies can cause distortion in mortality trends and, correspondingly, in international comparisons.

Usually it is difficult to detect whether there is any bias in the mortality data of a particular country as compared to other countries. However, one has to keep in mind this possibility while making international comparisons.

There are also several statistical aspects that have to be taken into account in order to avoid the possibility of misleading conclusions based on international comparisons. First of all, the absolute number of deaths, without taking into account the size of the population, should not be used. Mortality rates or other indices should normally be used. In cases in which mortality for all ages or for a wide age band is compared, appropriate mortality rates have to be age-standardized beforehand (*see* **Standardization Methods**). Comparisons of crude death rate (i.e. a simple ratio of the number of deaths to the population size) are often misleading, particularly when one compares countries with different population age structures. For example, the crude death rate is usually higher in developed countries compared to developing ones, although an opposite situation should be expected when considering the health of the population in general. This happens purely because of differences in population structure; that is, developed countries have a much higher proportion of older people with, naturally, high mortality. There are two methods (direct and indirect) to age-standardize mortality rates in order to eliminate the influence of differences in population age structure between countries. If there is a sufficient amount of data for each age group, usually the direct method is used. Mortality rates are calculated for each age group and then are combined into the one index, assuming that the given country has the "standard" population structure. There are two commonly used standards for international comparisons: the world and the European standard populations (see Table 1).

The indirect method of standardization is usually used in cases in which relatively rare causes of deaths are compared, or there are not enough data due to other reasons, to estimate mortality in each age group. This standardization is based on the assumption that the age-specific mortality is the same – that is, "standard" – in each country. These "standard" age-specific mortality rates are usually calculated using combined data from all countries included in the comparisons. The expected number of deaths is calculated on the basis of the above "standard" mortality rates and the actual age distribution of the population in a given country. The ratio of actually observed and calculated expected cases is used as the standardized mortality ratio.

Table 1   Standard populations (world and European)

Age group (years)	World	European
0	2 400	1 600
1–4	9 600	6 400
5–9	10 000	7 000
10–14	9 000	7 000
15–19	9 000	7 000
20–24	8 000	7 000
25–29	8 000	7 000
30–34	6 000	7 000
35–39	6 000	7 000
40–44	6 000	7 000
45–49	6 000	7 000
50–54	5 000	7 000
55–59	4 000	6 000
60–64	4 000	5 000
65–69	3 000	4 000
70–74	2 000	3 000
75–79	1 000	2 000
80–84	500	1 000
85+	500	1 000
Total	100 000	100 000

Sources: (a) Waterhouse et al. [1]; (b) *World Health Statistics Annual*, Geneva, WHO (any issue). Reproduced by permission of the International Agency for Research against Cancer (IARC) and the WHO.

One also has to be careful when comparing countries with small populations. Mortality indices for these countries are less stable, and the position of such countries may change significantly from one year to the next because of random variations.

For international comparisons, it is preferable to use mortality rates or other mortality based indices which are calculated centrally; for example, by the WHO. Indices calculated individually by each country may have some bias due to the different calculation methods and software used in each country. This may happen particularly in the case of **life expectancy** as there are several different mathematical methods and software packages to calculate this index from the raw, age-disaggregated mortality data.

Mortality data are collected by and are available from several international organizations and agencies (e.g. the United Nations, the WHO, the Statistical Office of the European Communities, and the Organization for Economic Cooperation and Development). The database maintained by the WHO is probably the most comprehensive and widely used. Detailed mortality data are published yearly in the *World Health Statistics Annual* [2]. Copies of the database with raw mortality data are available on request in computer-readable form from the WHO headquarters [3] or can be downloaded from the Internet (`www.who.int`). For European countries, this information in the form of age-standardized mortality rates is also available as a part of the "Health for All" statistical data base maintained by the WHO Regional Office for Europe in Copenhagen. These data, together with user-friendly data presentation software which facilitates international comparisons, can be downloaded from the Internet (`www.who.dk`).

References

[1]   Waterhouse, J., Muir, C., Correa, P. & Powell, J., eds (1976). *Cancer Incidence in Five Continents*, Vol. 3. IARC, Lyon, p. 456.

[2]   World Health Organization (1995). *World Health Statistics Annual 1994*. WHO, Geneva.

[3]   World Health Organization, Global Programme on Evidence for Health Policy, 20 Avenue Appia, CH-1211 Geneva 27, Switzerland.

(*See also* **Geographic Patterns of Disease**)

R. Prokhorskas

Mortality Odds Ratio *see* Standardization Methods

Multifactorial Threshold Models
see Genetic Epidemiology, Overview

Multiplicative Model

In epidemiology and biostatistics, **relative risk models** are often called *multiplicative models*. In a relative risk model the effect of an exposure or other factors is described as

$$R = R_0 \times RR(z),$$

where R_0 is the background (or baseline) risk and $RR(z)$ is the **relative risk** associated with a covariate vector z.

The most commonly used relative risk model is the loglinear model $RR(z) = \exp\left(\sum_i \beta_i z_i\right)$. This is a multiplicative function since the effect of each covariate is to multiply the **risk** by a factor proportional to the covariate value. However, additive functions are also useful in describing relative risks. For example, in the assessment of **dose–response** it is often reasonable to describe the relative risk of an exposure in terms of an **additive model** for the **excess relative risk**, i.e. $ERR = RR - 1 = \beta_1 z_1$. If there is an additional exposure of interest, then it is useful to consider additive relative risk models of the form:

$$RR = 1 + \beta_1 z_1 + \beta_2 z_2$$

or

$$RR = 1 + \beta_1 z_1 + \beta_2 z_2 + \beta_3 z_1 z_2.$$

The second of these models is a generalization of the multiplicative excess relative risk model

$$RR = (1 + \beta_1 z_1) \times (1 + \beta_2 z_2).$$

Thomas [2] and Breslow & Storer [1] describe general relative risk functions that include both additive and multiplicative models. The articles on **Relative** Risk Modeling and the **Cox Regression Model** contain additional discussion of relative risk models. The articles on Parametric Models in Survival Analysis and **Poisson Regression in Epidemiology** present general classes of additive and multiplicative models that are useful in describing excess and relative risks. These articles also discuss methods for parameter estimation and inference with such models.

References

[1]   Breslow, N.E. & Storer, B.E. (1985). General relative risk functions for case–control studies, *American Journal of Epidemiology* **122**, 149–162.

[2]   Thomas, D.C. (1981). General relative risk functions for survival time and matched case–control studies, *Biometrics* **37**, 673–686.

DALE PRESTON

Multistage Carcinogenesis Models

Cancer is a disorder of cells whereby a visible tumor is the end result of a whole series of changes which may have taken many years to develop. Cancers generally derive from the clonal expansion of a single cell (monoclonal) that is dramatically altered by the series of events.

To understand the process of carcinogenesis, the story must start at the beginning – normal cells. A normal cell has a well-defined shape and is organized within its environment of other normal cells. Growth (cell division or replication) is dictated by the stimulatory and inhibitory signals of the environment, which are normally in balance until a growth stimulus is required. In normal development and growth, growth control allows individual organs (e.g. heart, liver, lungs) to reach a specific size which is homeostatically maintained.

The process of replication brings with it the risk of mutations. Mutations may be thought of as permanent alterations in deoxyribonucleic acid (DNA) (occurring within all or part of the DNA of a cell) that can impair the regulatory communication between the cell and its environment. The most generally accepted mechanism is as follows. A single mutation alters the physical nature of the cell, making it less responsive to external stimuli, resulting in frequent cell division. As genetic damage accumulates, the damaged cell becomes deaf to external stimuli. Lack of external influence eventually results in uncontrolled replication, characteristic of malignancy, and the resulting tumor (clonal mass of mutated cells) damages healthy tissue in its neighborhood or metastasizes where it may establish new colonies at distant sites. Other mechanisms exist including loss of genetic material, alterations in cellular death, alterations in cellular communication not related to mutations, and alteration in mitochondrial DNA. The net effect in all cases is general loss of homeostatic control of cellular division, growth of a tumor, and resulting damage to surrounding tissue.

One hundred and forty years ago, Johannes Mueller, a German microscopist, demonstrated that cancers were made up of cells. This discovery initiated a search for the specific differences between normal and cancer cells. By 1914, the German cytologist, Theodor Boveri, concluded that malignant cells had atypical chromosomes and that any event leading to such abnormality would cause cancer. Advances in biological technology, especially in the fields of cellular and molecular biology, have identified many genes that take part in the progression from normalcy to cancer.

The process of carcinogenesis is inherently probabilistic, at least as long as it is unknown why certain individuals are afflicted with cancer under certain conditions and others are unaffected. Attention will be focused on stochastic models of carcinogenesis at the cellular level since one of the least understood aspects of tumor development is the **latent period** between cancer initiation and the appearance of tumors. Mathematical models of carcinogenesis strive to investigate the number and types of events in the progression from normalcy to malignancy and allow examination of hypothetical schemes that may be tested objectively.

There are two basic concepts that have been used in describing the events leading to carcinogenesis: hit theory and multistage theory. The biological hypothesis behind the hit theory of carcinogenesis is that a cell must be damaged a certain number of times before it loses growth control and becomes tumorigenic. The damage to the cell is thought to be caused by particles of the carcinogen hitting the nucleus of the cell. The damage incurred is dependent on the

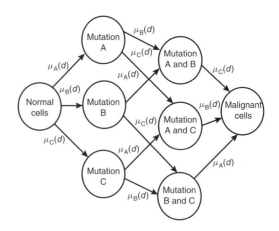

Figure 1 Three-hit model of carcinogenesis [16]. In this model, mutation rates are denoted by μ_i, $(\mu_A = \mu_B = \mu_C = \mu)$. All rates are expressed as number of mutations per unit dose of carcinogen (denoted by d) for a fixed period of time

number of hits the cell receives and the dose of the carcinogenic agent. A majority of the literature on hit theory modeling comes from the area of biophysics where interest has centered on the interaction between radiation and target cells with respect to mutagenicity. Hit theory directly related to modeling the process of carcinogenesis does not have a pronounced history. Figure 1 displays a three-hit model of carcinogenesis.

The first mathematical model of carcinogenesis was that of Iversen & Arley [5]. Their model postulated that carcinogenic "hits" are independently and randomly distributed among all normal cells of a tissue. Each normal cell hit by the carcinogen undergoes an irreparable change which marks the onset of the cancer process. This model is frequently referred to as the "one-hit" model of carcinogenesis because only a single hit is necessary for a cell to undergo a mutation which will eventually lead to malignancy. Once the cell becomes mutated, it is assumed to lose growth control and proliferates via replication. An observable tumor results when enough replicated cells have amassed to be clinically detectable.

Stochastic Models of Carcinogenesis

Many years after the development of Iversen & Arley's stochastic cancer model, Rai & Van Ryzin [16] resurrected the underlying theme of the one-hit model and adapted it to include more than a single hit, i.e. a multihit model. The biological hypothesis behind the multihit model is that a normal cell must be damaged a multiple number of times before it results in a malignant cell. The amount of damage that is incurred is dependent on the number of hits the cell receives and the dose of the carcinogenic agent. Rai & Van Ryzin further assumed that, once a cell has been subjected to at least j hits, it becomes malignant and will eventually result in a tumor. Unlike Iversen & Arley [5], they did not model the growth process of malignant cells. Mathematically, it was assumed that once a cell received j hits it instantaneously became an observable tumor.

The multihit model has been used to model the occurrence of cancer in a variety of tissues; however, it is not clear from Rai & Van Ryzin's mathematical derivation that their theory applies to entire tissues as it does to an individual cell. Disregarding this caveat, the "hit" theory of carcinogenesis was still not well received even after Rai & Van Ryzin's development of a generalized theory, and was generally abandoned at this point. This was most likely due to the perceived simplistic nature of the "hit" theory model and a lack of plausibility relative to the multistage theory of carcinogenesis.

The multistage theory of carcinogenesis also assumes several events leading to DNA damage; however, it is hypothesized that these events must occur in a particular sequence. In essence, the multistage model is an order-restricted multihit model. This theory was initially conceptualized by Muller [10] and Nordling [12] from the observation that for some carcinomas the cancer incidence rate rapidly increased with increasing age. Multistage theory continues to be a popular concept since current biological evidence suggests that genetic changes usually occur in a specific order. Figure 2 displays a two-stage model of carcinogenesis.

The two-stage model shown in Figure 2 assumes that a normal cell must pass through two unique, sequential stages before becoming malignant. This model has three types of cells: normal cells, stage-one cells, and stage-two (malignant) cells. In the small time interval $[t, t + \Delta t]$, the following events may occur:

1. A normal cell may acquire a mutation resulting in damage to a single strand of the DNA which results in one normal cell and one stage-one cell with probability $\mu_1 \Delta t + o(\Delta t)$.

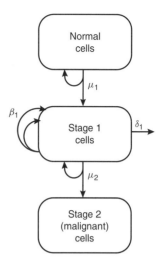

Figure 2 Two-stage model of carcinogenesis. In this model, mutation rates are denoted by μ_i, birth rates are denoted by β_i, and death/differentiation rates are denoted by δ_i. All rates are expressed as number of events per cell per unit of time

2. A stage-one cell may replicate, resulting in two stage-one cells with probability $\beta_1 \Delta t + o(\Delta t)$.
3. A stage-one cell may differentiate or die, i.e. leave the system, with probability $\delta_1 \Delta t + o(\Delta t)$.
4. A stage-one cell may acquire a mutation, resulting in damage to a single strand of the DNA which results in one stage-one cell and one stage-two (malignant) cell with probability $\mu_2 \Delta t + o(\Delta t)$.

The probability of more than one event occurring in this small time interval is $o(\Delta t)$.

For the model shown in Figure 2 (and most classes of multistage models used to date) the growth of normal cells is assumed to be constant or deterministic. In the context of the model, it is assumed that the number of normal cells at any time t is constant. All intermediate cell types (in this case, stage-one cells) are assumed to undergo growth kinetics via a linear birth–death process. A linear birth–death process implies that the rate of growth of a cell population is proportional to the number of cells in the tissue. Further modeling assumptions are that the birth–death processes and mutation processes are stochastic and independent of one another. In addition, each cell acts independently of other cells, the transformation process is irreversible, i.e. damage to the genome is "fixed", and once a malignant cell is produced it loses growth control and will eventually result in a tumor. Mathematically, these assumptions imply that the model portrays the process of carcinogenesis as a Markov process. A Markov process describes the fate of any cell at time t as depending only on the present state of the cell at time t and not on the past history of that cell. More precisely, this model may be described as a continuous-time multiple branching process since all cell types (with the exception of malignant cells) implement growth kinetics that spawn birth–death processes from which the progeny form branching processes.

Mathematically, the main outcome studied in the context of these mathematical models of carcinogenesis is the time-to-first-entry into the malignant state, generally referred to as the tumor incidence rate. Let T be the associated random variable, in which case tumor incidence is defined as

$$\lambda(t) = \lim_{\Delta \to 0} \frac{\Pr[T \in [t, t+\Delta)|(T \geq t)]}{\Delta}. \quad (1)$$

This is generally converted into a cumulative distribution function (CDF) for tumor onset by the formula

$$\Pr(T < t) = 1 - \exp\left[-\int_0^t \lambda(s)\,ds\right]. \quad (2)$$

For the simple two-stage model of carcinogenesis in Figure 2, several authors have derived a closed-form solution for the tumor incidence rate for time-constant rate parameters (Kopp–Schneider et al. [6] and Zheng [21]). The solution is given as

$$\Pr(T \leq t) = 1 - \exp[-\Lambda(t)], \quad (3)$$

where

$$\Lambda(t) = \left(\frac{X_0 \mu_1}{\beta}\right)\left[\frac{t}{2}(\beta - \delta - \mu_2 + R)\right.$$
$$\left. + \log\left(\frac{(\delta - \beta + \mu_2 + R) + (\beta - \delta}{-\mu_2 + R)\exp(-Rt)}{2R}\right)\right] \quad (4)$$

where

$$R = [(\beta + \delta + \mu_2)^2 - 4\beta\delta]^{1/2}. \quad (5)$$

The most general formulation for the CDF is derived by Portier et al. [15]. They use the Kolmogorov backwards equations to develop a system of ordinary differential equations (ODEs) which,

through a simple algebraic manipulation, can be used to derive (2) for any nonhomogeneous multistage model of carcinogenesis. The model is still required to be stochastically linear (the rate constants cannot depend upon the numbers of cells in each stage of the process). If we expand the two-stage model in Figure 2 to include a birth–death process on the normal cells (rates $\beta_0(t)$ and $\delta_0(t)$ for birth and death of normal cells, and rates $\beta_1(t)$ and $\delta_1(t)$ for stage-one cells), then the ODEs derived by Portier et al. [15] are

$$\frac{d}{ds}\Psi_0(s) = \beta_0(t - s)[\Psi_0(s)]^2 + \delta_0(t - s)$$
$$+ \mu_1(t - s)\Psi_0(s)\Psi_1(s) - [\beta_0(t - s)$$
$$+ \delta_0(t - s) + \mu_1(t - s)]\Psi_0(s)$$

and

$$\frac{d}{ds}\Psi_1(s) = \beta_1(t - s)[\Psi_1(s)]^2 + \delta_1(t - s)$$
$$- [\beta_1(t - s) + \delta_1(t - s)$$
$$+ \mu_2(t - s)]\Psi_1(s), \quad (6)$$

where the initial conditions are $\Psi_0(0) = 1$ and $\Psi_1(0) = 1$. The CDF for tumor incidence is calculated by solving this system from $s = 0$ to $s = T$ and plugging the solutions into the calculation

$$\Pr(T \leq t) = [\Psi_0(t)]^{m_0}[\Psi_1(t)]^{m_1}, \quad (7)$$

where m_i is the initial number of cells in stage i of the process at time $t = 0$. A detailed derivation of these ODEs would be inappropriate in this context; interested readers should refer to the manuscript by Portier et al. [15] for the details.

Even without the details, it is possible to develop systems of ODEs intuitively for more complex multistage models. Examining the form of system (7) relative to the form of the model in Figure 2, it is possible to illustrate the pattern of these equations. Starting with the end of (6) first, it is clear that in the equations pertaining to $\Psi_i(s)$, the rates of the process by which cells move out of state $i[\beta_i(t - s), \delta_i(t - s)$, and $\mu_{i+1}(t - s)]$ are summed, multiplied by $\Psi_i(s)$ and subtracted from the differential equation. The remaining terms in the differential equation for $\Psi_i(s)$ are the product of each rate for cells leaving the state i times the $\Psi_.(s)$ for the eventual location of the resulting cell(s). These terms are all added to the differential equation. For example, a birth results in two cells returning to the state in which the birth occurs. For state i, the resulting product to be added to the differential equation for $\Psi_i(s)$ is $\beta_i(t-s)\Psi_i(s)\Psi_i(s)$; that is the rate for the event of birth for the proper time, $\beta_i(t-s)$, times the generating functions for the states of the two resulting cells, $\Psi_i(s)$ and $\Psi_i(s)$. A mutation from state i results in one cell returning to state i and the next cell going on to state $(i+1)$ so the resulting product to be added to the differential equation for $\Psi_i(s)$ is $\mu_i(t-s)\Psi_i(s)\Psi_{i+1}(s)$. Note that, for the state just prior to the malignant state (state 1 in the two-stage model), since the function for the final state [$\Psi_2(s)$ in the two-stage model] is identically zero at all times, this term drops out of the system. Finally, since death/differentiation simply removes a cell and does not place it into any state being followed by the system, the proper term to add to $\Psi_i(s)$ for a death is simply $\delta_i(t-s)$. The calculation of the CDF is a direct extension of (7) to include all stages in the more complicated model.

The most important aspect of this modification to the determination of the CDF for tumor onset is the ability to consider much more complicated and realistic models (see below) and to incorporate biochemical and pharmacological events into the determination of rate constants for the model (see Portier et al. [15]).

Towards More Realistic Models

The hit theory and multistage theory have played dominant roles in the mathematical modeling of carcinogenesis. The history of carcinogenic modeling can be described as a hierarchy of models within a respective framework, i.e. hits or stages. Generally, each newly developed model encompasses the previously developed models. Thus, mathematical models attempt to include the evolution of biological evidence in cancer biology. A natural extension in the mathematical modeling of carcinogenesis is the development of a single model which incorporates concepts from both hit theory and multistage theory. This class of models still embodies all of the mathematical models constructed under the multihit and multistage paradigms, and thus the history of carcinogenesis modeling is preserved, while simultaneously current experimental evidence is being incorporated into this class of models. In essence, a natural extension in the continuum of the mathematical modeling

of carcinogenesis is being implemented. This class of models is referred to as the multipath/multistage models of carcinogenesis.

In fusing the hit theory and multistage theory of carcinogenesis, it is important to understand the notions of stages and hits in the context of the multipath/multistage model. Stages will be defined as necessary events for carcinogenesis that must occur in a specific order. Conversely, hits are defined as events that have no specific ordering and no direct bearing on carcinogenesis; however, they may augment the rate at which a stage occurs. Consequently, by definition, hits yield alternative pathways to cancer. Figure 3 displays a two-path/three-stage model of carcinogenesis. There are two possible scenarios for a normal cell to be transformed into a malignant cell:

1. A normal cell may undergo three mutational events: transformation from the normal state to stage one (rate μ_1), transformation from stage one to stage two (rate μ_2), and then transformation from stage two to the malignant state (rate μ_3). This is the most direct path to carcinogenesis where three stages are traversed.

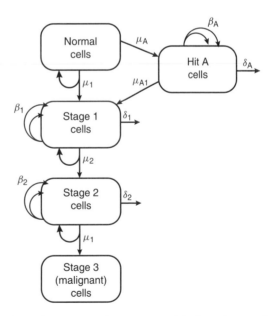

Figure 3 Two-path/three-stage model of carcinogenesis. In this model, mutation rates are denoted by μ_i, birth rates are denoted by β_i, and death/differentiation rates are denoted by δ_i. All rates are expressed as number of events per cell per unit of time

2. A normal cell may undergo four mutational events: transformation from the normal cells to hit A cells (rate μ_A), transformation to stage one (rate μ_{A1}), transformation from stage one to stage two (rate μ_2), and then transformation to the malignant state (rate μ_3).

In a modeling context, Figure 3 is a four-stage model added to a three-stage model since hits and stages are mathematically indistinguishable. However, biologically this is not simply a fourth stage added to a simple three-stage model, but a construct based on some observations regarding certain carcinogenic mechanisms. Because the hit A cells still lead to stage-one cells, this state does not really constitute a stage by the definition given. It is more closely related to a hit since passage through this stage in moving to stage one is not required, but does alter the overall mutation rate.

Experimental evidence for the multipath/multistage model is supported by current cancer research in the area of oncogenes and tumor suppressor genes. Oncogenes are thought to be genes whose activation accelerates replication. Tumor suppressor genes are thought to act in the opposite manner; they are genes whose deactivation removes some restrictions on the mechanism that regulates cell proliferation. Thus, if oncogenes are activated and tumor suppressor genes deactivated, the net result is believed to be a cell, and eventually a colony of cells, with little or no growth control (malignancy).

Current biological theory in the area of molecular carcinogenesis suggests that a malignant cell results from the accumulation of genetic damage to a single cell. The multipath/multistage model may possibly explain the underlying mechanisms involved in the transformation of the mechanisms by which the oncogenes and suppressor genes control replication. Three equally likely possibilities exist:

1. Oncogene activation and suppressor gene deactivation must occur in a sequential manner and induce carcinogenesis. This situation would fit the multistage theory of carcinogenesis. This theory includes models such as those by Armitage & Doll [1, 2], Neyman & Scott [11], Moolgavkar & Venzon [9], and Portier & Kopp-Schneider [14].
2. Oncogene activation and suppressor gene deactivation are not restricted to a particular order of occurrence. Thus, carcinogenesis is induced once both these events occur, regardless of order. This would directly relate to the multihit theory hypothesis. Models in this class have been proposed by Iversen & Arley [5] and Rai & Van Ryzin [16].
3. One of the events in the process, say oncogene activation, could have no direct bearing on carcinogenesis such that it is unnecessary for tumor formation. However, it may still alter the rate at which one of the other events, say suppressor gene deactivation, occurs. Thus, oncogene activation could be considered as a potential hit which augments suppressor gene deactivation. Because suppressor gene deactivation is necessary for carcinogenesis, it is a stage in the process. Models in this class have been proposed by Portier [13] and Tan [20], and developed by Sherman & Portier [17].

Estimation Considerations

Historically, mathematical models related to the cancer process have relied on tumor response data, i.e. the presence or absence of a tumor, for parameterization. However, tumor response data are not sufficient to uniquely parameterize the simplest of mathematical cancer models. Mathematical and statistical techniques have been derived over the past several years to take advantage of some of the intermediate cancer biomarker data currently being collected [3, 4, 6, 19]. Premalignant lesion data from rodent skin papilloma studies (number of skin papillomas) and hepatocarcinogenicity studies (number and size of enzyme-altered hepatic lesions) have been used to elucidate the underlying cancer mechanisms of a variety of chemical carcinogens.

Mathematical models have also been developed to focus strictly on the growth properties of premalignant lesions. From cell labeling studies carried out over a period of time (incidence labeling data), Moolgavkar & Luebeck [8] have developed methods to estimate the birth rate of premalignant cells. Lyles [7] incorporates incidence and prevalence cell labeling data (BrdU cell labeling data and PCNA cell labeling data, respectively) to estimate the rate parameters of the cell cycle. From these methods, one may test a variety of hypotheses which may elucidate aberrant cell growth typically characterized by premalignant cell populations.

Mathematical models of carcinogenesis are not limited to using a single type of data (i.e. tumor response data alone or labeling index data alone) in the modeling process. Several pieces of information may be incorporated into a single model to more fully describe the cancer process or fill in the gaps created by previous models. Important aspects of this approach are its close ties to the underlying biology of the cancer process and the enhancement of statistical power in hypothesis testing (due to the use of additional data). Once a model and data are chosen, one may use maximum likelihood techniques to arrive at parameter estimates and likelihood ratio tests to examine a broad range of hypotheses.

References

[1]   Armitage, P. & Doll, R. (1954). The age distribution of cancer and a multistage theory of carcinogenesis, *British Journal of Cancer* **8**, 1–12.

[2]   Armitage, P. & Doll, R. (1957). A two-stage theory of carcinogenesis in relation to the age distribution of human cancer, *British Journal of Cancer* **11**, 161–169.

[3]   Dewanji, A., Moolgavkar, S. & Luebeck, E. (1991). Two-mutation model for carcinogenesis: Joint analysis of premalignant and malignant lesions, *Mathematical Biosciences* **104**, 97–109.

[4]   Dewanji, A., Venzon, D. & Moolgavkar, S. (1989). A stochastic two-stage model for cancer risk assessment. II. The number and size of premalignant clones, *Risk Analysis* **9**, 179–187.

[5]   Iverson, S. & Arley, N. (1950). On the mechanism of experimental carcinogenesis, *Acta Pathologica et Microbiologica Scandinavica* **27**, 773–803.

[6]   Kopp-Schneider, A., Portier, C. & Sherman, C. (1994). The exact formula for tumor incidence in the two-stage model, *Risk Analysis* **14**, 1079–1080.

[7]   Lyles, C. (1996). The modeling of cell proliferation: Incorporating the cell cycle. *Unpublished doctoral dissertation*, Department of Biostatistics, University of North Carolina, Chapel Hill.

[8]   Moolgavkar, S. & Luebeck, E.G. (1992). Interpretation of labeling indices in the presence of cell death, *Carcinogenesis* **13**, 1007–1010.

[9]   Moolgavkar, S. & Venzon, D. (1979). Two-event models for carcinogenesis: Incidence curves for childhood and adult tumors, *Mathematical Biosciences* **47**, 55–77.

[10]   Muller, H. (1951). Radiation damage to the genetic material, *Science Progress* **7**, 93–493.

[11]   Neyman, J. & Scott, E. (1967). Statistical aspects of the problem of carcinogenesis, in *Proceedings of the Fifth Berkeley Symposium on Mathematical Statistics and Probability*. University of California Press, Berkeley, pp. 745–776.

[12]   Nordling, C. (1953). A new theory on the cancer inducing mechanism, *British Journal of Cancer* **7**, 68–72.

[13]   Portier, C. (1987). Statistical properties of a two-stage model of carcinogenesis, *Environmental Health Perspectives* **76**, 125–131.

[14]   Portier, C. & Kopp-Schneider, A. (1991). A multistage model of carcinogenesis incorporating DNA damage and repair, *Risk Analysis* **11**, 535–543.

[15]   Portier, C., Kopp-Schneider, A. & Sherman, C. (1996). Calculating tumor incidence rates in stochastic models of carcinogenesis, *Mathematical Biosciences* **135**, 129–146.

[16]   Rai, K. & Van Ryzin, J. (1981). A generalized multihit dose-response model for low dose extrapolation, *Biometrics* **37**, 341–352.

[17]   Sherman, C. & Portier, C. (1994). The multipath/multistage model of carcinogenesis, *Informatik Biometrie und Epidemiologie in Medizin und Biologie* **25**, 250–254.

[18]   Sherman, C. & Portier, C. (1995). Quantitative analysis of multiple phenotype enzyme-altered foci in rat hepatocarcinogenesis experiments: The multipath/multistage model of carcinogenesis, *Carcinogenesis* **16**, 2499–2506.

[19]   Sherman, C., Portier, C. & Kopp-Schneider, A. (1994). Multistage models of carcinogenesis: An approximation method for the size and number distribution of late-stage clones, *Risk Analysis* **14**, 1039–1048.

[20]   Tan, W. (1991). *Stochastic Models of Carcinogenesis*. Marcel Dekker, New York, pp. 135–212.

[21]   Zheng, Q. (1994). On the exact hazard and survival functions of the MVK stochastic carcinogenesis model, *Risk Analysis* **14**, 1081–1084.

CLAIRE D. SHERMAN &
CHRISTOPHER J. PORTIER

MVK Two Stage Model *see* Latent Period

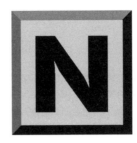

Nearest Neighbor Tests *see* Clustering

Net Probability of Death from a Cause *see* Competing Risks

Net Risk *see* Crude Risk

Nonconcurrent Cohort Study *see* Cohort Study, Historical

Nondifferential Bias *see* Bias, Nondifferential

Nondifferential Error

Suppose a response variable Y has a conditional distribution $F(y|x)$ given a true exposure measurement, $X = x$. Suppose that instead of measuring X, one measures an error-prone version of X, say Z. Then the error process is said to be nondifferential if $F(y|x, z) = F(y|x)$, namely if Y and Z are conditionally independent given X. In usual cases, though not in all cases, the effect of analyzing the model $F(y|x)$ by substituting Z for X will be to **bias** estimates of **exposure effect** toward the null hypothesis (*see* **Bias Toward the Null**) when the exposure error is nondifferential. However, if exposure measurements are differential, the bias can be in any direction.

The term nondifferential error can also be applied to errors in the outcome measure, Y. Suppose that one measures the error-prone version W of Y, rather than Y itself. Then the error process is nondifferential if W is conditionally independent of X given Y.

(*See also* **Bias in Observational Studies**; **Differential Error**; **Measurement Error in Epidemiologic Studies**; **Misclassification Error**; **Validity and Generalizability in Epidemiologic Studies**)

M.H. GAIL

Nondifferential Measurement Error *see* Measurement Error in Epidemiologic Studies

Noninformative Censoring *see* Biased Sampling of Cohorts in Epidemiology

Nonresponse

It would be preferred in virtually any **sample survey** to obtain an answer to every questionnaire item from every sample member who is eligible to participate. Unfortunately, almost all surveys fail to achieve that level of performance. Nonresponse may occur at the level of the sample unit (*unit nonresponse*) or in an individual questionnaire item *(item nonresponse)*. It is a potential source of error in survey estimates because it may cause some segments of a **target population** to be underrepresented. Also, nonresponse may reduce statistical power by resulting in a measured sample that is smaller than the desired sample size. Concern about nonresponse has increased over the past two decades as survey researchers have observed a general decline in response rates [4, 5, 11, 16–18]. This article reviews the causes of survey nonresponse, the nature of nonresponse error and its potential impact on survey estimates, and techniques for measuring and reporting nonresponse.

Causes of Nonresponse

Total Nonresponse

Some researchers categorize nonresponse as **non-sampling error**, considering it as a function only of the data collection process. However, as will be described below, at the unit level, nonresponse may be a function of the sampling process as well. Therefore, overall it is most appropriate to consider survey error attributable to nonresponse as *nonobservation error* [11]. This broader concept appropriately casts survey nonresponse as the failure of the survey process to obtain full participation from all eligible members of a sample.

The *total nonresponse* for any particular measured variable is the sum of the two levels of nonresponse: unit nonresponse and item nonresponse (both expressed as percentages). For example, if a survey fails to obtain participation from 20% of the eligible sample, and if among the 80% who participate no response is obtained from 10% for the variable of interest, total nonresponse for that variable is $0.20 + 0.10 \times 0.80 = 28\%$. Therefore, although in most surveys unit nonresponse accounts for the largest proportion of total nonresponse, it is important for

researchers to account for both levels of nonresponse, in combination as well as individually.

The above example applies to the typical **cross-sectional** sample survey. Total nonresponse is both more complicated and usually more serious in the case of sample attrition in a longitudinal panel study, a design in which repeated measures are to be obtained from the same respondents over two or more waves (observation points). Total nonresponse for any particular variable in a panel study is cumulative over the nonresponse at each wave. Therefore, it is important to account for overall nonresponse for the duration of a panel study as well as wave-specific nonresponse.

Unit Nonresponse

Unit nonresponse occurs when members of a sample who are eligible to participate in a survey either do not participate at all or participate only partially, such that sufficient data are not obtained to include them in the analysis. Depending on the survey design, a unit may be an individual, a household, an institution or organization (e.g. a school), or other group. Unit nonresponse is a function of two components. The first is failure to contact sample members (non-contacts), which appears to account for most cases of unit nonresponse [17]. Examples of this type of problem include cases where, for the entire survey period, persons are not at home (e.g. due to business or vacation travel) or constantly use a telephone answering machine or voice-mail system. The second component of unit nonresponse is failure to obtain participation. This includes two types of cases. One is where a sample member refuses to complete an interview/questionnaire. The other is where a sample member who otherwise would complete an interview/questionnaire is unable to do so, for example because of an illness or injury, or being too busy with other activities.

Although hard data are lacking, researchers have attributed recent increases in unit nonresponse to secular trends in the US, especially in urbanized areas [11, 18], whereby the population has become more mobile, resulting in people being available at their usual place of residence for shorter periods. In particular, the Council of American Survey Research Organizations (CASRO) [5] noted that is has become more difficult to contact women because of their increased participation in the labor force.

Kessler et al. [13] observed that there is an increased tendency for entire households to be away from home when interviewers call because of growing proportions of single-member households and dual-earning couples, increased commuting time, and an increase in evening activities outside the home. Moreover, people appear to be more protective of their more limited personal time at home, making them less receptive to requests to participate in a survey [4].

Two particular aspects of survey methodology may effect unit nonresponse. The first is the mode of initiating contact and collecting data. In general, unit nonresponse is lowest for face-to-face interviews, slightly larger for telephone interviews, and largest for mail (postal) surveys [1, 8]. The second is the burden participation places on respondents. For example, nonresponse tends to be larger for longer interviews/questionnaires, less salient survey topics, and sensitive or threatening survey topics. Additionally, nonresponse tends to vary among population subgroups. In particular, nonresponse tends to be greater among young adults, the elderly, the poor, persons with little education, and persons with certain disabilities such as impaired hearing [1, 11]. Other factors such as characteristics of the survey sponsor and the time of year also may effect unit nonresponse [12]. Finally, the sampling process may contribute to unit nonresponse in instances when problems with the sampling frame prevent the researcher from contacting a sample member, such as if the frame contains erroneous or out-of-date address and/or telephone information.

A special case of unit nonresponse is when a respondent begins to participate in a survey but fails to complete an interview/questionnaire. These *partial completes* occur more often in face-to-face and telephone interview surveys than in mail surveys, when the respondent "breaks off" from an interview before it is completed (for example, because of a lack of time or a refusal to answer any more questions). Further complicating the matter is that some so-called *complete* questionnaires may include unanswered questions (item nonresponse). Thus, although partial completes usually are categorized as a component of unit nonresponse, they are strongly related to item nonresponse. The larger the item nonresponse for a case, the more likely it is to be considered a partial complete. Because there is no standard definition of a partial complete, the researcher's decision about whether to include a case in the analysis or to count

it as a unit nonresponse usually is guided by two factors: the proportion of the questions answered by the respondent; and whether responses are obtained for questionnaire items measuring key variables for the analysis.

Item Nonresponse

Item nonresponse occurs when an eligible sample member participates in a survey but does not provide a usable response to one or more of the survey questionnaire items (questions). For a survey where the questionnaire contains some items that do not apply to all respondents, item nonresponse refers only to questions that apply to a particular respondent. Thus, the data record for some respondents regarded as "completes", because their overall participation in a survey was acceptable, may include **missing values** for some variables.

Item nonresponse is a function of two components. The first is failure to obtain an answer to a question, which may occur for several reasons. The most obvious one is when a question is presented but the respondent refuses to answer or is unable to provide the requested information. However, item "nonresponse" also includes cases where a question is not presented because a respondent or interviewer does not follow instructions correctly (e.g. does not understand that a question applies to the respondent, or records only one response to a multiple response question). Also, an interviewer may fail to present a question because the interviewer feels uncomfortable with the subject matter, or the interviewer may fail to encourage a respondent properly to answer a difficult question. Finally, item "nonresponse" also includes cases where a respondent "answers" a question but the response is not recorded (by the respondent or interviewer).

The second component of item nonresponse is failure to obtain a usable response to a question. In a mail survey or other type of self-administered questionnaire study a respondent's handwriting may be illegible, or a respondent may record two response choices where only one response is requested and/or logical (e.g. a respondent may record both "yes" and "no" for a dichotomous question). For an interview survey an interviewer may fail to probe properly to obtain a clear and complete response. This is particularly a problem for open-ended questions or "other – specify" type responses. Similar problems of lack of clarity and completeness are even more likely to occur in a mail survey or other type of self-administered questionnaire study.

A special issue for item nonresponse is when a respondent answers "don't know" to a question, which may or may not be a case of missing data. In some cases, a respondent may use this response as a convenient and polite way to refuse to answer. In others, it may indicate that a respondent is unable to answer because of inability to retrieve the necessary information (e.g. from memory or records), the respondent has no opinion about the subject of a question, or because none of the response choices is appropriate. In still other cases, "don't know" may indicate that the respondent has no knowledge about the subject. For example, "I don't know" may be a valid response to a question such as "Whom would you call if a member of your household needs emergency medical treatment?". Before data collection begins, the researcher should anticipate the possibility that a respondent may answer "don't know" to virtually any question and decide whether to treat it as a nonresponse or as a valid response to be included in the analysis. This decision, even for identical questions, may vary from one survey to another depending on the purposes of the study and how the data will be interpreted. In general, the issue is whether it is reasonable to expect respondents to have adequate knowledge (e.g. about their age) or hold an opinion (e.g. about their health status) so as to be able to answer a question, as opposed to a situation where "don't know" may be a relevant substantive response (e.g. indicating a lack of knowledge about a health service).

Nonresponse Error and its Potential Impact

Nonresponse error is a function of two components: the magnitude of nonresponse (i.e. nonresponse rate); and the extent to which nonrespondents systematically differ from respondents. Concern about survey nonresponse has been driven mainly by the increase in unit nonresponse rates, probably because unit nonresponse results in fewer cases in the analysis, reducing statistical power and the precision of survey estimates. All things being equal, a higher rather than lower survey response rate is preferred because a higher rate indicates that unit nonresponse

is lower. Moreover, when unit nonresponse is low, total nonresponse probably is low (for most variables) because item nonresponse is fairly low in most well-conducted surveys [6]. In general, the lower the total nonresponse rate the less concern about whether the participation of nonrespondents would have changed the survey estimates, simply because there are relatively few nonrespondents.

However, a high response rate does not mean that nonresponse error necessarily is trivial. For example, nonrespondents may differ substantially from respondents in terms of relatively rare characteristics [13] or if most nonrespondents are concentrated within one or two sample strata or population subgroups [20]. Also, nonresponse error may be substantial even when nonresponse is low if the factors causing nonresponse are associated strongly with important variables in the study. Ironically, as Kessler et al. [13] have observed, sometimes the techniques used to increase response rates and reduce nonresponse (e.g. special types of contact strategies or monetary incentives) can *increase* nonresponse error if they are more effective among some population subgroups than others, and if an underrepresented subgroup differs strongly from the others in terms of key study variables.

Nonresponse often is correlated with important demographic or other background characteristics (e.g. education in mail surveys, or health status in interview surveys) [4, 6]. But even if nonrespondents are similar to respondents on those characteristics, they may differ in terms of other important variables, such as attitudes and behaviors [20]. For example, persons who engage in risky behaviors may be less willing than others to participate in a survey about the epidemiology of the human immunodeficiency virus [19]. Therefore, the key nonresponse issue is *nonobservation* **bias**, whereby the absence of nonrespondents from the analysis causes one or more survey estimates to be consistently lower or higher than their population parameter (true value). This may substantially change the univariate and/or multivariate distributions of the survey data and result in erroneous interpretations of a study's findings.

The methods for taking account of sampling error in survey estimates (e.g. confidence intervals) assume that nonresponse error (as well as other nonsampling error) is zero. As nonresponse error increases, the model on which the computation and interpretation of inferential statistics are founded becomes less appropriate. Therefore, the investment in carefully designing and selecting a large, random sample of a target population to minimize sampling error may be subverted by a substantial nonresponse bias. In most cases when the potential for nonresponse bias is relatively large, a researcher should consider using data collection strategies that have been shown to obtain high response rates. Also, the researcher may consider employing various strategies for obtaining information about the nonrespondents that can be used to take nonresponse error into account in the analysis. These decisions about survey design must balance available resources with a study's objectives. For example, an exploratory study may be able to tolerate larger amounts of both nonsampling and sampling errors than a study that is intended to provide a rigorous test of an important hypothesis. In most cases a researcher will invest more resources in the latter type of study.

Measuring and Reporting Nonresponse

Unfortunately, no model exists for taking nonresponse error into account in a way similar to that for assessing statistical inferences based on probability theory. Moreover, in most cases it is very difficult or impossible to estimate nonresponse error because reliable knowledge, independent of the survey, about the population regarding the variables measured in the survey usually is not available. Tests for nonresponse bias usually are limited to comparisons of nonrespondents with respondents, or respondents with the target population, in terms of aggregate characteristics such as socioeconomic status and other demographic variables based on data from existing sources (sometimes with questionable reliability) such as the US Census, institutional records (e.g. from schools or clinics), information that may be available from the sampling frame (e.g. residential location), or interviewer observation (e.g. type of dwelling unit) [7, 11]. Such comparisons may be useful if the criterion variables are strongly associated with the main variables of interest in the survey. Although it rarely is possible to make comparisons directly regarding the main variables of interest, researchers sometimes try to approximate this by comparing early respondents with late respondents [15] or by conducting brief follow-up interviews with subsamples of nonrespondents [6, 11, 13].

In addition to using techniques that tend to reduce nonresponse, researchers also sometimes apply various *post hoc* adjustments to improve the representativeness of survey estimates. These include techniques such as poststratification and a variety of strategies to impute values for missing questionnaire items (*see* **Missing Data**).

Survey researchers usually report a *response rate* (or a similar rate that may go by another name, such as cooperation rate or completion rate) rather than a *nonresponse rate*. It seems reasonable to regard a survey nonresponse rate as the complement of its response rate, obtained by subtracting the percentage response rate from 100% [11]. Unfortunately, despite attempts to encourage survey researchers to adopt a standard definition of response rate, there is no universally accepted definition for either a survey response rate or nonresponse rate [3, 5, 11, 14, 17, 21]. Thus, there is considerable confusion in comparing the quality of survey data across studies (meta-analysis), time periods, and survey methods.

However, to provide some guidance on this important issue, the prevailing concept appears to be that a survey response rate should reflect the degree to which a survey succeeds in obtaining the cooperation of all potential respondents in the sample: Accordingly, the response rate may be calculated as the proportion of sample members known or estimated to be eligible for participation in the survey, from whom a complete/usable set of data is obtained. While there appears to be general agreement about the numerator for the response rate calculation (i.e. complete/usable cases), there is substantial variation in specifying the denominator, especially regarding the definition and estimation of eligible sample members [16, 17]. Moreover, the factors that effect eligibility vary with the sampling design and data collection procedures. In particular, this issue becomes quite complex in surveys using methods such as **random-digit dialing** telephone interviews, in which it is difficult and sometimes impossible to determine the eligibility of a substantial proportion of the initial sample.

Until standard definitions of response and nonresponse rates are adopted, it is recommended that survey reports state how the response rate (or similar term) is calculated, including the definition of eligible sample members [6, 14, 21]. Response rates rarely are reported for individual items. Item nonresponse usually is indicated by reporting the number of cases and/or degrees of freedom when presenting results in the text and/or tables of a survey report. However, when appropriate, it is recommended that an item nonresponse rate should be calculated as the proportion of respondents from whom a usable response was not obtained to a questionnaire item, from among the number of respondents who were eligible to answer that item.

Finally, because nonresponse error is not necessarily a direct function of the response rate, and because the definition and calculation of response rate are not consistent, it is not possible unequivocally to specify acceptable levels of survey response/nonresponse. However, some gross guidelines are that a survey with a response rate lower than 50% is very likely to contain a substantial nonresponse error [2, 8, 9]. A response rate greater than 75% generally may be regarded as good to excellent [8, 10]. However, it is strongly recommended that virtually any response rate should be compared with the response rate for other surveys addressing similar topics, dealing with similar populations, and using similar methods. Also, the study's goals should be considered: the more at stake in terms of the study's findings, the less the tolerance for nonresponse error.

References

[1]   Aday, L.A. (1989). *Designing and Conducting Health Surveys*. Jossey-Bass, San Francisco.
[2]   Babbie, E.R. (1973). *Survey Research Methods*. Wadsworth, Belmont.
[3]   Bailar, B. & Lanphier, C.M. (1978). *Development of Survey Methods to Assess Survey Practices*. American Statistical Association, Washington.
[4]   Bradburn, N.M. (1992). Presidential address: a response to the nonresponse problem, *Public Opinion Quarterly* **56**, 391–397.
[5]   Council of American Survey Research Organizations (1982). *On the Definition of Response Rates*. A Special Report of the CASRO Task Force on Completion Rates. CASRO, Port Jefferson.
[6]   Czaja, R. & Blair, J. (1996). *Designing Surveys: A Guide to Decisions and Procedures*. Pine Forge Press, Thousand Oaks.
[7]   de Vaus, D.A. (1986). *Surveys in Social Research*. George Allen & Unwin, London.
[8]   Dillman, D.A. (1978). *Mail and Telephone Surveys: The Total Design Method*. Wiley, New York.
[9]   Erdös, P.L. (1983). *Professional Mail Surveys*. Robert E. Krieger, Malabar.
[10] Fowler, F.J. Jr. (1988). *Survey Research Methods*. Sage, Beverly Hills.
[11] Groves, R.M. (1989). *Survey Errors and Survey Costs*. Wiley, New York.
[12] Heberlein, T.A. & Baumgartner, R. (1978). Factors affecting response rates to mailed questionnaires: a quantitative analysis of the published literature, *American Sociological Review* **43**, 447–462.
[13] Kessler, R.C., Little, R.J.A. & Groves, R.M. (1995). Advances in strategies for minimizing and adjusting for survey nonresponse, *Epidemiologic Reviews* **17**, 192–204.
[14] Kviz, F.J. (1977). Toward a standard definition of response rate, *Public Opinion Quarterly* **41**, 265–267.
[15] Lin, I.-F. & Schaeffer, N.C. (1995). Using survey participants to estimate the impact of nonparticipation, *Public Opinion Quarterly* **59**, 236–258.
[16] Slattery, M.L., Edwards, S.L., Caan, B.J., Kerber, R.A. & Potter, J.D. (1995). Response rates among control subjects in case–control studies, *Annals of Epidemiology* **5**, 245–249.
[17] Spaeth, M.A. (1992). Response rates at academic survey research organizations, *Survey Research* **23**, 18–20.
[18] Steeh, C.G. (1981). Trends in nonresponse rates, 1952–1979, *Public Opinion Quarterly* **45**, 40–57.
[19] Tourangeau, R. and Smith, T.W. (1996). Asking sensitive questions: the impact of data collection mode, question format, and question content, *Public Opinion Quarterly* **60**, 275–304.
[20] Warwick, D.P. & Lininger, C.A. (1975). *The Sample Survey: Theory and Practice*. McGraw-Hill, New York.
[21] Wiseman, F. & McDonald, P. (1980). *Toward the Development of Industry Standards for Response and Nonresponse Rates*. Marketing Science Institute, Cambridge, Mass.

F.J. KVIZ

Nonresponse Bias *see* Bias from Nonresponse

Nonsampling Errors

It has become conventional to partition the total survey error into components representing sampling and nonsampling errors. Sampling error arises from the sampling process itself, i.e. from the fact that we are making inferences from observations on a randomly chosen subset of units, rather than observing the whole population. Nonsampling errors include all the errors not attributable to this incomplete enumeration. Every step in the survey process is a potential source of nonsampling error, from imperfections in the initial specification and listing of the **target population**, through failure to obtain complete information from all units drawn in the sample (*see* **Nonresponse**) or to obtain correct information from the units that we do contact, to errors in recording and managing the data after the survey has been completed.

Sampling error is relatively easy to deal with, at least in principle. We can reduce its effect by increasing the sample size or by clever choice of design and estimator. Moreover, we can estimate its size internally from the sample measurements themselves. In contrast, nonsampling errors often increase as we increase the sample size or the complexity of the sampling procedure and, although special surveys can be designed to get information on some components, it is difficult to measure the size of most components without external information of some sort. Unfortunately, the nonsampling component of the total error is likely to be at least as large as the sampling component in a well-designed survey. Since the impact of this component of total survey error is not captured by conventional formulas for the standard error, published estimates of survey error almost always underestimate the true state of affairs.

In the following sections we look at some specific sources of nonsampling error, with special reference to health surveys, under three general headings: coverage errors (frame errors and nonresponse); **measurement errors** (question and format effects, respondent errors, interviewer effects); and processing errors. The choice of survey mode can have a substantial impact on all these components. In health research, this usually involves a choice among personal interviews, telephone interviews or mailed questionnaires. Some useful advice on the relationship between the survey mode and data quality for a variety of health outcomes is given by Van der Zouwen et al. [32], Siemiatydi [30], and Sibbald et al. [28]. Once the mode has been chosen, most methods aimed at reducing the nonsampling errors involve more resources being spent on preparation, pre-testing and piloting, training and supervision, and processing. These methods tend to be expensive and, with a limited budget, mean that the sample size will need to be reduced.

Coverage Errors

Coverage errors arise when the population from which the sample is really drawn differs from the target population. Two major sources of such errors are deficiencies in the sampling frame or listing from which the sample of units is drawn, and a failure to elicit responses from every unit that is drawn in the sample.

Frame Errors

A key requirement in the early stages of planning for any survey is the development of a frame, i.e. a list of units from which the sample will be drawn. In a telephone survey the frame will consist of a list of phone numbers, in a mail survey it will be a list of addresses, while in a personal interview survey it might be a list of households, area sampling units, hospitals or physicians' practices. Except in the very simplest situations, the population defined by the frame is likely to differ from the target population whose characteristics we really want to measure. For example, in a telephone survey any member of the target population who is not accessible by telephone will be excluded [7]. Similarly, in any survey based on a register or list of patients held by a health facility, such as a practice, a certain proportion will have either moved address or left the facility entirely [25].

Frame error can take the form of overcoverage. This can occur when the frame contains units that do not belong to the target population, or when there are multiple or duplicate listings such that single population units are identified with more than one frame element. However, the most common type of frame error takes the form of undercoverage (or incomplete coverage), with some units in the target population omitted from the frame. The effect of undercoverage depends both on the proportion of missing units and on the magnitude of the difference between the values of the missing units and those listed in the frame. For example, consider a simple mean or proportion, θ. If we use subscripts T, F, and NC to denote values for the target population, the frame, and the units not covered by the frame respectively, then we have

$$\theta_T = \theta_F + \pi_{NC}(\theta_{NC} - \theta_F),$$

where π_{NC} denotes the proportion of the target population units that are not covered by the frame. We see that the **bias** (i.e the difference between the target and frame population values) is the product of the proportion of undercoverage and the difference between the means of the units in the frame and the omitted units. Most health surveys are concerned with more complex quantities than means and proportions (**relative risks,** regression parameters, etc.). Here the effect cannot be expressed quite so simply, but the basic idea still applies; there is little bias from undercoverage if the proportion of units not covered by the frame is small or if parameter values for the omitted units are very similar to those of the frame units.

Unfortunately there is no way to detect the presence of undercoverage either from the frame or from the sample itself, and no simple way to overcome the problem completely. Some ways to help alleviate this and other frame problems are discussed by Lessler & Kalsbeek [19, pp. 80–102] and Groves [13, pp. 81–128].

Nonresponse

Even if we have a reasonably complete frame from which to draw our sample, we may not be able to elicit responses from every unit. People may not return mailed questionnaires, or they may be out when the interviewer calls. Some people may be unwilling or unable to respond even if they are contacted. Some units may not provide any information at all (*unit* nonresponse) while others may provide responses for some items but not others (*item* nonresponse). Nonresponse can be regarded as another aspect of undercoverage, and the effect is very similar to that for incomplete frames; the degree of bias depends both on the response rate and on the extent to which nonresponders differ from responders. The response bias will be small if the proportion of nonrespondents is small (i.e. a high response rate) or if there is little difference between responders and nonresponders. Differences between responders and nonresponders can be substantial in many health surveys. For example, readiness to respond may be influenced by recently experienced health events, which may engender greater interest in participating in a health survey [3], or by health status, with those having the symptoms under investigation more likely to respond [20, 31]. One difference between nonresponse and frame undercoverage is that we do at least know the proportion of nonrespondents so that the possibility of a problem is clearly signalled, even if we have no idea of its size. Perhaps for this reason,

there has been more attention paid to nonresponse than to any other source of nonsampling error.

As with most nonsampling errors, prevention is usually the best form of cure. It is hard to do much to control differences between responders and nonresponders, but it may be possible to increase the response rate. The choice of survey mode can have a big impact on response rates. In general, response rates for postal surveys tend to be lower, but older people who feel threatened by face-to-face interviews with a stranger may respond well to a mail survey [15]. The design of questions and the quality of interviewers can also affect the response rate [4]. Extra training and extensive piloting can improve things here. Once the survey is in progress, we can make vigorous attempts to contact initial nonrespondents. For example, we might get interviewers to call back several times if a person is not at home, or send several reminder letters with a mailed questionnaire. Providing incentives such as paying people to take part may also improve response rates in some circumstances (although this can accentuate differences between responders and nonresponders if, for example, low-income people are more likely to be attracted by the offer [27]). Most of these measures are costly and implementation will usually have to be at the expense of sample size. This tradeoff will be worthwhile if the extra responses are sufficiently different to alter the survey estimate.

Getting an indication of the size of the difference between responders and nonresponders is difficult. Direct subsampling of nonrespondents, although expensive, may be worthwhile in some circumstances. If we have auxiliary information on all units listed in the frame, then we can calculate differences between the means of the auxiliary variables for respondents and nonrespondents. If these variables are correlated with the study variables, this will give some indication of the potential problems. For example, Andersen et al. [1] compared respondent reports of care received with medical record data and derived adjustments. Frequently, however, such auxiliary information is not available. Another approach is possible if we are prepared to assume that willingness to respond lies on a continuum of cooperation. Then we may get some idea of the likely magnitude of problems by looking at differences between estimates for early and late responders, or those who respond only after additional prompting [15]. A number of studies have shown that nonresponders are more like late responders than early responders [9, 29].

One way of getting direct information on non-respondents which is particularly useful in health surveys is through the use of proxy (or surrogate) respondents. Questionnaires constructed using concrete items which require less interpretation by the proxy and a shorter range of possible responses are more likely to yield responses congruent with subject response. In health surveys, studies have shown that proxies are able to report accurately on areas of health and functioning, although they tend to rate patients as slightly more impaired than patients rate themselves [11, 22]. Agreement between subject and proxy tends to be lower for conditions that are not observable, relatively private and not likely to be discussed, such as mental conditions and general aches and pains [22]. The best agreement is achieved in subject–proxy pairs where the respondents live together; correlation is reduced as contact between subjects is reduced.

Finally, a whole range of statistical procedures have been proposed to mitigate the effects of unit nonresponse. These include post-stratification and weighting adjustments based on estimates of the probability of response. These estimates might be based on auxiliary information, for example, or on extra information collected from respondents. A common procedure uses data on how often each respondent has been available for interview in the past week. A good review of these procedures is given in Lessler & Kalsbeek [19, pp. 161–233]. The most common procedure of all, particularly for item nonresponse, is to impute the missing values from respondent data. Many different imputation procedures have been proposed and a good overview can be found in Kalton & Kasprzyk [16]. There can be problems making inferences, and particularly with estimating precision, if too many values are imputed. Rao [26] and the ensuing discussion give some idea of the problems (*see* **Missing Data**).

Measurement Errors

Measurement errors arise from complex interactions among the survey mode, the instrument (i.e. the questionnaire in most health surveys), the particular question, the respondent, and, in personal interview and telephone surveys, the interviewer. For convenience, we group common problems under three general headings, but most problems involve all of these components to some extent.

Question and Format Effects

It is obvious that asking the right questions is critical if we are to obtain good information about the quantities in which we are interested. Common sense tells us that questions should be clear and unambiguous and expressed in language that the respondent can understand. Unfortunately, the situation is much more complex than this. The survey mode (personal interview, telephone interview, mailed questionnaire) can have a big impact. For example, telephone respondents tend to indicate a more favorable health status than mail respondents [23]. Differences can be large; in a study reported in Moore [24], 44% of people interviewed personally answered "Yes" when asked if they favored contraceptives being made freely available to unmarried women, in contrast to 75% of those questioned by telephone or mail. Even for a given choice of mode, very subtle changes in the wording, context, format, and layout of a questionnaire can have a measurable effect on the survey response. The order in which questions are asked affects the way that people respond in all modes, but even seemingly inconsequential factors such as the placement of instructions and the color of print has been shown to affect the responses. Questionnaire design is a specialist subject with a huge literature of its own. A good introduction can be found in Kalton & Schuman [17] which is essential, if chastening, reading for anyone planning a survey for the first time.

Respondent Errors

The respondent is the ultimate source of information. Even if the question is understood clearly, he or she must have access to the information that is sought and must be able (and willing) to access this information accurately. Accuracy of recall is related to respondent motivation, the degree of detail required, the significance of the event and the time elapsed since it occurred, and also to the nature of the topic. For example, illness in healthy subjects may be underreported because it is not of current concern to the respondent (*see* **Recall Bias**).

Many surveys ask about events that occur in a specific time-period, such as the number of visits to a doctor over the past year. This requires respondents to place events in time, and a common distortion is "telescoping", where an event is remembered as having happened more recently than was actually the case. Fortunately, this has the opposite effect to loss of recall and the two errors may partially offset each other. Surveys asking for sensitive or personal information (e.g. about diet, sexual activity or alcohol consumption) may engender a "social desirability bias" resulting from the wish of a respondent to convey a positive image in keeping with social norms and to avoid criticism. This can distort the measurement of the variable of interest significantly [14, 33].

Methods to reduce respondent measurement errors require some understanding of their causes. The literature on this topic is wide-ranging, and includes work in cognitive psychology on memory and judgment as well as work in social psychology, survey methodology, and other disciplines. A good introduction is given by Groves [13, Chapter 9]. The Survey Research Center at Michigan has conducted a long-term study aimed at improving the quality of reporting of health events. Some of the results are summarized by Cannell et al. [5]. Successful techniques tried by Cannell and his colleagues at Michigan include the use of instructions to respondents asking them to think carefully about their responses and emphasizing that accurate and complete answers are important, the use of feedback, and securing a formal agreement of respondent commitment. Some of their findings are surprising. For example, they found that longer questions sometimes gave an increase in the number of health events reported, suggesting that the common advice to "keep the questions short" might be better phrased as "keep the questions simple" (see [17]).

Interviewer Effects

In personal interview and telephone surveys, the interviewer introduces a further source of measurement error. Some interviewers may simply not adhere to the survey protocol. Most problems stem from the interaction between the interviewer and respondent. The effect is likely to vary according to the type of question, with attitude questions, questions requiring probing, fixed-alternative and forced-choice items, together with poorly worded and ambiguous questions, being particularly susceptible to interviewer variability. When questions are unclear and consistently require additional interviewer input,

there is a greater likelihood that results may be influenced by the interviewer; different interviewers may interpret questions differently, or may rephrase questions in a directive manner [10]. "Acquiescence bias" arising from the disposition to answer "yes" (or, less commonly, "no") regardless of the question asked, may be more severe in interviews with respondents who are of low socioeconomic status, or belong to minority cultures, when the interviewer is perceived to be of higher status.

The impact of interviewer variability depends on several things. For simple means and proportions, the variance of the sample estimate in simple random sampling is inflated by a factor $1 + (n - 1)\rho_{int}$, where n is a weighted average of the interviewers' case-loads and ρ_{int} is the intra-interviewer correlation as defined by Kish [18]. This correlation is a scale-free measure of the size of the variability among interviewers. The effect is similar with more complex survey designs. The impact depends both on the interviewer variability, as measured by ρ_{int}, and on the size of the case-load. Even very small values of ρ_{int} can have a big impact on the precision of the estimate if the average case-load is large. Most medical and health surveys are interested in more complex issues such as making comparisons between subgroups, comparing **relative risks**, estimating regression coefficients, and so on. There is a general belief that the impact of interviewer variability is much less severe for more complex parameters. The special case of comparisons between subgroups is examined by Davis & Scott [8]. They show that the impact depends on the distribution of the case-loads between the subgroups and on the interaction between the interviewers and the members of the subgroups. The effect will usually be smaller than for a single mean but can be almost as large if the case-loads are very unbalanced and the interviewer effect differs between subgroups.

Most suggestions for reducing interviewer effects involve putting effort into the initial selection of interviewers, and into their training and supervision. A quality control protocol for checking interviewing consistency using audio tapes of randomly selected interviews has been shown to reduce interviewer variability [10]. The number of interviewers involved in a survey is an important factor since small differences between interviewers may give rise to appreciable reductions in the precision of sample estimates if each interviewer has a large case-load. With a constant ρ_{int}, the impact of interviewer variance can be reduced by increasing the number of interviewers and so reducing the number of individuals responding to each interviewer. However, this will usually result in a more heterogeneous pool of interviewers, particularly in heath surveys, where the interviewer often needs special expertise, and in less intensive training and supervision, all of which will tend to increase ρ_{int}. Data quality can sometimes be improved by careful deployment of the interviewers. We have seen above that making sure that interviewers see respondents from all subgroups can improve the precision of subgroup comparisons. Matching interviewers to respondents, such as using an interviewer of the same gender for examining sexual behavior [6], can also sometimes be effective. For example, older white male interviewers gained more reports of substance abuse in a study by Johnson & Parsons [15].

Processing Errors

Once the respondents have answered the questions, the responses have to be coded, edited and entered in a machine-readable form. Supplemental editing will usually be needed to clean the data. Finally, the raw data will be manipulated into a form suitable for analysis. Missing values may be imputed at this stage. The processing stage is the least glamorous but often the most important step in the whole survey process. Errors can creep in at every step; we may find coding errors, transcription errors, and errors introduced by the editing. However, we have an opportunity to remedy some of the nonsampling errors introduced earlier in the survey operation. All large survey organizations have their own specialized editing procedures for detecting inconsistencies and unlikely responses. In some cases we may have to check back with the original respondent to get clarification of responses that do not pass the editing checks.

Coding and transcription errors can be minimized by cutting down the human component of the process as far as possible with the use of computer-assisted data entry techniques. Computer assisted telephone interviewing (CATI) is one of these techniques. Providing interviewers with laptop computers so that data entry and editing can be carried out at the time of the original interview as with CATI is another. Most of the effective methods to control human errors involve careful selection, training, and supervision of

personnel, just as with other sources of nonsampling errors. A good survey of modern methods for process control in surveys is given by Lyberg et al. [23].

Further Reading

Good general surveys of the broad field of nonsampling errors can be found in the books by Groves [13] and Lessler & Kalsbeek [19] and in the collections edited by Biemer et al. [2] and Lyberg et al. [21].

References

[1] Andersen, R., Kasper, J. & Frankel, M.R. (1970). *Total Survey Error. Applications to Improve Health Surveys.* Jossey-Bass, San Francisco.

[2] Biemer, P.R., Groves, R.M., Groves, K.E.K., Lyberg, L.E., Mathiowetz, N.A. & Sudman, S. eds. (1991). *Measurement Errors in Surveys.* Wiley, New York.

[3] Brambilla, D.J. & McKinlay, S.M. (1987). The comparison of responses to mailed questionnaires and telephone interviews in a mixed mode health survey, *American Journal of Epidemiology* **126**, 962–971.

[4] Cannell, C.F., Miller, P.V. & Okesenberg, L. (1981). Research on interviewing techniques, *Sociological Methodology* **12**, 389–437.

[5] Cannell, C.F., Fowler, F.J., Kalton, G., Okesenberg, L. & Bischoping, K. (1989). New quantitaive techniques for presenting survey questions, *Bulletin of the International Statistical Institute* **53**, 481–495.

[6] Catania, J.A., Binson, D., Canchola, J., Pollack, L.M., Hauck, W. & Coates, T.J. (1996). Effects of interviewer gender, interviewer choice, and item wording on responses to questions concerning sexual behaviour, *Public Opinion Quarterly* **60**, 345–375.

[7] Davis, P.B., Lay Yee, R., Chetwynd, J. & McMillan, N. (1993). The New Zealand Partner Relations Survey: methodological results of a national telephone survey, *Journal of Acquired Immune Deficiency Syndome* **7**, 1509–1516.

[8] Davis, P. & Scott, A. (1995). The effect of interviewer variance on domain comparisons, *Survey Methodology* **21**, 99–106.

[9] de Marco, R., Verlato, G., Zanolin, E., Bugiani, M. & Drane, J.W. (1994). Nonresponse bias in an EC respiratory health survey in Italy, *European Respiratory Journal* **7**, 2139–2145.

[10] Edwards, S., Slattery, M.L., Mori, M., Berry, T.D., Caan, B.J., Palmer, P. & Potter, J.D. (1994). Objective system for interviewer performance evaluation for use in epidemiological studies, *American Journal of Epidemiology* **140**, 1020–1028.

[11] Epstein, A.M., Hall, J.A., Tognetti, J., Son, L.H. & Conant, L. (1989). Using proxies to evaluate quality of life, *Medical Care* **27**, 291–298.

[12] Groves, R.M. (1989). *Survey Errors and Survey Costs*. Wiley, New York.

[13] Hebert, J.R., Clemow, L., Pbert, L., Ockene, I.S. & Ockene, J.K. (1995). Social desirability bias in diet self-report may compromise the validity of dietary intake measures, *International Journal of Epidemiology* **2**, 389–398.

[14] Hebert, J.R., Bravo, G., Korner-Bitensky, N. & Voyer, L. (1996). Refusal and information bias associated with postal questionnaires and face-to-face interviews in very elderly subjects, *Journal of Clinical Epidemiology* **49**, 373–381.

[15] Johnson, T.P. & Parsons, J.A. (1994). Interviewer effects on self-reported substance use among homeless persons, *Addictive Behaviours* **19**, 83–93.

[16] Kalton, G. & Kasprzyk, D. (1986). The treatment of missing survey data, *Survey Methodology* **12**, 1–16.

[17] Kalton, G. & Schuman, H. (1982). The effect of the question on survey response: a review, *Journal of the Royal Statistical Society, Series A* **145**, 42–73.

[18] Kish, L. (1962). Studies of interviewer variance for attitudinal items, *Journal of the American Statistical Association* **57**, 92–115.

[19] Lessler, J.T. & Kalsbeek, W.D. (1992). *Nonsampling Error in Surveys*. Wiley, New York.

[20] Locker, D. & Grusher, M. (1988). Response trends and non-response bias in a mail survey of oral and facial pain, *Journal of Public Health* **48**, 20–25.

[21] Lyberg, L.E., Biemer, P.P., Collins, M., de Leeuw, E., Dippo, C., Scwarz, N. & Trewin, D. eds. (1997). *Survey Measurement and Process Quality*. Wiley, New York.

[22] Magaziner, J., Bassett, S.S., Hebel, J.R. & Gruber-Baldini, A. (1996). Use of proxies to measure health and functional status in epidemiological studies of community-dwelling women aged 65 years and older, *American Journal of Epidemiology* **143**, 283–292.

[23] McHorney, C.A., Kosinski, M. & Ware, J.E. (1994). Comparisons of the costs and quality of norms for the SF-36 health survey collected by mail versus telephone interview: results from a national survey, *Medical Care* **32**, 551–567.

[24] Moore, D.S. (1985). *Statistics: Concepts and Controversies*. Freeman, San Francisco.

[25] Pope, D. & Croft, P. (1996). Surveys using general practice registers: who are the non-responders?, *Journal of Public Health Medicine* **18**, 6–12.

[26] Rao, J.N.K. (1996). On variance estimation with imputed data, *Journal of the American Statistical Association* **91**, 499–506.

[27] Schweitzer, M. & Asch, D.A. (1995). Timing payments to subjects of mail surveys: cost effectiveness and bias, *Journal of Clinical Epidemiology* **48**, 1325–1329.

[28] Sibbald, B., Addington-Hall, J., Brenneman, D. & Freeling, P. (1994). Telephone versus postal surveys of general practitioners: methodological considerations, *British Journal of General Practice* **44**, 297–300.

[29] Siemiatydi, J. & Campbell, S. (1984). Nonresponse bias and early versus all responders in mail and telephone surveys, *American Journal of Epidemiology* **120**, 291–301.

[30] Siemiatydi, J. (1979). A comparison of mail, telephone and home interview strategies for household health surveys, *American Journal of Public Health* **69**, 238–245.

[31] Tennant, A. & Badley, E.M. (1991). Investigating nonresponse bias in a survey of disablement in the community: implications for survey methodology, *Journal of Epidemiology and Community Health* **45**, 247–250.

[32] Van der Zouwen, J. & De Leeuw, E. (1990). The relationship between mode of administration and quality of data in survey research, *International Sociological Association Paper* 90S23659.

[33] Welte, J.W. & Russell, M. (1993). Influence of socially desirable responding in a study of stress and substance abuse, *Alcoholism, Clinical and Experimental Research* **17**, 758–761.

A. SCOTT & P. DAVIS

Nutrient Density Model *see* Nutritional Epidemiology

Nutritional Epidemiology

Epidemiology is the study of the etiology of illness and related phenomena in human populations [38]. Nutritional epidemiology, a branch of epidemiology, seeks to unfold the causal relationship between aspects of the diet and occurrence of human illness (*see* **Causation**). Historically, nutritional epidemiology was concerned mainly with nutritional deficiency diseases where a gross deficiency in a particular food or nutrient caused an untoward condition to occur. An early example, which took place in 1753, was the observation that consumption of lemons and oranges prevented the occurrence of scurvy among sailors on British ships, and this has led to the discovery of vitamin C deficiency as a cause of scurvy.

In recent years, the focus of nutritional epidemiology has been shifted from nutritional deficiency syndromes to the dietary determinants of chronic diseases such as heart disease and cancer. The underlying premise in contemporary nutritional epidemiology is that a person's long-term habitual diet has an impact on the occurrence of chronic disease. However, because the etiology of chronic diseases is a great deal more complex than that of deficiency syndromes, this shift in focus has indeed presented immense challenges. Whereas the occurrence of a deficiency syndrome typically has a single cause (deficiency in a food or nutrient item), the risk of a chronic disease not only can be attributed to numerous causal factors, including genetic, environmental, personal lifestyle (e.g. smoking, drinking, physical exercise) as well as dietary, but also the factors exert varying effects with complex **interactions** on disease occurrence. Moreover, a person's diet is made up of a myriad of dietary components, all of which tend to be correlated with each other, and some of which may increase the risk of disease while others may have a protective effect. Whereas a deficiency syndrome has a short **latent period** of exposure to a single cause (the time interval between onset of deficiency and onset of disease), many chronic diseases have latent periods of exposure that are protracted and ill-defined. Because humans are exposed to most dietary factors for their entire lives, there is no clear standard for comparison. Unlike a deficiency syndrome, where the exposure variable can be categorized as "not deficient" or "deficient", the degree of risk for a chronic disease attributed to most dietary factors varies on a continuum. Also, choosing the most relevant time (person's age) at which to begin measuring diet relative to disease onset (the reference period) is difficult and subjective because the reference period is seldom known and may vary not only from one disease to another but also among persons. Additionally, diet can at any time affect the disease process, and its effects may vary over time. The greatest challenge of all which confronts nutritional epidemiology of chronic diseases is how to measure accurately and precisely a person's long-term diet. Clearly these factors make it difficult to attribute the occurrence of a chronic disease to any single food or nutrient item, and consequently any observed relationship between a food or nutrient item and chronic disease must be interpreted with care and replicated in multiple studies. Notwithstanding, nutritional epidemiology has made important contributions to our knowledge regarding the influence of diet on the etiology of human diseases. The intent of this article is to present a brief overview of nutritional epidemiology. A comprehensive and lucid treatise of the subject

is given by Willett [44]. Other general references on nutritional epidemiology include [20] and [25].

Types of Nutritional Epidemiologic Study

Different methods and procedures can be used to carry out a nutritional epidemiologic study on the dietary etiology of human disease occurrence, and comprehensive accounts on epidemiologic study designs are available in the literature [25, 38]. Most of the nutritional epidemiology studies conducted to date are **observational** in nature, in that the allocation of persons to dietary exposure group is not under the control of the investigator. Instead, disease frequency is observed and compared between groups of subjects with different dietary exposures. In this section, we select a sampling of research findings from the different types of nutritional epidemiologic studies.

Group-based correlational studies, which correlate the aggregate disease rate with the average dietary intake for different groups of people, provided the earliest clues that a person's diet may affect the risk of chronic disease. A *geographic correlational study* compares the disease rate and average food intake of groups of people living in diverse geographic areas (*see* **Ecologic Study**). As an example, Armstrong & Doll in 1975 [3] correlated the cancer **incidence** and mortality rates with the per capita consumption of foods and nutrients from various countries. The correlations ranged from 0.7 to 0.8 for meat and animal fat consumption with colon cancer incidence and mortality in men and women; for fat intake with breast cancer incidence and mortality in women; and for fat intake with mortality from cancer of the corpus uteri. These remarkably high correlations stimulated further research on intake of animal products and cancer risk.

Other group-based correlational studies that make use of experiments ongoing in nature are studies of migrants, time trend, and special populations. **Migrant studies** compare disease rates defined by migration status. The disease rates of the first and second generation migrants are compared with rates of people in the country of origin as well as people in the host country. Haenszel & Kurihara in 1968 [15] compared the mortality from cancer and other diseases of the first generation Japanese migrants (Issei), US born second generation Japanese (Nisei), the Japanese in

Table 1 SMR comparing male mortality rates with those of Japanese men in Japan, adapted from Haenszel et al. [15]

Cause of death	Japan	Issei	Nisei	US whites
Stomach cancer	100	74	38	17
Colon cancer	100	374	288	489
Intracranial lesions of vascular origin (CVA)	100	32	24	37
Arteriosclerotic heart disease	100	226	165	481

Japan, and US whites. Table 1 summarizes the results for selected causes of death for men. The standardized mortality ratio (SMR) is the ratio of the rate of each index group to the rate of the standard population (Japanese in Japan) statistically adjusted to the age distribution of the standard population. The rate of the standard population is re-expressed as 100 [38] (*see* **Standardization Methods**).

It can be seen that stomach cancer and cerebrovascular accident (CVA) mortality rates show steady progressions from those in the parent country, where rates are high, to those in the host country, where rates are low. Similarly for colon cancer and heart disease, the mortality experience of the Issei and Nisei increased dramatically towards that of the US whites. The mortality rates for all four sites are higher in the Issei than in the Nisei, and part of this difference can be attributed to the considerable age difference between the two groups with the Issei being older than the Nisei. (The SMR corrects for age differences between the index groups and the standard population, but not between index groups.)

Migrant studies have provided strong evidence for the existence of environmental causes for chronic disease by finding that disease rates of the migrant populations diverged from those of the people in their country of origin and approached the rates of the people in their host country. Since the migrant populations and the people in their country of origin share the same genetic background, the change in disease rates must be attributed to environmental and lifestyle factors.

Studies of time trends can also be helpful in determining the role of the environment in disease etiology. For instance, mortality from stomach cancer in the US declined by more than 30% between 1950 and 1960, and this decline is coincident with a dramatic increase in the per capita consumption of fresh fruits and vegetables (*see* **Morbidity and Mortality, Changing Patterns in the Twentieth Century**). *Studies of special populations* whose diet is restricted also provide a unique opportunity to evaluate the role of the environment and lifestyle factors on disease etiology. For example, disease rates may be compared between Mormons, who abstain from caffeine intake, and a similar group of non-Mormon individuals, to assess the role of caffeine on disease development.

Although useful for generating diet–disease hypotheses, group-based correlational studies have fundamental weaknesses. The most crucial drawback of group-based data is **confounding**. Exposure data are collected at the group rather than at the individual subject level, making confounding a virtual certainty because the high correlations between exposure variables at the individual subject level cannot be disentangled. For example, in many populations where meat intake is high, vegetable intake tends to be low, and consequently any apparent association between average meat consumption and disease rate would be confounded by vegetable intake. When comparing populations of different races (and genetic backgrounds), as in a geographic correlation study, confounding by different genetic predispositions to diseases also renders the findings equivocal. The quality of the **cause of death** data on the death certificates can also vary considerably among countries (*see* **Death Certification**), and this may render the disease rates not comparable.

The types of study described below record dietary exposure and disease status from individual subjects, thus avoiding many of the drawbacks inherent in group-based data. The most widely used study design in nutritional epidemiology is the **case–control study**. With this study design, people with the disease (cases) and comparable individuals without the disease in question (**controls**) are asked about their dietary and nondietary exposures. Nutritional factors associated with disease occurrence are determined by comparing the past diet of the cases with that of the controls.

Two case–control studies were undertaken, one in Hong Kong [23] and one in the UK [11], to assess the effect of dietary calcium on hip fracture in men and women. Dietary calcium intake was estimated based on the frequency of consumption of nine food items in the Hong Kong study and six food items in the British study. A total of 400 radiologically confirmed fracture cases, 400 hospital controls, and 400 community controls were recruited in Hong Kong, and 300 cases were compared with 600 community controls in the UK. A clear protective effect of calcium intake on hip fracture was found in all groups excepting the British women (Table 2).

Case–control studies have largely been consistent in demonstrating the adverse effect of dietary fat for prostate cancer. One of these studies, conducted in Hawaii, included 452 histologically confirmed prostate cancer cases diagnosed between 1977 and 1983, and 899 age-matched (*see* **Matching**) population controls [21]. The participants were administered a diet history questionnaire with over 100 food items. Table 3 shows a monotonic effect of saturated fat on the risk of prostate cancer in older cases (those diagnosed after age 69), and the finding is consistent in most of the ethnic groups.

The case–control study offers many strengths in the investigation of the dietary etiology of chronic diseases. It is relatively inexpensive and efficient, typically requiring several hundred study participants and 2–4 years to complete the study; individual diet is measured and related to the risk of disease; and confounding can be minimized through appropriate selection of controls, by using appropriate statistical analysis techniques, or both. The case–control study is often the only feasible choice of study design for rare diseases. The primary disadvantage

in all case–control studies is that the measurement of exposure data relies on recall. This is particularly a problem in nutritional studies where cases must remember their past diets before the onset of disease. The diet may also have changed as a result of the disease process, and the current diet has been found to influence the recall of past diet. The results from a case–control study will be invalid if the cases remember their past diets differently than the controls do (**recall bias** of exposure), and if the controls are not comparable with the cases (**selection bias**). Healthy control bias can be especially problematic in studies of nutritional epidemiology if only health-conscious volunteers serve as controls.

Cohort studies avoid the inherent problems which afflict the case–control study, namely recall bias and selection bias. In this study design, diet is measured on a large number of disease-free individuals who are then monitored for disease occurrence. To date, cohort studies in nutritional epidemiology have been few in number, primarily because of their considerable high cost in terms of resources and length of follow-up. More than a decade of follow-up on thousands or even hundreds of thousands of individuals may be required in a cohort study of diet and chronic disease. Because a person's diet is likely to change with age, it is important to record dietary intake on several occasions from each study subject throughout

Table 2 Relative risks for hip fracture by quintiles of calcium intake (mg/day), adapted from Lau et al. [23] and Cooper et al. [11]

	Hong Kong			Britain		
	Calcium intake	Relative risk		Calcium intake	Relative risk	
Quintile	Range	Women	Men	Range	Women	Men
Q1 (low)	<75	1.9	2.1	<433	1.2	6.2
Q2	75–82	1.9	1.4	433–566	1.4	5.8
Q3	83–128	1.1	1.7	567–683	1.1	3.3
Q4	129–243	1.2	1.5	684–837	1.2	6.2
Q5 (high)	≥244	1.0	1.0	≥838	1.0	1.0

Table 3 Odds ratios for prostate cancer by quantiles of dietary fat intake, for cases diagnosed after age 69 and their matched controls, adapted from Kolonel et al. [21]

Quantile[a]	Total	Caucasians	Japanese	Filipinos	Hawaiians	Chinese
Q1	1.0	1.0	1.0	1.0	1.0	1.0
Q2	1.1	2.0	0.6	4.0	1.2	1.1
Q3	1.5	2.3	0.8	5.8	1.3	1.6
Q4	1.7	2.6	1.2	2.8		

[a]Quartiles for total, Caucasians, Japanese, and Filipinos, and tertiles for Hawaiians and Chinese.

the follow-up period. Repeated measurements will provide more accurate information about the average long-term exposure. As noted earlier, nutritional epidemiology of chronic disease is based on the premise that long-term dietary exposure affects disease risk.

In one large cohort study, 43 757 male health professionals in the US were recruited to investigate the etiology of the intake of dietary fiber on the occurrence of myocardial infarction. The cohort members completed a mailed dietary questionnaire with over 100 food items; they were then followed for 6 years for the occurrence of heart disease. Intake of dietary fiber, particularly from cereal, was found to be statistically associated with a decreased risk for myocardial infarction [32]. Table 4 shows the **relative risks** adjusted for relevant covariates.

Another cohort study example is the Iowa Women's Health Study, used to investigate the postulation that aspects of the diet influence the occurrence of endometrial cancer [47]. A cohort of over 23 000 women was recruited and a questionnaire with 127 food items was administered to each participant. After 7 years of follow-up, dietary intake was correlated with the incidence of endometrial cancer. Although the findings are on the whole equivocal, caloric intake from animal sources and intake of processed meat appear to be associated with a slight increase in the risk of endometrial cancer, especially during the early years of follow-up (Table 5).

In an *intervention study* or *controlled trial*, study participants are randomly allocated to the different dietary regimens. If the subjects have the disease, the dietary component is tested as a therapeutic agent, and if the subjects are disease-free, the dietary component is tested as a chemopreventive agent. The controlled trial has one crucial advantage over the cohort study described above, and that is randomization. Because random allocation of subjects to different exposure groups tends to reduce confounding, the controlled trial is able to establish with greater confidence whether a dietary component is a causal factor. However, practical limitations concerning compliance, dosage, latency (*see* **Latent Period**), and cost seriously diminish the usefulness of intervention studies in nutritional epidemiology. Most free-living individuals will not strictly follow a dietary regimen, and the persons in the control group may adopt a diet similar to the test diet, particularly if it is perceived to be beneficial (a phenomenon known as control drift). These compliance issues will obscure the differences between the treatment groups, making it more difficult to ascertain a true effect of the diet on disease risk. An example of "control drift" was found in the Multiple Risk Factor Intervention Trial (MRFIT) which randomly allocated 12 866 men at high risk for coronary heart disease to either a special intervention program or usual care [27]. The intervention program was a three-pronged intervention aimed

Table 4   Relative risks for myocardial infarction by quintile of energy-adjusted dietary fiber, adapted from Rimm et al. [32]

Type of fiber	Q1 (low)	Q2	Q3	Q4	Q5
Total	1.00	1.01	0.96	0.92	0.64
Fruit	1.00	0.93	0.83	0.84	0.82
Vegetable	1.00	1.06	0.98	1.00	0.84
Cereal	1.00	0.98	0.90	0.88	0.73

Table 5   Relative risks for endometrial cancer by tertile of intake for selected dietary factors, adapted from Zheng et al. [47]

	≤4 years after cohort entry			≥5 years after cohort entry		
	T1 (low)	T2	T3	T1 (low)	T2	T3
Caloric intake from animal foods	1.0	1.3	1.2	1.0	0.9	0.9
Total meat	1.0	1.0	1.3	1.0	1.0	0.9
Red meat	1.0	0.9	1.2	1.0	0.9	0.9
Seafood	1.0	1.4	1.0	1.0	1.4	2.0
Processed meat	1.0	1.4	1.6	1.0	1.0	1.3
Dairy products	1.0	1.2	1.2	1.0	0.8	1.0
Eggs	1.0	1.2	1.4	1.0	1.4	1.3

at smoking cessation, blood pressure, and serum cholesterol reduction through lifestyle and dietary modification. Although serum cholesterol dropped from 254 to 236 mg/dl over 72 months in the intervention group, a similar reduction occurred in the nonintervention group: from 254 to 240 mg/dl.

A randomized, double blind, placebo controlled trial of 29 133 male smokers, the Alpha-Tocopherol, Beta-Carotene Cancer Prevention Study, was undertaken to determine whether supplementation of alpha-tocopherol and beta-carotene would prevent lung cancer [7]. The study failed to confirm results from observational studies that had found a protective effect for these dietary components. Lack of precise dosage and latency information have been postulated as factors in the results.

Community intervention trials are experimental studies carried out at the population level; they are generally concerned with the effectiveness of an education or incentive program on behavior. For example, a number of participating communities may be randomly allocated either to receive information about the benefits of low-fat diets (test) or to receive no such information (control). **Cross-sectional** surveys, based typically on a sample of subjects from each community, are conducted before and after the information campaign to determine if there is a greater change in diet in the test communities than in the control communities. "Contamination" between groups, where the control communities also receive the test information, can be a problem in community trials.

Variation in Dietary Intake

As noted previously, the underlying premise of nutritional epidemiology is that a person's true "average" diet affects the occurrence of chronic diseases. It would be an easy task to ascertain a person's true diet provided that a person eats the same foods and the same quantity of each food day in and day out (no day-to-day variation), and that a person's diet and its nutrient content can be measured perfectly (no measurement error). In reality, a person's diet varies not only from day to day, but food preference and quantity consumed may be altered as one ages and as circumstances change. In contrast to simple exposures such as smoking, a person's diet is a composite exposure consisting of many food and beverage items consumed in varying amounts, and each

food and beverage item contains numerous macro and micronutrients. It is unlikely that an instrument ever will ever be developed which will ascertain dietary intake exactly. Indeed, accurate assessment of a person's long-term average diet is a major concern of nutritional epidemiologic research today, and methods and procedures for estimating the long-term diet are still evolving. In this section we delineate the concepts and definitions of variation in dietary intakes. Measurement error will be discussed in the next section.

The day-to-day variation in a person's food and nutrient intake is assumed to be random, that is, a person's daily diet fluctuates randomly about his or her "average" diet. This assumption implies that the average dietary intake over a number of randomly selected days will approach a person's true habitual intake, and that any deviation of intake on a given day from the true average diet is a reflection of imprecision (sampling error) rather than **bias**.

Some dietary components have been found to be more variable than others. Macronutrients, such as fat which is present in most foods, tend to show less day-to-day variation than substances that are present in only a few foods or whose amount is very high in a particular food. For instance, eating a mango can drastically increase the intake of beta-carotene for that day. The day-to-day dietary intake variation for a given person is referred to as *within-person variance*. And the variation in dietary intake among different persons is called *between-person variance*. To estimate within-person variance, more than one measurement per person is required.

It might be useful to depict the within-person and between-person components of dietary variation by a statistical model. The random effects analysis of variance model, also called the variance components model, is given as:

$$Y_{ij} = \mu + \alpha_i X_i + \varepsilon_{ij},$$

where Y_{ij} is the nutrient or food of interest for the ith person and the jth day of measurement, μ is the mean intake across persons and days, X_i is a dummy variable that identifies person i, α_i represents the random effect due to person i, and ε_{ij} represents the random day-to-day variability, or the within-person variability.

The variance components model assumes that these conditions hold: the variance of ε_{ij}, designated by σ_ε^2, is constant across days and persons, and the covariance between ε_{ij} and $\varepsilon_{i'j}$ is zero when $i \neq i'$. The variance of α_i, designated by σ_α^2, is constant across persons, and the covariance between α_i and $\alpha_{i'}$ is zero when $i \neq i'$. Models of dietary components often violate the first variance homogeneity assumption because persons with higher intake tend to have a larger within-person variance (i.e. the variance of ε_{ij} is proportional to Y_{ij}). The assumption is usually upheld after a suitable transformation (usually log) is applied to the nutrient data Y_{ij}.

The total variance (σ_y^2) is the sum of the between-person variance (σ_α^2) and the within-person variance (σ_ε^2). (With m replicated observations per person, total variability is $\sigma_\alpha^2 + \sigma_\varepsilon^2/m$.) The ratio of these quantities ($\sigma_\varepsilon^2/\sigma_\alpha^2$) gives an indication of the relative importance of the within-person to the between-person variance components. A ratio close to zero indicates that most of the dietary intake variability occurs between persons, in which case the intake level for an individual would be fairly constant from day-to-day. A ratio around one indicates an equal split between the two components, and ratios greater than one indicate that the within-person variance exceeds between-person variance. Another useful statistic based on the variance components is the "intraclass correlation coefficient", which will be described later under **validation studies**.

Numerous investigators have estimated the within-person and between-person variance components for the daily intake of common nutrients based on repeated food records [5, 16, 24, 28, 39]. Table 6 presents a summary of the results in the form of ratios. Although between-person variation is substantial, within-person variability is the larger variance component, accounting for 55% (carbohydrate) to 82% (vitamin A) of the total variation.

Measurement Error

Error in measuring the exposure variable is a common concern in all etiologic research. Measurement error may be minimal in simple exposures such as smoking history, but it may be quite consequential in complex exposures such as long-term dietary cholesterol intake. **Measurement error** occurs when the true exposure value in the ith person, X_i, is not directly observable, but instead a surrogate value, Z_i, is measured. Measurement error, defined as ($Z_i - X_i$), may be *random* (unbiased) or *systematic* (biased). The error is random if the expected (long-range average) value of Z_i is X_i, and is systematic if the expected value of Z_i is not X_i. Random measurement error will occur if a person is just as likely to overreport as to underreport, by the same amount, the consumption of a food item. **Systematic error** will occur if a person is more likely to underreport than overreport, or vice versa, the consumption of an item.

Systematic measurement error of the exposure variable may or may not bias the exposure–disease association. If measurement error is constant for all persons (e.g. all persons underreport the use of cooking oil by the same amount), the exposure–disease association will not be biased, and the power will not be diminished. However,

Table 6 Ratio of within-person to between-person variance components, adapted from [5], [16], [24], [28], and [39]

Nutrient	Number of studies	Median ratio	Range of ratios
Energy (kcal)	12	1.4	0.8-2.2
Protein	10	1.4	1.2–3.9
Carbohydrate	9	1.2	0.8–2.0
Fat	9	1.3	0.9–2.8
Percent of calories from fat	8	2.4	1.3–4.8
Saturated fat	8	1.5	1.0–2.8
Cholesterol	11	4.4	1.8–6.8
Vitamin C	9	2.3	1.6–4.0
Vitamin A	7	4.6	1.6–>100
Iron	8	2.4	1.5–3.6
Calcium	10	1.6	1.0–2.6
Zinc	6	2.4	1.7–11.7
Dietary fiber	3	1.7	1.1–2.2

systematic measurement error is seldom, if ever, the same for all individuals.

Although systematic measurement error may not be constant for all persons, the overall average error in persons with disease (cases) may be the same as that in persons without disease (controls). This is called **nondifferential measurement error**. Nondifferential error will not bias the exposure–disease association, but it will reduce the statistical power. **Differential measurement error** occurs when the overall average error in the cases is not the same as that in the controls (e.g. the cases on average underestimated the use of cooking oil more so than the controls). Systematic errors which are differential between cases and controls will lead to invalid estimates of the exposure–disease association, and the extent and direction of the bias are difficult to predict.

The consequence of **random measurement error** in the exposure variable will depend on the specific situation. If the exposure variable is a single continuous or dichotomous variable, random measurement error will attenuate the exposure–disease association, that is, **bias towards the null** the correlation coefficient, regression coefficient or relative risk. Random measurement error also tends to inflate the standard deviation for the association, thereby reducing power of statistical tests. If the exposure variable is polytomous (with more than two exposure levels), the **odds ratio** or relative risk for the most extreme exposure level will be biased toward the null value, while those for the intermediate levels can be biased away from the null [6, 13, 26]. When confounding variables are measured with random error, the effect of the exposure variable on disease risk may be biased away from the null, even if the exposure variable were measured without error [22]. Also random measurement error in the exposure variable can lead to incomplete adjustment of confounding, resulting in residual confounding in the adjusted exposure–disease association estimates [2, 14].

It is a useful practice to estimate the extent of measurement error in the exposure variables so that more reliable exposure–disease associations can be ascertained by taking into account these errors. Correction of measurement error may help to clarify whether an observed null exposure–disease association is real or attenuated. A *reproducibility study* with repeated measurements of the exposure variables can be deployed to estimate random exposure

measurement error. To evaluate systematic measurement error, a **validation study** of the dietary instrument against a "gold standard", or at least a more superior instrument, is required.

The simplest approach to reduce random measurement error in the exposure variable is to use the average value obtained from repeated measurements of the exposure, as an average based on replicated values has less random error than a single measured value. For example, study subjects are asked to keep food records on several occasions. This approach may be feasible in a small etiologic study but is likely to be prohibitive in a large study.

An alternative strategy to minimize the effect of exposure measurement error on the exposure–disease association is to estimate the association correcting statistically, for the measurement error in the exposure variable. The general approach is to quantitate the statistical relationship between the measured value, Z_i, and the true value, X_i, of the exposure variable obtained from a "calibration" study and to use this relationship in the correction of measurement error (*see* **Measurement Error in Epidemiologic Studies**). The "calibration" study is either a reproducibility or validation substudy based on a sample of subjects taken from the main etiologic study. Statistical methods pertaining to the correction of exposure measurement error abound in the literature, and they are still evolving. Because of the broad nature of these methods, which encompass different statistical models and assumptions and different types of measurement error, the account given below is intended only to provide a brief and incomplete sketch of the topic, with a sampling of references for the reader to turn to for more information.

The basic concept underlying the measurement error correction methods can be depicted by a simplified model. The expected value of X, given the observed Z, is substituted for every study participant in the main etiologic study, based on the calibration substudy information. $E(X|Z)$ is then substituted for Z in the disease etiology model in the main study to obtain an estimate of the true exposure–disease association. A critical assumption of this model is that the relationship between X and Z in the main study is the same as that in the calibration substudy sample. Wacholder et al. [41] warn that the value from the "gold standard" in the calibration study is almost always measured with error, albeit with less error than the measurements used in the main study. They show that correction to such an "alloyed gold standard" only partially eliminates the bias when the measurement errors between the two methods are moderately to strongly positively correlated. But when the measurement errors are either inversely correlated, uncorrelated, or weakly positively correlated, the corrected exposure–disease association estimate will tend to be overcorrected (anticonservative). It is clear that care needs to be exercised in the application of these statistical correction techniques.

The two examples shown below illustrate the effect of exposure measurement errors on the exposure–disease association and the role of the statistical correction method. Both the examples assume that results from a calibration substudy are available, that the relationship between X and Z in the calibration substudy can be extrapolated to the main study, and that the exposure measurement error is nondifferential, that is, it does not depend on disease status.

Example 1

This example illustrates a statistical technique for correcting systematic and random measurement errors in a dichotomous exposure variable [12]. Results from a validation study are required. Table 7 shows the frequencies for the association between a "true" exposure (X) and disease status.

The relationship between the true exposure (X) and the observed exposure (Z) from the calibration substudy is given in Table 8. Even with a moderately high **sensitivity** of 0.60 and **specificity** of 0.70, the exposure–disease associations are severely attenuated. As shown in Table 9, the true odds ratio of 5.0 becomes 1.6 and the true relative risk of 2.3 becomes 1.2.

Table 7 Association between true exposure (X) and disease status

	True exposure		
Disease status	Yes	No	Total
Yes	300	100	400
No	150	250	400
Total	450	350	800

Case–control
study: odds ratio $= (300 \times 250)/(150 \times 100) = 5.00$
Cohort study: relative risk $= (300/450)/(100/350) = 2.33$

Table 8 Relationship between true exposure (X) and observed exposure (Z)

	True exposure		
Observed exposure	Yes	No	Total
Yes	60	30	90
No	40	70	110
Total	100	100	200

Sensitivity $= \xi = 60/(60 + 40) = 0.60$.
Specificity $= \psi = 70/(30 + 70) = 0.70$.

Table 9 Association between observed exposure (Z) and disease status

	Observed exposure		
Disease status	Yes	No	Total
Yes	210	190	400
No	165	235	400
Total	375	425	800

Case–control
study: odds ratio $= (210 \times 235)/(165 \times 190) = 1.57$
Cohort study: relative risk $= (210/375)/(190/425) = 1.25$

Table 10 Correction identities

	Exposure	
Disease	Yes	No
Yes	a	b	n_D
No	c	d	n_{ND}

$$a_{\text{true}} = \frac{n_D\,\psi - b_{\text{obs}}}{\xi + \psi - 1}, \qquad b_{\text{true}} = \frac{n_D\,\xi - a_{\text{obs}}}{\xi + \psi - 1}$$

$$c_{\text{true}} = \frac{n_{ND}\,\psi - d_{\text{obs}}}{\xi + \psi - 1}, \qquad d_{\text{true}} = \frac{n_{ND}\,\xi - c_{\text{obs}}}{\xi + \psi - 1}$$

The odds ratio or relative risk estimates can be corrected for measurement error when sensitivity (ξ) and specificity (ψ) estimates are available from a validation substudy, using the identities in Table 10.

In our example,

$$a_{\text{true}} = \frac{400(0.70) - 190}{0.6 + 0.7 - 1} = 300,$$

$$b_{\text{true}} = \frac{400(0.6) - 210}{0.6 + 0.7 - 1} = 100,$$

$$c_{\text{true}} = \frac{400(0.70) - 235}{0.6 + 0.7 - 1} = 150,$$

$$d_{\text{true}} = \frac{400(0.6) - 165}{0.6 + 0.7 - 1} = 250.$$

This technique can be generalized to correct for differential measurement error if sensitivity and specificity estimates are available separately for cases and controls. Note the standard error for the corrected association will be larger than that for the uncorrected value to account for the sampling error in the estimation of sensitivity and specificity. A corrected standard error is not available in the literature. Rarely are epidemiologic studies focused on one dichotomous exposure variable without other covariates.

Example 2

This example illustrates that random measurement error in two dietary exposures will tend to bias their correlation towards zero. If information is available from a reproducibility study for the two measurements W and U, and no systematic error is present, then the following variance components model hold,

$$W_{ij} = \mu_W + \alpha_i X_i + \varepsilon_{ij},$$

$$U_{ij} = \mu_U + v_i X_i + \zeta_{ij},$$

so that the overall variances are $\mathrm{var}\, W = s_b^2 + s_w^2/n$ and $\mathrm{var}\, U = v_b^2 + v_w^2/m$. All errors are assumed to be uncorrelated. The estimate of the "true" correlation can be computed as

$$r_{\mathrm{true}} = r_{\mathrm{obs}} \left[(1 + s_w^2/(s_b^2 n))(1 + v_w^2/(v_b^2 m)) \right]^{1/2}$$

where r_{obs} is the observed correlation between W_{obs} and U_{obs}, s_w^2 is the within-person variability of W from a reproducibility study, s_b^2 is the between-person variability of W from a reproducibility study, n is the number of replicated values of W from a reproducibility study, v_w^2 is the within-person variability of U from a reproducibility study, v_b^2 is the between-person variability of U from a reproducibility study, and m is the number of replicated values of U from a reproducibility study.

The proof is given below:

$$r_{\mathrm{obs}} = \frac{\mathrm{cov}(W_{\mathrm{obs}}, U_{\mathrm{obs}})}{[\mathrm{var}(W)\,\mathrm{var}(U)]^{1/2}}$$

$$= \frac{\mathrm{cov}(\mu_W + a_i X_i + \varepsilon_{ij}, \mu_U + v_i X_i + \zeta_{ij})}{[(s_b^2 + s_w^2/n)(v_b^2 + v_w^2/m)]^{1/2}}$$

$$= \frac{\mathrm{cov}(\mu_W, \mu_U)}{[s_b^2 v_b^2 (1 + s_w^2/(ns_b^2))(1 + v_w^2/(mv_b^2))]^{1/2}}$$

$$= \frac{\mathrm{cov}(\mu_W, \mu_U)}{(s_b^2 v_b^2)^{1/2}}$$

$$\times \frac{1}{[(1 + s_w^2/(ns_b^2))(1 + v_w^2/(mv_b^2))]^{1/2}}$$

$$= r_{\mathrm{true}} \frac{1}{[(1 + s_w^2/(ns_b^2))(1 + v_w^2/(mv_b^2))]^{1/2}}.$$

When only one variable U is measured with error, the formula relating the true and observed correlations becomes

$$r_{\mathrm{true}} = r_{\mathrm{obs}}(1 + v_w^2/(v_b^2 m))^{1/2}.$$

Similarly, if only random error is present in the exposure variable, the slope in a linear regression can be corrected as

$$b_{\mathrm{true}} = b_{\mathrm{obs}}(1 + v_w^2/(mv_b^2))^{1/2}.$$

As an example suppose a reproducibility study includes 14 food records from which fat and vitamin E intake were computed. Assume the within to between person variance ratios of 1.5 for fat and 4.0 for vitamin E. In a large epidemiologic study, the correlation between these two nutrients was found to be 0.55. An estimate of the correlation corrected for measurement error is

$$0.55 \times [(1 + 1.5/14)(1 + 4.0/14)]^{1/2} = 0.66.$$

Again, the standard deviation for the corrected correlation coefficient or regression coefficient must account for the variability in the estimation of s_b^2, s_w^2, v_b^2, and v_w^2. Rosner et al. [34] derived a standard deviation for the corrected correlation based on the delta method. Readers are referred to Beaton et al. [5] for a more general formula where the measurement errors cannot be assumed uncorrelated, and to Kupper [22] for the effect on partial correlations when a confounder is measured with error.

Statistical principles and procedures for the correction of exposure measurement errors in relative risk and odds ratio estimates under more complex models and assumptions are expounded in the following references: [1], [2], [4], [31], [33], [35]–[37], and [43]. These methods address multiple continuous or categorical exposure variables, confounding variables, both systematic and random measurement errors, and other situations often encountered in nutritional epidemiologic research.

Dietary Assessment Methods

As noted earlier, the day-to-day variation and the measurement errors inherent in ascertaining a person's long-term diet constitute the major challenge in modern day nutritional epidemiology. Continuing research efforts are still being devoted to developing better methods for measuring a person's "average" diet. All the instruments used for assessing dietary intake rely on information supplied directly by the study participants, usually in the form of a questionnaire. Selection of a dietary assessment instrument for a given nutritional epidemiologic study is motivated by the intended use of the dietary data, and considerations include whether the short-term or long-term "average" diet is relevant, what dietary components are most germane, and whether absolute intake or relative intake (i.e. the ranking of individuals by intake) is desired.

The most commonly used tools for dietary assessment are food records, 24-hour recalls, and food frequency questionnaires. Food records and 24-hour recalls, methods that assess recent diet, are generally not feasible for use in large-scale epidemiology studies. Both methods provide information on the total diet (daily calories) and can give information concerning patterns of food consumption.

Food records are arguably the most accurate method for assessing dietary intake. Participants are required to record in a diary all foods at the time they are eaten, as well as ingredients to all recipes. Weighing foods before eating and any leftovers afterward is a common method for evaluating the amount of food consumed. The record-keeping typically covers 3–7 days. Clearly, this technique puts a heavy demand on the participants and is suitable only for literate and motivated volunteers. Another disadvantage with food records is that the very act of recording of foods consumed can change dietary behavior, either by avoiding foods that are considered undesirable or by simplifying the diet to facilitate the transcription. However, food diaries are often the assessment method of choice when high accuracy in the measurement of diet is needed, as for example in validation studies (described later).

In the *24-hour recall* method, a trained interviewer elicits information about the foods consumed and their amounts, during the past day. This technique is rapid, typically taking 10–20 minutes to complete, and is not very burdensome to the study participants.

The quality of the 24-hour recall is directly related to the skill of the interviewer, who uses structured probes to facilitate an individual's memory, but who must be careful not to influence the responses. Interviews should be unannounced to avoid having the persons change their diets for ease of recall. Telephone administration of 24-hour recalls is feasible, although the estimation of amounts is more difficult.

The crucial drawback of food records and 24-hour recalls is that the large within-person variability in most dietary components causes such short-term dietary information to be highly imprecise, deviating substantially from a person's usual or average diet. We illustrate this with the variance components model. Person k has true mean intake of $\mu + \alpha_k$, but with a single record or recall the measured value would be $\mu + \alpha_k + \varepsilon_{kj}$ with variance σ_ε^2. Averaging data across multiple records improves the estimation of the person's true average diet; with m replicated days of collection, person k's measured value would be $\mu + \alpha_k + \sum_j (\varepsilon_{kj})/m$ with variance σ_ε^2/m. It can be seen that the within-person variation becomes negligible as m increases. The number of replicated days required to characterize a person's "true" long-term average diet with high precision has been estimated from numerous dietary variability studies. Briefly, the estimates range from 4 days to 15 days for energy intake, 6 to 14 for fat intake, 6 to 23 days for vitamin C intake, and 47 to 105 days for vitamin A intake. Adjustment for calories (described later) tends to decrease the number of days slightly. Because many different methods were used to estimate the required number of replicated measurements, interested readers are directed to the following selected references: [5], [16], [24], [28], and [39].

The dietary assessment method best suited for use in large-scale nutritional epidemiologic studies is the *food frequency questionnaire* (FFQ), also referred to as the *diet history method*. With the FFQ technique, the frequency (and sometimes amount) of consumption of a list of commonly eaten foods is obtained. The list may consist of only a few highly selected food items, or as many as 100–200 food items, depending on the etiologic hypothesis being tested. The questions may be open ended, where the respondent gives the frequency of consumption for each food item as times per day, week, month or year, or they may be close ended where several frequency categories are listed. Seasonal food items are incorporated by asking for their intake during the season they are available. Many of these questionnaires have "write-in" options where more detail is obtained about specific foods or where participants can add food items important to their diets that are not covered by the list. If the amount consumed is also estimated, typically by incorporating usual portion size or serving size of each food item, the questionnaire is then referred to as "quantitative". The serving sizes of foods with natural units such as eggs are relatively easy to assess. For other foods, aids such as household measures, food models, or photographs are often used to facilitate estimation.

The FFQ method is flexible in that it can be used for short-term or long-term dietary recall, and for estimating a partial or comprehensive diet; it can be administered by an interviewer or self-administered. When the long-term average diet is desired, as is the case with most nutritional epidemiologic research, it is important to inquire about a person's diet covering the relevant time frame or reference period. In a case–control study, the case is asked about his or her "usual" diet before the onset of symptoms, and the control is typically asked about last year's diet, provided there has not been a recent change in the diet. In a cohort study, it is important to administer the FFQ more than once to increase the precision of the estimate of a person's average diet.

A comprehensive diet (or total caloric intake) is sometimes required as overnutrition or undernutrition may have a direct effect on disease risk. Also, measurement of dietary components relative to the total diet may be of interest (see caloric adjustment below).

A drawback of the FFQ is that its list format makes it "population sensitive". A questionnaire that is well suited to one population (e.g. Caucasians) may not include the necessary items to cover adequately the diet in another group (e.g. Japanese). It is crucial to ensure that a FFQ covers all the commonly consumed food items in the population. The FFQ interview can be lengthy, typically requiring between 1 and 2 hours to complete, and this may adversely affect the response rate. Because the FFQ inquires only about consumption of selected foods, it measures relative rather than absolute dietary intake. Administration of different FFQs to the same person is likely to produce different absolute values on intakes, such as grams of fat consumed per day. However, the dietary intakes of a group of persons as assessed by the two FFQs should show comparable rankings. Measurement of relative intake is generally adequate

for etiologic research because comparison between cases and controls is of central interest.

Dietary Components

Diet consists of many substances, such as nutrients, additives, contaminants, and other unknown compounds. Information collected on a limited set of relevant foods may be adequate when the dietary component of interest is concentrated in those foods. In most studies on nutritional etiology of disease, however, a wide variety of dietary components are of interest, such as intake of total calories; macronutrients, including fat, protein, and carbohydrate; micronutrients, including vitamin A, vitamin E, and iron; and intake of particular foods or groups of food, such as red meat or fruits.

In many of the early studies, information on a brief list of foods was collected, and analysis was focused on food intake. More recently, questionnaires on comprehensive diet were introduced, and the emphasis was on nutrient rather than food intake. There is now some realization that both nutrients and foods are important. A nutrient may react in the same way biologically regardless of its food source, in which case the nutrient intake is relevant. Also, nutrient analyses allow comparison across studies from populations with different food intakes. An example where food intake may be the relevant exposure is the recent interest in the influence of soy product consumption on the risk of certain cancers. Analyses often incorporate both nutrients and food sources. For instance, fat from meat sources and fat from dairy products can be studied as separate exposures. Because food choices are correlated, it is desirable to study food patterns and disease risk. Analysis of food patterns with techniques such as factor analysis has been attempted but is very preliminary.

Use of dietary supplements can substantially alter a person's dietary profile, and information on supplement use should be collected. However, the nutrient data should be analyzed separately from food alone and from foods and supplements, as it is not known if a nutrient from a food and from a supplement behave the same way biologically.

Computation of Nutrients

Computation of nutrients requires information on the nutrient composition of the food. Information generally comes from published nutrient composition tables, but may be supplemented by food analysis. National nutrient composition data are available from many countries; the US Department of Agriculture (USDA) publishes information about the nutritional content of foods in the US. Investigators need to use food composition data from food sources similar to those under study whenever possible. Nutrient content can vary dramatically by locale. For example, the carotene content of plants is affected by soil type, and the iodine content of fish is affected by seawater content. The nutrient composition data in national tables usually represents an average value from analyses of that food from different sources and locales. The tables generally have information on hundreds of nutrients, given as units, such as grams and milligrams, per 100 grams of food. The nutrient composition data have varying degrees of accuracy. Macronutrients such as protein and fat content tend to vary less between food samples than micronutrients. Some nutrients, like selenium, are so variable between samples that usefulness of the nutrient composition data is questionable.

The algorithm for nutrient computation is to compute, for each food in the recall or FFQ, the daily grams of consumption. If portion size is asked, each serving size needs to be assigned a weight in grams. Otherwise, weight in grams should be assigned to a standard serving size. Daily grams are computed for each food as frequency of intake per day times the gram weight of that food. These quantities are compared against a food composition table, and daily nutrients from each food are computed as daily grams of consumption times the nutrient content of that food per 100 grams, multiplied by 100. These quantities are summed across foods for each person to obtain nutrients per day. Note that each food on the dietary assessment instrument must be associated with a food in the composition table. This assignment is very labor intensive for food records and 24-hour recalls and requires a person knowledgeable about nutrition, such as a dietitian. A questionnaire specific food composition table is required for FFQs where several foods are grouped into a single question. For example, an item for beef may include steak and roasts. The corresponding item in the food composition table will be a weighted average of nutrient composition data for each beef item. Complex questionnaires generally require initial preparation before comparison with food composition data, such as adjustment for oils added during cooking and fats eaten on meats.

Reproducibility and Validity

With FFQs, volunteers are asked to estimate their own usual diets. In the parlance of the variance components model, a participant is being asked to recall the true average intake $\mu + \alpha_k$, thereby "eliminating" the within-person day-to-day variability. It is of course essential to gauge how well the FFQ measures true average diet. Desirable qualities for a FFQ are reproducibility and validity.

A *reproducible*, or reliable, instrument will give consistent answers on repeated administrations. To study reliability, a FFQ is given to the same person at two or more points in time and their responses are compared. The time period between administrations cannot be too short so that participants remember what they reported earlier. It also cannot be too long as an intervening dietary change can affect responses. Therefore, a period of several months is typical. Correlations between multiple administrations of questionnaires have ranged from 0.5 to 0.7; these correlations compared favorably with the reproducibility for many biological measures, such as blood pressure, over similar time intervals.

A *valid* instrument measures what it is intended to measure. A valid instrument is reproducible, although the reverse is not necessarily true. To verify validity of an instrument, measurements are compared against accurate measurements from a "gold standard". Because no perfect gold standard exists for diet, FFQs are typically compared against superior dietary measurements, mostly commonly against repeated food records, Burke's dietary history, or repeated 24-hour recalls. Biological markers are also used. Generally, a random sample of subjects from the population of interest is asked to give information on their diets via multiple records or recalls. These records or recalls need to span different days of the week and different seasons for the average across measurements to match closely the person's true average diet. Timing of the administration of the FFQ is problematic. Administration prior to the recalls and records prevents the more detailed record keeping from altering the questionnaire responses, that is, a learning effect. However, the reference periods will be different, in that the questionnaire will ask about the year prior to the period of detailed dietary information. Administration several months after the last record or recall has the benefit that the reference periods will be similar. As the participants cannot be told at the beginning that a subsequent questionnaire will be requested, drop out can be a problem; the records or recalls of persons unwilling to do the subsequent questionnaire will be unusable. Also, fatigue may detrimentally affect the quality of responses to the FFQ. It is crucial that the same food composition table be used to compute the nutrient intakes from both dietary methods so that the difference between them cannot be attributed to differences in the nutrient computation methods.

Ideally, correlation between the test method (FFQ) and the gold standard should only reflect the extent to which the FFQ measures diet accurately. However, the food record, the 24-hour recall, and the FFQ methods all require the participants to record their diets, which may induce spurious correlations: a person who is a poor recorder of diet will tend to report low intake values on all instruments, regardless of true intake. In this regard, use of biomarkers as the gold standard in validation studies seems appealing, as the measurement procedure is completely unrelated to recording of the diet. However, there are serious limitations to their use, as few biomarkers exist and those that do, such as doubly-labeled water and 24-hour urine nitrogen, only measure current nutritional status, not "usual" status. In addition, biomarkers are not only inordinately expensive, but they can only validate one nutrient at a time, and are dependent on a person's metabolism as well as dietary intake.

Analysis of Validation Studies

Measurements of validity need to be adjusted or stratified (*see* **Stratification**) for variables that will be controlled for in the final epidemiologic analysis. For instance, validation should be performed separately for different gender, age, ethnic, and education groups if the questionnaire is intended for use in these groups. Inclusion of groups with diverse diets in the validation study will increase between-person variation which will inflate the correlation. The between-person variance will be reduced through stratification or adjustment in the epidemiologic analysis, and therefore the adjustment should be performed in the

validation study also. For instance, without adjustment for sex, a FFQ that poorly assesses calories could yield a high correlation with a "gold standard", simply because it is able to distinguish the substantial difference in caloric intake between men and women.

Several statistical methods can be used to compare the performance of a dietary questionnaire with that of a "gold standard". The choice of statistical method will depend on the intended use of the validation study. Means and standard deviations can be presented for both methods, and a paired *t* test used to compare the means. For most etiologic studies, it may be sufficient for a questionnaire simply to rank people correctly, in which case a systematic overestimation or underestimation in nutrient values will not bias the exposure–disease association. A single number comparing the two dietary methodologies for each nutrient is desirable as a moderate number of nutrients are generally compared in a validation study. The most frequently used agreement measure is Pearson's correlation coefficient r on log transformed nutrient data, which measures the linear relation between the two measurements. A disadvantage to this statistic is that it depends not only on the agreement between the methods, but also on between-person variability in the population. Use of r, however, allows for easy comparison with past studies. The intraclass correlation coefficient, defined as $r_I = (\sigma_\alpha^2 - \sigma_\varepsilon^2)/(\sigma_\alpha^2 + \sigma_\varepsilon^2)$ from the variance components model, measures **agreement**, rather than correlation, because it accounts for the between-person variability. The r_I can be thought of as the proportion of the total variation accounted for by between-person variability. Often in a validation study, an investigator would like to know if the questionnaire performs equally well for different groups. The correlation coefficients can be statistically compared between subgroups by converting the correlations to Fisher z statistics, which approximately have a normal distribution, and comparing the z' values by a chi-square statistic [40].

The **kappa** statistic is a measure of agreement for nominal variables that adjusts for chance agreement. To use kappa in validation studies of dietary questionnaires, the nutrients from each of the two measurements must be categorized. A disadvantage to this statistic is that the agreement depends on the categorization, and it must be decided whether to use different cutpoints for the food records and the questionnaire, in

Table 11   Pearson's correlation coefficients between FFQs and a superior dietary assessment method, adapted from [25]

Nutrient	Number of investigations	Median	Range	Interquartile range
Energy (kcal)	12	0.48	0.29–0.74	0.35–0.58
Protein	10	0.42	0.18–0.80	0.41–0.58
Carbohydrate	7	0.48	0.27–0.60	0.42–0.58
Fat	12	0.52	0.08–0.94	0.36–0.59
Cholesterol	6	0.50	0.42–0.67	0.46–0.60
Vitamin C	9	0.46	0.33–0.64	0.38–0.58
Vitamin A	6	0.40	0.21–0.63	0.33–0.51
Vitamin E	4	0.49	0.39–0.64	0.44–0.56
Calcium	3	0.63	0.61–0.66	–

which case the kappa measures correlation, or whether to use the same cutpoints, in which case agreement is measured. A weighted kappa is a generalization where cells other than those representing complete agreement are counted as partial agreements; with specific weights, the weighted kappa is related to the intraclass correlation coefficient. Regression coefficients cannot be used to measure the strength of the relationship, since the slope is not scale-free but depends on the standard deviations of the measurements.

Numerous studies have been conducted to validate the FFQ against repeated food records or 24-hour recalls, or Burke's diet history [25]. A summary of the results is presented in Table 11. It can be seen that the correlation varies substantially between studies, attributed to differences in the period between assessments, the number of repeated food records or recalls, and the populations studied. Most correlations appear to be in the range of 0.35 to 0.60. In one of the most detailed validation studies, women completed a FFQ at the beginning of the study, collected four 1-week food records at 3-month intervals, and then completed another FFQ [44]. In this study, the correlations ranged from 0.28 for iron to 0.61 for carbohydrate. Adjustment for caloric intake tended to improve the correlations. Questionnaires can be validated for food intake as well, although the correlations tend to be low because of the high within-person variability for foods.

Statistical Methods

As noted previously, nutritional epidemiology investigates the influence of the diet (exposure variable) on disease occurrence or death (outcome variable). Because nutritional epidemiology is a branch of chronic disease epidemiology, all of the statistical principles and methods for chronic disease epidemiology [8, 9, 38] are applicable to nutritional epidemiology. Thus, the exposure–disease association in nutritional epidemiology is quantified by the odds ratio, **risk** ratio, or hazard ratio, depending on the study design, and the statistical models used to estimate this association include the **logistic regression**, **Cox regression**, and **Poisson regression** models. What is unique about nutritional epidemiology is that the primary exposure variable (a person's long-term diet) is imprecisely measured, due to considerable within-person variation and measurement errors. As highlighted in the previous sections, many of the statistical methods were developed to address this problem. In this section, several other statistical topics that are especially germane to nutritional epidemiology will be highlighted.

Grouping of the Exposure Variable

In the statistical analysis of data from nutritional epidemiology, the exposure variable (food or nutrient intake) is often initally categorized into approximately evenly sized groups, such as tertiles, quartiles or quintiles, and then entered into the appropriate statistical model as indicator or dummy variables. The cutpoints are generally based on the distribution of the controls, although the joint distribution of cases and controls can also be used and provides the best dispersion of counts by exposure category. This grouping of continuous exposure variables serves several purposes: the distribution of a nutrient tends to be skewed to the right and categorization dampens the effect of the extreme values; the effect of measurement error is reduced in that the dietary questionnaire needs only to categorize people into broad categories of intake; and the relationship between exposure and risk of disease occurrence can be assessed for **dose–response** trend. If the exposure is to be used as a continuous variable, then it is important to check that the relationship is indeed monotonic prior to analysis. Statistical evaluation of trend can be performed in a number of ways, such as using a continuous predictor or assigning scores to categories [38].

Multiple Comparisons

Some dietary questionnaires have more than 100 food items, which are then converted to between 20 and 30 nutrients. Statistical analysis of exposure–disease associations for all of these exposure variables will give rise to many statistical tests of "significance". Moreover, statistical analysis if often repeated in subgroups defined by such factors as gender, race, age, or subcategory of disease (e.g. stage of disease). It is not uncommon to perform an overwhelmingly large number of statistical tests from a single study, giving a high likelihood of finding many "statistically significant" test results purely by chance. It is crucial that the investigator is aware of this problem. It is equally important to make clear in the research report which hypotheses constitute a priori or a posteriori tests. A stricter criterion for reporting "statistical significance" should be deployed for a posteriori tests.

Multicollinearity

Certain types of eating patterns are generally seen together in individual diets, such as high fat and low fiber diets. These eating patterns sometimes create very high correlations, or multicollinearity, between dietary exposures, leading to problems in model estimation. If two exposure variables, such as fat and dietary fiber, are highly inversely correlated, then the regression coefficient (and hence the effect measure) for fat will vary depending on whether dietary fiber is in the model. Therefore, with multicollinearity, the regression coefficient does not reflect any underlying effect of the variable on disease, but rather a marginal effect that depends on what other variables are included in the model. Additionally, standard errors of regression coefficients are inflated when the

independent variables in the model are highly correlated with each other, and the correlated variables may not individually be statistically significant even if there is a strong relationship between the set of predictor variables and the outcome variable. In nutritional epidemiologic studies, correlations between foods and nutrients need to be investiaged prior to building a model with multiple nutritional predictors. Remedial measures for multicollinearity, such as ridge regression, are available. However, effects of nutrients with near perfect correlation cannot be estimated separately.

Energy Adjustment Methods

Almost all of a person's total energy (caloric) intake is contributed by three macronutrients: intake of fat, protein, and carbohydrate. (Alcohol intake may also contribute substantially to some peoples' energy intake.) The current thinking of some nutritional epidemiologists is that it is not enough to estimate the effect of a food or nutrient on the risk of disease without giving due consideration to total energy intake [44]. For example, if high fat and energy intake were found to elevate the risk for colon cancer, then it is important to distinguish whether the apparent effect of fat intake on colon cancer actually acts through its contribution to the energy content (higher fat intakes results in higher energy content) or whether there is a specific effect of fat, independent of energy intake, on colon cancer. Statistically, what is needed is to estimate the association between fat intake and colon cancer adjusting for energy intake. Another justification for energy adjustment is that the same amount of a nutrient consumed will have less potency on a large person than on a smaller person (here, energy intake can be thought of as a surrogate for body size). Energy adjustment has also been advocated for micronutrients, such as vitamins and minerals, even though they have no appreciable energy content.

Not all nutritional epidemiologists agree with the need for energy adjustment in the estimation of nutrient-disease associations, and even though a variety of statistical methods have been proposed for energy adjustment, none is generally accepted as a standard. Indeed, energy adjustment is currently highly contentious [10, 17–19, 29, 30, 42, 44–46]. This section presents a brief sketch of the four proposed energy adjustment models. In these models, D denotes disease status, N denotes calories from the nutrient of interest, and T denotes total caloric intake. The exact specification of the regression model $M(\cdot)$ is not given, but the logistic and Cox **proportional hazards** models are the common choices.

Standard Model. $M(D) = \beta_{0S} + \beta_{1S}N + \beta_{2S}T + \varepsilon$, where the variables N and T are entered in the model simultaneously.

Residual Model. $M(D) = \beta_{0R} + \beta_{1R}R + \beta_{2R}T + \varepsilon$, where R is the residual from the linear regression model of N on $T : N = \alpha_0 + \alpha_1 T$.

Partition Model. $M(D) = \beta_{0P} + \beta_{1P}N + \beta_{2P}(T - N) + \varepsilon$, where the caloric intake is partitioned into calories from the nutrient of interest (N) and those from other sources ($T - N$).

Nutrient Density Model. $M(D) = \beta_{0N} + \beta_{1N} (N/T) + \beta_{2N}T + \varepsilon$, where the calories from the nutrient are divided by the total calories (N/T) to give the proportion of calories from the nutrient of interest.

The following identities show that the first three models are in fact equivalent when N and T are continuous. However, the models are not equivalent when either N or T or both are categorized and represented by indicator variables. Brown et al. [10] noted that the residual model is the most powerful and robust of the three models with categorized variables.

Relationship between standard and residual models:

$$\beta_{0S} = \beta_{0R} - \alpha_0 \beta_{1R},$$

$$\beta_{1S} = \beta_{1R},$$

$$\beta_{2S} = \beta_{2R} - \alpha_1 \beta_{1R}.$$

Relationship between standard and partition models:

$$\beta_{0S} = \beta_{0P},$$

$$\beta_{1S} = \beta_{1P} - \beta_{2P},$$

$$\beta_{2S} = \beta_{2P}.$$

Relationship between residual and partition models:

$$\beta_{0P} = \beta_{0R} - \alpha_0 \beta_{1R},$$

$$\beta_{1P} - \beta_{2P} = \beta_{1R},$$

$$\beta_{2P} = \beta_{2R} - \alpha_1 \beta_{1R}.$$

No one model appears clearly superior to another. The choice of model with continuous variables may be guided by the meaning of the parameters contained in each model. In the standard model, β_{1S} measures the effect on D of increasing N by 1 unit while keeping total calories constant, that is, the effect of substituting calories from sources other than N (denote by N') with calories from N. β_{2S} represents the effect on D of increasing T by 1 unit while keeping N constant, that is, the effect of increasing calories from N'.

In the residual model, the above identities show that β_{1R} also measures the effect of substituting calories from N' with calories from N. The parameter β_{2R} represents the effect on D of increasing T by 1 unit while holding R constant. Recall that $R = N - \alpha_0 - \alpha_1 T$. Substituting $T' = (N + N') + 1$ into the equation, R is constant only when an increase of 1 unit in N' is matched with a concomitant increase in N of $\alpha_1/(1 - \alpha_1)$ units.

The partition model parameter β_{1P} measures the effect of increasing N by 1 unit while holding N' constant, that is, the effect on D of adding 1 calorie from N. By the identity with β_{2S}, β_{2P} represents the effect of increasing calories from N' by 1 unit.

The nutrient density model has a more complex structure that involves the reciprocal of caloric intake, making its coefficients rather difficult to interpret.

The partition model appears to have the parameters with the most straightforward interpretation, although it cannot be used to energy-adjust food or micronutrient intake. Pike et al. [29, 30] point out that the interpretation of β_1 in all four models is complicated by the fact that N' is itself made up of many dietary components. Suppose the nutrient of interest is fat. A β_{1S} of 0 would indicate that a substitution of 1 nonfat calorie with 1 fat calorie has no effect, that is, that calories from different sources have the same influence on the risk of D. This conclusion would be incorrect if calories from carbohydrate have a protective effect and calories from protein and alcohol have a direct effect on risk. The effect of calories from fat is being compared against the average effect of calories from the other components in these models.

Wacholder et al. [42] argue that it is not possible to distinguish the generic effect on the delivery of energy from the nutrient of interest and any specific effect of that nutrient. They point out that the true model of interest is

$$M(D) = \beta_0 + \beta_N N + \beta_{N'} N' + \beta_T T + \varepsilon,$$

which is a nonidentifiable problem because $T = N + N'$. All four models given above are special cases of this model, where one of the parameters is excluded. Therefore, the parameters in the energy adjustment models are confounded by the missing parameter and cannot clearly distinguish between a generic caloric effect and a specific nutrient effect. It is clear that when energy and nutrient intakes are too highly correlated, the variables measure nearly the same function (highly collinear), and their effects on D cannot be segregated. In this case, the residuals from the regression of N on T will have limited variability, as most of it will have been explained by calories, and should not be used to represent an independent exposure variable.

Energy adjustment methods can be used as a tool to investigate the joint effects of energy and individual nutrients on disease risk, but it is clear that much care must be taken in its application and interpretation.

Acknowledgments

This project was supported in part by National Institutes of Health (NIH) grants P01-CA-33619 and P30-CA-71789 from the National Cancer Institute.

References

[1] Armstrong, B.G. (1985). Measurement error in the generalised linear model, *Communications in Statistics – Simulation and Computation* **14**, 529–544.

[2] Armstrong, B.G. (1990). The effects of measurement errors on relative risk regressions, *American Journal of Epidemiology* **132**, 1176–1184.

[3] Armstrong, B. & Doll, R. (1975). Environmental factors and cancer incidence and mortality in different countries, with special reference to dietary practices, *International Journal of Cancer* **15**, 617–631.

[4] Armstrong, B.G., Whittemore, A.S. & Howe, G.R. (1989). Analysis of case–control data with covariate measurement error: application to diet and colon cancer, *Statistics in Medicine* **8**, 1151–1163.

[5] Beaton, G.H., Milner, B.A., Corey, P., McGuire, V., Cousins, M., Stewart, E., de Ramos, M., Hewitt, D., Grambsch, P.V., Kassim, K. & Little, J.A. (1979). Sources of variance in 24-hour dietary recall data: implications for nutrition study design and interpretation, *American Journal of Clinical Nutrition* **32**, 2456–2259.

[6] Birkett, N.J. (1992). Effect of nondifferential misclassification on estimates of odds ratios with multiple levels of exposure, *American Journal of Epidemiology* **136**, 356–362.

[7] Blumberg, J. & Block, G. (1994). The alpha-tocopherol, beta-carotene cancer prevention study in Finland, *Nutrition Reviews* **54**, 242–250.

[8] Breslow, N.E. & Day, N.E. (1980). *Statistical Methods in Cancer Research*, Vol. I: *The Analysis of Case–Control Studies*. World Health Organization, International Agency for Research on Cancer, Lyon.

[9] Breslow, N.E. & Day, N.E. (1987). *Statistical Methods in Cancer Research*, Vol. II: *The Design and Analysis of Cohort Studies*. World Health Organization, International Agency for Research on Cancer, Lyon.

[10] Brown, C.C., Kipnis, V., Freedman, L.S., Hartman, A.M., Schatzin A. & Wacholder, S. (1994). Energy adjustment methods for nutritional epidemiology: the effects of categorization, *American Journal of Epidemiology* **139**, 323–338.

[11] Cooper, C., Barker, D.J.P. & Wickham, C. (1988). Physical activity, muscle strength, and calcium intake in fracture of the proximal femur in Britain, *British Medical Journal* **297**, 1443–1446.

[12] Copeland, K.T., Checkoway, H., McMichael, A.J. & Holbrook, R.H. (1977). Bias due to misclassification in the estimation of relative risk, *American Journal of Epidemiology* **105**, 488–495.

[13] Dosemeci, M., Wacholder, S. & Lubin, J. (1990). Does misclassification of exposure always bias a true effect toward the null value?, *American Journal of Epidemiology* **132**, 746–748.

[14] Greenland, S. (1980). The effect of misclassification in the presence of covariates, *American Journal of Epidemiology* **112**, 564–569.

[15] Haenszel, W. & Kurihara, M. (1968). Studies of Japanese migrants. I. Mortality from cancer and other diseases among Japanese in the United States, *Journal of the National Cancer Institute* **40**, 43–68.

[16] Hartman, A.M., Brown, C.C., Palmgren, J., Pietinen, P., Verkasalo, M., Myer, D. & Virtamo, J. (1990). Variability in nutrient and food intakes among older middle-aged men. Implications for design of epidemiologic and validation studies using food recording, *American Journal of Epidemiology* **132**, 999–1012.

[17] Howe, G.R. (1989). The first author replies. Re: Total energy intake: implications for epidemiologic analyses, *American Journal of Epidemiology* **129**, 1314–1315.

[18] Howe, G.R., Miller, A.M. & Jain, M. (1986). Re: Total energy intake: implications for epidemiologic analyses, *American Journal of Epidemiology* **124**, 157–159.

[19] Kipnis, V., Freedman, L.S., Brown, C.C., Hartman, A., Schatzkin, A. & Wacholder, S. (1993). Interpretation of energy adjustment models for nutritional epidemiology, *American Journal of Epidemiology* **137**, 1376–1380.

[20] Kohlmeier, L. & Helsing, E., eds (1989). *Epidemiology, Nutrition and Health: Proceedings of the First Berlin Meeting on Nutritional Epidemiology, Berlin, 1988*.

Smith-Gordon, London; Nishimura Company Niigata-Shi, Japan, pp. 1–109.

[21]   Kolonel, L.N., Yoshizawa, C.N. & Hankin, J.H. (1988). Diet and prostatic cancer: a case–control study in Hawaii, *American Journal of Epidemiology* **127**: 999–1012.

[22]   Kupper, L.L. (1984). Effects of the use of unreliable surrogate variables on the validity of epidemiologic research studies, *American Journal of Epidemiology* **120**, 643–648.

[23]   Lau, E., Donnan, S., Barker, D.J.P. & Cooper, C. (1988). Physical activity and calcium intake in fracture of the proximal femur in Hong Kong, *British Medical Journal* **297**, 1441–1443.

[24]   Liu, K., Stamler, J., Dyer, A., McKeever, J. & McKeever, P. (1978). Statistical methods to assess and minimize the role of intra-individual variability in obscuring the relationship between dietary lipids and serum cholesterol, *Journal of Chronic Diseases* **31**, 399–418.

[25]   Margetts, B.M. & Nelson, M., eds. (1991). *Design Concepts in Nutritional Epidemiology.* Oxford University Press, New York.

[26]   Marshall, J.R., Priore, R., Graham, S. & Brasure, J. (1981). On the distortion of risk estimates in multiple exposure level case–control studies, *American Journal of Epidemiology* **113**, 464–473.

[27]   Multiple Risk Factor Invention Trial Research Group (1982). Multiple risk factors intervention trial: risk factor changes and mortality results, *Journal of the American Medical Association* **248**, 1465–1477.

[28]   Nelson, M., Black, A.E., Morris, J. & Cole, T.J. (1989). Between and within subject variation in nutrient intake from infancy to old age: estimating the number of days required to rank dietary intakes with desired precision, *American Journal of Clinical Nutrition* **50**, 155–167.

[29]   Pike, M.C., Bernstein, L. & Peters, R.K. (1989). Re: Total energy intake: implications for epidemiologic analyses, *American Journal of Epidemiology* **129**, 1312–1313.

[30]   Pike, M.C., Peters, R.K. & Bernstein, L. (1993). Re: Total energy intake: implications for epidemiologic analyses, *American Journal of Epidemiology* **137**, 811–812.

[31]   Prentice, R.L. (1982). Covariate measurement errors and parameter estimation in a failure time regression model, *Biometrika* **69**, 331–342.

[32]   Rimm, E.B., Ascherio, A., Giovannucci, E., Spiegelman, D., Stampfer, M.J. & Willett, W.C. (1996). Vegetable, fruit, and cereal fiber intake and risk of coronary heart disease among men, *Journal of the American Medical Association* **275**, 447–451.

[33]   Rosner, B.A. (1996). Measurement error models for ordinal exposure variables measured with error, *Statistics in Medicine* **15**, 293–303.

[34]   Rosner, B. & Willett, W.C. (1988). Interval estimates for correlation coefficients corrected for within-person variation: implications for study design and hypothesis testing, *American Journal of Epidemiology* **127**, 377–386.

[35]   Rosner, B., Spiegelman, D. & Willett, W.C. (1990). Correction of logistic regression relative risk estimates and confidence intervals for measurement error: the case of multiple covariates measured with error, *American Journal of Epidemiology* **132**, 734–745.

[36]   Rosner, B., Spiegelman, D. & Willett, W.C. (1992). Correction of logistic regression relative risk estimates and confidence intervals for random within-person measurement error, *American Journal of Epidemiology* **136**, 1400–1413.

[37]   Rosner, B., Willett, W.C. & Spiegelman, D. (1989). Correction of logistic regression relative risk estimates and confidence intervals for systematic within-person measurement error, *Statistics in Medicine* **8**, 1051–1069.

[38]   Rothman, K.J. (1986). *Modern Epidemiology.* Little, Brown, & Company, Boston.

[39]   Sempos, C.T., Johnson, N.E., Smith, E.L. & Gilligan, C. (1985). Effects of intraindividual and interindividual variation in repeated dietary records, *American Journal of Epidemiology* **121**, 120–130.

[40]   Snedecor, G.W. & Cochran, W.G. (1989). *Statistical Methods*, 8th Ed. Iowa State University Press, Ames.

[41]   Wacholder, S., Armstrong, B. & Hartge, P. (1993). Validation studies using an alloyed gold standard, *American Journal of Epidemiology* **137**, 1251–1258.

[42]   Wacholder, S., Schatzkin, A., Freedman, L.S., Kipnis, V., Hartman, A. & Brown, C.C. (1994). Can energy adjustment separate the effects of energy from those of specific macronutrients?, *American Journal of Epidemiology* **140**, 848–855.

[43]   Willett, W. (1989). An overview of issues related to the correction of non-differential exposure measurement error in epidemiologic studies, *Statistics in Medicine* **8**, 1031–1040.

[44]   Willett, W. (1990). *Nutritional Epidemiology.* Oxford University Press, New York.

[45]   Willett, W. & Stampfer, M.J. (1986). Total energy intake: implications for epidemiologic analyses, *American Journal of Epidemiology* **124**, 17–27.

[46]   Willett, W.C. & Stampfer, M.J. (1993). Re: Total energy intake: implications for epidemiologic analyses, *American Journal of Epidemiology* **137**, 812–813.

[47]   Zheng, W., Kushi, L.H., Potter, J.D., Seller, T.A., Doyle, T.J., Bostick, R.M. & Folsom, A.R. (1995). Dietary intake of energy and animal foods and endometrial cancer incidence, *American Journal of Epidemiology* **142**, 388–394.

LYNNE R. WILKENS & JAMES LEE

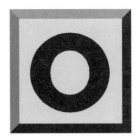

Observational Study

An observational study is a study in which conditions are not under the control of the investigator, unlike an **experimental study**. In particular, the exposures or treatments of interest are not assigned at random to experimental units by the investigator. Thus, associations between exposure and health outcome, say, may result from **confounding** by factors associated both with exposure and outcome.

Epidemiologic studies of disease etiology in humans are almost always observational because it is unethical to allocate people to receive potentially harmful exposures. Although the investigator does not control the allocation of exposure in observational studies, it is possible to mimic experimental designs in many respects and, by proper collection of observational data, to examine critically the hypothesis that the exposure has a causal impact (*see* **Causation**) on health outcome. The process of causal induction from observational data was brilliantly described by Hill [1, 2] (*see* **Hill's Criteria for Causality**).

Observational data are particularly subject to confounding in studies of therapeutic effects because factors that cause a doctor or patient to select a particular treatment are also often strongly related to health outcome. Such confounding has been called 'confounding by indication' [3]. Whenever possible, an experimental design, the controlled clinical trial, should be used to evaluate such treatments.

References

[1]   Hill, A.B. (1953). Observation and experiment, *New England Journal of Medicine* **248**, 995–1001.
[2]   Hill, A.B. (1965). The environment and disease: association or causation, *Proceedings of the Royal Society of Medicine* **58**, 295–300.
[3]   Miettinen, O.S. (1983). The need for randomization in the study of intended effects, *Statistics in Medicine* **2**, 267–271.

M.H. GAIL

Occupational Epidemiology

Especially since the late 1970s, numerous epidemiologic studies have revealed elevated **risks** of cancer, cardiovascular disease, and neurologic and other disorders among various occupational groups [110]. Strong evidence that many disorders are work-related was unobtainable from the clinical experiences or **case reports** that used to be the basis for identifying occupational risks. The introduction of modern, rigorous principles for epidemiologic research and the integration of epidemiologic courses in **occupational health** training have played an important role in this development. Many textbooks on epidemiologic methods have appeared since the early 1980s, and some of these have specifically focused on occupational epidemiology [40, 75, 119]. The availability of computers and statistical packages also has facilitated the progress.

It is hardly possible to predict the directions in occupational epidemiology that will lead to the most important future achievements. Only the more general aspects and principles of occupational epidemiology can be illustrated here by examples drawn from the several different subject matter areas. The challenge in occupational epidemiology has been, and will be, to identify adverse agent(s) or processes rather than to associate health risks with occupational groups or titles, because successful prevention can only be based on the elimination or reduction of specific exposures. The difficulties in this respect are often considerable, however, as occupational exposures tend to be mixed, and lifestyle factors may interfere.

The refinements of methods in epidemiologic research [63] came long after the first few epidemiologic studies of occupational disorders. In 1843, W.A. Guy studied "pulmonary consumption" in letter press printers and identified a higher risk among compositors than among pressmen [103]. The observation in 1879 of an increased occurrence of lung cancer among Schneeberg miners [71], and the excess of bladder cancer among German aniline workers reported around the turn of the century [138], are other examples of early occupational epidemiology.

A more recent example of occupational epidemiology, from 1948, demonstrated a high **proportional mortality** of lung cancer among British workers exposed to inorganic arsenic [79]. A few years later an increased risk of lung cancer was demonstrated among gas workers [48] and also bladder cancer in rubber workers [39]. Important studies of the risk of lung cancer in asbestos workers [145] and in underground miners were published in the 1960s [169, 170]. Studies on chemically induced cardiovascular disease also appeared relatively early – for example, among workers exposed to carbon disulfide [77, 159].

There is now, in the 1990s, an increasing interest in the effects of work stress and psychosocial determinants of the risk of cardiovascular disease [30]. Other recent studies concern neurologic disorders and their relationships to occupational exposures [12, 101], occupational studies of cancer in various countries [121], occupational hazards for women [65, 100, 175], for fetal loss and abnormalities

[97, 102], and for asthma [57, 96, 162]. Ergonomic risk factors and musculoskeletal disorders as well as reproductive hazards from occupational exposures are other aspects that have attracted interest since the 1980s. The health effects of electromagnetic fields have been among the most intriguing questions in occupational and **environmental epidemiology** during the 1990s [12, 92, 109, 144, 158], although the initiating study in this respect concerned cancer in children [172].

For the future, as for today, a central issue in occupational epidemiology will be the assessment of the effect of single as well as combined exposures. The recently developed tools of **molecular epidemiology** may increase the power of epidemiologic studies to detect risks at lower exposure levels and in smaller worker groups. These new tools are already being used in occupational epidemiology to define biomarkers of exposure or early effects, to identify susceptible individuals and to specify cancers by their mutational patterns [74, 150, 167].

Defining Research Questions for Occupational Epidemiology

New ideas for occupational studies have come from a variety of sources. A clinical observation has often suggested a connection between a disease and an exposure; sometimes toxicologic data from animal experiments have indicated a possible health hazard. Suggestions for a study may also have originated from observations or suspicions among workers about an adverse health effect. Still other leads for study derive from an examination of death records in various occupational groups (*see* **Occupational Mortality**) or from studies that link census data on job titles with cancer registry data or other **disease registries** or **causes of death**. Clues for new studies may also come from **case–control studies** that routinely tend to assess a number of exposures; should some unexpected associations appear, further studies are usually warranted.

The Role of Clinical Observations for Epidemiologic Research

The concerns about asbestos exposure as a cause of lung cancer and mesothelioma have probably generated more studies in occupational epidemiology than any other job-related health risk. The first suspicion of a lung cancer risk was raised by two case reports in 1935 [61, 106], and other such reports followed before the association between exposure and disease was clearly assessed in 1955, both in England [49] and California [34]. The risk of mesothelioma was not noticed until 1960; again the first suspicions arose from clinical observations [169].

The perception of possibly different risk patterns for the different types of asbestos may in part explain the numerous studies that have been conducted worldwide on asbestos exposure, but little gain in specific knowledge has been achieved in this respect. Indeed, between 1977, when the International Agency for Research Against Cancer (IARC) Monograph on asbestos exposure and cancer risk was published, and 1986, when this material was updated in the Monograph Supplement 7 [87], there was little new information regarding the effect of specific types of asbestos in spite of more than a doubling of the number of available studies. Several of these studies on asbestos in many countries have probably been motivated by the need to convince both the medical community and the authorities in each country with local studies on the health risk.

An even more clear-cut example of how a clinical observation initiated a large number of epidemiologic studies arose from the discovery of a cluster (*see* **Clustering**) of paranasal cancer cases among furniture workers in High Wycombe, UK [2, 108]. The many subsequent studies from various parts of the world have been convincingly consistent [87]. Similarly, a cluster of nasal cancers was traced to boot and shoe manufacturing [1], and again, this link was confirmed in many studies from several countries [87]. The rarity of this type of cancer certainly facilitated the recognition of a causal relationship (*see* **Causation**) to occupational exposures.

The report in 1974 of liver angiosarcomas among workers exposed to vinyl chloride provides still another example of how the observation of a cluster of cases of a rare tumor [45] gave rise to a number of further studies. Some of these included also other cancers and cardiovascular disease [50]. The first report on human liver angiosarcoma [45] referred to animal experiments that indicated the possibility of an oncogenic effect of vinyl chloride, but this knowledge seemed not to have reduced workplace exposures. A note added to the report on the human angiosarcomas

described unpublished data showing liver angiosarcoma and other tumors in animals exposed to vinyl chloride. The consistent findings in humans and animals convincingly established the risk of liver angiosarcoma from exposure to vinyl chloride.

Studies of the association of phenoxy herbicides with soft tissue sarcomas and lymphomas represent another theme in occupational epidemiology that arose from clinical observations and a case series report [68]. In contrast to the vinyl chloride case, there has been no convincing experimental evidence of a cancer risk from phenoxy herbicides. However, in particular, the 2,4,5-trichlorophenoxyacetic acid was known to contain varying amounts of 2,3,7,8-tetrachlorodibenzodioxin and other dioxins, for which there was growing evidence of cancer risks from animal data from 1977 onwards [85, 165]. Although there has been some inconsistency among the ensuing studies, it seems that soft tissue sarcomas are mainly related to dioxin exposure, whereas the lymphomas, especially the non-Hodgkin lymphomas, might be caused by phenoxy herbicides themselves [69]. Dioxin may also have cardiovascular effects [25, 55, 126].

Clinical observations also have stimulated epidemiologic studies in other areas than cancer. Painters with severe neurasthenic or psychoorganic syndromes in the 1970s raised the question of a role for long-term solvent exposure. Following some initial case–control and **cohort studies** in Sweden and Denmark indicating an effect [16, 116, 122], further epidemiologic research has been conducted and essentially confirmed both acute effects and the syndromes that may appear after long-term solvent exposure [32, 43, 166].

Animal Data Initiating Occupational Epidemiology

Sometimes the initial clue that precipitates epidemiologic research arises from animal studies. An example of strong animal evidence of a cancer risk preceding epidemiologic research concerns lung cancer among workers with exposure to chloromethyl methyl ether [53, 86]. The animal data existing in this case have apparently been so convincingly corroborating the epidemiologic findings that preventive actions were taken in many countries and few further human studies have followed.

Animal carcinogenesis studies of trichloroethylene also triggered epidemiologic investigations in the late 1970s [13, 160]. The early results were less convincing of a cancer risk, and only by aggregating the results from the later three most informative studies [5, 17, 153], and comparing the observed to expected numbers of liver and biliary tract cancers as well as non-Hodgkin's lymphomas, could an IARC Working Group conclude that there was limited evidence for a carcinogenic effect from trichloroethylene in humans [90].

Many epidemiologic studies also followed animal studies showing that formaldehyde caused cancer in the nasal cavity. An excess of nasal and nasopharyngeal cancers appeared as a fairly consistent finding in several of these ensuing studies [87]. Still, the IARC Working Group that evaluated this agent considered the available studies to provide only limited evidence for a carcinogenic effect in humans. This and the previous example indicate the problems and the latitude involved in trying to assess a cancer risk definitively. In the case of 1,3-butadiene, an IARC working group concluded that there was limited evidence of carcinogenicity in spite of strongly suggestive epidemiologic data [91].

Animal data suggest carcinogenic risks from lead, cadmium, and beryllium, but epidemiologic findings have been relatively weak, although finally convincing enough for cadmium and beryllium to permit a conclusion about sufficient evidence for a carcinogenic effect also in humans [88]. A more recent meta-analysis suggests also a cancer risk for workers exposed to lead [58].

These examples notwithstanding, it is perhaps surprising that relatively few epidemiologic studies have been initiated in response to animal studies, especially in view of the large number of chemicals tested. For diseases other than cancer, there are even fewer examples of animal studies leading to epidemiologic investigations, but there is also a relative lack of animal studies about other effects than cancer. Furthermore, the principles of occupational epidemiology have been less developed for such other diseases.

Record Linkage Studies

Epidemiologists have linked mortality or cancer registry data with census or **death certificate** information on occupation (*see* **Record Linkage**) in efforts to discover new occupational health hazards. Even when there is an increased risk of some disorder in an occupational group, the imprecise measure of exposure in such linkage studies attenuates the effect, however. This dilution problem may explain why the associations found have usually been weak and have contributed relatively little new knowledge. Census data reflect the occupational status at a point in time (e.g. during a particular week), and are therefore inherently poor measures of the occupational exposure that may, or may not, have occurred over many years.

A source of potential **confounding** (see discussion later) in registry linkage studies is the geographic variation in disease incidence, which may be real or may reflect local preferences in diagnostic practice (*see* **Geographic Patterns of Disease**). A common job in an area with a high incidence of some disease may therefore be associated with an artifactually increased occupational risk of the disease. For example, the linkage of registry data in Sweden indicated an excess of brain cancer in glass workers, but further evaluation showed that there was also a locally increased risk for others living in the relatively small area where the glassworks were located [176].

These limitations do not imply that registry studies are futile, however. For example, a Nordic registry linkage study has contributed essential information regarding the risk of lung cancer in connection with silica exposure [107]. A **proportional mortality study** linking causes of death to jobtitles on the death certificates also suggested an occupational risk for leukemia from exposure to electric and magnetic fields [117]. Similarly, record linkage studies gave an early indication that multiple sclerosis was associated with solvent exposure [118] – a connection that now seems rather likely in the light of a recent meta-analysis [101].

Concerns of Workers and Others

Sometimes workers perceive adverse health effects and attract the interest of epidemiologists. For example, a group of men exposed to bromochloropropane, a pesticide for nematodes, noted that none of them had fathered any children. This risk was later confirmed in epidemiologic studies [173, 174]. In contrast, suspicions that work with video display units could cause spontaneous abortions have created considerable concern and many studies, but no consistent effect has been demonstrated [109]. There are probably many small-size negative or nonpositive studies relating to workers' anxiety about a health hazard that are unpublished and unknown but that nevertheless reassure the workers involved.

Sometimes media reports have initiated a study, as for example reports of a cluster of childhood leukemia and non-Hodgkin's lymphoma in the vicinity of the Sellafield nuclear plant in England. A subsequent case–control study suggested that paternal exposure could have been the cause [60]; much controversy and other studies have followed, and the risks remain unclear.

Options in Study Design

Cohort Studies

Cohort studies are often regarded as the most valid and informative type of epidemiologic study. Cohorts are defined by a common event for its members. This event is usually of a somewhat complex nature, involving employment during a defined period at a particular industry; exposure to a specific agent may preferably also be required. Employment records or trade union registers are almost always the starting point for defining an occupational cohort. **Cross-sectional studies** of specific exposures in the past or data gathered as a consequence of biological monitoring programs may also define suitable cohorts for follow-up. For example, cohorts can be defined based on surveillance programs for lead in blood or some solvent metabolite, such as trichloroacetic acid or mandelic acid in urine (reflecting exposure to trichloroethylene and styrene, respectively (*see* **Surveillance of Diseases**)).

The analysis of occupational cohorts may be based on either **cumulative incidence** or **incidence density**, and these rates can be compared between the exposed and unexposed in terms of a rate ratio (**relative risk**) or, more rarely, a rate difference. In countries with sound mortality statistics and cancer registries, the observed numbers of specific causes of death or cancer types in a cohort are usually compared to expected numbers as based on the general population rates. These expected numbers are calculated by the "**person-years** method" from the national (or regional) rates, and the relative risk in the exposed cohort, compared to the general (or regional) population, is expressed as the standardized mortality ratio (SMR) [35, 59] (*see* **Standardization Methods**). In

cancer incidence studies the corresponding measure of effect is usually referred to as the standardized incidence ratio (SIR).

Occupational cohorts are usually historical or retrospective in character (*see* **Cohort Study, Historical**) but may also include some prospective follow-up. Still, the accuracy of the exposure assessment is usually limited by that in the retrospective phase of the study. A purely prospective cohort study would permit more accurate exposure assessment in principle, but this design is rarely used because it may take decades to complete. Many cohort studies fail to address adequately the changes in the pattern of exposure over time. Inaccuracies in exposure assessment can therefore be severe for those individuals who change jobs and who acquire new exposures, which in combination with the earlier exposures may enhance multistage development of diseases such as cancer.

It may be difficult to trace individuals of an occupational cohort in countries without registries of the living population and of deaths, or because of restrictions in the use of identifying information. In many countries tracing may therefore rely on driving license registries, telephone directories, and writing and calling people with similar family names living in the vicinity of a factory at issue.

A successful follow-up includes 95% or more of the cohort, as is possible in countries with good registries. Emigrants are difficult but not impossible to trace in contrast to "guest workers", who often come from less developed countries without population statistics. If the follow-up requires health examinations for assessing the health outcome, then a reference cohort usually needs to be established for sound comparisons; the participation rate may drop to 80% or less.

To account for a **latent period** between exposure and disease, especially in cancer studies, new cases and cumulative person-years may be ignored in the analysis for a certain period of time after the start of exposure. Alternatively, the cases and the person-years, along with the observed and expected number of cases, might be analyzed separately according to the time period since first exposure. Further aspects of the analysis of occupational cohort data are discussed below in connection with the healthy worker effect.

Cross-Sectional Studies

A traditional approach in occupational epidemiology has been the cross-sectional study, i.e. to examine an exposed and a nonexposed group at a particular point in time and to compare the **prevalence** of some disease or symptoms in the two groups according to degree of exposure. Cohort or case–control studies of incident disease are preferable, however, because they are not distorted by factors that influence survival or persistence of disease following disease onset. Nevertheless, many medically less serious health problems may be studied by a cross-sectional approach, especially as there is no other realistic possibility regarding, for example, lung or renal dysfunctions, neurobehavioral or neurophysiologic disturbances, or musculoskeletal and other nonlethal disorders. A problem with the cross-sectional design is, however, that the more severely affected workers might have left their jobs, resulting in an underestimate of the true health effects of a particular exposure.

Studies of pregnancy outcome, such as the occurrence of malformations or low birthweight may be regarded as cross-sectional. Also, the prevalence of pregnancies that terminate in spontaneous abortions may be compared between women with or without an exposure of interest. Similar to other cross-sectional studies in occupational epidemiology, the exposure information gathered in studies on reproduction may pertain to an entire period, e.g. pregnancy, or even before.

The prevalence **odds ratio** is sometimes used to measure risk in cross-sectional studies, but when the prevalence rate is large, as for abortions or musculoskeletal and other common disorders, the prevalence odds ratio poorly approximates the more intelligible **prevalence ratio**. Hence, when the prevalence rate is 10% in the unexposed and 40% in the exposed, the odds ratio is 6.0, whereas the prevalence ratio is only 4.0. Furthermore, a potentially confounding factor has different effects on the prevalence ratio than on the odds ratio. Thus, the use of **logistic regression** to adjust the odds ratio for confounding is of little utility in cross-sectional studies of common symptoms or disorders. Further details in this regard may be found elsewhere [15, 120, 177].

Cross-sectional studies in occupational health are usually applied also to data involving molecular markers such as deoxyribonucleic acid (DNA) or protein adducts to indicate an early effect of an exposure or a sort of subclinical disorder. There are both shorter overviews and extensive conference proceedings on adduct studies with a variety of examples in occupational and environmental health [22, 74, 167]. Some further aspects of the use of molecular biological data are raised in the section "Use of Molecular Epidemiology in Occupational Health" below.

Case–Control (Case–Referent) Studies

Etiologic factors for rare diseases are usually best studied by case–control designs, unless exposures are very unusual (or extremely common). Except when the case–control study is nested in a cohort (*see* **Case–Control Study, Nested**), the study population is open or dynamic in occupational case–control studies. Together with the time period involved, the **study population** forms the base for a study. An open base can be predetermined by defining the study population in geographic or administrative terms, but, alternatively, the boundaries may be secondarily laid down by the way the cases are recruited. That is, the study base can be either primary or secondary [113].

In a study with a primary base, all cases of the disease (or a representative sample of these cases) in an area are ascertained from cancer registries (or other disease registries when existent) or hospital files. The cases are compared in terms of various exposures with a sample of subjects from the study base, i.e. the **controls**. This approach implies that the general population is the reference for estimating the odds ratio. If the study base is secondary, then one would have to recruit the controls similarly to the cases, such as by taking patients with other diseases in a hospital to serve as controls for the cases with the disease of interest from that hospital [114] (*see* **Case–Control Study, Hospital-Based**). Results obtained from a secondary base tend to be less reliable than those derived from a primary base.

Especially since the 1980s, the case–control study has become widely used in occupational health for studying the effects of exposures that are not confined to any particular industry, as, for example, in studies of cancer risks from pesticide use in farming and forestry. The risk of exposure to a particular industrial process or agent can also be studied by locating the case–control study to a restricted population living in the area where a particular factory is located. Examples include studies of lung cancer risk from exposure to arsenic in copper smelter workers as well as in the general population [14, 131]. As an alternative to a cohort design, a **case–cohort study** may be useful by allowing multiple case–control comparisons against a common control group.

When other disease entities are used as controls, there is the possibility that these may be associated with exposure. In this case, the exposure frequency of the diseased controls does not reflect the exposure frequency in the base population and the risk ratio is **biased** (*see* **Bias in Case–Control Studies**). If a mix of other disorders are intended to be used as the controls, then some disease entities may be associated with the exposure and should therefore be excluded. Should unrelated disorders be misjudged and also excluded, no bias in the estimated rate ratio (odds ratio) would result, as the relation of exposed to nonexposed among the remaining, properly selected, controls is not affected. Appropriate exclusions may easily be misunderstood and lead to skeptical comments, however, unless clear arguments are given for leaving out some disorders from the control series. Since more than one occupational exposure might be of interest as influencing the occurrence of a disease, a refinement might be necessary in the selection of control disorders because some conditions might be related to some but not all exposures under consideration.

Nested Case–Control (Case–Referent) Studies

A nested case–control study is obtained if the cases as well as the sample of controls are drawn from a closed population, that is, within a cohort. The nested case–control study is usually applied to gather information on exposures and confounders not assessable for all cohort members in the main study. For example, the combined effect of an industrial exposure and smoking (or other exposure) might be of interest. Then, if the distribution of smoking is not known for the cohort members, smoking status need be determined only for the cases and for a sample of the base population, that is, a sample of the cohort members; see, for example, the nested case–control study of lymphohematopoietic cancer in a cohort of workers manufacturing styrene-butadiene rubber [143].

Proportional Mortality Studies and Mortality Odds Ratio Studies

As already mentioned, the proportional mortality study has been applied in occupational epidemiology

for many years [79] and may be seen as a kind of cross-sectional study at the time of death, even though the deaths considered are not simultaneous. The principle is to calculate the proportion of deaths from a particular disease out of all deaths and calculate the ratio of the proportions of cause-specific deaths for exposed and nonexposed individuals, the proportional mortality ratio (PMR). **Stratifications** and standardizations for age and other factors may be applied. Another possibility is to use national or regional proportions of specific causes of death for comparisons. The proportional mortality study tends to be somewhat insensitive because any excess mortality would not only affect the numerator but also increase the denominator.

Proportional mortality data may also be analyzed by a case–control approach – sometimes more specifically referred to as a mortality odds ratio study. Analogously to a hospital-based case–control study, other deaths than those from the disease of interest are used as controls [8, 115]. Thus, the ratio of odds of the cause of death of interest to the other deaths for the exposed and nonexposed, respectively, namely the mortality odds ratio, can be estimated as the exposure odds ratio for the cases and for the other deaths. Control diseases should be excluded if they are suspected to be related to the exposure as in case–control studies with hospital controls. The aforementioned copper smelter study may illustrate this approach as comparing various types of cancer and cardiovascular deaths against a common control group of deaths unlikely to be related to the exposure [14].

Correlational Studies

With a continuous census over time in an open study base, a comparison could even be made with regard to incidence rates in regions with a more or less concentrated representation of the type of industry and exposure under consideration. Although studies of this type have been presented in the field of occupational epidemiology, this design cannot be recommended because of the lack of information on exposures and confounders at the individual level and because of the dilution with nonexposed individuals. The design, also called an **ecologic study**, is perhaps more useful in environmental epidemiology, for example in studying health effects of air or water pollution.

Character of Exposed Populations and the Healthy Worker Effect

Being able to work usually requires good health, which means that there is some selection regarding who will enter a particular job as well as who is expelled from it. More skilled jobs tend to recruit workers with different lifestyles from workers in less skilled jobs, and health-related departures from the labor force may be concentrated among low socioeconomic groups [46]. A particular group of workers is therefore likely to be healthier than the general population and also tends to differ from other workers. This health-related selection process, called the "healthy worker effect" [111], makes it difficult to find proper comparison groups and explains why various worker groups often enjoy better health outcomes and have smaller risks than expected [6, 44]. For women employed in Sweden in both 1960 and 1970, however, a registry follow-up study found no evidence for a healthy worker effect [64].

One can distinguish between a healthy worker effect in the period shortly after hire and a healthy worker survivor effect operating on a long-term basis. The latter may cause cumulative exposure to become associated with good health among the long-term employees and have a tendency to depress the upper end of an exposure–response curve.

Cohort Studies

In cohort studies, the healthy worker effect is usually evidenced by a total mortality of about 90% or less than expected. A decrease in cardiovascular deaths tends to contribute most to the healthy worker effect, but other causes of death may also be below expected levels. Sometimes the observed number of deaths is as low as only about 50%–60% of the expected, as, for example, in some studies for cardiovascular disease [125], other noncancer deaths [24], as well as cancer [161].

When the healthy worker effect is strong, the comparison with expected numbers based on national or regional rates is questionable, but often there is no alternative reference population. One should be cautious, however, in concluding that there is no risk when national or regional rates are taken as the reference. Even with an appropriate reference, studies showing no effect should be looked upon as essentially uninformative or "nonpositive" rather

than "negative" unless there is a large number of cases [3, 76]. If a cohort is large enough, then internal comparisons regarding exposure–response relationships might offer the better comparability, but often there is no unexposed reference group in such studies. Regarding the early period of follow-up, preemployment measures such as health exams create strong selection for a healthy worker effect; a further concern is that cases might have been selectively lost to follow-up – for example, due to sorting out of deceased individuals from company registries.

The healthy worker effect has been relatively weak in many cohort studies from the Nordic countries. Possibly the low unemployment rate that prevailed for a long period of time made it necessary for employers to recruit even people with a marginal health prognosis. In contrast, a more pronounced healthy worker effect may occur in countries and time periods characterized by a high unemployment rate. Usually the healthy worker effect is greater in the younger age groups in a cohort and in the early phase of follow-up [130].

In many studies, the higher risk ratios have appeared among workers with short-time employment rather than among those who have been employed for a long time, and risk may decrease with increasing duration of employment and exposure. The reason for the poor health outcome in short-time employees is usually sought in certain lifestyle characteristics. Part of the explanation may also be that only those workers remaining healthy stay on the job long enough to achieve a higher degree of exposure measured as years of employment or as a product of exposure concentration and time [20]. Allowing for a time lag following initial employment tends to reduce this healthy worker survivor effect.

Adjustment for length of follow-up and employment status (if associated with the disease, independently of the exposure) may also reduce bias from the healthy survivor effect [54, 128, 154]. Computer programs are available that can provide appropriate person-time data for such adjustments [129]. Arrighi & Hertz-Picciotto [6] compared methods to deal with the healthy worker survivor effect in a study of exposure to arsenic on lung cancer risk. The so-called G method of Robins et al. [139] was thought to be most appropriate, but a lagged analysis worked relatively well except for diseases with a short induction-latency time.

Cross-Sectional Studies

A recent study of symptoms of the respiratory tract, lung function and airway responsiveness in relation to occupational and smoking histories in underground bituminous coal miners and nonmining controls illustrates selection problems in cross-sectional studies [135]. Miners with the longest duration of work at the coal face responded less often to methacholine than miners who had never worked at the coal face, and miners who responded to methacholine were less likely to have worked in dusty jobs than miners not responding. It was concluded that these findings probably resulted from health-related job selection. Similarly, a cross-sectional study of animal feed workers revealed a decreasing prevalence of most chronic respiratory symptoms with increasing years of exposure to dust and endotoxin [147]. Thus, the healthy worker effect may lead to underestimation of risk in cross-sectional studies and even obscure a risk altogether.

Case–Control Studies

The healthy worker effect can also influence the results of case–control studies if exposed individuals tend to be healthier than other members of the population constituting the study base. A more subtle, reversed, and less obvious healthy worker effect can occur in hospital-based case–control studies. If the working population with the exposure of interest is healthier than others in the study base, then the controls would less often be exposed, as many of them come from the unexposed part of the study population with less good health. The result of the healthy worker effect in such case–control studies using hospital (or deceased) controls would therefore be an exaggerated rate ratio (odds ratio). The same reasoning applies to proportional mortality studies. Park et al. [127] have presented parallel analyses showing that mortality odds ratios (MORs) and PMRs were higher than SMRs for some causes of death; it seems likely that "the truth" might be somewhere between the different estimates obtained. In case–control studies this reverse healthy worker effect is avoided when population controls are enrolled.

A related phenomenon in case–control studies may arise when controls are recruited by **random digit dialing**. Subjects answering the telephone are less likely to be working or to have an exposed job, especially if exposure is associated with a job that demands long working hours. Thus, the exposure frequency in the study base might be underestimated, resulting in an exaggerated estimate of the effect of the exposure.

Assessment of Exposure

Conferences held in the early 1990s reflect the efforts made to improve exposure assessment in occupational epidemiology [19, 73, 78]. Specific knowledge is required for preventive measures to reduce or eliminate hazardous agents or processes from the work environment. The proper assessment of exposure is therefore a key issue in any study of work-related adverse health effects. There are conceptual difficulties in defining exposure and dose, and further problems in accurately measuring or classifying the exposure. Errors in this regard can also affect adjustments for confounding.

Records showing the specific job tasks of the workers are available in many companies and usually form the basis for cohort studies, but can also be used for exposure assessment in case–control and proportional mortality studies. Case–control studies often rely on questionnaire information or interviews, however, and may therefore be subject to **recall bias** or **interviewer bias** (observer bias).

Measures of Exposure

Measures of exposure are usually either exposure intensity, exposure duration, or cumulative exposure. For acute diseases, peak exposure intensity is often particularly relevant. Cumulative exposure measured as duration or as time-integrated intensity are often used in studies of chronic disease. With ionizing radiation as the paradigm, cumulative exposure is commonly taken as a proper determinant of risk for genotoxic and carcinogenic agents, and there are specific arguments in support of such a measure [137]. These arguments are based on an assumption of linear kinetics in the metabolism. However, a literature survey on cancer studies has shown that intensity measures of exposure often yielded larger relative risks than duration of exposure, and intensity measures also often yield monotonically increasing exposure–response curves [28].

Furthermore, in a pharmacokinetic study relating cumulative exposure to tissue dose for insoluble, respirable dust particles and toxic metabolites of a nonpolar organic solvent, Smith [149] found no linear relationship between cumulative exposure and tissue dose. It was suggested that this observation could explain why a disproportionally high risk of pulmonary effects is commonly seen for workers with relatively short but intense dust exposures. Specific measures of exposure that result in large apparent risks and clear **dose–response** relationships have been suggested for particular diseases, such as silicosis [41].

Job–Exposure Matrices

Occupations or job tasks are easier to recall and report correctly than exposures to specific agents like metals, solvents, or pesticides. Hoar [80] proposed a **job–exposure matrix** to translate job task histories into estimates of exposure to specific agents. A job–exposure matrix consists of jobs on one axis and specific exposures to substances or other agents on the other, with the matrix elements describing the likelihood of an individual's exposure to a specific substance in a given job, either in binary or polytomous categories. A matrix may also dichotomize exposure on a probability basis [31].

However, it is necessary to adapt the job–exposure matrix to the country or region and the type of industry where it is to be used. A population-specific job–exposure matrix may therefore be preferable to general job–exposure matrices developed elsewhere. Such a matrix can be constructed from the results of in-depth interviews of a job-stratified sample of cohort members [98].

Ronneberg [141] used a job–exposure matrix in a study of Norwegian aluminum smelter workers. Jobs held by cohort members were identified from personnel records; work tasks and their locations were determined for all jobs, and information was gathered about changes in exposure conditions over time. Then the jobs were combined into categories thought to represent similar exposure conditions, and time-weighted average exposures were estimated on a relative scale.

A specific job–exposure matrix for chlorinated solvents assigned semiquantified estimates of the probability and intensity of exposure to each four-digit job category of the Standard Industrial Classification and Standard Occupational Classification codes in the US [62]. The matrix was also designed to account for the changing patterns of use of these solvents by decade from the 1920s to the 1980s. An algorithm was applied to assign each study subject a unique lifetime probability of exposure and an estimated score of cumulative exposure for each of the solvents. An important goal of the matrix was to reduce the number of false positive exposure assessments.

The latter principle is corroborated by a study of astrocytomas and exposure to methylene chloride showing that the odds ratios increased with increasing **specificity** of the exposure assessment [51]. The risk estimate more than tripled compared with the risk estimate obtained without taking probability of exposure and exposure by decades into account and coding for industries and occupations.

There have been many comparisons and evaluations of the validity of the various approaches to assess exposure. Structured questionnaire information is commonly used, but underreporting of exposure remains a problem [93, 132]. On the basis of a large-scale study from Canada [146], Dewar et al. [47] found that the assessment of exposure by an expert team was more efficient than the use of a job–exposure matrix. This may explain why interviews resulted in several increased odds ratios in a study of mental retardation and parental occupation, whereas the use of a job–exposure matrix did not [140].

Men and women with the same job title may have different exposure patterns, indicating a need for gender-specific job–exposure matrices [112]. A comparison of information on exposure to dusts, gases, and fumes from a job–exposure matrix with questionnaire data indicated a better agreement in men than in women and suggested that men had a more accurate recollection of exposure – especially well-educated men [82]. Smoking habits had no effect on the perception of exposure. For women, the perception of exposure did not vary significantly according to respiratory symptoms. In men, however, subjects without chronic cough or chronic bronchitis even had a significantly higher perception of exposure than the others, but no difference was shown for wheezing, dyspnoea, or asthma.

Stengel et al. [155] compared the performance of experts vs. job–exposure matrices in studies of glomerulonephritis and bladder cancer. Categories of exposure as obtained from both experts and job–exposure matrices were dichotomized, using different cutoff points for exposure and nonexposure. **Sensitivity** of the job–exposure matrices vis-à-vis the experts was low (23%–63%), whereas **specificity** was rather high (87%–98%). Assuming an odds ratio of 3 and an exposure prevalence of 10%, and taking the experts' classification of exposure to be completely correct, the use of a job–exposure matrix led to attenuation of the odds ratio by a factor of 1.5–2.1, and to a loss of power equivalent to a reduction in the number of subjects by a factor of 5–10. On the other hand, the job–exposure matrix performed better than self-reported exposure in discriminating high-risk subgroups in a study of lung cancer and asbestos exposure among construction workers [56].

Job–exposure matrices have also been applied to assess physical exposures such as electric and magnetic fields [21] as well as to study aspects of work organization such as work control, social support, and psychological and physical job demands [81, 94].

Some Other Aspects on Exposure Assessment

Data from biological monitoring programs may be helpful for exposure assessment in cohort studies. For example, when animal studies indicated a cancer risk from trichloroethylene in the late 1970s, existing data from routine monitoring of the metabolite trichloroacetic acid in urine could be used for defining cohorts for follow-up with regard to cancer [13, 160]. Although trichloroacetic acid in urine clearly indicated exposure, the proper measure of exposure (e.g. peak values or simple averages) was not evident.

Hygienists are needed not only for judgments about whether a particular exposure is likely to have occurred, but also to evaluate documents on previously measured exposures. Measurement strategies and methods of sampling and analysis have varied over the years. It is especially important to consider the sampling strategies when hygienists' measurements are used for epidemiologic purposes [163]. The reason is that such measurements usually have been made for control of the work environment after changes in an industrial process for hygienic or technical reasons and therefore tend to underestimate the average daily exposures. Hygienists also need to assess the potential for dermal absorption which was important, for example, for grape farmers exposed to the insecticide Phosmet [156].

Considerable differences in exposure may occur between workers from the same factory and with the same job titles [99]. Only one-quarter of some worker groups had individual mean exposures within a twofold range for 95% of the individuals. Furthermore, about one-third of the worker groups had a greater than 10-fold range for 95% of the individuals. There were also large day-to-day variations, especially for outdoor workers and when the process was intermittent. Indoor work in a continuous process led to more homogenous exposures.

Uncertainties are likely to affect any exposure assessment, causing some individuals to be taken as more exposed and others as less exposed than they really are. In principle, one should emphasize the need for a positive **predictive value** rather than sensitivity of a job-exposure matrix or a questionnaire for assessing exposure to agents of interest [136]; the reverse is true for confounding factors, however.

Sometimes the presence of recall bias or observer bias in case–control data can be revealed by comparing the odds ratio for those with and without reported exposure but within job categories with potential exposure. If the latter, who report no exposure, show a decreased risk in comparison to those in clearly unexposed jobs, it is likely that an increased odds ratio for those reported exposed reflects some bias in the assessment of exposure [9].

If there are no systematic influences on the exposure assessment, then the result is **nondifferential error**, which usually leads to risk estimates that are **biased towards the null** value (*see* **Misclassification Error**). Nondifferential missclassification makes it difficult to discover adverse health effects by attenuating the risk estimates. However, even in the presence of nondifferential error, chance sometimes may lead to exaggerated risk estimates. Little attention has been paid to this possibility in reporting of study results, but it has been well illustrated by computer simulations [151]. Dosemeci et al. [52] showed that discretizing continuous exposure data can lead to biases away from the null if nondifferential error acts on the continuous exposure measurement.

Assessment of exposure in limited time windows may yield particular insights. A time-window approach that is sensitive to recent exposures may enable one to detect a late stage effect for cancer or other diseases. For example, exposure to radon and radon progeny in mines in the 5–15 years before

Occupational Epidemiology

lung cancer seems to have had an important effect on risk [26].

Confounding in Occupational Epidemiology

Determinants of risk that are associated with the exposure under consideration can spuriously increase the apparent risk from this exposure. Such determinants are called "**confounders**". Confounders can also obscure an effect, either when the confounding risk factor tends to be more common in absence of the exposure or when it is protective. In principle, confounding may explain all or part of an association of a disease with an exposure, either because the control of a known confounding factor is incomplete, or because the confounder has not been identified. Mismeasurement or nondifferential missclassification of a confounder can lead to poor control for confounding [4, 136]. However, as long as the exposure under study has a quite strong effect, incomplete control of confounding is not too deleterious for risk estimation [18].

Often the concern about confounding in occupational epidemiology has been focused on lifestyle factors such as smoking and alcohol use or socioeconomic class. Even for a strong risk factor like smoking for lung cancer, the confounding influence is quite modest because smoking tends to be nearly equally prevalent among the occupationally exposed and the unexposed [7, 18].

The most important confounders to consider in occupational epidemiology are other work-related exposures and factors [42]. For example, it is difficult to investigate the role of welding fumes on lung cancer risk because asbestos has often been used in protective equipment in the welding process, and there is also considerable exposure to magnetic fields from electric arc welding, which may or may not be a risk factor. Likewise, in the artistic glass industry, there has been exposure to many different and potentially carcinogenic metals or metallic compounds, but again, asbestos has also been present to protect from the warm glass [88].

Sometimes various exposures are inextricably linked. For example, some phenoxy herbicides have contained impurities of chlorinated dibenzodioxins as a result of the manufacturing process. The association between exposures of this kind is so tight that there is no way to control properly for confounding of

one compound to find out the effect of another. Instead, one has to consider the effect of these exposures en bloc [7]. Similarly, occupational job titles might sometimes have to be viewed as blocs of exposures. The best possibilities for prevention occur, however, when specific exposures or processes can be identified as hazardous.

Since a worker may be exposed to a complex array of occupational and other agents of physical or psychosocial character, there is considerable potential for some mutually confounding effects in occupational studies. For this and other reasons, it has become increasingly common to consider many exposures, especially in case–control studies. For example, Blair et al. [27] considered some 150 occupations and about as many industrial categories in a study of lymphoma. When a great number of exposures are analyzed, false positive findings may result from the play of chance in the many comparisons. There is also the possibility that confounding from one or more of the exposures associated with increased risk may explain some other positive associations as well. More interest should probably be devoted to this possibility than to the consequences of multiple comparisons because exposures for consideration in a study are not randomly selected but are usually included on the basis of some evidence or suspicion of an adverse effect.

Interaction of Exposure Effects

When multiple exposures occur in occupational settings it would be useful to know whether synergistic or antagonistic **interactions** are present (*see* **Synergy of Exposure Effects**). Not many examples in this respect were found in a literature survey [10], but, for example, combined exposure to vinyl chloride and arsenic increased the risk of respiratory cancer, and the combined exposure to phenoxy herbicides and solvents seemed to increase the risk of lymphoma. This latter interaction has also been recently confirmed by other data in which the combination of phenoxy herbicides and solvent exposure gave an odds ratio of 8.6 vs. 2.6 and 1.4, respectively, for the two exposures alone [134]. Exposure to plastic and rubber chemicals resulted in an odds ratio of 2.2, which increased to 4.8 in the presence of solvents.

As in these examples, the sample sizes available for assessing such occupational interactions are usually small, resulting in considerable uncertainty in the estimates. A background of differently combined exposures may explain inconsistent findings obtained in different studies on the same agent, as can interactions with factors outside the work environment. In the latter respect, the strong synergistic effect of smoking and asbestos exposure on the risk of lung cancer is a classical example [67]. Arsenic and smoking also act synergistically to increase the risk of lung cancer [133]. A synergistic effect of smoking and exposure to radon progeny seems likely as well, although the results differ to some extent between studies [26].

Use of Molecular Epidemiology in Occupational Health

The great achievements in molecular biology over the past decade have also influenced occupational epidemiology [72, 74, 150, 167]. Chemical adducts to DNA or various proteins like hemoglobin and albumin have been used as either markers of exposure or taken as early adverse health effects. A somewhat later development has involved attempts to evaluate exposure effects in relation to metabolic polymorphism and to detect mutations, for example in the p53 gene. Specific mutations in the p53 gene in squamous skin cancers have been associated with ultra-violet (UV)-light exposure [33] and in liver tumors with widespread exposure to aflatoxin B_1 and hepatitis B virus [36, 83], and, by analogy, it is likely that characteristic mutations may result also from occupational exposures to carcinogens.

Studies involving adducts are usually of a cross-sectional design and tend to reflect rather recent exposures due to the turnover of cells and proteins in blood. There is a similarity in this respect to investigations based on chromosomal aberrations, sister chromatid exchanges or micronuclei. These latter type of studies became common in the late 1970s and early 1980s [152]. It has been unclear to what extent chromosomal damage implies any serious effect, but a cohort follow-up indicates that chromosomal aberrations might be predictive of cancer development [66]. In an evaluation of the cancer risk to humans from styrene exposure, an IARC Working Group took into special account the many studies indicating chromosomal damage [89]. Even so, there now seems to be a decreasing enthusiasm to use chromosomal damage as an outcome measure.

The case–control design is well suited to detecting exposures that can lead to mutations in oncogenes or tumor supressor genes [150]. The cases are divided into subentities defined by some mutational characteristic, and each such subentity of cases is compared with controls regarding exposure. For example, Taylor et al. [157] compared 62 cases of acute myeloid leukemia with 630 controls. The 10 leukemia patients who were positive for *ras*-mutation were found to have worked more often in high risk occupations. Odds ratios between 1.9 and 7.2 were obtained for the various exposure categorizations made. In contrast, the odds ratios for the *ras*-negative cases ranged from 0.6 to 0.9.

The case–control design is also useful for studying the impact of the genetically determined polymorphism of enzymatic activity and metabolic capacity that determines the susceptibility to risk from an occupational exposure. For example, individuals with one form of the polymorphic CYP1A1 gene appeared to be more susceptible to risks from smoking and occupational exposures such as asbestos than those with other alleles [38, 104]. Although these results have not been confirmed, the applied epidemiologic design used in these studies defines a valid approach for studying metabolic activity and occupational exposures as well as smoking. Efforts to identify individuals at increased occupational risk for bladder cancer because of a glutathione-S-transferase M1 deficiency can serve as another example of this type of study [37]. Glutathione-S-transferase polymorphism may also influence the susceptibility to nonmalignant asbestos-related disease [148].

Occupational exposures may even increase the risk for a clearly inherited disorder. Few individuals with the genetic trait for familial amyloid polyneuropathy develop the disease, suggesting that some other factors might have been involved in the clinically overt cases. In a case–control study of this disorder, solvent exposure appeared as a fairly strong risk factor, with an 11-fold risk for the more heavily exposed [70].

More time is needed to evaluate the role of **molecular epidemiology** for identifying health risks in the workplace [164]. The complexity and the costs involved in these studies will remain a major hindrance for future development, even though some interesting and important results are likely to appear. Identification of genetically determined susceptibility to occupational exposures raises ethical concerns because persons without elevated susceptibility may be selected for employment. Instead, the proper goal should be to create a safe work environment even for those individuals who are more susceptible.

The Etiologic Contribution of Occupational Exposures

The proportion of disease burden attributable to specific exposures or jobs is rather substantial. In Germany, for example, about 250 asbestos-associated lung cancers and 400 mesotheliomas have been recognized and compensated for each year [23]. Lung cancer claims among the underground uranium mine workers in Thuringia and Saxony ranked second to asbestos. Lung cancers related to silicotic scar tissue and to chromium (VI) and arsenic compounds and other chemicals were also subject to compensation.

Estimates of the etiologic contribution of occupational exposures to morbidity or mortality may be obtained by calculating the so-called population **attributable risk** or etiologic fraction. Any particular occupational exposure is quite rare in the general population, however, and can therefore cause only a limited proportion of disease. The overall burden of diseases related to various occupational exposures may nevertheless be considerable. A study of lung cancer in Norway indicated a population attributable risk of 22%–35% for occupations with definitely hazardous exposures [95]. The estimate rose to 37%–47% when jobs with "possibly exposed" categories were also included. Asbestos exposure was the main single risk factor. Attributable risks may add up to more than 100% due to interaction between risk factors. Not surprisingly, therefore, the contribution from smoking could still be estimated to be 82%.

The quantitative impact of working conditions on cardiovascular diseases in Denmark has been suggested to account for 16% of the premature cardiovascular mortality in men and 22% in women [123]. Including sedentary work as an occupational risk factor, the etiologic fractions rose to 51% and 55% for men and women, respectively. Monotonous high-paced work and shift work were considered the most important single factors, whereas the impact of rather rare chemical exposures to carbon disulfide, nitroglycol, lead, arsenic, carbon monoxide, and other agents was marginal.

Estimates of attributable risk for musculoskeletal and neurologic disorders can be calculated as well. Olsen et al. [124] estimated the population attributable risk for coxarthrosis, a degenerative condition of the hip joint, as 40% for physical workload on the job, 55% for sports, and 15% for excess weight. Overall these three risk factors could account for about 80% of the "idiopathic" coxarthrosis. Landtblom et al. [101] reviewed 10 studies of multiple sclerosis and found relative risks near two for exposure to solvents. Assuming the frequency of relevant solvent exposure to be in the range of 10%–20% in an industrialized country, one would estimate a population attributable risk of about 10% or more. These few examples indicate that the contribution of occupational exposures to cancer as well as other disorders is not negligible.

Concluding Remarks

Identification of risks from occupational exposures and quantification of the associated burden of diseases should lead to prevention efforts. Mandated and voluntary changes in the work environment and proper supervision to ensure compliance with regulations may be as beneficial to health as attempts to change personal habits and lifestyle. Continuous epidemiologic surveillance is important to obtain information about the long-term impact of preventive measures.

When an epidemiologic study indicates a health risk associated with an industrial process, required changes in the production process may be costly. Workers and the management often hold different views of the balance between the costs and health benefits of preventive measures. It is not unusual, however, that an improvement in the work environment also improves productivity; even so there is usually considerable resistance from an industry to accept epidemiologic evidence of a risk and to improve the work environment.

The method of presenting epidemiologic results is critical to a successful prevention strategy when serious health effects are indicated, such as excess cancer deaths or malformations. When the study pertains to a particular plant or company, it is advisable first to inform the management as well as the employees or their representatives. Mass media may be interested as well, but untimely information through the media can create controversy and hostility towards occupational health research. Press conferences in the presence of management and worker representatives can be useful for limiting negative publicity for a company, because, eventually, the mass media will get access to the information when a scientific report is published. It is therefore advisable to provide information in a more controlled manner [11].

In view of the technical difficulties of conducting epidemiologic studies and a natural reluctance to accept that an industrial process may be harmful, it is not surprising that interpretations of data may differ and serious controversies arise. For example, in 1966 Hueper [84] reconsidered his early warnings, in view of the European experiences, of lung cancer risk from exposure to radon progeny, and accused government officials of having impeded studies of this health hazard among uranium miners in the US. By 1966, Hueper's suspicions had been confirmed by the first report on an excess of lung cancer among these miners [171]. As late as 1971, B. MacMahon wrote in the preface to a comprehensive report on lung cancer in uranium miners [105]:

> The epidemic now in progress among American uranium miners could readily have been – and indeed was – predicted on the basis of past experience in other parts of the world. Less predictable was the extent of the scientific, legal and political controversy that the American experience would engender. Although ... few medical experiences have been so carefully documented, diametrically opposite opinions are still held and expressed not only regarding the interpretation of the facts that have emerged but as to the nature of the facts themselves.

When epidemiologic study results are weak or inconsistent it is indeed difficult to come up with a tenable judgment on the health risk involved. Some subjectivity is unavoidable in such situations, but decision makers may get some guidance from ethical considerations. Hence, it seems reasonable to give the benefit of the doubt to those suffering the risk [3], and in balancing benefits against risk one has to be clear about who takes the risk and who has the benefit. In occupational health, the situation is more complicated than in medical treatment, where the risk of adverse side-effects might be weighed against benefits for the same individual [168]. A comprehensive discussion of the ethical guidelines in occupational health can be found elsewhere [142].

References

[1]   Acheson, E.D., Cowdell, R.H. & Jolles, B. (1970). Nasal cancer in the Northamptonshire boot and shoe industry, *British Medical Journal* **1**, 385–393.

[2]   Acheson, E.D., Hadfield, E.H. & Macbeth, R.G. (1967). Carcinoma of the nasal cavity and accessory sinuses in woodworkers, *Lancet* **i**, 311–312.

[3]   Ahlbom, A., Axelson, O., Stöttrup Hansen, E., Hogstedt, C., Jensen, U. & Olsen J. (1990). Interpretation of "negative" studies in occupational epidemiology, *Scandinavian Journal of Work, Environment and Health* **16**, 153–157.

[4]   Ahlbom, A. & Steineck, G. (1992). Aspects of missclassification of confounding factors, *American Journal of Industrial Medicine* **21**, 107–112.

[5]   Anttila, A., Pukkala, E., Sallmen, M., Hernberg, S. & Hemminki, K. (1995). Cancer incidence among Finnish workers exposed to halogenated hydrocarbons, *Journal of Occupational Medicine* **37**, 797–806.

[6]   Arrhighi, H.M. & Hertz-Picciotto, I. (1993). The evolving concept of the healthy worker survivor effect, *Epidemiology* **5**, 189–196.

[7]   Axelson, O. (1978). Aspects on confounding in occupational health epidemiology, *Scandinavian Journal of Work, Environment and Health* **4**, 85–89.

[8]   Axelson, O. (1979). The case-referent (case control) study in occupational health epidemiology, *Scandinavian Journal of Work, Environment and Health* **5**, 91–99.

[9]   Axelson, O. (1980). A note on observational bias in case-referent studies in occupational health epidemiology, *Scandinavian Journal of Work, Environment and Health* **6**, 80–82.

[10] Axelson, O. (1991). Cancer and combined exposures to occupational and environmental factors, *Recent Results in Cancer Research* **122**, 60–70.

[11] Axelson, O. (1994). Dynamics of management and labor in dealing with occupational risks, in *The Identification and Control of Environmental and Occupational Disease*, M.A. Mehlman, ed. Princeton Scientific Publishing, Princeton.

[12] Axelson, O. (1996). Where do we go in occupational neuroepidemiology?, *Scandinavian Journal of Work, Environment and Health* **22**, 81–83.

[13] Axelson, O., Andersson, K., Hogstedt, C., Holmberg, B., Molina, G. & de Verdier, A. (1978). A cohort study on trichloroethylene exposure and cancer mortality, *Journal of Occupational Medicine* **20**, 194–196.

[14] Axelson, O., Dahlgren, E., Jansson, C.-D. & Rehnlund, S.O. (1978). Arsenic exposure and mortality, a case referent study from a Swedish copper smelter, *British Journal of Industrial Medicine* **35**, 8–15.

[15] Axelson, O., Fredriksson, M. & Ekberg, K. (1994). Use of prevalence ratio v the prevalence odds ratio as a measure of risk in cross sectional studies, *Occupational and Environmental Medicine* **51**, 574.

[16] Axelson, O., Hane, M. & Hogstedt, C. (1976). A case–referent study on neuropsychiatric disorders among workers exposed to solvents, *Scandinavian Journal of Work, Environment and Health* **2**, 14–20.

[17] Axelson, O., Seldén, A., Andersson, K. & Hogstedt, C. (1994). Updated and expanded Swedish cohort study

on trichloroethylene and cancer risk, *Journal of Occupational Medicine* **36**, 556–562.

[18] Axelson, O. & Steenland, K. (1988). Indirect methods of assessing the effect of tobacco use in occupational studies, *American Journal of Industrial Medicine* **13**, 105–118.

[19] Axelson, O. & Westberg, H. (1992). Introductory note to the concepts of exposure and dose in occupational epidemiology, *American Journal of Industrial Medicine* (Special issue) **21**, 3–4.

[20] Baillargeon, J. & Wilkinson, G.S. (1999). Characteristics of the healthy survivor effect among male and female Hanford workers, *American Journal of Industrial Medicine* **35**, 343–347.

[21] Baris, D., Armstrong, B.G., Deadman, J. & Theriault, G. (1996). A case cohort study of suicide in relation to exposure to electric and magnetic fields among electrical utility workers, *Occupational and Environmental Medicine* **53**, 17–24.

[22] Bartsch, H., Kadlubar, F. & O'Neill, I., eds. (1993). Biomarkers in human cancer – Part II. Exposure monitoring and molecular dosimetry, *Environmental Health Perspectives* **99**, 2–309.

[23] Baur, X., Marczynski, B., Rozynek, P. & Voss, B. (1994). Bronchopulmonale Prakanzerosen und Tumoren – Risikogruppen aus arbeitsmedizinischer Sicht (Bronchopulmonary precancerous conditions and tumors – risk groups from the occupational medicine viewpoint), *Pneumologie* **48**, 825–834.

[24] Beall, C., Delzell, E. & Macaluso, M. (1995). Mortality patterns among women in the motor vehicle manufacturing industry, *American Journal of Industrial Medicine* **28**, 325–337.

[25] Becher, H., Flesch-Janys, D., Kauppinen, T., Kogevinas, M., Steindorf, K., Manz, A. & Wahrendorf, J. (1996). Cancer mortality in German male workers exposed to phenoxy herbicides and dioxins, *Cancer, Causes and Control* **7**, 312–321.

[26] BEIR IV. Committee of Biological Effects of Ionizing Radiations, US National Research Council. (1988). *Health Risk of Radon and other Internally Deposited Alpha-Emitters*. National Academy Press, Washington.

[27] Blair, A., Linos, A., Stewart, P.A., Burmeister, L.F., Gibson, R., Everett, G., Schuman, L. & Cantor, K.P. (1993). Evaluation of risks for non-Hodgkin's lymphoma by occupation and industry exposures from a case-control study, *American Journal of Industrial Medicine* **23**, 301–312.

[28] Blair, A. & Stewart, P.A. (1992). Do quantitative exposure assessments improve risk estimates in occupational studies of cancer?, *American Journal of Industrial Medicine* **21**, 53–63.

[29] Boffetta, P. & Kogevinas, M. (1999). Introduction: epidemiologic research and prevention of occupational cancer in Europe, *Environmental Health Perspectives* **107**, Supplement 2, 229–231.

[30] Boggild, H. & Knutsson, A. (1999). Shift work, risk factors and cardiovascular disease, *Scandinavian Journal of Work, Environment and Health* **25**, 85–89.

[31] Bouyer, J. & Hemon, D. (1993). Comparison of three methods of estimating odds ratios from a job exposure matrix in occupational case–control studies, *American Journal of Epidemiology* **137**, 472–481.

[32] Brackbill, R.M., Maizlish, N. & Fischbach, T. (1990). Risk of neuropsychiatric disability among painters in the United States, *Scandinavian Journal of Work, Environment and Health* **16**, 182–188.

[33] Brash, D.E., Rudolph, J.A., Simon, J.A., Lin, A., McKenna, G.J., Baden, H.P., Halperin, A.J. & Ponten, J. (1991). A role of sunlight in skin cancer, UV-induced p53 mutations in squamous cell carcinoma, *Proceedings of the National Academy of Sciences* **88**, 10124–10128.

[34] Breslow, L. (1955). Industrial aspects of bronchogenic neoplasms, *Diseases of the Chest* **28**, 421–430.

[35] Breslow, N.E. (1984). Elementary methods of cohort analysis, *International Journal of Epidemiology* **13**, 112–115.

[36] Bressac, B., Kew, M., Wands, J. & Ozturk, M. (1991). Selective G to T mutations of p53 gene in hepatocellular carcinoma from southern Africa, *Nature* **350**, 429–431.

[37] Brockmoller, J., Kerb, R., Drakoulis, N., Staffeldt, B. & Roots, I. (1994). Glutathione S-transferase M1 and its variants A and B as host factors of bladder cancer susceptibility, a case–control study, *Cancer Research* **54**, 4103–4111.

[38] Caporaso, N., Hayes, R.B., Dosemeci, M., Hoover, R., Ayesh, R., Hetzel, M. & Idle, J. (1989). Lung cancer risk, occupational exposure, and the debrisoquine metabolic phenotype, *Cancer Research* **49**, 3675–3679.

[39] Case, R.A.M. & Hosker, M.E. (1954). Tumour on the urinary bladder as an occupational disease in the rubber industry in England and Wales, *British Journal of Preventive and Social Medicine* **8**, 39–50.

[40] Checkoway, H.A., Pearce, N.E. & Crawford-Brown, D.J. (1989). *Research Methods in Occupational Epidemiology*. Oxford University Press, New York.

[41] Checkoway, H. & Rice, C.H. (1992). Time-weighted averages, peaks, and other indices of exposure in occupational epidemiology, *American Journal of Industrial Medicine* **21**, 25–33.

[42] Checkoway, H., Savitz, D.A. & Heyer, N.J. (1991). Assessing the effects of nondifferential missclassification of exposures in occupational studies, *Applied Occupational and Environmental Hygiene* **6**, 528–533.

[43] Cherry, N.M., Labréche, F.P. & McDonald, J.C. (1992). Organic brain damage and occupational solvent exposure, *British Journal of Industrial Medicine* **49**, 776–781.

[44] Choi, B.C. (1992). Definition, sources, magnitude, effect modifiers, and strategies of reduction of the healthy worker effect, *Journal of Occupational Medicine* **34**, 979–988.

[45] Chreech, J.L. & Johnson, M.N. (1974). Angiosarcoma of liver in the manufacture of polyvinyl chloride, *Journal of Occupational Medicine* **16**, 150–151.

[46] Dahl, E. (1993). Social inequality in health – the role of the healthy worker effect, *Social Science and Medicine* **36**, 1077–1086.

[47] Dewar, R., Siemiatycki, J. & Gerin, M. (1991). Loss of statistical power associated with the use of a job-exposure matrix in occupational case-control studies, *Applied Occupational and Environmental Hygiene* **6**, 508–515.

[48] Doll, R. (1952). The causes of death among gas-workers with special reference to cancer of the lung, *British Journal of Industrial Medicine* **9**, 180–185.

[49] Doll, R. (1955). Mortality from lung cancer in asbestos workers, *British Journal of Industrial Medicine* **12**, 81–86.

[50] Doll, R. (1988). Effects of exposure to vinyl chloride. An assessment of the evidence, *Scandinavian Journal of Work, Environment and Health* **14**, 61–78.

[51] Dosemeci, M., Cocco, P., Gomez, M., Stewart, P.A. & Heineman, E.F. (1994). Effects of three features of a job-exposure matrix on risk estimates, *Epidemiology* **5**, 124–127.

[52] Dosemeci, M., Wacholder, S. & Lubin, J. (1990). Does non-differential missclassification of exposure always bias a true effect toward the null value?, *American Journal of Epidemiology* **132**, 746–748.

[53] Figueroa, W.G., Raszkowski, R. & Weiss, W. (1973). Lung cancer in chloromethyl ether workers, *New England Journal of Medicine* **288**, 1096–1097.

[54] Flanders, W.D., Cardenas, V.M. & Austin, H. (1993). Confounding by time since hire in internal comparisons of cumulative exposure in occupational cohort studies, *Epidemiology* **4**, 336–341.

[55] Flesch-Janys, D., Berger, J., Gurn, P., Manz, A., Nagel, S., Waltsgott, H. & Dwyer, J.H. (1995). Exposure to polychlorinated dioxins and furans (PCDD/F) and mortality in a cohort of workers from a herbicide-production plant in Hamburg, Federal Republic of Germany, *American Journal of Epidemiology* **142**, 1165–1175.

[56] Fletcher, A.C., Engholm, G. & Englund, A. (1993). The risk of lung cancer from asbestos among Swedish construction workers, self-reported exposure and a job exposure matrix compared, *International Journal of Epidemiology* **22**, Supplement 2, S29–S35.

[57] Forastiere, F., Balmes, J., Scarinci, M. & Tager, I.B. (1998). Occupation, asthma, and chronic respiratory symptoms in a community sample of older women, *American Journal of Respiratory and Critical Care Medicine* **157**, 1864–1870.

[58] Fu, H. & Bofetta, P. (1995). Cancer and occupational exposure to inorganic lead compounds, a meta-analysis of published data, *Occupational and Environmental Medicine* **52**, 73–81.

[59] Gardner, M.J. (1986). Considerations in the choice of expected numbers for appropriate comparisons in occupational cohort studies, *Medicina del Lavoro* **77**, 23–47.

[60] Gardner, M.J., Snee, M.P., Hall, A.J., Powell, C.A., Downes, S. & Terrell, J.D. (1990). Results of case-control study of leukaemia and lymphoma among young people near Sellafield nuclear plant in West Cumbria, *British Medical Journal* **300**, 423–429.

[61] Gloyne, S.R. (1935). Two cases of squamous carcinoma of the lung occurring in asbestosis, *Tubercle* **17**, 5–10.

[62] Gomez, M.R., Cocco, P., Dosemeci, M. & Stewart, P.A. (1994). Occupational exposure to chlorinated aliphatic hydrocarbons, job exposure matrix, *American Journal of Industrial Medicine* **26**, 171–183.

[63] Greenland, S., ed. (1987). *Evolution of Epidemiologic Ideas. Annotated Readings on Concepts and Methods.* Epidemiology Resources Inc., Chestnut Hill.

[64] Gridley, G., Nyren, O., Dosemeci, M., Moradi, T., Adami, H.O., Carroll, L. & Zahm, S.H. (1999). Is there a healthy worker effect for cancer incidence among women in Sweden?, *American Journal of Industrial Medicine* **36**, 193–199.

[65] Gunnarsdottir, H.K., Kjaerheim, K., Boffetta, P., Rafnsson, V. & Zahm, S.H. (1999). Women's health: occupation, cancer, and reproduction. A conference overview, *American Journal of Industrial Medicine* **36**, 1–5.

[66] Hagmar, L., Brögger, A., Hansteen, I.L., Heim, S., Högstedt, B., Knudsen, L., Lambert, B., Linnainmaa, K., Mitelman, F. & Nordenson, I. (1994). Cancer risk in humans predicted by increased levels of chromosomal aberrations in lymphocytes. Nordic study group on the health risk of chromosome damage, *Cancer Research* **54**, 2919–2922.

[67] Hammond, E.C., Selikoff, I.J. & Seidman, H. (1979). Asbestos exposure, cigarette smoking and death rates, *Annals of the New York Academy of Sciences* **330**, 473–490.

[68] Hardell, L. (1977). Soft-tissue sarcomas and exposure to phenoxyacetic acids – a clinical observation, *Läkartidningen* **74**, 2753–2754 (in Swedish).

[69] Hardell, L., Eriksson, M., Axelson, O. & Hoar Zahm, S. (1994). Cancer epidemiology, in *Dioxins and Health*, A. Schecter, ed., Plenum Press, New York, Chapter 16 pp. 525–547.

[70] Hardell, L., Holmgren, G., Steen, L., Fredrikson, M. & Axelson, O. (1995). Occupational and other risk factors for clinically overt familial amyloid polyneuropathy, *Epidemiology* **6**, 598–601.

[71] Härting, F.H. & Hesse, W. (1879). Der Lungenkrebs, die Bergkrankheit in den Schneeberger Gruben, *Vierteljahrsschrift für Gerichtliche Medicin und Öffentliches Gesundheitswesen* **30**, 296–307; **31**, 102–132; **31**, 313–337.

[72] Hayes, R.B. (1985). Genetic susceptibility and occupational cancer, *Medicina del Lavoro* **86**, 206–213.

[73] Heederik, D., Boleij, J.S.M., Kromhout, H. & Smid, T. (1991). Use and analysis of exposure monitoring data in occupational epidemiology; an example of an epidemiological study in the Dutch animal food industry, *Applied Occupational and Environmental Hygiene* **6**, 458–464.

[74] Hemminki, K. (1992). Use of molecular biology techniques in cancer epidemiology, *Scandinavian Journal of Work, Environment and Health* **18**, Supplement 1, 38–45.

[75] Hernberg, S. (1992). *Introduction to Occupational Epidemiology*. Lewis, Chelsea.

[76] Hernberg, S. (1981). "Negative" results in cohort studies. How to recognize fallacies, *Scandinavian Journal of Work, Environment and Health* **7**, Supplement 4, 121–126.

[77] Hernberg, S., Partanen, T., Nordman, C.H. & Sumari, P. (1970). Coronary heart disease among workers exposed to carbon disulphide, *British Journal of Industrial Medicine* **27**, 313–325.

[78] Herrick, R.F. & Stewart, P.A. (1991). International workshop on retrospective exposure assessment for occupational epidemiologic studies. Preface, *Applied Occupational and Environmental Hygiene* **6**, 417–420.

[79] Hill, A.B. & Faning, E.L. (1948). Studies in the incidence of cancer in a factory handling inorganic compounds of arsenic. I. Mortality experience in the factory, *British Journal of Industrial Medicine* **5**, 1–6.

[80] Hoar, S.K. (1982). Job-exposure matrices in occupational epidemiology, *Journal of the National Cancer Institute* **69**, 1419–1420.

[81] Hollmann, S., Klimmer, F., Schmidt, K.-H. & Kylian, H. (1999). Validation of a questionnaire for assessing physical work load, *Scandinavian Journal of Work, Environment and Health* **25**, 105–114.

[82] Hsairi, M., Kauffmann, F., Chavance, M. & Brochard, P. (1992). Personal factors related to the perception of occupational exposure, an application of a job exposure matrix, *International Journal of Epidemiology* **21**, 972–980.

[83] Hsu, I.C., Metcalf, R.A., Sun, T., Welsh, J.A., Wang, N.J. & Harris, C.C. (1991). Mutational hotspot in the p53 gene in human hepatocellular carcinomas, *Nature* **350**, 427–428.

[84] Hueper, W.C. (1966). *Occupational and Environmental Cancers of the Respiratory System*. Springer-Verlag, Berlin.

[85] Huff, J.E., Salmon, A.G., Hooper, N.K. & Zeise, L. (1991). Long-term carcinogenesis studies on 2, 3, 7, 8-tetrachlorodibenzo-p-dioxin and hexachlorodibenzo-p-dioxins, *Cell Biology and Toxicology* **7**, 67–94.

[86] IARC (1974). *Monographs on the Evaluation of Carcinogenic Risk of Chemicals to Man. Some Aromatic Amines, Hydrazine and Related Substances, N-Nitroso Compounds and Miscellaneous Alkylating Agents*, Vol. 4. International Agency for Research on Cancer, Lyon.

[87] IARC (1987). *Monographs on the Evaluation of Carcinogenic Risk to Humans. Overall Evaluations of Carcinogenicity. An Updating of IARC Monographs*, Vols 1–42, Suppl. 7. International Agency for Research on Cancer, Lyon.

[88] IARC (1993). *Monographs on the Evaluation of Carcinogenic Risks to Humans.* Vol. 58, *Beryllium, Cadmium, Mercury, and Exposures in the Glass Manufacturing Industry*. International Agency for Research on Cancer, Lyon.

[89] IARC (1994). *Monographs on the Evaluation of Carcinogenic Risks to Humans.* Vol. 60, *Some Industrial Chemicals*. International Agency for Research on Cancer, Lyon.

[90] IARC (1995). *Monographs on the Evaluation of Carcinogenic Risks to Humans.* Vol. 63, *Dry Cleaning, Some Chlorinated Solvents and Other Industrial Chemicals*. International Agency for Research on Cancer, Lyon.

[91] IARC (1999). *Monographs on the Evaluation of carcinogenic Risks to Humans.* Vol. 71, *Re-evaluation of some organic chemicals, hydrazine and hydrogen peroxide*. International Agency for Research on Cancer, Lyon.

[92] Jauchem, J.R. & Merritt, J.H. (1991). The epidemiology of exposure to electromagnetic fields; an overview of the recent literature, *Journal of Clinical Epidemiology* **44**, 895–906.

[93] Joffe M. (1992). Validity of exposure data derived from a structured questionnaire, *American Journal of Epidemiology* **135**, 564–570.

[94] Johnson, J.V. & Stewart, W.F. (1993). Measuring work organization exposure over the life course with a job-exposure matrix, *Scandinavian Journal of Work, Environment and Health* **19**, 21–28.

[95] Kjuus, H., Langård, S. & Skjaerven, R. (1986). A case-referent study of lung cancer, occupational exposures and smoking. III. Etiologic fraction of occupational exposures, *Scandinavian Journal of Work, Environment and Health* **12**, 210–215.

[96] Kogevinas, M., Anto, J.M., Sunyer, J., Tobias, A., Kromhout, H. & Burney, P. (1999). Occupational asthma in Europe and other industrialised areas: a population-based study. European Community Respiratory Health Survey Study Group, *Lancet* **353**, 1750–1754.

[97] Kogevinas, M. & Sala, M. (1998). Pesticides and congenital malformations – how many studies will it take to reach a conclusion?, *Scandinavian Journal of Work, Environment and Health* **24**, 445–447.

[98] Kromhout, H., Heederik, D., Dalderup, L.M. & Kromhout, D. (1992). Performance of two general job-exposure matrices in a study of lung cancer morbidity in the Zutphen cohort, *American Journal of Epidemiology* **136**, 698–711.

[99] Kromhout, H., Symanski, E. & Rappaport, S.M. (1993). A comprehensive evaluation of within- and between-worker components of occupational exposure to chemical agents, *Annals of Occupational Hygiene* **37**, 253–270.

[100] Lagerstrom, M., Hansson, T. & Hagberg, M. (1998). Work-related low-back problems in nursing, *Scandinavian Journal of Work, Environment and Health* **24**, 449–464.

[101] Landtblom, A.-M., Flodin, U., Söderfeldt, B., Wolfson, C. & Axelson, O. (1996). Organic solvents and

multiple sclerosis. A synthesis of the current evidence, *Epidemiology* **7**, 429–433.

[102] Lindbohm, M.L. (1999). Women's reproductive health: some recent developments in occupational epidemiology, *American Journal of Industrial Medicine* **36**, 18–24.

[103] Lilienfeld, A.M. & Lilienfeld, D.E. (1979). A century of case–control studies, progress?, *Journal of Chronic Diseases* **32**, 5–13.

[104] London, S.J., Daly, A.K., Fairbrother, K.S., Holmes, C., Carpenter, C.L., Navidi, W.C. & Idle, J.R. (1995). Lung cancer risk in African-Americans in relation to a race-specific CYP1A1 polymorphism, *Cancer Research* **55**, 6035–6037.

[105] Lundin, F.E., Wagoner, J.K. & Archer, V.E. (1971). *Radon Daughter Exposure and Respiratory Cancer; Quantitative and Temporal Aspects*. NIOSH and NIEHS Joint Monograph No. 1. Department of Health, Education and Welfare, Public Health Service, Washington.

[106] Lynch, K.M. & Smith, W.A. (1935). Pulmonary asbestosis III. Carcinoma of the lung in asbestos-silicosis, *American Journal of Cancer* **24**, 56–64.

[107] Lynge, E., Kurppa, K., Kristofersen, L., Malker, H. & Sauli, H. (1986). Silica dust and lung cancer, results from the Nordic occupational mortality and cancer incidence registers, *Journal of the National Cancer Institute* **77**, 883–889.

[108] Macbeth, R. (1965). Malignant disease of the paranasal sinuses, *Journal of Laryngology* **79**, 592–612.

[109] McDonald, A. (1995). Work and pregnancy, in *Epidemiology of Work Related Diseases*, J.C. McDonald, ed. British Medical Journal Publishing Group, London.

[110] McDonald, J.C. ed. (1995). *Epidemiology of Work Related Diseases*. British Medical Journal Publishing Group, London.

[111] McMichael, A.J. (1976). Standardized mortality ratios and the "healthy worker effect", scratching beneath the surface, *Journal of Occupational Medicine* **18**, 165–168.

[112] Messing, K., Dumais, L., Courville, J., Seifert, A.M. & Boucher, M. (1994). Evaluation of exposure data from men and women with the same job title, *Journal of Occupational Medicine* **36**, 913–917.

[113] Miettinen, O.S. (1985). *Theoretical Epidemiology, Principles of Occurrence Research in Medicine*. Wiley, New York.

[114] Miettinen, O.S. (1985). The "case–control" study: valid selection of subjects (with dissents, comment and response), *Journal of Chronic Diseases* **38**, 543–558.

[115] Miettinen, O.S. & Wang, J.-D. (1981). An alternative to the proportionate mortality ratio, *American Journal of Epidemiology* **114**, 144–148.

[116] Mikkelsen, S. (1980). A cohort study of disability pension and death among painters with special regard to disabling presenile dementia as an occupational disease, *Scandinavian Journal of Social Medicine* **16**, Supplement, 34–43.

[117] Milham, S. (1982). Mortality from leukaemia in workers exposed to electrical and magnetic fields, *New England Journal of Medicine* **307**, 249.

[118] Milham, S., Jr. (1983). *Occupational Mortality in Washington State 1950–1979*. DHHS Pub. No. (NIOSH) 83–116. Centers for Disease Control and Prevention, Cincinnati, pp. 1663–1664.

[119] Monson, R.R. (1990). *Occupational Epidemiology*. CRC Press, Boca Raton.

[120] Nurminen, M. (1995). To use or not to use the odds ratio in epidemiologic analyses?, *European Journal of Epidemiology* **11**, 365–371.

[121] Occupational Cancer in Europe (1999). *Environmental Health Perspectives* **107**, Supplement 2.

[122] Olsen, J. & Sabroe, S. (1980). A case–reference study of neuropsychiatric disorders among workers exposed to solvents in the Danish wood and furniture industry, *Scandinavian Journal of Social Medicine* **16**, Supplement, 44–49.

[123] Olsen, O. & Kristensen, T.S. (1991). Impact of work environment on cardiovascular diseases in Denmark, *Journal of Epidemiology and Community Health* **45**, 4–10.

[124] Olsen, O., Vingård, E., Köster, M. & Alfredsson, L. (1994). Etiologic fractions for physical work load, sports and overweight in the occurrence of coxarthrosis, *Scandinavian Journal of Work, Environment and Health* **20**, 184–188.

[125] Ott, M.G., Skory, L.K., Holder, B.B., Bronson, J.M. & Williams, P.R. (1983). Health evaluation of employees occupationally exposed to methylene chloride. Mortality, *Scandinavian Journal of Work, Environment and Health* **9**, Supplement 1, 8–16.

[126] Ott, M.G. & Zober, A. (1996). Cause specific mortality and cancer incidence among employees exposed to 2,3,7,8-TCDD after a 1953 Reactor accident, *Occupational and Environmental Medicine* **53**, 606–612.

[127] Park, R., Krebs, J. & Mirer, F. (1994). Mortality at an automotive stamping and assembly complex, *American Journal of Industrial Medicine* **26**, 449–463.

[128] Pearce, N. (1992). Methodological problems in time-related variables in occupational cohort studies, *Revue d'Épidemiologie et de Santé Publique* **40**, S43–S54.

[129] Pearce, N. & Checkoway, H. (1987). Epidemiologic programs for computers and calculators. A simple computer program for generating person-time data in cohort studies involving time-related factors, *American Journal of Epidemiology* **125**, 1085–1091.

[130] Pearce, N.E., Checkoway, H. & Shy, C.M. (1986). Time-related factors as potential confounders and effect modifiers in studies on an occupational cohort, *Scandinavian Journal of Work, Environment and Health* **112**, 97–107.

[131] Pershagen, G. (1985). Lung cancer mortality among men living near an arsenic-emitting smelter, *American Journal of Epidemiology* **122**, 684–694.

[132] Pershagen, G. & Axelson, O. (1982). A validation of questionnaire information on occupational exposure and

smoking, *Scandinavian Journal of Work, Environment and Health* **8**, 24–28.

[133] Pershagen, G., Wall, S., Taube, A. & Linnman, L. (1981). On the interaction between occupational arsenic exposure and smoking and its relationship to lung cancer, *Scandinavian Journal of Work, Environment and Health* **7**, 302–309.

[134] Persson, B. & Fredrikson, M. (1995). A pooled analysis of non-Hodgkin's lymphoma and the role of rare occupational exposures and interaction of risk factors, in *Occupational Exposures and Malignant Lymphoma*, B. Persson, ed. Linköping University Medical Dissertations No. 475. Faculty of Health Sciences, Linköping University, Linköping.

[135] Petsonk, E.L., Daniloff, E.M., Mannino, D.M., Wang, M.L., Short, S.R. & Wagner, G.R. (1995). Airway responsiveness and job selection; a study in coal miners and non-mining controls, *Occupational and Environmental Medicine* **52**, 745–749.

[136] Plato, N. & Steineck, G. (1993). Methodology and utility of a job-exposure matrix, *American Journal of Industrial Medicine* **23**, 491–502.

[137] Rappaport, S.M. (1993). Biological considerations in assessing exposures to genotoxic and carcinogenic agents, *International Archives of Occupational and Environmental Health* **65**, S29–S35.

[138] Rehn, L. (1906). Blasenkrankungn bei Anilinarbeitern, *Verhandlungen der Deutschen Gesellschaft für Chirurgie* **35**, 313–318.

[139] Robins, J.M., Blevins, D., Ritter, G. & Wulfsohn, M. (1992). G-estimation of the effect of prophylaxis therapy for pneumocystis carinii pneumonia on the survival of AIDS patients, *Epidemiology* **3**, 319–336.

[140] Roeleveld, N., Zielhuis, G.A. & Gabreëls, F. (1993). Mental retardation and parental occupation, a study on the applicability of job exposure matrices, *British Journal of Industrial Medicine* **50**, 945–954.

[141] Ronneberg, A. (1995). Mortality and cancer morbidity in workers from an aluminium smelter with prebaked carbon anodes. Part I, Exposure assessment, *Occupational and Environmental Medicine* **52**, 242–249.

[142] Samuels, S.W., ed. (1986). The environment of the work place and human values, *American Journal of Industrial Medicine* **9**, 1–113.

[143] Santos-Burgoa, C., Matanoski, G.M., Seger, S. & Schwartz, L. (1992). Lymphohematopoietic cancer in styrene-butadiene polymerization workers, *American Journal of Epidemiology* **136**, 843–854.

[144] Savitz, D.A., Pearce, N.E. & Poole, C. (1989). Methodological issues in the epidemiology of electromagnetic fields and cancer, *Epidemiological Reviews* **11**, 59–78.

[145] Selikoff, I.J., Churg, J. & Hammond, E.C. (1964). Asbestos exposure and neoplasia, *Journal of the American Medical Association* **188**, 22–26.

[146] Siemiatycki, J., ed. (1991). *Risk Factors for Cancer in the Workplace*. CRC Press, Boca Raton.

[147] Smid, T., Heederik, D., Houba, R. & Quanjer, P.H. (1992). Dust- and endotoxin-related respiratory effects in the animal feed industry, *American Review of Respiratory Disease* **146**, 1474–1479.

[148] Smith, C.M., Kelsey, K.T., Wiencke, J.K., Leyden, K., Levin, S. & Christiani, D.C. (1994). Inherited glutathione-S-transferase deficiency is a risk factor for pulmonary asbestosis, *Cancer Epidemiology, Biomarkers and Prevention* **3**, 471–477.

[149] Smith, T.J. (1992). Occupational exposure and dose over time, limitations of cumulative exposure, *American Journal of Industrial Medicine* **21**, 35–51.

[150] Söderkvist, P. & Axelson, O. (1995). On the use of molecular biology data in occupational and environmental epidemiology, *Journal of Occupational and Environmental Medicine* **37**, 84–90.

[151] Sohrahan, T. & Gilthorpe, M.S. (1994). Non-differential missclassification of exposure always leads to an underestimate of risk, an incorrect conclusion, *Occupational and Environmental Medicine* **51**, 839–840.

[152] Sorsa, M. (1980). Cytogenetic methods in the detection of chemical carcinogens, *Journal of Toxicology and Environmental Health* **6**, 1077–1080.

[153] Spirtas, R., Stewart, P.A., Lee, J.S., Marano, D.E., Forbes, C.D., Grauman, D.J., Pettigrew, H.M., Blair, A., Hoover, R.N. & Cohen, J.L. (1991). Retrospective cohort mortality study of workers at an aircraft maintenance facility. I. Epidemiological results, *British Journal of Industrial Medicine* **48**, 515–530.

[154] Steenland, K. & Stayner, L. (1991). The importance of employment status in occupational cohort mortality studies, *Epidemiology* **2**, 418–423.

[155] Stengel, B., Pisani, P., Limasset, J.C., Bouyer, J., Berrino, F. & Hemon, D. (1993). Retrospective evaluation of occupational exposure to organic solvents, questionnaire and job exposure matrix, *International Journal of Epidemiology* **22**, Supplement 2, S72–S82.

[156] Stewart, P.A., Fears, T., Kross, B., Ogilvie, L. & Blair, A. (1999). Exposure of farmers to phosmet, a swine insecticide, *Scandinavian Journal of Work, Environment and Health* **25**, 33–38.

[157] Taylor, J.A., Sandler, D.P., Bloomfield, C.D., Shore, D.L., Ball, E.D., Neubauer, A., McIntyre, O.R. & Liu, E. (1992). *ras* Oncogene activation and occupational exposures in acute myeloid leukemia, *Journal of the National Cancer Institute* **84**, 1626–1632.

[158] Theriault, G. (1992). Electromagnetic fields and cancer risks, *Revue d'Épidemiologie et de Santé Publique* **40**, S55–S62.

[159] Tiller, J.R., Schilling, R.S.F. & Morris, J.N. (1968). Occupational toxic factor in mortality from coronary heart disease, *British Medical Journal* **4**, 407–411.

[160] Tola, S., Vilhunen, R., Järvinen, E. & Korkola, M.-L. (1980). A cohort study of workers exposed to trichloroethylene, *Journal of Occupational Medicine* **22**, 737–740.

[161] Torchio, P., Lepore, A.R., Corrao, G., Comba, P., Settimi, L., Belli, S., Magnani, C. & di Orio, F. (1994). Mortality study on a cohort of Italian licensed pesticide users, *Science of the Total Environment* **149**, 183–191.

[162] Toren, K., Balder, B., Brisman, J., Lindholm, N., Low-hagen, O., Palmqvist, M. & Tunsater, A. (1999). The risk of asthma in relation to occupational exposures: a case–control study from a Swedish city, *European Respiratory Journal* **13**, 496–501.

[163] Ulfvarson, U. (1992). Validation of exposure information in occupational epidemiology, *American Journal of Industrial Medicine* **21**, 125–132.

[164] Vainio, H. (1999). Biomarkers in the identification of risks, especially with regard to susceptible persons and subgroups, *Scandinavian Journal of Work, Environment and Health* **25**, 1–3.

[165] van Miller, J.P., Lalich, J.J. & Allen, J.R. (1977). Increased incidence of neoplasms in rats exposed to low levels of tetrachlorodibenzo-p-dioxin, *Chemosphere* **6**, 537–544.

[166] van Vliet, C., Swaen, G.M., Volovics, A., Tweehuysen, M., Meijers, J.M., de Boorder, T. & Sturmans, F. (1990). Neuropsychiatric disorders among solvent-exposed workers. First results from a Dutch case-control study, *International Archives of Occupational and Environmental Health* **62**, 127–132.

[167] Vineis, P. (1992). Uses of biochemical and biological markers in occupational epidemiology, *Revue d'Épidemiologie et de Santé Publique* **40**, S63–S69.

[168] Vineis, P. & Soskolne, C.L. (1993). Cancer risk assessment and management. An ethical perspective, *Journal of Occupational Medicine* **35**, 902–908.

[169] Wagner, J.C., Sleggs, C.A. & Marchand, P. (1960). Diffuse pleural mesothelioma and asbestos exposure in North Western Cape Province, *British Journal of Industrial Medicine* **17**, 260–271.

[170] Wagoner, J.K., Miller, R.W., Lundin, Jr, F.E., Fraumeni, J.F. & Haij, N.E. (1963). Unusual mortality among a group of underground metal miners, *New England Journal of Medicine* **269**, 281–289.

[171] Wagoner, J.K., Archer, V.E., Carrol, B.E., Holaday, D.A. & Lawrence, P.A. (1964). Cancer mortality patterns among U.S. uranium miners and millers, 1950 through 1962, *Journal of the National Cancer Institute* **32**, 787–801.

[172] Wertheimer, N. & Leeper, E. (1979). Electrical wiring configurations and childhood cancer, *American Journal of Epidemiology* **109**, 273–284.

[173] Whorton, M.D. (1980). Recovery of testicular function among DBCP workers, *Journal of Occupational Medicine* **22**, 177–179.

[174] Whorton, M.D., Krauss, R.M., Marshall, S. & Milby, T.H. (1977). Infertility in male pesticide workers, *Lancet* **ii**, 1259–1261.

[175] Women's health: occupation, cancer and reproduction. Special issue (1999). *American Journal of Industrial Medicine* **36**, 1–224.

[176] Wingren, G. & Axelson, O. (1992). Cluster of brain cancer spuriously suggesting occupational risk among glassworkers, *Scandinavian Journal of Work, Environment and Health* **18**, 85–89.

[177] Zocchetti, C., Consonni, D. & Bertazzi, P.A. *versus* Lee, J. (1995). Letters to the Editor. Estimation of prevalence rate ratios from cross-sectional data, *International Journal of Epidemiology* **5**, 1064–1067.

OLAV AXELSON

Occupational Health and Medicine

Occupational health is an activity organized to protect the health of employees from harmful consequences arising out of their work. It includes industrial medicine and occupational medicine which also provides medical **surveillance** services. The aims are to reduce the frequency and severity of occupational diseases, i.e. diseases caused or exacerbated by the occupational environment, and hence to reduce premature death and disability. The prevention or reduction of occupational disease is emphasized, and this involves changes in the occupational environment that may be achieved by those practicing occupational hygiene. The importance given to occupational health is dependent on the social attitudes of the population in which it is based, and many of the occupational health questions now considered would have seemed of trivial concern a few decades ago. Occupational health includes safety, sometimes emphasized by the use of the term "health and safety", which is concerned with the reduction of accidents in the workplace.

Important elements are first the identification of adverse health effects of occupational exposure to a pollutant (*see* **Occupational Epidemiology**) and, secondly, the implementation of measures to reduce exposure and hence the frequency or severity of adverse health effects. This second step may involve standard setting, i.e. the setting of exposure limits predicted to lead to minimal adverse health effects. The setting of such limits may utilize **dose–response** data but also takes into account practicality and the milieu in which employers and workers interact.

Historical Development

The Italian physician, Bernardino Ramazzini (1633–1714), has been referred to as the "father of occupational medicine" [13]. He was professor of medicine at the Universities of Modena and Padua. He stressed the importance of direct examination of workers and introduced the concept of the taking of an occupational history. He described diseases associated with a wide range of occupations and their causes [24], including diseases caused by the inhalation of dusts and gases and those caused by poor ergonomic practices. Ramazzini's publications were the main source on illnesses caused by work for over a century [18]. Popper [22] drew the distinction between "occupational diseases" and "workers diseases", the former restricted to diseases caused directly by some intrinsic feature of the occupation, such as exposure to a chemical, while the latter also includes diseases occurring for socioeconomic reasons associated with the occupation. Ramazzini had noted that breast cancer was more prevalent in nuns than other women, and attributed this to celibacy.

In the eighteenth century there was a growing concern on the effects of industrialization. Guy [10] analyzed the proportion of deaths due to pulmonary consumption in broad occupational groupings and attributed an excess of such deaths to poor conditions, such as inadequate drainage and ventilation, an inadequate water supply, and overcrowding, in both dwellings and workshops. William Farr (1807–1883), the first compiler of Abstracts in the General Register Office of England and Wales, introduced a classification of occupations in 1851 that was used for the analysis of **occupational mortality** from official **vital statistics.** Later, Hill [12] used national insurance statistics to examine sickness absences of printers, cotton weavers, and spinners. From about this time, and particularly after the end of World War II, there was increasing attention to research into the extent and causes of occupational diseases, and this research necessitated the application of statistical concepts and methods into the design and analysis of studies.

Types of Study

The relationship between the occupational environment and health has been studied in a variety of ways. Insofar as occupational diseases may be caused by industrial pollutants, then basic studies of the interaction between pollutants and biological systems have been carried out in toxicology, by *in vitro* experiments, and by animal experimentation.

Studies of humans have involved experimentation, looking at acute effects, but such studies are infeasible, and unethical, for chronic effects. Such effects have been studied by epidemiologic investigations (*see* **Observational Study**). The outcome variables include mortality, the occurrence or presence of a disease, and the value of a variable that measures some function of health. For example, measures of lung function, such as the forced expiratory volume, are indicators of health but do not indicate disease unless grossly abnormal. Disease outcomes include diseases specific to occupational exposure, e.g. the pneumoconioses are caused by the inhalation of dust or fibers. They also include nonspecific diseases, the incidence of which may be increased by occupational exposure. For example, the frequency of lung cancer is increased by exposure to asbestos and a number of chemicals, but it occurs also in the absence of such exposures.

The main study designs employed have been:

1. **Cross-sectional study** – a study examining the relationship between disease, or a measure of health, and occupational conditions at a given time.
2. **Cohort study** – a study in which subjects are selected and followed-up over time to observe their mortality, morbidity, or changes in some functional measure of health, and to relate these to the exposure within the occupation. Cohort studies have been used particularly in the study of cancer, and frequently are *historical cohort studies* in which the cohort is defined in terms of existing historical data, such as records of employees. Follow-up is then from some time in the past – often many years or decades – to the present (*see* **Cohort Study, Historical**).
3. **Case–control (case-referent) study** – A study in which cases of disease are identified and noncases are chosen as **controls** or referents. The previous occupational exposure history of cases and controls are then ascertained and compared to give estimates of the association between the occupational environment and the disease. Case–control studies may be nested within a cohort study so that the cohort study is used to identify cases of disease in an occupational population and the case–control study is used to obtain more detailed information on exposure on a smaller number of cases and controls than would be practical for all members of a large cohort (*see* **Case–Control Study, Nested**) [16, 14].

Landmark Studies

One of the earliest controlled clinical trials took place in the area of occupational health. J. Lind, a naval surgeon on the *Salisbury*, divided a group of 12 seamen suffering from scurvy into six groups of 2. One of the treatments was two oranges and a lemon a day, and the "most sudden and visible good effects" were observed in the two seamen receiving this treatment. Regrettably it took another 50 years before lemon juice was supplied as a dietary supplement on British naval vessels [15; 21, pp. 14, 15].

The association between exposure to occupational environments and cancer has been a constant theme. The first malignant disease to be associated with a particular occupation was cancer of the scrotum in chimney sweeps, described by Percivall Pott [23]; see [20] and [27]. Härting & Hesse [11] reported an excess of respiratory cancers in underground metal miners, later shown to be due to radon daughters. This was the first association between an external agent and an internal cancer. The studies of Doll [6] on lung cancer amongst gas-workers, and of Case et al. [2] on bladder cancer and exposure to chemicals, were important studies, not only with respect to the identification of occupational carcinogens, but also in the early use of historical prospective cohort studies and the use of the **person-years at risk** method of mortality analysis. The risk of exposure to asbestos in producing lung cancer has been identified and confirmed using historical prospective studies [7, 25, 19], and the strong link between amphibole asbestos exposure and mesothelioma has been evaluated using similar studies following the identification of the link by Wagner et al. [26].

Particular Statistical Concepts, Problems, and Techniques

Most of the statistical methods used in occupational health are not unique to that area. Problems of potential **bias** due to **confounding** are often present in epidemiologic studies since the workers in groups to be compared may differ systematically in other characteristics. The confounding effect of smoking in studies on occupational respiratory diseases is a particular problem because of the large effect on health of the smoking habit. A particular type of bias, which may be considered as due to confounding, but is more

usefully considered separately, is the "healthy worker effect", which may arise in any epidemiologic study in which a workforce is compared with the general population or different workforces are compared with one another. A second problem is that due to the *latency* of occupational cancers, i.e. an excess of cancer due to occupational exposure does not occur until many years after the exposure (*see* **Latent Period**). Related to this, during a follow-up study of current workers the extent of exposure is constantly changing during the period of follow-up when adverse health effects are being noted. This makes the linking of the extent of exposure to the health effect difficult. A full account of many of the statistical methods used in occupational health is given by Checkoway et al. [3].

Healthy Worker Effect

Studies of occupational health are carried out in groups of workers who select themselves, and are selected by employers, into particular occupations. These selection processes lead to the "healthy worker effect", which occurs because they are likely to eliminate the most unhealthy from entering the workforce and also may mean that those developing ill health are less likely to remain in the job. As noted by McMichael [17], these selection effects lead to lower mortality rates than would be expected. Fox & Collier [9] noted that the healthy worker effect consisted of three components, which they attributed to selection (*see* **Selection Bias**), survival, and length of follow-up. They found that the effect was particularly marked in the first 10 years after the start of employment in which there was exposure to vinyl chloride. The consequence of the healthy worker effect is that comparisons of mortality between employed groups and the general population may be biased unless workers are followed-up after they have left the employed group and unless comparisons take account of time since the start of employment. Methods of analysis using internal comparisons may take account of the initial selection criteria provided that these were applied similarly to the groups under comparison.

The Analysis of Mortality – External Comparisons

One method of analysis of follow-up studies where the outcome is mortality consists of the comparison of the observed number of deaths due to all or specific causes with the number that would be expected taking into account the age distribution of the cohort studied, the period during which follow-up occurred, and the varying lengths of follow-up of the different subjects in the study. The indirect method of standardization is the basis of the method, referred to as the *person-years* method (*see* **Standardization Methods**). This method was first used by Doll [6] and has been commonly applied in occupational mortality studies. The total follow-up period is divided into periods, usually of 5 years, and within each of these periods the ages of those persons followed within that period of time are similarly subdivided, again usually into 5-year groups. The expected number of deaths is calculated by multiplying the person-years at risk in each of the age–period intervals by the age- and period-specific death rates of a standard population. The standard population is a national or regional population for which death rates are available. The usual measure of effect is the ratio of observed to expected deaths which, in analogy with indirect standardization, is often referred to as a standardized mortality ratio (SMR).

The method has usually been applied to single groups or descriptively to a few subgroups, but may be extended to take account of other variables recorded for the persons followed-up using **Poisson regression** [1].

The Analysis of Mortality – Internal Comparisons

A disadvantage of the person-years method is the implicit assumption that the death rates in the occupational group would be the same as in the standard population except for factors within the occupational environment. While this assumption is not strictly necessary, the healthy worker effect has to be taken into account in the interpretation of the results. The method does assume that the death rates in the occupational group and the standard population are in a fixed proportion in all the age–period groups, i.e. that the standard death rates apply to the occupational group at least proportionally. The approach may be modified by working internally within the occupational group and avoiding the use of a standard population for comparison. This leads to internally calculated SMRs, and comparison of more than two of these depends on **proportional hazards** of the subgroups across the age-period strata. This problem may

be overcome by the use of directly standardized rates, which leads to the *standardized rate ratio* (SRR).

All these methods involve **stratification** and become imprecise when there are several variables to take into account. Stratification can be avoided by using the most general method, i.e. Poisson modeling (*see* **Poisson Regression**).

As it is often required to assess the mortality of an occupational group in the context of the population of which the workers are a part and also to assess dose–response relationships within the occupational group, or to compare subgroups within the whole occupational group, a combination of external and internal methods is appropriate. For example, Checkoway et al. [4], in a study of workers employed in the mining and processing of diatomaceous earth, analysed the mortality due to lung cancer in the whole group. The methods of analysis included comparison with US national death rates using the SMR and internal analyses using Poisson regression to examine the trend with extent of exposure. The combination of methods led to the conclusion that there was an excess of deaths due to lung cancer in the workforce, compared with the US population, and that this excess was in those with the highest cumulative exposure in dust-exposed jobs.

Time-Related Exposure and Covariates

A measure of exposure to an occupational agent that may be used is cumulative exposure, i.e. the intensity of exposure accumulated to give a time-weighted cumulative measure. Clearly this measure will continue to increase as long as exposure is occurring. Methods of analysis relating health outcomes to exposure have to take this into account, not only with respect to the appropriate exposure to link with the outcome event, but also, equally importantly, to allocate the earlier years, when the event did not take place, to the lower cumulative exposure; failure to do this results in biased results [8]. Other variables that may be included in the analysis as covariates (confounders) may also be time-dependent – for example, smoking and age. One way of dealing with this problem is through a proportional hazards model [5] with time-related variables. Another way when there are no covariates is to use the person-years method, or corresponding internal methods, with each individual transferring from one cumulative exposure category to the next when the cumulative exposure reaches the appropriate values.

Latency

Many diseases do not occur until some time after the exposure that has caused the disease. In particular, occupational cancers usually do not occur, i.e. they cannot be diagnosed, until at least 10 years after exposure. This feature should be incorporated into the analysis since, otherwise, very recent exposure, that cannot be relevant to the disease, is included as if that exposure were relevant. One method of dealing with this problem is to begin the follow-up after an interval, of say 10 years, since the start of exposure, and to ignore deaths and person-years at risk within this interval. This method does not allow regression-type methods including cumulative exposure but may be extended for this situation by defining a lagged cumulative exposure; for example, the lagged cumulative exposure relevant to the disease risk of a 45-year-old worker would be the cumulative exposure at age 35.

Allowing for latency also helps to reduce the influence of the healthy worker effect.

Future Developments

The perceived importance of occupational diseases is dependent on societal attitudes. The major occupational effects of early industrialization have been eliminated, and the large excess death rates due to exposure to asbestos and other occupational pollutants have been identified and preventive measures taken, although the **excess mortality** continues to occur because of the long latency effects. Concern has moved to the possibility or suspicion of smaller effects. Methods will need to be developed to identify small effects of occupational pollutants. As the estimation of small effects may not be achievable by epidemiologic studies, there is likely to be an increasing emphasis on biological methods and on the translation of biological findings into meaningful **risk assessments** for exposed populations.

The concept of individual susceptibility to disease has been a long-standing concept, but there has been insufficient knowledge for most occupational diseases on how to identify those who would be most susceptible to occupational exposure. This means that it has not been practical to screen out of the exposed

workforce those most likely to develop disease due to exposure to a pollutant. Advances in **molecular epidemiology** may contribute to this area by leading to the possible identification of susceptible individuals, who could be advised to avoid employment in particular industries.

References

[1] Berry, G. (1983). The analysis of mortality by the subject-years method, *Biometrics* **39**, 173–184.

[2] Case, R.A.M., Hosker, M.E., McDonald, D.B. & Pearson, J.T. (1954). Tumours of the urinary bladder in workmen engaged in the manufacture and use of certain dyestuff intermediates in the British chemical industry. Part I, *British Journal of Industrial Medicine* **11**, 75–104.

[3] Checkoway, H., Pearce, N. & Crawford-Brown, D.J. (1989). *Research Methods in Occupational Epidemiology*. Oxford University Press, New York.

[4] Checkoway, H., Heyer, N.J., Seixas, N.S., Welp, E.A.E., Demers, P.A., Hughes, J.M. & Weill, H. (1997). Dose-response associations of silica with nonmalignant respiratory disease and lung cancer mortality in the diatomaceous earth industry. *American Journal of Epidemiology* **145**, 680–688.

[5] Cox, D.R. (1972). Regression models and life-tables (with discussion), *Journal of the Royal Statistical Society, Series B* **34**, 187–220.

[6] Doll, R. (1952). The causes of death among gas-workers with special reference to cancer of the lung, *British Journal of Industrial Medicine* **9**, 180–185.

[7] Doll, R. (1955). Mortality from lung cancer in asbestos workers, *British Journal of Industrial Medicine* **12**, 81–86.

[8] Enterline, P.E. (1976). Pitfalls in epidemiologic research: an examination of the asbestos literature, *Journal of Occupational Medicine* **18**, 150–156.

[9] Fox, A.J. & Collier, P.F. (1976). Low mortality rates in industrial cohort studies due to selection for work and survival in the industry, *British Journal of Preventive and Social Medicine* **30**, 225–230.

[10] Guy, W.A. (1844). A third contribution to a knowledge of the influence of employments upon health, *Journal of the Statistical Society of London* **7**, 232–243.

[11] Härting, F.H. & Hesse, W. (1879). Der Lungenkrebs, die Bergkrankheit in den Schneeberger Kobaltgruben, *Vjschr Gericht Med Offentl Gesundheitswesen* **31**, 102–132, 313–337.

[12] Hill, A.B. (1929). An investigation of sickness in various industrial occupations, *Journal of the Royal Statistical Society* **92**, 183–238.

[13] Koelsch, F., ed. (1912). *Bernardo Ramazzini, der Vater der Gewerbehygiene*. Stuttgart.

[14] Liddell, F.D.K., McDonald, J.C. & Thomas, D.C. (1977). Methods of cohort analysis: appraisal by

application to asbestos mining (with discussion), *Journal of the Royal Statistical Society, Series A* **140**, 469–491.

[15] Lind, J. (1753). *A Treatise of the Scurvy*. Sands, Murray & Cochran, Edinburgh.

[16] Mantel, N. (1973). Synthetic retrospective studies and related topics, *Biometrics* **29**, 479–486.

[17] McMichael, A.J. (1976). Standardized mortality ratios and the "healthy worker effect": scratching below the surface, *Journal of Occupational Medicine* **18**, 165–168.

[18] Milles, D. (1985). From workers' diseases to occupational diseases: the impact of experts' concepts on workers' attitudes, in *The Social History of Occupational Health*, P. Weindling, ed. Croom Helm, London, pp. 55–77.

[19] Newhouse, M.L. (1969). A study of the mortality of workers in an asbestos factory, *British Journal of Industrial Medicine* **26**, 294–301.

[20] Ogle, W. (1885). Letter to the Registrar-General on the mortality in the registration districts of England and Wales during the ten years 1871–80, in *Supplement to the 45th Annual Report of the Registrar General of Births. Deaths, and Marriages, in England*, p. xxiii.

[21] Pocock, S.J. (1983). *Clinical Trials: A Practical Approach*. Wiley, Chichester.

[22] Popper, M. (1882). *Lehrbuch der Arbeiterkrankheiten und Gewerbehygiene*. Zwanzig Vorlesungen, Stuttgart.

[23] Pott, P. (1775). *Chirurgical Observations*, Vol. 3. L. Hawes, W. Clark, and R. Collins, London, pp. 177–183.

[24] Ramazzini, B. (1700). *De Morbis Artificum* (translated by W.C. Wright as *Diseases of Workers*. Hafner, New York, 1964).

[25] Selikoff, I.J., Churg, J. & Hammond, E.C. (1964). Asbestos exposure and neoplasia, *Journal of the American Medical Association* **188**, 22–26.

[26] Wagner, J.C., Sleggs, C.A. & Marchand, P. (1960). Diffuse pleural mesothelioma and asbestos exposure in the North Western Cape Province, *British Journal of Industrial Medicine* **17**, 260–271.

[27] Waldron, H.A. (1983). A brief history of scrotal cancer, *British Journal of Industrial Medicine* **40**, 390–401.

G. BERRY

Occupational Mortality

The study of occupational mortality involves the systematic tabulation of mortality by occupational groups or by socioeconomic groups when these are defined by occupation. Three main methods are used to conduct these studies.

The first method, **cross-sectional studies**, utilizes the number of deaths occurring to persons in a given occupation during a given time period divided by the number of persons in that occupation in the middle of the period. The source for the numerator is usually **death certificates**; the denominator is usually based on the census. As the age distribution varies considerably between the occupational groups, an age **standardization** is needed in order to compare the mortality of different occupational groups. In the cross-sectional studies, the comparative mortality figure (CMF, direct standardization) or the standardized mortality ratio (SMR, indirect standardization) are used as summary measures of an occupational group's relative mortality.

The second method, death certificate studies, involves the distribution of deaths by cause for a given occupational group compared with the distribution for a total population without regard to occupation. Such studies are often sex-specific or limited to the male population. Here **proportional mortality ratios (PMRs)** are used as summary measures for each occupational group's relative mortality from a given cause of death.

The third method, follow-up studies (*see* **Cohort Study**), is based on individually matched records and typically on census data. A census population is followed up for deaths and emigrations, and maybe also for new census data, which allows separate analyses of persons who stayed in an occupation from one census to the next. In these studies various methods are used for the matching of individual records (*see* **Record Linkage**). In the UK, for example, the study population is flagged in the National Health Service Central Register; whereas in the Nordic countries the matching is based on the personal identification numbers used in both censuses and death and emigration registrations. In the follow-up studies, the CMFs and SMRs are often used as summary measures for an occupational group's mortality. However, each individual in these studies has a record containing the census characteristics, the number of **person-years at risk**, and the eventual **cause of death**. It is therefore possible to use these data sets also for internal comparisons of the mortality between occupational groups; for example, controlled for sex, age, marital status, and region.

Cross-Sectional Studies

The study of occupational mortality is closely linked to procedures developed in England and Wales, where the first cross-sectional study was published in 1855 [38]. Since then, occupational mortality studies have been published every ten years; no other country has a similar record. The potentials and limitations of cross-sectional studies are therefore best illustrated by this series of data.

It was realized in England in the late 1840s that

if the age of the various classes of society ... are abstracted from the census returns ... and if the deaths are abstracted in the same classes ... the relative mortality ... can be satisfactorily deduced ... and much light will be thrown upon the causes which really influence the health and well being of the working, middle and higher classes [37].

Farr used this method to tabulate the mortality for 1851 by occupation, and commented that

the professions and occupations of men open a new field of inquiry, on which we are now prepared to enter, not unconscious, however, of the peculiar difficulties that beset all inquiries into the mortality of limited, fluctuating, and sometimes ill-defined sections of the population [38].

The methodological problems entailed in occupational mortality studies were thus realized from the very beginning. In 1851, miners, bakers, butchers, and inn and beershop keepers experienced the heaviest rates of mortality.

CMFs were first calculated for the 1880–1882 data. The 1900–1902 data showed a variation in the CMF from 600 or below for clergyman, priest, minister; gardener, nurseryman, seeds-man; gamekeeper; and farmer, grazier, farmer's son, etc.; to 1800 or above for inn-, hotel-servant; costermonger, hawker; tin miner; and general laborer [39].

In the 1910–1912 decennial supplement, Stevenson "included for the first time an attempted grading of the male working population into eight social classes as determined by occupation", where "I represented as far as possible the middle and upper classes ... III skilled labour, and V unskilled labour" [47]. The social classes II and IV were intermediate classes, and textile workers, miners, and agricultural workers formed separate classes. **Infant mortality** showed a steep gradient from 76 deaths per 1000 births in social class I to 153 in social class V. The CMFs for men aged 25–65 for the classes I–V were 88, 94, 96, 93, and 142. Commercial clerks with a CMF of 108 formed 28% of class I and thus inflated the overall

CMF for class I. This gave rise to a discussion about criteria for grouping of occupations into social classes, a discussion which has persisted ever since.

The changing composition of the labor force made it necessary to shift from an industry based classification to one in which it was "no longer necessary to assign the head of a tinplate etc. works to the same social class as his labourers" [40]. In 1921–1923, the relative mortality for occupations and social classes were presented both by the CMFs and by summary measures similar to SMRs. The CMFs for social classes I–V were 821, 942, 951, 1007, and 1258; and the SMRs were 82, 94, 95, 101, and 125. The two methods of calculation gave similar results, illustrating a subsequently often observed robustness of occupational mortality data.

From a previous holistic view of occupation as encompassing both occupational risks and living conditions, an interest in separating the two aspects emerged in the 1930s. To address this question, the 1930–1932 decennial supplement added tables on the mortality of married women by the social class of their husbands. Similar gradients of SMRs from social classes I–V were found; for men 90, 94, 97, 102, and 111; and for women 81, 89, 99, 103, and 113; and it was concluded "that the contribution made by actual work done to men's social mortality gradient from all causes must be small compared with the contribution made by the accompanying environmental, economic and selective factors" [48].

The 1951 classification included 600 occupations. However, the more detailed classification increased the risk for discordance between numerators and denominators. There was a tendency for people to be given more prestigious occupational titles on death certificates than they had in the census: in 1949–1953, for example, 1443 deaths were registered among company directors compared with only 98 expected deaths based on the number of company directors registered at the census and the mortality rates for all men. As a supplement to the SMRs for deaths in persons aged 20–64, PMRs were therefore presented for deaths in persons aged 65–74 to avoid the problem of discordance between the numerators and denominators. The post-war concern about equity was reflected in systematic tabulations of trends in social class differences in the 1949–1953 decennial supplement. The SMRs for men from social classes I–V were 98, 88, 101, 104, and 118 [41], showing that the English society still had a disadvantaged social class V. The relatively high SMR for social class I was partly due to **misclassification** [25]. A new observation was that the social class gradient of some diseases changed as they became more frequent. The mortality from lung cancer almost tripled in men under 65 years from 1921–1923 to 1930–1932, and the social class gradient changed from an excess risk in social class I in 1921–1923, to equal risks across social classes in 1931–1932, and to a clear excess risk in social class V in 1949–1953. Coronary heart disease increased rapidly in men after the war. In 1930–1932 it was a disease of "the better classes" [11], with an SMR gradient from 237 in social class I to 67 in social class V, but the gradient in 1949–1953 was from 150 in social class I to 89 in social class V.

"The most disturbing feature of the [1959–1963 decennial supplement] when compared with earlier analyses [was] the apparent deterioration in social class V" [42]. The SMRs for the five social classes were 76, 81, 100, 103, and 143. A new and shorter occupational classification was used in 1960, but the results for social class V remained "even when the rates were adjusted to the 1950 classification" [42]. The social class gradient in lung cancer had become even steeper, with SMRs of 53 in social class I and 148 in social class V. The change in the social distribution of coronary heart disease had continued, and the SMRs were now 98 for social class I and 112 for social class V.

When it came to results for specific occupations in 1959–1963, the concern about discordance between numerators and denominators clearly influenced the interpretation. Following a review of occupational cancers, Adelstein wrote that "although the exercise known as occupational mortality is not a useful tool as an early warning system, it remains a valuable analysis of mortality of groupings of occupations as a back-up and reference system" [1]; a modest aim compared with the expectations a hundred years earlier.

The social class III was in 1970–1972 divided into nonmanual and manual workers. The SMRs for men over the six social classes were 77, 81, 99, 106, 114, and 137. Similar patterns were seen for women and for stillbirths, and mortality of infants and children. Gradients across social classes showed, for example, that social class V had an almost fourfold risk of respiratory diseases but the same risk of pancreatic cancer as social class I. Some occupations stood out with high risks for specific diseases; for example, butchers with

cancer of the lung and maxillary sinus, and electro- and dip platers with cancer of the lung [34].

The 1972 smoking rates for men by occupational order showed a high positive correlation with the lung cancer mortality. Under these circumstances the previous concern about the influence of living conditions on occupational mortality became a concern about "life-styles of persons" [34]. In a paper on "work or way of life", Fox & Adelstein found that only 18% of the variation in mortality between occupational orders remained when the mortality was standardized for social class [12].

In 1979–1983, the social gradient in mortality for men went from an SMR of 66 in social class I to 165 in social class V; the official comment being that "these data are subject to serious bias and do not represent usable estimates of mortality by social class" [35]. However, aggregated into nonmanual workers (social classes I, II, and IIIN) and manual workers (social classes IIIM, IV, and V), where a serious misclassification would not be expected, the data showed "an overall fall in all-cause mortality from 1970–1972 to 1979–1983 for both manual and non-manual occupational classes, but the rate of decline [had] been greater in non-manual groups. Thus the social gap [had] widened" [27].

As a consequence of concern about biases, the 150 year old practice of combining census and death certificate data was abolished with the next decennial supplement, that for 1990.

Cross-sectional studies of occupational mortality were undertaken in several other countries – for example, in France in 1907–1908 [19], and in the US in 1930 [51] and 1950 [14–16, 20] – but in no other country did these studies have the same importance for the social debate as in England and Wales.

Death Certificate Studies

At the time of the 1990 decennial supplement for England and Wales, advancement in technology had rendered the cross-sectional method obsolete, as the overall mortality of an occupational group could now be estimated from the individually matched records of a follow-up study known as the Longitudinal Study (see below). However, the death certificate data were used for search of specific associations between detailed occupations and causes of deaths using only PMRs. This analysis included 1.8 million deaths from 1979–1980 and 1982–1990. New observations were, for example, an excess risk of leukemia, lymphoma, aplastic anemia, and agranulocytosis in teachers, "suggesting a possible hazard from exposure to childhood infections" [8].

In the US, large-scale death certificate studies started in the 1970s. The first study was from Washington State and covered deaths from 1950 to 1971 [28]. An update included deaths from 1950 to 1979. The systematic tabulation of PMRs for detailed occupation and cause of death revealed, for example, an increased risk of leukemia in workers exposed to electric and magnetic fields and a deficit of multiple sclerosis among outdoor workers [29].

Similar studies were undertaken in California [36], Massachusetts [10], Utah [3], and Rhode Island [21]. A detailed analysis of the large number of solvent exposed jewelry workers from Rhode Island revealed an excess mortality from mental disorders, kidney diseases, liver, and kidney cancer [9].

A standardized reporting, coding, and registration scheme for occupation on death certificates from 12 states started in the US in 1984. A PMR analysis for broad groups has been published for the 270 000 deaths occurring in 1984 for persons above the age of 20 [43]. Data from death certificates from 1985 to 1991 are available on public-use data tapes [32].

Follow-Up Studies

That the numerator/denominator bias in cross-sectional studies could be overcome in follow-up studies of census populations was realized as early as the 1920s in the Nordic countries, among others [7]. It was, however, 50 years later that such studies started to emerge. The earliest studies were a 4 month follow-up of the 1960 census population from the US [22], a 5 year follow-up of the Norwegian 1960 census population [49], a 17 year follow-up of a sample of the French 1954 census population [5], and a 10 year follow-up of the Swedish 1960 census population [46].

The 1970 censuses were used for follow-up studies of the national populations In Denmark [2, 4], Finland [26, 45], and Norway [23], and a joint analysis was made of the occupational mortality in Norway, Sweden, Finland, and Denmark for the 10 year period 1971–1980 [33]. The Longitudinal Study from the UK is a follow-up study of a 1% sample of the 1971 census population, where the sample is, in addition, continuously supplemented with 1% of births and immigrations [13]. A 6 month follow-up of the Italian 1980 census population was published in 1995 [44]. In addition to sex, age, and occupation, these studies often also include other census variables such as marital status, housing conditions, region, family composition, etc.

Some important and fairly consistent observations have been made from the follow-up studies of census populations, such as:

1. All marginal groups of the labor market have an excess overall mortality compared with the working population. In the Nordic countries in 1971–1980, the SMR for economically inactive men was 233, when the economically active men were used as the standard. The SMR for economically inactive women, the majority being housewives, was 151 [33]. In England and Wales in 1971–1975, the SMRs for unemployed men or men with an inadequately described occupation were 306 and 185, respectively, when all men were used as the standard [13].

2. There is a social class gradient in the overall mortality. The SMRs for men in England and Wales in 1971–1975 varied from 80 in social class I to 115 in social class V [13]. The short follow-up of the US 1960 census showed for white men aged 25–64 a mortality ratio of 0.92 for white-collar workers and of 1.07 for blue-collar workers, when the mortality of all men was used as the standard [22].

3. Farmers have a low overall mortality in many countries. The mortality ratio for white male agricultural workers was 0.76 in the US study [22], the SMR for farmers in the Nordic countries was 87 [33], and farm workers in Italy had a 20% deficit in overall mortality compared with all economically active men [44].

4. When studied, the social class gradient in mortality seems to have widened. In Finland in 1971–1983, the overall mortality for men aged 35–49 declined for all occupational classes, but in 1984–1990 it increased for workers and farmers while declining further for white-collar employees [50]. In France, the overall mortality for men aged 35–60 decreased by 28%–30% for professionals, foremen, and salaried employees, but by only 7%–12%

for skilled, unskilled, and farm workers from 1955–1959 to 1975–1980 [6].

5. For men, the social gradient is universally steeper for external causes of death and other diseases than for neoplasms and cardiovascular diseases [24].

The follow-up studies of census data are often criticized for lack of information on personal habits, especially tobacco smoking. Such data are available in a follow-up study of 300 000 US veterans who were interviewed about their smoking habits in 1954 and 1957. A follow-up study of this cohort provides smoking adjusted **relative risks** [17, 18], but the number of deaths for a given combination of occupation and cause of death is often small.

However, data from smaller cohorts with a broad range of recorded variables may often provide useful supplementary information to the census studies. Data from the Longitudinal Study have shown, for example, that men unemployed at the time of the census have an excess mortality in the subsequent years [31]. Very useful supplementary data came from the British Regional Heart Study, where unemployed men had an excess mortality even when controlled for age, town, social class, smoking, alcohol intake, and pre-existing diseases [30].

However, at present follow-up studies of census populations provide the most comprehensive data on overall mortality by occupational groups in unselected populations.

References

[1]   Adelstein, A.M. (1972). Occupational mortality: cancer, *Annals of Occupational Hygiene* **15**, 53–57.

[2]   Andersen, O. (1985). *Mortality and Occupation 1970–80*. Statistical Studies No. 41. Danmarks Statistik, København (in Danish).

[3]   Bangerter, N.H., Dandoy, S., Elison, G. & Brockert, J.E. (1985). *Utah's Occupational Health Surveillance System, 1980–82. Collection of Technical Reports.* Utah Department of Health, Salt Lake City.

[4]   Danmarks Statistik (1979). *Mortality and Occupation*. Statistical Studies No. 37. Danmarks Statistik, København (in Danish).

[5]   Desplanques, G. (1976). *Adult Mortality by Social Environment 1955–1971*. No. 195 des Collections de l'INSEE, Série D, No. 44 (in French).

[6]   Desplanques, G. (1985). *Adult Mortality. Results of Two Longitudinal Studies (Period 1955–1980)*. No. 479 des Collections de l'INSEE, Série D, No. 102 (in French).

[7]   Det Statistiske Departement (1921). *Meeting of Nordic Statisticians, København, 29–31 August 1921*. SM 4:

64: 3. Det Statistiske Departement, København (in Danish).

[8]   Drever, F., ed. (1995). *Occupational Health. Decennial Supplement*. Office of Population Censuses and Surveys. HMSO, London.

[9]   Dubrow, R. & Gute, D.M. (1987). Cause-specific mortality among Rhode Island jewelry workers, *American Journal of Industrial Medicine* **12**, 579–593.

[10] Dubrow, R. & Wegman, D.H. (1982). *Occupational Characteristics of White Male Cancer Victims in Massachusetts 1971–73*. National Institute for Occupational Health, US Department of Health and Human Services, Cincinnati.

[11] Editorial (1959). Health and social class, *Lancet* **i**, 303–305.

[12] Fox, A.J. & Adelstein, A.M. (1978). Occupational mortality: work or way of life?, *Journal of Epidemiology and Community Medicine* **32**, 73–78.

[13] Goldblatt, P., ed. (1990). *Longitudinal Study. Mortality and Social Organization*. Office of Population Censuses and Surveys. HMSO, London.

[14] Guralnick, L. (1962). *Mortality by Occupation and Industry among Men 20 to 64 Years of Age: United States, 1950*. Vital Statistics, Special Reports, Vol. 53, No. 2. National Center for Health Statistics, Washington.

[15] Guralnick, L. (1963). *Mortality by Occupation and Industry among Men 20 to 64 Years of Age: United States, 1950*. Vital Statistics, Special Reports, Vol. 53, No. 4. National Center for Health Statistics, Washington.

[16] Guralnick, L. (1963). *Mortality by Occupation and Industry among Men 20 to 64 Years of Age: United States, 1950*. Vital Statistics, Special Reports, Vol. 53, No. 5. National Center for Health Statistics, Washington.

[17] Hrubec, Z., Blair A.E. & Vaught, J. (1995). *Mortality Risks by Industry among U.S. Veterans of Known Smoking Status. 1954–1980*. Vol. 2. Department of Health and Human Services, Public Health Service, National Cancer Institute, NIH Publication No. 95–2747.

[18] Hrubec, Z. Blair, A.E., Rogot, E. & Vaught, J. (1992). *Mortality Risks by Occupation among U.S. Veterans of Known Smoking Status. 1954–1980*. Vol. 1. Department of Health and Human Services, Public Health Service, National Cancer Institutes, NIH Publication No. 92–3407.

[19] Huber, M. (1912). Occupational mortality, *Bulletine de la Statistique Générale de la France*, **1**, 402. Librairie Félix Alcan, Paris (in French).

[20] Kaplan, D.L., Parkhurst, E. & Whelpton, P.K. (1961). *Comparability of Reports on Occupation from Vital Records and the 1950 Census*. Vital Statistics, Special Reports, Vol. 53, No. 1. National Center for Health Statistics, Washington.

[21] Kelley, B.C. & Gute, D.M. (1986). *Surveillance Cooperative Agreement between NIOSH and States (Scans) Program. Rhode Island 1980–82*. National Institute for

Occupational Health, US Department of Health and Human Services, Cincinnati.

[22] Kitagawa, E.M. & Hauser, P.M. (1973). *Differential Mortality in the United States: a Study in Socioeconomic Epidemiology*. Harvard University Press, Cambridge, Mass.

[23] Kristofersen, L. (1979). *Occupational Mortality*. Reports from Statistical Central Bureau 79/19. Statistical Central Bureau, Oslo (in Norwegian).

[24] Kunst, A.E., Groenhof, F., Mackenbach, J.P. & The EU Working Group on Socioeconomic Inequalities in Health (1988). Occupational class and cause specific mortality in middle aged men in 11 European countries: comparison of population based studies, *British Medical Journal* **316**, 1636–1642.

[25] Logan, W.P.D. (1959). Occupational mortality, *Proceedings of the Royal Society of Medicine* **52**, 463–468.

[26] Marin, R. (1986). *Occupational Mortality 1971–80*. Series no. 129, Central Statistical Office of Finland, Helsinki.

[27] Marmot, M.G. & McDowall, M.E. (1986). Mortality decline and widening social inequalities, *Lancet* **ii**, 274–276.

[28] Milham, S. (1976). *Occupational Mortality in Washington State 1950–71*. Vols. I–III. National Institute for Occupational Safety and Health, US Department of Health and Human Services, Cincinnati.

[29] Milham, S. (1983). *Occupational Mortality in Washington State 1950–79*. National Institute for Occupational Safety and Health, US Department of Health and Human Services, Cincinnati.

[30] Morris, J.K., Cook, D.G. & Shaper, A.G. (1994). Loss of employment and mortality, *British Medical Journal* **308**, 1135–1139.

[31] Moser, K.A., Goldblatt, P.O., Fox, A.J. & Jones, D.R. (1987). Unemployment and mortality: comparison of the 1971 and 1981 longitudinal study census samples, *British Medical Journal* **294**, 86–90.

[32] National Center for Health Statistics (1993). Mortality by occupation, industry, and cause of death: 12 reporting states, in *Final Data from the Centers for Disease Control and Prevention/National Center for Health Statistics. Public-use Data Tapes 1985–91*.

[33] Nordic Statistical Secretariat (1988). *Occupational Mortality in the Nordic Countries 1971–1980*. Statistical Reports of the Nordic Countries, No. 49, Nordic Statistical Secretariat, Copenhagen.

[34] Office of Population Censuses and Surveys (1978). *Occupational Mortality 1970–72. Decennial Supplement. England and Wales*. HMSO, London.

[35] Office of Population Censuses and Surveys (1986). *Occupational Mortality 1979–80, 1982–83. Decennial Supplement. Great Britain. Part I. Commentary*. HMSO, London.

[36] Petersen, G.R. & Milham, S. (1980) *Occupational Mortality in the State of California 1959–61*. National Institute for Occupational Health, US Department of Health and Human Services, Cincinnati.

[37] Registrar-General (1846). *Seventh Annual Report on Births, Deaths, and Marriages in England*. HMSO, London.

[38] Registrar-General (1855). *Fourteenth Annual Report on Births, Deaths, and Marriages in England*. HMSO, London.

[39] Registrar-General (1908). *Supplement to the Sixty-fifth Annual Report on Births, Deaths, and Marriages in England. Part II*. HMSO, London.

[40] Registrar-General (1927). *Report on Occupational Mortality during 1921–23. Decennial Supplement. Part II*. HMSO, London.

[41] Registrar-General (1954). *Occupational Mortality. Decennial Supplement. England and Wales. Part I*. HMSO, London.

[42] Registrar-General (1971). *Occupational Mortality Tables. Decennial Supplement. England and Wales*. HMSO, London.

[43] Rosenberg, H.M., Burnett, C., Maurer, J. & Spirtas, R. (1993). Mortality by occupation, industry, and cause of death: 12 reporting states, 1984, in *National Center for Health Statistics. Monthly Vital Statistics Report 42*, no. 4, supplement, pp. 1–63.

[44] Roseo, G., ed. (1995). *Occupational Mortality in Italy in the 1980s*. Istituto Superiore per la Prevenzione e la Sicurezza del Lavoro, Roma (in Italian).

[45] Sauli, H. (1979). Mortality, in *Occupational Mortality in 1971–75*. Studies No. 54, Central Statistical Office of Finland, Helsinki.

[46] Statistiska Centralbyrån (1981). *Mortality Register 1961–1970*. Promemorior från SCB 81:5, Örebro (in Swedish).

[47] Stevenson, T.H.C. (1923). The social distribution of mortality from different causes in England and Wales, 1910–12, *Biometrika* **15**, 382–400.

[48] Stocks, P. (1938). The effects of occupation and of its accompanying environment on mortality, *Journal of the Royal Statistical Society* **101**, 669–708.

[49] Tønnesen, B.L. (1974). *Selected Aspects of the Mortality in Norway 1960–64 Compared with Other Countries*, Statistical Central Bureau, Oslo (in Norwegian).

[50] Valkonen, T., Martelin, T., Rimpalä, A., Notkala, V. & Savela, S. (1993). *Socio-economic Mortality Differences in Finland 1981–90. Population 1993:1*. Statistics Finland, Helsinki.

[51] Whitney, J.S. (1934). *Deaths Rates by Occupation, Based on Data of the U.S. Census Bureau, 1930*. National Tuberculosis Association, New York.

(*See also* **Occupational Epidemiology**; **Occupational Health and Medicine**; **Vital Statistics, Overview**)

ELSEBETH LYNGE

Odds

If an event E has probability $\Pr(E)$, the odds of the event is defined as $\Pr(E)/\{1 - \Pr(E)\}$.

M.H. GAIL

Odds Ratio

If two events, E_1 and E_2, have respective probabilities $\Pr(E_1)$ and $\Pr(E_2)$, the odds ratio comparing E_1 with E_2 is $[\Pr(E_1)/\{1 - \Pr(E_1)\}]/[\Pr(E_2)/\{1 - \Pr(E_2)\}]$, namely the ratio of the **odds** of E_1 to the odds of E_2.

M.H. GAIL

Onset Confounding *see* Biased Sampling of Cohorts in Epidemiology

Over Adjustment *see* Cohort Study

Overmatching

Overmatching refers to the unnecessary or inappropriate use of **matching** in a **cohort** or **case–control study**. Matching on intermediate factors on the causal pathway (*see* **Causation**) can inappropriately attenuate estimates of exposure effect, and matching on factors that are not **confounders** can needlessly reduce the power of the study [1, pp. 104–106]. Overmatching is also sometimes used to describe elaborate matching schemes that make it difficult to find suitable **controls** satisfying all matching criteria (*see* **Matched Analysis**).

Reference

[1]   Breslow, N.E. & Day, N.E. (1980). *Statistical Methods in Cancer Research*, Vol. 1. *The Analysis of Case-Control Studies*. International Agency for Research on Cancer, Lyon.

M.H. GAIL

Overt Bias *see* Propensity Score

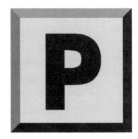

Pair Matching *see* Matching

Parasitic Diseases *see* Epidemic Models, Deterministic

Partial Crude Probability of Death from a Cause *see* Competing Risks

Partition Model *see* Nutritional Epidemiology

Perinatal Period *see* Infant and Perinatal Mortality

Person-Time Incidence Rate *see* Hazard Rate

Person-Years At Risk

In follow-up studies of subjects subsequent to various treatments or exposures and in the study of chronic disease where the **incubation period** or length of illness may be months or years, consideration must be given to the time the subjects were under observation or to the time intervening between the initial exposure and the eventual outcome, e.g. recovery, onset of disease, or death. If the probability of a given outcome is related to time, outcome measures are affected by the length of the observational period [1].

Person-years at risk are units of measurement which combine persons and time by summing individual units of time (years and fractions of years) during which subjects in a study population have been exposed to the risk of the outcome under study. A person-year is defined as the equivalent of the experience of one individual for one year [2]. Each subject contributes only as many years as he or she has been actually observed (or exposed); a subject under observation for one year contributes one person-year; six months would contribute one-half person-year, etc. Person-years at risk frequently comprise the denominator of calculations of **incidence rates** measured over extended and variable time periods or of measures of morbidity and mortality resulting from chronic exposure to environmental hazards such as industrial toxic waste materials or cigarette smoke.

References

[1]   Kahn, H.A. & Sempos, C.T. (1989). *Statistical Methods in Epidemiology*. Oxford University Press, New York.
[2]   Last, J.M., ed. (1983). *A Dictionary of Epidemiology*. Oxford University Press, New York.

R.A. ISRAEL

Person-Years Method *see* Expected Number of Deaths

Pharmacoepidemiology, Overview

Pharmacoepidemiology, the study of patterns of medication use in the population and their effects on disease, is a new field. The need for this area of research became evident in 1961, during the thalidomide catastrophe, when it was realized that drugs prescribed for therapeutic purposes could produce unexpected risks. The entry of thalidomide, a new hypnotic drug, on the market was accompanied by a sudden sharp increase in the frequency of rare birth defects, characterized by the partial or complete absence of limbs [29, 31]. Consequently, several countries either instituted agencies to regulate drugs or expanded the mandate of existing agencies [52]. These agencies were previously interested only in the demonstration of a drug's efficacy, but now required proof of a drug's safety before it was tested in humans let alone before it was marketed for use by the general population. These proofs of safety, based on toxicologic and pharmacologic studies, were necessary before randomized controlled trials (RCTs) could be conducted on human subjects, primarily to demonstrate the efficacy of a drug.

The use of the epidemiologic approach to characterize population patterns of medication use and to assess their effects developed as a complement to RCTs for several reasons. First, RCTs were designed to assess the efficacy and effectiveness of a drug, providing as well some data on its safety with respect to commonly arising side-effects. However,

rare side-effects typically cannot be identified in clinical trials because of their small size. For example, to detect a **relative risk** of 2, for a side-effect having an **incidence** of 1 per 100, we would require a two-arm trial with over 3000 subjects per arm ($\alpha = 0.05$, $\beta = 0.1$). If the incidence of the side-effect is 1 per 10 000, the sample size per arm would need to be over 300 000. Clearly, these sample sizes are rarely if ever used in RCTs, yet the number of people who will be using these drugs will be in the millions.

Secondly, RCTs usually restrict the study subjects to people without coexisting disease, who are therefore not taking other medications that could interact with the study medication. They are also restricted with respect to age, rarely including children and elderly subjects. Yet, the elderly will be major consumers of most of these medications, along with other medications they are using for coexisting diseases.

Thirdly, RCTs will usually be based on a short follow-up that typically assesses medication use for a period of 3–12 months. Yet, again, subjects may be using these medications for years, so that the effect of the prolonged use of these medications remains clearly unknown from the RCT data. Finally, there are situations where the RCT is either unethical or inapplicable. For example, it would be ethically unacceptable today in North America or Europe to assess the long-term effects of a new anti-hypertensive agent against placebo in an RCT, although this has been done in China [12]. Yet, a large number of hypertensive patients from the general population are either untreated or do not comply with their treatment. They could be used as the reference group for a nonrandomized study based on a **cohort study** design.

Although pharmacoepidemiology can be simply regarded as an application of epidemiologic principles and methods to the field of medications, it is now developing as a discipline of its own because of the special nature of drugs. Indeed, the ways by which drugs are prescribed, employed, marketed and regulated impose certain constraints on epidemiologic research into their use and effects. This field poses challenges that often require special solutions not found in other domains of application, such as cancer, cardiovascular, occupational or infectious disease epidemiology; medications are marketed rapidly, practice patterns of prescribing by physicians are variable and profiles of drug use by patients are complicated by varying compliance patterns. This complex and dynamic context in which pharmacoepidemiology is situated, as well as the available sources of data, have given rise to unique statistical challenges. The fact that the lifetime of a drug on the market is relatively short and can suddenly be shortened still further by a regulatory or corporate withdrawal, often imposes major constraints on studies of its effects. These studies must be conducted rapidly and use existing data in an efficient way without compromising validity (*see* **Validity and Generalizability in Epidemiologic Studies**).

In this article we describe several areas where biostatistical input has served to advance pharmacoepidemiology. Although the last two decades have witnessed an explosion of methodologic advances put forward by biostatistics in the design and analysis of epidemiologic studies, most of these have been fundamental to the field of epidemiology in general. We do not discuss these areas here since they are dealt with extensively elsewhere (*see* **Analytic Epidemiology**; **Descriptive Epidemiology**). Instead, we focus on the biostatistical aspects that produced unique methodologic advances, specific to problems posed by pharmacoepidemiologic research.

The Case–Crossover Design

When conducting a **case–control study**, the selection of **controls** is usually the most challenging task. The fundamental principle is that selected controls should be representative of the source population which gave rise to the cases [33] a principle often difficult to implement in practice, especially when dealing with acute adverse events and transient exposures.

For example, we may wish to study the **risk** of ventricular tachycardia in association with the use of inhaled beta agonists in asthma. This possible effect has been hypothesized on the basis of clinical study observations of hypokalemia and prolonged Q-T intervals as measured on the electrocardiogram in patients after beta agonist exposure [1]. These unusual cardiac deviations were observed only in the 4-hour period following drug absorption. Thus, a case–control study of this issue would first select cases with this adverse event and investigate whether the drug was taken during the 4-hour span preceding the event. For **controls**, on the other hand, the investigator must define a time point of reference for which to ask the question about use of this drug in the "past 4 hours". However, if, for example, the drug is more

likely to be required during the day, but controls can only be reached at home in the evening, the **relative risk** estimate will be **biased** by the differential timing of responses for cases and controls.

Consequently, when dealing with the study of transient drug effects on the risk of acute adverse events, Maclure [30] proposed the *case–crossover design*, which uses the cases as their own controls. The case–crossover design is simply a crossover study in the cases only. The subjects alternate at varying frequencies between exposure and nonexposure to the drug of interest until the adverse event occurs, which does for all subjects in the study since all are cases by definition. Each case is investigated to determine whether exposure occurred within the predetermined effect period, namely within the 4 hours previous to the adverse event in our example. This occurrence is then classified as having arisen either under drug exposure or nonexposure on the basis of the effect period. Thus, each case is either exposed or unexposed. For the reference information, data on the average drug use pattern are necessary to determine the probability of exposure in the time window of effect. This is done by obtaining data for a sufficiently long period of time to derive a stable estimate. In our example, we might determine the average number of times a day each case has been using beta agonists (two inhalations of 100 µg each) in the past year. This will allow us to estimate the proportion of time that each asthmatic is usually spending as "exposed" in the 4-hour effect period. This proportion is then used to obtain the number of cases expected on the basis of time spent in these "at-risk" periods, for comparison with the number of cases observed during such periods. This is done by forming a two-by-two table for each case, with the corresponding control data as defined above, and combining the tables using the **Mantel–Haenszel** technique as described in detail by Maclure [30]. The resulting **odds ratio** is then given by $OR = \sum a_i N_{0i} / \sum (1 - a_i) N_{1i}$, where a_i is 1 if case i is exposed, 0 if not, N_{0i} is the expected number of unexposed periods and N_{1i} the expected number of exposed periods during the reference time span.

Table 1 displays hypothetical data from a case–crossover study of 10 asthmatics who experienced ventricular tachycardia. These were all queried regarding their use of two puffs of inhaled beta agonist in the last 4 hours and on average over the past year. The fact of drug use within the effect period is defined

Table 1 Hypothetical data for a case–crossover study of beta agonist exposure in last 4 hours and the risk of ventricular tachycardia in asthma

Case no.	Beta agonist use[a] in last 4 hours (a_i)	Usual beta agonist use in last year	Periods of exposure (N_{1i})	Periods of non-exposure (N_{0i})
1	0	1/day	365	1825
2	1	6/year	3	2184
3	0	2/day	730	1460
4	1	1/month	12	2178
5	0	4/week	208	1982
6	0	1/week	52	2138
7	0	1/month	12	2178
8	1	2/month	24	2166
9	0	2/day	730	1460
10	0	2/week	104	2086

[a]Inhalations of 200 μg: 1 = yes, 0 = no

by a_i with three cases having used beta agonists in the 4-hour period prior to the adverse event. The usual frequency of drug use per year is converted to a ratio of the number of exposed periods to the number of unexposed periods, the total number of 4-hour periods being 2190 in one year. Using the Mantel–Haenszel formula to combine the 10 two-by-two tables, the estimate of the odds ratio is 3.0, and the 95% confidence interval (1.2, 7.6).

The case–crossover design depends on several assumptions to produce unbiased estimates of the odds ratio. Greenland [14] presented examples where the odds ratio estimates from this approach can be biased. For example, the probability of exposure cannot vary over the time. Similarly, **confounding** factors must be constant over time. Finally, there cannot be **interaction** between unmeasured subject characteristics and the exposure. Nevertheless, this approach is being used successfully in several studies [38, 43]. It has also been adapted for application to the **risk assessment** of vaccines [11].

Confounding Bias

Because of the lack of randomization, the most important limitation of **observational studies** in pharmacoepidemiology is whether an important confounding factor is biasing the reported relative risk estimate. A factor is considered a confounder if it is associated, at each level of drug exposure, with the adverse event, and with exposure to the drug

itself. Two approaches exist to address the problem of confounding variables, which we describe in the context of the case–control design, although they apply equally well to a cohort design. The first is to select controls that are matched to the cases with respect to all confounding factors and to use the appropriate corresponding techniques of analysis for matched data, usually **conditional logistic regression** (*see* **Matched Analysis**; **Matching**). This approach, although often appropriate, has been shown to be susceptible to bias from residual confounding due to coarse matching [5]. The second solution is to select controls unmatched with respect to these confounding factors, but to measure these confounders for all study subjects and use statistical techniques based on either **stratification** or multiple regression, permitting removal of their effect on the risk from the effect of the drug under study. This approach can also lead to residual confounding if the confounder data are not analyzed properly. For example, the risk of venous thromboembolism has been found to be higher among users of newer oral contraceptive drugs than users of older formulations [22, 41, 53], after controlling for the effect of age. A recent study, however, showed that when confounding by the woman's age is analyzed using finer age bands, the relative risk is substantially reduced [10].

Beyond such difficulties generic to epidemiology, the context of pharmacoepidemiology has produced several situations where confounding requires particular statistical treatment. Some are described in this section.

Missing Confounder Data

It is at times impossible to obtain data on certain important confounding variables. A frequent situation encountered in pharmacoepidemiology is that of complete data for the cases and incomplete data for the controls of a case–control study. This is often encountered in "computerized database" studies based on administrative databases where cases have likely been hospitalized and thus have an extensive medical dossier. For these cases, the investigator will thus have access to ample information on potential confounding variables. However, if the controls are population-based (*see* **Case–Control Study, Population-Based**), it is unlikely they were hospitalized and will not provide comparable data on confounders in the absence of medical charts.

Consequently, confounder data will only be available in the cases, and not in the controls.

We can assess whether a factor is a confounder on the basis of data available solely for the cases, so that if the factor is deemed not to be a confounder, then the final analysis of the risk of the drug under study will not need to be adjusted. The approach is described by Ray & Griffin [37] and was used in the context of a study of nonsteroidal anti-inflammatory drug (NSAID) use and the risk of fatal peptic ulcer disease [15]. The strategy is based on the definition [5] of a confounder C (C+ and C− denote presence and absence) in the assessment of the association between a drug exposure E (E+ and E− denote exposure or not to the drug) and an adverse condition D (D+ and D− denote cases and controls, respectively). Confounding is present if both following conditions are satisfied:

1. C and E are associated in the control group (in D−).
2. C and D are associated in E+ and in E−.

Assuming, in the absence of **effect modification**, a common odds ratio between E and D (OR_{ED}) in C+ and in C−, condition 1 becomes equivalent to: C and E are associated in the case group (D+). Thus, if in the cases we find no association between the potential confounder and drug exposure, confounding by this factor can be excluded outright, without having to verify condition 2. In this instance, the analysis involving drug exposure in cases and controls can be performed directly without any concern for the confounding variable. This strategy for assessing confounding is extremely valuable for several case–control studies in pharmacoepidemiology, since if confounding is excluded by this technique, crude methods of analysis can be used to obtain a valid estimate of the odds ratio. However, this is not often the case.

As an example, we use data from a case–control study conducted using the Saskatchewan computerized databases to assess whether theophylline, a drug used to treat asthma, increases the risk of acute cardiac death [47]. In this study, the 30 cases provided data on theophylline use, as well as on smoking, possibly an important confounder. However, the 4080 controls only had data available on theophylline use and not on smoking. Table 2 displays the data from this study. The crude odds ratio between theophylline use and cardiac death is 4.3((17/13)/(956/3124)).

Table 2 Data from a case–control study of theophylline use and cardiac death in asthma, with the smoking confounder data missing for controls

	Cases		Controls	
	E	Ē	E	Ē
Notation:				
Combined	a	c	b	d
Stratified by smoking:				
Smokers	a_0	c_0	a	a
Nonsmokers	a_1	c_1	a	a
Data:				
Combined	17	13	956	3124
Stratified by smoking:				
Smokers	14	5	a	a
Nonsmokers	3	8	a	a

[a]These frequencies are missing for controls.

Because of the **missing data** on smoking, it is only possible to partition the cases, but not the controls, according to smoking. The odds ratio between theophylline use and smoking among the cases is estimable and found to be 7.5((14/5)/(3/8)), thus indicating that smoking is indeed a strong confounder.

An approach was recently developed to permit the estimation of the *adjusted* odds ratio of the theophylline by cardiac death association, in the absence of confounder data among the controls [46]. The adjusted odds ratio is given by

$$OR_{adj} = P_0(w - y)/[(1 - P_0)y], \qquad (1)$$

where $y = \{v - [v^2 - 4(r - 1)rwx]^{1/2}\}/[2(r - 1)]$, $v = 1 + (r - 1)(w + x)$ when $r \neq 1$ (and $y = wx$ when $r = 1$), r is the odds ratio between exposure and confounder among the cases, x is the probability of exposure among the controls, P_0 is estimated by $a_0(a_0 + c_0)$, and w is the **prevalence** of the confounder among the controls [46]; w is the only unknown and must be estimated from external sources. An estimate of the variance of OR_{adj} in (1) exists in closed form. For the illustrative data, an external estimate of smoking prevalence among asthmatics, obtained from a Canadian general population health survey, is 24%. Using this estimate, the adjusted odds ratio is 2.4, much lower than the crude estimate of 4.3, with 95% confidence interval (1.0, 5.8).

This statistical approach was developed specifically to address the frequent problem of missing confounder data in pharmacoepidemiology. When using computerized databases, these data are more often missing only in the control series of a case–control study. This technique, based on statistical reasoning, allows us to derive adjusted estimates of relative risk with few assumptions. Extensions of this type of approach to a regression context will expand its usefulness.

The Case–Time–Control Design

Case–control studies in pharmacoepidemiology that assess the intended effects of drugs are often limited by their inability to obtain a precise measure of the indication of drug exposure. Adjustment for this crucial confounding factor becomes impossible and an unbiased estimate of the drug effect is unattainable [50]. This bias, arising from confounding by indication, is a major source of limitation in pharmacoepidemiology [32]. Here again, a within-subject approach, similar to the case–crossover design, has been developed. By using cases and controls of a conventional case–control study as their own referents, the *case–time–control design* eliminates the biasing effect of unmeasured confounding factors such as drug indication [44]. This approach is applicable only in situations where exposure varies over time, which is typically often the case for medications.

The correct application of the case–time–control design is based on a specific model for the data, a model that entails inherent assumptions and imposes certain conditions for the approach to be valid. The model, based on a case–control sampling design, is presented for a dichotomous exposure that varies over time and that is measured only for two consecutive time periods, the current period and the reference period. The logit of exposure $L_{ijkl} = \text{logit}\{\Pr(E_{ijkl} = 1)\}$, is given by

$$L_{ijkl} = \mu + S_{il} + \pi_j + \Theta_k \qquad (2)$$

where E_{ijkl} represents the binary exposure for group i, period j, outcome k and subject l within group i, μ represents the overall exposure logit, S_{il} is the effect of study subject l in group i, π_j is the effect of period j and Θ_k is the effect of event occurrence k. More specifically, $i = 0$, 1 denotes the case–control group (1 = case subjects, 0 = control subjects), $j = 0$, 1 denotes the period (1 = current period, 0 = reference period), $k = 0$, 1 denotes the event occurrence (1 = event, 0 = no event) and $l = 1, \ldots, n_i$ designates the study subject within group i, with n_1 case subjects and n_0 control subjects. The confounding effect of unmeasured severity or indication is inherently accounted for by S_{il}.

The period effect, measured by the log of the odds ratio, is given by $\delta_\pi = \pi_1 - \pi_0$ and estimated from the control subjects. The net effect of exposure on event occurrence is given by $\delta_\Theta = \Theta_1 - \Theta_0$. The case subjects permit one to estimate the sum $\delta_\Theta + \delta_\pi$ so that the effect of exposure on event occurrence δ_Θ, is estimable by subtraction. The estimation of the odds ratio is based on any appropriate technique for matched data, such as conditional logistic regression.

Three basic assumptions are inherently made by this logit model. The first is the absence of effect modification of the exposure–outcome association by the unmeasured confounder, i.e. the exclusion of the $S_{il}\Theta_k$ interaction term in model (2). The second is the absence of effect modification of the exposure–outcome association by period, i.e. a null value for the $\pi\Theta_k$ interaction term. The third is the lack of effect modification of the exposure–period association by the confounder, represented by the absence of an $S_{il}\pi_j$ interaction term in model (2). Greenland [14] presented examples of the bias that can occur with this approach when the model contains the latter interaction, as explained in Suissa [45].

The approach is illustrated with data from the Saskatchewan Asthma Epidemiologic Project [40], a study conducted to investigate the risks associated with the use of inhaled beta agonists in the treatment of asthma. Using databases from Saskatchewan, Canada, a cohort of 12 301 asthmatics was followed during 1980–87. All 129 cases of fatal or near-fatal asthma and 655 controls were selected. The amount of beta agonist used in the year prior to the index date was found to be associated with the adverse event. In comparing low (12 or less canisters per year) with high (more than 12) use of beta agonists. The crude odds ratio for high beta-agonist use is 4.4, with 95% confidence interval (2.9, 6.7). Adjustment for all available markers of severity, such as oral corticosteroids and prior asthma hospitalizations as confounding factors, lowers the odds ratio to 3.1, with 95% confidence interval (1.8, 5.4), the "best" estimate one can derive from these case–control data using conventional tools.

The use of inhaled beta agonists, however, is known to increase with asthma severity which also increases the risk of fatal or near-fatal asthma. It is therefore not possible to separate the risk effect of the drug from that of disease severity. To apply the case–time–control design, exposure to beta agonists was obtained for the 1-year current period and the 1-year reference period. Among the 129 cases, 29 were currently high users of beta agonists and were low users in the reference period, while 9 cases were currently low users of beta agonists and were high users previously. Among the 655 controls, 65 were currently high users of beta agonists and were low users in the reference period, while 25 were currently low users of beta agonists and were high users previously. The case–time–control odds ratio, using these discordant pairs frequencies for a matched pairs analysis, is given by $(29/9)/(65/25) = 1.2$, with 95% confidence interval $(0.5, 3.0)$. This estimate, which excludes the effect of unmeasured confounding by disease severity, indicates a minimal risk for these drugs.

The case–time–control approach provides an unbiased estimate of the odds ratio in the presence of confounding by indication, a common obstacle in pharmacoepidemiology. This is possible despite the fact that the indication for drug use (in our example, disease severity) is not measured, because of the within-subject analysis. Nevertheless, as mentioned above, its validity is subject to several strict assumptions. This approach must therefore be used with caution.

Risk Functions Over Time

Most epidemiologic studies assessing a risk over time routinely assume that the hazards are constant or proportional. Rate ratios are then estimated by **Poisson regression** models or Cox's **proportional hazards** model [6]. Often, deviations from these simplifying assumptions are addressed at the design stage, by restricting the study to a specific follow-up period where the assumptions are satisfied. For instance, to study the risk of cancer associated with an agent considered to be an initiator of the disease, the first few years of follow-up after the initiation of exposure will not be accounted for in the analysis, to allow for a reasonable **latency period**. On the other hand, if the agent is suspected to be a cancer promoter, these same first years will be used in the

analysis. Since such considerations are mostly dealt with at the design stage, little attention has been paid to the analytic considerations of this issue.

In pharmacoepidemiology, the risk of an adverse event often varies strongly with the duration of use of a drug. Figure 1 shows three different risk profiles, typical of drug exposure. Figure 1(a) displays the usual profile of risk associated with an acute effect. The drug will affect susceptible subjects early, reflected by the early sharp rise in the curve, and once these subjects are eliminated from the cohort, the remaining subjects will return to some lower constant baseline risk. The peak can occur almost

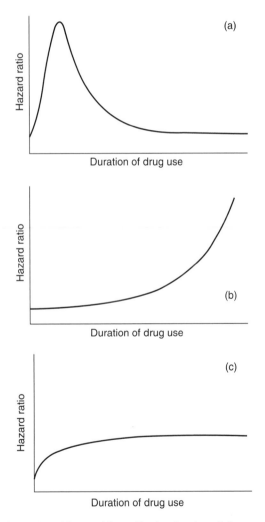

Figure 1 Different risk profiles by duration of drug use: (a) acute effect; (b) increasing risk; (c) constant risk

immediately, as with allergic reactions to antibiotics, or may take a certain time to affect the organ, as with gastrointestinal hemorrhage subsequent to NSAID use. This profile of risk was used to explain variations in the risk of agranulocytosis associated with the use of the analgesic dipyrone [16]. It has recently been used to assess the risk profile of oral contraceptives [48]. Figure 1(b) shows a gradually increasing model of risk, associated with diseases of longer latency such as cancer. Figure 1(c) displays the constant hazard model, after a rapid rise in the risk level.

Unfortunately, such graphs are not part of the analysis plan of most pharmacoepidemiologic studies at this point, despite the existence of appropriate techniques [9, 16]. The next few years should see an increasing use of spline functions and other similar tools to model the risk of drugs by their duration of use. The wider access to newer statistical software such as S-PLUS [42] among researchers in pharmacoepidemiology, as well as the publication of papers that simplify the understanding of these sophisticated approaches [13, 16], will encourage their wider use in a field where they are clearly pertinent.

Probabilistic Approach for Causality Assessment

The traditional epidemiologic approach to assess whether a drug causes an adverse reaction is based on the Hill criteria [18], that require the association to be biologically plausible, strong, specific, consistent and temporally valid (*see* **Hill's Criteria for Causality**). These criteria are applied to the results of pharmacoepidemiologic studies and, depending on the number of criteria satisfied, provide a level of confidence regarding causality of the drug (*see* **Causation**). The result of this exercise will be, if a drug is judged to cause an adverse reaction, that all exposed cases, or at least some etiologic proportion of these cases [39], are due to the drug. This approach is valuable for inferences to the population, but does not allow cases to be assessed individually, does not incorporate the specifics of the case, and does not entirely address the unique features of drugs as an exposure entity in epidemiology.

The study of individual cases of adverse reactions has been the mainstay of national pharmacovigilance centers throughout the world for several decades [3, 52]. When a case report of a suspected drug-associated adverse event is received, the natural question is whether the drug actually caused the event. Several qualitative approaches have been proposed to answer this question [20, 25]. Recently, however, a formal quantitative approach using biostatistical foundations has been put forward [26–28]. It is based on Bayes' theorem, which can be used in the following way:

$$\Pr(D \to E|B, C)$$
$$= \Pr(D \to E|B)\Pr(C|D \to E, B)/\Pr(C),$$

where $D \to E$ denotes that the drug D causes the adverse event E, B represents the background characteristics of the case that are known to affect the risk, while C represents the case information.

This Bayes' theorem approach allows us to estimate the posterior probability that an adverse event was caused by a drug by separating the problem into two components. The first component is the prior probability of the event given the baseline characteristics of the patients. This is estimated from existing data obtained from clinical trials or epidemiologic studies. The second component is the probability of case information given that the drug caused the event.

The primary limitation of this approach is the scarcity of data available to estimate the two components. In many instances, it is difficult to find the clinical and epidemiologic data necessary to estimate the prior probability, especially for rare clinical conditions that have not been the object of extensive population-based research. The same limitation applies to the second probability component because of the problems of finding cases relevant to proven drug causation. **Case series** that apply directly to the case being assessed are often difficult to find. These limitations are real but not limited to the Bayesian approach – they are a general problem in the assessment of individual cases. The authors of these methods suggest that the primary purpose of the Bayesian approach is to provide a framework in which subjective judgments relevant to assessment of an individual case are coherently combined.

To facilitate the use of the Bayesian method, the equation is usually expressed in terms of **odds** rather than probabilities. This formulation simplifies somewhat the need for data, since epidemiologic studies more frequently report odds ratios than absolute probabilities. The relative likelihood may also be easier to estimate subjectively. This equation formulated in terms of odds is given as

$$\text{posterior odds} = \Pr(D \to E|B, C)/\Pr(D \nrightarrow E|B, C)$$
$$= [\Pr(D \to E|B)/\Pr(D \nrightarrow E|B)]$$
$$\text{prior odds}$$
$$\times [\Pr(C|D \to E, B)/\Pr(C|D \nrightarrow E, B)]$$
$$\text{likelihood ratio.}$$

This approach was applied on several occasions [19, 23, 24, 34] and was recently made user-friendly by computerizing [21]. The increasing amount of new epidemiologic data on disease distribution and risk factors combined with new clinical and pharmacologic insights on drug effects will make this probabilistic approach more effective in future uses.

Methods Based on Prescription Data

One of the distinguishing features of pharmacoepidemiology is the use of computerized administrative health databases to answer research questions reliably and with sufficient rapidity. The usual urgency of concerns related to drug safety makes these databases essential to perform such risk assessment studies. In particular, databases containing only information on prescriptions dispensed to patients, and no outcome information on disease diagnoses, hospitalizations or vital status, have been the object of interesting statistical developments. These standalone prescription drug databases, that do not require to be linked to outcomes databases, are more numerous and usually more easily accessible than the fully linked databases. They provide a source of data that allows the investigation of patterns of drug use that can yield some insight into the validity of risk assessment studies as well as generate and test hypotheses about these risks. In this section we briefly review some of the resourceful uses of these drug prescription databases in pharmacoepidemiology.

A technique that was developed specifically for the context of drug databases is prescription sequence analysis [36]. Prescription sequence analysis is based on the situation when a certain drug A is suspected of causing an adverse event that itself is treated by a drug B. To apply this technique, the computerized drug database is searched for all patients using drug A. For these subjects, all patients prescribed drug B in the course of using drug A are identified

and counted. Under the null hypothesis that drug A does not cause the adverse event treated by drug B, this number of subjects should be proportional to the duration of use of drug A relative to the total period of observation. This extremely rapid method of assessing the association between drug A and drug B is assessed for its **random error** with a Monte Carlo simulation analysis. This technique was applied to assess whether patients using the antivertigo or antimigraine drug flunarizine (drug A) causes mental depression, as measured by the use of antidepressant drugs (drug B). The authors found that the number of patients starting on antidepressant drugs during flunarizine use was in fact lower than expected [36]. They thus concluded, using this rapid approach based solely on drug prescription data, that this drug probably does not cause mental depression. An extension of prescription sequence analysis, called prescription sequence symmetry analysis, was recently proposed [17]. Using a population of new users of either drug A or B, this approach compares the number of subjects who used drug A before drug B to that using B before A. Under the null hypothesis, this distribution should be symmetrical and the numbers should be equal.

Another function of these databases is to use the prescriptions as covariate information to explain possible confounding patterns. The concept of *channeling* of drugs was put forward as an explanation of unusual risk findings [49]. For example, a case–control study conducted in New Zealand found that fenoterol, a beta agonist bronchodilator used to treat asthma attacks, was associated with an increased risk of death from asthma [8]. Using a prescription drugs database, it was found that severe asthmatics, as deemed from their use of other asthma medications prescribed for severe forms of the disease, were in fact channeled to fenoterol, probably because fenoterol was felt by prescribers to be a more potent bronchodilator than other beta agonists [35]. This phenomenon of channeling can be assessed rapidly in such databases, provided medications can be used as proxies for disease severity. This approach can be subject to bias, however, as it has been used with **cross-sectional** designs that cannot differentiate the directionality of the association. An application of channeling using a longitudinal design was recently presented [4]. It indicated that channeling can vary according to the timing of exposure, i.e. that disease severity was not associated with first-time use of a drug, but subsequently severe patients were more likely to be switched to that drug. This type of research into patterns of drug prescribing and drug use can be very useful in understanding the results of case–control studies with limited data on drug exposures and subject to confounding by indication.

These prescription drug databases have also been used to study patterns of interchange in the dispensing of NSAIDs. Such research is important because switching patterns permits the identification of brands that may not be well tolerated and result in the prescription of another agent. By using a stochastic approach, Walker et al. [51] estimated the transition probabilities from one NSAID to another. For a set of k different brands of NSAID, they derived the expected marginal distributions of the transition matrix that corresponds to a global equilibrium state by solving a system of $k + 1$ equations with $k + 1$ unknowns. By comparing these expected values with the observed marginals of the transition matrix, it was possible to assess whether this population had reached this stable state and for which drugs. Such models can be used rapidly to assess patterns of interchange and identify potentially harmful agents.

Finally, these prescription drugs databases may in certain situations provide all the necessary data for a conventional cohort or case–control study. For instance, the use of beta blockers to treat hypertension and other cardiac diseases has been hypothesized to cause depression. A prescription for an antidepressant drug can be used as a proxy for the outcome of depression. In this way, a standalone prescription drug database can provide data on exposure to beta blockers, on the outcome of depression, as well as on covariate information from other medications [2, 7].

Acknowledgments

Samy Suissa is the recipient the Senior Scientist Award from the Medical Research Council (MRC) of Canada. The McGill Pharmacoepidemiology Research Unit is funded by the Fonds de la Recherche en Santé du Quebec (FRSQ) and grants from the National Health Research and Development Programme (NHRDP) and the MRC.

References

[1]   Aelony, Y., Laks, M.M. & Beall, G. (1975). An electrocardiographic pattern of acute myocardial infarction associated with excessive use of aerosolized isoproterenol, *Chest* **68**, 107–110.

[2]   Avorn, J., Everitt, D.E. & Weiss, S. (1986). Increased antidepressant use in patients prescribed beta-blockers. *Journal of the American Medical Association* **255**, 357–360.

[3]   Baum, C., Kweder, S.L. & Anello, C. (1994). The spontaneous reporting system in the United States, in *Pharmacoepidemiology*, 2nd Ed, B.L. Strom, ed. Wiley, New York, pp. 125–138.

[4]   Blais, L., Ernst, P. & Suissa, S. (1996). Confounding by indication and channeling over time: the risks of beta-agonists, *American Journal of Epidemiology* **144**, 1161–1169.

[5]   Breslow, N. & Day, N.E. (1980). *Statistical Methods in Cancer Research*. Vol. I: *The Analysis of Case–Control Studies*. International Agency for Research on Cancer, Lyon.

[6]   Breslow, N. & Day, N.E. (1987). *Statistical Methods in Cancer Research*, Vol. II: *The Design and Analysis of Cohort Studies*, 2nd Ed. International Agency for Research on Cancer, Lyon.

[7]   Bright, R.A. & Everitt, D.E. (1992). Beta-blockers and depression: evidence against an association, *Journal of the American Medical Association* **267**, 1783–1787.

[8]   Crane, J., Pearce, N., Flatt, A., Burgess, C., Jackson, R., Kwong, T., Ball, M. & Beasley, R. (1989). Prescribed fenoterol and death from asthma in New Zealand 1981–1983: case–control study, *Lancet* **1**, 917–922.

[9]   Efron, B. (1988). Logistic regression, survival analysis, and the Kaplan–Meier curve, *Journal of the American Statistical Association* **83**, 414–425.

[10] Farmer, R.D.T., Lawrenson, R.A., Thompson, C.R., Kennedy, J.G. & Hambleton, I.R. (1997). Population-based study of risk of venous thromboembolism associated with various oral contraceptives, *Lancet* **349**, 83–88.

[11] Farrington, C.P., Nash, J. & Miller, E. (1996). Case series analysis of adverse reactions to vaccines: a comparative evaluation, *American Journal of Epidemiology* **143**, 1165–1173.

[12] Gong, L., Zhang, W., Zhu, Y., Zhu, J., Kong, D., Page, V., Ghadirian, P., Lehorier, J. & Hamet, P. (1996). Shanghai trial of Nifedipine in the elderly (STONE), *Journal of Hypertension* **19**, 1–9.

[13] Greenland, S. (1995). Dose-response and trend analysis in epidemiology: alternatives to categorical analysis, *Epidemiology* **6**, 356–365.

[14] Greenland, S. (1996). Confounding and exposure trends in case–crossover and case–time–control design, *Epidemiology* **7**, 231–239.

[15] Griffin, M.R., Ray, W.A. & Schaffner, W. (1988). Non-steroidal anti-inflammatory drug use and death from peptic ulcer in elderly persons, *Annals of Internal Medicine* **109**, 359–363.

[16] Guess, H.A. (1989). Behavior of the exposure odds ratio in a case–control study when the hazard function is not constant over time, *Journal of Clinical Epidemiology* **42**, 1179–1184.

[17] Hallas, J. (1996). Evidence of depression provoked by cardiovascular medication – a prescription sequence symmetry analysis, *Epidemiology* **7**, 478–484.

[18] Hill, A.B. (1965). The environment and disease: association or causation?, *Proceedings of the Royal Society of Medicine* **58**, 295–300.

[19] Hutchinson, T.A. (1986). A Bayesian approach to assessment of adverse drug reactions: evaluation of a case of acute renal failure, *Drug Information Journal* **20**, 475–482.

[20] Hutchinson, T.A., Leventhal, J.M., Kramer, M.S., Karch, F.E., Lipman, A.G. & Feinstein, A.R. (1979). An algorithm for the operational assessment of adverse drug reactions. II. Demonstration of reproducibility and validity, *Journal of the American Medical Association* **242**, 633–638.

[21] Hutchinson, T.A., Dawid, A.P., Spiegelhalter, D.J., Cowell, R.G. & Roden, S. (1991). Computer aids for probabilistic assessment of drug safety I: A spread-sheet program, *Drug Information Journal* **25**, 29–39.

[22] Jick, H., Jick, S.S., Gurewich, V., Myers, M.W. & Vasilakis, C. (1995). Risk of idiopathic cardiovascular death and nonfatal venous thromboembolism in women using oral contraceptives with differing progestogen components, *Lancet* **346**, 1589–1593.

[23] Jones, J.K. (1986). Evaluation of a case of Stevens–Johnson syndrome, *Drug Information Journal* **20**, 487–502.

[24] Kramer, M.S. (1986). A Bayesian approach to assessment of adverse drug reactions: evaluation of a case of fatal anaphylaxis, *Drug Information Journal* **20**, 505–518.

[25] Kramer, M.S. Leventhal, J.M., Hutchinson, T.A. & Feinstein, A.R. (1979). An algorithm for the operational assessment of adverse drug reactions. I. Background, description, and instructions for use, *Journal of the American Medical Association* **242**, 623–632.

[26] Lane, D.A. (1984). A probabilist's view of causality assessment, *Drug Information Journal* **18**, 323–330.

[27] Lane, D.A. (1986). The Bayesian approach to causality assessment, *Drug Information Journal* **20**, 455–461.

[28] Lane, D.A., Kramer, M.S., Hutchinson, T.A., Jones, J.K. & Naranjo, C.A. (1987). The causality assessment of adverse drug reactions using a Bayesian approach, *Journal of Pharmaceutical Medicine* **2**, 265–283.

[29] Lenz, W. (1966). Malformations caused by drugs in pregnancy, *American Journal of Diseases of Children* **112**, 99–106.

[30] Maclure, M. (1991). The case–crossover design: a method for studying transient effects on the risk of acute events, *American Journal of Epidemiology* **133**, 144–153.

[31] McBride, W.G. (1961). Thalidomide and congenital abnormalities, *Lancet* **ii**, 1358.

[32] Miettinen, O.S. (1983). The need for randomization in the study of intended effects, *Statistics in Medicine* **2**, 267–271.

[33] Miettinen, O.S. (1985). *Theoretical Epidemiology: Principles of Occurrence Research in Medicine*. Wiley, New York.

[34] Naranjo, C.A., Lanctot, K.L. & Lane, D.A. (1990). The Bayesian differential diagnosis of neutropenia associated with antiarrhythmic agents, *Journal of Clinical Pharmacology* **30**, 1120–1127.

[35] Petri, H. & Urquhart, J. (1991). Channeling bias in the interpretation of drug effects, *Statistics in Medicine* **10**, 577–581.

[36] Petri, H., De Vet, H.C.W., Naus, J. & Urquhart, J. (1988). Prescription sequence analysis: a new and fast method for assessing certain adverse reactions of prescription drugs in large populations, *Statistics in Medicine* **7**, 1171–1175.

[37] Ray, W.A. & Griffin, M.R. (1989). Use of Medicaid data for pharmacoepidemiology, *American Journal of Epidemiology* **129**, 837–849.

[38] Ray, W.A., Fought, R.L. & Decker, M.D. (1992). Psychoactive drugs and the risk of injurious motor vehicle crashes in elderly drivers, *American Journal of Epidemiology* **136**, 873–883.

[39] Rothman, K.J. (1986). *Modern Epidemiology*. Little, Brown, & Company, Boston.

[40] Spitzer, W.O., Suissa, S., Ernst, P., Horwitz, R.I., Habbick, B., Cockcroft, D., Boivin, J.F., McNutt, M., Buist, A.S. & Rebuck, A.S. The use of beta-agonists and the risk of death and near death from asthma, *New England Journal of Medicine* **326**, 501–506.

[41] Spitzer, W.O., Lewis, M.A., Heinemann, L.A., Thorogood, M. & MacRae, K.D. (1996). Third generation oral contraceptives and risk of venous thromboembolic disorders: an international case–control study. Transactional Research Group on Oral Contraceptives and the Health of Young Women, *British Medical Journal* **312**, 83–88.

[42] StatSci (1995). *S-PLUS Version 3.3*. StatSci, a division of MathSoft, Inc., Seattle.

[43] Sturkenboom, M.C., Middelbeek, A., de Jong, L.T., van den Berg, P.B., Stricker, B.H. & Wesseling, H. (1995). Vulvo-vaginal candidiasis associated with acitretin, *Journal of Clinical Epidemiology* **48**, 991–997.

[44] Suissa, S. (1995). The case–time–control design, *Epidemiology* **6**, 248–253.

[45] Suissa, S. (1998). The case–time–control design: further assumptions and conditions, *Epidemiology* **9**, 441–445.

[46] Suissa, S. & Edwardes, M. (1997). Adjusted odds ratios for case–control studies with missing confounder data in controls. *Epidemiology* **8**, 275–280.

[47] Suissa, S., Hemmelgarn, B., Blais, L. & Ernst, P. (1996). Bronchodilators and acute cardiac death, *Journal of Respiratory and Critical Care Medicine* **154**, 1598–1602.

[48] Suissa, S., Blais, L., Spitzer, W.O., Cusson, J., Lewis, M. & Heinemann, L. (1997). First-time use of newer oral contraceptives and the risk of venous thromboembolism, *Contraception* **56**, 141–146.

[49]   Urquhart, J. (1989). ADR crisis management, *Scrip* **1388**, 19–21.

[50]   Walker, A.M. (1996). Confounding by indication, *Epidemiology* **7**, 335–336.

[51]   Walker, A.M., Chan, K.W.A. & Yood, R.A. (1992). Patterns of interchange in the dispensing of non-steroidal anti-inflammatory drugs, *American Journal of Epidemiology* **45**, 187–195.

[52]   Wiholm, B.E., Olsson, S., Moore, N. & Wood, S. (1994). Spontaneous reporting systems outside the United States, in *Pharmacoepidemiology*, 2nd Ed., B.L. Strom, ed. Wiley, New York, pp. 139–156.

[53]   World Health Organization Collaborative Study of Cardiovascular Disease and Steroid Hormone Contraception, (1995). Venous thromboembolic disease and combined oral contraceptives: results of international multicentre case–control study. World Health Organization Collaborative Study of Cardiovascular Disease and Steroid Hormone Contraception, *Lancet* **346**, 1575–1582.

(*See also* **Pharmacoepidemiology, Study Designs**)

S. SUISSA

Pharmacoepidemiology, Study Designs

The field of **pharmacoepidemiology** includes the study of the use of and effects of pharmaceuticals in populations [10]. In general, the study designs used in pharmacoepidemiology are the same as those used in other areas of **clinical epidemiology**. There are three key differences, however.

First, because pharmacoepidemiology studies are usually performed after drug marketing, and because 500–3000 patients are generally studied prior to drug marketing, pharmacoepidemiology studies usually must include substantially larger numbers of patients in a **cohort study** or, alternatively, tap an equivalently sized population for a **case–control study**, in order to contribute new useful information.

Secondly, because at least one randomized clinical trial was already performed prior to drug marketing, pharmacoepidemiology studies are less likely to use randomized clinical trial study designs; many of the same limitations which the premarketing randomized clinical trials were subject to would apply as well to any postmarketing randomized clinical trial, and so they would not be able to contribute new useful information. For example, because of the need for huge sample sizes, randomized clinical trials are not an efficient means of studying uncommon adverse effects, or the effects of drugs in types of patients commonly excluded from such trials.

Thirdly, because pharmacoepidemiology questions often arise as regulatory, commercial and public health crises, answers must often be obtained very quickly.

This need for rapidly performed studies of massive sample size has led to a series of special approaches which have characterized the field of pharmacoepidemiology, and will be the primary focus of this article. Other analytic issues which are special to pharmacoepidemiology include the need for special attention to the drug regimen. In many other areas of clinical epidemiology, "exposure" is frequently treated as a dichotomous variable. Even when studying drugs, most randomized clinical trials specify a single fixed dose of the drug of interest. In contrast, once a drug is on the market, questions of how its effects vary with different doses, different durations of therapy, and different regimens (e.g. intermittent vs. continuous administration) are often the questions which are of greatest clinical importance. For reasons of space, these have not been discussed here. The reader is referred elsewhere for such considerations [2].

Data Resources Used in Pharmacoepidemiology

Historically, the primary data resource used in pharmacoepidemiology was the spontaneous reporting system [1, 18]. This is a nonsystematic collection of case reports (*see* **Case Series, Case Reports**) of adverse events following use of drugs, considered by the treating physician as possibly due to the drug. These are reports to the medical literature but, more voluminously, to regulatory bodies. As case reports, they are useful primarily for generating rather than testing hypotheses. For example, case reports of acute flank pain following the use of suprofen generated formal studies which tested and confirmed the resulting hypothesis [14], while analogous spontaneous reports of anaphylactic reactions to tolmetin were not confirmed when these hypotheses were formally tested [13].

Another approach to pharmacoepidemiology studies uses **vital statistics** data and drug utilization data to perform analyses of secular trends, searching for whether trends in drug exposure over time or across geographic areas correlate with trends in disease occurrence [9]. For example, with the marketing of oral contraceptives, mortality rates from pulmonary embolism increased, but only in women of reproductive age [5]. While this type of study is easy to perform, it obviously is prone to many difficulties, including the limitations inherent in vital statistics data as well as identifying which of the possible correlations truly reflect cause vs. simply coincidence (*see* **Hill's Criteria for Causality**). For example, in a study using data from 18 different cancer registries around the world to investigate the relationship between sales of methyldopa and the development of biliary carcinoma [12], the results from one of the cancer registries showed an artifactual association, caused by changes in coding practices in that registry.

Over the past two decades, pharmacoepidemiology has been to the fore in scientific fields using automated databases of claims information for its research [7, 11]. In clinical epidemiology studies, the largest expense of the study is generally that of data collection, and this is particularly problematic in the very large studies of pharmacoepidemiology. However, using these automated databases, the substantial cost of data collection for these very large studies is borne by the underlying insurance system, rather than the study. A large proportion of pharmacoepidemiology studies are now using such systems. However, given the relatively small number of exposed diseased individuals relative to unexposed diseased individuals, in using an automated database to implement such a study one needs to obtain a huge number of medical records of diseased individuals, relatively few of whom are exposed. Inasmuch as most of the cost of this type of study is the cost of obtaining these medical records, this is inefficient, and new methods are needed to enable one to sample from unexposed diseased individuals. The major weakness of these systems is the uncertain validity of the data, especially the diagnosis data [11]. Furthermore, these systems can lack information about key potential **confounding** variables, if they do not come to medical attention. Thus, there is increasing interest in the exploration of medical record databases, as opposed to claims databases, for such research [3].

Historically, there have been a few ongoing systems of *ad hoc* data collection, tailored for pharmacoepidemiology research. One of these has been a hospital-based system of collecting drug exposures and outcomes in hospitals, pioneered by the Boston Collaborative Drug Surveillance Program [4]. This system has the advantage of known **incidence rates** and high-quality data collected on site in the hospital, but an inability to study either the many important drugs used in outpatients, or uncommon adverse reactions, even if serious. New data collection in this system was abandoned many years ago, although a few hospitals have mounted analogous systems elsewhere.

Another such system has been the system of case–control surveillance developed by the Drug Epidemiology Unit, now the Slone Epidemiology Unit at Boston University [8]. This also focuses on hospitals, but collects information on prior drug exposures as possible causes of the hospitalization, performing **hospital-based case–control studies**. This system suffers from the uncertain validity of the drug exposure data obtained from patients and from restriction to hospital-based case–control studies, with the inherent problems of **selection bias**. In recent years, data collection for this system has been curtailed.

Finally, many pharmacoepidemiology studies are still designed as *ad hoc* clinical epidemiology studies, whether cohort or case–control. The choices among these designs are discussed elsewhere.

Special Methodological Approaches Used to Apply These Resources

In applying the special resources described above, unique challenges are confronted by pharmacoepidemiologists, in part because of the nature of the information being collected, and in part because of the large sample sizes required. These are each discussed in turn below.

Validity of Exposure and Outcome Data

In order to perform a valid epidemiologic study, one obviously must have valid information on both exposure and outcome. This can be very problematic in pharmacoepidemiologic studies. The best measures of disease occurrence are medical records, as patients often do not understand the details of the diseases which they have. Case–control studies have a major advantage here, as patients can be identified from their health care providers. However, medical records are very poor sources of information about prior drug use, as drugs tend to be recorded very incompletely [15]. Obtaining drug histories directly from patients can be problematic, however, as most patients cannot identify the drugs they are on now, even less the drugs they took in the past. Special techniques have been developed by pharmacoepidemiologists in order to maximize the validity of the drug data collected from patients as part of case–control studies, e.g. the use of indicator prompts and pictorial handouts. The details of these approaches are beyond the scope of this article, but the reader is referred elsewhere for them [17]. However, suffice it to say that much work remains to be done on these issues.

In contrast, data on drug exposure from claims databases are extremely valid, as they represent documentation of the exact drugs dispensed to patients. Reimbursement by insurance carriers varies according to the identity and amount of the drug [11]. While this does not assure compliance with the dispensed drug, it is a level better than prescribing information, as many prescribed drugs are never dispensed. In contrast, however, the diagnosis information in these databases is of uncertain validity, as reimbursement generally does not depend on diagnosis and, especially, on correct and precise diagnoses [11]. As such, in studies using these databases, considerable attention needs to be paid to obtaining validation of these diagnoses.

Special Study Designs Used to Increase Efficiency

Because of the large numbers of individuals included in many pharmacoepidemiology studies, even when using claims databases, pharmacoepidemiologists seek special study designs to enable the data processing and, especially, any medical record review to be more efficient. In general, pharmacoepidemiologists are studying diseases of low incidence. Furthermore, any given drug is used by a small proportion of the population. As such, one is investigating a low **prevalence** of exposure and a low **incidence** of disease. To the degree one includes general population samples, therefore, one collects information on a large number of people who do not contribute much additional statistical information to the investigation. Case–control studies can be useful toward this end,

when the prevalence of exposure is high. However, for many drugs this is not applicable.

Another approach which is used is the **nested case–control study**. In this design, an investigator first creates a cohort of exposed individuals and then, within that cohort, identifies cases and a random sample of noncases for the study. This design is efficient and allows one to use conventional statistical methods for the analysis of case–control studies, which is a major advantage. However, it can result in logistical problems in identifying the sample of noncases, as they must be at risk of developing the disease at the same time as the case, and identifying these risk sets can be difficult [16].

Another design beginning to be used by pharmacoepidemiologists is the **case–cohort study**, an approach pioneered in **occupational epidemiology** [6]. In this situation, one identifies a cohort of exposed subjects in advance, and the subset of people who are cases, as with the nested case–control study. However, instead of sampling randomly from the known noncases those at risk of developing the disease at the same time as the case, one randomly samples from the entire cohort, creating a subcohort, which also can include some of the cases. Then, the distribution of exposures and **confounders** in the case group can be compared for analytic purposes to the distribution in the subcohort. This approach has the advantage of achieving much smaller sample sizes with a simple sampling scheme. Also, one can study multiple outcomes within the same study. It has the disadvantage of requiring analyses different from those of normal case–control studies. Instead, a modified Cox **proportional hazards** approach is used and, until recently, software was not available to implement this.

Conclusions

In conclusion, pharmacoepidemiologists use the same methods of study design as do other clinical epidemiologists. However, because of the special characteristics of the field, there are special issues of study design and analysis which arise. These have been discussed briefly in this article.

References

[1]   Baum, C., Kweder, S.L. & Anello, C. (1994). The spontaneous reporting system in the United States,

in *Pharmacoepidemiology*, 2nd Ed., B.L. Strom, ed. Wiley, Chichester, pp. 125–138.

[2]   Guess, H.A. (1989). Behavior of the exposure odds ratio in a case–control study when the hazard function is not constant over time, *Journal of Clinical Epidemiology* **42**, 1179–1184.

[3]   Hall, G. (1992). Pharmacoepidemiology using a UK database of primary care records, *Pharmacoepidemiology and Drug Safety* **1**, 33–37.

[4]   Lawson, D.H. & Beard, K. (1994). Intensive hospital-based cohort studies, in *Pharmacoepidemiology*, 2nd Ed., B.L. Strom, ed. Wiley, Chichester, pp. 157–170.

[5]   Markush, R.E. & Seigel, D.G. (1969). Oral contraceptives and mortality from thromboembolism in the United States, *American Journal of Public Health* **59**, 418–434.

[6]   Prentice, R.L. (1986). A case–cohort design for epidemiologic cohort studies and disease prevention trials, *Biometrika* **73**, 1–11.

[7]   Ray, W.A. & Griffin, M.R. (1989). The use of Medicaid data for pharmacoepidemiology, *American Journal of Epidemiology* **129**, 837–849.

[8]   Shapiro, S. (1994). Case–control surveillance, in *Pharmacoepidemiology*, 2nd Ed., B.L. Strom, ed. Wiley, Chichester, pp. 301–322.

[9]   Stolley, P.D. (1982). The use of vital and morbidity statistics for the detection of adverse drug reactions and for monitoring of drug safety, *Journal of Clinical Pharmacology* **22**, 499–504.

[10] Strom, B.L. (1994). What is pharmacoepidemiology?, in *Pharmacoepidemiology*, 2nd Ed., B.L. Strom, ed. Wiley, Chichester, pp. 3–14.

[11] Strom, B.L. & Carson, J.L. (1990). Use of automated databases for pharmacoepidemiology research, *Epidemiologic Reviews* **12**, 87–107.

[12] Strom, B.L., Hibberd, P.L. & Stolley, P.D. (1985). No evidence of association-between methyldopa and biliary carcinoma, *International Journal of Epidemiology* **14**, 86–90.

[13] Strom, B.L., Carson, J.L., Schinnar, R., Sim, E. & Morse, M.L. (1988). The effect of indication on the risk of hypersensitivity reactions associated with tolmetin sodium vs. other nonsteroidal antiinflammatory drugs, *Journal of Rheumatology* **15**, 695–699.

[14] Strom, B.L., West, S.L., Sim, E. & Carson, J.L. (1989). The epidemiology of the acute flank pain syndrome from suprofen, *Clinical Pharmacologic Therapy* **46**, 693–699.

[15] Strom, B.L, Carson, J.L., Halpern, A.C., Schinnar, R., Snyder, E.S., Stolley, P.D., Shaw, M., Tilson, H.H., Joseph, M., Dai, W.S., Chen, D., Stern, R.S., Bergman, U. & Lundin, F. (1991). Using a claims database to investigate drug-induced Stevens-Johnson syndrome, *Statistics in Medicine* **10**, 565–576.

[16] Suissa, S. (1994). Novel approaches to pharmacoepidemiology study design and statistical analysis, in *Pharmacoepidemiology*, 2nd Ed., B.L. Strom, ed. Wiley, Chichester, pp. 629–646.

[17] West, S.L. & Strom, B.L. (1994). Validity of pharmacoepidemiology drug and diagnosis data, in *Pharmacoepidemiology*, 2nd Ed., B.L. Strom, ed. Wiley, Chichester, pp. 549–580.

[18] Wiholm, B.-E., Olsson, S., Moore, N. & Wood, S. (1994). Spontaneous reporting systems outside the United States, in *Pharmacoepidemiology*, 2nd Ed., B.L. Strom, ed. Wiley, Chichester, pp. 139–156.

B.L. Strom

Plus Digit Dialing *see* Telephone Sampling

Poisson Regression

For response variables that have counts or frequencies as outcomes it is often reasonable to assume an underlying Poisson distribution and describe the impact of explanatory variables on their means by some regression function. Poisson regression models, as a widely applicable class of models particularly useful in biostatistics, emerged in the late 1970s; see, for example, [6], [11], [21]–[25], [28], [29], [31], and [32].

As an example consider the data given in Table 1, taken from [27]. Randomly chosen household members from a probability sample of Oakland, CA, were asked to note which stressful events had occurred within the last 18 months and to report the month of occurrence of these events. A scattergram of the data indicates a decline of recalls as events lie farther in the past, possibly due to the fallibility of human memory (see Figure 1). To define a Poisson regression model, assume that (i) the number of recalls is a random variable Y distributed as Poisson with mean μ, and (ii) μ is some function of X, the number of months before interview. Plotting logarithms of frequencies against months suggests a linear relationship

$$\log \mu = \alpha + \beta x.$$

For this loglinear model, the mean satisfies the exponential relationship,

$$\mu = \exp(\alpha + \beta x) = e^{\alpha}(e^{\beta})^{x}.$$

Table 1 Distribution by months prior to interview of stressful events reported from subjects: 147 subjects reporting exactly one stressful event in the period from 1 to 18 months prior to interview. Reprinted from [27, p. 3] by permission of Academic Press, Inc.

Months	1	2	3	4	5	6	7	8	9	10	11	12	13	14	15	16	17	18
Number	15	11	14	17	5	11	10	4	8	10	7	9	11	3	6	1	1	4

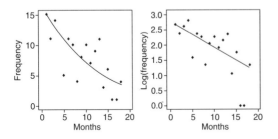

Figure 1 Scattergram of observed frequencies and their logarithms against months before interview. Solid lines represent fitted means and respective values for the linear predictor for the Poisson regression model mentioned in the text

A one-unit increase in X has a multiplicative effect of e^β on μ, i.e. the mean of Y at $x + 1$ equals the mean of Y at x multiplied by e^β.

Most of the widely available software packages are capable of fitting generalized linear models, and can be used to obtain maximum likelihood estimates for the parameters of Poisson regression models as well. For these data one finds $\hat{\alpha} = 2.803$ and $\hat{\beta} = -0.0838$; hence

$$\hat{\mu} = 16.5 \times 0.920^x,$$

indicating a negative trend in time.

Using the relationship between the multinomial and conditional Poisson distributions, this is shown to be equivalent to an exponential decay model for the probability of remembering an event. For a more detailed discussion, see [27] or [33].

Definition

To define the basic version of a Poisson regression model, suppose that we have observations $y_1, \ldots, y_n$ for the response variable $Y_1, \ldots, Y_n$, assumed to be independently distributed Poisson variates with means $\mu_1, \ldots, \mu_n$, i.e.

$$f(y_i|\mu_i) = \frac{\mu_i^{y_i}}{y_i!} \exp(-\mu_i). \qquad (1)$$

The systematic component of the model is specified by some regression function η, depending on regression parameters $\beta_1, \ldots, \beta_k$, with each component relating values $x_{i1}, \ldots, x_{ik}$ of explanatory variables to respective means, i.e.

$$\mu_i = \eta_i(\beta) = \eta_i(x_{i1}, \ldots, x_{ik}; \beta_1, \ldots, \beta_k). \qquad (2)$$

Often, this relationship is such that some monotone transformation g of the means is connected to a *linear predictor* of explanatory variables,

$$g(\mu_i) = \sum_{j=1}^{k} x_{ij}\beta_j.$$

In this situation g is called the *link function* and the model defined in this manner is an instance of a generalized linear model (see [35] and [36] or, for an introductory text, [18]). For $\eta_i(\beta) = \exp\left(\sum_{j=1}^{k} x_{ij}\beta_j\right)$ we have the familiar loglinear model,

$$\log \mu_i = \sum_{j=1}^{k} x_{ij}\beta_j.$$

For the model specified by the stochastic component (1) and regression function (2), the log likelihood function is written as

$$\ell_y(\beta) = \sum_{i=1}^{n} \{y_i \log[\eta_i(\beta)] - \eta_i(\beta) - \log(y_i!)\}. \qquad (3)$$

It may be worthwhile noting that this reduces to a k-parameter exponential family log likelihood,

$$\ell_y(\beta) = \sum_{j=1}^{k} \left(\sum_{i=1}^{n} x_{ij}y_i\right) \beta_j - \sum_{i=1}^{n} \exp\left(\sum_{j=1}^{k} x_{ij}\beta_j\right)$$
$$- \sum_{i=1}^{n} \log(y_i!), \qquad (4)$$

with jointly sufficient statistics $\sum_{i=1}^{n} x_{ij}y_i$, $j = 1, \ldots, k$, if the model is log linear.

Some Special Cases

Loglinear Models for Contingency Tables

Suppose, in obvious notation, y_{ij} with indices $i = 1, \ldots, I$ and $j = 1, \ldots, J$ form a two-dimensional contingency table, according to some classifying factors A and B having I and J categories, respectively. A common method for analyzing data of this kind is to assume that cell frequencies Y_{ij} are independently distributed as Poisson and to use loglinear models, where in an analysis-of-variance-like fashion logarithms of expected cell frequencies μ_{ij} are assumed to be sums of several effects, e.g. for the **multiplicative model**,

$$\log(\mu_{ij}) = \beta_o + \beta_i^A + \beta_j^B, \qquad (5)$$

subject to some constraints on the βs. Sums of independent Poisson variates are again distributed as Poisson with means equal to the sum of respective means. Row totals Y_{i+}, column totals Y_{+j}, and grand total Y_{++} are, therefore, Poisson variates with means $\mu_{i+} = \mu_{i1} + \cdots + \mu_{iJ}$, $\mu_{+j} = \mu_{1j} + \cdots + \mu_{Ij}$, and $\mu_{++} = \sum_{i,j} \mu_{ij}$, respectively. Under the assumption of the multiplicative model these quantities are related by

$$\mu_{ij} = \frac{\mu_{i+}\mu_{+j}}{\mu_{++}},$$

showing that the joint distribution of the contingency table is, in a multiplicative manner, completely determined by the marginal distributions.

The Poisson model assumption implies that marginals are random. If, instead, the total is fixed by the sampling design, it may be more appropriate to assume a multinomial distribution for the table. Formally, the multinomial model can be inferred from the Poisson model by conditioning on the total y_{++}. For the probability π_{ij} of an observation falling into row i and column j, we then have $\pi_{ij} = \mu_{ij}/\mu_{++}$, and from assuming the multiplicative model (5), it follows that

$$\pi_{ij} = \pi_{i+}\pi_{+j}, \qquad (6)$$

where π_{i+} and π_{+j} are the marginal probabilities of an observation falling into row i and column j, respectively. Hence, row and column variables A and B are independently distributed.

Likewise, if row totals are fixed, then each row may be assumed to be multinomially distributed. Again, this can be inferred from the Poisson model by conditioning on the row totals, and the multiplicative model (5) implies identical distributions for the rows – a condition usually called *homogeneity*. It may be worthwhile noting that maximum-likelihood estimates for the parameters in the Poisson models are identical to those obtained for some other sampling designs, such as the multinomial designs just mentioned, making this class of model particularly interesting and useful.

Loglinear models for two- and higher-dimensional contingency tables, used to describe the association and interaction structure connecting the variables, are discussed in the article on Loglinear Models in the *Encyclopedia of Biostatistics*. Usually, the goal is to find a parsimonious model that fits the data well and allows meaningful substantive interpretation. Most commonly, this search is restricted to hierarchical models.

Multiplicative Rate Models

If occurrences of some kind of event are counted over time, then often interest lies in the rate at which events occur. The rate describes the instantaneous risk for an event to happen at a given point in time. To be more specific, the probability of observing exactly one event in the interval ranging from t to $t + h$, divided by its length h, is assumed to tend to some value $\lambda(t)$, as h tends to 0. $\lambda(t)$, as a function of time t, is called the *rate* or *intensity function*.

An important special case, termed the Poisson process, assumes that waiting times between successive events are independent and exponentially distributed with common mean $1/\lambda$. Here, the rate function is constant over time, $\lambda(t) \equiv \lambda$. Furthermore, the number $Y(t)$ of events that occur up to time t is distributed as Poisson with mean $\mu = \lambda t$. Note that the mean of $Y(t)/t$ equals the rate λ. This suggests a Poisson regression approach

$$\log \lambda = \log(\mu/t) = \alpha + \beta x$$

for modeling the dependence of the rate function on an explanatory variable X. This can be rewritten as

$$\log \mu = \alpha + \beta x + \log t,$$

with $\log(t)$ as an *offset*, i.e. a variable in the linear predictor, the corresponding regression parameter of which is set equal to 1. Observe that this defines a multiplicative model for the rate function,

$$\lambda = e^\alpha (e^\beta)^x, \qquad (7)$$

Table 2 Number of recurrences of superficial bladder cancer for 31 male patients with grade 2, stage T_1, solitary primary tumours and respective times under observation (in months) by size of primary tumour. Subset of data analyzed in [38]

Size	Recurrences	Time under observation
≤3 cm	1	2, 3, 6, 8, 9, 10, 11, 13, 14, 16, 21, 22, 24, 26, 27
	2	7, 13, 15, 18, 23
	3	20
	4	24
>3 cm	1	1, 5, 17, 18, 25
	2	18, 25
	3	4
	4	19

with a *baseline rate* $\lambda_0 = \exp(\alpha)$ and proportionality factor $\exp(\beta x)$.

For illustrative purposes a subset of the data analyzed in [38] is reprinted in Table 2. For 31 male patients, who have been treated for superficial bladder cancer, the number of recurrent tumours has been recorded for some time after removal of the primary tumour. Defining X to be 1 for larger primary tumours (>3 cm) and 0 otherwise, and assuming a Poisson process with rate (7), yields parameter estimates $\hat\alpha = -1.95$ and $\hat\beta = 0.385$. The (baseline) rate for smaller tumours is (estimated as) 0.142, the rate for larger tumours being 1.47 times larger. In terms of waiting times between recurrences, means are estimated as 7.06 and 4.80 months, respectively.

Now suppose that we have recorded, for n individuals, time under observation, t_i, and the number y_i of events occurred. Observation times are assumed to be nonrandom and counts to be mutually independent. We also have a set of explanatory variables $x_{i1}, \ldots, x_{ik}$ available for each subject. Under the assumption of *proportional rates*, $\lambda_i = \lambda_0 \exp\left(\sum_{j=1}^k x_{ij}\beta_j\right)$, we have

$$\mu_i = \lambda_i \times t_i = \lambda_0 \exp\left[\log(t_i) + \sum_{j=1}^k x_{ij}\beta_j\right]$$

$$= \lambda_0 t_i \prod_{j=1}^k \exp(x_{ij}\beta_j), \qquad (8)$$

i.e. a loglinear model for the mean of the Poisson process, involving the logarithm of observation times as an "explanatory" variable, with the associated regression parameter fixed at a value of 1.

If the process is such that it can be characterized by a time-varying rate function $\lambda(t)$, it is called a

nonhomogeneous Poisson process. Writing

$$\Lambda(t) = \int_0^t \lambda(u)\mathrm{d}u$$

for the *integrated rate* or *intensity function*, the number of occurrences of the event in period until time point t is again distributed as Poisson, but with mean equal to $\Lambda(t)$. Note that events in nonoverlapping time intervals are independent, but waiting times between successive events are, contrary to the homogeneous process with constant rate, neither identically distributed nor independent. In this situation model (8) can be modified, using a *baseline rate* function $\lambda_0(t|\alpha)$, possibly depending on some additional parameter α, to give

$$\mu_i = \exp\left\{\log[\Lambda_0(t_i|\alpha)] + \sum_{j=1}^k x_{ij}\beta_j\right\}.$$

Choosing $\Lambda_0(t|\alpha)$ to be t, t^α, or $\exp(\alpha t)$ corresponds to an exponential, a Weibull, or an extreme value intensity function, respectively, and results in a loglinear model for the Y_is. Disregarding constant terms, the likelihood function for this model is

$$L(\alpha, \beta) = \prod_{i=1}^n \left[\Lambda_0(t_i|\alpha)\exp\left(\sum_{j=1}^k x_{ij}\beta_j\right)\right]^{y_i}$$

$$\times \exp\left[-\Lambda_0(t_i|\alpha)\exp\left(\sum_{j=1}^k x_{ij}\beta_j\right)\right]. \quad (9)$$

If times for occurrences of each event were known, a multiplicative term, depending on the parameter α, would be added to (9); see [32].

There is a close connection to **relative risk models**, which are very frequently used in epidemiology.

This class of models assumes that risk factors interact in a multiplicative way. See [9] and [12], and, for a critical review, [26].

Proportional Hazard Models for Censored Survival Times

Now suppose that individuals are under observation until either a single event of interest occurs or the period of observations ends for some other reason. For each subject the data are of the form (y_i, c_i), where y_i is the time under observation, and c_i is an indicator variable for censoring, taking the value 1 if the event has occurred at time y_i, and the value 0 if the event has not occurred until time y_i. This is a similar situation to the one in the previous example, but with one terminal event that stops the process; interest, however, lies in the analysis of the *survival times* y_i (*see* **Survival Analysis, Overview**).

The distribution of the survival time can be uniquely described by the rate function, in the context of survival analysis usually called **hazard rate** or *force of mortality*. As before, a common approach assumes **proportional hazard** rates,

$$\lambda(y_i | \alpha, \beta) = \lambda_0(y_i | \alpha) \exp\left(\sum_{j=1}^{k} x_{ij}\beta_j\right),$$

with a *baseline hazard* $\lambda_0(y_i | \alpha)$.

Assuming a noninformative censoring mechanism (and continuous survival times), the kernel of the likelihood function is $\prod_{i=1}^{n} f(y_i)^{c_i} \times S(y_i)^{1-c_i}$, where $f(y_i)$ denotes the density for the ith survival time, and $S(y_i) = 1 - F(y_i)$, the *survival function*, i.e. the probability for the ith survival time to exceed y_i. The ratio $f(y_i)/S(y_i)$ is identical to the hazard function. For proportional hazard rates, the likelihood function can therefore be expressed as

$$L_{y,c}(\alpha, \beta)$$

$$= \prod_{i=1}^{n} \left[\Lambda_0(y_i | \alpha) \exp\left(\sum_{j=1}^{k} x_{ij}\beta_j\right) \right]^{c_i}$$

$$\times \exp\left[-\Lambda_0(y_i | \alpha) \exp\left(\sum_{j=1}^{k} x_{ij}\beta_j\right) \right],$$

where $\Lambda_0(y_i | \alpha) = \int_0^{y_i} \lambda_0(u | \alpha) \mathrm{d}u$ denotes the cumulative baseline hazard rate. Writing, as we did before,

$\mu_i = \exp\left\{ \log[\Lambda_0(y_i | \alpha)] + \sum_{j=1}^{k} x_{ij}\beta_j \right\}$, $L(\alpha, \beta)$ is the likelihood function for n independent Poisson variates C_i with means μ_i. Aitkin & Clayton [2] used this fact to bring survival analysis into the framework of generalized linear models (see also [7], [28], and [31]).

If no assumptions on the functional form of the baseline hazard function are made, then this is Cox's proportional hazards model [13, 14] that can be fitted by maximizing a "partial likelihood" (*see* **Cox Regression Model**). Another semiparametric model, due to Breslow [7], assumes a piecewise exponential distribution for the survival times, the baseline hazard function in this case is constant over prespecified intervals of time. To be more specific, suppose that the time axis is split into intervals $(a_{p-1}, a_p]$, $p = 1, \ldots, P$, with $0 = a_0 < a_1 < \cdots < a_P < a_{P+1} = \infty$. The baseline hazard can now be written as

$$\lambda_0(y | \alpha) = \exp(\alpha_p), \quad \text{if } a_{p-1} < y \le a_p.$$

To simplify notation, for individual i and interval $(a_{p-1}, a_p]$ the proportional hazard assumption can be expressed in terms of a constant λ_{ip}, where

$$\lambda_{ip} = \exp\left(\alpha_p + \sum_{j=1}^{k} x_{ij}\beta_j\right). \tag{10}$$

Define P_i to be such that y_i is contained in interval $(a_{P_i-1}, a_{P_i}]$ and e_{ip} to be the exposure time of individual i in the pth interval, i.e.

$$e_{ip} = \begin{cases} a_p - a_{p-1}, & \text{if } p = 1, \ldots, P_i - 1, \\ y_i - a_{P_i-1}, & \text{if } p = P_i \end{cases}.$$

Also, introduce an extended censoring indicator variable to be

$$c_{ip} = \begin{cases} 1, & \text{if } p = 1, \ldots, P_i - 1, \\ c_i, & \text{if } p = P_i. \end{cases}$$

Disregarding constant terms, the likelihood function is then

$$L_{y,c}(\alpha, \beta) = \prod_{i=1}^{n} \prod_{p=1}^{P_i} (\lambda_{ip} e_{ip})^{c_{ip}} \exp(-\lambda_{ip} e_{ip}),$$

where λ_{ip} is defined by (10). Since this is a Poisson likelihood for the "counts" c_{ip}, the *piecewise exponential model* reduces to a loglinear model. If intervals are chosen such that their endpoints correspond

Table 3 Survival times: Time in years, Cens (= 0 for censored), Gender (1 for male), and Age for 33 patients treated for papillary thyroid carcinoma. Subset of data analyzed in [30]

Time	Cens	Gender	Age	Time	Cens	Gender	Age
27.42	0	1	21	2.33	0	1	76
8.50	1	2	31	1.33	0	1	46
0.13	1	1	62	0.08	1	2	84
0.83	1	1	53	2.83	0	2	69
5.92	0	2	52	2.25	1	2	90
1.92	0	2	67	0.25	1	2	52
0.92	1	1	73	3.42	0	2	71
11.67	0	2	56	1.92	1	2	75
0.17	1	1	57	3.00	1	1	69
5.00	1	2	71	1.00	1	1	75
0.08	1	1	53	8.50	1	2	73
0.08	1	2	53	4.17	0	2	36
0.92	1	2	48	3.50	1	1	38
5.08	1	2	65	1.25	1	2	69
5.42	1	2	49	0.33	1	2	77
0.25	0	1	61	0.67	1	1	87
0.17	1	1	71				

to observed times of death, i.e. t_is with $c_i = 1$, then maximum likelihood estimates for the regression parameters β are found to be close to those obtained from the Cox model; see [3] and [39].

For an example consider the data printed in Table 3. For 33 patients treated for papillary thyroid carcinoma, survival time, censoring indicator (Cens), Age, and Gender are reported. This is a small subset of the data analyzed in [30]. For cutpoints $a_1 = 0.5$, $a_2 = 1$, $a_3 = 2$, and $a_4 = 3$, the piecewise-constant baseline hazard function is, up to a constant, estimated as

$$\lambda_0(y) = \begin{cases} 0.45, & \text{if } y \leq 0.5, \\ 0.36, & \text{if } 0.5 < y \leq 1, \\ 0.11, & \text{if } 1 < y \leq 2, \\ 0.16, & \text{if } 2 < y \leq 3, \\ 0.20, & \text{if } 3 < y. \end{cases}$$

Regression parameters, estimated for gender and age, are -0.70 and 0.04, respectively.

Log-nonlinear Models

While loglinear models do have some desirable properties, it may not always be possible to find a parameterization such that the regression function is linear on the log scale. An example of this is given in [20], using a log-logistic regression function. The data come from a radioimmunoassay, a widely used technique to measure the quantity of a given biological substance

by identifying the amount of a radioactive labeled antibody from a reagent by subsamples of increasing concentration. The response variable is the amount of radioactive material remaining measured in counts per minute. If these are very large, a normal distribution for the counts may be assumed, but if this is not the case, an underlying Poisson distribution seems to be more appropriate. For counts $y_1, \ldots, y_n$ and concentrations $x_1, \ldots, x_n$ a regression function of the form

$$\eta_i(\beta_1, \ldots, \beta_4)$$
$$= \beta_1 + \frac{\beta_2}{1 + \exp\{-[\beta_3 + \beta_4 \log(x_i)]\}} \quad (11)$$

can be used to describe the relationship between mean counts and concentrations. Note that this model cannot be transformed into a loglinear one.

Other examples of log-nonlinear models arise frequently in the analysis of contingency tables, when specific structure in the data suggests inclusion of nonlinear **interaction** effects into the regression function. See, for instance, [1, pp. 287–293].

Likelihood Inference

When adopting a modeling approach it seems to be natural to estimate the parameters of a model by maximizing the likelihood function, or, equivalently, its logarithm. The likelihood function contains all the relevant information about the mechanism that generated the data as well as the data actually observed. The larger its value the stronger the support given, by the data, to the corresponding value of the parameters. When dealing with Poisson regression models, maximum-likelihood estimation is, by far, the most often used method to obtain estimates for the unknown parameters.

Poisson regression models as defined above are instances of curved exponential family models; even if the model is loglinear, it is an exponential family model. So a much more general theory applies to this class of models. Here, only the special case will be considered. Readers interested in a general and detailed treatment are referred to, for example, Barndorff-Nielsen & Cox [5].

To maximize the log likelihood function one usually calculates partial derivatives with respect to all the parameters, sets them equal to 0, and solves this system of equations for the unknowns. For a Poisson regression model with log likelihood (3), the *estimating equations*

$$u_j(\beta) = \sum_{i=1}^{n} \frac{\partial}{\partial \beta_j} \eta_i(\beta) \frac{1}{\eta_i(\beta)} [y_i - \eta_i(\beta)] = 0$$

need to be solved. If the model is loglinear, then this simplifies to

$$u_j(\beta) = \sum_{i=1}^{n} x_{ij} \left[y_i - \exp\left(\sum_{h=1}^{k} x_{ih} \beta_h \right) \right] = 0.$$

A generally applicable method for obtaining estimates numerically is provided by the *Fisher scoring algorithm*. In the present case, this is seen to be an *iteratively reweighted least squares procedure*, where, in each step of the iterative algorithm, a weighted least squares problem is to be solved. As a particular consequence to this fact, methods developed for diagnosing linear regression models can be modified for generalized linear models. To define *leverage* and *influence* one only needs to refer to respective quantities calculated from the last iteration step. Formulas needed to do so are lengthy to write down, but most of the widely used software packages provide, at least as an option, the figures. For more on diagnostics for generalized linear models see [15]. Software packages found useful for fitting Poisson regression models include GLIM [20] and S-PLUS [10].

Not much is known about existence and uniqueness of maximum likelihood estimators in the general case. For loglinear models, however, if all observed sufficient statistics involved are larger than 0, then maximum likelihood estimates for the means, i.e. $\hat{\mu}_i = \eta_i(\hat{\beta})$, do exist and are unique, which is also true for $\hat{\beta}$, if the design matrix is of full rank. For a more detailed discussion, see [1] and the references therein.

A statistic capable of measuring the amount of support given by the data to a particular value of the parameter compared to its maximum likelihood estimate is the *deviance*, defined as minus two times the logarithm of the *normed likelihood*:

$$\begin{aligned} D_y(\beta) &= -2 \log \left(\frac{L_y(\beta)}{L_y(\hat{\beta})} \right) \\ &= -2[\ell_y(\beta) - \ell_y(\hat{\beta})] \\ &= -2 \sum_{i=1}^{n} \left\{ y_i \log \left[\frac{\eta_i(\beta)}{\eta_i(\hat{\beta})} \right] \right. \\ &\quad \left. - [\eta_i(\beta) - \eta_i(\hat{\beta})] \right\}. \end{aligned}$$

The deviance cannot be negative. It provides a measure of distance between the model described by β and the model characterized by the most likely parameter $\hat{\beta}$ and can, thus, be used to construct likelihood regions. Assuming β to be the "true" parameter, the deviance has an asymptotic χ^2 distribution with k degrees of freedom, where k is the dimension of the parameter β. This admits an interpretation of likelihood regions as confidence sets.

To obtain a measure of goodness of fit similar to the residual sum of squares in normal linear regression, the likelihood for the *maximal model* that perfectly fits the data can be compared to the likelihood of the model under consideration. This statistic is usually written as

$$\text{dev}_y = 2 \sum_{i=1}^{n} \left\{ y_i \log \left[\frac{y_i}{\eta_i(\hat{\beta})} \right] - [y_i - \eta_i(\hat{\beta})] \right\}, \tag{12}$$

and termed *deviance* as well. Assuming the null model to be correct, the expected value for the latter statistic is approximately equal to the number of residual degrees of freedom, i.e. the number of observations minus the number of parameters in the model.

The deviance is a very important tool in searching for a "good", i.e. a parsimonious and well fitting, model, as it can be used to compare nested hierarchical models. Suppose we have a model with parameter β and a smaller one with a parameter γ, which can be obtained from β by setting r components to 0. Then, assuming the smaller model to be the correct one, the difference of deviances (12) is asymptotically χ^2 distributed with r degrees of freedom. Note that this is a likelihood ratio test for the smaller model with the null hypothesis against the larger model as the alternative.

The deviance is a useful measure of discrepancy, frequently supposed to have an approximate χ^2 distribution. However, this is to be taken with care, as χ^2 is not, in general, guaranteed to be a large sample distribution of (12). The deviance itself can be approximated by

$$X^2 = \sum_{i=1}^{n} \frac{[y_i - \eta_i(\hat{\beta})]^2}{\eta_i(\hat{\beta})}, \qquad (13)$$

which is known as the *Pearson goodness-of-fit statistic*.

Another way of performing significance tests of hypotheses about single parameters is by applying a *Wald test*. This uses the approximate normality of the maximum likelihood estimates and computes, as the test statistic, the ratio of the estimate of the parameter of interest and its asymptotic standard error. The formula is complex, but, again, many statistical packages provide the figures for the Wald test, sometimes under the heading *t-test*, as well as observed significance values. For more detailed accounts on likelihood inference for a generalized linear model with some emphasis on the Poisson regression model see [1], [19], [34] and [35] and the references therein.

An obvious way of defining residual quantities is to use square roots of contributions to the sums in (12) or (13), and attach the appropriate signs. Denoting raw residuals by $r_i = y_i - \eta_i(\hat{\beta})$, we have

$$r_i^D = \text{sgn}(r_i)(-2\{y_i \log[y_i/\eta_i(\hat{\beta})] - [y_i - \eta_i(\hat{\beta})]\})^{1/2} \qquad (14)$$

for the *deviance residuals* and

$$r_i^P = \frac{y_i - \eta_i(\hat{\beta})}{[\eta_i(\hat{\beta})]^{1/2}} \qquad (15)$$

for the *Pearson residuals*. In any case, large residuals indicate large contributions to the respective goodness-of-fit statistics. Both deviance and Pearson residuals can (and should) be standardized.

This requires computation of leverages for all observations. See [37] and [15] for more on residuals in generalized linear models.

For the time trend model fitted to the Stress Recall Data one calculates a deviance of 24.57 with 16 degrees of freedom. The deviance is 1.5 times larger than its approximate expected value, indicating a moderate amount of *overdispersion* (see [8], [16], and [17] for more on the phenomenon of overdispersion in Poisson regression models). Compared to a model with only the constant term included, we see a difference of deviances of 26.67. Referring to its approximate chi-square distribution (with 1 degree of freedom) clearly confirms the time trend. The regression parameter for the explanatory variable "months before interview" has been estimated as -0.0837, with an asymptotic standard error of 0.017, resulting in a t-value of -4.99, which is definitely large enough to reject the hypothesis of no time trend. The smallest deviance residual is -1.99, the largest 2.04, and there is no obvious pattern suggesting any specific inadequacies in the model.

References

[1]   Agresti, A. (1990). *Categorical Data Analysis*. Wiley, New York.

[2]   Aitkin, M. & Clayton, D. (1980). The fitting of exponential, Weibull and extreme value distributions to complex censored survival data using GLIM, *Applied Statistics* **29**, 156–163.

[3]   Aitkin, M., Laird, N. Francis, B. (1983). A reanalysis of the Stanford heart transplant data (with comments and rejoinder), *Journal of the American Statistical Association* **78**, 264–292.

[4]   Aitkin, M., Anderson, D., Francis, B. & Hinde. J. (1989). *Statistical Modeling in GLIM*. Clarendon Press, Oxford.

[5]   Barndorff-Nielsen, O.E. & Cox, D.R. (1994). *Inference and Asymptotics*. Chapman & Hall, London.

[6]   Bishop, Y.M.M., Fienberg, S.E. & Holland, P. (1975). *Discrete Multivariate Analysis*. MIT Press, Cambridge, Mass.

[7]   Breslow, N. (1974). Covariance analysis of censored survival data, *Biometrics* **30**, 89–100.

[8]   Breslow, N. (1990). Tests of hypotheses in overdispersed Poisson regression and other quasi-likelihood models, *Journal of the American Statistical Association* **85**, 565–571.

[9]   Breslow, N.E. & Day, N.E. (1980). *Statistical Methods in Cancer Research*, Vol. 1. *The Analysis of Case–Control Studies*. International Agency for Research on Cancer, Lyon.

[10] Chambers, J.M. & Hastie, T.J. (1992). *Statistical Models in S*. Wadsworth & Brooks, Pacific Gove.

[11] Charnes, A., Frome, E.L. & Yu, P.L. (1976). The equivalence of generalized least squares and maximum likelihood estimates in the exponential family, *Journal of the American Statistical Association* **71**, 169–172.

[12] Clayton, D. & Hills, M. (1993). *Statistical Models in Epidemiology*. Oxford University Press, Oxford.

[13] Cox, D.R. (1972). Regression models and life tables (with discussion), *Journal of the Royal Statistical Society, Series B* **34**, 187–220.

[14] Cox, D.R. (1975). Partial likelihood, *Biometrika* **62**, 269–276.

[15] Davison, A.C. & Snell, E.J. (1991). Residuals and diagnostics, in *Statistical Theory and Modelling. In Honour of Sir David Cox*, D.V. Hinkley, N. Reid & E.J. Snell, eds. Chapman & Hall, London, pp. 83–106.

[16] Dean, C.B. (1992). Testing for overdispersion in Poisson and binomial regression models, *Journal of the American Statistical Association* **87**, 451–457.

[17] Dean, C. & Lawless, J.F. (1989). Tests for detecting overdispersion in Poisson regression models, *Journal of the American Statistical Association* **84**, 467–472.

[18] Dobson, A. (1990). *An Introduction to Generalized Linear Models*, 2nd Ed. Chapman & Hall, London.

[19] Firth, D. (1991). Generalized linear models, in *Statistical Theory and Modelling. In Honour of Sir David Cox*, D.V. Hinkley, N. Reid & E.J. Snell, eds. Chapman & Hall, London, pp. 55–82.

[20] Francis, B., Green, M. & Payne, C., eds (1993). *The GLIM System. Release 4 Manual*. Clarendon Press, Oxford.

[21] Frome, E.L. (1981). Poisson regression analysis, *American Statistician* **35**, 262–263.

[22] Frome, E.L. (1983). The analysis of rates using Poisson regression models, *Biometrics* **39**, 665–674.

[23] Frome, E.L. & DuFrain, R.J. (1986). Maximum likelihood estimation for cytogenic dose–response curves, *Biometrics* **42**, 73–84.

[24] Frome, E.L. & Morris, M.D. (1989). Evaluating goodness of fit of Poisson regression models in cohort studies, *American Statistician* **43**, 144–147.

[25] Frome, E.L., Kutner, M.H. & Beauchamp, J.J. (1973). Regression analysis of Poisson-distributed data, *Journal of the American Statistical Association* **68**, 935–940.

[26] Greenland, S. & Maldonado, G. (1994). The interpretation of multiplicative-model parameters as standardized parameters, *Statistics in Medicine* **13**, 989–999.

[27] Haberman, S. (1978). *Analysis of Qualitative Data*. Vol. 1. *Introductory Topics*. Academic Press, New York.

[28] Holford, T.R. (1980). The analysis of rates and survivorship using log-linear models, *Biometrics* **36**, 299–306.

[29] Koch, G.G., Atkinson, S.S. & Stokes, M.E. (1986). Poisson regression, in *Encyclopedia of Statistics*, Vol. 7, S. Kotz & N.L. Johnson, eds. Wiley, New York, pp. 32–41.

[30] Ladurner, D. & Seeber, G. (1984). Das papilläre Schilddrüsenkarzinom–Prognose und prognostische Faktoren, *Langenbeck's Archiv für Chirurgie* **363**, 43–55.

[31] Laird, N. & Olivier, D. (1981). Covariance analysis of censored survival data using log-linear analysis techniques, *Journal of the American Statistical Association* **76**, 231–240.

[32] Lawless, J.F. (1987). Regression methods for Poisson process data, *Journal of the American Statistical Association* **82**, 808–815.

[33] Lindsey, J.K. (1995). *Modelling Frequency and Count Data*. Clarendon Press, Oxford.

[34] Lindsey, J.K. (1996). *Parametric Statistical Inference*. Clarendon Press, Oxford.

[35] McCullagh, P. & Nelder, J.A. (1989). *Generalized Linear Models*, 2nd Ed. Chapman & Hall, London.

[36] Nelder, J.A. & Wedderburn, R.W. (1972). Generalized linear models, *Journal of the Royal Statistical Society, Series A* **135**, 370–384.

[37] Pierce, D.A. & Schafer, D.W. (1986). Residuals in generalized linear models, *Journal of the American Statistical Association* **81**, 977–986.

[38] Seeber, G.U.H. (1989). On the regression analysis of tumour recurrence rates, *Statistics in Medicine* **8**, 1363–1369.

[39] Selmer, R. (1990). A comparison of Poisson regression models fitted to multiway summary tables and Cox's survival model using data from a blood pressure screening in the city of Bergen, Norway, *Statistics in Medicine* **9**, 1157–1165.

G.U.H. Seber

Poisson Regression for Survival Data in Epidemiology

Various authors [3, 9, 11, 12] have noted that **Poisson regression** can be used to analyze cohort survival data (*see* **Cohort Study**). This formulation also leads to a unification of **risk** estimation based on internal comparison of rates among members of a cohort with various exposure levels and classical epidemiologic methods based on external rates that yield standardized mortality ratios or standardized incidence ratios [2, 5] (*see* **Standardization Methods**).

Poisson regression is an important alternative to partial-likelihood-based analysis of the **proportional**

hazards model (*see* **Cox Regression Model**) and to parametric analyses of such models (*see* **Survival Analysis, Overview**) for two main reasons. First, it provides an efficient and intuitive method for dealing with cumulative exposures and other time-dependent covariates and for allowing risk to depend on multiple time scales (e.g. attained age, time since exposure, or calendar time). Secondly, it facilitates the consideration of a broad range of risk models including those that allow for the direct parametric description of baseline rates, absolute excess rates, and **relative risks**.

Breslow & Day [4] offer a general discussion of the use of Poisson regression in the analysis of cohort survival data. Some of the most extensive applications of these methods have involved studies of radiation effects on mortality and cancer incidence in the atomic bomb survivors [14].

Poisson Regression of Survival Data

The data from cohort survival studies typically consist of information on whether or not the event of interest occurred, the event or censoring time, t, and a vector of possibly time-dependent covariates, $\mathbf{z}$, for each cohort member. Since interest centers on **hazard rates** it is natural and useful for the purposes of analysis or summarization to reorganize such data into an event–time table defined by a cross-classification over a set of time intervals and covariate categories. The data for each cell in such a table include the total number of events, c_{is}, the total time (person-years) at risk, R_{is}, and representative values of the covariates, z_{is} for time period i and category s. For each cell the ratio of the number of events to the time at risk is a crude hazard rate. The analysis involves regression methods to smooth these rates as a function of time and other covariates.

When such tables are produced as simple summaries of a data set, it is common to limit the number of time periods and other factors used to define the table. However, for modeling rates it is appropriate to use detailed tables with many cells based on a relatively fine **stratification** over time and other factors. For example, a rate table to be used in an analysis of an occupational cohort study (*see* **Occupational Epidemiology**) might be defined in terms of age, year, age at first exposure, sex, and cumulative exposure with hundreds or even thousands of cells. An event–time table for a clinical trial might involve

follow-up time, age at entry, sex, and treatment. Although not usually necessary in practice, the methods can be applied to a table based on individual subjects where the only grouping is on time. This suggests the close connection between the use of Poisson regression methods for the analysis of rates and the Andersen–Gill counting process method [1] for analysis of hazard functions.

If it is assumed that the hazard, λ_{is} is constant within each cell, then the expected number of events in the cell is given by

$$\mathrm{E}(c_{is}) = R_{is} \times \lambda_{is}.$$

In terms of a parametric function, $\lambda(t_i, z_{is}, \theta)$ for the rates, the log likelihood for the survival data under the piecewise constant hazard assumption is

$$\sum_{l,s} c_{is} \ln(\lambda(t_l, z_{is}, \theta)) - R_{is} \times \lambda(t_i, z_{is}, \theta),$$

which is equivalent to the log likelihood that would arise if the event counts in the table were independent Poisson random variables. Thus, Poisson regression can be used to estimate the parameters in this model.

With this approach, modeling rates in terms of time is straightforward since, in contrast to Cox regression, there is no distinction between time-dependent and time-independent covariates. This is because the time-dependent computations are carried out when the event – time table is constructed and are not repeated each time a model is fitted.

Using External Rates or Expected Cases

In some situations one has external data on the expected rates λ_q^e stratified by time and other factors (e.g. age, calendar time period, and sex but not exposure or treatment related factors). In this case, it is possible to compute the expected number of cases for each cell in the table as $C_{is}^e = R_{is} \times \lambda_q^e$, where $q = q(is)$ denotes the external rate strata corresponding to cell is. In this case, Poisson regression can be used to model the relative hazard, ρ_{is}, since

$$\mathrm{E}(c_{is}) = C_{is}^e \times \rho_{is} = R_{is} \times \lambda_q^e \times \rho_{is}.$$

When **person-years** are replaced by expected numbers of cases, this type of analysis is known as the subject-years method or standardized mortality ratio (SMR) regression [4].

Models for Rate Regression

Following the pioneering work of Cox [8], the most commonly used hazard function model is the loglinear proportional hazards model

$$\lambda(t, z, \theta) = \lambda_0(t, \alpha) \times \exp(\beta z). \qquad (1)$$

Here λ_0 is a baseline hazard for an individual with covariate $z = 0$.

Other models are also important, however. For example, in **dose–response** studies it is often useful to consider models in which the **excess relative risk** is a linear function of dose d; that is

$$\lambda(t, z, \theta) = \lambda_0(t, \alpha) \times (1 + \beta d).$$

Preston [16] has described a flexible general class of parametric additive hazard models of the basic form

$$\lambda_0(t, \alpha, z_0) + \lambda_{\text{EAR}}(t, \beta, z_1) \qquad (2)$$

and

$$\lambda_0(t, \alpha, z_0)[1 + \lambda_{\text{ERR}}(t, \beta, z_1)], \qquad (3)$$

in which λ_0 represents the baseline or background rates and λ_{EAR} and λ_{ERR} describe the excess absolute risks or excess relative risks. In these models baseline rates are usually assumed to be loglinear functions of the covariates while the excess risks are modeled as linear or products of linear and loglinear functions of the covariates.

One reason for the popularity of the Cox regression model is that it allows one to focus (perhaps too much) on the **relative risk** while treating the baseline hazard as completely unspecified. A similar simplification is possible in the analysis of **relative risk models** for rates using Poisson regression. This is accomplished by the inclusion of a **multiplicative** parameter for each time interval leading to models such as

$$\tau_i \exp(\beta z) \quad \text{or} \quad \tau_i(1 + \beta d). \qquad (4)$$

This approach can also be extended to allow stratification over additional factors, in which case the model is similar to the stratified Cox regression model. Preston et al. [17] describe an efficient algorithm for models with large numbers of stratum parameters.

Parameter Estimation and Inference

Parameter estimates for Poisson regression models are computed using maximum likelihood methods. Models in which the rates depend on the parameters through a linear function βz, are Generalized Linear Models (GLMs). Parameter estimates for GLMs can be computed using iteratively reweighted least squares with person-years (or cases for subject-years analysis or standardized mortality/incidence ratio regression) as an "offset". These methods are available in all of the major statistical packages including GLIM, SAS, and S-PLUS (*see* **Software, Biostatistical**). However, the more general rate function models such as (3) and (4) are not GLMs. In this case, it is necessary to make use of special software to define the likelihood and possibly its derivatives. The Epicure package [17] is designed to work with models in the general class described by (1)–(4) above.

Inference about parameters of interest can be carried out using the standard asymptotic methods, including Wald, score, and likelihood ratio tests. However, because of the nonlinear nature of the models and, in many applications, the limited information on **excess risks**, asymptotic standard errors and hence hypothesis tests and confidence intervals based on Wald tests can be misleading. Score or likelihood ratio tests and profile-likelihood-based confidence intervals should be emphasized when working with additive hazard models.

An important issue concerns the assessment of goodness of fit for Poisson regression models derived from detailed event–time tables. Because rate modeling often involves relatively rare events and event–time tables with many cells, the rates or the number of events in each cell of the table can be quite small. In this case, neither the global deviance nor the Pearson chi-square statistic provides reasonable guidance as to goodness of fit. The total deviance is often much smaller than the putative degrees of freedom (the number of cells in the table minus the number of free parameters in the model). Pregibon [15] developed generalized regression diagnostics that can be used for regression models in exponential families. While such diagnostics may be useful in looking for lack of fit and other problems with fitted models [10], they should be interpreted with caution since the underlying data are not independent Poisson counts. In view of these issues, the most effective general method for the assessment of goodness of fit when using Poisson regression to analyze rates is to make use of likelihood ratio tests designed to detect specific departures from models of interest, such as time dependence or nonlinearity, or to make use of Akaike's criterion or related statistics to compare alternative (possibly nonnested) models.

Creating Event–Time Tables

The creation of an adequate event–time table is often the most difficult aspect of carrying out analyses of rates using Poisson regression. Among other features, an ideal program for the construction of event–time tables would:

1. allow for categorization on multiple time scales (age, year, length of follow-up, etc.), as well as multiple time-independent and time-dependent factors with variable length intervals in each of these scales;
2. allow for late entry, disjoint follow-up intervals, and multiple events;
3. include procedures for the computation of and categorization on time-dependent quantities;
4. allow computation and storage of counts for multiple event types along with representative values (often time-at-risk weighted means) for covariates of interest for each cell in the table;
5. have efficient procedures for handling the large, sparse tables that can arise when one stratifies on multiple time scales;
6. be able to deal with the data structures that can arise in describing complex exposure histories; and
7. facilitate the incorporation of external rates.

Several computer programs are currently available for the creation of event–time tables. However, many of these programs, e.g. OCMAP [6] and O/E [13], are designed for specific applications and are of limited use in more general problems. Procedures for the creation of such tables in the major statistical programs are extremely limited or nonexistent. The DATAB module in Epicure [17] and "Person-years" [7] are probably the most flexible general-purpose programs for event–time tabulation available at this time. Hopefully, there will be major improvements in this area over the next few years.

Summary

Poisson regression is a powerful tool for the analysis of rates from cohort survival studies that facilitates simple, straightforward analyses of temporal patterns, baseline risks, excess relative or **absolute risks**, and other aspects of hazard functions that may be difficult to assess with other methods. The application of Poisson regression requires that data on individual subjects be organized into event–time tables stratified on time and other factors of interest and, for the most interesting models, specialized software capable of dealing with nonlinear Poisson regression models is also required. The tools needed to conduct these analyses are available today but it is likely that they will be more fully developed in the years to come.

References

[1]   Andersen, P.K., Borgan, Ø., Gill, R.D. & Keiding, N. (1993). *Statistical Models Based on Counting Processes*. Springer-Verlag, New York.

[2]   Berry, G. (1983). The analysis of mortality by the subjects years method, *Biometrics* **39**, 173–184.

[3]   Breslow, N.E. (1974). Covariance analysis of censored survival data, *Biometrics* **30**, 89–99.

[4]   Breslow, N.E. & Day, N.E. (1987). *Statistical Methods in Cancer Research*, Vol. II: *The Design and Analysis of Cohort Studies*. IARC Scientific Publications 82, International Agency for Research on Cancer, Lyon.

[5]   Breslow, N.E., Lubin, J.H., Marek, P. & Langholz, B. (1983). Multiplicative models and cohort analysis, *Journal of the American Statistical Association* **78**, 1–12.

[6]   Caplan, R.J., Marsh, G.M. & Enterline, P.E. (1983). A generalized effective exposure modeling program for assessing dose-response in epidemiologic investigations, *Computers in Biomedical Research* **16**, 587–596.

[7]   Coleman, M. (1986). Cohort study analysis with a FORTRAN computer program, *International Journal of Epidemiology* **15**, 134–137.

[8]   Cox, D.R. (1972). Regression models and life tables (with discussion), *Journal of the Royal Statistical Society, Series B* **34**, 187–220.

[9]   Frome, E. (1983). The analysis of rates using Poisson regression models, *Biometrics* **39**, 665–675.

[10]   Frome, E. & Morris, M.D. (1989). Evaluating goodness of fit of Poisson regression models in cohort studies, *American Statistician* **43**, 144–147.

[11]   Holford, T.R. (1980). The analysis of rates and survivorship using log-linear models, *Biometrics* **36**, 299–305.

[12]   Laird, N. & Oliver, D. (1981). Covariance analysis of censored survival data using log-linear models, *Journal of the American Statistical Association* **76**, 231–240.

[13]   Monson, R.R. (1974). Analysis of relative survival and proportional mortality, *Computers in Biomedical Research* **7**, 325–332.

[14]   Pierce, D.A., Shimizu, Y., Preston, D.L., Vaeth, M. & Mabuchi, K. (1996). Studies of the mortality of atomic bomb survivors. Report 12, Part I. Cancer Mortality 1950–1990, *Radiation Research* **146**, 1–27.

[15]   Pregibon, D. (1981). Logistic regression diagnostics, *Annals of Statistics* **9**, 705–724.

[16]   Preston, D.L. (1990). Modeling radiation effects on disease incidence, *Radiation Research* **124**, 343–344.

[17]   Preston, D.L., Lubin, J., Pierce, D.A. & McConney, M.E. (1993). *Epicure, Users' Guide*. Hirosoft International, Seattle.

D. PRESTON

Population-Based Study

A population-based study is a study of properties of a well-defined population, such as individuals residing in a defined geographic region in a given time period. The size of such a population can be estimated, and, if all cases of a disease arising from such a population are identified, **rates** of disease can be calculated. Valid sampling frames can be constructed for estimating the **prevalence** of risk factors and other characteristics of such a population. **Population-based case–control studies** yield not only estimates of **relative risk** for given exposures but also estimates of exposure-specific **absolute risk**. The latter are obtained by combining information on the overall **risk** of disease in the population with information on the prevalences and relative risks of various exposure levels.

M.H. GAIL

Potthoff and Whittinghill Test *see* Clustering

Potthoff Design for Telephone Sampling *see* Telephone Sampling

Predictive Values

The positive predictive value of a diagnostic or **screening** test refers to the proportion of individuals with positive test results who actually have the target disease or disorder, i.e. Pr(disease|positive test result). In the diagram in the article on **Sensitivity**, the positive predictive value is $a/(a+b)$. A synonym is the post-test or posterior probability of disease, given a positive test result.

Correspondingly, the negative predictive value is the proportion of individuals with negative test results who do not actually have the disease or disorder in question. This is Pr(no disease|negative test result), or $d/(c+d)$ in the diagram. A synonym is the post-test or posterior probability of no disease, given a negative test result. There is also some interest in the complement of this quantity, $c/(c+d)$, which is the post-test probability of disease, given a negative test result.

The predictive values are useful clinically, and may influence therapeutic decisions. An individual with a positive result from a test with high positive predictive value is a relatively good candidate for therapeutic intervention. Conversely, there is relatively little justification for intervention for an individual with a negative result from a test that has high negative predictive value for no disease.

Predictive values are functions both of the test characteristics, in particular sensitivity and **specificity**, and of the **prevalence** of disease in the population. For instance, if the testing is done in a high-risk population, where the prevalence (or, equivalently, the pretest probability of disease) is high, then one would expect the predictive values of disease to be relatively high. Conversely, if the disease is rare, then the predictive values for disease are relatively low; in an extreme case, even the positive predictive value may be sufficiently small that therapy cannot be justified on the basis of the test alone, particularly if the therapy is expensive or hazardous.

(*See also* **Clinical Epidemiology, Overview**; **Diagnostic Tests, Evaluation of**)

S.D. WALTER

Prescription Sequence Analysis *see* Pharmacoepidemiology, Overview

Prevalence

Prevalence is the number of persons who have a disease or condition at a given point in time in a defined population. Sometimes prevalence refers to persons who either have currently or have previously had a disease, e.g. the prevalence of persons with a cancer diagnosis at any time up to the present. The term *prevalence* is used also to refer to the proportion of individuals with disease in the population, namely the **prevalence rate or ratio**.

M.H. GAIL

Prevalence–Incidence Bias

Bias in epidemiologic studies is a form of "systematic error in the design, conduct, or analysis of a study that results in a mistaken estimate of an exposure's effect on the risk of disease" [5]. While biases have been categorized in many ways, Rothman describes three general types: **selection bias,** *information bias*, and **confounding** [3]. Selection bias results from improper specification or selection of the study sample and leads to a distortion of the effect measured [3, 4].

Jerzy Neyman identified a form of bias in analytic epidemiologic studies which is in essence the result of the use of prevalent rather than incident cases of disease to assess etiologic relationships [2] (*see* **Causation**). *Prevalence–incidence bias* is a

form of selection or sampling bias that results in part from evaluating the exposure–disease association well after the exposure first occurs. During that time interval, cases of short duration, due to death or short course of illness, cases mild in severity or asymptomatic, and cases in which the presence of disease alters or entirely removes the exposure, are missed [4].

Neyman developed a fictitious example that assessed the impact of differential survival on an etiologic association [2]. This example, which assessed the relationship between cigarette smoking and lung cancer, is shown in Table 1.

In this example, a comparison of the development of lung cancer between time 0 and time T in smokers and nonsmokers indicates a reduced risk among smokers (relative **odds ratio** = 0.44). If one assumes, however, that 95% of the lung cancer cases in nonsmokers died before time T, as opposed to only 10% of the lung cancer cases in smokers, and that lung cancer was the only source of mortality in this population, then a **case-control study** applied to those alive at time T would produce a large putative effect for smoking (relative odds = 8.0).

While clearly fictitious in terms of the known risk of smoking on lung cancer, this example serves to demonstrate the effect of using prevalent cases, at time T, to describe the risk of disease development. If an exposure, as in this example, results in selective survival and prevalent cases are used, then the estimate of the risk of disease is an overestimate. If an exposure results in selective mortality, then the estimate of the risk of disease associated with that exposure is an underestimate.

Prevalence–incidence bias is a particular problem in evaluating associations between selected risk factors and coronary heart disease (CHD) [1, 4]. Many cases of CHD are rapidly fatal and some are clinically mild or asymptomatic. Each of these situations can

Table 1   An example of prevalence–incidence bias using fictitious data on smoking and lung cancer [2]

	Number at time 0	Lung cancer by time T	Case-control study at time T	
			Number	Lung cancer cases
Smokers	10 000	1000[a]	9900	900
Nonsmokers	10 000	2000[b]	8100	100
Relative odds ratios		0.44		8.00

[a]Includes 100 deaths from lung cancer.
[b]Includes 1900 deaths from lung cancer.

Table 2 Prospective versus retrospective study estimates of the relative odds of CHD among Framingham men with and without high cholesterol [1, 4]

Cholesterol	Prospective study[a]		Retrospective study[b]	
	CHD	No CHD	CHD	No CHD
High[c]	85	462	38	34
Low	116	1511	113	117
Relative odds ratio	2.40		1.16	

[a]Developed CHD by time T.
[b]CHD present at time T.
[c]Cholesterol measured at exam. 1 in prospective study and at exam. 6 in retrospective study.

lead a study of prevalent cases to a faulty conclusion due to an under-representation of cases. In addition, in CHD, and in perhaps other diseases, it is possible that the presence of the disease will result in a modification of the exposure being evaluated. This could make the association between an exposure and disease appear either larger or smaller than it really is. Such an example is shown in Table 2.

Here, the true risk of the development of CHD associated with high serum cholesterol, evident in the prospective study (relative odds = 2.40), is not seen in a case-control study using prevalent cases of CHD and assessment of serum cholesterol at the same time (relative odds = 1.16) [1, 4]. It is likely that persons with diagnosed CHD have altered their dietary patterns and reduced both their intake of foods high in cholesterol and their weight. It should be noted that this same change in relative odds was evident when analyses by Friedman et al. of the prospective component were restricted to persons who survived the full time period, lending further credence to the possibility that prevalent cases of CHD may have altered their lifestyles, which resulted in lower serum cholesterol [1, 4].

In summary, prevalence–incidence bias is likely to exert its effect when a considerable amount of time elapses between exposure and selection of subjects for a study [4]. It is a bias that can result in either an overestimate or underestimate of the true risk of disease associated with a particular factor and is evident in case-control studies where prevalent, rather than incident, cases are selected as subjects.

The ability to correct, or even measure, the spurious effect caused by this bias is limited at best [4].

Avoidance of this form of bias is not simply achieved through the use of incident rather than prevalent cases in a case-control study. Ascertaining the true association between the exposure and the disease can only be achieved through the use of a prospective study of incident disease (*see* **Cohort Study**).

References

[1]   Friedman, G.D., Kannel, W.B., Dawber, T.R. & McNamara, P.M. (1966). Comparison of prevalence, case history, and incidence data in assessing the potency of risk factors in coronary heart disease, *American Journal of Epidemiology* **83**, 366–377.

[2]   Neyman, J. (1955). Statistics – servant of all sciences, *Science* **122**, 401–406.

[3]   Rothman, K.J. (1986). *Modern Epidemiology*. Little, Brown, & Company, Boston.

[4]   Sackett, D.L. (1979). Bias in analytical research, *Journal of Chronic Diseases* **32**, 51–63.

[5]   Schlesselman, J.J. (1982). *Case-Control Studies: Design, Conduct, Analysis*. Oxford University Press, New York.

(*See also* **Case–Control Study, Prevalent**)

SYLVIA. E. FURNER

Prevalence of Disease, Estimation from Screening Data

Consider a large **sample survey** in which the investigators have used a simple, cheap but fallible indicator of morbidity in order to assess the **prevalence** of one or more illnesses. If morbidity is estimated solely on the basis of this fallible information, then there is a possibility that the results will be **biased**. A common refinement of this sample design (particularly in psychiatric epidemiology) is to use the fallible information as a *screen* to stratify the original sample into two or more groups (usually referred to as screen positives and screen negatives), and then to subsample from these strata for a more thorough diagnostic investigation that is assumed to reveal the correct status of the subject (the gold standard). The results of this second phase of investigation are then used to calibrate the fallible screening instrument and to develop an unbiased estimator of prevalence from the whole sample. This design is an example of *two-phase sampling*. An alternative, related design involves supplementing the large screened sample by a completely independent *calibration* or **validation** sample of comparable subjects who are assessed using both the screen and the gold standard (*see* **Screening, Overview**; **Screening, Models of**).

Two-phase or multiphase sampling is also often referred to as double sampling by survey statisticians and it is extensively used in industry as one design for lot quality assurance sampling (LQAS). In the health field it is also commonly but less satisfactorily referred to as *two-stage* or *multistage sampling*. The latter terminology is more properly and more usually applied to circumstances in which the sampling units at each stage are different (i.e. *nested* sampling designs). For example, one might take a random sample of clinics or health regions in the first stage of the survey and then randomly sample patients from within each of the selected clinics or regions. In two-phase sampling the sampling units remain the same at both phases of the survey.

The use of a randomization procedure while "in the field" to determine second-phase sample membership offers the possibility of concatenating initial and later phases of data collection into a single assessment of each subject. However, it is more common for first and later phases of data collection to involve both different measurement techniques and different research staff, and to take place on different occasions and in different locations. Of increasing interest is the use of registry (*see* **Disease Registers**) or other bureaucratic information systems, such as hospital birth records, as the source of first-phase "screening" data.

The terminology of first-phase "screening" implies the purposeful application of a screening test: a cheap, robust and often noninvasive test that is, however, recognized as being fallible or less accurate than the gold standard. This is how the idea of screening was introduced in the first paragraph of the present article. From a statistical perspective, however, this is a needless limitation to this sampling design. The statistical problem remains essentially the same whether a true screening test is used to assess morbidity, or whether the screen in fact attempts to measure risk factors rather than ill health, or whether the strata in the two-phase design arise "naturalistically", say, through the operation of a patient referral process. An example of the latter would be an epidemiological study

of children sampled from all hospital birth records but stratified by hospital. The critical element of the design is not the use of a screening test, but the stratification of the sampling design on a variable or variables for which inference about the outcome variable should be made marginal to the strata rather than conditional on them. Simple prevalence estimation, being marginal to all other variables, is the obvious example, but the point also applies to more general analyses. To the extent that second-phase sampling results in data missing by design, the methods to be discussed also relate to methods for data *missing at random* [19] (*see* **Missing Data**) and to the use of *surrogate* or *auxiliary* measures [22].

One final note on terminology: here we use the term "screening" to indicate the provision of a simple fallible indicator of the subjects' state in order to stratify the first-phase sample prior to subsampling and further investigation. The term "screening" is also commonly used to describe the first phase of the process of *case detection*. Suspected cases, who have been identified by the screening procedure, are then further investigated with a view to treatment (in a clinical setting) or entry into a research study, a clinical trial for example. In this situation interest in the screen negatives is more limited, typically to concerns relating to false negative patients who ought to be receiving treatment or other forms of help, and to the costs and possible risks associated with the screening process itself. Screening for caseness is not the subject of this article, but is discussed elsewhere (*see* **Screening, Overview**).

The Analysis of Two-Phase ("Screened") Samples

Prevalence Estimation Using Simple Conditional Probabilities

Figure 1 illustrates the sample selection process. From a first-phase sample of size N, $N(s+)$ are screen positive and $N(s-)$ are screen negative (where $N(s-) = N - N(s+)$). Of those subjects who are screen positive, a subsample of size $N_{v+}(s+)$ are selected at random for a full diagnostic assessment (validation). These subjects will have complete data on all variables. Of these, $N_{v+}(s+, d+)$ are found to have a positive diagnosis and $N_{v+}(s+, d-)$ to have a negative diagnosis. Similarly, among the $N(s-)$ screen negatives a random sample of size

Phase 1   Screen   Phase 2   Diagnosis
Sampling   Sampling

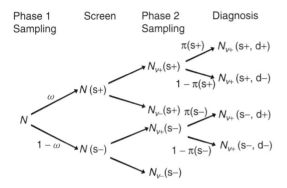

Figure 1 Two-phase data collection

$N_{v+}(s-)$ is also selected for validation. Of these second-phase subjects, $N_{v+}(s-, d+)$ are found to have a positive diagnosis (despite the screening information) and $N_{v+}(s-, d-)$ are negative. Note that the $N_{v+}(s+, d-)$ subjects are false positives (with respect to the screening information) and the $N_{v+}(s-, d+)$ are false negatives. Finally there are $N_{v-}(s+)$ and $N_{v-}(s-)$ subjects for which there are missing second-phase diagnostic data.

The proportion of cases in the screen-positive and screen-negative strata are denoted by $\pi(s+)$ and $\pi(s-)$, respectively. The proportion of screen positives in the first phase is ω and the proportion of screen negatives is therefore $1 - \omega$. Using simple conditional probabilities, the overall prevalence, π, is given by

$$\pi = \omega\pi(s+) + [1 - \omega]\pi(s-) \qquad (1)$$

and can be estimated by inserting sample estimates of each of the components on the right-hand side of the expression. That is, ω, $\pi(s+)$ and $\pi(s-)$ are estimated by $n(s+)/n$, $n_{v+}(s+, d+)/n_{v+}(s+)$ and $n_{v+}(s-, d+)/n_{v+}(s-)$, respectively.

Using the well-known delta method, the variance of π is given by

$$\mathrm{var}(\pi) = \omega^2\pi(s+)[1 - \pi(s+)]/N_{v+}(s+)$$
$$+ (1 - \omega^2)\pi(s-)[1 - \pi(s-)]/N_{v+}(s-)$$
$$+ [\pi(s+) - \pi(s-)]^2\omega(1 - \omega)/N. \qquad (2)$$

This variance is estimated by insertion of the sample estimates of ω, $\pi(s+)$ and $\pi(s-)$, as before.

This simple approach [6] is very straightforward and that most commonly used in two-phase prevalence estimation studies. If, however, the investigator wishes

to consider multiple subpopulations and/or investigate the effects of risk exposures on the prevalence of disease, then there are less cumbersome methods.

Prevalence Estimation Using Inverse Probability (Expansion) Weights

For the ith subject with complete data a *probability weight* or *expansion weight*, w_i, can be defined as the reciprocal of the sampling fraction (probability of selection) for the second-phase sample. In the simplest design the weight takes on just two distinct values, one for the screen-positive subjects and another for the screen negatives. The estimates of the sampling fractions are $n_{v+}(s+)/n(s+)$ and $n_{v+}(s-)/n(s-)$, yielding inverse probability weights of $n(s+)/n_{v+}(s+)$ and $n(s-)/n_{v+}(s-)$, respectively. The sum of the weights over the subjects in the second-phase sample will be the first-phase sample size. The sum of the products, w_iY_i, where $Y_i = 1$ for validated cases and $Y_i = 0$ for the nonvalidated cases, again over the subjects of the second phase, provides an estimate of the number of cases in the first-phase sample. An estimate of the prevalence of disorder is therefore provided by the ratio

$$\pi = \frac{\sum w_iY_i}{\sum w_i}. \qquad (3)$$

This estimator is the Horvitz–Thompson estimator familiar to survey methodologists (see, for example, [18]). As in the use of conditional probabilities, it is straightforward to use a *Taylor series* linearization method (the delta method) to estimate the variance of this ratio. Other methods of variance estimation, including the jackknife or bootstrap sampling, can also be used in the case of either of the prevalence estimation methods [18, Chapter 5].

Note that, although conditional probabilities and inverse probability weighting look superficially very different – the weighting method seeming to estimate directly the marginal model of interest while the conditional probability approach derives the marginal rate from the "uninteresting" conditional model for disease given the screen score – in this simple case the two methods of prevalence estimation are algebraically equivalent. The variance estimates, however, being based on different Taylor expansions, may differ slightly, but this is of no practical significance in large samples.

A More General Framework

Let X denote risk exposures assessed at phase 1, Z the screen score and Y the measure of true case status. If complete information were available on all subjects, the maximum likelihood estimator of β, the vector of coefficients for the effects of risk exposures, would be found by maximizing the log-likelihood $\sum_i \log \operatorname{Pr}_\beta(Y_i|X_i)$. In the context of two-phase sampling, and letting i index subjects with complete data and j index subjects not selected for the second phase, then the expectation-maximization (EM) algorithm for finding the maximum likelihood estimator would involve the iterative solution of

$$l(\beta) = \sum_{i \in V+} \log \operatorname{Pr}_\beta(Y_i|X_i)$$
$$+ \sum_{j \in V-} \operatorname{E}[\log \operatorname{Pr}_\beta(Y|X_j)\}|\beta^c, X_j, Z_j], \quad (4)$$

where β^c is the current estimate. Various authors have discussed the solution of such equations, primarily for categorical risk factors [4, 5, 10, 35]. Eq. (4) suggests a number of alternative estimators based on different approximations or sample-based estimates of the expectation term, including various forms of imputation. In the *mean score* method of Pepe and others [22, 23, 26], the expectation is estimated by the sample average. This is equivalent to solving score equations of the form

$$\sum_{i \in V+} S_\beta(Y_i|X_i)$$

$$+ \sum_{j \in V-} \left\{ \sum_{i \in \left\{ \begin{array}{l} X_i = X_j \\ Z_i = Z_j \end{array} \right.} \frac{S_\beta(Y_i|X_j)}{N_{V+}(X_i = X_j, Z_i = Z_j)} \right\} = 0,$$
$$(5)$$

which may be rewritten as

$$\sum_{i \in V+} \left[1 + \frac{N_{V-}(X_i, Z_i)}{N_{V+}(X_i, Z_i)} \right] S_\beta(Y_i|X_i)$$
$$= \sum_{i \in V+} w_i S_\beta(Y_i|X_i) = 0. \quad (6)$$

The w_i here correspond to the expansion weight of the previous section. Hence, the estimating equations can be easily solved by means of weighted regression,

with weighted **logistic regression** being the common choice.

Weighted regression estimators similar to (6) have been derived within the survey research field [2, 3]. Flanders & Greenland [11] derive the same estimator using pseudo-likelihood arguments, proposing the use of the variously termed "empirical", "robust", "information sandwich," "heteroscedastistic consistent," and "Huberized" parameter covariance matrix [14]. In this case the parameter covariance matrix obtained assumes the weights W_i to be known. In practice, the weights are usually estimated and often adjusted using a variety of methods quite separate from the analysis for prevalence estimation. The weights can be "poststratified" [16] to conform to known population rates, or "raked" [9] to conform to some known margins, or they may be smoothed using parametric or nonparametric regression methods [17], or even trimmed [25] or shrunken [7]. Whatever the weights chosen, the subsequent analysis of the prevalence data can include any risk exposure measures, continuous or discrete, from either phase.

Perhaps contrary to intuition, Pepe et al. [23] illustrate how if weights are estimated by simple sample cell frequencies, then subjects in the nonvalidation set contribute information through the variation in these random weights, and worthwhile efficiency gains can be made by fully exploiting this variation rather than assuming the weights to be known. However, where some cells are empty or where one or more risk exposures or surrogate measures are continuous, the mean score method cannot be applied directly. Although under such circumstances some estimator based on smoothing might be attempted, a series of papers by Robins and others [27–29] argue that such estimators may not approach their asymptotic distribution in the moderate samples of typical studies. Instead they draw on the ideas of semi-parametric regression estimators to propose a modified score function of the form

$$\sum_{i \in V+} [w_i h(X_i)\varepsilon_i(\beta) + (1 - w_i)\phi(W_i)]$$
$$+ \sum_{j \in V-} \phi(W_j) = 0, \quad (7)$$

where w_i is the usual expansion weight, $\varepsilon_i(\beta)$ is the simple observed minus model expected residual, and $h(X)$ and $\phi(W)$ are functions of the data and parameters that can be chosen to achieve optimal efficiency.

Though of considerable interest, there is currently little practical experience with such estimators.

Many of the issues already discussed have parallels in Bayesian methods for multiphase sampling, including the choice as to the direction in which to model the graph [24]. Estimation is typically carried out using Markov chain Monte Carlo methods and *Gibbs sampling* in particular (see, for example, [12]). Although the ability to incorporate prior information may be of particular value where some screen strata may not have been subsampled, a particular focus of Bayesian work in this area has been in model choice and *model averaging* [36]. This typically arises where the data from the two phases are linked by happenstance rather than by formal design, for example as occurs in the overlapping samples obtained from bureaucratic systems and capture–recapture sampling methods, and thus where there are a number of plausible probability models that could describe the dependencies within the data. Recently, Robins & Ritov [27] have criticized the use of independent prior distributions for the parameters of the screen and of the diagnostic measure that have typically been used.

Comparisons of Methods

The Bayesian, conditional probability, weighting, and EM methods for a simple prevalence study are compared in Pickles et al. [24]. Schill & Drescher [30] present some comparisons for the related design where the screen is for risk exposure.

Statistical Software

In general, users of commercial statistical packages should take great care in the use of any weighting procedures provided. The use of weights within most packages (such as SPSS [20]; *see* **Software, Biostatistical**) will give the correct estimates of prevalence and **odds ratios**, but unfortunately, for the most part, will not use the appropriate variance estimator. Estimates for confidence intervals, for example, and associated significance tests will be invalid. This arises from the fact that the weights are typically interpreted as *frequency weights* (an indicator of the number of observations with identical data to that provided in a given record). The package accordingly treats the ith subject in the second-phase sample as if it had actually been recorded w_i times. The appropriate use of a probability weight, however, recognizes that the observation has only occurred once, but that the observed second-phase subject is representative of w_i first-phase subjects, all but one of which have not provided second-phase data. Programs such as SUDAAN [31] and STATA [34] will deal satisfactorily with weights assumed known. In general, though with substantial variation in ease of use, almost any statistical program can be persuaded to draw appropriate samples for bootstrap estimation of the variance of weighted estimates. Software for mean score and semi-parametric regression methods is not widely available, although implementation is claimed to be straightforward. Bayesian models can now be easily fitted using Gibbs sampling programs such as Bayesian inference Using Gibbs Sampling (BUGS) [33].

Design Considerations

The relative advantages and disadvantages of screening in a two-phase survey, and also considerations of optimal designs, have been discussed by, among others, Deming [8] and Shrout & Newman [32]. Clearly the use of a preliminary screening instrument has potential advantages when it is both expensive, time-consuming and difficult to carry out an accurate diagnostic assessment. It is intuitively appealing (particularly for clinically trained researchers contemplating a series of long and detailed psychiatric interviews, for example) to consider some way of excluding the majority of subjects who do not have a problem in order that valuable diagnostic resources can be expended on those that do. The rarer the illness, the more appealing this idea becomes. The approach is only practically viable, however, if the potential screening procedures are cheap (relative to the full diagnostic assessment), accurate, easily administered, and accepted by the survey participants. Here accuracy implies both a high **sensitivity** and a high **specificity**, with high sensitivity being the more important of the two screening test characteristics. Clearly, we do not want a screening test which misses a relatively high proportion of our rare cases of illness. Hand [13] discusses the determination of the cut-off for a screening questionnaire that gives optimal sensitivity and specificity, and how different cut-offs may be appropriate for either prevalence estimation or case detection. Begg & Greenes [1] discuss the estimation of screen error rates from two-phase studies.

The costs involved in collecting survey data using a two-phase design come from three areas of activity: recruitment, screening, and diagnostic assessment. If it is difficult and/or expensive to recruit subjects, then the two-phase design becomes less attractive, and a better strategy might be to lower the cost of diagnostic assessment procedures. An example of the latter would be the development of fully structured interviews for use by lay interviewers. In many situations the relative gains in efficiency from two-phase sampling seem to be rather slight. In summary, in relation to single-phase designs, two-phase designs will be more efficient when the prevalence is low, and are likely to be less efficient if the screen costs more than half of the cost of the diagnostic assessment [32]. Deming [8] has argued that unless there are clear gains in terms of relative efficiency, many of the disadvantages of the design would lead us to decide not to adopt it in survey work. These include the extra administrative problems related to conducting a survey in two phases, the logistical problems in recontacting respondents selected for the second phase, scheduling their second-phase assessment and minimizing **nonresponse** and noncompliance. There are also the problems for the management of the more complex databases and the increased complexity in the analysis of the results. Despite all of these problems, the design seems to be growing in popularity. One suspects that investigators pay too little attention to them at the design stage of a study or, if they do, give them less weight than the obvious attractions of the design. Clinicians (and others) clearly consider that it is a waste of valuable resources to spend time assessing people without problems. The idea of only assessing a very small proportion of those likely to be well is possibly the strongest motivation for a two-phase study. Even if we accept this view we should be very wary of assessing too small a proportion of screen negatives and should definitely resist the temptation to assess none of them!

Little work has been done on the design of two-phase studies for estimating the effects of risk exposure. Design possibilities include **stratification** by potential risk factors. Palmgren [21] considers optimal design for estimating an **odds ratio** for comparing two prevalences. Reilly [26] also considers optimal two-phase designs.

Other Areas of Application

Although the purpose of this article is to discuss screening procedures for prevalence estimation, it is also useful to consider other areas of application in which either screening or two-phase sampling might be of potential value. The first is in studies specifically designed to evaluate the performance of new screening instruments or **diagnostic tests** [1]. In a prospective design all the first-phase subjects are assessed using the screen and then selected subsamples are evaluated using the gold standard. In a **retrospective study** all of the first-phase subjects are given (or already have) a definitive diagnosis and in this design the selected subsamples are the ones who then get an assessment using the new test or screening procedure. Note that it is particularly important that the assessments made within the two phases (irrespective of whether the study is prospective or retrospective) are made independently, i.e. the assessors are blind to previous results. The value of maintaining blindness is another reason why both first-phase strata should be subsampled in a simple two-phase prevalence study (assuming, as should be the case, that first-phase results are not made available to the second-phase assessor). Similar designs might also be used in studies of diagnostic **agreement**: a trainee clinician or research student, for example, diagnosing all available patients and then their supervisor validating the diagnoses by independent assessment of subsamples of the first-phase diagnostic groups [15]. The final area of application to be mentioned here is in the use of surrogate endpoint measures (i.e. screens) in lengthy follow-up studies and, in particular, randomized controlled trials. This is an area of application that is in infancy but has been discussed in the context of mean score [23] and regression methods [28].

References

[1]   Begg, C.B. & Greenes, R.A. (1983). Assessment of diagnostic tests when disease verification is subject to selection bias, *Biometrics* **39**, 207–215.

[2]   Binder, D.A. (1983). On the variances of asymptotically normal estimators from complex surveys, *International Statistical Review* **51**, 279–292.

[3]   Binder, D.A. (1996). Linearization methods for single and two-phase samples: a cookbook approach, *Survey Methodology* **22**, 17–22.

[4]   Chambless, L.E. & Boyle, K.E. (1985). Maximum likelihood methods for complex sample data: logistic regression and discrete proportional hazards models,

Communications in Statistics – Theory and Methods **14**, 1377–1392.

[5] Chen, T.T. (1979). Log-linear models for categorical data with misclassification and double-sampling, *Journal of the American Statistical Association* **74**, 481–487.

[6] Cochran, W.G. (1977). *Sampling Techniques*, 3rd Ed. Wiley, New York.

[7] Cohen, T. & Spencer, B.D. (1991). Shrinkage weights for unequal probability samples, in *American Statistical Association 1991 Proceedings of the Survey Research Methods Section*. American Statistical Association, Alexandria, pp. 625–630.

[8] Deming, W.E. (1977). An essay on screening, or two-phase sampling, applied to surveys of a community, *International Statistical Review* **45**, 29–37.

[9] Deming, W.E. & Stephan, F.F. (1940). On a least squares adjustment of a simple frequency table, when the expected margin totals are known, *Annals of Statistics* **11**, 427–444.

[10] Espeland, M.A. & Hui, S.L. (1987). A general approach to analyzing epidemiological data that contain misclassification errors, *Biometrics* **43**, 1001–1012.

[11] Flanders, W.D. & Greenland, S. (1991). Analytic methods for two stage case–control studies and other stratified designs, *Statistics in Medicine* **10**, 739–747.

[12] Gilks, W.R. Clayton, D.G., Spiegelhalter, D.J., Best, N.G., McNeil, A.J., Sharples, L.D. & Kirby, A.J. (1993). Modelling complexity: applications of Gibbs sampling in medicine (with discussion), *Journal of the Royal Statistical Society, Series B* **55**, 39–102.

[13] Hand, D. (1987). Screening versus prevalence estimation, *Applied Statistics* **36**, 1–7.

[14] Huber, P.J. (1967). The behaviour of maximum likelihood estimates under non-standard conditions, in *Proceedings of the Fifth Berkeley Symposium on Mathematical Statistics and Probability*, vol. 1, L. LeCam & J. Neyman, eds. University of California Press, Berkeley, pp. 221–233.

[15] Jannarone, R.J., Macera, C.A. & Garrison, C.Z. (1987). Evaluation of inter-rater agreement through "case–control" sampling, *Biometrics* **43**, 433–437.

[16] Kish, L. (1965). *Survey Sampling*. Wiley, New York.

[17] Lazzeroni, L.C. & Little, R.J.A. (1993). Models for smoothing post-stratification weights, in *American Statistical Association 1993 Proceedings of the Survey Research Methods Section*. American Statistical Association, Alexandria, pp. 764–769.

[18] Lehtonen, R. & Pakkinen, E.J. (1995). *Practical Methods for the Design and Analysis of Complex Surveys*. Wiley, Chichester.

[19] Little, R.J.A. & Rubin, D.B. (1987). *Statistical Analysis with Missing Data*. Wiley, Chichester.

[20] Norusis, M.J. (1993). *SPSS for Windows*. SPSS Inc., Chicago.

[21] Palmgren, J. (1987). Precision of double sampling estimators for comparing two probabilities, *Biometrika* **74**, 687–694.

[22] Pepe. M.S. (1992). Inference using surrogate outcome data and a validation sample, *Biometrika* **79**, 355–365.

[23] Pepe, M.S., Reilly, M. & Fleming, T.R. (1994). Auxiliary outcome data and the mean score method, *Journal of Statistical Planning and Inference* **42**, 137–160.

[24] Pickles, A., Dunn, G. & Vazquez-Barquero, J.L. (1995). Screening for stratification in two-phrase (two-stage) epidemiological surveys, *Statistical Methods in Medical Research* **4**, 73–89.

[25] Potter, F.J. (1990). A study of procedures to identify and trim extreme sampling weights, in *American Statistical Association 1990 Proceedings of the Survey Research Methods Section*. American Statistical Association, Alexandria, pp. 225–230.

[26] Reilly, M. (1996). Optimal sampling strategies for two-stage studies, *American Journal of Epidemiology* **143**, 92–100.

[27] Robins, J.M. & Ritov, Y. (1997). A curse of dimensionality appropriate (CODA) asymptotic theory for semi-parametric models, *Statistics in Medicine* **16**, 285–319.

[28] Rotnitzky, A. & Robins, J.M. (1995). Semiparametric regression estimation in the presence of dependent censoring, *Biometrika* **82**, 805–820.

[29] Rotnitzky, A. & Robins, J.M. (1997). Semi-parametric regression models with non-ignorable non-response, *Statistics in Medicine* **16**, 81–102.

[30] Schill, W. & Drescher, K. (1997). Logistic analysis of studies with two-stage sampling: a comparison of four approaches, *Statistics in Medicine* **16**, 117–132.

[31] Shah, B.V., Folsom, R.E., Lavange, L.M., Wheeless, S.C., Boyle, K.E. & Williams, R.L. (1995). *SUDAAN: Software for the Statistical Analysis of Correlated Data*. Research Triangle Institute, Research Triangle Park.

[32] Shrout, P.E. & Newman, S.C. (1989). Design of two-phase prevalence surveys of rare disorders, *Biometrics* **45**, 549–555.

[33] Spiegelhalter, D.J., Thomas, A., Best, N.G. & Gilks, W.R. (1995). *BUGS: Bayesian Inference Using Gibbs Sampling, Version 5.0*. Medical Research Council Biostatistics Unit, Institute of Public Health, University Forvie Site, Cambridge,

[34] StataCorp (1997). *Stata Statistical Software: Release 5.0*. Stata Corporation, College Station.

[35] Tenenbaum, A. (1970). A double sampling scheme for estimating from binomial data with misclassification, *Journal of the American Statistical Association* **65**, 1350–1361.

[36] York, J., Madigan, D., Heuch, I. & Lie, R.T. (1995). Birth defects registered by double sampling: a Bayesian approach incorporating covariates and model uncertainty, *Applied Statistics* **44**, 227–242.

(*See also* **Diagnostic Tests, Evaluation of**)

A. PICKLES & G. DUNN

Prevalence Rate or Ratio

The prevalence rate or ratio refers to the number of people who have a disease or condition at a given point in time in a given population divided by the number of people in that population. This quantity is also known as the *prevalence proportion*.
(*See also* **Prevalence**)

M.H. GAIL

Prevalent Case

A prevalent case is a subject with a given disease or condition who is alive in a defined population at a given time. Sometimes the condition may refer to the previous occurrence of an illness, as for persons who now have or who previously have had cancer. Thus, prevalent cases include subjects who developed disease previously as well as **incident cases** who just developed disease.

(*See also* **Biased Sampling of Cohorts in Epidemiology**; **Case–Control Study, Prevalent**; **Cross-Sectional Study**)

M.H. GAIL

Prevalent Cohort Studies *see* Biased Sampling of Cohorts in Epidemiology

Preventable Fraction

When considering a protective exposure or intervention, an intuitively appealing alternative to **attributable risk** (AR) is the preventable fraction (PF). The preventable or prevented fraction measures the impact of an association between a protective exposure and a disease at the population level. It is defined as the proportion of disease cases averted by a protective exposure or intervention [5]. It can be

formally written as:

$$PF = \{Pr(D|\overline{E}) - Pr(D)\}/Pr(D|\overline{E}), \quad (1)$$

where $Pr(D)$ is the probability of disease in the population, which may have some exposed (E) and some unexposed ($\overline{E}$) individuals, and $Pr(D|\overline{E})$ is the hypothetical probability of disease in the same population but with all (protective) exposure eliminated. Another formulation of the PF is the proportion of cases prevented by the (protective) factor or intervention among the totality of cases that would have developed in the absence of the factor or intervention [5], which is why the denominator in (1) is the hypothetical probability of disease in the population in the absence of the protective factor.

The PF can be rewritten as:

$$PF = Pr(E)(1 - RR), \quad (2)$$

where $Pr(E)$ denotes the **prevalence** of the protective exposure in the population and RR the **relative risk**. As is apparent from (2), the PF depends both on the prevalence of the protective exposure and the strength of the association between the protective exposure and disease, in a similar fashion as for AR. A strong association between exposure and disease (marked by a low RR) may therefore correspond to a high or low value of the PF, depending on the prevalence of exposure, and portability from population to population is not a common property of the PF.

For a protective factor (RR < 1), the PF lies between 0 and 1 and is usually expressed as a percentage. The PF increases with the prevalence of exposure and the strength of the association between exposure and disease. The PF is null in the absence of association between exposure and disease (RR = 1) and negative when the exposure factor is a risk factor (RR > 1), in which case there is no rationale for using the PF as a measure of impact.

Counter to what intuition might suggest, the PF is not a mere negative AR; that is, the PF does not equal − AR (unless RR = 1). The relationship between AR and the PF was worked out by Walter [6] and is given by

$$1 - PF = 1/(1 - AR). \quad (3)$$

For a protective factor, AR is negative but can be made positive by reversing the coding of exposure. Under reverse coding, the exposed (protective) level is relabeled as the reference level and the unexposed level as the "exposed", which leads to a positive value of AR. This value is interpreted as the proportion of cases attributable to lack of exposure to the protective factor and which could therefore potentially be prevented by generalizing exposure in the population. This valid interpretation of AR under reverse coding has been used in the literature. For example, a positive AR for protective dietary factors was estimated in a **case–control study** of gastric cancer [3]. AR under this interpretation is sometimes called the preventable fraction [2, 4], which may introduce some confusion.

It is important to note that the value of AR under reverse coding differs from the value of the PF. For instance, if RR and Pr(E) are both equal to 0.5, then the PF is equal to 0.25 (or 25%), and the value of AR obtained by reversing the coding is 0.33 (or 33%). This difference is not surprising in view of the differing definitions of AR and the PF. AR, with reverse coding, measures the potential reduction in disease cases if all subjects in the current population became exposed (if the absence of exposure were eliminated from the population), while the PF measures the reduction in disease cases obtained by moving from a totally unexposed population to the current population with exposure prevalence given by Pr(E).

Given their close relationship, AR and the PF share the same properties. Regarding the interpretation of the PF, the above definition implies that the PF measures the actual reduction in disease load due to exposure. This interpretation is fully warranted only under the same conditions that ensure the validity of the interpretation of AR as the actual reduction of disease corresponding to the elimination of exposure. These conditions are unbiased estimations of the PF, a causal role for the exposure (*see* **Causation**), and invariance of the distribution of the other factors influencing disease occurrence under a change in the exposure distribution. It might therefore be wiser to define the PF as the *potential* reduction in disease load *associated with* exposure.

The PF can not only be defined with regard to a protective exposure factor, but also to the *de novo* introduction of a prevention program in the target population (e.g. an intervention designed to reduce smoking). In such a case, since the prevalence of the program is equal to zero before its implementation, one can assess the impact of its introduction through the estimation of PF. Clearly,

the impact depends both on the effectiveness of the program and its diffusion in the population (i.e. the prevalence of "exposure" to the program), which is reflected in the estimate of PF. This has been suggested as an analytic tool for assessing the effects of interventions [1].

It follows from (3) that estimability and estimation issues are similar for AR and the PF. Adjusted PF estimates based on the **Mantel–Haenszel** approach have been derived for **cohort**, case–control and **cross-sectional studies** [2]. Unadjusted estimates and adjusted estimates based on the weighted-sum approach have been derived for cross-sectional studies, and corresponding sample size calculations are available for using a test that the PF equals 0 to assess interventions [1].

References

[1] Gargiullo, P.M., Rothenberg, R. & Wilson, H.G. (1995). Confidence intervals, hypothesis tests, and sample sizes for the prevented fraction in cross-sectional studies, *Statistics in Medicine* **14**, 51–72. (Erratum in *Statistics in Medicine* **14**, 841, 1995).

[2] Greenland, S. (1987). Variance estimators for attributable fraction estimates, consistent in both large strata and sparse data, *Statistics in Medicine* **6**, 701–708.

[3] La Vecchia C., D'Avanzo, B., Negri, E., Decarli, A. & Benichou, J. (1995). Attributable risk for stomach cancer in Northern Italy, *International Journal of Cancer* **60**, 748–752.

[4] Last, J.M., ed. (1983). *A Dictionary of Epidemiology*. Oxford University Press, New York.

[5] Miettinen, O.S. (1974). Proportion of disease caused or prevented by a given exposure, *American Journal of Epidemiology* **99**, 325–332.

[6] Walter, S.D. (1976). The estimation and interpretation of attributable risk in health research, *Biometrics* **32**, 829–849.

JACQUES BENICHOU

Primary Base Case–Control Study
see Case–Control Study

Probability of Causation *see* Attributable Risk

Prognostic Scores *see* Confounder Summary Score

Propensity Score

The propensity score is the conditional probability of exposure to treatment rather than control given observed covariates or, more generally, the conditional probability of selection given observed covariates. It is used to adjust for nonrandom treatment assignment or nonrandom selection. As a scalar summary of multidimensional covariates, the propensity score is often used for matching, **stratification**, or weighting adjustments. **Matching** and stratification are common in **observational studies**; that is, in studies of the effects of treatments not randomly assigned to subjects as they would be in a randomized clinical trial. Weighting adjustments are common in adjusting for **nonresponse** in surveys. Propensity scores have also been used as part of permutation inference and Bayesian inference, and have been incorporated as a variable in a model. Propensity scores were proposed by Rosenbaum & Rubin [23].

In thinking about what propensity scores may reasonably be expected to accomplish, it is useful to distinguish overt and hidden **biases**. An overt bias is visible in the data at hand. For instance, suppose that in comparing smokers and nonsmokers with recorded ages, one observes that smokers are somewhat older than nonsmokers. Then, a direct comparison of the mortality of smokers and nonsmokers ignoring age would be affected by an overt bias due to age. A hidden bias is similar, but it is not visible in the data at hand, though it may be suspected to exist. Adjustments for the propensity score reduce or eliminate overt biases, but the adjustments do little to address hidden biases, which must be investigated by other means; see Rosenbaum [22, Sections 4–8].

In an observational study, N subjects are observed, of whom n receive the treatment and $N-n$ receive the control. Each subject has a vector $\mathbf{X}$ of observed covariates that describe the condition of subjects prior to treatment, so $\mathbf{X}$ is not affected by the treatment. Write $Z = 1$ if the subject receives the treatment and $Z = 0$ if the subject receives the control, so $n = \sum_{i=1}^{N} Z_i$. The propensity score $e(\mathbf{X})$ is the conditional probability of receiving the treatment

given the covariates $\mathbf{X}$; that is, $e(\mathbf{X}) = \Pr(Z = 1|\mathbf{X})$. Although the propensity score will be discussed in the context of nonrandom treatment assignment in observational studies, it may be applied in other contexts, such as nonresponse in **sample surveys**; see [14].

The propensity score has several properties, the first of which is its balancing property. Pick a value of the propensity score $e(\mathbf{X})$, and sample at random treated subjects, those with $Z = 1$, and control subjects, those with $Z = 0$, having this same value of $e(\mathbf{X})$. Then these treated and control subjects with the same $e(\mathbf{X})$ have the same distribution of $\mathbf{X}$. To express this formally, follow Dawid [6] in writing $A \perp\!\!\!\perp B|C$ for A is conditionally independent of B given C. Then the balancing property of the propensity score says:

$$\mathbf{X} \perp\!\!\!\perp Z|e(\mathbf{X}) \qquad (1)$$

or, equivalently,

$$\Pr[\mathbf{X}|Z = 1, e(\mathbf{X})] = \Pr[\mathbf{X}|Z = 0, e(\mathbf{X})].$$

The proof of (1) is straightforward; see [23, Theorem 1].

The balancing property is used in the following way. For each treated subject, find a **control** with approximately the same $e(\mathbf{X})$ forming a matched pair. Then the resulting matched sample will comprise a treated and control group with similar distributions for $\mathbf{X}$. If $\mathbf{X}$ is of high dimension, then matching exactly on $\mathbf{X}$ is difficult, but matching on a scalar $e(\mathbf{X})$ is straightforward. For instance, if $\mathbf{X}$ is a 20-dimensional vector of binary covariates, then there are 2^{20} or about a million possible values of $\mathbf{X}$, so finding controls that exactly match for all of $\mathbf{X}$ is infeasible with samples of reasonable size. In practice, one must estimate $e(\mathbf{X})$; for instance, using **logistic regression** of Z on $\mathbf{X}$. This is illustrated in [25] and [26]. There, 221 children with prenatal exposures to barbiturates were matched to 221 unexposed children drawn from a reservoir of 7027 potential controls. The vector $\mathbf{X}$ contained 20 covariates, such as gender, mother's socioeconomic status, mother's education, mother's cigarette use, etc. In this particular example, matching on the scalar estimate of the propensity score balanced all 20 covariates. Generally, after matching, the distributions of $\mathbf{X}$ in matched treated and control groups are compared to check that matching on the estimate of $e(\mathbf{X})$ has succeeded in balancing $\mathbf{X}$.

Alternatively, divide subjects into strata that are homogeneous in $e(\mathbf{X})$. Within strata, treated and control subjects tend to have similar distributions of **X**. This is illustrated in [24] where five strata formed from an estimated propensity score balance a 74-dimensional **X** of covariates in a study of coronary bypass surgery.

It is useful to compare and contrast the balancing property of propensity scores with the balancing property of randomization in a randomized experiment. Like randomization, strata that are homogeneous in the propensity score $e(\mathbf{X})$ may be quite heterogeneous in **X**; however, within strata, the heterogeneity in **X** is not systematically related to the treatment group Z. For instance, in the coronary bypass example in [24], patients were denied bypass surgery if they were quite healthy and did not need it or if they were extremely ill and were unlikely to survive surgery. The stratum with the lowest probabilities of surgery, the lowest $e(\mathbf{X})$s, was extremely heterogeneous, containing both the healthiest and the sickest patients; however, within that stratum, the bypass patients and the controls had similar distributions of **X**. Balancing does not eliminate heterogeneity; rather, it leaves the heterogeneity intact, but makes it nearly orthogonal to the treatment Z. Unlike randomization, adjustments for the propensity score balance the observed covariates **X** used in calculating $e(\mathbf{X})$, but they do not generally balance unobserved covariates. Randomization balances both observed and unobserved covariates, so randomization removes both overt and hidden biases, whereas adjustments for propensity scores reduce or eliminate only overt biases.

Each subject has two potential responses, a response r_T that would be observed if the subject received the treatment and a response r_C that would be observed if the subject received the control (see [16], [28], [29]). In fact, r_T is observed only if the subject receives the treatment, $Z = 1$, and r_C is observed only if the subject received the control, $Z = 0$. The effect caused by the treatment is a comparison of r_T and r_C, such as $r_T - r_C$; that is, a comparison of what the response would have been under treatment and under control. Because r_T and r_C cannot be observed jointly for one subject, causal effects cannot be calculated for individual subjects. Nonetheless, there are consistent and sometimes unbiased estimates of population summaries of causal effects under certain circumstances. For instance, in a randomized experiment the average response of treated subjects minus the average response of control

subjects is an unbiased estimate of the average treatment effect, $\tau = \mathrm{E}(r_T - r_C) = \mathrm{E}(r_T) - \mathrm{E}(r_C)$, and for binary responses, the sample **odds ratio** is a consistent estimate of the population odds ratio

$$\Psi = [\Pr(r_T = 1)\Pr(r_C = 0)]/[\Pr(r_T = 0)\Pr(r_C = 1)];$$

see Holland & Rubin [11]. Later in this discussion, it will be important to distinguish the odds ratio Ψ from the conditional odds ratio,

$$\omega_{\mathbf{X}} = \frac{\Pr(r_T = 1|\mathbf{X} = \mathbf{x})\Pr(r_C = 0|\mathbf{X} = \mathbf{x})}{\Pr(r_T = 0|\mathbf{X} = \mathbf{x})\Pr(r_C = 1|\mathbf{X} = \mathbf{x})}$$

given $\mathbf{X} = \mathbf{x}$,

which is generally a function of **x**. Even when $\omega_{\mathbf{X}}$ is constant, not varying with **x**, it does not typically equal the odds ratio Ψ that would be calculated in a randomized experiment without reference to covariates.

Adjustment for a covariate **X** in an observational study will yield consistent or unbiased estimates of population treatment effects if treatment assignment is ignorable, a term that will now be defined. Treatment assignment is said to be ignorable given **X** if

$$Z \perp\!\!\!\perp (r_T, r_C)|\mathbf{X}$$

and $\qquad\qquad\qquad\qquad\qquad\qquad$ (2)

$$0 < \Pr(Z = 1|\mathbf{X}) < 1, \quad \text{for all } \mathbf{X}.$$

This says that subjects may have unequal probabilities of receiving the treatment Z, but conditionally given the covariates **X**, the assignment of subjects to treatment groups is equitable in the sense that it is unrelated to the responses subjects will later exhibit; that is, $\Pr(Z = 1|r_T, r_C, \mathbf{X}) = \Pr(Z = 1|\mathbf{X}) = e(\mathbf{X})$. It is not difficult to show that, if treatment assignment is ignorable, then exact matching or stratification or correct model-based adjustment for **X** can be used to estimate population causal effects such as τ or ψ; see [29] and [23, Theorem 4], with their $b(\mathbf{X}) = \mathbf{X}$. For instance, with ignorable assignment, an unbiased estimate of τ is obtained by sampling **X** at random, sampling a treated and a control subject at random with this same **X**, and differencing their responses. The average of such differences is consistent for τ. With ignorable assignment, the odds ratio ψ is consistently estimated in an analogous way by first obtaining unbiased estimates of the four probabilities, $\Pr(r_T = 1)$, $\Pr(r_C = 0)$, $\Pr(r_T = 0)$, and $\Pr(r_C = 1)$, and, secondly, calculating the odds ratio of the unbiased estimates. Hamilton [10], Little [14], Sobel [34], and Stone [36] discuss related issues.

The second fact about the propensity score is that if treatment assignment is ignorable given $\mathbf{X}$, then it is also ignorable given just the propensity score $e(\mathbf{X})$, so if it suffices to adjust for $\mathbf{X}$ in estimating τ or ψ, then it suffices to adjust for the scalar $e(\mathbf{X})$. Formally, it may be shown [23, Theorem 3] that (2) implies

$$Z \perp\!\!\!\perp (r_{\mathrm{T}}, r_{\mathrm{C}}) | e(\mathbf{X})$$

and   (3)

$$0 < \Pr[Z = 1 | e(\mathbf{X})] < 1, \quad \text{for all } e(\mathbf{X}).$$

In short, the propensity score tends to balance observed covariates $\mathbf{X}$ whether or not treatment assignment is ignorable. If treatment assignment is ignorable, then there is overt bias but no hidden bias, so it suffices to adjust for the observed covariates $\mathbf{X}$; but in this case, it suffices to adjust for the scalar $e(\mathbf{X})$. Specifically, if treatment assignment is ignorable, then parameters such as the average treatment effect τ or the odds ratio ψ can be consistently estimated by adjusting for the scalar $e(\mathbf{X})$ rather than the multivariate $\mathbf{X}$.

The performance of the propensity score in matching or stratification has been studied by simulation. Drake [7] compared propensity score adjustments and model-based adjustments when the propensity score or the model for the responses is incorrect. Gu & Rosenbaum [9] compared various matching techniques, in particular, concluding that matching on the propensity score was better than certain distance-based matching procedures when there are many covariates; say 20 or more covariates. Rubin & Thomas [32, 33] examine propensity score methods when covariates have multivariate normal distributions, ellipsoidal distributions, and empirical distributions derived from an example.

An alternative to matching or stratification for the propensity score is weighting adjustments. Although r_{T} is observed only if $Z = 1$ and r_{C} is observed only if $Z = 0$, the quantities Zr_{T} and $(1 - Z)r_{\mathrm{C}}$ are always observed, although they are often zero. With a known propensity score, the quantity

$$\frac{Zr_{\mathrm{T}}}{e(\mathbf{X})} - \frac{(1 - Z)r_{\mathrm{C}}}{1 - e(\mathbf{X})}$$ (4)

may be computed for all N subjects. If treatment assignment is ignorable, then the average value of (4) may be shown to be unbiased for the average treatment effect τ; see [20]. In practice, estimated

propensity scores are used in place of known propensity scores in (4), so the estimator becomes, in effect, the difference of two Horvitz–Thompson estimators [12] with estimated weights. As it turns out, the use of estimated weights is beneficial. The estimator based on (4) using estimated propensity scores is often superior to the analogous estimator based on true propensity scores for much the same reason that a poststratified estimator is often better than a sample mean; see [20] for specifics.

The propensity score is also used in various other ways. If the propensity score follows a linear logit model, then conditioning on a sufficient statistic for the parameters of the logit model eliminates unknown parameters in the propensity score, and yields exact permutation tests under the assumption that treatment assignment is ignorable; see [18]. For instance, this may be used to adjust matched pairs for imbalances in covariates that were not fully controlled by the matching; see [21]. The use of propensity scores in Bayesian inference is discussed by Rubin [31]. The propensity score may be used as a variable in a model-based adjustment; see [23, Corollary 4.3] for theory, and see [2] and Solomon et al. [35] for applications. Robins et al. [17] develop a novel semiparametric estimate of a regression coefficient using estimated propensity scores and various generalizations. See also [3] and [4]. Joffe & Rosenbaum [13] discuss the use of propensity scores with ordered doses and their use in case–cohort studies.

It is important to distinguish adjustment by balancing $\mathbf{X}$ from adjustment by control for $\mathbf{X}$. In a randomized experiment, random assignment of treatments would balance $\mathbf{X}$, while blocking, matching, or model-based adjustment, such as covariance adjustment, for $\mathbf{X}$ would control for $\mathbf{X}$. In experiments, balancing by randomization would permit estimation of the average treatment effect τ or the odds ratio ψ based on averaged proportions, but control for $\mathbf{X}$ would be required to estimate the conditional odds ratio $\omega_{\mathbf{x}}$ and other parameters that condition on a particular value of $\mathbf{X}$. Gail et al. [8] carefully develop some consequences of the distinction between balance and control in randomized experiments. Similarly, in an observational study with ignorable treatment assignment, matching or stratification for the propensity score $e(\mathbf{X})$ balances $\mathbf{X}$ permitting estimation of τ or ψ, but control for $\mathbf{X}$ would be required to estimate conditional parameters such as $\omega_{\mathbf{x}}$. Balancing and control may be combined. In experiments, this is done, for instance, using a randomized complete blocks design. In observational studies, this is done by combining matching or stratification $e(\mathbf{X})$ with further adjustments and for $\mathbf{X}$. See [19], [21], [24], [27], and [30] for discussion of various aspects of combining matching or stratification with model-based adjustments.

For several applications of propensity scores, see [1], [2], [5], [15], [19], [35], and [37].

References

[1] Aiken, L., Smith, H. & Lake, E. (1994). Lower medicare mortality among a set of hospitals known for good nursing care, *Medical Care* **32**, 771–787.

[2] Berk, R. & Newton, P. (1985). Does arrest really deter wife battery?, *American Sociological Review* **50**, 253–262.

[3] Cook, E. & Goldman, L. (1988). Asymmetric stratification. An outline for an efficient method for controlling confounding in cohort studies, *American Journal of Epidemiology* **127**, 626–639.

[4] Cook, E.F. & Goldman, L. (1989). Performance of tests of significance based on stratification by a multivariate confounder score or by a propensity score, *Journal of Clinical Epidemiology* **42**, 317–324.

[5] Czajka, J., Hirabayashi, S., Little, R.J.A. & Rubin, D.B. (1992). Projecting from advanced data using propensity modeling: an application to income tax statistics, *Journal of Business and Economic Statistics* **10**, 117–131.

[6] Dawid, A.P. (1979). Conditional independence in statistical theory (with discussion), *Journal of the Royal Statistical Society, Series B* **41**, 1–31.

[7] Drake, C. (1993). Effects of misspecification of the propensity score on estimators of treatment effect, *Biometrics* **49**, 1231–1236.

[8] Gail, M., Wieand, S. & Piantadosi, S. (1984). Biased estimates of treatment effect in randomized experiments with nonlinear regressions and missing covariates, *Biometrika* **71**, 431–444.

[9] Gu, X.S. & Rosenbaum, P.R. (1993). Comparison of multivariate matching methods: structures, distances and algorithms, *Journal of Computational and Graphical Statistics* **2**, 405–420.

[10] Hamilton, M. (1979). Choosing a parameter for 2×2 table or $2 \times 2 \times 2$ table analysis, *American Journal of Epidemiology* **109**, 362–375.

[11] Holland, P. & Rubin, D. (1988). Causal inference in retrospective studies, *Evaluation Review* **12**, 203–231.

[12] Horvitz, D. & Thompson, D. (1952). A generalization of sampling without replacement from a finite universe, *Journal of the American Statistical Association* **47**, 663–685.

[13] Joffe, M.M. & Rosenbaum, P.R. (1999). Propensity scores, *American Journal of Epidemiology* **150**, to appear.

[14] Little, R.J.A. (1986). Survey nonresponse adjustments for estimates of means, *International Statistical Review* **54**, 139–157.

[15] Myers, W., Gersh, B., Fisher, L., Mock, M., Holmes, D., Schaff, H., Gillispie, S., Ryan, T. & Kaiser, G. (1987). Time to first new myocardial infarction in patients with mild angina and three-vessel disease comparing medicine and early surgery: a CASS registry study of survival, *Annals of Thoracic Surgery* **43**, 599–612.

[16] Neyman, J. (1923). On the application of probability theory to agricultural experiments. Essay on principles. Section 9 (in Polish). *Roczniki Nank Roiniczych Tom X*, 1–51. Reprinted in *Statistical Science* **5**, (1990), 463–480, with discussion by T. Speed and D. Rubin.

[17] Robins, J., Mark, S. & Newey, W. (1992) Estimating exposure effects by modelling the expectation of exposure conditional on confounders, *Biometrics* **48**, 479–495.

[18] Rosenbaum, P.R. (1984). Conditional permutation tests and the propensity score in observational studies, *Journal of the American Statistical Association* **79**, 565–574.

[19] Rosenbaum, P. (1986). Dropping out of high school in the United States: an observational study, *Journal of Educational Statistics* **11**, 207–224.

[20] Rosenbaum, P.R. (1987). Model-based direct adjustment, *Journal of the American Statistical Association* **82**, 387–394.

[21] Rosenbaum, P.R. (1988). Permutation tests for matched pairs with adjustments for covariates, *Applied Statistics* **37**, 401–411.

[22] Rosenbaum, P.R. (1995) *Observational Studies.* Springer-Verlag, New York.

[23] Rosenbaum, P. & Rubin, D. (1983). The central role of the propensity score in observational studies for causal effects, *Biometrika* **70**, 41–55.

[24] Rosenbaum, P. & Rubin, D. (1984). Reducing bias in observational studies using subclassification on the propensity score, *Journal of the American Statistical Association* **79**, 516–524.

[25] Rosenbaum, P. & Rubin, D. (1985). Constructing a control group using multivariate matched sampling methods that incorporate the propensity score, *American Statistician* **39**, 33–38.

[26] Rosenbaum, P. & Rubin, D. (1985). The bias due to incomplete matching, *Biometrics* **41**, 106–116.

[27] Rubin, D.B. (1973). The use of matched sampling and regression adjustment to remove bias in observational studies, *Biometrics* **29**, 185–203.

[28] Rubin, D.B. (1974). Estimating the causal effects of treatments in randomized and nonrandomized studies, *Journal of Educational Psychology* **66**, 688–701.

[29] Rubin, D.B. (1977). Assignment to treatment group on the basis of a covariate, *Journal of Educational Statistics* **2**, 1–26.

[30] Rubin, D.B. (1979). Using multivariate matched sampling and regression adjustment to control bias in observational studies, *Journal of the American Statistical Association* **74**, 318–328.

[31] Rubin, D.B. (1985). The use of propensity scores in applied Bayesian inference, in *Bayesian Statistics*, Vol. 2, J. Bernardo, M. DeGroot, D. Lindley & A. Smith, eds. Elsevier, New York, pp. 463–472.

[32] Rubin, D.B. & Thomas, N. (1992). Characterizing the effect of matching using linear propensity score methods with Normal distributions, *Biometrika* **79**, 797–809.

[33] Rubin, D.B. & Thomas, N. (1996). Matching using estimated propensity scores–relating theory to practice, *Biometrics* **52**, 249–264.

[34] Sobel, M. (1992). Causal inference in the social and behavioral sciences, in *A Handbook for Statistical Modelling in the Social and Behavioral Sciences*, G. Arminger, C. Clogg & M. Sobel, eds. Plenum, New York, Chapter 1, pp. 1–38.

[35] Solomon, P., Draine, J. & Mannion, E. (1996). The impact of individualized consultation and group workshop family education interventions on ill relative outcomes, *Journal of Nervous and Mental Disease* **184**, 252–254.

[36] Stone, R. (1993). The assumptions on which causal inference rest, *Journal of the Royal Statistical Society, Series B* **55**, 455–466.

[37] Stone, R., Obrosky, D., Singer, D., Kapoor, W., Fine, M., Hough, L., Karpf, M., Lave, J., Li, Y., Medsger, A., Redmond, C. & Ricci, E. (1995). Propensity score adjustment for pretreatment differences between hospitalized and ambulatory patients with community acquired pneumonia, *Medical Care* **33**, 56–66.

PAUL R. ROSENBAUM

Proportional Hazards, Overview

In survival analysis, statistical models are frequently specified via the hazard function $\alpha(t)$. A simple model for the relation between the hazard functions in two groups (e.g. a treatment group 1 and a control group 0) is the *proportional hazards model*, where

$$\alpha_1(t) = \theta\alpha_0(t), \qquad (1)$$

θ being the treatment effect. The relation (1) between the two hazards implies that the corresponding *survival functions* are related by the equation

$$S_1(t) = S_0(t)^\theta,$$

the so-called Lehmann alternatives.

To test the hypothesis $\alpha_1(t) = \alpha_0(t)$, several nonparametric tests are available. Among these, the logrank test is locally most powerful against proportional hazards alternatives.

In the semiparametric model (1), where "the baseline hazard" $\alpha_0(t)$ is left completely unspecified, there exist several estimators for the hazard ratio θ. Among these, the estimator based on the **Cox regression model** is the most frequently used; in fact, using this model, it is possible to adjust the treatment effect θ for effects of other prognostic factors. This proportional hazards model has gained widespread popularity in biostatistics.

In some epidemiologic applications, the hazard function $\alpha_1(t)$ in an exposed group is compared with a *known* hazard function; say, $\alpha_0(t)$. In this case, the maximum likelihood estimator $\hat{\theta}$ in the model (1) is the so-called *standardized mortality ratio*, which is the ratio between the observed number of deaths in the exposed group and the number of deaths one would expect if the hazard in the exposed group were $\alpha_0(t)$ (*see* **Standardization Methods**). Furthermore, the score test for the hypothesis $\theta = 0$ is the one-sample logrank test.

In conclusion, for survival data, proportional hazards has become the structure of choice, much like linearity in models for the mean of a quantitative outcome variable. However, other models are, indeed, available, including additive hazard models and accelerated failure time models.

PER KRAGH ANDERSEN

Proportional Incidence Ratio (PIR)
see Standardization Methods

Proportional Mortality Ratio (PMR)

With mortality data classified by **cause of death**, the PMR consists of a numerator that is the number of deaths from a particular cause and a denominator of total deaths from all causes. Thus, a PMR is simply the fraction (or percentage) of deaths from a particular cause.

In **descriptive epidemiology** involving characterization of PMRs by person, place, and time, it is customary to calculate standardized proportional mortality ratios (SPMRs) that use indirect standardization to adjust for age and often for age, gender, and race. See **standardization methods** for details of these calculations as well as for a historical description of the use of PMRs in vital statistics, the limitations of PMR analyses, and the relationships between PMRs and standardized mortality ratios (SMRs).

Particularly in **occupational epidemiology**, situations arise where the first and only available data consist of deaths classified by cause among persons who share a common occupational exposure. In these situations, a **proportional mortality study** is undertaken. Despite its major limitations and its often erroneous interpretation as an indicator of risk of mortality, PMR analysis can serve a useful role in descriptive epidemiology. A simple and low-cost proportional mortality study can suggest etiologic hypotheses and lead to a chain of increasingly complex analytic epidemiologic studies that ultimately establishes **causation**.

T. COLTON

Proportional Mortality Study

Sometimes the only information available for an epidemiologic **observational study** consists of mortality records (usually death certificates) among a particular group of individuals who share some common exposure. This often occurs in occupational studies where the group consists of workers with a particular job classification, all workers in some industry, or employees at a particular installation or plant (*see* **Occupational Epidemiology; Occupational Mortality**). Examples of each of these are: nuclear shipyard workers, US Army veterans who served in Vietnam, and employees at a factory where inorganic arsenic compounds are handled. The intent is to see whether an exposure that the workers or group share is associated with increased risk of disease. Since the available information is only on deaths, it is mortality rather than morbidity that can be studied.

The key feature that characterizes a proportional mortality study is that there are no denominator data available that allow for the calculation of mortality risk or death rates. With information on causes of death among the group of decedents, one can calculate the proportion of *all* deaths due to a specific cause, namely the proportional mortality.

The essential strategy in a proportional mortality study is to compare the proportional mortality in the group of interest with proportional mortality in a comparison group. The comparison group can consist of an external **control** group, such as the general population for which **vital statistics** are available, or an internal control group; namely, a group of decedents from the same source population who do not share the exposure of interest. Thus, the essential comparison in a proportional mortality study is the ratio of proportional mortality in the study group to that in the comparison group, in other words, the **proportional mortality ratio (PMR)**.

The basic premise of a proportional mortality study is that if exposure is associated with increased risk of a specific disease, then with the available data on deaths by cause one should find proportionally more deaths from that cause among the exposed than among a comparison group of deaths, whether the comparison group consists of an external or an internal control group. Obviously, proportional mortality studies apply only to fatal diseases. For example, the common diseases of vision such as cataract, glaucoma, and age-related macular degeneration are each nonfatal and, hence, there is no place for proportional mortality studies of such disorders.

Of course, since mortality for virtually every disease has some relationship with age, there is the possibility that the decedents in the study and comparison groups have different age distributions. Consequently, age constitutes a potential **confounding** variable in virtually every proportional mortality study. To adjust for such potential confounding, it is customary to use **standardization methods** – in particular, indirect standardization – and to calculate a standardized proportional mortality ratio (SPMR). (Although standardization is usually by age, one can also standardize on other characteristics such as gender, race, and calendar time.)

Thus, using the three examples of occupational exposure described above, there have been proportional mortality studies conducted with calculation of SPMRs that have examined the following:

(i) proportional mortality for leukemia and hematopoietic malignancies among shipyard nuclear workers vs. an internal comparison group of workers at these same shipyards but who were not involved in nuclear work [11]; (ii) proportional mortality from accidents and violent causes among US Army veterans who served in Vietnam vs. an internal comparison group of US Army veterans of the Vietnam era but who did not serve in Vietnam [2]; and (iii) proportional mortality from cancer – in particular, lung and skin – among employees at an arsenical factory in the UK vs. an external comparison group of population deaths (obtained from the death register of the area in which the factory was located) [7].

Interpretation of Proportional Mortality Studies

Proportional mortality studies need particularly cautious interpretation. A common and naive misinterpretation is to view the PMR or SPMR as equivalent to a **relative risk** as obtained in a **cohort study** or an **odds ratio** as obtained in a **case–control study**. Proportional mortality does *not* measure the *risk* of death from that cause. As defined, it measures only the relative frequency of that particular cause among all causes of death.

The basic limitation of a proportional mortality study is that one cannot determine whether an increase in proportional mortality for a particular cause of interest resulted from an increase in the risk of death from that cause (the basic premise underlying the study design), or from a deficit in mortality; namely, a lowering of risk of mortality, for various causes other than that of particular interest. For example, if a proportional mortality analysis resulted in an increased proportional mortality for some specific cancer, then one could not tell whether there was indeed an increased risk of death from that particular cancer, or whether the increased proportional mortality might have resulted from a lower risk of, say, mortality from cardiovascular diseases and accidents.

Even if there is increased risk of mortality from a particular cause, another limitation of proportional mortality is that one cannot distinguish whether such an increase resulted from an increase in the **incidence rate** of the disease or a worsening of the prognosis among existing (prevalent) cases of the disease.

The aforementioned basic limitations of the proportional mortality study severely limit its analytic potential. Proportional mortality studies are often the first, or an early, attempt to explore an association epidemiologically. Why are proportional mortality studies undertaken? In comparison with **analytic epidemiologic** studies, proportional mortality studies can be completed much more rapidly and with considerably less expenditure of resources. Often, it is the findings of a proportional mortality study that lead to a cascade of analytic epidemiologic studies of increasing complexity and cost that ultimately result in establishing a causal relationship between exposure and disease (*see* **Causation**). However, there have been proportional mortality studies with equivocal and controversial findings that have led to considerable efforts and expenditure of resources in subsequent analytic epidemiologic studies that ultimately result in the assurance to an alarmed public that there is no association between exposure and disease. An example of the latter is a proportional mortality study of the association of low-level occupational exposure to radiation among nuclear workers at Portsmouth Naval Shipyard, UK, with leukemia and hematopoietic cancers; a subsequent large-scale and expensive historical cohort study of mortality failed to find increased cancer mortality risks from radiation exposure [12]. In fact, a further analysis of more detailed and complete data at Portsmouth Naval Shipyard revealed **misclassification** bias in designating the causes of death in the initial proportional mortality study [5].

An important point in interpretation is that the same concerns with chance, bias (*see* **Bias in Observational Studies**), and confounding that apply to cohort and case–control studies apply also to proportional mortality studies. Of particular concern in proportional mortality studies are: the completeness of ascertainment of deaths; the accuracy of the coding of **causes of death**; the definition of exposure and its possible misclassification; and proper accounting for relevant confounding variables.

Most epidemiology textbooks, such as Henenkens & Buring [6] and Rothman & Greenland [14], describe proportional mortality studies, their characteristics, and limitations. More details about study design and analysis appear in occupational epidemiology texts such as Checkoway et al. [3] and Monson [10]. Considerable details on the statistical analysis and modeling of proportional mortality data appear in

Breslow & Day [1]. One can also view a proportional mortality study as a special type of case–control study, as pointed out by Miettinen & Wang [9], and deploy the relevant design and analysis strategies for that design, in particular the calculation of a mortality odds ratio (MOR). This latter view of proportional mortality is discussed in the next section.

Design and Analysis of Proportional Mortality Studies

External Controls

The design of a proportional mortality study with external controls is indeed simple and straightforward. The basic material consists of deaths by cause among a particular group who share some exposure. One must take care that there is reasonably complete ascertainment of deaths in the series and that exposure classification is valid. As an example of an incomplete series, consider the situation of examining the employment records of an industrial plant and identifying all those instances where an employee had died. A proportional mortality analysis based on these existing records would likely find increased proportional mortality for diseases such as acute myocardial infarction and accidents, deaths that are likely to occur during employment, and deficits in diseases such as cancer, which are likely to occur subsequent to employment and during retirement. Ideally, an appropriate proportional mortality study would include *all* deaths among those employed at the plant and would require ascertainment of deaths among former plant workers and retirees. Such ascertainment of postemployment deaths, presuming that there has not been widespread migration from the area, might entail searches of death certificates among the local health agencies, presuming that these sources can readily identify prior plant employees. Similarly, with the group of decedents assembled for analysis, one has to consider carefully the definition of exposure and have reasonable certainty that the group of deaths was indeed exposed to the agent under consideration. For example, a proportional mortality analysis of *all* employees at a plant would necessarily include office workers and others who might have minimal or no exposure to the agent under consideration. Such inclusions would tend to dilute the effects that exposure to the agent might have on proportional mortality.

The choice of the external reference standard population is also important, although one's possible choices are often extremely limited. If, for example, the group of decedents under study consists of almost exclusively white males who died during the period 1960–1975 (which was the case with the proportional mortality study of nuclear workers at Portsmouth Naval Shipyard), then one would ideally choose a reference population of white male decedents during this same calendar time. Anticipating age standardization, one needs a reference population of decedents classified by cause of death and by age, race, and calendar period. In this particular situation, although one might have preferred to use deaths from New England for the reference population, the only available proportional mortality data with this amount of detail were those for the entire US.

Once the reference population has been chosen, the calculation of the SPMR is straightforward, with details of the calculations described in the article on **standardization methods**. Determination of the standard error of proportional mortality appears in Breslow & Day [1], although the authors warn against the conduct of statistical inference methods on PMRs.

Internal Controls

For a proportional mortality analysis with internal controls, one needs a group of deaths from unexposed subjects who are in other ways "comparable" with the exposed study group. For example, in a proportional mortality study of US soldiers who served in Vietnam, an obvious internal control group consists of deaths during the same time period among US soldiers who did not serve in Vietnam. In the example of shipyard nuclear workers at Portsmouth Naval Shipyard, the internal control group consisted of deaths among shipyard employees who were nonnuclear workers.

One common method for analysis of these data is to employ the methods for external controls described above to each of the exposed and unexposed groups of decedents and then to compare qualitatively the resulting SPMRs in the two groups. For example, in the initial proportional mortality study at Portsmouth Naval Shipyard [11], the SPMRs for leukemia were 5.62 for the nuclear workers (nearly a sixfold increase) and 0.71 for nonnuclear workers (close to the null value of 1.00). It is noted, however, that this initial study was particularly prone to bias in that there was (i) incomplete ascertainment of deaths; (ii) gross opportunity for misclassification of exposure (nuclear worker or not), since this was based on the recall of next of kin as to whether or not the decedent wore a radiation monitoring badge at work; and (iii) misclassification of cause of death, since the study's principal investigator determined, from his review of the data, the underlying cause of death for each decedent.

Another approach, as mentioned above, is to regard a proportional mortality study with internal controls as a variant of a case–control study. Cases consist of deaths from the cause of interest among both exposed and unexposed and controls consist of deaths from all other causes among both exposed and unexposed. Within this framework, one can analyze the data by the methods applicable to case–control studies; namely, to calculate an odds ratio. In this instance, such a calculation yields what is called a standardized mortality odds ratio (SMOR). Adjustment for confounding by age, or by other characteristics, can be accomplished with use of **Mantel–Haenszel methods**.

Viewed within the case–control framework, one might wish to be more careful in the choice of controls in the design of such a proportional mortality study. Following the basic principle underlying the choice of controls in a case–control study; namely, that the controls should represent the source population from which the cases came, one would not necessarily choose all other deaths as controls. Instead, one would choose controls more carefully from a limited group of causes of death where there was a known lack of association of each cause with the exposure of interest. Thus, one would exclude from the control series those causes of death where there was a known or suspected association with the exposure of interest. Similar considerations apply in **hospital-based case–control studies**, in which one seeks to avoid selecting control diseases that may be associated with exposure.

Other Considerations

In some instances, one can categorize exposure according to duration and/or intensity and examine **dose–response** relationships in proportional mortality. Duration of employment often serves this purpose and, for the nuclear worker illustration, cumulative

recorded radiation exposure by means of badge-monitoring constitutes an ideal dose measure. Methods for dose–response modeling with proportional mortality, based on **logistic regression**, are described by Breslow & Day [1].

There has been considerable investigation of the relationship between the PMR and the standardized mortality ratio (SMR) analyses of the same set of data. In fact, if one takes cause-specific SMRs and divides each by the all-causes SMR, then theoretically these should agree with the corresponding cause-specific PMRs. Kupper et al. [8] call this ratio of cause-specific to all-cause SMRs a relative standardized mortality ratio (RSMR). Zwerling et al. [15] give a recent example comparing the PMR and RSMR approaches with injury mortality among Iowa farmers. Decoufle et al. [4] and Roman et al. [13] also compared the PMR and SMR.

References

[1]   Breslow, N.E. & Day, N.E. (1987). *Statistical Methods in Cancer Research*, Vol. II. *The Design and Analysis of Cohort Studies*. International Agency for Research on Cancer, Lyon.

[2]   Bullman, T.A., Kang, H.K. & Watanabe, K.K. (1990). Proportionate mortality among US Army Vietnam veterans who served in Military Region I, *American Journal of Epidemiology* **132**, 670–674.

[3]   Checkoway, H., Pearce, N.E. & Crawford-Brown, D.J. (1989). *Research Methods in Occupational Epidemiology*. Oxford University Press, Oxford.

[4]   Decoufle, P., Thomas, T.L. & Pickle, L.W. (1980). Comparison of the proportionate mortality ratio and standardized mortality ratio risk measures, *American Journal of Epidemiology* **111**, 263–269.

[5]   Greenberg, R.G., Rosner, B., Hennekens, C., Rinsky, R. & Colton, T. (1985). An investigation of bias in a study of nuclear shipyard workers, *American Journal of Epidemiology* **121**, 1301–1308.

[6]   Hennekens, C.H. & Buring, J. (1987). *Epidemiology in Medicine*. Little, Brown, & Company, Boston.

[7]   Hill, A.B. & Fanning, E.L. (1948). Studies in the incidence of cancer in a factory handling inorganic compounds of arsenic. I. Mortality experience in the factory, *British Journal of Industrial Medicine* **5**, 1–6.

[8]   Kupper, L.L., McMichael, A.J., Symons, M.J. & Most, B.M. (1978). On the utility of proportional mortality analysis, *Journal of Chronic Diseases* **31**, 15–22.

[9]   Miettinen, O. & Wang, J.D. (1981). An alternative to the proportionate mortality ratio, *American Journal of Epidemiology* **114**, 144–148.

[10]   Monson, R.R. (1990). *Occupational Epidemiology*, 2nd Ed. CRC Press, Boca Raton.

[11]   Najarian, T. & Colton, T. (1978). Mortality from leukemia and cancer in shipyard nuclear workers, *Lancet* **i**, 1018–1020.

[12]   Rinsky, R.A., Zumwalde, R.D., Waxweiler, R.J., Murray, W.E., Jr, Bierbaum, P.J., Landrigan, P.J., Terpilak, M. & Cox, C. (1981). Cancer mortality at a naval nuclear shipyard, *Lancet* **i**, 231–235.

[13]   Roman, E., Beral, V., Inskip, H., McDowall, M. & Adelstein, A. (1984). A comparison of standardized and proportional mortality ratios, *Statistics in Medicine* **3**, 7–14.

[14]   Rothman, K.J. & Greenland, S. (1997). *Modern Epidemiology*, 2nd Ed. Raven–Lippincott, Philadelphia.

[15]   Zwerling, C., Burmeister, L.F. & Jensen, C.M. (1995). Injury mortality among Iowa farmers, 1980–1988: comparison of PMR and SMR approaches, *American Journal of Epidemiology* **141**, 878–882.

T. COLTON & R.W. CLAPP

Prospective Method *see* Expected Number of Deaths

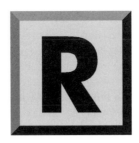

Random Digit Dialing Sampling for Case–Control Studies

Random digit dialing (RDD) is a method of sampling households through the selection of telephone numbers by a random choice of the digits in the telephone numbers. RDD was initially developed as a sampling method for household surveys, but it is now considered a useful tool in epidemiologic research, particularly for selecting **controls** in a **population-based case–control study**, i.e. studies using controls selected from the general population, as distinct from hospital controls or other specialized lists. In countries with high levels of telephone coverage, RDD can provide an almost unbiased sample of the household population for use as controls. Furthermore, once the households are contacted by telephone, there is a relatively low cost of screening to locate persons with the demographic and health characteristics that match the cases for the disease being studied.

RDD obviously omits residents of households that do not have telephones. In the US only about 5% are without telephones, but they are mainly very low-income households, and if the causal factors for the disease are believed to be heavily influenced by income, the results could be seriously **biased**. For such studies the researcher should consider whether RDD is appropriate. However, in most case–control studies, the exclusion of nontelephone households is not believed to have any appreciable effect. It is prudent to exclude cases who do not have home telephones from the analysis so that cases and controls have similar socioeconomic characteristics.

In the US each telephone contains 10 digits, consisting of a three-digit area code, a three-digit central office code (generally referred to as an exchange), and a four-digit suffix. There are presently 35 000–40 000 active area code/central office code combinations in use in the US. Since 10 000 possible number combinations exist in the four-digit suffixes attached to each area code/central office, there are a little over 350 000 000 possible telephone numbers that can be dialed in RDD, about four times the approximately 90 000 000 households with telephones. Most of the 75% of telephone numbers that do not connect to households are unassigned numbers; others are connected to businesses, government offices, institutions, pay phones, computers, faxes, etc.

With simple random sampling, about three-quarters of the calls will be completely unproductive, consisting of nonworking or nonhousehold numbers. The costs of such unproductive calls are quite high, and statisticians have examined the properties of a number of sampling methods designed to reduce the number of excess calls. The general consensus among sampling and survey statisticians is that currently one of two available methods should be used – what is referred to as the *Mitofsky–Waksberg Procedure* [13], or the *List-Assisted Method* [3, 8]. Both methods increase the proportion of household numbers in the sample from about 25% to 50%–60%. Brick et al. [2] note that although the list-assisted method is slightly biased, the bias is trivial for most practical purposes. The Mitofsky–Waksberg procedure provides a completely unbiased sample of households but has several operational complications that can affect the timing and the required record-keeping. (*See* **Telephone Sampling** for a description of the two sampling methods and a list of references.)

The cheapest method of sampling is to use *directory sampling*, that is, select a simple random sample from a sampling frame of all telephone numbers listed in the white pages of current telephone directories for the geographic area of interest. In the US, this procedure will produce a highly biased sample since only about two-thirds of telephone households have their current numbers listed. It is not recommended by knowledgeable statisticians. If used, the biases can be reduced, although not eliminated, by restricting the cases in the study to those whose telephone numbers are listed in telephone directories. It should be noted that although restricting both cases and controls to households listed in telephone directories appears to be similar to RDD in that the cases and controls come from similar populations, the population eligible for the study with RDD is about 95% of all households as compared with about 60% for directory sampling. The potential for bias is thus generally quite small for RDD studies but can be substantial for directory sampling. For this reason, directory sampling is usually not recommended.

There are, at present, at least two commercial firms that maintain up-to-date records on existing area codes/central office codes in the US (GENESYS Sampling Systems and Survey Sampling Inc.). These companies can select samples using either of the two recommended methods, or following other procedures specified by the client. Both companies have extensive resources for geographic coding and can help identify the area codes/central office codes in the geographic area designated for a study. Statisticians and epidemiologists who have not had extensive experiences with RDD studies would probably benefit by consulting one of these companies for assistance in sampling.

Potthoff [9] has described the steps in selecting controls. We summarize and extend his discussion. The cases are all of the eligible ones that occur in a given geographical region in a given time period. RDD controls are sampled from the same region, typically by strata (demographic categories such as sex, age, race). Frequently, geographic subareas are included in the matching criteria; the subareas may be defined by census tracts, zip codes, telephone exchanges, or broader geography such as counties or central cities vs. suburbs. The areas may serve as proxies for environmental or socioeconomic matching, but they should be broad enough to produce the required number of controls. In general, everyone within a stratum (often referred to as a matching cell) is given the same chance of selection. The sample sizes are designated in advance for the strata, the size being based on the desired number of controls per case, the available budget, and possibly logistical considerations. Most population-based case–control studies use **frequency matching** of controls to cases within strata rather than individual matching. Frequency matching involves defining matching cells, for example, white females 40–44 years of age, and locating the desired number of controls in each matching cell. RDD selection can be used for both individual and frequency matching.

Telephone contacts can be used to select controls and to conduct interviews, or only for the sample selection, in which case subsequent interviews may be carried out in personal visits to the households or, more rarely, by mail. The decision on which approach to use depends on the length and content of the interview, e.g. whether physical measurements or laboratory tests are necessary, whether observation of such items as prescription drugs is required, etc. The same general principles are used for both types of studies. If personal visits will be required, then the researcher should take this into account in establishing the geographic area in which the study will be conducted in order to avoid excessive interviewer travel. Methods of sampling that tend to cluster the sampling units, e.g. the Mitofsky–Waksberg method, should be considered.

With telephone interviewing, the selection and enlistment of controls and the interviewing can be done in a single telephone contact [5, 6]. Alternatively, a two-step process can be used in which the first call is restricted to taking a household census with sample selection carried out as an office operation, and a second telephone call made for a telephone interview or to arrange for a visit [6]. If the time schedule permits, then the two-step process is usually preferable since it provides a tighter control on sample size. There is difficulty in achieving the exact sample sizes in a one-step process without incurring biases from loss of persons who are infrequently at home and require multiple attempts to reach. However, some researchers prefer the one-step method because it usually produces a somewhat higher response rate. In addition, if there is a long lapse of time between the two contacts, then a nontrivial part of the sample will have moved, introducing the potential for important biases in the study as well as some uncertainty in the number of controls that will be interviewed. If a two-step process is used, then the time period between the two steps should be kept as short as possible.

A number of issues arise in the sample selection via RDD. They are discussed briefly below. More complete discussions can be found in the references, particularly [5]–[7], [11], and [12].

1. RDD covers only persons living in households with telephones. It is normal practice to exclude from the analysis the cases that do not have telephones or who do not reside in ordinary households, e.g. institutions or the military. A clear definition of households and household members needs to be established to treat such ambiguous cases as college students, persons in the military, etc.

2. The geographic areas that are used to determine the boundaries of the study, or the matching cells, frequently consist of political units (counties or cities) or census tracts. These areas may not conform to telephone exchanges, leading to a considerable amount of screening to identify persons within the designated geographic area. To avoid this excessive screening, the researcher should consider the possibility of defining the study area as the set of telephone exchanges that approximates the geography desired. Matching cells can also be defined by telephone exchanges. The same geographic rules need to be applied to cases as to controls.

3. If the boundaries of the study area are political or census-defined geography, then it is necessary to include all telephone exchanges that cover the area. If the geographic location is not obvious from the telephone exchange, then each respondent should be asked whether the residence is within the boundaries of the study area.

4. In case–control studies, it is usually desirable to select controls with equal probability. Two problems occur in RDD sampling. The first is that households with two or more telephone numbers have greater chances of selection than those with one number. The higher probability of selection of such households can be avoided by subsampling them, i.e. retaining one-half of households with two telephone numbers, one-third of those with three numbers, etc. This adds somewhat to the number of households that need to be screened to reach the required sample size (about 4% of US, households have more than one telephone number), but the resulting simplification in the analyses usually makes it worthwhile. The second problem arises when it is considered undesirable to choose more than one person in a household, either to avoid a heavy response burden in any household or because the intraclass correlations within a household would appear to complicate analyses of the data. Subsampling within households will create considerable variation in probabilities of selection and is not recommended. Many case–control studies are restricted to the adult population, or to a subset, such as ages 45–69. In such cases it is possible to reduce sharply the number of households with multiple controls by designating in advance half of the sample for male controls and half for female controls. In any household, only the males, or females, are then eligible for the sample. Depending on the distribution of the desired number of controls by sex, instead of designating 50% of the sample for male controls and 50% for females, a 60–40, 70–30, or some other ratio could be used. This sex designation of the sample greatly increases the amount of screening necessary to locate the controls, and a researcher should weigh this fact against the desirability of simpler analytic methods. Potthoff [9] has described another method of choosing only one control per household with an equal probability sample, but this method also increases the required screening.

5. With frequency matching, the amount of screening that will be required can be estimated by calculating the number of households that need to be screened to locate one required control in each of the matching cells (strata), and multiplying it by the number of desired controls. The stratum with the largest value determines the screening sample size. This result should be increased to account for the percentage of refusals or those who are out of scope (e.g. persons with some types of chronic diseases may be considered ineligible for the study). It may also be necessary to increase the screening if

no more than one person per household is chosen and one of the devices described earlier for doing this is used.

6. It is frequently difficult to determine the total number of households that will need to be screened to provide the desired number of controls, and the subsampling rates for the various strata. Some of the difficulty comes from the small samples desired per matching cell and the consequent large sampling errors on the household yield. Another reason may be uncertainty of the population size of the various strata when geographic matching is required. When time permits, it is useful to do the sampling in waves, (e.g. divide the workload into monthly subsamples) with each wave a random sample of the population. The sample sizes and subsampling rates in each wave can be based on experience in previous waves. Since the waves are all random samples, the data can be pooled without the need to take the different sample sizes and rates into account.

7. It is necessary to inquire whether the telephone number reached is for a home, business, institution, or some other nonhousehold facility. This is normally one of the first questions asked. Some small businesses operate in residential units and the telephones are used both for business and personal use. The questions asked should be able to identify such cases and retain them in the sample. Both companies previously referred to that supply telephone samples can match the sample numbers with yellow page directory listings to reduce the number of business numbers that need to be dialed. There is a small loss of households that operate small businesses, but the bias is generally considered trivial.

8. A policy needs to be established on how to treat answering machines, that is, whether to leave messages or simply to hang up and try again. Answering machines are quite common in the US, and the method of dealing with them could have an important effect on response rates.

9. The study should include provision for a considerable number of callbacks to insure that persons who are infrequently at home have the same chance of selection as the rest of the population. Many researchers make eight to 12 calls for the hard-to-get population spread throughout

daylight and evening hours and weekdays and weekends, and some researchers use larger numbers. As a result of the large number of households in which all adults are employed and the number containing only a single adult, it is necessary to mount a major follow up operation to attain a reasonable response rate. There have been a number of studies of the differences between persons who can be easily reached by telephone and those requiring more effort, and they have revealed important differences in occupational status and life styles. There are also likely to be differences in exposure and in background variables affecting many diseases. Failure to achieve reasonably consistent response rates among persons who are easily reached and those who require more callbacks could lead to serious biases that are not possible to detect and correct for. Although a main purpose of the callbacks is to make first contact with the household residents, it can also be used to try to convince potential respondents who initially refused to cooperate and to change their minds. Conversion of about one-third of those who initially refused is not uncommon.

10. Evening calls are necessary in a large number of households, and researchers should recognize that most of the interviewing will have to be done after normal working hours. A common practice is to start off with one round of daytime calls to the entire sample which will usually identify almost all of the nonworking, business, and institutional numbers, and a minority of the households. The remaining calls – mostly to households – are then made in the evening.

Under some circumstances, weighting the data may be necessary to avoid biases in the analysis. Weighting will be needed if all persons within a matching cell did not receive the same chance of selection, e.g. if there was subsampling of household members within the same matching cell, or if all households with more than one telephone number were retained in the sample. For example, if households with multiple telephones were not subsampled, then households with two telephone numbers should be given a weight of one-half, those with three numbers given a weight of one-third, etc. Similarly, with subsampling within households so that only one person within a cell was chosen, the weight should be the number of household members within the matching cell. If the subsampling went further so that only one person per household was selected for the control regardless of the number of matching cells represented in a household, then a more complex system of weighting will be required. Such subsampling should be avoided if at all possible since it will complicate the study operations and may have a serious effect on the precision of the results.

Standard **odds ratio** analysis is not strictly applicable in case–control studies that use cluster sampling such as the Mitofsky–Waksberg method or that require weighting. Modifications in the analysis that account for clustering are described by Graubard et al. [4]. Appropriate confidence intervals for odds ratios can also be obtained through use of either of two software packages originally developed for analyses of surveys using complex sample designs but that also contain provision for estimating the precision of odds ratios, WESVAR [1] and SUDAAN [10]. If there are only minor deviations from an unclustered, equal-probability sample selection scheme, then it is probably satisfactory to use the more common methods of establishing confidence intervals around odds ratios.

References

[1]   Brick, J.M., Broene, P., James, P. & Severynse, J. (1996). *A User's Guide to WesVarPC*. Westat, Rockville.

[2]   Brick, J.M., Waksberg, J., Kulp, D. & Starer, A. (1995). Bias in list-assisted telephone samples, *Public Opinion Quarterly* **59**, 218–235.

[3]   Casady, R.J. & Lepkowski, J.M. (1993). Stratified telephone survey designs, *Survey Methodology* **19**, 103–113.

[4]   Graubard, B.I., Fears, T.R. & Gail, M.H. (1989). Effects of cluster sampling on epidemiologic analysis in population-based case–control studies, *Biometrics* **45**, 1053–1071.

[5]   Harlow, D.L. & Davis, S. (1988). Two one-step methods for household screening and interviewing using random digit dialing, *American Journal of Epidemiology* **127**, 857–863.

[6]   Hartge, P., Brinton, L.A., Rosenthal, J.F., Cahill, J.I., Hoover, R.N. & Waksberg, J. (1984). Random digit dialing in selecting a population-based control group, *American Journal of Epidemiology* **120**, 825–833.

[7]   Hartge, P., Cahill, J.I., West, D., Hauck, M., Austin, D., Silverman, D. & Hoover, R. (1984). Design and methods in a multi-center case–control interview study, *American Journal of Public Health* **74**, 52–56.

[8]   Lepkowski, J.M. (1988). Telephone sampling methods in the United States, in *Telephone Survey Methodology*,

R.M. Groves, P.P. Biemer, L.E. Lyberg et al., eds. Wiley, New York, pp. 73–98.

[9]   Potthoff, R.F. (1994). Telephone sampling in epidemiologic research: to reap the benefits, avoid the pitfalls, *American Journal of Epidemiology* **139**, 967–978.

[10]   Shah, B.V., Barnwell, B.G., Hunt, P.N. & LaVange, L.M. (1992). *SUDAAN User's Manual*. Research Triangle Institute, Research Triangle Park.

[11]   Wacholder, S., McLaughlin, J.K., Silverman, D.T. & Mandel, J.S. (1992). Selection of controls in case–control studies. I. Principles, *American Journal of Epidemiology* **135**, 1019–1028.

[12]   Wacholder, S., Silverman, D.T., McLaughlin, J.K. & Mandel, J.S. (1992). Selection of controls in case–control studies III. Design options, *American Journal of Epidemiology* **135**, 1042–1050.

[13]   Waksberg, J. (1978). Sampling methods for random digit dialing, *Journal of the American Statistical Association* **73**, 40–46.

(*See also* **Sample Surveys**)

JOSEPH WAKSBERG

Random Error

Suppose one seeks to measure the width of a table by repeatedly applying a ruler to obtain a series of measurements. One assumes that the true table width, μ, remains constant and that any given measurement, $y_i = \mu + e_i$, represents the sum of a systematic component and an error component, $e_i = y_i - \mu$. In this simple model, μ is called the systematic part, and, if the expectation of e_i is zero, e_i is called the random error. If it is assumed that the random errors are independent, then the mean value $\bar{y} = \mu + n^{-1}\sum e_i$ converges (almost surely) to the true value. As the sample size, n, increases, the effects of random error diminish, and, in particular, if the e_i have a common variance, σ^2, $\text{var}(\bar{y}) = \sigma^2/n$. The diminishing influence of random error with increasing sample size is also found in more general models with systematic and random components.

Suppose, however, we subsequently learn that our ruler had been worn down so that the putative interval [0, 1] cm was only 0.9 cm long. Then, the errors $e_i = y_i - \mu$ have expectation $(\mu - 0.1) - \mu = -0.1$ cm, and $\bar{y}$ gets closer and closer to the **biased** answer,

$\mu - 0.1$, as n increases. Thus, increasing the sample size offers no protection against **systematic error** and only leads to more precise biased estimates.

M.H. GAIL

Randomized Recruitment Method
see Case–Control Study, Two-Phase

Rate

Rate refers to a limiting ratio of the changes in two quantities as these changes tend to zero. The denominator often involves time, t, as for the **hazard rate**, $\lambda(t) = \lim_{\Delta\downarrow} \Delta^{-1}\mathrm{Pr}$ (disease first occurs in $[t, t + \Delta)$|disease first occurs at or after t). The notation $[t, t + \Delta)$ means that the event occurs at or after t but before $t + \Delta$.

Sometimes rate refers to a proportion, as in neonatal mortality rate and **prevalence rate**.

M.H. GAIL

Rater Agreement *see* Agreement, Measurement of

Recall Bias

Recall bias occurs in **case–control studies** and refers to the **bias** that results when cases with the disease of interest tend to over- or underestimate their previous exposures, compared with controls without disease. For example, a woman who has just given birth to a malformed infant may more assiduously recall her antenatal drug exposures than a **control** woman who had a normal infant. Recall bias induces **differential error** and can seriously distort the results of a case–control study.

(*See also* **Bias in Case–Control Studies**; **Bias in Observational Studies**; **Bias, Overview**).

M.H. GAIL

Record Linkage

At the core of all **descriptive epidemiology** studies lies a data set, with many variables, which has been gathered to answer a specific hypothesis. Often it is only as the project develops that the researcher realizes the potential of exploring alternate study endpoints by adding in other data about the same respondents. The tried and tested technique is for a clerk to look at the individual records, sorted in some logical order, and put the records together, applying intuitive decision rules based on human judgment. As record systems have been computerized over the past 20 years, one of the greatest impacts of increased processing power has been to facilitate linkages between related data sets, even when they do not share a unique identifier.

Three main techniques are used for record linkage, Newcombe [13] and Jamieson et al. [9] describe in detail the technical issues relating to exact matching and probability linkage. They can be summarized as follows:

1. *Unique.* Records are linked together where unique identifiers such as insurance number or health service number match exactly. The files of records are computer sorted into the same order, and matched together within blocks. It is a fairly simple process, but may only identify 80%–85% of true matches due to errors in recording of identifiers.

2. *Fuzzy.* For data sets which do not have unique identifiers, key identifiers such as surname, date of birth, sex, date of interview/treatment, and postal district are used for linkage. To cope with coding errors, fuzzy matching identifies records which are "almost" the same, such as surname spelling incorrect, or year and month of birth correct, but day wrong. Computer programs either present a choice of matches for the user to choose the best match, or have incorporated a simple scoring system and determine the best match from the score. Computer algorithms are well

developed for matching on individual variables, and this technique provides 85%–90% of true matches. It requires human intervention and there may be operator **bias**.

3. *Probability*. This is the most sophisticated form of linkage, in which decision rules on records matching are programmed based on the probability of two records being from different people having the same identifier. These probabilities are aggregated to a score and checked against a threshold to determine whether a match is made. The computer system needs to be tailored for the data sets to be matched and is processor intensive, but provides linkages of 95%–99% true matches with false positive rates of 1%–2%.

The following are examples of the uses made of record linkage within healthcare systems and demonstrate the value of this powerful technique. Many of the examples come from uses made of the Scottish Medical Record Linkage Database [7], which contains morbidity records from Scottish hospitals, and mortality records from the General Register Office (Scotland) from 1968 onwards – almost 4 million people with 12 million episodes.

Medical record linkage poses problems of data confidentiality and privacy, because the linked data are comprehensive and the techniques use personal identifying data. Most analytic studies do not require access to patient identifiable data once the linkages have been made. For administrative data sets, strict controls need to be in place to ensure that the data are not released to individuals and used for purposes other than those registered in government legislation.

The issue of infringing civil liberties, by invasion of privacy through wrongful use of information, is currently taxing most governments. Researchers need to be aware of legislation and appropriate use of data. For example, in Scotland, access to identifiable data is controlled by medically qualified data holders, and a Privacy Advisory Committee [10] has been established, with membership drawn from senior medical officers, legal professions, and the public, to ensure that ethical approval is in place for record linkage studies.

Evidence-Based Medicine

The perception remains that descriptive epidemiology has little to contribute to the development of evidence-based medicine with its focus on randomized clinical trials (see McPherson [12]). Probability-based record linkage techniques can make a major contribution in assessing the efficacy of treatment regimes at the macro level. For example, using exact matching on health service administration numbers, Evans et al. [4] at the Tayside Medicines Monitoring Unit are able to use **case–control** methodology to review the association of topical nonsteroidal anti-inflammatory drugs with hospital admission for upper gastrointestinal bleeding and perforation. The Scottish Health Service are now automating the linkage between prescribing data, patient hospitalization, and death profiles. This will establish a facility for post-marketing surveillance, in which possible adverse drug reactions can be quickly analyzed and assessed before the public are alarmed by the media (*see* **Pharmacoepidemiology, Overview**).

Another area in which linkage is being used effectively is the follow-up of very low birthweight children and the impact of their improved survival on health care costs. In California [2], probability-linked data from the California Birth Cohort and Medicaid claims in years after birth have been used to evaluate competing hypotheses for racial and ethnic differences in mortality and health care costs, and to assess the need for hospital services from the improved neonatal survival of these children.

Outcome Measurement

Evaluating the effects of medical care is not a new idea, but it has received increased emphasis over the past decade because of concerns for the quality and cost of medical care. While most attention has been placed on determining the effectiveness of new treatment regimes through randomized control trials, the inclusion criterion for patients can be so selective that the true efficacy of the treatment can only be assessed when it comes into general usage. Application of record linkage techniques using administrative databases for follow-up of cohorts of patients with specific disease patterns, or procedures, permits analysis of outcomes measures which would otherwise be prohibitively expensive.

The Clinical Resource and Audit Group of the Scottish Office Department of Health have pioneered the publication of routine clinical outcome measures in the UK since 1993. The three reports [17] to date have been produced following detailed consultation with health service professionals, to gain consensus on the measures and to assess the feasibility of using them to monitor the effectiveness and appropriateness of health purchasing strategies. Without a unique patient identifier, probability linkage is the key to determining readmission rates, including to other institutions, and postoperation survival after discharge.

While the measures tend to be presented as interval estimates, standardized for **confounding** factors, such as age, sex, deprivation, and co-morbidities, administrative data do not yet contain robust measures of severity of disease. As with all descriptive epidemiology techniques, the outcome measures highlight topics for more detailed investigation via randomized controlled trials or clinical audit.

Survival Rates

As the search continues for new, meaningful outcome measures, one of the main uses of record linkage has been analysis of survival patterns for disease, especially for cancer (*see* **Survival Analysis, Overview**). Most civil registration authorities provide an exact matching service for bona fide researchers. However, increased computing power has meant that this process can now be automated to include probability or "fuzzy" matching techniques, which increase the reliability of the links. Within the Scottish Cancer Registry, we found that exact matching with manual techniques under-ascertained almost 5% of deaths [16], because the procedures were built on zero tolerance of false positive rates. This resulted in one study for the nuclear industry showing a "healthy worker" effect (*see* **Occupational Epidemiology**), until another three deaths were determined by automated probability linkage among the cohort of employees.

The availability of population-based data in specific **diseases registers**, such as cancer, diabetes, and renal failure, with linkage to death registrations enables the development of survival tables [16] (*see* **Life Table**), which are of use not only to the professional dealing with individual patients but also to the patients and their carers. Society is becoming more attuned to the concepts of **risk**, and one of the most common questions asked when life-threatening disease is diagnosed is "What is my chance of surviving 1 year, 5 years, or 10 years?". Insurance companies are very interested in improved estimates of actuarial risk for health care policies.

Changing Treatment Patterns in Hospital Care

Access to databases containing linked patient episodes over long time periods (15+ years) helps to identify the changing treatment patterns and use of hospital resources by cohorts of patients with specific disease. For example, the protocol for clinical treatment of asthma in children has changed considerably over the past 20 years, and Strachan et al. [18] used linked data for children with their first hospital admission for asthma between 1980 and 1984 to explore the increase in subsequent emergency admissions for the disease during the following 10 years.

In mental health the impact of policies for shifting care from the acute sector to the community can be monitored from linked data sets. Geddes & Juszczak [5] argue that trends in increased suicide rates for recently discharged female psychiatric patients may well be related to changes in discharge protocols due to implementation of government policy and new clinical practice. In a similar vein, the Scottish Health Service is currently linking mental health discharge records to the general hospital patient database, to investigate if the policy of early discharge from psychiatric institutions has resulted in psychiatric patients being readmitted to acute care after a short period in the community.

The effect on emergency readmission rates from early hospital discharge and associated quality of care have been identified by Henderson et al. [8] and Thomas & Holloway [19]. Investigation of Scottish data demonstrates "like" Trusts which have significantly different medical emergency readmission rates, with inversely related bed occupancy rates and lengths of continuous inpatient stay. Instead of focusing on efficiency (high throughput, and short length of hospital stay) commissioners of health care can consider the effect of a 50% variation in the risk of emergency readmissions: Does this provide acceptable levels of value for money versus quality of care for the patient?

One of the roles of descriptive epidemiology is to aid the understanding of uncertainty. McPherson [12] uses the example of 5 year mortalities following treatments for prostatectomy, reported from analysis of large linked databases, to highlight the impact of changing clinical practice without the rigors of assessment trials, and the concerns raised amongst patients when consensus cannot be reached amongst clinicians on the effect of different treatments.

Health Service Planning

The potential of taking data created routinely as part of a government's system for paying for medical care and turning it into information on health needs and the health of the population is well demonstrated by the work of Roos & Shapiro [14] and Roos et al. [15] and his team at the Manitoba Center for Health Policy and Evaluation. The research attempts to move beyond medical care policy initiatives (e.g. insuring availability, quality of care, and efficiency) to health policy initiatives of improving longevity and quality of life. As pressures grow, throughout Europe and North America, to contain the costs of health care by reducing investment in acute sectors, health planners are looking to such population health information systems for quantitative trend data on which to base their decisions. Evidence is needed to answer questions such as:

1. Are high risk populations poorly served or do they have poor health outcomes despite availability of services?
2. Can we shift resources from acute care to primary care?
3. What services can be rationed without jeopardizing at-risk populations?

Lack of population morbidity information leads epidemiologists to use hospitalization rates as proxy measures for underlying morbidity. Improved availability of general practice diagnosis and treatment data from administrative systems in the surgery allows estimation of the true level of demand in communities, which can be linked with hospital discharge data at a patient level. This is invaluable for needs assessment work in public health, where commissioners of services attempt to balance supply with demand within small geographic areas.

Longitudinal and Cohort Studies

Many of the most renowned epidemiologic studies, such as Framingham [20] and Whitehall [11], used the manual tracking systems available from civil death registries. The advent of computer technology has made automated follow-up of survey data for alternative endpoints other than death a simple process – provided that informed consent is obtained by the subject for access to computerized medical records.

In 1973–76, a cohort of the population in the west of Scotland towns of Paisley and Renfrew, aged 45–64 years, took part in a cardiovascular survey of mid-life health, the MIDSPAN [6] project. Participants gave written consent to their medical records being used for follow-up, and the data set now includes details of all episodes of hospital care and death registrations for participants as they have aged over the past 20 years. It can be used for prospective **case–control studies** to investigate determinants of good and poor health from baseline lifestyle variables and clinical measurements.

The West of Scotland Coronary Prevention Study (WOSCOPS) [21] demonstrated the value of automated linkage in a randomized–controlled trial compared to prospective follow-up using direct contact with patients. An accuracy check of the study's own independent records of deaths and hospitalizations for the study population with data available from the Scottish Medical Record Linkage Database showed that while almost 100% accuracy was achieved for deaths, the study records under-ascertained hospitalizations for cardiovascular disease.

In the US, the Veterans Affairs database [1] has formed the source for multicenter randomized and quasi-randomized health service trials, which are much easier to plan and conduct in a centralized state system than in the private sector.

The UK Case–Control Study for Childhood Cancers will report findings in 1997. One of the methodological issues which has arisen from the study, access to case notes, has demonstrated the value of conducting applied research within the health administration system of the country rather than solely in an academic environment. The study is investigating hypotheses for cause and effect of cancer in children, covering ionizing radiation, chemical exposure, preconception and *in utero* exposure, parental occupational hazards, electromagnetic fields, and infectious exposure.

Summary

This article has described the main applications of record linkage techniques in epidemiology: from follow-up studies in randomized controlled trials and surveys to outcome measurement and survival following hospital care in the general population.

The Chief Medical Officer of the UK government [3] recently identified the need to use better descriptions of public health risk. We have demonstrated that, within health administration systems, much of the data already exists. When integrated using linkage techniques, these data can be used to build the knowledge base to identify these risks and to quantify them in both relative and attributable ways.

The use of such linked databases for descriptive epidemiology brings the following benefits:

1. data ascertainment, validity, and quality are documented within the administrative system;
2. linkage can be performed by computer at low cost relative to staff costs;
3. completeness of linkage is greater than by manual methods;
4. research efforts can focus on the analyses and interpretation of the data rather than data collection.

Provided that privacy and confidentiality rules are strictly applied, and users remember that in any linkage system, be it exact match or probability-based, one cannot be 100% certain that the correct data have been linked, there are vast data repositories available waiting to unlock the answers to key epidemiologic questions.

References

[1] Ashton, C.M., Menke, T.J., Deykin, D., Camberg, L.C. & Charns, M.P. (1996). A state-of-the-art conference on databases pertaining to veterans' health, *Medical Care* **34**, MS1–MS234.

[2] Bell, R.M., Keesey, J. & Richards, T. (1994). The urge to merge: linking vital statistics records and medicaid claims, *Medical Care* **32**, 1004–1018.

[3] Department of Health (1996). *"On the State of Public Health" – Annual Report of the Chief Medical Officer*. HMSO, London.

[4] Evans, J.M.M., McMahon, A.D., McGilchrist, A.D., White, G., Murray, F.E., McDevitt, D.G. & McDonald, T.M. (1995). Topical non-steroidal anti-inflammatory drugs and admission to hospital for upper gastrointestinal bleeding and perforation: a record-linkage case control study, *British Medical Journal* **311**, 22–26.

[5] Geddes, J.R. & Juszczak, E. (1995). Period trends in rates of suicide in first 28 days after discharge from psychiatric hospital in Scotland, 1968–92, *British Medical Journal* **311**, 357–360.

[6] Hawthorne, V.M., Beevers, D.G. & Greaves, D.A. (1974). Blood pressure in a Scottish town, *British Medical Journal* **3**, 600–603.

[7] Heasman, M.A. (1968). The use of record linkage in long-term prospective studies, in *Record Linkage in Medicine, Proceedings of the International Symposium, Oxford*, E.D. Acheson, ed. Oxford University Press, Oxford.

[8] Henderson, J., Evans, J.G. & Goldacre, M.J. (1991). Use of medical records linkage to study readmission rates, *British Medical Journal* **303**, 389–393.

[9] Jamieson, E., Roberts, J. & Browne, G. (1995). The feasibility and accuracy of anonymised record linkage to estimate shared clientele among three health and social service agencies, *Methods of Information in Medicine* **34**, 371–377.

[10] Kendrick, S. & Clarke, J. (1993). The Scottish Record Linkage System, *Health Bulletin* **51**, 72–79.

[11] Marmot, M.G., Rose, G., Shipley, M. & Hamilton, P.J.S. (1978). Employment grade and coronary heart disease in British civil servants, *Journal of Epidemiology and Community Health* **32**, 244–249.

[12] McPherson, K. (1994). The best and the enemy of the good: randomized controlled trials, uncertainty, and assessing the role of patient choice in medical decision making, *Journal of Epidemiology and Community Health* **48**, 6–15.

[13] Newcombe, H.B. (1988). *Handbook of Record Linkage: Methods for Health and Statistical Studies, Administration and Business*. Oxford University Press, Oxford.

[14] Roos, N.P. & Shapiro, E. (1995). A productive experiment with administrative data, *Medical Care* **33**, DS7–DS12.

[15] Roos, N.P., Black, C.D., Frehlich, N., Decoster, C., Cohen, N., Tataryn, D., Mustard, C.A., Toil, F., Carriere, K.C., Burchill, C.A., MacWilliam, M. & Bogdanovic, B. (1995). A population-based health information system, *Medical Care* **33**, DS13–DS20.

[16] Scottish Health Service, Information & Statistics Division (1993). *Trends in Cancer Survival in Scotland: 1968–1990*. Common Services Agency, Edinburgh.

[17] Scottish Office Department of Health (1996). *Clinical Outcome Measures – CRAG Report*. HMSO, Edinburgh.

[18] Strachan, D.P., Seagroatt, V. & Cook, D.G. (1994). Chest illness in infancy and chronic respiratory disease in later life – an analysis of month of birth, *International Journal of Epidemiology* **23**, 1060–1068.

[19] Thomas, J.W. & Holloway, J.J. (1991). Investigating early readmission as an indicator for quality of care studies, *Medical Care* **29**, 377–394.

[20] Truett, J., Cornfield, J. & Kannel, W.A. (1967). A multivariate analysis of the risk of coronary heart disease in Framingham, *Journal of Chronic Diseases* **20**, 167–179.

[21]   West of Scotland Coronary Prevention Study Group (1995). Computerized records linkage compared with traditional patient follow-up methods in clinical trials and illustrated in a prospective epidemiological study, *Journal of Clinical Epidemiology* **48**, 1441–1452.

MARY SMALLS & STEVE KENDRICK

Regression Calibration *see* Measurement Error in Epidemiologic Studies

Relative Hazard

The relative hazard is the ratio of two **hazard rate** functions at a given time. If this hazard ratio is constant, as is assumed in the **proportional hazards model**, it can be consistently estimated both from **cohort** and from time-matched **case–control studies** (*see* **Density Sampling**). Over a small time interval, the relative hazard can be estimated as the **incidence density** ratio, also known as the **incidence rate** ratio.

M.H. GAIL

Relative Odds

The relative odds, or **odds ratio**, is the ratio of the **odds** of disease in an exposed cohort divided by that in an unexposed cohort. The relative odds can be estimated not only from **cohort** data but also from **case–control** data, because the relative odds of exposure comparing cases with disease-free controls equals the relative odds of disease comparing exposed with unexposed [1]. For rare diseases, the odds ratio approximates the **relative risk**.

Reference

[1]   Cornfield, J. (1951). A method of estimating comparative rates from clinical data. Application to cancer of the lung, breast and cervix, *Journal of the National Cancer Institute* **11**, 1269–1275.

M.H. GAIL

Relative Risk

The relative risk is the ratio of the **risk** of disease in an exposed **cohort** over a defined time interval to the risk of disease in an unexposed cohort over this same time interval. Relative risk is synonymous with **cumulative incidence ratio**. Relative risk can be estimated both from cohort studies, and, for rare diseases, from **case–control studies**.

M.H. GAIL

Relative Risk Function (RRF) *see* Geographical Analysis

Relative Risk Modeling

Risk models are used to describe the hazard function (*see* **Hazard Rate**; **Survival Analysis, Overview**) $\lambda(t, z)$ for time-to-failure data as a function of time t and covariates $\mathbf{Z} = Z_1, \ldots, Z_p$, which may themselves be time dependent. The term "relative risk models" is used to refer to the covariate part $r(\cdot)$ of a risk model in a **proportional hazards** form

$$\lambda(t, \mathbf{Z}) = \lambda_0(t)\, r[\mathbf{Z}(t); \boldsymbol{\beta}], \qquad (1)$$

where $\boldsymbol{\beta}$ represents a vector of parameters to be estimated. In the standard proportional hazards model, the **relative risk** term takes the loglinear form $r(\mathbf{Z}, \boldsymbol{\beta}) = \exp(\mathbf{Z}'\boldsymbol{\beta})$. This has the convenient property that it is positive for all possible covariate and parameter values, since the hazard rate itself must be nonnegative. However, in particular applications, some alternative form of relative risk model may be more appropriate.

First, an aside on the subject of time is warranted. Time can be measured on a number of different scales, such as age, calendar time, or time since start of observation. One of these must be selected as the time axis t for use of the proportional hazards model. In clinical trials, time since diagnosis or start of treatment is commonly used for this purpose, since one of the major objectives of such studies is to make statements about prognosis. In epidemiologic studies, however, age is the preferred time axis, because it is usually a powerful determinant of disease rates, but it is not of primary interest; thus, it is essential that its **confounding** effects be eliminated. However, other temporal factors, such as calendar date, or time since exposure began may still be relevant and can be handled either by treating them as covariates or by **stratification**.

Why Model Relative Risks?

Before proceeding further, it is worth pausing to inquire why one might wish to adopt the proportional hazards model at all. Certainly, there are examples of situations where some other form of model provides a better description of the underlying biologic process. Two alternative models that have received some attention are the additive hazards model $\lambda(t, \mathbf{Z}) = \lambda_0(t) + \mathbf{Z}'\boldsymbol{\beta}$ and the accelerated failure-time model $S(t, \mathbf{Z}) = S_0[t \exp(\mathbf{Z}'\boldsymbol{\beta})]$, where $S(t) = \exp[-\int_0^t \lambda(u)du]$ is the survival function. Although any risk model can be reparameterized in proportional hazards form, it may be that a more parsimonious model can be found using some alternative formulation. For example, the additive risk model could be written as $\lambda(t, \mathbf{Z}) = \lambda_0(t)(1 + \tilde{\mathbf{Z}}'\boldsymbol{\beta})$, where $\tilde{\mathbf{Z}} = \mathbf{Z}/\lambda_0(t)$ if the baseline hazard $\lambda_0(t)$ were some known parametric function, such as a set of external rates for an unexposed population. In this case, whether the proportional hazards or additive hazards model provides a more parsimonious description of the data depends on whether relative risk or the **excess risk** is more nearly constant over time (or requires the fewest time-dependent **interaction** effects).

The advantages of relative risk models are both mathematical and empirical. Mathematically, the proportional hazards model allows "semiparametric" estimation of covariate effects via partial likelihood without requiring parametric assumptions about the

form of the baseline hazard. Furthermore, at least with the standard loglinear form of the relative risk model, asymptotic normality seems to be achieved faster in many applications than for most alternative models. Empirically, it appears that many failure-time processes do indeed show rough proportionality of the hazard to time and covariate effects, at least with appropriate specification of the covariates. Evidence of this phenomenon for cancer incidence is reviewed in Breslow & Day [2, Chapter 2]: age-specific **incidence rates** from a variety of populations have more nearly constant ratios than differences.

Data Structures and Likelihoods

Failure-time data arise in many situations in biology and medicine. In clinical trials, time-to-death or time-to-disease-recurrence are frequently used endpoints. In epidemiology, **cohort studies** are often concerned with disease incidence or mortality in some exposed population, and **case–control studies** can be viewed as a form of sampling within a general population cohort. All these designs involve the collection of a set of data for each individual $i = 1, \ldots, I$ comprising a failure or censoring time t_i, a censoring indicator $d_i = 1$ if the failure time is observed (i.e. the subject is affected), zero otherwise, and a vector of covariates $\mathbf{z}_i$, possibly time dependent.

The appropriate likelihood depends on the sampling design and data structure. For a clinical trial or cohort study with the same period of observation for all subjects, but where only the disease status, not the failure-time itself, is observed, a **logistic model** for the probability of failure of the form $\Pr(D = 0|\mathbf{Z}) = [1 + \alpha r(\mathbf{Z}, \boldsymbol{\beta})]^{-1}$ might be used, where α is the odds of failure for a subject with $\mathbf{Z} \equiv 0$. Again, the standard form is obtained using $r(\mathbf{Z}, \boldsymbol{\beta}) = \exp(\mathbf{Z}'\boldsymbol{\beta})$. The likelihood for this design would then be

$$L(\alpha, \boldsymbol{\beta}) = \prod_i \Pr(D = d_i|\mathbf{Z} = \mathbf{z}_i; \alpha, \boldsymbol{\beta})$$

$$= \prod_i \frac{[\alpha r(\mathbf{z}_i; \boldsymbol{\beta})]^{d_i}}{1 + \alpha r(\mathbf{z}_i; \boldsymbol{\beta})}. \qquad (2)$$

The same model and likelihood function would be used for an unmatched case–control study, except that α now involves the control sampling fractions as well as the baseline disease risk.

In a clinical trial or cohort study in which the failure times are observed, the proportional hazards model (1) leads to a full likelihood of the form

$$L[\lambda_0(\cdot), \boldsymbol{\beta}] = \prod_i \lambda_0(t_i)^{d_i} r[\mathbf{z}_i(t_i); \boldsymbol{\beta}]^{d_i}$$

$$\times \exp\left\{ -\int_{s_i}^{t_i} \lambda_0(t)\, r[\mathbf{z}_i(t); \boldsymbol{\beta}]\mathrm{d}t \right\}, \quad (3)$$

where s_i denotes the entry time of subject i. Use of the full likelihood requires specification of the form of the baseline hazard. Cox [6] proposed instead a "partial likelihood" of the form

$$L(\boldsymbol{\beta}) = \prod_{n=1}^{N} \frac{r[z_{i_n}(t_n); \boldsymbol{\beta}]}{\sum_{j \in R_n} r[z_j(t_n); \boldsymbol{\beta}]}, \quad (4)$$

where $n = 1, \ldots, N$ indexes the observed failure times, i_n denotes the individual who fails at time t_n and R_n denotes the set of subjects at risk at time t_n. This likelihood does not require any specification of the form of the baseline hazard; the estimation of $\boldsymbol{\beta}$ is said to be "semiparametric", as the relative risk factor is still specified parametrically (e.g. the loglinear model in the standard form). This partial likelihood can also be used to fit relative risk models for matched case–control studies (including **nested case–control studies** within a cohort), where n now indexes the cases and R_n indicates the set comprising the nth case and his matched controls.

For very large data sets, it may be more convenient to analyze the data in grouped form using **Poisson regression**. For this purpose, the total person-time of follow-up is grouped into $k = 1, \ldots, K$ categories on the basis of time and covariates, and the number of events N_k and person-time T_k in each category is recorded, together with the corresponding values of the (average) time t_k and covariates $\mathbf{z}_k$. The proportional hazards model now leads to a Poisson likelihood for the grouped data of the form

$$L(\lambda, \boldsymbol{\beta}) = \prod_{k=1}^{K} [-\lambda_k T_k r(\mathbf{z}_k; \boldsymbol{\beta})]^{N_k}$$

$$\times \exp[-\lambda_k T_k r(\mathbf{z}_k; \boldsymbol{\beta})]/N_k!, \quad (5)$$

where $\lambda_k = \lambda_0(t_k)$ denotes a set of baseline hazard parameters that must be estimated together with $\boldsymbol{\beta}$.

Approaches to Model Specification

For any of these likelihoods, it suffices to substitute some appropriate function for $r(\mathbf{Z}; \boldsymbol{\beta})$ and then use the standard methods of maximum likelihood to estimate its parameters and test hypotheses. In the remainder of this article, we discuss various approaches to specifying this function. The major distinction we make is between empiric and mechanistic approaches. Empiric models are not based on any particular biologic theory for the underlying failure process, but simply attempt to provide a parsimonious description of it, particularly to identify and quantify the effects of covariates that affect the relative hazard. Perhaps the best known empiric model is the loglinear model for relative risks, but other forms may be appropriate for testing particular hypotheses or for more parsimonious modeling in particular data sets, as discussed in the following section. With a small number of covariates, it may also be possible to model the relative risk nonparametrically. Mechanistic models, on the other hand, aim to describe the observed data in terms of some unobservable underlying disease process, such as the **multistage theory of carcinogenesis**. We touch on such models briefly at the end.

Before proceeding further, it should be noted that what follows is predicated on the assumption that the covariates $\mathbf{Z}$ are accurately measured (or that the exposure–response relationship that will be estimated refers to the measured value of the covariates, not to their true values). There is a large and growing literature on methods of adjustment of relative risk models for measurement error (*see* **Measurement Error in Epidemiologic Studies**).

Empiric Models

The loglinear model, $\ln r(\mathbf{Z}; \boldsymbol{\beta}) = \mathbf{Z}'\boldsymbol{\beta}$, is probably the most widely used empiric model and is the standard form included in all statistical packages for logistic, Cox, and Poisson regression (*see* **Software, Biostatistical**). As noted earlier, it is nonnegative and it produces a nonzero likelihood for all possible parameter values, which doubtless contributes to the observation that in most applications, parameter estimates are reasonably normally distributed, even with relatively sparse data. However, the model involves two key assumptions that merit testing in any particular application:

1. for a continuous covariate Z, the relative risk depends exponentially on the value of Z; and
2. for a pair of covariates, Z_1 and Z_2, the relative risk depends multiplicatively on the marginal risks from each covariate separately (i.e. $r(\mathbf{Z}; \boldsymbol{\beta}) = r(Z_1; \beta_1) r(Z_2; \beta_2)$).

Neither of these assumptions is relevant for a single categorical covariate with K levels, for which one forms a set of $K - 1$ indicator variables corresponding to all levels other than the "referent" category. In other cases, the two assumptions can be tested by nesting the model in some more general model that includes the fitted model as a special case. This test can be accomplished without leaving the general class of loglinear models. For example, to test the first assumption, it may suffice to add one or more transformations of the covariate (such as its square) to the model and test the significance of its additional contribution. To test the second assumption, one could add a single product term (for two continuous or binary covariates) or a set of $(K - 1)(L - 1)$ products for two categorical variables with K and L levels respectively.

If these tests reveal significant lack of fit of the original model, one might nevertheless be satisfied with the expanded model as a reasonable description of the data (after appropriately testing the fit of that expanded model). However, one should then also consider the possibility that the data might be more parsimoniously described by some completely different form of model. In choosing such an alternative, one would naturally be guided by what the tests of fit of the earlier models had revealed, as well as by categorical analyses. For example, if a quadratic term produced a negative estimate, that might suggest that a linear rather than loglinear model might fit better; similarly, a negative estimate for an interaction term might suggest an **additive** rather than **multiplicative** form of model for joint effects. In this case, one might consider fitting a model of the form $r(\mathbf{Z}; \boldsymbol{\beta}) = 1 + \mathbf{Z}'\boldsymbol{\beta}$. Alternatively, one might prefer a model that is linear in each component, but multiplicative in their joint effects, $r(\mathbf{Z}; \boldsymbol{\beta}) = \prod_p (1 + Z_p \beta_p)$, or one that is loglinear in each component but additive jointly, $r(\mathbf{Z}; \boldsymbol{\beta}) = 1 + \sum_p [\exp(Z_p \beta_p) - 1]$.

In a rich data set, the number of possible alternative models can quickly get out of hand, so some structured approach to model building is needed. The key is to adopt a general class of models that would include all the alternatives one might be interested in as special cases, allowing specific submodels to be tested within nested alternatives. A general model that has achieved some popularity recently consists of a mixture of linear and loglinear terms of the form

$$r(\mathbf{Z}, \mathbf{W}; \boldsymbol{\beta}, \boldsymbol{\gamma})$$
$$= \exp(\mathbf{W}_0'\boldsymbol{\gamma}_0)\left[1 + \sum_{m=1}^{M} \mathbf{Z}_m'\boldsymbol{\beta}_m \exp(\mathbf{W}_m'\boldsymbol{\gamma}_m)\right], (6)$$

where $\boldsymbol{\beta}_m$ and $\boldsymbol{\gamma}_m$ denote vectors of regression coefficients corresponding to the subsets of covariates $\mathbf{Z}_m$ and $\mathbf{W}_m$ included in the mth linear and loglinear terms, respectively. Thus, for example, the standard loglinear model would comprise the single term $m = 0$, while the linear model would comprise a single term $m = 1$ with no covariates in the loglinear terms. A special case that has been widely used in radiobiology is of the form

$$r(\mathbf{Z}, \mathbf{W}; \boldsymbol{\beta}; \boldsymbol{\gamma}) = 1 + (\beta_1 Z + \beta_2 Z^2)$$
$$\times \exp(-\beta_3 Z + \mathbf{W}'\boldsymbol{\gamma}),$$

where Z represents radiation dose (believed from microdosimetry considerations to have a linear-quadratic effect on mutation rates at low doses multiplied by a negative exponential survival term to account for cell killing at high doses) and $\mathbf{W}$ comprises modifiers of the slope of the **dose–response** relationship, such as attained age, sex, latency, or age at exposure. For example, including the log of latency and its square in $\mathbf{W}$ allows for a lognormal dependence of excess relative risk on latency (*see* **Poisson Regression for Survival Data in Epidemiology** for a discussion of software for fitting such models).

Combining linear and loglinear terms, using the same p covariates, would produce a model of the form $r(\mathbf{Z}; \boldsymbol{\beta}, \boldsymbol{\gamma}) = \exp(\mathbf{Z}'\boldsymbol{\gamma})(1 + \mathbf{Z}'\boldsymbol{\beta})$ against which the fit of the linear and loglinear models could be tested with p df. Although useful as a test of fit of these two specific models, the interpretation of the parameters is not straightforward since the effect of the covariates is essentially split between the two components. It would be of greater interest to form a model with a single set of regression coefficients and an additional mixing parameter for the combination of the submodels. Conceptually the simplest such model is the exponential mixture [28]

$$r(\mathbf{Z}; \boldsymbol{\beta}; \theta) = (1 + \mathbf{Z}'\boldsymbol{\beta})^{1-\theta} \exp(\theta \mathbf{Z}'\boldsymbol{\beta}), \quad (7)$$

which produces the linear model when $\theta = 0$ and the loglinear model with $\theta = 1$. An alternative, based on the Box–Cox transformation, was proposed by Breslow & Storer [3], which also includes the linear and loglinear models as special cases. However, Moolgavkar & Venzon [20] pointed out both of these mixture models are sensitive to the coding of the covariates: for example, for binary covariates, relabelling the two possible values leads to different models, leading to different inferences both about the mixing parameter and the relative importance of the component risk factors. Guerro & Johnson [12] developed a variant of the Box–Cox model of the form

$$r(\mathbf{Z}; \boldsymbol{\beta}, \theta) = \begin{cases} \exp(\mathbf{Z}'\boldsymbol{\beta}), & \theta = 0, \\ (1 + \theta \mathbf{Z}'\boldsymbol{\beta})^{1/\theta}, & \theta \neq 0, \end{cases} \quad (8)$$

which appears to be the only model in the literature to date that does not suffer from this difficulty. These kinds of mixtures could in principle also be used to compare relative risk with additive (excess) risk models, although the interpretation of the β coefficient becomes problematic because it has different units under the different submodels.

Although suitable for testing multiplicativity vs. additivity with multidimensional categorical data, these mixtures are less useful for continuous covariates because they combine two quite different comparisons (the form of the dose–response relationship for each covariate and the form of their joint effects) into a single mixing parameter. One way around this difficulty is to compare linear and loglinear models for each covariate separately first to determine the best form of model, then to fit joint models, testing additivity vs. multiplicativity. Alternatively, one could form mixtures of more than two submodels with different mixing parameters for the different aspects.

A word of warning is needed concerning inference on the parameters of most nonstandard models. Moolgavkar & Venzon [20] pointed out that for nonstandard models, convergence to asymptotic normality can be very slow indeed. Thus, the log-likelihoods are generally far from quadratic, leading to highly skewed confidence regions. For this reason, Wald tests and confidence limits should generally be avoided. Furthermore, as the parameter moves away from the null, the standard error increases more quickly than the mean, so that the Wald test can appear to become less and less significant the larger the value of the parameter [13, 34]. These problems are particularly important for the mixing parameters θ, for which

inference should be based on the likelihood ratio test and likelihood-based confidence limits. For example, Lubin & Gaffey [15] describe an application of the exponential mixture of linear-additive and linear-multiplicative models [28] to testing the joint effect of radon and smoking on lung cancer risk in uranium miners; the point estimate of θ was 0.4, apparently closer to additivity than multiplicativity, but the likelihood ratio tests rejected the additive model ($\chi_1^2 = 9.8$) but not the multiplicative model ($\chi_1^2 = 1.1$). A linear mixture showed an even more skewed likelihood, with $\hat{\theta} = 0.1$ (apparently nearly additive) but with very similar likelihood ratio tests that rejected the additive but not the multiplicative model.

Models for Extended Exposure Histories

Chronic disease epidemiology often involves measurement of an entire history of exposure $\{X(u), u < t\}$ which we wish to incorporate into a relative risk model through one or more time-dependent covariates $\mathbf{Z}(t)$. How this is done depends upon one's assumptions about the underlying disease mechanism. We defer for the moment the possibility of modeling such a disease process directly and instead continue in the vein of empiric modeling, now focusing on eliciting information about the temporal modifiers of the exposure–response relationship.

Most approaches to exposure–response modeling in epidemiology are based on an implicit assumption of *dose additivity*, i.e. that the excess relative risk at time t is a sum of independent contributions from each increment of exposure at earlier times u, possibly modified in some fashion by temporal factors. This hypothesis can be expressed mathematically as

$$r[t, X(\cdot); \boldsymbol{\beta}; \boldsymbol{\gamma}] = R[Z(t); \boldsymbol{\beta}],$$

where

$$Z(t) = \int_0^t f[X(u); \alpha] \, g(t, u; \boldsymbol{\gamma}) \, du, \quad (9)$$

and where $R(Z; \boldsymbol{\beta})$ is some known relative risk function such as the linear or loglinear models discussed above, f is a known function describing the modifying effect of dose rate, and g is a known function describing the modifying effect of temporal factors. The simplest weighting functions would be $f(X) = X$ and $g(t, u) = 1$, for which $Z(t)$ becomes cumulative exposure, probably the most widely used exposure index in epidemiology. For many diseases with long latency, such as cancer, it is common to use lagged cumulative exposure, corresponding to a weighting function of the form $g(t, u; \gamma) = 1$ if $t - u > \gamma$, zero otherwise. Other simple exposure indices might include time-weighted exposure $\int_0^t X(u) (t - u) \, du$ or age-weighted exposure $\int_0^{t-\gamma} X(u) u \, du$, which could be added as additional covariates to $R(\mathbf{Z}; \boldsymbol{\beta})$ to test the modifying effects of latency or age at exposure. The function f can be used to test dose-rate effects (the phenomenon that a long, low-intensity exposure has a different risk from a short, high-intensity exposure for the same cumulative dose). For example, one might adopt a model of the form $f(X) = X^\alpha$ or $f(X) = X \exp(-\alpha X)$ for this purpose.

Models that do not involve unknown parameters α and γ are easily fitted using standard software by the device of computing the time-dependent covariate(s) for each subject in advance. Relatively simple functions of γ (such as the choice of lagging interval in the simple latency model) might be fitted by evaluating the likelihood over a grid of values of the parameter. For more complex functions $g(t, u; \boldsymbol{\gamma})$, such as a lognormal density in $t - u$ with unknown mean and variance (and perhaps additional dependence of these parameters on age, exposure rate, or other factors), it is preferable to use a package with the capability of computing $Z(t; \alpha, \boldsymbol{\gamma})$ at each iteration. This generally requires some programming by the user, whereas most of the likelihood calculations and iterative estimation are handled by the package. For example, using SAS procedure NLIN, one can recompute the covariates at each iteration by the appropriate commands inside the procedure.

Unfortunately, the additivity assumption has seldom been tested. In principle, this could be done by nesting the dose-additive model in some more general model that includes interactive effects between the dose increments received at different times. The obvious alternative model would simply add further covariates of the form

$$Z^*(t) = \int_0^t \int_0^u F[X(u)X(v); \alpha]$$
$$\times \, G(t, u, v; \boldsymbol{\gamma}, \delta) \, dv \, du, \qquad (10)$$

where F and G are some known weighting functions. However, one should take care to see that the dose-additive model is well fitted first before testing the

additivity assumption (e.g. by testing for nonlinearities and temporal modifiers).

Nonparametric Models

The appeal of Cox's partial likelihood is that no assumptions are needed about the form of the dependence of risk on time, but it remains parametric in modeling covariate effects. Even more appealing would be a nonparametric model for both time and covariate effects. For categorical data, no parametric assumptions are needed, of course, although the effects of multiple covariates are commonly estimated using the loglinear (i.e. multiplicative) model, with additional interaction terms as needed. Similarly, continuous covariates are frequently categorized to provide a visual impression of the exposure–response relationship, but the choice of cutpoints is arbitrary. However, nonparametric smoothing techniques are now available to allow covariate effects to be estimated without such arbitrary grouping.

One approach relies only on an assumption of monotonicity. Thomas [29] adapted the technique of isotonic regression to relative risk modeling, and showed that the maximum-likelihood estimator (MLE) of the exposure–response relationship under this constraint was a step function with jumps at the observed covariate values of a subset of the cases. The technique has been extended to two dimensions by Ulm [33], but in higher dimensions the resulting function is difficult to visualize and can be quite unstable.

Cubic splines and other means of smoothing provide attractive alternatives which produce smooth, but not necessarily monotonic, relationships. The generalized additive model [14] has been widely used for this purpose. For example, Schwartz [26] described the effect of air pollution on daily mortality rates using a generalized additive model, after controlling for weather variables and other factors using similar models. A complex dependence on dew point temperature was found, with multiple maxima and minima, whereas the smoothed plot of the particulate air pollution was seen to be almost perfectly linear over the entire range of concentrations.

With the advent of Markov chain Monte Carlo methods, Bayesian techniques for model selection and smoothing have become feasible and are currently an active area of research. A full treatment of these methods is beyond the scope of this article; see Gilks et al. [11] for recent reviews of this literature.

Mechanistic Models

In contrast with the empiric models discussed above, there are circumstances where the underlying disease process is well enough understood to allow it to be characterized mathematically. Probably the greatest activity along these lines has been in the field of cancer epidemiology. Two models in particular have dominated this development, the multistage model of Armitage & Doll [1] and the two-event model of Moolgavkar & Knudson [18] (*see* **Multistage Carcinogenesis Models**). For thorough reviews of this literature, see [17], [31], and [36]; here, we merely sketch the basic ideas.

The Armitage–Doll multistage model postulates that cancer arises from a single cell that undergoes a sequence of k heritable changes, such as point mutations, chromosomal rearrangements, or deletions, in a particular sequence. The model further postulates that the rate of one or more of these changes may depend on exposure to carcinogens. Then the model predicts that the hazard rate for the incidence of cancer (or more precisely, the appearance of the first truly malignant cell) following continuous exposure at rate X is of the form

$$\lambda(t, Z) = \alpha t^{k-1} \prod_{i=1}^{k} (1 + \beta_i X). \qquad (11)$$

Thus, the hazard has a power function dependence on age and a polynomial dependence on exposure rate with order equal to the number of dose-dependent stages. It further implies that two carcinogens would produce an additive effect if they act at the same stage and a multiplicative effect if they act at different stages. If exposure is instantaneous with intensity $X(u)$, its effect is modified by the age at and time since exposure: if it acts at a single stage i, then the excess relative risk at time t is proportional to $Z_{ik}(t) = X(u)u^{i-1}(t - u)^{k-i-1}/t^{k-1}$ and for an extended exposure at varying dose rates, the **excess relative risk** is obtained by integrating this expression over u [8, 35]. More complex expressions are available for time-dependent exposures to multiple agents acting at multiple stages [30]. These models can be fitted relatively easily using standard software by first evaluating the covariates $Z_{ik}(t)$ for each possible combination of $i < k$ and then fitting the linear relative risk model, as described above. Note, however, that the expressions given above are only approximations to the exact solution of the stochastic differential equations [16], which are valid when the mutation rates are all small.

The Moolgavkar–Knudson two-stage model postulates that cancer results from a clone of cells of which one descendant has undergone two mutational events, either or both of which may depend on exposure to carcinogens. The clone of intermediate cells is subject to a birth-and-death process with rates that may also depend on carcinogenic exposures. The number of normal stem cells at risk varies with age, depending on the development of the particular tissue. Finally, in genetically susceptible individuals, all cells carry the first mutation at birth. The predicted risk under this model (in nonsusceptible individuals) is then approximately

$$\lambda[t, X(u)] = \mu_1 \mu_2 [1 + \beta_2 X(t)] \int_0^t [1 + \beta_1 X(u)]$$
$$\times \exp[\rho(t - u)] du, \qquad (12)$$

where μ_k are the baseline rates of the first and second mutations, β_k are the slope of the dependence of the mutation rates on exposure, and ρ is the net proliferation rate (birth minus death rates) of intermediate cells. For the more complex exact solution, see [24].

There have been a number of interesting applications of these models to various carcinogenic exposures. For example, the multistage model has been fitted to data on lung cancer in relation to asbestos and smoking [30], arsenic [4], coke oven emissions [9], and smoking [5, 10], as well as to data on leukemia and benzene [7] and nonleukemic cancers and radiation [32]. The two-stage model has been fitted to data on lung cancer in relation to smoking [23], radon [21, 25], and cadmium [27], as well as to data on breast [22] and colon cancers [19]. For further discussion of some of these applications, see [31].

As in any other form of statistical modeling, the analyst should be cautious in interpretation. A good fit to a particular model does not of course establish the truth of the model. Instead the value of models, whether descriptive or mechanistic, lies in their ability to organize a range of hypotheses into a systematic framework in which simpler models can be tested against more complex alternatives. The usefulness of the multistage model of carcinogenesis, for example, lies not in our belief that it is an accurate description of the process, but rather in its ability to distinguish whether a carcinogen appears to act early or late in the process or at more than one stage. Similarly, the importance of the Moolgavkar–Knudson model lies in its ability to test whether a carcinogen acts as an "initiator" (i.e. on the mutation rates) or a "promoter" (i.e. on proliferation rates). Such inferences can be valuable, even if the model itself is an incomplete description of the process, as must always be the case.

References

[1]   Armitage, P. & Doll, R. (1961). Stochastic models of carcinogenesis, in *Proceedings of the Fourth Berkeley Symposium on Mathematics, Statistics and Probability*, J. Neyman, ed. University of California Press, Berkeley, pp. 18–32.

[2]   Breslow, N.E. & Day, N.E. (1980). *Statistical Methods in Cancer Research*, Vol. I. *The Analysis of Case–Control Studies*. IARC Scientific Publications, No. 32, Lyon.

[3]   Breslow, N.E. & Storer, B.E. (1985). General relative risk functions for case–control studies, *American Journal of Epidemiology* **122**, 149–162.

[4]   Brown, C.C. & Chu, K. (1983). A new method for the analysis of cohort studies: implications of the multistage theory of carcinogenesis applied to occupational arsenic exposure, *Environmental Health Perspectives* **50**, 293–308.

[5]   Brown, C.C. & Chu, K. (1987). Use of multistage models to infer stage affected by carcinogenic exposure: example of lung cancer and cigarette smoking, *Journal of Chronic Diseases* **40**, 171–179.

[6]   Cox, D.R. (1972). Regression models and life tables, *Journal of the Royal Statistical Society, Series B* **34**, 187–220.

[7]   Crump, K.S., Allen, B.C., Howe, R.B. & Crockett, P.W. (1987). Time factors in quantitative risk assessment, *Journal of Chronic Diseases* **40**, 101–111.

[8]   Day, N.E. & Brown, C.C. (1980). Multistage models and primary prevention of cancer. *Journal of the National Cancer Institute* **64**, 977–89.

[9]   Dong, M.H., Redmond, C.K., Maxumdar, S. & Costantion, J.P. (1988). A multistage approach to the cohort analysis of lifetime lung cancer risk among steelworkers exposed to coke oven emission, *American Journal of Epidemiology* **128**, 860–873.

[10] Freedman, D.A. & Navidi, W.C. (1989). Multistage models for carcinogenesis, *Environmental Health Perspectives* **81**, 169–188.

[11] Gilks, W.R., Richardson, S. & Spiegelhalter, D.J., eds (1996). *Markov Chain Monte Carlo in Practice*. Chapman & Hall, London.

[12] Guerro, V.M. & Johnson, R.A. (1982). Use of the Box–Cox transformation with binary response models, *Biometrika* **69**, 309–314.

[13] Hauck, W.W. & Donner, A. (1977). Wald's test as applied to hypotheses in logit analysis, *Journal of the American Statistical Association* **72**, 851–853.

[14] Hastie, T.J. & Tibshirani, R.J. (1990). *Generalized Additive Models*. Chapman & Hall, New York.

[15] Lubin, J.H. & Gaffey, W. (1988). Relative risk models for assessing the joint effects of multiple factors, *American Journal of Industrial Medicine* **13**, 149–167.

[16] Moolgavkar, S.H. (1978). The multistage theory of carcinogenesis and the age distribution of cancer in man, *Journal of the National Cancer Institute* **61**, 49–52.

[17] Moolgavkar, S.H. (1986). Carcinogenesis modelling: from molecular biology to epidemiology, *Annual Review of Public Health* **7**, 151–169.

[18] Moolgavkar, S. & Knudson, A. (1980). Mutation and cancer: a model for human carcinogenesis, *Journal of the National Cancer Institute* **66**, 1037–1052.

[19] Moolgavkar, S.H. & Luebeck, E.G. (1992). Multistage carcinogenesis: population-based model for colon cancer, *Journal of the National Cancer Institute* **84**, 610–618.

[20] Moolgavkar, S. & Venzon, D.J. (1987). General relative risk regression models for epidemiologic studies, *American Journal of Epidemiology* **126**, 949–961.

[21] Moolgavkar, S.H., Cross, F.T., Luebeck, G. & Dagle, G.D. (1990). A two-mutation model for radon-induced lung tumors in rats, *Radiation Research* **121**, 28–37.

[22] Moolgavkar, S.H., Day, N.E. & Stevens, R.G. (1980). Two-stage model for carcinogenesis: epidemiology of breast cancer in females, *Journal of the National Cancer Institute* **65**, 559–569.

[23] Moolgavkar, S.H., Dewanji, A. & Luebeck, G. (1989). Cigarette smoking and lung cancer: reanalysis of the British doctors' data, *Journal of the National Cancer Institute* **81**, 415–420.

[24] Moolgavkar, S.H., Dewanji, A. & Venzon, D.J. (1988). A stochastic two-stage model for cancer risk assessment. I. The hazard function and the probability of tumor, *Risk Analysis* **8**, 383–392.

[25] Moolgavkar, S.H., Luebeck, E.G., Krewski, D. & Zielinski, J.M. (1993). Radon, cigarette smoke, and lung cancer: a re-analysis of the Colorado Plateau uranium miners' data, *Epidemiology* **4**, 204–217.

[26] Schwartz, J. (1993). Air pollution and daily mortality in Birmingham, Alabama, *American Journal of Epidemiology* **137**, 1136–1147.

[27] Stayner, L., Smith, R., Bailer, A.J., Luebeck, E.G. & Moolgavkar, S.H. (1995). Modeling epidemiologic studies of occupational cohorts for the quantitative assessment of carcinogenic hazards, *American Journal of Industrial Medicine* **27**, 155–170.

[28] Thomas, D.C. (1981). General relative risk models for survival time and matched case–control studies, *Biometrics* **37**, 673–686.

[29] Thomas, D.C. (1983). Nonparametric estimation and tests of fit for dose–response relations, *Biometrics* **39**, 263–268.

[30] Thomas, D.C. (1983). Statistical methods for analyzing effects of temporal patterns of exposure on cancer risks, *Scandinavian Journal of Work and Environmental Health* **9**, 353–366.

[31]   Thomas, D.C. (1988). Models for exposure–time–response relationships with applications in cancer epidemiology, *Annual Review of Public Health* **9**, 451–482.

[32]   Thomas, D.C. (1990). A model for dose rate and duration of exposure effects in radiation carcinogenesis, *Environmental Health Perspectives* **87**, 163–171.

[33]   Ulm, K. (1983). Dose–response-models in epidemiology, in *Mathematics in Biology and Medicine: An International Conference.* Bari, Italy.

[34]   Vaeth, M. (1985) On the use of Wald's test in exponential families, *International Statistical Review* **53**, 199–214.

[35]   Whittemore, A.S. (1977). The age distribution of human cancers for carcinogenic exposures of varying intensity, *American Journal of Epidemiology* **106**, 418–32.

[36]   Whittemore, A. & Keller, J.B. (1978). Quantitative theories of carcinogenesis, *SIAM Review* **20**, 1–30.

DUNCAN C. THOMAS

Relative Standardized Mortality Ratio (RSMR) *see* Standardization Methods

Relative Survival *see* Excess Mortality

Reliability, Observers *see* Agreement, Measurement of

Reliability Ratio *see* Measurement Error in Epidemiologic Studies

Reliability Study

Reliability studies and **validation studies** provide information on **measurement error** in exposures or other covariates used in epidemiologic studies. Such information on the measurement error process is needed to obtain valid estimates and inference using methods such as regression calibration or maximum likelihood (*see* **Misclassification Error**). Reliability studies are based on repeating an error-prone measurement, and the validity of this method depends on a model for the errors given by (1) below. Validation studies are applicable to a broader class of error models, including models admitting **differential error**, but validation studies require that one be able to measure correct ("gold standard") covariate values on some subjects.

To define reliability sampling plans more precisely, let $\mathbf{Y}$ be the response variable, and let $\mathbf{X}$ be the true values of the variable which may be misclassified or measured with error. In some cases, $\mathbf{X}$ can never be observed and can be thought of as a *latent* variable. In other cases, $\mathbf{X}$ is a "gold standard" method of covariate assessment which is infeasible and/or expensive to administer to large numbers of study participants. Instead of observing $\mathbf{X}$, we observe $\mathbf{W}$, which is subject to error. Finally, there may be covariates $\mathbf{Z}$ upon which the model for response depends that are measured without error. In main study/reliability study designs, the main study consists of the data $(\mathbf{Y}_i, \mathbf{W}_i, \mathbf{Z}_i)$, $i = 1, \ldots, n_1$. If the reliability study is *internal*, it consists of $(\mathbf{Y}_i, \mathbf{W}_{ij}, \mathbf{Z}_i)$, $j = 1, \ldots, n_i$, $i = n_1 + 1, \ldots, n_1 + n_2$ observations, and if the reliability study is *external*, it consists of $(\mathbf{W}_{ij})$, $j = 1, \ldots, n_i$, $i = n_1 + 1, \ldots, n_1 + n_2$ observations. Thus, there is only a single measurement for each main study subject, but replicate measurements for each subject in the reliability study.

The measurement error model for which a reliability study can be used is

$$\mathbf{W} = \mathbf{X} + \mathbf{U}, \qquad (1)$$

where $\mathbf{U}$ is a mean zero error term with some variance–covariance Σ. The error $\mathbf{U}$ is assumed independent of $\mathbf{X}$. Note that model (1) implies that the error is **nondifferential**, not only with respect to $\mathbf{Y}$ but also with respect to $\mathbf{Z}$ because $f(\mathbf{W}|\mathbf{X}, \mathbf{Y}, \mathbf{Z}) = f(\mathbf{W}|\mathbf{X})$.

Under model (1), replicate data from a reliability study can be used for valid estimation and inference. This model has been applied to the analysis of blood pressure, serum hormones, and other serum biomarkers such as vitamin concentrations, viral load measurements, and CD4 cell counts.

We assume that subjects in an internal reliability study are selected completely at random. That is, if V

is an indicator variable that equals 1 if a participant is in the validation study and 0 otherwise, then $\Pr(V = 1 | \mathbf{Y}, \mathbf{X}, \mathbf{Z}, \mathbf{W}) = \Pr(V = 1) = \pi$.

To correct point and interval estimates relating **Y** to **X** for **bias** from measurement error in **W**, it is necessary to estimate Σ and $\text{var}(\mathbf{X}) = \Sigma_{\mathbf{X}}$ using model (1). Estimates of the quantities, Σ and $\Sigma_{\mathbf{X}}$, are needed to correct the estimate of the parameter of interest describing the association between **Y** and **X**, β, for bias due to measurement error. If an internal reliability sample is used one can estimate Σ from it. The quantity $\text{var}(\mathbf{W}) = \Sigma_{\mathbf{W}}$ can be estimated from the combined main study/internal reliability study data, and $\Sigma_{\mathbf{X}}$ can be estimated by $\hat{\Sigma}_{\mathbf{X}} = \hat{\Sigma}_{\mathbf{W}} - \hat{\Sigma}$. The same approach can be used if an external reliability sample is used except, in this case, $\Sigma_{\mathbf{W}}$ should be estimated from the main study only. This is because, under model (1), it is reasonable to assume that Σ may be transportable from one population to another, whereas $\Sigma_{\mathbf{X}}$, and hence $\Sigma_{\mathbf{W}}$, are likely to vary across populations. Because an internal reliability study ensures that Σ is correctly estimated and yields more efficient estimates of $\Sigma_{\mathbf{X}}$, it is preferred to an external reliability study.

In some applications, the goal of the research is simply estimation of the reliability coefficient, also known as the intraclass correlation coefficient, ρ, equal to $\Sigma_{\mathbf{X}}[\Sigma_{\mathbf{W}}]^{-1}$. These applications arise, for example, in the evaluation of new medical diagnostic procedures such as new technology for ascertaining the load of human immunodeficiency virus (HIV) in body tissue, or in assessing the consistency of different clinicians in evaluating the functional status of their patients. Designs of studies whose purpose is to estimate the reliability coefficient have $n_1 = 0$ and no data on **Y**. In what follows, we will first discuss design of such reliability studies. Then, we will discuss the main study/reliability study design, where $n_1 > 0$ and **Y** is observed in the main study and possibly in the reliability study.

Design of Reliability Studies

A nontechnical introduction to reliability study design considerations appeared in a recent epidemiology textbook by Armstrong et al. [1]. A series of papers by Donner and colleagues [3, 4, 8] investigated design of reliability studies in considerable detail. The first and last of these provided formulas for the power

to test $H_0 : \rho = \rho_0$, vs. $H_a: \rho = \rho A$, where ρ is the intraclass correlation or reliability coefficient, equal to $\Sigma_{\mathbf{X}} / \Sigma_{\mathbf{W}}$, for a given (n_2, R), and where R is the number of replicates per subject. In addition, tables were given for power for fixed values of n_2 and R. The first paper was based upon exact calculations, and the last paper developed a less computationally intensive approximation to the exact formula which appears to work quite well. The total number of observations ($n_2 \times R$) is minimized with a relatively small value for R, as long as the reliability is 40% or higher. In these cases, $R = 2$ or 3 is sufficient. Eliasziw & Donner [4] minimized reliability study cost with respect to n_2 and R, subject to fixed power to test H_0 vs. H_a as given above using the formula for power derived in [3]. Cost was taken as a function of the unit cost of replicating data within subjects, the unit cost of accruing subjects, and the unit cost related jointly to the number of replicates and the number of subjects. Tables were given for the optimal values of n_2 and R, for different unit cost ratios and different values of ρ_0. They found that for $\rho > 0.2$, the cost per subject is more influential than the cost per measurement. In addition, they found that the optimal n_2 and R were highly stable despite moderate changes in unit cost ratios.

Freedman et al. [5] investigated the design of reliability studies when **X** and **W** are binary. Reliability of W as a surrogate for X was parameterized by the probability of disagreement between the two replicate measures of X, W_1, and W_2, corresponding to the values obtained from two different raters (*see* **Agreement, Measurement of**). They gave tables for n_2 which assured a fixed confidence interval width around the estimated probability of disagreement when $R = 2$. For probability of disagreement between 0.05 and 0.40 and confidence interval widths of 0.1 to 0.2, sample sizes between 50 and 350 are needed. These authors also considered study design when the goal is to estimate the within-rater probability of disagreement as well as the between-rater probability of disagreement, and provided tables of power for scenarios in which there are two raters and two replicates per rater.

Design of Main Study/Reliability Studies

One can select various main study sizes (n_1), reliability study sizes (n_2), and numbers of replicate

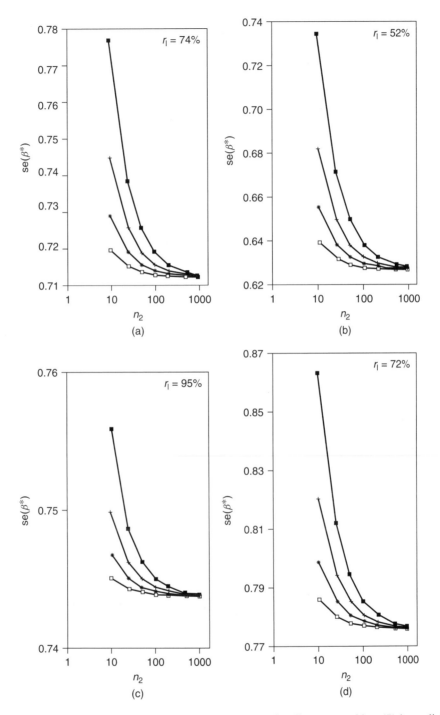

Figure 1   The relationship between the sample size (n_2) and the number of replicates per subject (R) in a reliability study, and the standard error of the measurement-error corrected logistic regression coefficient, β^*. Abbreviations and symbols used are: se for standard error and r_1 for the reliability coefficient $var(x)/var(w)$. Number of replicates, R: $\bullet = 2$; $+ = 3$; $* = 5$; $\square = 10$. (a) Cholesterol; (b) glucose; (c) body mass index; (d) systolic blood pressure

measurements (R) for each subject in the reliability substudy. An "optimal" main study/reliability study design will find (n_1, n_2, R) to achieve some design goal. One may wish to minimize the variance of an important parameter estimate, such as the log **relative risk**, β, subject to a fixed total cost. Alternatively, one may wish to minimize the overall cost of the study, subject to specified power constraints on the parameter of interest (*see* **Validation Study** for further discussion of choices of design optimization criteria). Liu & Liang [6] considered the optimal choice of R for internal reliability designs with $n_1 = 0$, that is, designs in which all subjects are in the reliability study. They studied generalized linear models for $f(\mathbf{Y}|\mathbf{X}, \mathbf{Z}; \beta)$ with the identity, log, probit, and logit link functions. They assumed the measurement error model for $\mathbf{X}$ described by (1) with $\mathbf{X}$ following a multivariate normal distribution MVN ($\mu_{\mathbf{X}}$, $\Sigma\mathbf{X}$). The validity of their results required an additional approximation in the case of the logistic link function, which is the link function most commonly used in epidemiology. For scalar $\mathbf{X}$ and $\mathbf{W}$, these authors derived a formula for asymptotic relative efficiency of β^*, the measurement-error corrected parameter describing the relationship between $\mathbf{Y}$ and $\mathbf{X}$, as a function of $\Sigma/\Sigma_{\mathbf{X}}$ and R. They found that the precision of β^*, relative to the precision which would be obtained for estimating β if $\mathbf{X}$ were never measured with error, is little improved by increasing R above 4.

Rosner et al. [7] investigated the effect of changing n_2 and R on the variance of elements of a nine-dimensional vector β, where β is the log **odds ratio** relating coronary heart disease incidence to the model covariates in data from the Framingham Heart Study [2]. Four of the model covariates were measured with error (Figure 1). In this figure, n_1 was 1731, and Σ and Σ_x were assigned the values estimated in the analysis. When n_2 was greater than or equal to 100, the standard error of the four measurement-error corrected estimates reached an asymptote, indicating little or no gain in efficiency from increasing n_2 beyond that value. At that point, the gain in efficiency ranges between a 10%–20% reduction in the variance for the three variables measured with some error (BMI has little error, as evidenced by the high reliability coefficient, $r_1 = 95\%$). Increasing the number of replicates decreased the standard errors of the estimates substantially when n_2 was

small, but made little difference for larger reliability studies. For the three variables measured with error (cholesterol, glucose, and systolic blood pressure), the design ($n_2 = 10$, $R = 10$) was equally efficient as the design ($n_2 = 100$, $R = 2$). Although the former requires fewer measurements, the latter may be more feasible, as it only requires two visits per subject.

Conclusions

Although model (1) is restrictive, there are many instances in biomedical research where it is considered reasonable. Methods of analysis under this model are well developed, but more research is needed on optimal design, and there is a need for user-friendly software for finding optimal designs.

Acknowledgements

This work was supported by National Cancer Institute grants CA50587 and CA03416.

References

[1] Armstong, B.K., White, E. & Saracci, R. (1992). *Principles of Exposure Measurement in Epidemiology*. Oxford University Press, Oxford, pp. 89–94.

[2] Dawber, T.R. (1980). *The Framingham Study*. Harvard University Press, Cambridge, Mass.

[3] Donner, A.P. & Eliasziw, M. (1987). Sample size requirements for reliability studies, *Statistics in Medicine* **6**, 441–448.

[4] Eliasziw, M. & Donner, A.P. (1987). A cost–function approach to the design of reliability studies, *Statistics in Medicine* **6**, 647–655.

[5] Freedman, L.S., Parmar, M.K.B. & Baker, S.G. (1993). The design of observer agreement studies with binary assessments, *Statistics in Medicine* **12**, 165–179.

[6] Liu, X. & Liang, K.Y. (1992). Efficacy of repeated measurements in regression models with measurement error, *Biometrics* **48**, 645–654.

[7] Rosner, B., Spiegelman, D. & Willett, W. (1992). Correction of logistic regression relative risk estimates and confidence intervals for random within-person measurement error, *American Journal of Epidemiology* **136**, 1400–1413.

[8] Walter, S.D., Eliasziw, M. & Donner, A.P. (1998). Sample size and optimal designs for reliability studies, *Statistics in Medicine* **17**, 101–110.

DONNA SPIEGELMAN

Replication Data *see* Measurement Error in Epidemiologic Studies

Retrospective Cohort Study *see* Cohort Study, Historical

Retrospective Study

Retrospective study is a term originally used to describe a **case–control study**, in which the previous exposures and other characteristics of cases with the disease of interest are compared with the previous exposures and other characteristics of disease-free **controls**. More generally, the term is applied to studies in which the relevant exposures and/or disease incidences have occurred before the time of the study data collection. For example, a **historical cohort study**, in which historical records of occupational exposures (*see* **Occupational Epidemiology**) and disease occurrence are analyzed just as in a prospective follow-up study, is sometimes called a retrospective study.

M.H. GAIL

Risk

Risk is the probability that an individual without disease will develop disease over a defined age or time interval. If risk is estimated as the proportion of members of a fixed cohort who develop disease in a defined time period, it corresponds to an average individual-specific risk (*see* **Cumulative Incidence**). This proportion is an estimate of a **crude risk** or **absolute risk** because it is reduced by the chance that subjects will die of other diseases before they develop the disease of interest (*see* **Competing Risks**).

Often the risk for the interval $[0, t)$ is calculated from $1 - \exp(-\int_0^t \lambda(u)\mathrm{d}u$, where $\lambda(u)$ is the cause-specific **hazard rate**. For small hazard rates, this expression is approximately equal to the **cumulative hazard**, $\int_0^t \lambda(u)\mathrm{d}u$. These expressions correspond to pure probabilities of disease and estimate the probability of developing disease in the absence of other causes of death under the assumption that the various causes of death act independently.

M.H. GAIL

Risk Assessment

The various usages of the term *risk* all concern the possible occurrence of events or situations, called *hazards*, the consequences of which are uncertain, but may be harmful. Informal usages of **risk** may indicate the nature, or merely the existence, of the possible danger ("There is a risk of post-operative infection"; "I never take risks"). In technical discussions the term is used quantitatively, but even there the usage is not standard.

There are two principal, and mutually incompatible, interpretations:

1. The probability, or chance, of an adverse event. Clearly, this must be put in context: it should refer to a defined set of circumstances, and, for hazards continuing over time, the rate per time unit, or for a unit of exposure, is normally used.
2. A combination of the chance of an adverse effect and its severity. There are obvious difficulties with this type of definition: How is severity measured, and how are the two components combined?

The extensive literature on risk covers many aspects, which are commonly collectively termed *risk assessment* or *risk analysis*. The first of these terms is sometimes used more restrictively, to include the concepts of *risk estimation, risk evaluation*, and *risk perception*, as defined below. The study of risk brings together engineers, behavioral and social scientists, statisticians, and others, and to some extent usage of terms varies amongst these groups. For example, engineers and other technologists tend to favor approach 2, statisticians and biologists tend to favor 1, and behavioral and social scientists tend often to use a mutifaceted approach. Reference [7] contains chapters by groups of writers from different backgrounds, and has extensive bibliographies. See also [1] for a popular exposition.

Risk theory has a specialized meaning, being concerned with the financial integrity of an insurance company in the light of random fluctuations in claims. It forms an application of the theory of stochastic processes [8].

Statisticians will note that usage 2 above is closely related to the concept of a *risk function* in decision theory. There, uncertain events, the distribution of which depends on an unknown scenario, have consequences measured by a loss function; a particular decision function, defining the action to be taken when the event is observed, has an average loss for any given scenario; and the *risk* (or *integrated risk*) is the mean of the average loss when taken over the prior distribution of the scenarios. Application of this approach is hampered by the difficulty of determining losses in financial terms, and of defining the various probability distributions.

Attention has been focused on various interrelated aspects of risk, including the following:

1. *Risk estimation*: the estimation of the probabilities of the adverse outcomes, and of the nature and magnitude of their consequences.
2. *Risk evaluation*: determination of the significance of the hazards for individuals and communities. This depends importantly on the next aspect.
3. *Risk perception*: the extent to which individuals assess risks and the severity of possible outcomes, assessments that may differ from those made by "experts".
4. *Risk management*: the measures taken by individuals and societies to prevent the adverse effects of hazards and to ameliorate their consequences.

We deal briefly with these topics in turn. The articles in [7], and their bibliographies, provide a much broader picture. Many of these topics are discussed fully elsewhere, in relation to risk assessment for environmental chemicals.

Health Hazards

There are several clearly distinct categories of hazards that give rise to health risks.

First, there are hazards that arise from the physical and biological environment. Many of the hazards in the physical environment are man-made. It is our own choice, collectively, to pollute the atmosphere with emissions from domestic fires, power stations, or burning oil wells, and to treat water supplies with disrespect. These are examples of damage *to* the environment, and damage to ourselves *from* the environment. The biological environment presents a hazard to us mainly in the form of microorganisms causing infectious disease.

Other hazards arise from personal, rather than societal, choice. These include habits with adverse consequences, such as the consumption of tobacco, alcohol, and narcotic drugs. The category includes also indulgence in sport and travel; and our often unwise dietary choices. We tend to shrug off the hazards that we ourselves incur, by understating the risks or overstating the benefits, while deprecating the folly of others.

Finally, there are hazards that cannot be prevented by personal decisions. They follow inexorably from our innate or ingrained characteristics – our genetic makeup or our experiences in early life. In some instances, medical science can reduce the risk to which susceptible individuals are subject: in others, the burden has to be endured.

Risk Estimation

The risks from many prominent health hazards can be estimated reliably from objective statistical information. In other instances, in which numeric information is lacking, risks may be guessed by informed experts (as in the setting of insurance premiums for nonstandard risks). There are, for instance, no reliable data on the frequency of explosions at nuclear power installations, and estimates of risk would have to rely on expert judgments, or on careful estimation of risks of failure at individual links in the chain of connected events.

Even when statistical information is available, an individual may argue that his or her risk is not properly represented by the population estimate. There is a long-standing debate as to whether medical statistical information necessarily applies to an individual in the population concerned; in the nineteenth century, for instance, opposite views were held by P.C.A. Louis and by C. Bernard. Clearly, if the individual has known characteristics that can be shown to affect the risk, they should be taken into account. If no such characteristics can be identified, it seems reasonable to apply the population estimate to the individual. The point is important in emphasizing that risk estimation is far from being an objective matter.

Statistical information on the risk of mortality from different diseases is widely available, for individuals of each sex at different ages, in different occupational (*see* **Occupational Epidemiology**) and social groups and for different countries (*see* **Mortality, International Comparisons**). Information on the risks of morbidity is less comprehensive. Such information, based on data for large populations, is of some value for the estimation of risks for random members of the populations, but gives little or no indication of risks for individuals exposed to certain specified hazards; such as environmental pollution (*see* **Environmental Epidemiology**), social habits, or the onset of disease.

For questions of this type, special investigations are required. The whole range of types of epidemiologic study is available, including **case–control studies, cohort studies**, and **case–cohort studies**. The risks of adverse progression of disease may be estimated by a study of prognosis. See [4] for an example of various investigatory methods employed in a study of the apparent excess risks of childhood leukemia due to contamination of water supplies in a town.

In many "high-profile" public health problems, it is not possible to mount epidemiologic studies to give unambiguous estimates of risk. The mechanism giving rise to the risk may not be fully understood, or the dangers may arise from a complex chain, the risks for which are difficult to measure. In such instances, the risks may be estimable only within very broad bands. For instance, in the crisis in the British beef industry, due to the outbreak of bovine spongiform encephalopathy (BSE), leading to an apparent risk of Creutzfeldt–Jakob disease (CJD), it was very difficult to estimate precisely the risk of CJD to a person eating beef. Since the cessation of use of suspect cattle feed, and the culling of relevant herds, it is probably reasonable to say that the risk is "extremely low", and perhaps to put some upper bound on it, but such estimates would rely on somewhat shaky data, and on the personal judgments of experts.

Another example is that of prolonged exposure to low levels of possibly carcinogenic chemicals. Carcinogenicity experiments, with the administration of high doses to animals, may give quite precise estimates of a median effective dose. However, risk estimation for low-level exposure to humans involves extrapolation to low doses (using models that are not necessarily correct [6]), and from the animal to the human species. The result of such extrapolation may well be reassuring, but it is unlikely to be quantitatively precise.

The quantification of risk, involving both the probabilities of adverse events and the severity of their effects, is clearly a complex matter. Many commentators would argue that the consequences of adverse events are multidimensional and cannot usefully be represented more simply. Others have argued in favor of a single scale. Duckworth [2], for instance, has constructed a scale for potentially fatal hazards. His index is the expected proportional shortening of life after the age at which the harzard is encountered, suitably discounted and expressed as a proportion of normal expectation of residual life. Nonfatal consequences could, more subjectively, be assessed as being equivalent to fractions of deaths. A logarithmic transformation is convenient for purposes of presentation.

Risk Evaluation and Perception

The evaluation of risk, either by individuals or by societies, should in principle involve a balancing of the costs and benefits: the potential occurrence of adverse effects, arising from exposure to a hazard, should be balanced against the potential benefits in physical or psychological rewards. Cost–benefit analysis is, however, a somewhat idealized concept. Apart from the difficulties of risk estimation, outlined above, both the potentially adverse effects and the supposed benefits may be difficult to evaluate on commensurate scales.

The benefits may in part be assessable as direct economic gains to a community. They may also include amenities, such as palatable food or attractive cosmetics, the value of which may be estimable by enquiry as to the prices that people are willing to pay for them.

The costs may be even more elusive. They include direct financial losses; for instance, in productivity. They include also disbenefits of pain and other symptoms. One might enquire how much people would be willing to pay to avoid such discomforts, but this would be a difficult exercise for people who had never experienced the symptoms in question.

Then, there is the crucial question of the value of human life. There are various approaches to this task, such as: (i) calculation of lost earning capacity; (ii) implicit evaluation based on societal practice, such as compensation awards or expenditure on specific safety measures; or (iii) the size of insurance premiums.

None of these possible approaches is likely to be simple, but it seems important to encourage further discussion and research, especially for the evaluation of risks for which community decisions, such as the imposition of government regulations, are required.

Evaluation by individuals of risks incurred by possible individual choices, again in principle involves the balancing of costs and benefits, but these may be very subjective and even more difficult to quantify than those involved in community action. In a sense, the decisions actually taken by individuals, sometimes without appreciable introspection, carry implications about the values attached by those individuals to the various elements in the equation. From this point of view, the relevant estimates of risk may be the subjective perceptions of the individuals themselves, rather than more "objective" estimates provided by experts. These two forms of estimate may be quite disparate. We tend to be more concerned about infrequent but dramatic events, such as major air crashes, than about frequent but less dramatic series of events such as the regular toll of road accident deaths. In one study [5], people thought that accidents caused as many deaths as disease, whereas in fact disease causes 15 times as many. The incidences of death from spectacular causes such as murder, botulism, tornadoes, and floods were all overestimated, whereas those for cancer, stroke, and heart disease were underestimated.

The importance of the "benefit" side of the equation is illustrated by the varying acceptability of activities with comparable risks. People are generally prepared to accept much higher risks of death from activities in which they participate voluntarily, such as sports, than from those encountered involuntarily.

Risk Management

This term covers the decisions, taken by individuals and communities, to accept or forego hazardous situations after assessment of risks, or to reduce exposure to the hazards and/or their adverse consequences.

As noted above, decisions by individuals are highly personal, and to a detached observer they may often seem irrational. A rational study of teenage smoking may conclude that the hazardous practice

should be avoided, but its conclusions may carry little weight with a young person who is ill-informed about risks, and whose "benefits" include the pleasures of conformity with peer practice. Nevertheless, in such situations, improved information about risks and adverse consequences is highly desirable, and the provision of risk information forms one of the major roles of government and other public bodies concerned with risks.

Institutions with a role in risk management include international, national, and regional governments, and a variety of public and private organizations. Apart from the provision of information, governments may issue regulations to reduce or control the use of hazardous substances. Their decisions may be guided by advisory committees, perhaps internationally based. For instance, in the assessment of evidence of carcinogenicity of chemicals, authoritative advice is provided by the program of the International Agency for Research on Cancer (IARC) Monographs on the Evaluation of the Carcinogenic Risk of Chemicals to Humans [3].

Institutions concerned with mitigation of the adverse effects of hazards include the judiciary (through compensation awarded in the law courts), insurance companies, and a variety of community bodies concerned with social welfare.

Conclusions

The interdisciplinary nature of all the aspects of risk assessment discussed here has encouraged lively discussion and research. Biostatistics forms only one component in the mixture, but it is an essential ingredient. Publications are spread widely in the technical press, but special note should be taken of the journal *Risk Analysis*.

References

[1]   British Medical Association (1987, 1990). *The BMA Guide to Living with Risk*. Penguin, London.
[2]   Duckworth, F. (1998). The quantification of risk, *RSS News* **26**(2), 10–12.
[3]   International Agency for Research on Cancer (IARC) (1982). *IARC Monographs on the Evaluation of the Carcinogenic Risk of Chemicals to Humans, Supplement 4, Chemicals, Industrial Processes and Industries Associated with Cancer in Humans. IARC Monographs*, Vols. 1–29. International Agency for Research on Cancer, Lyon.

[4] Lagakos, S.W., Wessen, B.J. & Zelen, M. (1986). An analysis of contaminated well water and health effects in Woburn, Massachusetts (with discussion), *Journal of the American Statistical Association* **81**, 583–614.

[5] Lichtenstein, S., Slovic, P., Fischhoff, B., Layman, M. & Combs, B. (1978). Judged frequency of lethal events, *Journal of Experimental Psychology: Human Learning and Memory* **4**, 551–578.

[6] Lovell, D.P. & Thomas, G. (1996). Quantitative risk assessment and the limitations of the linearized multistage model, *Human and Experimental Toxicity* **15**, 87–104.

[7] Royal Society (1992). *Risk: Analysis, Perception and Management*. Report of a Royal Society Study Group. Royal Society, London.

[8] Seal, H.L. (1988). Risk theory, in *Encyclopedia of Statistical Sciences*, Vol. 8, S. Kotz & N.L. Johnson, eds. Wiley, New York, pp. 152–156.

P. ARMITAGE

Risk Scores *see* Confounder Summary Score

Risk Set *see* Case–Control Study

Rosner's Method *see* Measurement Error in Epidemiologic Studies

***R*-to-1 Matching** *see* Matching

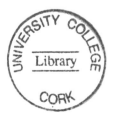

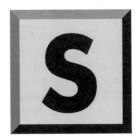

Sample Size for Epidemiologic Studies

Determining the number of subjects to be included in a study is a crucial step in designing the study and writing the protocol. To determine sample size, the study objectives have to be clearly defined, the general design (e.g. cohort, case–control) (*see* **Case–Control Study**; **Cohort Study**) and specific design options have to be selected, the main outcome and exposure variables have to be specified, the planned analysis strategy (i.e. hypothesis testing or estimation) and statistical methods have to be determined. Therefore, sample size determination is a very important aspect of design and cannot be carried out without a thorough and quantitative understanding of the planned study.

The study sample size should be large enough that the estimates will be sufficiently precise and the difference of interest is likely to be detected. It is usually true that the more subjects that are included in the study, the better the precision of the estimates, and the more likely the difference of interest will be detected. However, an oversized study may not always be the best choice because of economic and study time (sometimes ethical) considerations.

Hypothesis Testing and Power: The Case of a Normally Distributed Outcome

The principle of sample size and power considerations can be illustrated by a simple hypothesis test for normally distributed data. The normal case study will build the concepts and form the mathematical basis for most other sample size procedures, which will be discussed in later sections.

Suppose n samples are drawn from a population that has a normal distribution $N(\mu, \sigma^2)$. To test a null hypothesis H_0: $\mu = \mu_0$ vs. an alternative hypothesis H_a: $\mu = \mu_a (> \mu_0)$, we use a test statistic $Z = \sqrt{n}(\overline{X} - \mu_0)/\sigma_0$, which follows a standard normal distribution under H_0. For simplicity, we assume that the variances are known: under H_0, $\sigma^2 = \sigma_0^2$ and under H_a, $\sigma^2 = \sigma_a^2$. The null hypothesis will be rejected if the observed value of Z falls in an extreme region, i.e. $Z > c$, where c is a constant to be determined (see below).

Two types of error can be made with the test. First, a type I error is that the null hypothesis is true but the observed Z falls in the rejection region (i.e. $Z > c$) such that the null hypothesis is rejected. The type I error is also called the significance level of the test. It is often protected by setting an upper limit, e.g. 0.10 or 0.05, for the significance level. Secondly, a type II error is the probability of failing to reject the null hypothesis when the alternative hypothesis is true. Both error rates depend on the sample size, test statistic Z, and the critical value c. In the normal distribution, for a given H_a: $\mu = \mu_a > \mu_0$ (one-sided test),

$$\text{Type I error}: \alpha = P(Z > c | H_0) = 1 - \Phi(c),$$

$$\text{Type II error}: \beta = P(Z \leq c | H_a),$$

where $\Phi(\cdot)$ is the standard normal distribution function. Solving the first equation, we have $c = z_{1-\alpha}$, the $(1 - \alpha)$th percentile of the standard normal distribution.

The power of a statistical test is defined as the probability that a statistically significant test statistic will be obtained (i.e. reject the null hypothesis), given that the alternative hypothesis is true. It equals one minus the type II error. In the above example,

$$\text{Power} = 1 - \beta = P(Z > c | H_a)$$

$$= 1 - \Phi \left(\frac{z_{1-\alpha}\sigma_0 - \sqrt{n}(\mu_a - \mu_0)}{\sigma_a} \right).$$

Solving the equation, we obtain the required sample size to ensure a $1 - \beta$ power on detecting the difference of $\mu_a - \mu_0$; that is,

$$n = \left(\frac{z_{1-\alpha}\sigma_0 + z_{1-\beta}\sigma_a}{\mu_a - \mu_0} \right)^2.$$

This equation can also be used to find the minimum detectable difference for given statistical power $1 - \beta$ and sample size n; that is,

$$\Delta = \mu_a - \mu_0 = (z_{1-\alpha}\sigma_0 + z_{1-\beta}\sigma_a)/\sqrt{n}.$$

This is the smallest difference that can be detected with given sample size and power.

Although the sample size formula is obtained from a normal distribution, the relationship among the parameters of sample size, significance level α, power $1 - \beta$, variances, and effect-size Δ is generally true for any type of study and distribution. As the significance level α is getting smaller, or the power is getting higher, or the variances are getting larger, or the effect size is getting smaller, a larger sample size will be required. While the significance level is usually 5% and the power is usually 80% or 90%, it is very important to select suitable values for effect size and variances in designing a study. Investigators should not use overoptimistic values for the effect size or variances to avoid having an underpowered study.

The calculations of sample size, power and minimum detectable difference can be generalized to the case of $\mu_a < \mu_0$ by replacing $\mu_a - \mu_0$ with $|\mu_a - \mu_0|$ in the above formula. The above formulas are based on one-sided tests. For a two-sided alternative hypothesis, $H_a: \mu_a \neq \mu_0$, the sample size formula is essentially the same but $z_{1-\alpha}$ is replaced by $z_{1-\alpha/2}$.

The choice of a one-sided or two-sided test will depend on the problem of interest. If one wants to test only one direction, e.g. $\mu = \mu_0$ against $\mu > \mu_0$, or

test whether the population mean is greater than μ_0, then a one-sided test is appropriate. If the interest is to test the deviation from μ_0 from either direction, then a two-sided test is to be used. In this case, the null hypothesis will be rejected when the population mean is either too small or too large statistically compared with μ_0.

Estimation and Precision

In epidemiologic studies, researchers may be interested in estimating the magnitude of the effect from exposure instead of testing the hypothesis of no effect. The precision of an estimate can be measured by the width of a confidence interval that is designed to cover the true parameter of interest with a specified probability (coverage probability), $1 - \alpha$. In the normal distribution example, if we want to estimate the mean μ with known variance σ^2, then the $1 - \alpha$ confidence interval is $(\overline{X} - z_{1-\alpha/2}\sigma/\sqrt{n}, \overline{X} + z_{1-\alpha/2}\sigma/\sqrt{n})$. With regard to replications of sampling, we have a $1 - \alpha$ probability that the true mean μ will be included in this interval. The larger the sample size, the narrower the confidence interval, and therefore the higher the precision of the parameter estimate (*see* **Random Error**).

Over the last decades some researchers have been stressing the advantage of using confidence intervals rather than testing p-values to present study results and make statistical inferences. One reason is that a confidence interval conveys not only information on the point estimation but also an impression of the precision of the estimate. Some further discussions of the pros and cons of hypothesis testing and confidence intervals can be found in Rothman & Greenland [29].

The sample size calculated from the confidence interval viewpoint will depend on the objective of the study. If a study is solely to estimate the effect of a parameter of interest with a given precision, then the sample size can be calculated from the width of the confidence interval. For the normal mean example, if one wants the width of the $1 - \alpha$ confidence interval to be no more than 2δ, that is $2z_{1-\alpha/2}\sigma/\sqrt{n} \leq 2\delta$, then $n \geq (z_{1-\alpha/2}\sigma/\delta)^2$.

When the objective of a study is effectively to distinguish the parameter of interest from a specified value or distinguish among specified values, the sample size calculation should consider the expected location of the confidence interval. The sample size based on the width of the confidence interval alone will be insufficient [13]. In this case, the sample size obtained from confidence interval estimation will be similar to the sample size from hypothesis testing. In fact, hypothesis testing (two-sided) and confidence interval estimation are closely related. A study that yields a test p-value (two-sided) of precisely α for testing H_0: $\mu = \mu_0$ will have a $1 - \alpha$ confidence interval that has one end at μ_0. In other words, if the $1 - \alpha$ confidence interval of μ contains μ_0, then the null hypothesis H_0 will not be rejected with the significance level of α (two-sided).

Practical Considerations and Outline

In this article we will focus our presentation on the determination of sample size from the traditional hypothesis testing approach and present some limited results based on estimation and precision. For the actual study, the sample size, test significance level, variability, power and minimum detectable difference (effect size) have to be considered at the design stage. The relationship among these parameters will allow investigators to calculate one parameter given the others.

In practice, the test significance level is often 5% and the statistical power is usually 80% or 90%. The variability and expected difference are often obtained from previous studies. Special consideration may be given to the choice of the minimal difference to be detected. The difference should be reasonable and suitable, such that it is practically meaningful and the study can be planned and conducted feasibly. If the assumed difference is too large and the sample size is consequently underestimated, then the study may fail to detect the true difference due to insufficient power. On the other hand, an oversized study may be costly to conduct and sometimes may detect a "tiny" difference that is not practically meaningful. The factors of time, cost and recruitment of subjects from the study population should all be considered, together with the selection of the study sample size, power and expected difference.

In general, the required sample size for a study depends not only on the parameters such as α, power $1 - \beta$, and minimal detectable difference but also on the statistical procedures to be applied in the analysis and the study design. For epidemiologic studies,

typically cohort studies and case–control studies, many papers and review articles have been published for sample size and power determinations (e.g. [2], [21], [22], [32], [39]). In this article we give a broad overview of sample size determination methods for a variety of epidemiologic designs. The methodologic details are skipped and relegated to the references. In the second section, sample size determination methods for studies with a binomial outcome (in **cohort** and unmatched **case–control studies**) are discussed. Methods for matched case–control studies are discussed in the next section. For cohort studies with Poisson outcomes, the sample size determination methods are presented in the fourth section. The fifth section discusses sample size determination for cohort studies when the outcome of interest is time to event. The sample size required for cohort studies with longitudinal or correlated outcomes is discussed in the sixth section, while the following section highlights some sample size calculations when the problem of interest is estimation and precision. The final section presents some further considerations on sample size and power determination followed by a discussion.

Without loss of generality, we will present the sample size formulas for one-sided tests in the following sections. The two-sided formulas can be obtained by replacing $z_{1-\alpha}$ with $z_{1-\alpha/2}$ in all instances unless otherwise specified.

Studies with Binomial Outcomes

Dichotomous Exposure: Cohort Study

In **cohort studies** with a fixed follow-up time, the main outcome is typically disease occurrence. Let p_0 and p_1 be the proportion of subjects who develop the disease in the unexposed and exposed populations, respectively. For a one-sided test H_0: $p_1 = p_0$ vs. H_a: $p_1 > p_0$, assuming an equal number of subjects n in the exposed and unexposed groups, the required sample size is given as follows (e.g. [32]):

$$n = \frac{\left(z_{1-\alpha}\sqrt{(2\overline{p}\overline{q})} + z_{1-\beta}\sqrt{(p_1 q_1 + p_0 q_0)}\right)^2}{(p_1 - p_0)^2}, (1)$$

where $q_1 = 1 - p_1$, $q_0 = 1 - p_0$, $\overline{p} = (p_0 + p_1)/2$, and $\overline{q} = 1 - \overline{p}$. The above formula is obtained from a normal approximation to the test statistic for comparing two binomial proportions. The formula can be represented as

$$n = \frac{\left[z_{1-\alpha}\sqrt{(2\overline{p}\overline{q})} +z_{1-\beta}\sqrt{(p_0(1+r) - p_0(1+r^2))} \right]^2}{[p_0(1-r)]^2} \quad (2)$$

in terms of the risk ratio $r = p_1/p_0$ (see **Relative Risk**) to test H_0: $r = 1$ vs. H_a: $r > 1$.

In general, let π_e be the proportion of subjects in the exposed group. Then the total sample size required is given by

$$N = \frac{\left[z_{1-\alpha}\sqrt{(\overline{p}\overline{q}/\pi_e(1 - \pi_e))} +z_{1-\beta}\sqrt{(p_1 q_1/\pi_e + p_0 q_0/(1 - \pi_e))} \right]^2}{(p_1 - p_0)^2}. \quad (3)$$

Dichotomous Exposure: Case–Control Study

The sample size required for an unmatched **case–control study** is similar to that for a cohort study. Let p_1 and p_0 now denote the proportions of subjects exposed in the case and control groups, respectively. For a study with one control per case, the sample size required can be calculated by eqs (1) and (2). For a study with k controls per case, the number of cases required is given by [32]

$$n = \frac{\left(z_{1-\alpha}\sqrt{((1 + 1/k)\overline{p}'\overline{q}')} +z_{1-\beta}\sqrt{(p_1 q_1 + p_0 q_0)} \right)^2}{(p_1 - p_0)^2},$$

where $\overline{p}' = (p_1 + kp_0)/(1 + k)$ and $\overline{q}' = 1 - \overline{p}'$.

In practice, the exposure rate among controls, p_0, is usually obtained from previous studies and estimated from the general population. The **relative risk** $r = p_1/p_0$ or the **odds ratio** (OR) $= p_1 q_0/p_0 q_1$ is then specified under the alternative hypothesis to calculate the power of the study. For example, consider a case–control study of a potential association between congenital heart defects and oral contraceptives used around the time of conception. An estimate of the exposure rate among controls is 30%. Given $\alpha = 0.05$ and $\beta = 0.10$, in order to detect a relative risk of $r = 1.5$ (so $p_1 = 0.45$), and based on (2), the sample size required is $n = 177$ (per group).

When an OR is specified, the exposure rate among cases can be solved as follows:

$$p_1 = \frac{p_0 \text{OR}}{[1 + p_0(\text{OR} - 1)]}.$$

For the above example, the sample size required to detect an $\text{OR} = 2$ (so $p_1 = 0.462$), given $\alpha = 0.05$ (two-sided) and $\beta = 0.10$, will be $n = 153$ (per group).

Continuous Exposure: Cohort Study

For a continuous exposure variable, sample size estimation methods for cohort studies have been derived by several authors (e.g. [21] and [40]). Let $p(x)$ be the probability of developing a disease with exposure level $X = x$ over a fixed follow-up time. Within the framework of **logistic regression**, the association between $p(x)$ and the continuous exposure variable X can be modeled as

$$\log\left[\frac{p(x)}{(1 - p(x))}\right] = \delta + \theta x, \quad (4)$$

where θ is the log OR for a unit increase in X. Testing the null hypothesis of no association is equivalent to testing H_0: $\theta = 0$.

Whittemore [40] derived sample size requirements for Wald tests based on maximum likelihood methods. To approximate the variance of the maximum likelihood estimate of θ, the disease probability is assumed to be small, i.e. $p(x) \approx 0$. Under this assumption, the total sample size for testing $\theta = 0$ with significant level α and power $1 - \beta$ is estimated by

$$N = \frac{\left[z_{1-\alpha}\sqrt{v(0)} + z_{1-\beta}\sqrt{v(\theta_a)} \right]^2}{[\theta_a^2 e^\delta]}. \quad (5)$$

In formula (5), $v(\theta) = [m/(mm_{11} - m_1^2)](\theta)$ and $m(t) = E[\exp(tX)]$ is the moment-generating function of X, and m_1 and m_{11} are the first and second partial derivatives of $m(t)$ with respect to t, respectively. The term e^δ is the odds of disease corresponding to $X = 0$ and θ_a is the log OR under the alternative hypothesis for a unit increase in the exposure X. Formula (5) is suitable to use when the sample size N is large. Tables for various distributions of exposure are given in Whittemore [40]. For example, when X has an $N(0, 1)$ distribution, with $p(0) = 0.07$ (the disease probability in controls), $\exp(\delta) = p(0)/(1 - p(0)) = 0.075$, $\alpha = 0.05$ and power $= 0.90$, approximately

$N = 543$ observations are needed to detect an OR of $\exp(0.5) = 1.65$ for a unit increase in the exposure X.

Lubin & Gail [21] studied a general method based on the score test statistic

$$U(\theta_0) = \partial \log L / \partial \theta = \sum_i x_i(d_i - p(x_i)) \qquad (6)$$

evaluated under the null hypothesis H_0: $\theta = \theta_0$, where L is the likelihood function for the logistic model (4) and d_i is a disease indicator (i.e. $d_i = 1$ and $d_i = 0$ for disease and nondisease, respectively). The total sample size required to test the null hypothesis with a significance level α and power $1 - \beta$ is given by

$$N = \frac{\left[z_{1-\alpha}\sqrt{v_0(U(\theta_0))} + z_{1-\beta}\sqrt{v_a(U(\theta_0))}\right]^2}{[\Delta(\theta)]^2}, \qquad (7)$$

where $v_0(U(\theta_0))$ and $v_a(U(\theta_0))$ are the variances of $U(\theta_0)$ under H_0: $\theta = \theta_0$ and H_a: $\theta = \theta_a$, respectively; and $\Delta(\theta) = E_a[U(\theta_0)]/N$. The evaluation will depend on the hypothesized parameters θ_0 and θ_a, as well as the statistical distribution of the exposure variable X. In general, special numerical calculation is needed to estimate the sample size. Details and some examples are given in Lubin & Gail [21].

Continuous Exposure: Case–Control Study

Lubin et al. [22] have derived sample size formulas for **case–control studies** with continuous exposure variables based on the logistic model (4) and score test (6). Let $F_1(x)$ and $F_0(x)$ be the distributions of exposure among cases and **controls**, respectively. It is shown that the number of cases required for a one-sided test with significance level α and power $1 - \beta$ is given by

$$n = \frac{(k+1)}{k} \frac{\left[z_{1-\alpha}\sigma_x + z_{1-\beta}\sqrt{\left(\dfrac{k\sigma_1^2 + \sigma_0^2}{k+1}\right)}\right]^2}{(\mu_1 - \mu_0)^2}, \qquad (8)$$

where k is the number of controls for each case (so total sample size $N = (k+1)n$), and (μ_1, σ_1^2) and (μ_0, σ_0^2) are the mean and variance of the exposure variable under F_1 and F_0, respectively; and

$$\sigma_x = \frac{(\sigma_1^2 + k\sigma_0^2)}{(k+1)} + \frac{(\mu_1 - \mu_0)^2 k}{(k+1)^2}.$$

The quantities μ_0, μ_1, σ_0^2 and σ_1^2 may be obtained from preliminary data such as previous studies that give estimates of the distributions of the exposure variable among cases and controls, or calculated from specifying the distribution functions of exposure in cases and controls, in which case numerical integration may be needed. The details are given in Lubin et al. [22].

When continuous exposure variables are dichotomized in the study (cohort or case–control), the required sample size will be increased due to loss of information from dichotomization. The efficacy losses will depend on the nature of the exposure distribution and the choice of the cutoff points for the dichotomization, as discussed in Lubin et al. [22].

Adjustment for Confounding Variables

Whittemore [40] extended the sample size formula (5) to adjust for **confounding** variables. When the joint multivariate variables $\mathbf{X}$ (a vector of the variable of interest X_1 and the confounding variables $X_2, \ldots, X_k$) follow an exponential family distribution, the variance term $v(\theta)$ can be obtained from the moment-generating function for $\mathbf{X}$. For example, when $\mathbf{X}$ has a multivariate normal distribution with mean μ and positive covariance matrix Σ, Whittemore showed that

$$v(\theta) = \left[\text{var}(X_1)\exp\left(\theta'\mu + \frac{\theta'\Sigma\theta}{2}\right)(1 - \rho_{1\cdot2\ldots k}^2)\right]^{-1}$$

where X_1 is the exposure variable of interest, $\rho_{1\cdot2\ldots k}$ is the multiple correlation coefficient relating X_1 to $X_2, \ldots, X_k$, and k is the total number of variables.

Lubin & Gail [21] proposed a general method for determining the sample size required to test whether exposure is associated with disease outcome, while adjusting for potential confounding variables. The method is based on a regression model and can be applied to both **cohort studies** and **case–control studies**. Let $\mathbf{X}$ be the joint multivariate variables of exposure and potential **confounders**. It is assumed that the probability of disease for $\mathbf{X} = \mathbf{x}$ is given by

$$p(\mathbf{x}; \delta, \theta, \lambda) = \frac{r(\mathbf{x})}{[1 + r(\mathbf{x})]} \text{ and } r(\mathbf{x}) = e^{\delta}R(\mathbf{x}; \theta, \lambda),$$

where $R(\mathbf{x}; \theta, \lambda)$ is a smooth, positive function satisfying $R(\mathbf{0}; \theta, \lambda) = 1$, θ is the parameter of interest and λ is a vector of parameters (nuisance parameters) associated with the confounding variables. Thus, the

logistic regression model (4) is a special case of this model when $R(\mathbf{x}; \theta, \lambda) = \exp(\mathbf{x}\theta)$. In fact, the function $R(\mathbf{x}; \theta, \lambda)$ can assume a multiplicative or additive form (*see* **Additive Model**; **Multiplicative Model**). For a one-sided test of the null hypothesis $\theta = \theta_0$ vs. the alternative $\theta = \theta_a$, a score test statistic is again given in (6). The total sample size required for a significance level α and power $1 - \beta$ is given in (7). However, $\nu_0(U(\theta_0))$, $\nu_a(U(\theta_0))$ and $\Delta(\theta) = E_a[U(\theta_0)]/N$ contain the nuisance parameters δ and λ. For statistical analysis after data are collected, these parameters can be estimated by maximum likelihood. For sample size evaluation at the design stage, these parameters are replaced by δ_0 and λ_0 to which the maximum likelihood estimates $\hat{\delta}$ and $\hat{\lambda}$ (obtained under H_0: $\theta = \theta_0$) converge when the alternative hypothesis is true. The method works in general for both continuous or categorical variables as long as a joint distribution of $\mathbf{X}$ is specified. However, the sample size formula needs specialized numerical calculations based on the model specification for $R(\mathbf{x}; \theta, \lambda)$ and the joint distribution of $\mathbf{X}$.

An example discussed in Lubin & Gail [21] is to test the effect of radon exposure on lung cancer after adjusting for smoking. They considered a multiplicative joint OR model,

$$R(\text{WLM}, \text{SMOK}) = (1 + \theta \, \text{WLM})(1 + \lambda \, \text{SMOK}),$$

where SMOK denotes the mean number of cigarettes smoked per day and WLM denotes exposure to radon decay products measured in working level months. They illustrated the use of this model to test the null hypothesis $\theta_0 = 0$, against the alternative hypothesis $\theta_a = 0.015$ for a five-year study assuming $\lambda_a = 0.3$. Based on prior knowledge, a five-year lung cancer mortality rate among nonsmokers is 0.00471. Therefore, $\delta = \log[0.00471/(1 - 0.00471)] = -5.354$. For a case–control study with $k = 5$ (number of **controls** per case), $\alpha = 0.05$ and power $1 - \beta = 0.90$, they showed that $n = 251$ cases are needed (number of controls $= 5n = 1255$). This is slightly larger than the 218 cases and 1086 controls required when the SMOK factor is ignored. This is because the confounding variable SMOK brings additional variability into the **multiplicative model**. The calculation assumes independence of the radon and smoking exposure distributions. Lubin & Gail [21] showed that the required sample size would be much larger if the radon and smoking exposures were highly and negatively correlated.

Adjustment for Stratification Factors

When samples are drawn from several strata, the **stratification** factors should be considered in the data analysis as well as in the sample size calculation at the design stage. When the probability of disease can be modeled in a **logistic regression**, the method for adjusting for **confounding** variables described above [21] can be used to estimate sample size. Smith & Day [36] provided extensive tabulation for the required sample size. They concluded that if the stratification factor is not strongly related to the exposure or disease status, then an increase of more than 10% in the sample size is unlikely to be needed.

Logistic regression is a special case of generalized linear models. Therefore, the methods proposed by Self & Mauritsen [34] and Self et al. [35] for generalized linear models can be used for sample size and power calculations. The methods are based on a score test and a likelihood ratio statistic, respectively. The sample size is estimated by treating the **stratification** factors as nuisance parameters. Their methods require, in general, specialized numerical calculations based on a specified joint distribution for the covariates in the model. See the section on a **cohort study** with Poisson outcomes for further discussion.

Other methods for sample size estimation for stratified studies can be found in the literature. For testing unity of a common OR for a collection of several 2×2 tables, Munoz & Rosner [25] studied sample size determination based on the Mantel–Haenszel test for stratified data (*see* **Mantel–Haenszel Methods**). Their method is appropriate when all margins of each table are fixed. Woolson et al. [41] and Nam [26] considered sample size calculations based on Cochran's test that do not require fixed margins of the 2×2 tables in each stratum. Nam used a continuity correction to guarantee that the actual type I error rate of the test does not exceed the nominal level.

Test for Interaction and Trend

When the question of interest is whether the relative risks among different strata (or levels of **confounding** factors) are equal, the problem becomes a test of **interaction** between exposure and the **stratification** factors (or confounding factors). Smith & Day [36] presented methods for evaluating power and sample size for testing the interaction between a dichotomous stratification variable and a categorical exposure. They showed that in order to detect an interaction effect of the same magnitude as a specified main effect, a sample size at least four times as large as for testing the main effect is required.

In general, tests for interaction can be addressed by testing appropriate coefficients in a **logistic regression** model. Within this framework, the methods developed by Lubin & Gail [21] and Self et al. [34, 35] can be used to estimate the required sample size. The methods will treat the interaction terms as the parameters of interest and treat all other factors as nuisance parameters. Usually, the methods need specialized numerical calculations.

Testing for trend can also be addressed (*see* **Dose–Response**) within the framework of generalized linear models. For example, when an exposure variable X is ordered categorical, a trend test is to test whether the disease odds are proportionally increased as the exposure level increases. This is equivalent to testing for a nonzero value of parameter θ in the logistic model (4). The methods developed by Lubin & Gail [21] and Self et al. [34, 35] can be used to estimate the required sample size.

Matched Case–Control Study

To improve comparability and efficiency in **case–control studies**, one may match **controls** with cases on potential **confounders**. A pair-matched study matches one control with each case, which is the simplest matched case–control design. When the number of cases is limited, more than one control can be matched to each case to increase statistical precision. For the matched case–control studies, the matching should be considered in the data analysis as well as in the sample size and power calculations (*see* **Matched Analysis**).

Pair-Matched Study

The probabilities of outcomes of a pair-matched case–control study are laid out in the following 2×2 table:

	Control		
Case	$+$	$-$	
$+$	π_{11}	π_{10}	$\pi_{1.}$
$-$	π_{01}	π_{00}	$\pi_{0.}$
	$\pi_{.1}$	$\pi_{.0}$	1

The "+" and "−" signs denote exposure and nonexposure status, respectively. Let m_{01} and m_{10} denote the number of $(-+)$ and $(+-)$ pairs for (case, control), and $m = m_{01} + m_{10}$ be the total number of discordant pairs. Conditional on m, the observation m_{10} has a binary distribution with $p = \pi_{10}/(\pi_{01} + \pi_{10}) = \psi/(1 + \psi)$, where $\psi = \pi_{10}/\pi_{01}$ denotes the disease–exposure OR.

The test of no disease–exposure association, i.e. H_0: $\pi_{01} = \pi_{10}$, is equivalent to testing H_0: $p = 1/2$. Schlesselman [32] gave a formula for the total number of discordant pairs m required to detect a relative risk R based on a normal approximation to McNemar's test,

$$m = \frac{\left[z_{1-\alpha}/2 + z_{1-\beta}\sqrt{(p(1-p))}\right]^2}{[p - 1/2]^2}. \tag{9}$$

Suppose $\pi_{\mathrm{d}} = \pi_{01} + \pi_{10}$ is the probability of obtaining discordant pairs. Then the total number of pairs for the study is estimated by

$$n = m/\pi_{\mathrm{d}}. \tag{10}$$

To estimate π_{d}, some additional information is required other than the OR ψ and the marginal exposure rate for **controls**, $\pi_{.1}$. When exposure for cases and controls within each pair is statistically independent, Schlesselman gives the following estimate:

$$\pi_{\mathrm{d}} = \pi_{.1}(1 - \pi_{1.}) + \pi_{1.}(1 - \pi_{.1}),$$

where $\pi_{1.} = \psi\pi_{.1}/[1 + (\psi - 1)\pi_{.1}]$.

For example, Schlesselman shows that to detect an OR of $\psi = 2$, from (9) one requires $m = 90.3$ discordant pairs for $\alpha = 0.05$ (two-sided) and $\beta = 0.10$. For a control exposure rate $\pi_{.1} = 0.30$, assuming independent exposures, $\pi_{1.} = 0.46$, $\pi_{\mathrm{d}} = 0.485$, and the total number of pairs required for the study is $n = 187$.

When the independence assumption does not hold, Schlesselman's sample size estimate may be severely biased (often underestimated). Several corrections have been proposed to allow for correlation between the exposure status within pairs that is often induced in the case of efficient matching. To allow for exposure association, Fleiss & Levin [7] used the exposure OR $\omega = \pi_{11}\pi_{00}/\pi_{01}\pi_{10}$ and corrected the estimation of discordant probability π_{d} given by Schlesselman. Under the independence assumption, $\omega = 1$. In the case of $\omega \neq 1$, the corrected estimate of the discordant probability is

$$\pi'_d = \pi_d \frac{\sqrt{(1 + 4(\omega - 1)\pi_1(1 - \pi_{1.})) - 1}}{2(\omega - 1)\pi_{1.}(1 - \pi_{1.})}.$$

In the above example, if $\omega = 2.5$, then the corrected $\pi_d = 0.376$. Therefore, the required number of pairs for the study is $n = 241$ rather than 187.

Dupont [6] presented another correction based on the contingency coefficient

$$\phi = \frac{\pi_{11}\pi_{00} - \pi_{10}\pi_{01}}{\sqrt{(\pi_{1.}(1 - \pi_{1.})\pi_{.1}(1 - \pi_{.1}))}}$$

for the case–control exposure association within a pair. The discordant probability π_d is adjusted as follows for specified ψ, $\pi_{.1}$ and ϕ,

$$\pi'_d = \pi_d - 2\phi\sqrt{(\pi_{1.}(1 - \pi_{1.})\pi_{.1}(1 - \pi_{.1}))},$$

where

$$\pi_{1.} = \frac{\left[\begin{array}{c} 2\psi\pi_{.1}(\psi\pi_{.1} + 1 - \pi_{.1}) \\ +(\psi - 1)^2\pi_{.1}(1 - \pi_{.1})\phi^2 \\ -(\psi - 1)\pi_{.1}(1 - \pi_{.1})\phi\sqrt{(\phi^2(\psi - 1)^2 + 4\psi)} \end{array} \right]}{2[\psi\pi_{.1} + 1 - \pi_{.1})^2 + (\psi - 1)^2\pi_{.1}(1 - \pi_{.1})\phi^2]}.$$

Several other methods are discussed and reviewed by Lachin [15] and Wickramaratne [35]. Lachin recommended always using a corrected procedure for sample size estimation. He pointed out that Dupont's correction and Fleiss & Levin's correction give very similar results.

Multiple Control per Case Study

For studies calling for k matched **controls** for each case (i.e. $1:k$ **matching**), Schlesselman gave an approximation for the required number of matched sets, $n' = (k + 1)n/2k$, where n is calculated from (10) with given $\pi_{.1}$, ψ, test level α and power $1 - \beta$. This approximation is valid when the exposure rates in cases and controls are similar.

Taylor [37] and Lui [23] studied other approximations that do not assume that the exposure rates in cases and controls are similar. Lui provided simulation results showing that when the OR of exposure between cases and controls is small (≤ 4), his method gives more accurate results than that of Taylor; when ORs are large, the formula given by Taylor is recommended.

All three approximations (i.e. Schlesselman, Taylor and Lui) are based on the assumption of homogeneity of exposure among different matched sets. That is, the probabilities of exposure for cases and controls are constant across matched sets. Tables for the required number of case–control sets are given in Breslow & Day [2] for different values of power, significance level, relative risk and different matching ratios.

Two remarks are given as follows. First, a matched **case–control study** can be regarded as a special case of general stratified study in which each matching category is treated as a unique stratum. The methods discussed in the previous sections for unmatched case–control studies with confounding or **stratification** variables can therefore be used for sample size estimation. However, the methods may break down when the number of strata is large and data in each strata are sparse. Secondly, selection of the number of controls per case is more of a practical consideration (e.g. availability, time and cost) than a statistical power concern. In fact, the power gain is diminished when the number of controls is increased to beyond four controls per case (see [2]).

Cohort Study with Poisson Outcomes

When the number of events for a **cohort study** (e.g. diseases or deaths) is relatively small compared with the total number of subjects, the probability of events occurring may be modeled by a Poisson distribution (*see* **Poisson Regression**; **Poisson Regression for Survival Data in Epidemiology**). In such studies, it is often interesting to test the rate of event incidence rather than the overall probability of events.

Dichotomous Exposure

In a cohort study with dichotomous exposure, Gail [9] presents methods to calculate power for studies with Poisson outcomes when the number of exposed and unexposed samples are equal. Let μ_1 and μ_0 be the incidence rate per unit time for the exposed and unexposed groups, respectively. We want to test $H_0: \mu_0 = \mu_1$ vs. $H_a: \mu_1 > \mu_0$. Two study designs are considered by Gail. Design A is to follow subjects until a predetermined total number of events is observed. Design B is to follow subjects up to a predetermined length of time. For design A, Gail provides a table for the total number of events for given **relative risk** $r = \mu_1/\mu_0$, significance level α and power $1 - \beta$.

Brown & Green [4] extend the method to the case of unequal group sizes. Tables are provided for the total number of events. For Design B, the event rate for the unexposed group, λ_0, is estimated from given relative risk, significance level α and power $1 - \beta$. Tables are provided in Brown & Green [4]. Then, the expected duration of a study can be estimated as $t = \lambda_0/(\mu_0 n_0)$, where n_0 is the number of subjects in the unexposed group for the study that is specified by investigators.

When the expected number of events in the study is large, approximation formulas are presented in Gail [9], Brown & Green [4], as well as in Breslow & Day [2]. Let k be the ratio between the numbers of subjects in the exposed and unexposed groups. For design A, subjects are followed until a certain number of events, say m, is observed. Conditioning on m, the number of events observed in the exposed group, follows a binomial distribution with probability $k\mu_1/(k\mu_1 + \mu_0) = rk/(rk + 1)$. Based on a normal approximation to the arcsine transformation of the square root of a binomial proportion, Brown & Green [4] give

$$m = \frac{[z_{1-\alpha} + z_{1-\beta}]^2}{4\left[\sin^{-1}\sqrt{(rk/(rk+1))} - \sin^{-1}\sqrt{(k/(k+1))}\right]^2},$$

where r is the relative risk between exposed and unexposed groups.

On the basis of a normal approximation to a binomial proportion, Breslow & Day [2] give

$$m = \frac{\left[z_{1-\alpha}\sqrt{k/(k+1)} + z_{1-\beta}\sqrt{(rk)/(rk+1)}\right]^2}{[rk/(rk+1) - k/(k+1)]^2}. \tag{11}$$

A more accurate estimate is obtained by using Yates' correction to the chi-squared significance test [38], which results in multiplying the right-hand side of (11) by $(1 + \sqrt{(1 + A)})^2/4$, where

$$A = \frac{2[rk/(rk+1) - k/(k+1)]}{\left[z_{1-\alpha}\sqrt{k/(k+1)} + z_{1-\beta}\sqrt{(rk)/(rk+1)}\right]^2}.$$

Brown & Green [4] present an example of a study to compare **incidence rates** of congenital malformations among children born in a specific town. A control population is identified that is twice as large as the town under study ($k = 0.5$). To have 90% power to detect a fourfold relative risk, $r = 4$, it is estimated

that a total of $m = 20$ events will be needed (based on the table given in Brown & Green with $\alpha = 0.05$). Similar results are obtained from the approximation formulas. With Brown & Green's approximation, one obtains $m = 19$. With Breslow & Day's approximation, one obtains $m = 18$ without Yates' correction, and $m = 20$ with Yates' correction.

Loglinear Models

A loglinear model may be used to associate the event rate $\lambda(x)$ with the exposure level x; namely

$$\log[\lambda(x)] = \delta + \theta x. \tag{12}$$

A test of no association is equivalent to testing H_0: $\theta = 0$.

Sample size and power calculations for this model have been studied by Self et al. [34,35]. They developed methods for generalized linear models based on the score test in their first paper and based on the likelihood ratio test in their second paper. The loglinear model for Poisson outcomes is a special case of the models they discussed. For a categorical exposure variable X (or a finite number of categorized configurations for a continuous variable), the required sample size is estimated from a noncentral chi-square approximation to the test statistic. However, there is no explicit sample size or power formula in general. Sample size determination is performed numerically for given nuisance parameters and distribution of X. Simulations are recommended to check the accuracy of the estimated sample size. Simulation results [35] show that the method based on the likelihood ratio statistic usually gives better results than that based on the score test.

Test for Trend with Categorical Variable

When the exposure variable X is ordered categorical with K levels ($K > 2$), a trend test can be used to assess whether the event rate $\lambda(x)$ changes monotonically with exposure (*see* **Dose–Response**). Breslow & Day [2] presented a method to estimate the sample size based on a chi-square trend test statistic. The test is based on a score statistic under a loglinear model for a Poisson distribution (*see* **Poisson Regression**; **Poisson Regression for Survival Data in Epidemiology**). It contrasts the observed number of events, O_k, with the expected number of events, E_k, calculated from external rates. Let x_k be the kth exposure level of X. Then the power of the test is the probability such that

$$\sum_{k=1}^{k} O_k \left[x_k - \frac{\sum_j x_j E_j}{\sum_j E_j} \right] - z_{1-\alpha} \sqrt{V} \geq 0,$$

where $z_{1-\alpha}$ is the $(1 - \alpha)$th percentile of the standard normal distribution and

$$V = W \sum_k O_k$$

and

$$al W = \frac{\left[\sum_k x_k^2 E_k - \left(\sum_k x_k E_k \right)^2 \right]}{\sum_k E_k}.$$

Under an alternative of a linear trend in relative risk such that $r(x) = 1 + \theta x$, the left-hand side of the probability equation will have mean μ approximated by

$$\mu = \sum_k \theta x_k E_k \left[x_k - \frac{\sum_j x_j E_j}{\sum_j E_j} \right]$$

$$- z_{1-\alpha} \sqrt{\left(W \sum_k (E_k + \theta x_k E_k) \right)}$$

and variance σ^2 approximated by

$$\sigma^2 = \sum_k (1 + \theta x_k) E_k \left[x_k - \frac{\sum_j x_j E_j}{\sum_j E_j} \right]^2$$

$$- z_{1-\alpha} \sum_k \theta x_k E_k \left[x_k - \frac{\sum_j x_j E_j}{\sum_j E_j} \right]$$

$$\times \sqrt{\frac{W}{\sum_k E_k} + \frac{z_{1-\alpha}^2 W}{4}}.$$

Therefore, the expected number of events for given test level α and power $1 - \beta$ should satisfy $\mu = \sigma z_{1-\beta}$. This equation can be used to solve for the

number of events required for the study under a given distribution for the exposure variable X and alternative hypothesis $\theta = \theta_a$. Numerical methods are needed, in general, except for some special cases; see [2] for details and examples.

Survival Study

In a cohort study, when the time to an event (e.g. disease or death) is observed exactly or within a certain interval, survival analysis can be used for the comparison of incidence rates (*see* **Survival Analysis, Overview**; **Proportional Hazards, Overview**; **Cox Regression Model**). Survival analysis uses not only the number of events but also the time when an event occurs. This often brings more information for comparing event rates than a method using the number of events alone. The survival function $S(t)$ is a probability function that an individual will survive or be disease free up to a certain time point t. The hazard function is defined as

$$\lambda(t) = -\frac{dS(t)/dt}{S(t)}.$$

It measures an instantaneous mortality or morbidity risk relative to a survival probability at that time. A commonly used model for survival analysis is the proportional hazard model, which assumes that hazard functions for two groups satisfy

$$\lambda_1(t) = \psi \lambda_2(t).$$

It is of interest to test the constant hazard ratio $\psi = 1$ or the constant log hazard ratio $\theta = \log(\psi) = 0$ (*see* **Hazard Rate**; **Relative Hazard**).

In a survival study, it is uncommon to observe the actual event time for all subjects. Usually, for some subjects, time to event is censored by the end of the study or at some time point when the subject is lost to follow-up. The statistical power of testing $\theta = 0$ depends principally on the number of events actually observed.

Calculating the Number of Events

For a given alternative on the log hazard ratio, $\theta = \theta_a$, test significance level α and statistical power $1 - \beta$, the required total number of events is estimated as

$$D = \frac{4(z_{1-\alpha} + z_\beta)^2}{\theta_a^2} \qquad (13)$$

based on a score test under the proportional hazard model [33]. For example, to detect a hazard ratio of

1.5 with $\alpha = 0.05$ (two-sided) and $1 - \beta = 0.90$, the required number of events is $D = 256$.

An alternative approximation to the required total number of events based on a normal approximation to the log rank statistic, assuming constant hazard ratio $\psi_a = \exp(\theta_a)$, is given by Freedman [8] as

$$D = \frac{(z_{1-\alpha} + z_\beta)^2 (\psi_a + 1)^2}{(\psi_a - 1)^2}. \tag{14}$$

Simulation results show that this approximation usually provides a slight overestimate for the total number of events [8]. When θ_a is small (close to 0), expressions (13) and (14) will give similar estimates for the total number of events. For the above example, $\psi_a = 1.5$, the required number of events based on (14) is $D = 263$ instead of $D = 256$ from formula (13).

The sample size formulas (13) and (14) are obtained assuming an equal number of subjects allocated in the two study groups. If this is not the case, then the required total number of events corresponding to formula (13) is

$$D = \frac{(z_{1-\alpha} + z_\beta)^2}{\pi_1 \pi_0 \theta_a^2},$$

where π_1 and $\pi_0 = 1 - \pi_1$ are the proportions of subjects to be allocated to the two groups. The corresponding formula for (14) under unequal number of subjects in the two groups is

$$D = \frac{(z_{1-\alpha} + z_\beta)^2 (\pi_1 \psi_a + \pi_0)^2}{\pi_1 (\psi_a - 1)^2}.$$

Calculating the Number of Subjects

Suppose P is the average probability of an individual having an event in the study population. Then the total number of subjects required for the study is approximately $N = D/P$, where D is the total number of events required for the study.

If a study enrolls all subjects at once (e.g. a **cohort study**) and follows every subject up to time f, then the probability P can be estimated by $P = 1 - S(f)$, where S is an average of the two survival functions for the two study groups; that is, $S(t) = [S_0(t) + S_1(t)]/2$ at any time t.

In many cases, the survival function is approximated by an exponential distribution; that is, $S_0(t) = \exp(-\lambda_0 t)$ and $S_1(t) = \exp(-\lambda_1 t)$. The parameters λ_0 and λ_1 can be obtained from the specified median survival time for the corresponding survival functions. Continuing from the example above, where the hazard ratio to be detected is 1.5, suppose the median survival times for the unexposed and exposed subjects are two and three years, respectively. Then $\lambda_0 = 0.347$, $\lambda_1 = 0.231$ and $S(t) = [\exp(-0.347t) + \exp(-0.231t)]/2$. If the study has a three-year follow-up, then the required total sample size can be estimated as $N = 256/0.573 = 447$ based on (13), and $N = 263/0.573 = 459$ based on (14).

In experimental and cohort studies, subjects may be enrolled within a period of time, say from 0 to time T (see **Cohort Study**; **Experimental Study**). The follow-up time for subjects in the study can be anywhere between f (for the last recruited subject) and $T + f$ (for the first subject in the study). The probability of events for the study can be approximated by an average using Simpson's rule [33]; that is,

$$P = 1 - \tfrac{1}{6}[S(f) + 4S(0.5T + f) + S(T + f)],$$

where $S(t)$ is again the average of the two survival functions.

Lachin & Foulkes [16] presented a sample size and power calculation method based on exponential distributions. Their method allows for adjustment on the staggered entry of subjects, loss to follow-up (including deaths from **competing risks**), **stratification**, drop-in and lag in the effectiveness (or exposure effect) during the course of study. Lakatos [17] extended the method using the log rank statistic. Simulation studies show that Lakatos's method [17] is robust even when the proportionality assumption is not satisfied [18]. Other factors can influence sample size, including lack of **sensitivity** in making diagnoses and alternative methods of analysis such as comparison of two Kaplan–Meier curves (see, for example, [10]).

Longitudinal Studies

Longitudinal studies have become popular as the methods for longitudinal data analysis became available (see, for example, [5]). In a longitudinal study, repeated measures are taken from a subject over a period of time. A longitudinal study will provide information (e.g. time effect for individuals) that cannot be obtained by a **cross-sectional study**. This type of study can be used for time-dependent exposures (e.g. smoking, alcohol use, diet, stress, blood pressure) and/or recurrence outcomes (e.g. pain, allergy, asthma, depression). Data from a longitudinal study require special statistical methods because the repeated measures from the same subject tend to be correlated. It is therefore required to consider the correlation among repeated measures while planning the sample size and power for a longitudinal study.

Dichotomous Exposure

The impact of repeated measures on sample size calculations can be illustrated by comparing the average differences in a continuous response. Suppose k repeated measures are taken from each subject, assume the correlation coefficient between any two measures is ρ, then the average of the k measures has variance

$$\text{var}(\overline{Y}) = \frac{1}{k}[1 + (k-1)\rho]\sigma^2,$$

where σ^2 is the variance of each response measure. Assume the variance and correlation are the same under the null and alternative hypotheses. Then the sample size required to detect a difference Δ with significance level α (one-sided) and power $1 - \beta$ is

$$n = \frac{2(z_{1-\alpha} + z_{1-\beta})^2[1 + (k-1)\rho]\sigma^2}{k\Delta^2} \quad (15)$$

for each group [5, Chapter 2]. The correlation ρ will usually be positive. Therefore, the larger the value of ρ, the larger the required sample size for the study. This is because there is less independent information gained from each repeated measurement as ρ approaches 1. When $\rho = 1$, the number of subjects required is the same as in a study with one measurement per subject.

For example, consider a **cohort** (or **experimental**) **study** to investigate the association of a certain diet with total cholesterol level. Subjects in the study will have their total cholesterol measured quarterly for a period of a year. Suppose a standard deviation of 80 is assumed for each measure and the correlation between any two measures is $\rho = 0.5$. With $\alpha = 0.05$ and power = 90% to detect a 20-point difference, we will need $n = 172$ per group based on (15).

For a binary response variable, the sample size for a longitudinal study with repeated measures can be obtained similarly. Suppose p_0 and p_1 are the

proportions of subjects who develop the disease in the unexposed and exposed groups, respectively. Then the required sample size for a longitudinal study with k repeated measures is estimated as [5, Chapter 2]

$$n = \left(z_{1-\alpha}\sqrt{(2\overline{pq})} + z_{1-\beta}\sqrt{(p_1q_1 + p_0q_0)}\right)^2$$
$$\times \frac{[1 + (k-1)\rho]}{[k(p_1 - p_0)^2]}, \quad (16)$$

where $q_1 = 1 - p_1$, $q_0 = 1 - p_0$, $\overline{p} = (p_0 + p_1)/2$, and $\overline{q} = 1 - \overline{p}$. The quantity ρ is the correlation coefficient of the binomial response variable between any two repeated measures. It is assumed to be the same for all subjects under the null and alternative hypotheses. Because the binomial response takes values of 0 or 1, unlike for normal distributed data, the correlation coefficient ρ is constrained in complicated ways (see [5]). For repeated measures, the correlation ρ is usually positive and its value may range in $[0, b]$, where b can be less than 1.

In the above example, if the total cholesterol is dichotomized and the threshold for elevated total cholesterol is 200, then the response will be binomial (yes/no). If one assumes a correlation of 0.5 between any two responses, with $k = 4$ repeated measures, $p_1 = 60\%$ and $p_0 = 70\%$, a sample size of $n = 243$ per group is required to detect a 10 percentage point difference in elevated total cholesterol, with $\alpha = 0.05$ and power = 90%.

Generalized Estimating Equation Method

In general, Liu & Liang [20] presented a method for computing sample size and power for studies with longitudinal observations using the generalized estimating equation (GEE) method. Suppose μ_{ij} is the mean of the ith subject at the jth measure. The generalized linear model with a link function of g is given as

$$g(\mu_{ij}) = X_{ij}\theta + Z_{ij}\lambda,$$

where θ is a vector of parameters of interest, λ is a vector of nuisance parameters, and X_{ij} and Z_{ij} are covariates related to study design. The sample size required for testing H_0: $\theta = \theta_0$ vs. H_a: $\theta = \theta_a$ is derived based on a quasi-score test statistic.

The method can be applied to generalized linear models with longitudinal observations such as linear models for continuous responses, logistic models for binomial response, and loglinear models for Poisson responses. However, there is no explicit sample size formula except for some simple special cases, for which the sample size formulas are provided in Liu & Liang [20]. The sample size or power values are estimated numerically, in general.

To calculate sample size and power, we have to specify the values of the parameters of interest as well as the nuisance parameters under the alternative hypothesis. In addition, the element of the correlation matrix for the longitudinal observations has to be specified, and this is usually the most difficult part. Information about correlation may be obtained from previous studies. In the case of no prior information about the correlation, a sensitivity analysis may be performed using various correlation values based on the investigator's judgment. The sample size for the study may be taken conservatively based on the sensitivity analysis.

Estimation and Precision

The sample size determinations discussed so far are based on achieving a certain probability (power) to detect a given alternative for a specified statistical hypothesis test. When the problem of interest is to estimate the magnitude of the effect, e.g. the disease–exposure **odds ratio**, the study planning must focus on the precision of the estimate, which is often measured by the width of a confidence interval. In general, the sample size required for the study should be increased if the confidence level is increased, the variability associated with the measure is increased, or the total width of the confidence interval is reduced.

There are two different approaches to determining sample size based on the width of a confidence interval. One is to have the expected width of the confidence interval sufficiently small. Another is to have a tolerance level to guarantee that the width of the confidence interval will be within a given precision limit. In the latter case, the width of a confidence interval is regarded as a random variable. The latter approach usually requires larger sample sizes than the former. In this section we illustrate the two approaches to determining sample size for estimating ORs and **standardized mortality ratios**.

OR

Consider a 2 × 2 table generated from an unmatched case–control study:

Exposure	Case	Control	
Yes	n_{11}	n_{10}	$n_{1.}$
No	n_{01}	n_{00}	$n_{0.}$
	$n_{0.1}$	$n_{0.0}$	n

The OR is estimated by

$$OR = (n_{11}n_{00})/(n_{01}n_{10}).$$

For the first approach, O'Neill [28] derived a sample size equation by replacing the cell counts with their expected values and then using a logit method to calculate the confidence interval width. To have the expected width of the $1 - \alpha$ confidence interval less than 2δ, for given values of true OR, exposure rate π_0 for the control group, and the case–control ratio k (i.e. $k = n_{.0}/n_{.1}$), the number of cases required is

$$n_{.1} = \left[\frac{1}{\pi_1(1 - \pi_1)} + \frac{1}{\pi_0(1 - \pi_0)} \right] \left[\frac{z_{1-\alpha/2}}{\delta} \right]^2,$$

where π_1 is the exposure rate for the case group, which can be calculated as $\pi_1 = \pi_0 OR/[1 + \pi_0 (OR - 1)]$.

For the second approach, a $1 - \alpha$ confidence interval for $\ln(OR)$ is obtained from the normal approximation (e.g. [1, Chapter IV]),

$$\ln(OR) \pm z_{1-\alpha/2} \left[\frac{1}{n_{11}} + \frac{1}{n_{00}} + \frac{1}{n_{10}} + \frac{1}{n_{01}} \right]^{1/2}.$$

The precision of the estimate can be evaluated by the probability of the confidence interval being within $[-\delta, \delta]$. That is,

$$P \left(z_{1-\alpha/2} \left[\frac{1}{n_{11}} + \frac{1}{n_{00}} + \frac{1}{n_{10}} + \frac{1}{n_{01}} \right]^{1/2} \leq \delta \right)$$
$$= 1 - \beta.$$

The probability $1 - \beta$ is called the tolerance probability. The sample size required for the study is obtained by solving this equation for given values of the true OR, α, β, δ, the exposure rate π_0 for the control group, and the case–control ratio k. Numerical computation is needed to solve the equation for n. Satten & Kupper [31] provided tables (as well as a computer program) for the minimum sample size required to produce a 95% confidence interval of total width not greater than 2δ with probability $1 - \beta$ for various values of δ, k, OR, and π_0.

Satten & Kupper [31] also gave an example for a case–control study. The anticipated OR for the study population is no smaller than 3. For a probability of exposure in controls $\pi_0 = 0.05$, with tolerance probability $1 - \beta = 0.90$, $k = 1$, and in order to have the width of the 95% confidence interval no more than 1.5, $n = 271$ cases are required (with $k = 1$, the number of controls is the same). With O'Neill's method, the required number of cases is $n = 202$.

Standardized Mortality Ratio

The **standardized mortality ratio** (SMR) is the ratio between the observed number of events and the expected number of events. The latter quantity is usually derived from external studies or vital statistics and is assumed to be known and fixed (*see* **Vital Statistics, Overview**). The SMR is a common measure of **relative risk** in occupational epidemiologic studies (*see* **Occupational Epidemiology**).

Assume the observed number of events d in a cohort study follows a Poisson distribution with mean λ. The confidence interval of the SMR is obtained by finding the corresponding confidence limits for λ and then dividing these limits by the expected number of events. Using the relation between the Poisson distribution and the chi-squared distribution, Gordon [11] derived the $1 - \alpha$ confidence interval for λ as

$$(\lambda_L, \lambda_U) = \left[\tfrac{1}{2}c_{\alpha/2}(2d), \tfrac{1}{2}c_{1-\alpha/2}(2d + 1) \right],$$

where $c_\alpha(k)$ is the αth quantile of a chi-squared distribution with k degrees of freedom.

The expectations of λ_L and λ_U, and the expected width of the interval are

$$E(\lambda_L) = \sum_{d=1}^{\infty} \tfrac{1}{2}c_{\alpha/2}(2d)\frac{\lambda^d}{d!} \exp(-\lambda),$$

$$E(\lambda_U) = \sum_{d=0}^{\infty} \tfrac{1}{2}c_{1-\alpha/2}(2d + 1)\frac{\lambda^d}{d!} \exp(-\lambda),$$

$$E(w) = E(\lambda_U) - E(\lambda_L).$$

Tables are given by Gordon [11] for these expected values for various values of λ, which can be used to determine the expected number of events given the

true SMR and an upper limit, a lower limit or the width of the confidence interval.

The sample size obtained by Gordon is based on the first approach without having a tolerance level to guarantee the precision. The estimated sample size will be too small to distinguish the SMR from a specified value [13]. For example, to have the upper bound of the 95% confidence interval no more than 1.0 when the true SMR is 0.7, the expected number of events estimated by Gordon's method is 42.9. However, this sample size will have only a 50% chance of yielding a 95% confidence interval, which will exclude the value 1.0 when the true SMR is 0.7.

Based on the second approach, Greenland [13] provided a method to estimate the sample size needed so that the confidence interval can reliably distinguish between two different values of the SMR. He concluded that the sample size obtained will be similar to that based on a hypothesis test to compare the two specified SMR values. For the above example, in order to have a 90% chance that the upper 95% confidence interval be smaller than 1.0 when the true SMR is 0.7, the required number of events is 98.4. This sample size can also be obtained from a hypothesis test that compares SMR = 0.7 vs. SMR = 1.0, with significance level 0.05 and power of 90%.

Further Issues and Discussion

Exact Methods

As computing technology advanced in recent years, exact methods were developed for analyses of studies with categorical observations. These methods provide exact test p-values that may be quite different from the asymptotic p-values when the sample size and/or the probability of events is small. If it is planned to use exact methods for the analysis, then it is preferable to estimate the sample size for the study based on the same exact approach.

For pair-matched **case–control studies**, a number of papers have been published for calculating sample size and power based on McNemar's test. Lachin [15] compared several unconditional sample size and power calculation methods (*see* **Matched Analysis**). Royston [30] published tables of sample sizes based on the conditional and unconditional approaches.

For ordered categorical data, Hilton & Mehta [14] developed an algorithm for computing sample size and exact power. They also considered a Monte Carlo method for power estimation. They pointed out that the asymptotic power function works well when the number of categories is not too small (e.g. more than five categories).

Lui [24] considered sample size estimation for the exact conditional test under inverse sampling, in which one continues to sample subjects until one obtains a predetermined number of index subjects (e.g. events). Under inverse sampling, the number of events to be observed for each exposure group is fixed, and the number of subjects to be sampled follows a negative binomial distribution. Conditional on the total number of subjects, a conditional test is used to compare event rates for the two groups. Based on a numerical approximation, tables are provided for the minimum required number of events given events rates, significance level = 0.05 and power = 0.80 or 0.90.

Adjustment for Loss to Follow-up and Missing Data

In studies where loss to follow-up or **missing data** occur, the planned sample size should reflect the information loss to maintain the desired statistical power. If loss to follow-up or missing data are purely by chance (missing completely at random), then a simple adjustment on the sample size is to enlarge the required sample size by the proportion of information loss. For example, suppose the required sample size for a cohort study is 400 subjects per group and a 20% loss to follow-up rate is assumed, then the total number of subjects for the study may be enlarged to 500 ($= 400/(1-0.2)$) per group. This simple adjustment provides a conservative sample size estimate if the partial data obtained from the lost to follow-up subjects can be used in the statistical analysis (e.g. in longitudinal analysis models). If we know that 25% data from the 20% lost to follow-up subjects can be used in the analysis, then a refined sample size adjustment is $n = 400/(1-0.15) = 471$.

This simple adjustment can also be used for the case when missing data are missing at random, i.e. the probability of missingness depends on at most the data already observed but not on the missing data [19]. However, when data are not missing at random (nonignorable missingness), the probability of missingness will depend on the missing data. In this case, it can be difficult to compute the proportion of missing information. Further discussion of missing

data is beyond the scope of this article and can be found in Little & Rubin [19] (*see* **Missing Data in Epidemiologic Studies**).

Computation and Software

Several commercial software packages are currently available for sample size and power calculations (*see* **Software, Biostatistical**; **Software, Epidemiological**). They include EGRET-SIZ by Cytel Software Corporation, SamplePower by SPSS Inc., nQuery Advisor by Statistical Solutions, and PASS by Number Cruncher Statistical Systems. EGRET-SIZ is the only package for sample size and power calculations with the main focus on epidemiologic studies. It provides sample size estimates for four specialized statistical models including **logistic regression** (for **cohort** and unmatched **case–control studies**), **Poisson regression**, **conditional logistic regression** and **Cox** proportional hazards **regression**. A good feature of EGRET-SIZ is that there is a Monte Carlo procedure for one to verify the estimated sample size and obtain empirical power. SamplePower, nQuery Advisor and PASS provide sample size estimates for a broad range of statistical models including tests for means, proportions, analysis of variance (ANOVA), regression and survival analysis. Most of the software packages can be used to estimate one of the parameters among sample size, power, minimum detectable effect, variances, and test significance level, provided the other parameters are specified. Some of the packages (e.g. nQuery, SamplePower) have modules to estimate sample size from the given width of a confidence interval.

Other "freeware" may be found in public health service organizations or from individual statisticians. For example, "Epi info" from the Centers for Disease Control and Prevention provides some sample size estimation routines for cohort and case–control studies. A SAS module/macro for sample size analysis, "UnifyPow", has been developed and distributed by O'Brien [27]. Many computer codes for some specific and complex statistical methods may be obtained directly from the authors who developed these methods. For example, a power and sample size module for testing **interaction** has been developed by Lubin and colleagues at the National Cancer Institute based on a paper by Lubin & Gail [21]. A sample size calculation module is included in EPITOME, an epidemiologic data analysis package developed at the National Cancer Institute.

Although many approaches and software packages can be used to calculate sample size, care should always be taken to formulate the study problem in the framework that the computer software requires. It is necessary to follow the program instructions or user's manual to provide input parameters for the computer packages. In all cases, it is important to understand the statistical procedures for which the computer package is calculating the sample size or power. Otherwise, the calculated sample size can be erroneous and lead to an underpowered or overpowered study.

Discussion

Sample size determination is a very important aspect of the design of any study. It often helps to clarify important features of a study protocol. Investigators will not be able to calculate sample size without fully understanding the nature of the measurements to be taken, specifying the planned analysis (test statistic or estimation procedure, significance level and study power), and obtaining preliminary information on the effect to be detected and the variability of the measurements. Some important information can often be obtained from reviewing the literature or discussions with other investigators who conducted previous studies.

In practice, sample size and power evaluation may be an iterative learning process. The parameters and distribution characteristics obtained from previous studies can be used to estimate the required sample size for planning the current study. If there is no previous information for a new investigation, then a pilot study may be designed to gain some knowledge about the parameters and distribution. The results from this pilot study will then provide information for designing the main study. The iterative process may be integrated to form a two-stage design in which the results from the pilot study (first stage) will be used to guide the sample size estimation for the second stage. The data from both stages will be used for the final data analysis. For instance, the impact of additional follow-up in cohort studies was investigated by Brookmeyer et al. [3]. In randomized clinical trials, Gould & Shih [12] presented methods to adjust the sample size during the course of a study.

Group sequential procedures have been considered for experimental studies by health researchers, in which investigators are allowed to have several interim analyses. Each interim analysis not only provides a preliminary estimation of the parameters of interest before the completion of the study, but also offers a chance to terminate the study early when there is sufficient evidence to reach a conclusion (either positive or negative). Although this sequential approach has mainly been used and advocated for **experimental** and **case–control studies** (*see* **Case–Control Study, Sequential**), the idea can be used in **cohort studies** by performing interim analyses when partial follow-up data are available. However, there is usually less ethical pressure for early termination of **observational** epidemiologic studies than **experimental studies** such as randomized clinical trials. Furthermore, the need for a large sample size is often stressed in epidemiologic studies in order to estimate the parameters of interest with precision. For these reasons, sequential methods have not gained widespread acceptance and use in epidemiologic studies.

Usually, new statistical methods are developed for data analysis before they are considered in sample size estimation for designing studies. For some complicated study designs and statistical models, sample size estimation methods may not be available (e.g. case–cohort design, two-stage case–control studies, and structural models for causal inference; see [29]). Further research will be needed on sample size estimation for these specialized study designs and statistical models (*see* **Case–Cohort Study**; **Case–Control Study, Two-Phase**).

Two approaches may be considered to estimate sample size for a complicated study when there is no sample size estimation method available. First, a Monte Carlo simulation may be conducted to estimate the power empirically for several fixed sample sizes and thus to find the sample size that yields the required power. Today's powerful computation tools make this approach feasible. The second approach is to approximate the sample size by using a simplified study design and/or statistical model for which a sample size estimation method is available. The simple model should be chosen so that it requires at least as large a sample size as would be required by the more complex and presumably more efficient analysis. There is a tradeoff between using simpler methods and using more sophisticated models for sample size estimation. At the design stage, prior information about the parameters of the statistical models may be limited. Sample size estimation requires fewer assumptions with simplified statistical models than with more sophisticated models. Unless the assumed values of parameters and forms of distributions are accurate for the designed study, the sample size estimated from the sophisticated models may be inaccurate due to misleading assumptions. Simplified methods, on the other hand, can be more robust because of fewer assumptions.

Acknowledgment

The author would like to thank Dr Jacques Benichou for his detailed review, comments and suggestions. Thanks also to Dr Mitchell Gail for his valuable comments and some additional references.

References

[1] Breslow, N.E. & Day, N.E. (1980). *Statistical Methods in Cancer Research, Volume I – The Analysis of Case–Control Studies.* International Agency for Research on Cancer, Lyon.

[2] Breslow, N.E. & Day, N.E. (1987). *Statistical Methods in Cancer Research, Volume II – The Design and Analysis of Cohort Studies.* International Agency for Research on Cancer, Lyon.

[3] Brookmeyer, R., Day, N. & Pompe-Kirn, V. (1985). Assessing the impact of additional follow-up in cohort studies, *American Journal of Epidemiology* **121**, 611–619.

[4] Brown, C.C. & Green, S.B. (1982). Additional power computations for designing comparative Poisson trials, *American Journal of Epidemiology* **115**, 752–758.

[5] Diggle, P.J., Liang, K.Y. & Zeger, S.L. (1994). *Analysis of Longitudinal Data.* Oxford University Press, Oxford.

[6] Dupont, W.D. (1988). Power calculations for matched case–control studies, *Biometrics* **44**, 1157–1168.

[7] Fleiss, J.L. & Levin, B. (1988). Sample size determination in studies with matched pairs, *Journal of Clinical Epidemiology* **41**, 727–730.

[8] Freedman, L.S. (1982). Tables of the number of patients required in clinical trials using the logrank test, *Statistics in Medicine* **1**, 121–129.

[9] Gail, M. (1974). Power computations for designing comparative Poisson trials, *Biometrics* **30**, 231–237.

[10] Gail, M. (1994). Sample size estimation when time-to-event is the primary endpoint, *Drug Information Journal* **28**, 865–877.

[11] Gordon, I. (1987). Sample size estimation in occupational mortality studies with use of confidence interval theory, *American Journal of Epidemiology* **125**, 158–162.

[12] Gould, A.L. & Shih, W.J. (1992). Sample size re-estimation without unblinding for normally distributed outcomes with unknown variance, *Communications in Statistics A – Theory and Methods* **21**, 2833–2853.

[13] Greenland, S. (1988). On sample-size and power calculations for studies using confidence intervals, *American Journal of Epidemiology* **128**, 231–237.

[14] Hilton, J.F. & Mehta, C.R. (1993). Power and sample size calculations for exact conditional tests with ordered categorical data, *Biometrics* **49**, 609–616.

[15] Lachin, J.M. (1992). Power and sample size evaluation for the McNemar test with application to matched case–control studies, *Statistics in Medicine* **11**, 1239–1251.

[16] Lachin, J.M. & Foulkes, M.A. (1986). Evaluation of sample size and power for analysis of survival with allowance for nonuniform patient entry, losses to follow-up, noncompliance, and stratification, *Biometrics* **42**, 507–519.

[17] Lakatos, E. (1988). Sample sizes based on the logrank statistics in complex clinical trials, *Biometrics* **44**, 229–241.

[18] Lakatos, E. & Lan, K.K.G. (1992). A comparison of sample size methods for the logrank statistic. *Statistics in Medicine* **11**, 179–191.

[19] Little, R.J. & Rubin, D.B. (1987). *Statistical Analysis with Missing Data.* Wiley, New York.

[20] Liu, G. & Liang, K.Y. (1997). Sample size calculations for studies with correlated observations, *Biometrics* **53**, 937–947.

[21] Lubin, J.H. & Gail, M.H. (1990). On power and sample size for studying features of the relative odds of disease, *American Journal of Epidemiology* **131**, 552–566.

[22] Lubin, J.H., Gail, M.H. & Ershow, A.G. (1988). Sample size and power for case–control studies when exposures are continuous, *Statistics in Medicine* **7**, 363–376.

[23] Lui, K.J. (1988). Estimation of sample sizes in case–control studies with multiple controls per case, dichotomous data, *American Journal of Epidemiology* **127**, 1064–1070.

[24] Lui, K.J. (1996). Sample size for the exact conditional test under inverse sampling, *Statistics in Medicine* **15**, 671–678.

[25] Munoz, A. & Rosner, B. (1984). Power and sample size for a collection of 2×2 tables, *Biometrics* **40**, 995–1004.

[26] Nam, J. (1992). Sample size determination for case–control studies and the comparison of stratified and unstratified analyses, *Biometrics* **48**, 389–395.

[27] O'Brien, R.G. (1998). A tour of UnifyPow: A SAS module/macro for sample size analysis, *Proceedings of the Twenty-third SAS Users Group International Conference*, Cary, NC, 1346–1355.

[28] O'Neill, R.R. (1984). Sample sizes for estimation of the odds ratio in unmatched case–control studies, *American Journal of Epidemiology* **120**, 145–153.

[29] Rothman, K.J. & Greenland, S. (1998). *Modern Epidemiology.* Lippincott-Raven, Philadelphia.

[30] Royston, P. (1993). Exact conditional and unconditional sample size for pair-matched studies with binary

outcome: a practical guide, *Statistics in Medicine* **12**, 699–712.

[31]   Satten, G.A. & Kupper, L.L. (1990). Sample size requirements for interval estimation of the odds ratio, *American Journal of Epidemiology* **131**, 177–184.

[32]   Schlesselman, J.J. (1982). *Case–control Studies: Design, Conduct, Analysis*. Oxford University Press, Oxford.

[33]   Schoenfeld, D.A. (1983). Sample size formula for the proportional-hazards regression model, *Biometrics* **39**, 499–503.

[34]   Self, S.G. & Mauritsen, R.H. (1988). Power/sample size calculations for generalized linear models, *Biometrics* **44**, 79–86.

[35]   Self, S.G., Mauritsen, R.H. & Ohara, J. (1992). Power calculations for likelihood ratio tests in generalized linear models, *Biometrics* **48**, 31–39.

[36]   Smith, P.G. & Day, N.E. (1984). The design of case–control studies: the influence of confounding and interaction, *International Journal of Epidemiology* **13**, 87–93.

[37]   Taylor, J.M.G. (1986). Choosing the number of controls in a matched case–control study: some sample size, power and efficiency calculations, *Statistics in Medicine* **5**, 29–36.

[38]   Ury, H.K. & Fleiss, J.L. (1980). On approximate sample sizes for comparing two independent proportions with the use of Yates' correction, *Biometrics* **36**, 347–351.

[39]   Wickramaratne, P.J. (1995). Sample size determination in epidemiologic studies, *Statistical Methods in Medical Research* **4**, 311–337.

[40]   Whittemore, A.S. (1981). Sample size for logistic regression with small response probability, *Journal of the American Statistical Association* **76**, 27–32.

[41]   Woolson, R.F., Bean, J.A. & Rojas P.B. (1986). Sample size for case–control studies using Cochran's statistic, *Biometrics* **42**, 927–932.

GUANGHAN LIU

Sample Surveys

The use of sample surveys in biostatistics arises from the need to answer questions about health issues in the community. The earliest uses of survey methodology in health research in the US were motivated more by policy issues than by epidemiologic questions, and paralleled the use of surveys by the Census Bureau and other Federal agencies to address social and economic concerns. More recently, it has been recognized that research into the causes and outcomes of disease can benefit from studies in the entire community, rather than just in the formal health care system, particularly in countries like the US, where access to health care is not uniform. A number of practical concerns about conducting studies in the community then lead to the use of sample surveys, rather than complete enumeration.

Reasons for Conducting Sample Surveys

Perhaps the most compelling argument for using a sample survey rather than complete enumeration is that for the same cost a sample survey can provide results more accurately, with greater scope, and faster. Studying a well-chosen sample can increase accuracy by reducing **bias** and by increasing precision of the results. By reducing the number of people to be studied, a sample survey can devote more resources to finding and persuading nonresponders to participate, thus reducing **nonresponse** bias. Fewer interviewers are required, so that more effort can be devoted to training and monitoring them for accuracy. Replicate measurements may be made to increase the precision. Sample surveys can also take advantage of the smaller sample size and more intensive effort for each person to ask more questions or make more detailed measurements, thus broadening the scope of the questions addressed. Finally, sample surveys may be able to reduce the total time to collect and analyze the data, thus providing more timely answers to important questions.

A second important reason for the use of sample surveys is feasibility. When the **target population** is very large, such as the entire population of the US, a moderate-sized sample survey, if well designed, can provide highly accurate results at substantially less cost than a complete enumeration. The cost of a complete enumeration can be substantial both for the researchers and for the participants; one motivation for using sample surveys is when the respondents are institutions such as hospitals.

The desire to study certain subgroups in more depth also leads people to use sample surveys. Policy issues may require valid estimates for children, people age 65 and older, women, African-Americans, Hispanics, rural residents, or other subgroups in the population. A sampling design can oversample from important subgroups to increase precision and to ensure that their health can be characterized accurately.

Recently, epidemiologic studies have begun to take advantage of the ability of sample survey designs to increase power and reduce bias in studies of risk factors for disease onset and progression (*see* **Observational Study**). The power in comparative analyses of risk factors is largely determined by the number of **prevalent** or **incident** disease cases identified for study. To increase the number of cases, researchers can increase the sample size or the length of follow-up, an expensive strategy, or try to increase the proportion of disease cases in the sample by over-sampling groups at high risk. A clever design can improve power substantially. Sample surveys also help to reduce bias for epidemiologic studies by providing a truly comparable group of unaffected people, sampled from exactly the same population in which the affected group was identified (*see* **Controls**). A recent study of Alzheimer's disease in people 65 and older in the community in East Boston, Massachusetts, used a stratified sample design to over-sample from the oldest age groups and those with poor performance on a simple memory test. When a neurologist examined the resulting sample, about 35% were found to have clinical Alzheimer's disease, compared with an estimated **prevalence** of 10% in the community. In addition, the mean age of the unaffected comparison group was much closer to that of the Alzheimer's group in this sample than in the community, and both diseased and disease-free participants had received the same interviews and clinical evaluation [11].

Some History of Sample Surveys

Early Developments at the US Bureau of the Census

In the early part of the twentieth century, the importance of using random sampling in surveys was not generally recognized. Units to be canvassed were still selected purposively, with the survey managers deciding which units would be most "representative" of the population of interest. Probability theory had yet to be applied. In the 1930s, more attention was being paid to R.A. Fisher's work on the importance of randomization in experimental design, and in 1934 J. Neyman's paper [40] arguing in favor of random sampling and establishing the theoretical foundation for it appeared in the *Journal of the Royal Statistical Society* (also see Tschuprow [52]). These developments in statistical theory laid the groundwork for modern sample surveys. However, the key catalyst

for the incorporation of probabilistic sampling into the selection of units in sample surveys was the increasing need for reliable estimates to use in policy-making.

At the US Bureau of the Census, the first application of probabilistic sampling was in a 1937 "check census" of unemployment. The Bureau used postmen as canvassers, choosing two out of every 100 postal routes. The success of this early foray into probabilistic sampling was possibly a decisive moment for those decision-makers who were skeptical of the value of nonpurposive methods [9].

In the 1940 decennial census of population and housing, the first "long form" sample was introduced: 5% of the population was asked a set of questions in addition to the key census battery. This approach is still an integral part of the decennial census, enabling the Census Bureau to collect more detailed data without overburdening all respondents, and at a moderate cost [1, 16, 46].

In 1942 the Bureau was given the Work Projects Administration's Monthly Report on the Labor Force (MRLF), from which were derived unemployment estimates. In order to develop an efficient sample design for this survey, the Bureau statisticians under the direction of Morris Hansen and William Hurwitz found that they had to develop totally new theory for the design of sample surveys. Major new developments included sampling with unequal probabilities, cluster sampling, optimization in multistage sampling, and estimation methods. These are now considered standard sampling methods for face-to-face household surveys. Under the direction of Hansen and Hurwitz, a relatively small research staff made further contributions to sampling methods. One of the more public products of this work, a two-volume text by Hansen, Hurwitz, and William G. Madow published in 1953 [18], still stands as a classic work in statistics.

The MRLF, later named the Current Population Survey, provided a laboratory for research into sampling and other statistical aspects of survey methods. It also became a model for household surveys all over the world. Other current US demographic surveys have used the same basic design, including: The National Crime Survey (now The National Crime Victimization Survey), The National Health Interview Survey, The Survey of Income and Program Participation, The American Housing Survey (formerly The Annual Housing Survey), and The Consumer

Expenditure Quarterly and Diary Surveys. Data for all of these surveys are collected by the Bureau of the Census, typically for sponsoring agencies who publish the estimates from the surveys. Most of these surveys use as their basic frame the list of housing units obtained from the decennial census; this list is supplemented by frames for new construction and other special categories. Characteristics of those housing units and their occupants are used to stratify units within counties and to group counties within primary strata.

Extensions of the Survey Methodology to Other Fields of Study

The combination of the success of the sample survey method developed and used by the Census Bureau in the 1940s and 1950s in providing population, housing and economic data and the need for new data on health characteristics of the population led to the adoption of sampling techniques in conducting national health surveys, beginning in 1957 and continuing until the present time.

It had been established in the 1920s that community studies of illness and disability were feasible, and a major health survey to obtain data on diseases, injuries and impairments in the general population of the United States was conducted in 1935–1936 [38]. Following that survey, additional community studies on morbidity led to the formation of the US National Committee on Vital and Health Statistics in 1949, which ultimately recommended "That a continuing national morbidity survey be conducted.... Its purpose would be to obtain data on the prevalence and incidence of disease, injuries and impairments, on the nature and duration of the resulting disability, and on the amount and type of medical care received. The data would be obtained from a probability sample of households" [38]. Thus, what is now known as the National Health Interview Survey (NHIS) was begun.

The data from these continuing surveys have been used extensively by the US Federal government in setting policy and developing programs for the continued benefit of the population. Perhaps the largest such program ever enacted is the national health insurance program for the elderly, known as Medicare, which came into existence some eight years after the NHIS began producing relevant data on the health of the general population. In addition, data derived from the NHIS were used in developing the 1964 recommendations of the US Surgeon General regarding smoking and health.

Today, data from both national surveys and community population studies are being used to understand causes and prevention of disease. For example, most of what we know about the risk factors for coronary heart disease came from the results of the long-standing community study known as the Framingham Heart Study. Currently, community studies utilizing sampling techniques are being conducted in Hawaii, Illinois, Washington (state) and other areas to determine risk factors for Alzheimer's disease and other dementing illnesses, which may aid researchers in developing preventive strategies for the future. Data from a longitudinal supplement to the NHIS and from a national long-term care survey have suggested that a decline in disability among older people has been taking place over time [30]. These data will be useful for planning health care services for the elderly for the future.

Design and Objectives of Sample Surveys in Health and Medical Studies

The specification of the design and objectives of a sample survey form a very important part of the planning of the study. A clear statement of objectives is essential for the researcher to be able to stay on track and design the study effectively. One can become so engrossed in the details of planning that one loses sight of the overall purpose for the study, and perhaps makes decisions which may contradict the objectives which were originally set.

Objectives of Sample Surveys

As surveys are usually of two types, descriptive and analytic, the statement of objectives should include the main purpose. Most large-scale surveys are usually of the descriptive type, although analytic uses of the data may ultimately be made. An example of a statement of objectives which follows comes from a publication of the National Center for Health Statistics (NCHS) regarding the redesign of the NHIS in 1985 [31]:

> To continue to produce descriptive statistics about the health and health-related parameters of the civilian noninstitutionalized population of the United

States, and to monitor change in those variables over time. ...

To put more emphasis on measures of change in the NHIS. ...

To improve the precision of NHIS statistics for special small domains, such as black and Hispanic, of the population.

To improve the efficiency and analytical utility of NCHS's combined population survey program. ...

To investigate methods that would provide the NHIS greater flexibility to oversample subgroups of the population, oversample geographic areas of the United States, conduct follow back surveys, and respond more rapidly in the collection and production of statistics on special health topics.

To make the NHIS design more cost efficient while maintaining the same overall level of precision.

To incorporate health and health-related variables into the redesign of the NHIS. ...

These objectives were used in developing the criteria for the redesign of the survey, and, while they serve as an example for us, the careful statements enabled the NCHS statisticians to work through the design phase without losing sight of where they should be going.

Major Design Features of Sample Surveys

While there are numerous features of sample surveys which could be discussed in this article, space dictates that we limit our discussion to only a few of the main features seen in most sample surveys executed in practice. Recall the textbook definition of simple random sampling in a finite population, namely a method of selecting n units out of N such that each of the possible combinations of N units taken n at a time has an equal chance of being chosen (see, for example, [4]). In addition to simple random sampling, survey statisticians often employ methods of sampling including, but not limited to, **stratification** and **clustering**, and compute estimates using techniques such as ratio estimation and post-stratification. Following discussion of these topics, we will conclude the section with some information about sources of error in surveys.

Stratification. Use of **stratification** in sample surveys involves first the division of the population of N units into L nonoverlapping subpopulations, called strata, of size $N_1, N_2, \ldots, N_L$. In order to obtain

maximum benefit from selecting a stratified sample, the number of units, N_i, in each stratum must be known. The sample is then drawn independently from each stratum.

There are numerous reasons for using stratification in sample surveys. As stated in the introductory section, one reason for stratification is to insure that one can make estimates of a certain level of precision for subgroups of the population under study, by fixing sample sizes separately for each subgroup. Secondly, if it is known in advance of conducting the survey that characteristics to be estimated from the survey vary at substantially different rates from one subgroup to another, it is possible to achieve increased precision in the overall population estimates by creating strata in which within-stratum variability is small and between-stratum variability is large. For example, in the National Hospital Discharge Survey [15], larger hospitals (in terms of number of beds) tend to be more alike among themselves than they are like smaller hospitals, and similarly for the smaller hospitals. The variance of within-stratum estimates of a discharge rate may be quite small compared to the variance of rates among strata. A third reason for stratification is that the population may have natural divisions that lend themselves to stratification, or layering. For example, field offices for a given survey may be scattered throughout a large geographic area, thus dictating that the sample be stratified according to the geographic breakdowns inherent in the total population.

To illustrate the computations involved in estimating a population mean from a stratified sample and its sampling variance, consider a population that is divided into two strata with N_1 units in the first stratum and N_2 units in the second. The unbiased estimator of the mean is $\bar{x}_{\text{st}} = F\bar{x}_1 + (1 - F)\bar{x}_2$, where $\bar{x}_1$ and $\bar{x}_2$ are the respective within-stratum sample means and $F = N_1/N$ and $1 - F = N_2/N$. The variance of the estimate of the sample mean is

$$s_{\bar{x}_{\text{st}}}^2 = F^2 s_1^2 (1/n_1 - 1/N_1) + (1 - F)^2 s_2^2$$
$$\times (1/n_2 - 1/N_2),$$

where s_1^2 and s_2^2 are the sample variances within the two strata, and n_1 and n_2 are sample sizes within the strata. If the within-stratum variances are sufficiently small, the overall variance of the estimated mean could turn out to be smaller than the mean of a simple random sample. Finally, the results shown here can be extended to estimation of population totals, proportions, or other characteristics by algebraically manipulating the formulas given here for the mean.

As an example of the increased precision that can be achieved through stratification, consider the following data set taken from the Honolulu Asia Aging Study (HAAS), a study of dementing illness among Japanese-American men living in Hawaii [53]. The sample to be studied was selected from three groups based on the individuals' performance on a cognitive function screening test. Those persons who performed the poorest – and therefore were at highest risk of dementia – were chosen at the highest rate. The "good" performers were selected at the lowest rate, and those in the middle at an intermediate rate, the objective being to obtain the largest number of diseased cases possible while not ruling out the possibility that at least a few of the "good" performers may also have been at risk for dementia. The overall estimate of the prevalence of dementia among these men was 9.3% with a standard error of 1.6% when a simple binomial model was used to calculate the variance. However, when the stratified sampling assumptions were taken into account, as above, the standard error estimate was reduced to 0.83%. Thus, the stratified design in this case led to a standard error slightly more than half that of a simple random sample.

Clustering.   Clustering, or sampling in which the units sampled are chosen in groups or *clusters* of smaller units, called elements, is used for two reasons. First, for many surveys a *sampling frame*, or list of population units to be sampled, does not exist. For example, if one were asked to design a sampling plan for estimating the number of trees in a given geographic area, say the state of California, clearly no list of population units exists. Furthermore, the construction of such lists might be impossible for some studies, while for others it might be feasible but prohibitively expensive. However, from maps of geographic regions or lakes or whatever areas are to be sampled, it is possible to divide the region into subregions with definable boundaries. These subregions, which contain clusters of the sampling units of interest, are selected for study because they solve the problem of constructing a list of sampling units.

The second reason for selecting cluster samples is purely economic. Suppose that one were interested

in studying the characteristics of physicians in office-based practices in the United States. It is known that the American Medical Association maintains an up-to-date listing of all such physicians for the US. However, if one were to select a simple random sample of these physicians and send interviewers to collect the data from them, the interviewers would be traveling all over the country at tremendous expense to reach what would undoubtedly be a widely scattered sample of physicians. A more practical approach to conducting the study would be to select a relatively small sample of geographic areas around the nation and conduct interviews with a sample of physicians limited to those selected areas. Clearly, a simple random sample of 3000 physicians would cover the nation more evenly than 100 counties or metropolitan areas containing an average of 30 physicians each, but greater field costs in locating the doctors and traveling from place to place to interview them would outweigh the precision obtainable with the simple random sample.

The choice of cluster size involves balancing costs versus precision for a given survey and can become rather complicated, especially if the design involves several stages of sampling. Rather than becoming engrossed in an overly complicated analysis regarding cluster sampling, let us look at a simple design in which a simple random sample of n clusters is selected from N clusters in the population, with simple random selection of m elements (out of M) within each cluster. Let x_{ij} represent the observed value for the jth element in the ith cluster and let x_i be the cluster total. Here we need to distinguish between two kinds of means: the mean per cluster $\overline{X} = \sum x_i/N$ and the mean per element $\overline{X}/M = \sum x_i/NM$. Sampling at two levels thus introduces variance components for the effect of sampling clusters and elements within clusters. The between-cluster component can be calculated from the sample as

$$s_{\mathrm{b}}^2 = \sum_{i=1}^{n} \frac{(x_i - \bar{x})^2}{n-1}$$

and the within-cluster component as

$$s_{\mathrm{w}}^2 = \sum_{i=1}^{n} \frac{1}{m-1} \sum_{j=1}^{m} (x_{ij} - \bar{x}_i)^2,$$

where $\bar{x}_i$ is the cluster mean for the ith cluster. Then an unbiased estimator of the variance among all elements in the population is

$$V = \frac{(N-1)s_b^2 + N(M-1)s_w^2}{NM-1}.$$

As stated earlier, these considerations can be extended to multiple levels of sampling, unequal numbers of elements within the clusters and stratification of clusters prior to sampling, and stratification of elements within clusters before sampling.

One other aspect of cluster sampling deserves mention here; namely, the concept of intracluster, or intraclass, correlation. Characteristics of individuals occupying the same cluster are often likely to be correlated. For example, in a household health survey it would not be unusual to find correlated responses among members of a household. The intracluster correlation coefficient is defined to be

$$\rho = \frac{\mathrm{E}(x_{ij} - \bar{x})(x_{ik} - \bar{x})}{\mathrm{E}(x_{ij} - \bar{x})^2}.$$

Then, for the sampling design described above, the variance of the sample mean per element can be written in terms of the intracluster correlation coefficient as:

$$V(\bar{x}) = \frac{1-f}{n} \frac{NM-1}{M^2(N-1)} V[1 + (M-1)\rho],$$

where $f = n/N$, the sampling fraction, and ρ is the intracluster correlation coefficient. As a final note, intracluster correlation is closely related to the idea of overdispersion. For further information on cluster sampling and related topics, the reader is referred to classic sampling texts such as Cochran [4] or Hansen et al. [18].

Ratio Estimation and Post-Stratification.   Ratio estimation is a method in which the statistician takes advantage of known correlation between a characteristic to be estimated from a survey and an auxiliary variable available from a source independent of the survey in order to increase the precision of the survey estimate. Suppose that a variable y_i is available for every unit in the sample and that y_i is correlated with x_i, the variable of interest in the survey. Suppose further that the population total Y of the auxiliary variable is known. Then the ratio estimator of X, the population total of the xs, is

$$\hat{X}_R = \frac{x}{y}Y = \frac{\bar{x}}{\bar{y}}Y,$$

where x and y are the totals of the x_i and y_i, respectively. Similarly, the population mean could be estimated by replacing the total Y by the population mean of the auxiliary variable. The gain in precision obtained by calculating a ratio estimate can be seen in the approximate formula for the variance of the ratio, given by

$$V(\hat{X}_R) = \frac{N^2(1-f)}{n}(S_x^2 + R^2 S_y^2 - 2R\rho S_x S_y),$$

where ρ is the correlation between x and y and $R = X/Y$. Notice that if x and y are highly positively correlated, the variance of the ratio estimator is diminished by the large value of that correlation. The ratio estimator is also biased in most applications, but in large samples the bias is negligible.

Sources of Error in Surveys.   In what we have presented so far, the only errors ascribed to sample surveys have been those arising from the fact that only a sample of units are measured instead of the entire population. However, in complex surveys that involve multiple measures of quantities which may be difficult to measure, additional errors not related to sampling may be present. In what follows, we describe four sources of such errors, sometimes referred to as **nonsampling errors**.

First, the sample may not adequately cover the universe of units of interest. Secondly, it may not be possible to measure some of the units in the population chosen for the sample. This may occur for a variety of reasons, including inability of the fieldwork team to locate certain individuals selected for the sample, or the respondents' refusal to answer some or all of the questions being asked in the survey. Thirdly, the measuring device may not be able to determine accurately the characteristics being measured, or sample individuals may not understand the question or may not know the correct answer to the question. Finally, errors may arise in the recording, coding, editing, and tabulation of the data. The statistician may find it necessary to modify standard statistical procedures to account for the occurrence of such errors in order to make valid inferences from the data when nonsampling errors are present.

Errors of *coverage* arise when the sampling frame does not fully cover the universe of units to which the sample estimates are to be generalized (i.e. the target population). For example, suppose that in 1996 one uses the list of housing units from the 1990 decennial census as a frame for a sample of households for a US survey. Without supplemental frames, this list would exclude housing units constructed since the census. Thus, any estimates based on the sample would be generalizable only to the list of units, whereas the true population of interest is "all housing units in the US in 1996". Such coverage error could bias the results, because the people living in the newly constructed units might be different, on the variables of interest, than those living in the older housing units. Even if we supplemented the list with a frame that captured new construction since the census (for example, based on an ongoing survey of building permits or new construction), we might still have coverage error. This is because even the best lists are subject to errors. Lists constructed from door-to-door canvassing and listing of units could be incomplete if some unusual housing units were missed (e.g. a carriage house turned into a rental unit). Some lists, such as those constructed from a census, may not be complete if there were nonresponse to the census. And commercial providers of lists, such as professional associations, will only be able to supply lists that are as complete as the information their members provide.

A related problem is the potential discrepancy between the true population of inference, such as "all people in the US over the age of 18", and the target population, which might be "all people in the US over the age of 18 at a particular point in time". Although not a coverage error *per se*, it is an important issue to consider when defining the research question.

Both types of problems are related to the concept of "external validity".

Nonresponse, or failure to measure some of the units in the sample, is probably the most common nonsampling error incurred in survey practice. There are few, if any, surveys that do not experience at least some level of nonresponse. In the case of household surveys or surveys involving human respondents, one way of dealing with nonresponse is recontact with the nonrespondents in an attempt to obtain the required data. This may take the form of repeated visits to the household or repeated telephone calls. In some cases it is possible to make a valid estimate of the characteristic under study by recontacting a sample of the nonrespondents. Whatever method is used to obtain complete data, it is likely that a "hard core" of nonrespondents will persist in failing

to provide the requested data. If the percentage of nonresponse is relatively large, say greater than 5%, it is quite likely that the results of the study will be biased an unknown amount by the exclusion of those individuals who did not provide complete data. As an example, consider a disability survey in which persons are asked about their ability to perform certain activities of daily living. Studies have shown that the people who have the most difficulty in performing those activities are the ones who are most likely to refuse to answer the questions. Therefore, estimates of the prevalence of disability based on complete responses to the questions are lower than they would be if the more disabled individuals had answered the questions. Also, because the sample size is smaller than if complete response had been obtained, the standard errors of the estimates will be correspondingly larger. This, however, can be remedied if the statistician anticipates the loss of sample size and increases the sample size accordingly at the design stage.

A considerable body of literature on the adjustment of survey estimates for **missing data** exists. These techniques mostly involve weighting adjustments and so-called imputation procedures, which have been studied by numerous authors. For a useful summary of these methods, see Little & Rubin [29].

Analysis of variance models have been applied in the study of **measurement errors** in sample surveys in much the same way as in **experimental studies**. The simplest models assume that a measurement includes the true value of what is being measured plus an error term. However, when the errors depend in some way on the value of the characteristic or are correlated with the item being measured, the models must necessarily become more complicated. One way to attempt to determine the correct value for an item is to re-measure it by an independent method that is more accurate than the original method. In many surveys, for example, a subsample of respondents will be reinterviewed by the best interviewers to assess the correctness of the data obtained in the original interview. Other methods might involve embedding controlled experiments in surveys or subdividing the sample into groups so that there is no correlation between the groups. Many of these topics have been carefully reviewed in articles in the literature, such as Hansen et al. [17, 20].

The fourth area of nonsampling errors dealing with recording, coding, editing, and tabulating data will be discussed in the section on data management, later in this article.

Examples of Large-Scale Surveys in Current Use in Health Research

Surveys of the US NCHS

The NHIS.   As stated previously in this article, the NHIS was begun by the US Public Health Service in 1957, and has continued on an annual basis since that time. It is one of the major components of the NCHS of the Centers for Disease Control and Prevention. The NHIS produces information on the health of the US civilian noninstitutionalized population, collected by the US Bureau of the Census in household interviews throughout the United States. The sample design for this study has been evaluated and modified after each succeeding census during the survey's existence. The description which follows pertains to the design used to collect data, following the 1980 decennial census.

In concept, the design of the NHIS has remained essentially the same since 1957. That is, the sampling plan follows a stratified multistage probability design which permits continuous sampling of the target population. The sample of households interviewed each week is representative of the nation and the weekly samples are additive over time. This allows great flexibility in the agency's ability to respond to rapidly changing data needs.

The basic features of the design include a first-stage selection of 198 primary sampling units (PSUs) by sampling with probability proportional to size (pps) from an area frame supplemented by a frame of building permits to enable the inclusion of housing units constructed since the completion of the previous census. Approximately one-quarter of the PSUs are self-representing; that is, they are chosen with certainty. These PSUs are primarily metropolitan statistical areas which usually consist of a large city and its suburban areas. The nonself-representing PSUs are single counties, or groups of contiguous counties. Within the PSUs clusters of approximately eight households are selected in the area frame and four households in the permit frame. This results in a yearly expected number of interviewed households of about 49 000 and about 132 000 interviewed persons.

The respondent rules for the NHIS allow a single individual over the age of 17 to respond for all

persons dwelling in the household. However, if other persons over age 17 are available, they are invited to respond for themselves. Historically, between 65% and 70% of adults have been self-respondents. They answer questions for a set of basic health and demographic items. In addition, one or more sets of questions on current health topics are typically asked. Also, a random subsample of adult respondents are generally asked to respond to additional questions on current health topics, which vary from year to year.

Questionnaire topics include demographic characteristics such as age, sex, race, education, marital status, and family income. Health characteristics measured include disability days, physician visits, acute and chronic conditions, long-term limitations of activity, and short-stay hospital utilization. In addition, subsets of households are asked about selected chronic conditions. In the supplements that vary from year to year, special health items are asked in such areas as alcohol use, dental care, health insurance, aging, health promotion and disease prevention, vitamin and mineral intake, functional limitations, and risk factors for certain chronic diseases. Data from the survey are regularly published in the NCHS Vital and Health Statistics Series 10 reports, as well as in professional journals in the scientific literature. Standardized public use micro data tapes and compact disk-read-only memory (CD-ROMs) are also made available for purchase.

As a final word on the NHIS, it should be pointed out that the redesign developed and implemented in 1985 incorporated a feature that enabled the NCHS to integrate the survey designs of several of its population surveys. This was accomplished by using the NHIS sample as a sampling frame for the other surveys. In this way, the surveys could be linked analytically and possibly duplication of data collection could be avoided. Also, NHIS information could be used to oversample subgroups of the population in order to achieve sufficient sample size for studying groups which otherwise would have been underrepresented in the surveys. The successful application of this method to the design of the NHIS has led to considerably increased efficiency in the overall designs of NCHS surveys in recent years. For more details on the research leading to the development of this integrated design concept, the reader is referred to Massey [31]. An updated sampling design was put in place in the 1995 data year and will be used until 2004.

The National Health and Nutrition Examination Survey (NHANES). The NHANES is one of the NCHS surveys now linked to the NHIS through the integrated survey design concept. At its inception in 1971, however, the NHANES was conducted using an independent design. The purpose of the initial cycle of the NHANES, now known as NHANES I, was to measure the nutritional status of the US population and monitor changes in that status over time. The nutrition component represented an expansion of a previous series of three cycles of national health examination surveys which had been completed on subsets of the US population between 1959 and 1970. As in the previous cycles and in the NHIS, the target population was the civilian noninstitutionalized population of the US, only for this survey the population was limited to ages 1–74 because of a belief that older individuals would not respond to an examination survey as readily as younger people. It was also determined at the outset that emphasis should be placed on studying individuals believed to be at increased risk of having poor nutritional status, including segments of the population classified as at or below the poverty level, young children, and the aged. Hence oversampling of these segments of the population yielded a sample with sufficient numbers to study these characteristics.

Examinations were carried out in three mobile examination centers which traveled to the PSUs chosen in the first stage of sampling for the survey. Within each PSU, a sample of households was drawn – as in the NHIS – but a single individual from each household was selected to be examined in the mobile clinic. Because of the limited time frame of two years for completing a cycle of the NHANES, the number of PSUs was limited to 65. Approximately 30 000 persons were selected to be examined.

Data collection included both questionnaires and examinations. All sample persons received general medical history and dietary intake (both 24-hour recall and food frequency) questionnaires. A subsample received supplementary questionnaires selected on medical conditions, health care needs, and general well-being. The nutritional component examination included general medical and dental examinations, dermatological and ophthalmic examinations, anthropometric measurements, hand–wrist X-rays, and an extensive battery of laboratory determinations. In addition, a subset of sample persons in the so-called

"detailed" component received an extended medical examination, X-rays of major joints, audiometry, electrocardiography, goniometry, spirometry, pulmonary diffusion, a tuberculin test, and additional laboratory determinations. Additional details of the design and content of NHANES I are available in Miller [35].

A second cycle of the NHANES was conducted between 1976 and 1980. A major purpose for NHANES II was to monitor changes in health and nutritional status since the first cycle. The assessment of nutritional status was carried out using methods that were essentially the same as those used in the first cycle, with some modification. Again high-risk segments of the population were oversampled. The most important change in nutritional assessment in NHANES II concerned anemia, which was discovered to be a significant health problem for the US population. The approach included additional questionnaire items on symptoms, signs and causes of anemia, and additional laboratory measurements.

In the realm of the detailed health examination, new emphases were placed on diabetes, kidney pathology, liver disease, osteoarthritis and disk degeneration, cardiovascular conditions, and the effects of environmental exposures on health, as measured by pulmonary function and blood levels of carbon monoxide, lead, and pesticides. As with NHANES I, details of the design and content of this cycle are available in McDowell et al. [34].

A third cycle of NHANES was competed between 1988 and 1994, but since 1999 the NHANES is being conducted on a continuous basis. More information on NHANES III is contained in NCHS [39] and Harris et al. [21].

One other aspect of the NHANES deserves mention here. Several components of the National Institutes of Health, led by the National Institute on Aging, combined resources to fund a re-contact of the original NHANES I respondents in 1982, thus invoking a longitudinal component to the study. Of approximately 21 000 sample persons examined in NHANES I, some 14 000 were either located and reinterviewed or their vital status was determined. This longitudinal follow-up allowed one of the first nationally representative epidemiologic studies of its type to be conducted. A wide variety of data analyses have been completed and published in both the epidemiologic journal literature and in government publications. For more information concerning the design and objectives of this follow-up, see Cohen et al. [5].

The National Hospital Discharge Survey (NHDS). The NCHS has conducted the NHDS continuously since 1965. The original sample was selected from a sampling frame consisting of a listing of health facilities known as the National Master Facility Inventory. The basic design of the NHDS, with minor periodic updates, was followed until a major redesign in 1988. Hospitals were stratified by bed size and were sampled with probabilities ranging from certainty in the largest hospitals to 1 in 40 in the smallest. Eligible hospitals included those with an average length of stay of less than 30 days and excluded Federal, military and Veterans Administration hospitals. Within each hospital, discharges were selected using a systematic random sampling plan. Until 1985, information was abstracted manually at each sample facility, at which time the NCHS began using dual methods for collecting the in-hospital data, purchasing data tapes from commercial abstracting services, and sampling from those data tapes for hospitals where such services were used, and continuing the manual abstracting of the data in those hospitals that did not use the abstracting services.

The NHDS was redesigned in 1988 to conform to the integrated survey design paradigm described earlier for the NHIS. The new sampling frame consisted of hospitals listed in the SMG Hospital Market Data Tape [15]. As in the past, large hospitals (i.e. those with 1000 or more beds or 40 000 or more discharges per year) were sampled with certainty. The remaining strata were sampled using a three-stage design, which began with a sample of PSUs as in the NHIS, selected proportional to the projected 1985 population in the PSU, and a subsample of hospitals within the PSUs. Hospitals in the PSUs were then stratified by geographic region and ordered by PSU, abstracting service status, and hospital specialty-size group. A systematic sample was selected with a probability proportional to SMG annual numbers of 1987 discharges. Finally, a systematic random sample of discharges was selected according to the hospital's stratum, and to whether the manual or automated abstracting system was used in the hospital. This procedure resulted in a 1989 sample of 542 hospitals, of which 408 were eligible and responded to the survey. The number of patient records in the 1989 sample was approximately 233 000 discharge medical record abstracts. Currently the NHDS has been merged with other record-based surveys and expanded into one integrated survey of health care providers, including ambulatory surgical centers, hospital outpatient departments, emergency rooms, hospices and home health agencies.

Data collected in the survey include personal characteristics of the patients, including date of birth, sex, race, ethnicity, marital status, and expected sources of payment; administrative data, including admission and discharge dates, and discharge status; and medical information, including diagnoses, surgical and nonsurgical operations and procedures, and dates of surgery. Medical information is coded using the **International Classification of Diseases (ICD)**, 9th Revision, Clinical Modification (CM) (ICD-9-CM). The large number of medical records in the sample each year makes possible the study of relatively rare conditions, particularly when it is feasible to combine several years of NHDS data.

The National Ambulatory Medical Care Survey (NAMCS). The NCHS conducted the NAMCS from 1973 to 1990 as a survey of nonfederal office-based physicians in private and group practices throughout the United States. The purpose of the surveys was to provide national estimates of the characteristics of patient visits to physicians' offices, where the overwhelming majority of ambulatory care is rendered. A multistage stratified probability sample of approximately 3 000 physicians was selected to be interviewed each year. The design consisted of a first-stage selection of geographically defined primary sampling units, as in the NHIS and other surveys. Within each PSU, a sample of physicians was selected from frames provided by the American Medical Association and the American Osteopathic Association, stratified by specialty type. During a randomly selected week of the year, an interviewer visited the physicians assigned to that week and selected a sample of patients seen that week. Typically, about 65 000 patient records were sampled for the year. Interviewers – sometimes with the aid of the physician's staff – collected information on such topics as the patient's reason for the visit, relevant diagnoses made in the office, laboratory procedures performed, treatment(s) received, and disposition of the visit. National estimates of the characteristics of interest were computed by weighting the weekly estimates from the sample physicians and aggregating over time.

One of the limitations of the NAMCS is that it does not cover visits to hospital emergency and outpatient departments, the second largest segment of the ambulatory care system. In 1991, the NCHS began the National Hospital Ambulatory Medical Care Survey (NHAMCS) to fill a gap in the coverage of ambulatory medical care data. It is known, for example, that hospital ambulatory patients differ from office patients not only in their demographic characteristics but likely in their medical characteristics as well. The need for the new study was also related to increased efforts at medical care cost containment, the burgeoning aging population, large numbers of persons without health insurance, and emerging medical technologies. The result of a series of planning efforts by the NCHS and its contractors was a sample design that involved four stages of sampling. The first stage was a subsample of the NHIS PSUs chosen for the integrated sample design described above. Within PSUs, samples of hospitals were selected, then clinics within hospitals, and finally patient visits within clinics. The resulting sample included 474 eligible hospitals, 854 clinics from outpatient departments, 462 emergency service areas, 35 114 outpatient visits, and 36 271 emergency service visits. Data were collected by hospital staff who had been trained by survey field staff and recorded the information on one of two patient record forms designed to account for the differences in emergency and outpatient care. The items on the forms included the demographic characteristics of the patient and medical items relating to the patient's reason for the visit and physician diagnoses. The outpatient form resembles that used in the original NAMCS, whereas the emergency service form was designed to reflect the types of services provided in that setting. Finally, medical coding follows the ICD-9-CM classification, and reason for visit is coded according to the NAMCS reason for visit classification. For further information on the NHAMCS, see [32].

The National Nursing Home Survey (NNHS). What is now known as the NNHS began in 1963 with the first Institutional Population Survey conducted by the NCHS. This was originally intended to complement the NHIS, which covered only the noninstitutional population. The sampling frame for the study was the 1962 Master Facility Inventory (MFI) maintained by the NCHS and described earlier in this article. The sample contained institutions of four types: nursing care homes, personal care homes with nursing, personal care homes without nursing, and domiciliary care homes. The sample design was a multistage stratified design on which strata were defined by type of service and bed size. The sample was selected systematically within each of the basic strata. The second stage of sample was a systematic selection of residents or patients living in the sample establishments. A number of published reports have provided information on the characteristics of the homes and of the residents. For a more complete reading of the data, see, for example, Bryant [3].

A second cycle of the NNHS was conducted in 1973–1974 by the NCHS. The design was similar in nature to that of the first cycle, but emphasis was placed on the certification status of the homes; that is, whether the facility was certified to admit patients whose care was covered by the Medicare or Medicaid programs, which were not in existence at the time of the first survey. Thus, the design was changed to include certification status as a stratification variable. As one might expect, only nursing care homes were certified by Medicare for reimbursement.

The third cycle of the NNHS was conducted in 1977. Again, the design was constructed to reflect Medicare and Medicaid certification status. Many of the reports published using the data from this cycle involved trends in characteristics of the homes as well as the patients, comparing results from 1977 and the 1973–1974 cycle. A fourth cycle was completed in 1985 and provided additional trend data on the use of long-term care.

A new cycle of the NNHS was conducted in 1995. New preliminary data from this study have only recently been released. They suggest that a movement away from institutional care has begun, with more older and disabled persons utilizing newer forms of long-term care, including home-based care, visiting nurses, and the like. However, as the aging population continues to grow, it is expected that additional demands on the long-term care delivery system will grow as well. For further information on the new survey results, see Strahan [51].

Surveys of Other Health Agencies

The National Medical Expenditure Surveys.   To meet the growing demand for data on current health policy issues, the US government has sponsored three national household surveys of the utilization of health care services received and the expenditures related to use of those services. First, in 1977 the National Center for Health Services Research (later named the Agency for Health Care Policy and Research) and the NCHS conducted a National Medical Care Expenditure Survey (NMCES). A second survey, co-sponsored by the NCHS and the Health Care Financing Administration and named the National Medical Care Utilization and Expenditure Survey (NMCUES), was completed in 1980. Both surveys were based on multistage stratified probability designs, and both were panel surveys in the sense that the data were collected by a series of periodic interviews with the initial sample of households during the year of interest. The principal data items of interest included each dental, doctor, clinic, or emergency room visit, and each hospital stay, including dates and services received; charges for the services received; prescribed medicines purchased and their costs; other medical expenses, and finally sources of payment, including out-of-pocket and insurance amounts, both public and private. For more detailed information on the methodological issues involved in conducting these surveys, see Horvitz & Folsom [24].

A third survey, the National Medical Expenditure Survey (NMES), was conducted by the Agency for Health Care Policy and Research in 1987. Many of its characteristics were similar to the NMCES and NMCUES (see above), but a second component was added to include information on the population residing in or admitted to nursing homes and facilities for the mentally retarded. Furthermore, oversampling was used to insure greater representation of population groups of special policy interest including poor and low income families, the elderly, the functionally impaired, and black and Hispanic minorities. A detailed description of the design of this survey is given in Cohen et al. [6].

The National Long Term Care Survey (NLTCS). The 1982, 1984, 1989, and 1994 NLTCSs were designed to measure the point prevalence of chronic (90 days or more) disability in the US elderly Medicare enrolled population, as well as changes in chronic disability and institutionalization over time. The 1982 design was a list sample randomly drawn from Medicare administrative files. Screening interviews identified 6393 individuals with at least one chronic impairment in seven Instrumental Activities of Daily Living (IADL) or nine Activities of Daily

Living (ADL). Interviews were completed with 95% of the sample individuals.

The 1984, 1989, and 1994 surveys included both **cross-sectional** and longitudinal components, since new samples of persons who had reached age 65 and survived since the last interview were drawn from the Medicare files and screened. The three later surveys also included an institutionalization component for those persons who were admitted to nursing homes during the course of follow-up. A striking and somewhat unexpected finding from these surveys was that a slight decline in age-standardized disability and mortality (*see* **Standardization Methods**) was observed between the 1982 and 1989 surveys [30].

The National Longitudinal Mortality Study (NLMS). The NLMS is a long-term prospective study of mortality in the US. The study is funded and directed by the National Heart, Lung, and Blood Institute, is maintained at the Bureau of the Census, and obtains mortality information from the NCHS. The basic objective of the study is to investigate socioeconomic, demographic, and occupational differentials in mortality within the US.

The main study population consists of 13 cohorts of data of roughly 1.3 million records, drawn from the Census Bureau's Current Population Survey and from the 1980 census. The data records were matched to the National Death Index (NDI), a centralized, computerized index of death records in the US, to obtain mortality information for the period 1979–1989. The NDI is maintained by the NCHS and was begun in 1979. A public-use file of the NLMS data is available. For more information, see Rogot et al. [43, 44].

Sample Surveys in Other Countries

Sample surveys in health research are not limited to the US, although many of the methodologies presented here stemmed from work done in the US. Probably the best known international effort in sample survey work is the World Fertility Survey (WFS), conducted in several countries, including developing countries beginning in the mid-1970s and continuing into the 1980s. The studies have been described in several publications, including a large number dealing with the results of individual countries themselves. For an overall description, see WFS [55]. A description of the use of hand-held computers in conducting surveys in developing countries is provided by Forster & Snow [14]. Other aspects of the WFS, including implications for future such studies, are discussed by Cornelius [7].

Health surveys are also conducted in developed countries. Two examples from Canada include the heart health surveys [37] and the Canadian Health Survey [22, 23]. Other studies relate to drinking behavior [8]. Still other countries, such as the UK, Sweden, the Netherlands, Israel, and others, maintain national central bureaus of statistics, many of which are responsible for designing, conducting, and analyzing social surveys, which often include questionnaire items pertaining to health and well-being.

Data Collection and Management

In many studies, biostatisticians play a very active role in the collection and management of data. At a minimum, the statistical group needs to be represented as the data collection and data management systems are designed and implemented, so that the statisticians know how the data reached them for analysis. Decisions made at the data collection stage can have substantial impact on the analytic process.

Data Collection

Two key decisions about data collection will affect the statistician directly: how will the participant communicate responses to the researcher, and how will the researcher record and transmit the responses? Sample surveys can collect data by mail, by telephone, or in person; each approach has both advantages and drawbacks. Furthermore, data can be recorded on paper forms and keyed in later, or directly entered into a computer at the time of the interview. Another means of recording data that has been in more common use in recent years for some surveys is to have the respondents record answers to questions directly using a touchtone telephone.

Contact with Participant.   Mail questionnaires are used for some sample surveys because they offer a simple and economical way to request data. However, they have serious drawbacks. The most crucial one is the possibility of sampling bias. Bias can occur because the mailing list used as a frame may not

adequately reflect the target population, or because of poor response rates in some or all of the communities, or because of difficulty in interpreting and filling out the forms. A second serious problem is that some health issues cannot be addressed without in-person assessment of the participant. Blood pressure, for example, needs to be measured in person, and self-reported diagnosis of hypertension is a far less reliable alternative. Mail questionnaires may be useful for some highly motivated and sophisticated populations; mail surveys of physicians and nurses have been used successfully to study many chronic diseases of major public health importance (stroke, breast cancer, myocardial infarction, and so on). In addition, mail surveys may be useful for interim tracking of participants in longitudinal studies.

Telephone interviews avoid some of the problems of mail questionnaires, in that direct conversation may help to clarify concerns or confusion of the participants (*see* **Telephone Sampling**). Bias remains a problem, both because some people in the population do not have telephones and because response rates may be low and may be different for important subgroups. In addition, data requiring direct measurement of the participant cannot be collected over the telephone. In one particular survey of the National Institute on Aging, the Survey of the Last Days of Life, the use of the telephone was instrumental in securing an acceptable overall response rate for the study because many of the participants – recently bereaved individuals following the death of a spouse or other family member – were reluctant to be interviewed in person. In spite of a sometimes lengthy interview, lasting as long as between 45 minutes and one hour, the response rate and the overall quality of the data remained good [2].

In-person interviews allow the greatest variety of data to be collected on a participant. Direct measurements, performance tests, and blood samples for laboratory work can all be carried out even in participants' homes. Developing a suitable frame may be challenging, and participation rates may be low. In addition, in-person interviews are the most costly to conduct. Some studies use a combination of telephone interviews with in-person interviews of a subsample.

Data Recording and Transfer.   Recording the data and transferring to the computer are key steps, on which much of the data quality will depend. Perhaps the simplest approach is to record the answers on a preprinted form and have the forms keyed in to the computer at a later date. In this procedure there is no way to check data at the time of collection and prompt for correction of implausible answers. Some data checking can (and probably should) be programmed into the data entry keying program. Turnaround time depends on the data entry service. If the number of questions is small and the possible responses simple, a scanner form can be filled out by the participant or the interviewer, but this is practical only for the briefest of questionnaires. Careful design of a paper form is essential to make it clear and easy to fill out, and to key for data entry. It is useful to have a standardized header for paper forms, identifying the study, the batch, and sequence to record when a form was sent to data entry for keying, the staff member filling out the form and the date on which it was filled out. This information can be vital for data management.

Computer-assisted interviews in person (CAPI) and computer-assisted telephone interviews (CATI) are becoming more widely used, especially for large-scale sample surveys, where they offer pre-programmed checks for accuracy and rapid turnaround of data. The greatest drawbacks are the cost of the equipment and its support and maintenance, the need to train interviewers in use of the computer and the program, and the initial investment in time and effort for programming. It is important to recognize that a CAPI or CATI instrument is a program, and as such needs close attention to the overall architecture as well as to the details of branches, range checks, and logic checks. Developing a computer-assisted data collection instrument requires close collaboration between the programmer, the subject-matter specialist, and someone who is familiar both with computing and with forms design.

Data Management

Data management is the process that takes the data for the study from the point of its entry into the computer system to the time of analysis. The goal in data management is to build a system that handles quality control, tracking of study progress, linking of study components, and access for statistical analysis. In addition, the data management system needs to protect the data against loss, corruption, and unauthorized access. Each participant in the study should be assigned a study Identification Number (ID) at the time of sample selection, and the data management

process should track and refer to participants by ID rather than by any personal identifier such as name, social security number, or address.

Quality Control.   The goal of quality control is to ensure that the data to be analyzed are as faithful as possible a representation of the participant's true responses, and that any errors in responding, transcribing, uploading, or processing the data are identified and corrected. One common and potentially disastrous error is having a wrong ID on a form. IDs can be generated to include one or more "check digits", so that an invalid ID can be caught at the time of data keying or, if computer-assisted data collection is used, at the time of the interview. Other checks that can be carried out at the time of the first computer entry of the form are range checks (Is the value of the variable within the permitted limits for that question?), logic checks (Is the value for this variable logically consistent with the value entered for a previous related variable?), and branch checks (Has an answer been given for a question that should not have been asked or, conversely, has a question been skipped that should not have been skipped?). CATI and CAPI systems can be programmed to prompt the interviewer to correct the error at the time of data entry or, in some cases, to override the prompt if the response was unlikely but nonetheless correct. However, these checks can only be carried out within a single form collected at the same time – not across multiple forms. Thus, additional checks are probably needed at the time the data are uploaded into the main computer in which they are to be stored for analysis.

The quality control process also needs to include a standardized procedure for error correction. This should include both global corrections, where all records with a given value are changed to a new value, and person-specific corrections. It is useful to keep a system log of corrections, including the staff ID of the person who made the correction.

Database Management.   Until fairly recently, data were usually stored on the computer in American Standard Code for Information Interchange (ASCII) files or flat files, which were simply records in which each variable was identified by the columns that it occupied (a legacy from an era when data were stored on punch cards.) More sophisticated options now range from spreadsheets, to add-ons for statistical packages, to relational databases. The greatest advantage of a relational database is the ability to link data across studies and across forms within a study. The database chosen should be able to meet both operational and analytic needs, as well as being large and flexible enough to handle all the data collected in a given study. Operational needs include tracking completion of data for participants, tracking performance of interviewers, generating routine reports, and providing authorized people with interim access to the data. For statistical analysis, a friendly link to the statistical package is helpful. Some relational databases have a feature permitting some statistical packages to access the study directly, including variable labels. Again, it is crucial that the participant be identified by a study ID across all forms in the study.

Use of the database requires that the statistician know all the forms used in the study, the variable names for each form and the question to which they correspond, and the meaning of all possible values of the response, including missing value codes. One useful format for this information is a codebook – having on-line codebooks can be extremely helpful. The importance of good documentation of the database and the management process cannot be overemphasized.

A final word on maintaining and managing data files for a survey involves keeping backup files for each type of record created for the study. An example of a disaster that occurred at one statistical agency serves as a reminder of the importance of keeping the data properly backed up. Some years ago, seven cartons containing data tapes from a multi-million-dollar survey were being moved from one location to another for "safe keeping". In the course of this movement, the cartons were inadvertently left on the building's loading dock and were taken by trash collectors to the city's sanitary landfill. In spite of a valiant effort on the part of the agency to recover, clean, and reprocess the tapes, more than half of the total data set could not be recovered. Had the data been properly backed up prior to the movement of the tapes, such a disaster could have been avoided. Attention to such details is of utmost importance.

Analysis

Two considerations should determine the analytic strategy: What is the scientific question to be addressed? How was the sample obtained? Surveys conducted primarily for policy purposes often have as their primary goal the description of the health status of the country or state and important component groups. Examples would include the types of statistics described in the section on the NHIS: frequency distributions and cross tabulations of disability days, prevalence and incidence of acute and chronic conditions, physician visits, hospital utilization, and so on. Other examples might include national norms for certain measured quantities such as cholesterol level, blood pressure, height, and weight. Epidemiologic surveys, on the other hand, often are designed with the goal of analyzing the relationship between characteristics of the population and the risk of prevalent or incident disease or disease prognosis. The analytic strategies for accounting for the sample design in epidemiologic studies may differ from those in studies the main goal of which is to characterize a specific population.

Descriptive Analyses

These analyses usually consist of the presentation of population estimates of the characteristics under study and some indication of the sampling variability of the estimates. Most standard texts on survey sampling (e.g. Cochran [4]) provide the necessary information to construct the desired estimates. Typical analytic reports from descriptive surveys include a variety of standard tables containing estimates of means, totals and percentages, or proportions. If the survey designs are relatively simple, estimates of sampling variance can be computed using algebraic formulas. For more complicated designs, however, approximation techniques such as Taylor series representations (see, for example, Shah et al. [47]) or pseudo-replication methods (Kish & Frankel [26] and Efron [10]) are usually used to estimate sampling variability. In the estimation of variances, one needs to be aware of the possible necessity of applying a finite population correction factor, if the sampling rate for the survey is, say, more than 5%–10% in a given stratum, even though the overall sampling rate is much lower than that.

Two other areas of descriptive analysis deserve mention. First, a considerable amount of work has been done on the topic of small domain, or small area estimation. Here one is interested in providing estimates of health characteristics for either small strata (such as a subgroup of the population at high risk for disease) or for small geographic areas which are subgroups of the larger area covered by a given survey. When the sample sizes in the small area are too small to allow the computation of direct estimates from the survey, some researchers have proposed the use of so-called synthetic estimators, based on regression relationships between the characteristic of interest and ancillary variables available from the survey. Others have proposed the use of composite, or "shrinkage" estimators that combine direct and synthetic components. For additional information on this topic, see Fay & Herriott [13] and Purcell & Kish [41].

The final topic on descriptive analysis concerns the description of change from one time period to another. Estimates of change are usually desired to study the effects of forces that are known to have acted on the population under study. For example, if a hypertension intervention is initiated in a community, we would like to know whether the intervention has influenced the prevalence of hypertension in the community. In such an instance, it is necessary to estimate the prevalence both before and after the intervention, and it is best to retain the same sample for both occasions. On the other hand, if the goal is to estimate the average blood pressure level at the two occasions, it is best to select a new sample each time. Each of these alternatives has advantages and drawbacks. The first alternative requires careful maintenance of the sample over the time period for the study and the statistician must deal with dropouts and other losses to follow-up. The second alternative necessitates the drawing of a second sample and all the work required to educate and recruit new sample members. More information on this topic is available in Cochran [4].

Epidemiologic Studies

Studies of potential risk factors for the onset and progression of health problems, in contrast to descriptive studies, are likely to rely on regression models to measure the association between risk factors and disease and to adjust for other factors thought to affect the risk. There is general agreement that descriptive summaries based on survey data must adjust for the sample design, but there has been less of a consensus on how to estimate regression parameters and calculate standard errors for regression analysis of survey data. One possible approach for estimation is to analyze the data by a standard approach such

as maximum likelihood estimation, treating them as if they arose from a simple random sample (ignoring the sampling design). A second approach is to assume that the design influences the results primarily though key variables related to the sampling design, such as age, sex, or race, and to adjust for those by including coefficients for those variables as predicators in the model. In a stratified design, the variables chosen are typically the stratum definitions, at minimum. A third approach, more complicated to implement and thus used less frequently, is to modify the basic approach to reflect all features of the design, for example maximizing the likelihood over the complete probability distribution associated with the sampling design (design-based analysis). Finally, a more widely used approach is to modify the estimation approach to reflect the sampling weights in particular, for example by weighting the score function components to obtain so-called pseudo-maximum-likelihood estimates (model-based analysis). The estimation of standard errors associated with the point estimates is challenging and usually relies on some asymptotic assumptions. In the past, the ability of some researchers to adjust for complex sampling was limited by the lack of commercial software. Software is now available, however, to adjust for complex samples for many different kinds of regression models.

Some researchers have argued that adjustment is important when describing the parent population from which the survey sample was drawn, but not for estimating regression parameters for comparing risk groups [50]. For example, for standard linear regression, the usual estimator

$$\hat{\beta} = (X'X)^{-1}X'Y$$

is shown in standard texts to have commendable properties. If the sampling design is ignored, the estimator is the best linear unbiased estimator. In the survey data setting, however, as Sarndal et al. [45] point out, there are distinct theoretical drawbacks to the usual estimator. First, its optimal properties only hold if the model is correct. Secondly, obtaining standard error estimates that reflect the true variability from the sampling design is difficult. These authors recommend using a sample-weighted estimator. Other authors [19] have also stated that "the design is relevant, including especially the effects of intraclass correlations from cluster sampling, and perhaps also variable sampling fractions and other aspects of design. Failure to recognize such effects may lead to serious understatement of confidence intervals and overstatements of precision in inferences to the causal system".

The sample-weighted estimator for likelihood-based estimators from regression models makes use of the sampling weights, reflecting how much larger a segment of the population an individual would represent than in the sample. In a simple random sample, the log likelihood would just be the sum of the score contributions from each individual in the sample. The sample-weighted estimators assume that each individual should contribute to the total log likelihood by an amount reflecting the composition of the whole population; thus, the estimated log likelihood is a weighted sum of the individuals' contributions. This weighted sum is not typically the exact log likelihood for the full sample design. In fact, the design likelihood can rarely be calculated explicitly. However, the weighted sum can be thought of as an unbiased estimate of the log likelihood for the population from which the sample was drawn, and thus its root is called the pseudo maximum likelihood [42]. For linear regression, the sample weighted estimator or pseudo maximum-likelihood estimator (MLE) is given by

$$\hat{\beta}_w = (X'WX)^{-1}X'WY.$$

Pseudo maximum likelihood estimators have been worked out for a number of standard procedures including **logistic regression**. The correct point estimators can be obtained by using weights in standard software packages (*see* **Software, Biostatistical**), but the standard error estimates obtained by simply adding weights to a procedure for simple random samples will not be correct. More complicated standard error estimates, described below, must be used for pseudo-MLEs.

The sample-weighted estimates typically give different parameter estimates for stratified designs with unequal sampling weights than do the unweighted estimates, but are not affected by clustering. The conventional standard errors based on the usual estimates, however, may systematically underestimate the true sampling variability in the presence of clustering if there is within-cluster correlation. In this case, the usual regression estimators assume independent and identically distributed errors, and overestimate the effective sample size. A more conservative approach is to take account of the clustering by using a Taylor series approximation to the design-adjusted variance, as described in Skinner et al. [48] or Sarndal et al. [45]. Such estimates can also take account

of the sample weights used in the sample-weighted estimators. Commercial software is now available that calculates sample-weighted regression estimators, and calculates the Taylor series approximation for the standard error for linear regression, logistic regression, and so on [47].

Another approach to standard error estimation for sample surveys is resampling or replication. Balanced repeated replication and jackknife methods have been used for some time in survey sampling [26, 33]; more recently, these methods have been extended and, additionally, bootstrap methods have been applied [10, 25, 28, 42, 54]. These methods differ from the Taylor series approach in two key ways: first, unlike the Taylor series approximation, it is not necessary to write down an explicit differentiable expression for the variance; second, they may perform better in small samples than the Taylor series approximation [45]. Owing to recent improvements in computing, software is now available to implement replication-based methods (e.g. WesVar [36, 49]; VPLX [12]). A widely-used computer software package, SAS (SAS Institute, Cary, NC), will be adding a procedure for analyzing survey data in its next release.

The effect of clustering on the variance can be substantial if the number of primary sampling units is not large relative to the number of strata, but clustering does not affect the parameter estimates. Sample weighting can affect both the parameter estimates and the variance. If sampling weights are very unequal, the standard error of the sample-weighted estimates is typically substantially larger than that of the unweighted estimates, reflecting the uncertainty in weighting a small number of observations very heavily in the analysis. Korn & Graubard [27] have examined these effects for a study based on the NHANES I survey, and found that different analyses led to very different conclusions. They suggest that the clustering should generally not be ignored, but that if extremely unequal sampling fractions were used, one way to obtain reasonable point estimates without greatly increasing the standard error and thus decreasing the power of the study is to include those factors related both to the design and to the regression variables as covariates in the analysis. They note in conclusion, however, that a better solution might be to plan studies in advance to have adequate sample sizes in all strata to permit regression models to use the design in the analysis – the more conservative approach, and one that addresses directly the difficulties of making inferences about risk factors in a population using data from a complex survey design.

References

[1] Anderson, M. (1988). *The American Census: a Social History*. Yale University Press, New Haven.

[2] Brock, D.B., Holmes, M.B., Foley, D.J. & Holmes, D. (1992). Methodological issues in a survey of the last days of life, in *The Epidemiologic Study of the Elderly*, R.B. Wallace & R.F. Woolson, eds. Oxford University Press, New York, pp. 315–332.

[3] Bryant, E.E. (1965). Institutions for the Aged and Chronically Ill, *Vital and Health Statistics*, Series 12, No. 1, National Center for Health Statistics, Hyattsville.

[4] Cochran, W.G. (1977). *Sampling Techniques*, 3rd Ed. Wiley, New York.

[5] Cohen, B.B., Barbano, H.E., Cox, C.S., Feldman, J.J., Finucane, F.F., Kleinman, J.C. & Madans, J.H. (1987). Plan and Operation of the NHANES I Epidemiologic Followup Study: 1982–84, *Vital and Health Statistics*, Series 1, No. 22, National Center for Health Statistics, Hyattsville.

[6] Cohen, S., DiGaetano, R. & Waksberg, J. (1991). *Sample Design of the 1987 Household Survey*. Publication No. 91–0037, Agency for Health Care Policy and Research, Rockville.

[7] Cornelius, R.M. (1985). The world fertility survey and its implications for future surveys, *Journal of Official Statistics (Sweden)* 1, 427–433.

[8] Duffy, J.C. (1985). Questionnaire measurement of drinking behavior in sample surveys, *Journal of Official Statistics (Sweden)* 1, 229–234.

[9] Eckler, A.R. (1972). *The Bureau of the Census*. Praeger, New York.

[10] Efron, B. (1982). *The Jackknife, the Bootstrap, and Other Resampling Plans*. SIAM, Philadelphia.

[11] Evans, D.A., Funkenstein, H.H., Albert, M.S., Scherr, P.A., Cook, N.R., Chown, M.J., Hebert, L.E., Hennekens, C.H. & Taylor, J.O. (1989). Prevalence of Alzheimer's disease in a community population of older persons: higher than previously reported, *Journal of the American Medical Association* 262, 2251–2256.

[12] Fay, R.E. (1990). VPLX: variance estimates for complex samples, *American Statistical Association 1990 Proceedings of the Survey Research Methods Section*, American Statistical Association, Alexandria, pp. 266–271.

[13] Fay, R.E. & Herriott, R.A. (1979). Estimates of income for small places: an application of James–Stein procedures to Census data, *Journal of the American Statistical Association* 74, 269–277.

[14] Forster, D. & Snow, R.W. (1995). An assessment of the use of hand-held computers during demographic surveys in developing countries, *Survey Methodology* 21, 179–184.

[15] Graves, E.J. & Kozak, L.J. (1992). National Hospital Discharge Survey: Annual Summary, 1989, *Vital and Health Statistics*, Series 13, No. 109, National Center for Health Statistics, Hyattsville.

[16] Halacy, D. (1980). *Census: 190 Years of Counting America*. Elsevier/Nelson Books, New York.

[17] Hansen, M.H., Hurwitz, W.N. & Bershad, M. (1961). Measurement errors in censuses and surveys, *Bulletin of the International Statistical Institute* 38, 359–374.

[18] Hansen, M.H., Hurwitz, W.N. & Madow, W.G. (1953). *Sample Survey Methods and Theory*, Vols I & II. Wiley, New York.

[19] Hansen, M.H., Madow, W.G. & Tepping, B.J. (1983). An evaluation of model-dependent and probability-sampling inferences in sample surveys, *Journal of the American Statistical Association* 78, 776–808.

[20] Hansen, M.H., Hurwitz, W.N., Marks, E.S. & Mauldin, W.P. (1951). Response errors in surveys, *Journal of the American Statistical Association* 46, 147–190.

[21] Harris, T., Woteki, C., Briefel, R.R. & Kleinman, J.C. (1989). NHANES III for older persons: nutrition content and methodological considerations, *American Journal of Clinical Nutrition* 50, 1145–1149.

[22] Hidiroglou, M.A. & Rao, J.N.K. (1987). Chi-squared tests with categorical data from complex surveys: part I – simple goodness-of-fit, homogeneity and independence in a two-way table with applications to the Canada Health Survey (1978–1979), *Journal of Official Statistics (Sweden)* 3, 117–132.

[23] Hidiroglou, M.A. & Rao, J.N.K. (1987). Chi-squared tests with categorical data from complex surveys: part II – independence in a three-way table with applications to the Canada Health Survey (1978–1979), *Journal of Official Statistics (Sweden)* 3, 133–140.

[24] Horvitz, D.G. & Folsom, R.E. (1980). Methodological issues in medical care expenditure surveys, *American Statistical Association 1980 Proceedings of the Survey Research Methods Section*. American Statistical Association, Alexandria, pp. 21–27.

[25] Judkins, D. (1990). Fay's method for variance estimation, *Journal of Official Statistics (Sweden)* 6, 223–240.

[26] Kish, L. & Frankel, M. (1974). Inference from complex samples (with discussion), *Journal of the Royal Statistical Society, Series B* 36, 1–37.

[27] Korn, E.L. & Graubard, B.I. (1991). Epidemiologic studies utilizing surveys: accounting for the sampling design, *American Journal of Public Health* 81, 1166–1173.

[28] Kovar, J.G., Rao, J.N.K. & Wu, C.F.J. (1988). Bootstrap and other methods to measure errors in survey estimates, *Canadian Journal of Statistics* 16, Supplement, 25–45.

[29] Little, R.J.A. & Rubin, D.B. (1987). *Statistical Analysis with Missing Data*. Wiley, New York.

[30] Manton, K.G., Corder, L.S. & Stallard, E. (1993). Estimates of change in chronic disability and institutional incidence and prevalence rates in the U.S. elderly population from the 1982, 1984 and 1989 National Long Term Care Survey, *Journal of Gerontology* 48, S153–S164.

[31] Massey, J.T. (1989). Design and Estimation for the National Health Interview Survey, 1985–94, *Vital and Health Statistics*, Series 2, No. 110, National Center for Health Statistics, Hyattsville.

[32] McCaig, L.F. & McLemore, T. (1994). Plan and Operation of the National Hospital Ambulatory Medical Care Survey, *Vital and Health Statistics*, Series 1, No. 34, National Center for Health Statistics, Hyattsville.

[33] McCarthy, P.J. (1966). Replication: an approach to the analysis of data from complex surveys, *Vital and Health Statistics*, Series 2, No. 14. U.S. Government Printing Office, Washington.

[34] McDowell, A., Engel, A., Massey, J.T. & Maurer, K. (1981). Plan and Operation of the Second National Health and Nutrition Examination Survey: 1976–80, *Vital and Health Statistics*, Series 1, No. 15, National Center for Health Statistics, Hyattsville.

[35] Miller, H.W. (1973). Plan and Operation of the Health and Nutrition Examination Survey, *Vital and Health Statistics*, Series 1, No. 10a, National Center for Health Statistics, Hyattsville.

[36] Morgenstein, D.R. & Brick, J.M. (1966). WesVarPC: software for computing variance estimates from complex designs, *Proceedings of the Bureau of the Census 1996 Annual Research Conference*. Bureau of the Census, Washington, pp. 861–866.

[37] Nargundkar, M.S., Balram, C., Hogan, K., Joffres, M., MacLean, D., MacLeod, E.B., O'Connor, B. Petrasovits, A., Reeder, B. & Stechenko, S. (1990). Heart health surveys in Canada, *American Statistical Association 1990 Proceedings of the Social Statistics Section*, American Statistical Association, Alexandria, pp. 61–65.

[38] National Center for Health Statistics (1964). Health Survey Procedure, *Vital and Health Statistics*, Series 1, No. 2, Hyattsville.

[39] National Center for Health Statistics (1994). Plan and Operation of the Third National Health and Nutrition Examination Survey, 1988–94, *Vital and Health Statistics*, Series 1, No. 32, Hyattsville.

[40] Neyman, J. (1934). On the two different aspects of the representative method: the method of stratified sampling and the method of purposive selection, *Journal of the Royal Statistical Society* **97**, 558–606.

[41] Purcell, N.J. & Kish, L. (1979). Estimation for small domains, *Biometrics* **35**, 365–384.

[42] Rao, J.N.K., Wu, C.F.J. & Yue, K. (1992). Some recent work on resampling methods for complex surveys, *Survey Methodology* **18**, 209–217.

[43] Rogot, E., Sorlie, P.D., Johnson, N.J., & Schmitt, C. (1992). *A Mortality Study of One Million Persons by Demographic, Social, and Economic Factors: 1979–1985 Follow-up*, NIH Publication 92-3297, National Institutes of Health, National Heart, Lung & Blood Institute, Bethesda.

[44] Rogot, E., Sorlie, P.D., Johnson, N.J., Glover, C.S. & Treasure, D.W. (1988). *A Mortality Study of One Million Persons by Demographic, Social, and Economic*

Factors: 1979–1981 Follow-up, NIH Publication 88-2896, National Institutes of Health, National Heart, Lung & Blood Institute, Bethesda.

[45] Sarndal, C.E., Swensson, B. & Wretman, J. (1992). *Model Assisted Survey Sampling*. Springer-Verlag, New York.

[46] Scott, A.H. (1968). *Census, U.S.A.: Fact Finding for the American People, 1790–1970*. Seabury Press, New York.

[47] Shah, B.V., Folsom, R.A. & LaVange, L. (1991). *SUDAAN User's Manual*, Research Triangle Institute, Research Triangle Park.

[48] Skinner, C.J., Holt, D. & Smith, T.M.F., eds. (1989). *Analysis of Complex Surveys*. Wiley, New York.

[49] SPSS, Inc. (1998). *WesVar Complex Samples 3.0 Users Guide*. Westat, Rockville.

[50] Stevens, R.G., Jones, D.Y., Micozzi, M.S. & Taylor, P.R. (1989). Body iron stores and the risk of cancer (comment), *New England Journal of Medicine* **320**, 1012–1014.

[51] Strahan, G.W. (1997). An Overview of Nursing Homes and Their Current Residents: Data from the 1995 National Nursing Home Survey, *Advance Data*, No. 280, Centers for Disease Control and Prevention/National Center for Health Statistics, Hyattsville.

[52] Tschuprow, A.A. (1923). On the mathematical expectation of the moments of frequency distributions in the case of correlated observations, *Metron* **2**, 461–493, 646–683.

[53] White, L.R., Petrovich, H., Ross, G.W., Masaki, K.H., Abbott, R.D., Teng, E.L. Rodriguez, B.L., Blanchette, P.L., Havlik, R.J., Wergowske, G., Chiu, D., Foley, D.J., Murdaugh, C. & Curb, J.D. (1996). Prevalence of dementia in older Japanese-American men in Hawaii: the Honolulu–Asia Aging Study, *Journal of the American Medical Association* **276**, 955–960.

[54] Wolter, K.M. (1985). *Introduction to Variance Estimation*. Springer-Verlag, New York.

[55] World Fertility Survey (1986). *Final Report*, International Statistical Institute, Netherlands.

DWIGHT B. BROCK, LAUREL A. BECKETT &
JULIA L. BIENIAS

Sampled Population *see* Target Population

SAS *see* Software, Biostatistical

Scan Statistics for Disease Surveillance

Epidemiologists investigating disease incidence are drawn to clusters of cases occurring within a short period of time (*see* **Clustering**). Public health specialists as well as the media focus on clusters of cases of birth defects, cancer or suicides. Investigators seek to determine whether such clusters are more than just chance bunching, and search for common causative factors. Statistical tests are used to provide the researcher with a measure of the unusualness (statistical significance) of the cluster relative to chance bunching. A popular statistic used in **disease surveillance**, first investigated in detail by Naus [33], is the scan statistic, the maximum number of events in a window of predetermined width, w. Formally, if we rescale time to $[0, 1]$, and let $Y_w(t)$ be the number of events in time $[t, t + w]$, then the scan statistic, S_w, is

$$S_w = \max_{0 \le t < 1-w} Y_w(t). \qquad (1)$$

(Alternatively, without rescaling time, set T to be the time frame of interest, r the duration of the window in actual time units, $w = r/T$, and let S_w be the maximum of $Y_r(t)$ over $0 \le t \le T - r$.)

The most common application of the scan statistic is testing for clustering conditional on N, the total number of events observed. Under the null hypothesis, H_0, the times of the N events have a uniform distribution on the unit interval. Rejection of H_0 for large values of the scan statistics is a generalized likelihood ratio test [34] for testing against the pulse alternative H_a: that for some unknown τ, representing the start of the increase, $0 \le \tau \le 1 - w$, and some **relative risk** $\theta > 1$, the density is given by

$$f(t) = \begin{cases} \theta/(1 - w + w\theta), & \tau \le t < \tau + w, \\ 1/(1 - w + w\theta), & \text{otherwise.} \end{cases} \qquad (2)$$

The scan statistic has been used to detect clustering of a wide variety of reproductive and other outcomes, including congenital heart disease [37] and poisonings [19], and is used routinely in the Ontario Cancer Registry [26].

The unconditional version of the statistic could be used to sound an alarm in real time in prospective surveillance applications, and requires the investigator to specify, a priori, the duration of the interval under study, and λ, the expected number of events over the entire time period. The null hypothesis for this model assumes that events occur at random according to a Poisson process. An analogous pulse-type alternative is that for some unknown τ, and unknown $\theta > 1$, $E[Y_w(\tau)] = \theta\lambda w$, while for $t < \tau - w$ or $t > \tau + w$, $E[Y_w(t)] = \lambda w$. However, since, in practice, the purpose of monitoring is to stop when a cluster is observed, the test could be applied when there are two intensities with an unknown change point.

Often the scan statistic cannot be exploited fully since the precise times of the events are not known, but rather the data are grouped in discrete intervals. The most frequent application is when data are tabulated monthly, but clustering over 3, 6 or 12 months is of interest. The ratchet scan statistic [28, 45] maximizes $Y_w(t)$ when t can only take on values starting at the beginning of a calendar month.

Weinstock [48] modifies the scan so it can be used even when there is some underlying temporal trend to the disease specified by the density $f_0(t)$, or if the population at risk changes. He tests the hypothesis $H_0 : f(t) = f_0(t)$ by replacing the constant window, w, by a variable window width $\omega(t)$, where

$$\int_t^{t+\omega(t)} f_0(s) \, ds = w.$$

The statistic, however, thus loses its simple interpretation, and the associated optimal properties related to detecting pulses of length w.

A defect of the scan statistic is that w must be specified before the data are observed and should not be based on examination of the data. (For the surveillance model, both w and the time frame must be specified in advance.) Cressie [8] notes that it is better to choose an interval slightly larger than the true pulse rather than one slightly smaller. Some protection against missing a cluster can be achieved by choosing two window widths and utilizing the Bonferroni bounds to test each at the $\alpha/2$ level. Loader [31] and Nagarwalla [32] present a statistic for testing H_0 against (2) in the case when w is unknown.

Applications to the related problem of spatial clustering are given by Anderson & Titterington [3], and by Kulldorff [29]. Various current research topics concerning the scan statistic are described in [15].

The Exact Distribution

Since the scan statistic does not have a normal distribution even for large N, and, furthermore, moments are unavailable, most of the literature has focused on finding critical values, k, so that under H_0 the occurrence of k or more events in any window of width w is unlikely to be due to chance. Naus [33] calculates $\Pr(S_{1/2} \geq k), \Pr(S_{1/3} \geq k)$, and $\Pr(S_w \geq k), w \geq 1/2$, under the null distribution of no clustering. General formulas for the exact distribution under both the null and the alternative are based on a generalized ballot problem [6] dealing with the amount of lead among L candidates. Naus [34] applies the result to express the distribution under the null, when $w = 1/L, L$ an integer, as the sum of $L \times L$ determinants. The result was extended to arbitrary w [22], and to the distribution under a pulse alternative [8]. In general, these exact formulas are difficult to implement for moderate or large samples and small w, except in specialized cases, because they involve a large number of summations over many large determinants.

Approximations and Bounds

Many approximations or bounds are based on generalized Bonferroni-type inequalities involving intersections of up to J events, or on tighter versions of these inequalities for $J = 1$ [21] or $J = 2$ [26]. Especially for $J = 1$ and 2, these methods yield good approximations for small values of $\Pr(S_w \geq k)$, but are generally poorer for approximating the median of S_w or upper tail probabilities. Wallenstein [42] applies the simple bounds with $J = 1$ and 2 to $D_i = \sup_{0 \leq s \leq w} Y_w(iw + s) \geq k, i = 0, 1, \ldots, [1/w]$, to tabulate probabilities for a range of values of w common in disease surveillance applications. Berman & Eagelson [7] apply the upper bound with $J = 1$ based on $E_i = \{X_{(k+i-1)} - X_{(i)} < w\}, i = 1, \ldots N - k$, where $X_{(1)}, X_{(2)}, \ldots, X_{(N)}$ are the order statistics for the N events. An approximation that is both simple and accurate, involving sums and alternating sums of binomial coefficients, is given by Glaz et al. [17]. Other approximations are given by Glaz [13,14].

Naus [36] develops a highly accurate formula for type I error for several types of scan statistic, by noting that conditioning on the recent past is approximately the same as conditioning on the entire past, or

formally that $\Pr(D_i^c | D_1^c, \ldots, D_{i-1}^c) \cong \Pr(D_i^c | D_{i-1}^c)$. Thus, $\Pr(S_w \geq k)$ can be approximated based only on $\Pr(S_{1/2} \geq k)$ and $\Pr(S_{1/3} \geq k)$. Huffer & Lin [20] define M_k to be the number of k-clusters of length w, note that $\Pr(S_w \geq k) = \Pr(M_k \geq 1)$, and approximate this probability using the method of moments.

Applying the Hunter [21] bounds to $\Pr(\cup D_i)$, and then performing further approximations, a simple approximation for the null distribution of the scan statistic is [43]

$$\Pr(S_w \geq k) \cong (k/w - N + 1)\Pr(Z = k) + 2\Pr(Z > k), \qquad (3)$$

where $Z \sim \text{bin}(N, w)$, i.e. Z is a binomial random variable based on N trials with probability of success, w. The first term (with coefficient $(k/w - N)$) in this approximation is implicit in asymptotic work by Cressie [9], while Loader [31], based on large deviation theory, gives an analogous but slightly more complicated approximation which, at least for $w = 1/2$, improves precision.

For the conditional scan, Alm [2] uses asymptotic theory to find that under the null hypothesis, given $E(N) = \lambda$,

$$\Pr(S_w \leq k) \cong \Pr(Z \leq k) \exp\{-\lambda(k + 1 - \lambda w) \\ \times (1 - w)\Pr(Z = k)/(k + 1)\}, \qquad (4)$$

where Z has a Poisson distribution with mean value λw.

Wallenstein et al. [46] approximate the power of the scan statistic against a pulse alternative for the conditional and unconditional cases. A further approximation for the conditional case yields that for relative risk $\theta >> 1$,

$$\text{power} \cong \Pr(Z \geq k) + 2\Pr(Z = k)/(\theta - 1), \qquad (5)$$

where $Z \sim \text{bin}(N, \theta w/(1 - w + \theta w))$. Based on simulation results, Sahu et al. [39] suggest sample sizes to achieve adequate power and compare power for triangular and rectangular pulses.

Space–Time Clustering, Moments

The scan statistic can be modified [44] to test for space–time clustering, for the case where "space" consists of g discrete geographical areas (towns, schools, cities, etc.) and there is no overall time trend. The statistic can be viewed as a variant of the Ederer–Myers–Mantel [10] statistic, where the maximum number of events within a calendar year is replaced by the maximum within any 365-day interval. The numerator of the statistic is the difference between the scan statistic for each geographical area and its expected value, and the denominator is the square root of the sum of the variances. When the number of geographic regions is moderately large, the central limit theorem indicates that the statistic has approximately a normal distribution.

Using both exact probabilities ($N < 19$) and simulation, the first two moments of the scan are tabulated [44] for six window widths and a range of Ns from 2 to 1000. Values of N not tabulated can be obtained from interpolation, or by use of the suggested linear approximations $E[S_w(N)] = wN + b_wN$, where the coefficients, b_w, are estimated from the tabulated data. Other methods of approximating or computing moments are given by Glaz [14].

Seasonal Clustering

For detecting seasonal clustering, data from several years are merged. The resulting 365-day period is viewed as a circle, with December 31 adjacent to January 1. The circular scan statistic, C_w, is the maximum number of events in a fraction, w, of the year. Ajne [1] finds $\Pr(C_{1/2} \geq k)$ in terms of an infinite sum, in contrast to the much simpler expression for the line [33]. He also points out that $C_{1/2}$ is the most powerful invariant test for the pulse alternative as θ approaches infinity, while Cressie [8] extends this result to general w and finds some interesting asymptotic results.

The pulse alternative differs from the sinusoidal alternative (peak followed by a trough 6 months later) for which Edwards' statistic [11] is often used as a test of seasonal clustering. The statistic $C_{1/2}$ is related to Hewitt's statistic [18] in which the monthly totals are replaced by their **ranks**, and the test statistic is the maximum over the sums of six consecutive monthly ranks. Rogerson [38] compares the statistics $C_{1/4}$, $C_{1/3}$, and $C_{5/12}$ with his generalizations of Hewitt's statistic based on the maximum of the sum of the ranks over 3, 4 or 5 consecutive months.

Except for special cases, the exact distribution of the circular scan statistic is very difficult to obtain

since it cannot be cast in the form of a ballot problem, as the first and last "candidates" are the same. Nevertheless, the computation of $\Pr(C_w > k)$ can be reformulated so that the single probability that cannot be derived, involving an intersection of $[1/w]$ events, is very small, and approximations [45] can be obtained using methods similar to those described for the line.

Wallenstein et al. [45] propose a modification of the circular scan, termed the ratchet scan, which is applicable when only monthly totals are available and give a figure plotting P values against values of the statistic. Krauth [27] gives bounds based on the Bonferroni inequality, so that the P values need not be read off a figure.

A Generalized Scan Statistic, with Application to Assessment of Inhomogeneities in DNA Sequence Data

Glaz & Naus [16] generalize the scan statistic to the case of N independent random variables, $X_1, X_2, \ldots, X_N$, where N could be fixed or a random variable. They let $Y_m(t)$ be the sum of m consecutive random variables X_t to X_{t+m-1}, and define the scan statistic, S_m, as the maximum of $Y_m(t)$ over the integers $t = 1$ to $N - m + 1$.

The special case where X is a binary random variable could be applied in the context of clustering of disease. For example, letting $X = 1$ denote the event that a birth is associated with a congenital malformation, and $X = 0$ otherwise, the statistic S_m is the maximum number of cases of congenital malformations in a series of m consecutive births. Fu & Curnow [12] show that S_m is a function of the log likelihood ratio for testing the hypothesis of a constant probability of disease, against the pulse alternative of a higher probability for m consecutive trials and a lower one elsewhere. Under both the null and pulse alternatives, they give a method to obtain exact probabilities, which, however, is difficult to implement for $m > 20$. Saperstein [40] and Naus [35] relate the distribution of S_m to a generalization of the birthday problem, and give results concerning the null distribution conditional on N. Wallenstein et al. [47] give an approximation for the power against a pulse alternative.

Recently, the generalized scan statistic has been applied to problems in deoxyribonucleic acid (DNA) sequencing in which DNA can be viewed as a sequence of letters from a four-letter alphabet of nucleotides, a 20-letter alphabet of amino acids derived from triplets of these four nucleotides, or a three-letter alphabet of charges of amino acids. Exact or approximate probabilities for the length of the longest almost matching subsequence, or the largest net charge within any series of m consecutive amino acids, are given by Glaz & Naus [16], Sheng & Naus [41], and Karwe & Naus [25]. Asymptotic results for the distribution of the generalized scan statistic, based on methods such as the Chen–Stein method of Poisson approximation, are given by Arratia et al. [4, 5], Karlin & Macken [24], and Karlin & Brendel [23].

References

[1]   Ajne, B. (1968). A simple test for uniformity of a circular distribution, *Biometrika* **55**, 343–354.

[2]   Alm, S.E. (1983). On the distribution of the scan statistic of a Poisson process, in *Probability and Mathematical Statistics. Essays in Honour of Carl-Gustave Esseen*, A. Gut & L. Holst, eds. Uppsala University Press, Uppsala, pp. 1–10.

[3]   Anderson, N.H. & Titterington, D.M. (1997). Some methods for investigating spatial clustering, with epidemiological applications, *Journal of the Royal Statistical Society* **160**, 87–105.

[4]   Arratia, R., Goldstein, L. & Gordon, L. (1990). Poisson approximation and the Chen Stein method, *Statistical Science* **5**, 403–434.

[5]   Arratia, R., Gordon, L. & Waterman, M.S. (1990). The Erdös Rényi law in distribution for coin tossing and sequence matching, *Annals of Statistics* **18**, 539–570.

[6]   Barton, D.E. & Mallows, C.L. (1965). Some aspects of the random sequence, *Annals of Mathematical Statistics* **36**, 236–260.

[7]   Berman, M. & Eagelson, G.K. (1985). A useful upper bound for the tail probabilities of the scan statistic when the sample size is large, *Journal of the American Statistical Association* **80**, 886–889.

[8]   Cressie, N. (1977). On some properties of the scan statistic on the circle and the line, *Journal of Applied Probability* **14**, 272–283.

[9]   Cressie, N. (1980). The asymptotic distribution of the scan statistic under uniformity, *Annals of Probability* **8**, 828–840.

[10]   Ederer, F., Myers, M.H. & Mantel, N. (1964). A statistical problem in space and time: do leukemia cases come in clusters?, *Biometrics* **20**, 626–636.

[11]   Edwards, J.H. (1961). The recognition and estimation of cyclic trends, *Annals of Human Genetics* **25**, 83–86.

[12]   Fu, Y. & Curnow R.N. (1990). Locating a changed segment in a sequence of Bernoulli variables, *Biometrika* **77**, 295–304.

[13]   Glaz, J. (1989). Approximations and bounds for the distribution of the scan statistic, *Journal of the American Statistical Association* **84**, 560–566.

[14]   Glaz, J. (1992). Approximations for tail probabilities and moments of the scan statistic, *Computational Statistics and Data Analysis* **14**, 213–227.

[15]   Glaz, J. & Balakrishnan, N., eds. (1999). *Scan Statistics and Applications*. Birkhauser, Boston.

[16]   Glaz, J. & Naus J. (1991). Tight bounds and approximations for scan statistic probabilities for discrete data, *Annals of Applied Probability* **1**, 306–318.

[17]   Glaz, J., Nans, J., Roos, M. & Wallenstein, S. (1994). Poisson approximations for the distribution and moments of ordered m-spacings, *Journal of Applied Probability* **31a**, 271–281.

[18]   Hewitt, D., Milner, J., Csima, A. & Pakuyla, A. (1971). On Edwards' criterion of seasonality and a nonparametric alternative, *British Journal of Preventive and Social Medicine* **25**, 174–176.

[19]   Hryhorczuk, D.O., Frateschi, L.J., Lipscomb, J.W. & Zhang, R. (1992). Use of the scan statistic to detect temporal clustering of poisonings, *Journal of Toxicology – Clinical Toxicology* **30**, 459–465.

[20]   Huffer, F.W. & Lin C.T. (1997). Approximating the distribution of the scan statistic using moments of the number of clumps, *Journal of the American Statistical Association* **92**, 1466–1475.

[21]   Hunter, D. (1976). An upper bound for the probability of a union, *Journal of Applied Probability* **13**, 597–603.

[22]   Huntington, R. & Naus, J.I. (1975). A simpler expression for kth nearest neighbor coincidence probabilities, *Annals of Probability* **3**, 894–896.

[23]   Karlin, S. & Brendel, V. (1992). Chance and statistical significance in protein and DNA sequence analysis, *Science* **257**, 39–49.

[24]   Karlin, S. & Macken C. (1991) Some statistical problems in the assessment of inhomogeneities of DNA sequence data, *Journal of the American Statistical Association* **86**, 27–35.

[25]   Karwe, V.V. & Naus, J. (1997). New recursive methods for scan statistic probabilities, *Computational Statistics and Data Analysis* **23**, 389–402.

[26]   King, W.D., Darlington, G.A., Kreiger, N. & Fehringer, G. (1993). Response of a cancer registry to reports of disease clusters, *European Journal of Cancer, Series A* **29**, 1414–1418.

[27]   Krauth, J. (1991). Bounds for the linear probabilities of the linear ratchet scan statistic, in *Analyzing and Modeling Data and Knowledge*, M. Schader, ed. Springer-Verlag, Berlin, pp. 55–61.

[28]   Krauth, J. (1992). Bounds for the upper tail probabilities of the circular ratchet scan statistic, *Biometrics* **48**, 1177–1185.

[29]   Kulldorff, M. (1997). A spatial scan statistic, *Communications in Statistics, A: Theory and Methods* **26**, 1481–1496.

[30] Kwerl, S.M. (1975). Most stringent bounds on aggregated probabilities of partially specified dependent probability systems, *Journal of the American Statistical Association* **70**, 472–479.

[31] Loader, C. (1991). Large deviation approximations to the distribution of scan statistics, *Advances in Applied Probability* **23**, 751–771.

[32] Nagarwalla, N. (1996). A scan statistic with a variable window, *Statistics in Medicine* **15**, 845–850.

[33] Naus, J. (1965). The distribution of the size of the maximum cluster of points on a line, *Journal of the American Statistical Association* **60**, 532–538.

[34] Naus, J. (1966). Some probabilities, expectations, and variances for the size of the largest clusters and smallest intervals, *Journal of the American Statistical Association* **61**, 1191–1199.

[35] Naus, J. (1974). Probabilities for a generalized birthday problem, *Journal of the American Statistical Association* **69**, 810–815.

[36] Naus, J. (1982). Approximations for distributions of scan statistics, *Journal of the American Statistical Association* **77**, 177–183.

[37] Paneth, N., Kiely, M., Hegyi, T. & Hiatt, I. (1984). Investigation of a temporal cluster of congenital heart disease, *Journal of Epidemiology and Community Health* **38**, 340–344.

[38] Rogerson, P.A. (1996). A generalization of Hewitt's test for seasonality, *International Journal of Epidemiology* **25**, 644–648.

[39] Sahu, S.K, Bendel, R.B. & Sison, C.P. (1993). Effect of relative risk and cluster configuration on the power of the one dimensional scan statistic, *Statistics in Medicine* **12**, 1853–1865.

[40] Saperstein, B. (1972). The generalized birthday problem, *Journal of the American Statistical Association* **67**, 425–428.

[41] Sheng, K. & Naus J. (1994). Pattern matching between two nonaligned random sequences, *Bulletin of Mathematical Biology* **56**, 1143–1162.

[42] Wallenstein, S. (1980). A test for detection of clustering over time, *American Journal of Epidemiology* **111**, 367–372.

[43] Wallenstein, S. & Neff, N. (1987). An approximation for the distribution of the scan statistic, *Statistics in Medicine* **6**, 197–207.

[44] Wallenstein, S., Gould, M.S. & Kleinman, M. (1989). Use of the scan statistic to detect time-space clustering, *American Journal of Epidemiology* **130**, 1057–1064.

[45] Wallenstein, S., Weinberg, C.R. & Gould, M. (1989). Testing for a pulse in seasonal event data, *Biometrics* **45**, 817–830.

[46] Wallenstein, S., Naus, J. & Glaz, J. (1993). Power of the scan statistic for the detection of clustering, *Statistics in Medicine* **12**, 1829–1843.

[47] Wallenstein, S., Naus, J. & Glaz, J. (1994). Power of the scan statistic in detecting a changed segment in a Bernoulli sequence, *Biometrika* **81**, 595–601.

[48] Weinstock, M. (1981). A generalized scan statistic for the detection of clusters, *International Journal of Epidemiology* **10**, 289–293.

S. WALLENSTEIN

Screening, Models of

Screening asymptomatic people to allow the early detection and treatment of chronic diseases is an important part of modern medicine and public health. For screening to be both an efficient and cost-effective medical intervention, it must be carefully targeted and evaluated. Mathematical models of disease screening constitute one of the major tools in the design and evaluation of screening programs.

The purpose of this article is to describe models for disease screening and how they have developed in recent years. The discussion will focus on screening for cancer, because most of the methodologic advances in screening design and evaluation have concerned cancer screening. In the first part of the article we will describe the characteristics of these models and illustrate them with a discussion of a simple screening model. In the second part we will describe the development of the two main types of model. In the third part we will discuss model fitting and validation, and in the final part we will briefly describe models for diseases other than cancer and discuss the current state and possible future directions for models of disease screening.

This is not intended to be an exhaustive study of all modeling of disease screening. Rather, it is intended to be a description of the main approaches used and their strengths and weaknesses. For more detailed reviews of modeling disease screening, see Eddy & Shwartz [30], Shwartz & Plough [56], Prorok [50, 51], Alexander [5], and Baker et al. [9].

What is Screening?

Screening for disease control can be defined as the examination of asymptomatic people in order to classify them as likely or unlikely to have the disease that is the object of screening. People identified by a screening test as likely to have the disease are then further investigated to arrive at a final diagnosis [45].

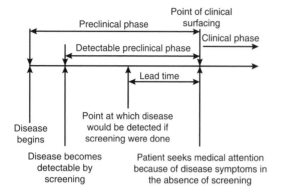

Figure 1   The natural history of a disease with and without screening

The objective of screening is the early detection of a disease where early treatment is either easier or more effective than later treatment.

Figure 1 is a schematic representation of the main features of the natural history of a disease which are relevant to screening. The *preclinical* phase of the disease is the phase in which a person has the disease but does not have any clinical symptoms and is not yet aware of having it. Screening aims to detect the disease during this phase. In principle, the preclinical phase starts with the beginning of the disease, but, in practice, modeling focuses on the phase commencing at the earliest point at which the disease is detectable with a screening test. This is known as the *detectable preclinical phase*.

The preclinical phase finishes with the *clinical surfacing* of the disease. This is the point at which the person develops clinical symptoms of the disease, seeks medical attention for these symptoms, and the disease is diagnosed. The disease then enters the *clinical phase*, where the person has a diagnosable case of the disease.

The outcome of a screening test is designated either *positive*, if the person is identified as likely to have the disease, or *negative* if they are not. All screening tests are open to error either from the test itself or its interpretation. These errors are designated as false positive, where a person without the disease has a positive screening result, and false negative, where a person with the disease has a negative screening result. The **sensitivity** of a screening test is the probability that a person with the disease has a positive screening result. The **specificity** of a screening test is the probability that a person without

the disease has a negative screening result. Cases of the disease which clinically surface following a false negative result (i.e. where the screening test missed the disease) are known as *interval cases*.

It is important to note that sensitivity and specificity are not properties of the test alone. For example, mammography is used to screen for breast cancer in women. In this case the sensitivity and specificity will depend on characteristics of the test, such as the nature of the mammography machine and the number of views taken, as well as on factors such as the skill of the person interpreting the mammogram, the size of any tumor in the woman being screened, the density of her breast tissue, and so on.

The *reliability* of a test is its capacity to give the same result, either positive or negative, on repeated application in a person with a given level of the disease. The *survival time* is the length of time between disease diagnosis, either by clinical surfacing or detection by screening, and death. The *lead time* is the time between the detection of a disease by screening and the point at which it would have clinically surfaced in the absence of screening.

The lead time is an important issue in the examination of screening benefits. The immediate focus of screening is to detect an early form of the disease. Hence the lead time can be used as an index of benefit in its own right. It is also important in examining survival benefits conferred by screening. A simple comparison of survival times between screened and unscreened populations is likely to show spurious screening benefits, since the survival time for a screen detected disease includes the lead time while that for a disease which surfaced clinically does not.

There is another, more subtle, reason why such survival comparisons may be spurious, even if adjusted for lead time. Screening will tend to detect people with a longer preclinical phase. This is known as **length-biased** sampling. Usually this will equate to a more slowly progressing disease. Since the disease behavior before clinically surfacing is likely to be correlated with that after surfacing, this is likely to result in screen detected diseases having a longer survival time than clinically surfacing diseases.

Why Use Modeling?

The evaluation of screening usually focuses on whether or not the screening program has led to a fall in mortality from the disease in question. As with most medical interventions, randomized controlled trials (RCTs) provide the most satisfactory empirical basis for evaluating screening programs. However, they do have significant limitations.

RCTs for screening are expensive and time-consuming to run – typically requiring very large sample sizes and having long time lags until benefits are apparent. For example, the RCT of mammography screening carried out in the two Swedish counties of Kopparberg and Ostergotland had a total sample size of 134 867. A statistically significant mortality differential between the control and study groups did not appear until after six years of follow-up, with a further four years of follow-up before the results could be considered definitive [58]. Twenty years of data would be required to yield results on some aspects of screening program design [21].

Any one trial cannot address all the issues involved in designing a screening program. For example, the Minnesota Colon Cancer Control Study used an RCT to demonstrate a statistically significant fall in mortality due to screening with a Fecal Occult Blood Test (FOBT), followed by colonoscopy in those with a positive screen [43]. However, Lang & Ransohoff [39] have subsequently suggested that the sensitivity of the FOBT is considerably less than that reported in the Minnesota study. The FOBT has a high false positive rate, and they argue that one-third to one-half of the fall in mortality could be due to chance selection for colonoscopy where an early cancer or large adenomatous polyp is present but not bleeding and the FOBT is positive for other reasons. The original RCT provides no basis for deciding on the role of the FOBT separately from that of colonoscopy.

Models are one way in which the information on the disease and screening tests from a number of different sources – including RCTs and other clinical and epidemiologic research – can be combined with known and hypothesized features of the specific population to be screened. They can be used to investigate the effect of different screening regimes on different subgroups of the population, both on disease mortality and program costs. For example, one use of modeling has been to investigate the inclusion of different age groups in the population to be screened. They can also be used to project the future course of the disease and screening program, to evaluate the changes in costs and benefits over time.

The modeling approach does have limitations. The extra information is obtained from models only by imposing assumptions about the screening process. These include assumptions about the natural history of the disease, about the characteristics of the screening test and about the behavior of the population under study. These assumptions can only rarely be verified, although they can be evaluated as part of the modeling process.

A further complication in making these assumptions is that the natural history of most diseases is not completely understood, particularly in the asymptomatic preclinical phase, which is the main focus of screening. This means that one may hypothesize a disease model that meets the constraints of current knowledge but which is still ultimately misleading.

Characteristics of Screening Models

Types of Model

Bross et al. [14] proposed a classification of models used to analyze screening strategies into two types: *surface models* and *deep models*. Surface models consider only those events that can be directly observed, such as disease incidence, prevalence, and mortality. Deep models, on the other hand, incorporate hypotheses about the disease process that generates the observed events. Their intent is to use the surface events as a basis for understanding the underlying disease dynamics. This implies models that explicitly describe the disease natural history underlying the observed incidence and mortality.

Deep modeling permits generalization from the particular set of circumstances that generated the surface events. As a result, whereas surface models provide a basis for interpreting the observable effects of screening, deep models provide an explicit basis for determining the outcomes of screening scenarios that have not been directly studied in clinical trials [56]. This article will focus on the application of deep models to population screening.

These models can be further grouped into two broad categories – those that describe the system dynamics mathematically and those that entail computer simulation. The first of these, designated *analytic* models, uses a model of the disease to derive direct estimates of characteristics of the screening procedure and its consequent benefits. The second, designated simulation models, uses the disease model to simulate the course of the disease in a hypothetical population with and without screening and derives measures of the benefit of screening from the simulation outcomes.

Markov Framework for Modeling

Most screening models use an illness–death model for the disease which is developed within the framework of a Markov chain. A sequence of random variables $\{X_k, k = 0, 1, \ldots\}$ is called a Markov chain if, for every collection of integers $k_0 < k_1 < \cdots < k_n < v$,

$$\Pr(X_v = i | X_{k_0}, \ldots, X_{k_n}) = \Pr(X_v = i | X_{k_n}),$$

$$\text{for all } i. \qquad (1)$$

In other words, given the present state (X_{k_n}), the outcome in the future $(X_v = i)$ is not dependent on the past $(X_{k_0}, \ldots, X_{k_{n-1}})$.

The Markov chain formulation is applied to an illness–death model in the following way [16]. The population under study is classified into n states, the first m of which are *illness states* and the remaining $n - m$ of which are *death states*. An *illness* state can be broadly defined to be the absence of illness (a *healthy state*), a single specific disease or stage of disease, or any combination of diseases. In modeling screening, these states typically refer to a healthy state and preclinical and clinical phases of the disease.

A *death* state is defined by **cause of death**, either single or multiple. Emigration or loss to follow-up may also be treated as a death state. In modeling screening, typically there will be one death state due to death from the disease and another due to death from any other competing cause (*see* **Competing Risks**). Entry to a terminal stage of the disease is also sometimes treated as a death state. Transition from one state to another is determined by the *transition probabilities*, p_{ij}, where

$$p_{ij} = \Pr(X_{k+1} = j | X_k = i),$$

$$i, j = 1, 2, \ldots, n; \quad k = 1, 2, \ldots. \quad (2)$$

Death states are *absorbing* states, since once one reaches that state, transition to any other state is impossible (i.e. $p_{ij} = 0$, for $i = m + 1, \ldots, n$, and $j \neq i$). The disease model is said to be *progressive* if, once one enters the first stage of the disease, in the absence of interventions (such as screening) and

competing risks, the only valid transitions are through the remaining disease stages. Because the disease is modeled using a Markov chain, the future path of an individual through the illness and death states depends only on his or her current state, and the future distribution of individuals between illness and death states depends only on the present distribution and not on any past distributions.

This basic model can be varied in a number of ways. The Markov chain treats time as increasing in discrete steps corresponding to the index k. Thus a transition between states can only occur at discrete time intervals. Most screening models extend this to allow transitions to occur in continuous time. In this case, the transition probabilities for any two points in time t_1 and t_2 are

$$p_{ij}(t_1, t_2) = \Pr(X(t_2) = j | X(t_1) = i),$$

$$i, j = 1, 2, \ldots, n. \qquad (3)$$

If $p_{ij}(t_1, t_2)$ only depends on the difference $t_2 - t_1$ but not on t_1 or t_2 separately, the model is *time homogeneous*. The simple Markov chain described above is time homogeneous. This can be varied to allow the transition probabilities to vary with time. The probabilities can also be allowed to vary with age and other relevant characteristics of the individual. Some of the model formulations also allow the probability of transition out of a state to depend on the sojourn time in that state.

A Simple Disease and Screening Model

In this section we describe a simple model presented (and discussed in greater detail) by Shwartz & Plough [56], based on a characterization of the disease process proposed by Zelen & Feinleib [65]. We assume that a person can be in one of three states – a healthy state, the preclinical phase of the disease, or its clinical phase. This characterization also implicitly assumes a death state following the clinical phase, but since the focus of the analysis is on the preclinical phase, the death state is not explicitly used.

The model is progressive in that once a person enters the preclinical state, in the absence of screening or death from another cause, the disease will ultimately surface and enter the clinical phase. If the person is screened while in the preclinical state, then the disease may be detected with a probability depending on the sensitivity of the screening test.

The main assumption underlying this model (and the whole screening process) is that the earlier in the preclinical phase the disease is found, the better will be the prognosis. Hence, the screening benefit is directly related to the lead time.

For this model we define the following:

1. L is the lead time;
2. $g(y)$ is the **hazard rate** for entering the preclinical state at age y;
3. $p(t)$ is the hazard rate for clinical surfacing after the disease has been in the preclinical phase for time t;
4. $f(t)$ is the false negative rate of the screen when the disease has been present for time t; and
5. $b(t)$ is the probability of ultimately dying from the disease if it is detected when it has been present for time t.

For simplicity, we ignore the possibility of death from other causes.

If we let m and σ^2 be the mean and variance of the sojourn time distribution, then Zelen & Feinleib [65] show that if we assume a constant hazard rate for disease initiation (i.e. $g(t) = g$) we obtain the following expression for the mean lead time:

$$\mathrm{E}(L) = \frac{m^2 + \sigma^2}{2m} = \frac{m}{2}\left[1 + \left(\frac{\sigma^2}{m}\right)\right]. \quad (4)$$

Note that $\mathrm{E}(L) > m/2$ for $\sigma^2 > 0$. This illustrates the effect of length-biased sampling, since, if the screen detected cases were selected at random from all of the cases, one would expect the mean lead time to be $m/2$.

This expression also illustrates one of the central difficulties with this form of modeling. The lead time, which is the main index of screening benefit, is a function of the distribution of the sojourn time in the preclinical phase. However, the preclinical phase is, by definition, unobservable. The question of how to estimate characteristics of the sojourn time distribution has been at the center of most of the work done in this area.

For a person to be in the preclinical state at age a, then they must have entered the preclinical state before age a and not leave it until after age a. Hence the probability of this is a function of the hazard rates

$g(\cdot)$ and $p(\cdot)$. Thus

$\mathrm{Pr}(\text{preclinical phase at age } a)$

$$= \int_0^a g(u) \exp[-G(u)] \exp[-P(a - u)]\, \mathrm{d}u. \quad (5)$$

Furthermore, the probability that the disease clinically surfaces in some time interval δa following a is

$\mathrm{Pr}(\text{clinical surfacing in } (a, \delta a))$

$$= \int_0^a g(u) \exp[-G(u)] \exp[-P(a - u)]$$
$$\times p(a - u)\delta a\, \mathrm{d}u. \quad (6)$$

We combine this with the prognosis measure $b(\cdot)$ to calculate a baseline probability of death from the disease in the absence of screening:

$\mathrm{Pr}(\text{death in the absence of screening})$

$$= \int_0^\infty \int_0^a g(u) \exp[-G(u)] \exp[-P(a - u)]$$
$$\times p(a - u)\delta a b(a - u)\, \mathrm{d}u\, \mathrm{d}a. \quad (7)$$

Now we introduce the effect of screening. We will consider the case of one screening test performed at age s. There are four possibilities:

1. the disease is detected by the screening test;
2. the disease clinically surfaces before the test (i.e. at age $a < s$);
3. the disease is missed by the screening test and clinically surfaces after the screen (i.e. it is an interval case); or
4. the disease both enters the preclinical phase and clinically surfaces after the screening test.

For the disease to be detected by this test, it must be in the preclinical phase and the test must not give rise to a false negative. The probability of this is

$\mathrm{Pr}(\text{disease detection at age } s)$

$$= \int_0^s g(u) \exp[-G(u)] \exp[-P(s - u)]$$
$$\times (1 - f(s - u))\, \mathrm{d}u. \quad (8)$$

We have already calculated the probability that the disease clinically surfaces at age $a < s$ in (6). For the disease to have been missed by the screen, the person must be in the preclinical state at age s, the test must have produced a false negative, and the disease must have clinically surfaced after the screen. The probability of this is

Pr(disease missed by test)

$$= \int_s^\infty \int_0^s g(u) \exp[-G(u)] \exp[-P(a-u)]$$
$$\times f(s-u)p(a-u)\delta a \, du \, da. \qquad (9)$$

The probability that the disease both enters the preclinical phase and clinically surfaces after the screening test is

Pr(disease both develops and surfaces

$$\text{after the screen}) = \int_s^\infty \int_s^\infty g(u) \exp[-G(u)]$$
$$\times \exp[-P(a-u)]p(a-u)\delta a \, du \, da. \qquad (10)$$

Once again we can combine these probabilities with our prognosis measure to obtain the probability of death from the disease in the presence of screening:

Pr(death in the presence of screening)

$$= \int_0^s g(u) \exp[-G(u)] \exp[-P(s-u)]$$
$$\times (1 - f(s-u))b(s-u) \, du$$
$$+ \int_0^s \int_0^a g(u) \exp[-G(u)] \exp[-P(a-u)]$$
$$\times p(a-u)\delta ab(a-u) \, du \, da$$
$$+ \int_s^\infty \int_0^s g(u) \exp[-G(u)] \exp[-P(a-u)]$$
$$\times f(s-u)p(a-u)\delta ab(a-u) \, du \, da$$
$$+ \int_s^\infty \int_s^\infty g(u) \exp[-G(u)] \exp[-P(a-u)]$$
$$\times p(a-u)\delta ab(a-u) \, du \, da. \qquad (11)$$

This expression gives us our screening figure to compare with the baseline figure in (7).

Although none of the models used for disease screening is exactly like the simple model presented here, they all incorporate its fundamental ideas. In particular, they all depend on knowing in one form or another the transition probabilities into and out of the preclinical state, the distribution of the sojourn time in the preclinical state, the sensitivity of the screening test, and the disease prognosis as a function of the development of the disease.

Analytic Models for Cancer

A mathematical disease model with two states was first proposed by Du Pasquier [24], but it was Fix & Neyman [32] who introduced the stochastic version and resolved many problems associated with the model. Their model has two illness states – the state of "leading a normal life" and the state of being under treatment for cancer – and two death states – deaths from cancer and deaths from other causes or cases lost to observation. Chiang [15] subsequently developed a general illness–death stochastic model which could accommodate any finite number of illness and death states. Some of the major analytic models developed for cancer screening are listed in Table 1.

Lincoln & Weiss [41] were the first to propose a model of cancer as a basis for analyzing serial screening, in this case screening for cervical cancer. They did not explicitly use a Markov framework, but their model implicitly uses a classification of the disease into illness states.

Zelen & Feinleib [65] proposed the simple three-state, continuous-time, progressive disease characterization described in the previous section and used it in model screening for breast cancer. In a modification to this basic model, the authors further divide the preclinical state into two parts, defined as:

1. a preclinical state in which the disease never progresses to the clinical state (i.e. the sojourn time is allowed to be infinite); and
2. a preclinical state in which the disease is progressive and will eventually progress to the clinical state.

These are used to allow for the possibility that some individuals with the disease in a preclinical state will never have the disease progressing to a clinical state. This approach has been generalized in a number of ways by subsequent authors, with most focusing on simple disease models and the estimation of specific screening characteristics.

Prorok [48, 49] extended the lead time estimation to multiple screens. Blumenson [10–12] calculated the probability of terminal disease as a function of disease duration to date, and used this as a prognostic measure to evaluate screening strategies. Shwartz [54, 55] modeled disease progression for breast cancer using tumor size and number of axillary lymph nodes involved to define the preclinical and clinical states. He then determined screening benefit

Table 1 Selected analytic models of cancer screening

Literature references for model	Model inputs	Key features	Model output/measures of screening benefit
Lincoln & Weiss [41]	The probability density for the beginning of the detectable preclinical phase and the probability of a false negative screen at time t after entering the detectable preclinical phase – calculated by assuming specific functional forms rather than by direct estimation	Two illness states – a "healthy" state, in which the disease is not detectable, and a state covering the time between when the disease is first detectable and when it is actually detected by a screening examination	Distribution of time to discovery of tumor
Zelen & Feinleib [65]	Disease prevalence and incidence data	Symptoms assumed never to appear, with all disease detected by screening Model applied to cervical cancer screening Progressive three-state illness model – a healthy state, the preclinical phase, and the clinical phase Assumes single screen Applied to breast cancer screening	Mean lead time
Prorok [48, 49]	Preclinical state sojourn time distribution and disease prevalence and incidence data	Uses the Zelen & Feinleib illness model and develops theory for application to multiple screens	Mean lead time and proportion of preclinical cases detected
Blumenson [10–12]	Disease incidence data Preclinical state sojourn time distribution Screening parameters including age at first screen, screening sensitivity, and screening interval	Similar three-state illness model to Zelen & Feinleib, with a point occurring in either the preclinical or clinical phase where the disease becomes incurable Applied to breast cancer screening	Number of cases of diseases becoming incurable before detection
Shwartz [54, 55]	Specific functional forms and associated parameters governing tumor growth rate and lymph node involvement – chosen to be consistent with published results and available data Breast cancer incidence and death rates and death rates from other causes Screening parameters	Model developed specifically for breast cancer Progressive illness model with a healthy state, 21 disease states defined in terms of the tumor size and lymph node involvement and two death states – death from breast cancer and death from any other cause Transition from preclinical phase to clinical phase possible in any disease state, with probability dependent on tumor size and tumor rate of growth	Changes in life expectancy as a result of screening The probability that there will be no disease recurrence and the probability of detection before nodal involvement The probability of disease detection before death from other causes

(continued overleaf)

Table 1 (*continued*)

Literature references for model	Model inputs	Key features	Model output/measures of screening benefit
Albert et al. [3, 4], Louis et al. [42]	Maximum likelihood estimation of model parameters based on screening data and model assumption	Model predictions validated against independent data source (third-order validation)	
		Progressive illness model with preclinical phase classified into states corresponding with prognostic tumor staging schemes, and two "death" states – one corresponding to clinical surfacing and one to death from a competing cause	Percentage reduction due to screening in observed cases of late disease
		Model of screening strategy with probability of positive screen depending on person's age and disease state	Percentage decrease in lost salvageables due to screening
		Applied to breast and cervical cancer screening	
Dubin [25, 26]	Age and stage-specific disease incidence	Aimed at maintaining comparability between the model and observable characteristics of a screened population	Increase in life expectancy
	Survival times in the presence and absence of screening – derived from screening data by assuming particular functional forms for survival distributions	Progressive illness model consisting of disease stages corresponding with prognostic tumor staging schemes	Reduction in probability of dying of breast cancer
		Applied to breast cancer	Reduction in life years lost to women dying of breast cancer
Day & Walter [22], Walter & Day [63], Walter & Stitt [64]	Disease incidence derived from screening data	Progressive three-state illness model – a "healthy" state with no detectable disease, the detectable preclinical phase, and the clinical phase	Mean lead time
	Probability distribution specified for preclinical state sojourn time and survival time	Focus on sojourn time in detectable preclinical phase and survival times after detection	Lead time
		Applied to breast cancer	Survival time after detection by screening
Coppleson & Brown [20]	Age-specific clinical incidence data and prevalence data derived from detection rates at first Pap smear	Four-state illness model developed for cervical cancer	Not applicable (model focused on examination of disease natural history)
		Found that observed data could not be explained without allowing for cancer regression in the illness model	
Albert [2]	Transition probability matrix for movement between model states estimated from numbers of cancers detected for each stage in a screening program	Four-state illness model developed for cervical cancer – a healthy state, two preclinical states, and a clinical state.	Not applicable (model focused on examination of disease natural history)
		Cancer regression allowed in the two preclinical states	

Model	Estimation / data	Description	Output
Brookmeyer & Day [13]	Parameters of sojourn distribution estimated from screening data and data on interval cancer cases	Extends Day & Walter model. Preclinical phase divided into two states – one in which the disease may progress or regress and a second in which the disease always progresses. Applied to cervical cancer	Total preclinical phase sojourn distribution. Screening false negative rate
van Oortmarssen & Habbema [59]	Parameters of sojourn distribution estimated from screening data and data on interval cancer cases	Similar illness model to Brookmeyer & Day. Applied to cervical cancer	Not applicable (model focused on examination of disease natural history)
Eddy [27, 29, 30]	Model parameters derived from published results of disease studies and screening programs	Five-stage combined disease and screening model – one healthy state, three preclinical states defined by detectability by screening, and one clinical state. Assumes that once a disease is detectable by a screening modality, then any screen using that modality will detect the disease. Applied to breast, cervix, lung, bladder, and colon cancer	Probability of disease detection. Probability of death following detection. Increase of life expectancy due to screening
Connor et al. [19], Chu & Connor [17]	Stage shifts estimated from analysis of a RCT of screening	Multi-stage progressive disease model. Focus is on estimation of the shift of the disease at detection to an earlier stage or an earlier point in the same stage as a result of screening. Applied to breast cancer screening	Reduction of deaths at a given stage due to screening. Death prognosis of screen detected cancers
Baker et al. [9]	Peak time period for mortality comparison selected from results of a RCT of screening.	Focuses analysis on period when screening has maximum effect and hence analysis of screening trial results gives rise to more powerful statistical tests. Applied to proportional hazards model for survival analysis	Ratio of cancer mortality between screened and control groups
Day & Duffy [21]	Uses known prognostic factors which are available early in a RCT of screening to predict subsequent mortality differentials	Users surrogate endpoints for RCT of screening to shorten the duration of the trial and increase its power. Applied to breast cancer	Tumor size at cancer detection used as a basis for predicting subsequent mortality differentials

measures, from data on five year survival rate and five year disease recurrence rate for patients, as a function of tumor size and lymph node involvement.

Albert and his co-workers [3, 4, 42] developed a comprehensive model for the evolution of the natural history of cancer in a population subject to screening and natural demographic forces. In its general formulation, the model uses Zelen & Feinleib's classification of the disease into preclinical and clinical phases, but divides the preclinical phase into states corresponding with prognostic tumor staging schemes. It also has two death states which correspond to clinical surfacing of the disease or death from a competing risk. The model is progressive, but allowance is made for staying indefinitely in any given state.

This model is then applied to breast and cervical cancer. Breast cancer is modeled with two illness states, state 1 corresponding to disease with no lymphatic involvement and state 2 corresponding to disseminated disease (the contrary case). Cervical cancer is modeled with three illness states, state 1 corresponding to neoplasms *in situ*, state 2 corresponding to occult invasive lesions, and state 3 corresponding to frankly invasive lesions. The authors then impose on this model a screening strategy with a particular probability of a positive screen, depending on a person's age and disease state. Using this, they derive equations describing how the natural history of cancer (depicted by the distribution of numbers in each state and associated sojourn times) evolves over time in the presence of screening. These, in turn, are used to derive equations for measures of benefit from screening in terms of the disease status. These benefit measures include the percentage reduction in the cumulative number of observed cases of late disease due to screening and the percentage decrease in lost "salvageables" due to screening. A salvageable is a person who would have benefited from screening but who, in the absence of screening, progresses to a late stage of the disease before discovery.

Dubin [25, 26] developed a general multi-stage disease model similar to that of Chiang [15], and applied this to breast cancer using the same two stage classification as Albert et al. [4]. He noted the difficulty in estimating parameter values for detailed disease models from existing data from screening programs. His model aimed to avoid these difficulties by maintaining comparability between the model and the observable characteristics of a screened population.

He did this by focusing on age and stage-specific incidence and survival times in the presence and absence of screening. He derived formulas for the proportion of disease incidence which had been diagnosed earlier due to screening than it would have been in the absence of screening, and used these to derive various measures of screening benefit. Dubin's model is not strictly a deep model as defined above. However, although he makes no explicit hypotheses about the rate of disease progression, such hypotheses are implicit in his model.

Day & Walter [22] developed a variation on the simple three-stage model which has been used extensively. The focus of this model is the sojourn time in the detectable preclinical phase, for which a probability distribution is specified. For example, Walter & Day [63], in applying the model to breast cancer, used several alternate distributions, including the exponential, the Weibull, and a nonparametric step function. Under the model assumptions, one may derive expressions for the anticipated **incidence rates** of clinical disease among groups with particular screening histories and for the anticipated **prevalence** of preclinical disease found at the various screening times. One advantage of this model is that it is relatively simple to obtain approximate confidence intervals for parameter values. The model was extended by Walter & Stitt [64] to permit evaluation of survival of cancer cases detected by screening.

A useful synthesis of the analytic models described above applied to breast cancer is presented by O'Neill et al. [46].

All of the above are progressive models, but there are some forms of cancer for which the assumption of progression is not appropriate and for which some form of regression is required. These are cancers, such as large bowel cancer and particularly cervical cancer, where screening detects preinvasive or even precancerous lesions [13].

A number of models have attempted to address this. Coppleson & Brown [20] developed a model for cervical cancer and found that the observed data could not be explained without allowing for regression. Albert [2] developed a variation of his earlier model for cervical cancer which allowed for regression from the carcinoma *in situ* stage back to the healthy state. Brookmeyer & Day [13] and van Oortmarssen & Habbema [59] both developed similar extensions to the Day & Walter model to divide the preclinical phase into two. The first stage allows regression to a healthy state, but once a cancer reaches the second stage only progression is allowed.

The Coppleson & Brown, Albert, and van Oortmarssen & Habbema studies provide an interesting variation on the use of these models, in that the aim of the model was not to study cancer screening directly. Rather, the model was used to study the disease dynamics and, in particular, to examine the epidemiologic evidence for the existence of regression in preinvasive cervical cancer.

The models described above follow a common theme of characterizing the disease as a series of states (corresponding to health, the various disease stages, and death), with people moving between the states with certain transition probabilities and/or certain sojourn times. Screening is then evaluated by superimposing on the disease process a screening process with particular screening regimes and screen sensitivity. This is in contrast to the next model, due to Eddy [27], which uses a different strategy.

Eddy's modeling strategy uses a time varying Markov framework. However, he models the **interaction** between the screen and the disease in his basic model. This is a five-stage model defined in terms of three time points. The first is a reference time point t_p. The way in which this is defined varies with the cancer under discussion but, as an example, for breast cancer it is the point at which the disease can first be detected by physical examination. The *occult interval* is then defined as the time interval between this and the point t_M at which the disease is first detectable by screening (e.g. by mammography). The *patient interval* is defined as the time between t_p and the time t_Π at which the patient would actually seek medical care for the lesion. With Eddy's model, t_Π, t_p, and t_M can occur in any order. The important assumption is that once a disease is detectable by a screening modality (i.e. after t_M), then any screen using that modality will always detect the disease. This assumption replaces the assumption commonly made in models of screening that successive screens are independent.

The other two states are a "healthy" state (which includes any preclinical disease which is still undetectable by screening) and a clinical disease state. Eddy models the probability distributions of the occult and patient intervals and uses these to derive formulas for the probabilities of discovering a malignant lesion by screening and by other methods.

Eddy's model has been applied to several breast cancer screening data sets as well as to cervical, gastrointestinal, lung, and bladder cancer. It has also been extended to the case in which there is more than one type of screening test [31].

Finally, there are three recent analytic models which provide interesting variations on screening modeling.

The first of these is the stage shift model [19]. This assumes that the effect of screening is to shift the diagnosis of a cancer from a higher to a lower stage or within a given stage to an earlier time of diagnosis. Connor et al. develop the theory for a RCT with equal sized intervention and control groups, but the equations can be modified to allow for proportional number of cases if unequal groups are used. The method of fitting this model requires a completed trial with follow-up that has reached the point at which comparable sets of cancer cases have accumulated in the study and control groups. For most of the discussion, Connor et al. ignore variability associated with the estimation process and the determination of the point at which comparability is reached in order to emphasize the exploratory nature of the analysis. However, they do present simple variance estimates based on the assumption that their data follow a Poisson distribution. The need for a completed trial and long follow-up period limits the model's applicability, but it has been used to analyze breast cancer screening data [17].

The second is the peak analysis model [9]. This uses data from an RCT to determine the time period during which screening has the maximum effect on mortality. The results of the trial can then be analyzed restricting attention to that time period, providing more powerful statistical tests. For breast cancer screening, for example, this could mean excluding the mortality experience of the first few years after the initiation of screening. A disadvantage of this model is that the selection of the peak time period for the mortality comparison could be regarded as "data-driven" and subject to the usual problems of a *post hoc* analysis [44].

The third is the use of surrogate endpoints for RCTs to shorten the duration of the trial and to increase the power [21]. Day & Duffy apply this approach to a study comparing breast cancer screening at three yearly and one yearly intervals. Tumor size is the most important variable in predicting survival from breast cancer in the screening context, so they consider the difference in tumor size distribution between the study groups. They show that using this as an index of benefit and projecting expected mortality allows a result after only five years, compared with the 15–20 years required for a trial based on observed mortality. Furthermore, they demonstrate the rather surprising result that the use of surrogate endpoints leads to an increase in the power of the RCT compared with using the observed mortality. While completed trials remain necessary to establish the primary benefits of screening, this approach allows faster and more efficient resolution of subsidiary issues.

Simulation Models for Cancer

Some of the major simulation models developed for cancer screening are listed in Table 2. Knox [34] developed the earliest and most comprehensive simulation model. As with the analytic models, Knox uses a healthy state, a number of illness states and two death states. However, the model involves considerably more illness states, including classifying the disease as a preclinical, early clinical, or late clinical cancer, and further classifying each of these as treated or not treated and each cancer as high or low grade.

Knox defines a transition matrix containing the estimated transfer rates between the various pathological states, modified according to the age of the individual or the duration of the state. He then simulates the evolution of the disease in a hypothetical cohort of study subjects which has similar characteristics to the population that he wishes to study (which, in this case, is the adult female population of England and Wales) using the transition matrix and a standard **life table** to provide the risks of competing causes of death.

Finally, he adds details of the screening procedures to be considered, specifying the clinico-pathological states to which they apply, and their sensitivities and specificities in relation to each, and the transfers between model states which will occur following detection or nondetection. The screening policies are arranged in incremental series, and the results compared with each other and with the results of providing no screening at all. This allows the appraisal of benefits and costs in both absolute and marginal terms.

This model has been applied to both cervical cancer [34] and breast cancer [35]. It illustrates one major difference between the analytic and simulation approaches – the greater complexity of the disease and screening models in the simulation case. However, this extra complexity requires more detailed information on the disease dynamics in order to specify the model and this information is often not readily available. Knox [36] says of his earlier work that

> The chief problem of applying the predictions stemmed from uncertainties about the clinical course of the early stages of cancer.

In this and in all his subsequent analyses, he simplified his model to one with only two illness states. This two-state model is worth discussing in detail because of its different approach to the population under study. Whereas the usual approach is to consider all people at risk of a cancer and to use the model to project mortality with and without screening, Knox's approach is to consider only those who have died from cancer, and to use the model to estimate how many would have been saved if screening had been offered. He refers to it as "tearing down" a graph of age-distributed deaths in successive steps through the insertion of screening procedures at selected ages [37]. This means that Knox does not need to consider variations in the course of the disease, such as lesions which never clinically surface or which regress to a healthy state, because all members of his population have, by definition, a progressive form of the disease.

The two illness states are designated A and B. During state A the disease is susceptible to early detection and full or partial cure. During state B, the disease is incurable. The sojourn time in each state varies around an age-specific mean. The screening procedure has a probability of detecting the lesion which rises linearly during period A, while the probability of curing the disease falls linearly during A.

This model has the advantage of simplicity, which means that it is relatively easy to find plausible parameter values for it. However, this simplicity has disadvantages. The model only considers the situation of a fully established screening program, so that it cannot be used to investigate issues surrounding setting up a new program. Also, because it is focused on mortality reduction, it cannot be used to consider issues relating to costs of screening programs.

Table 2 Selected simulation models of cancer screening

Literature references for model	Model inputs	Key features	Model output/measures of screening benefit
Knox [34, 35]	Model parameters derived from published results of disease studies and screening programs and from the known characteristics of population under study	Cohort simulation model	Simulated mortality and morbidity in the presence of screening under various screening regimes
		Illness model with 26 defined states	
		Transition matrix defined for movements between these states following detection or nondetection of disease in the presence of specified screening procedures	
		Model applied to a hypothetical cohort of study subjects with similar characteristics to the population under study	
		Model applied to both breast and cervical cancer screening	
Knox [36], Knox & Woodman [37]	Model parameters derived from published results of disease studies and screening programs and from the known characteristics of population under study	Cohort simulation model	Simulated reduction in mortality due to screening
		Illness model with two disease states – one in which the disease is susceptible to early detection and full or partial cure and a second in which the disease is incurable	
		Model applied to subjects who have died from cancer but may have been saved if screening had been offered	
		Applied to breast and cervical cancer screening	
Parkin [47]	Model parameters derived from published results of disease studies and screening programs and from the known characteristics of population under study	Microsimulation model developed for cervical cancer screening	Simulated mortality and morbidity in the presence of screening under various screening regimes
		Illness model has nine states – a healthy state, three preclinical states, one clinical state, two death states, and a hysterectomy state (in which a woman is no longer at risk of cervical cancer)	
		Model applied to a hypothetical population with age structure similar to that of the population under study	
Habbema et al. [33], van Oortmarssen et al. [61]	Model parameters derived from published results of disease studies and screening programs and from the known characteristics of population under study	General framework for microsimulation modeling	Simulated mortality and morbidity in the presence of screening under various screening regimes
		Follows similar approach to Parkin	
		Applied to breast and cervical cancer screening	

Researchers at the Australian Institute of Health and Welfare have extended this approach by combining Knox's disease model with a costs model to evaluate the introduction of breast and cervical cancer screening programs in Australia [6, 7]. They have also combined the disease model with mortality projections to investigate the timing of mortality reductions due to the introduction of a breast cancer screening program [8].

Parkin [47] identifies a number of advantages of the *cohort simulation* approach of transferring year by year specified proportions of a single cohort in a deterministic fashion between model states. These include the model's ability to:

1. demonstrate the relationships between variables;
2. explore the effects of different acceptance rates and test characteristics on outcome measures;
3. examine the net cost-effectiveness of different screening policies by imputing costs to the different outcomes of screening tests; and
4. explore the effect of different theoretic natural histories on the outcome of screening.

However, he also identifies some of the disadvantages of this approach. First, services have to be planned, not for a single cohort over an entire lifespan, but for a very heterogenous population over relatively short time periods. When a screening program providing for testing at certain fixed ages is introduced into a community, only people younger than the starting age for the screening policy can possibly receive the full schedule of tests. Thus, benefits from screening will at first be small, but will increase progressively as more of the population receives a series of examinations. Furthermore, many people will have already had previous examinations, so the results of the screening policy will depend on the existing screening status of the population. This cannot be simulated by a single cohort model; nor can differences in the risk of disease in different birth cohorts.

Secondly, it may be desirable to use characteristics other than age to identify subgroups of the population for selective screening. This is less often of practical use, since such subgroups are usually not readily identifiable, but a planning model should be able to explore the effectiveness of policies involving differential screening of such subpopulations. In addition, population subgroups often have different rates of attendance at screening programs which may be correlated with different disease risks.

Finally, screening programs do not exist in isolation from the rest of the health care system. Much screening activity can take place outside a screening program. Most models usually treat this activity as "diagnostic" and ignore it. However, a planning model should take account of all relevant screening activity.

Parkin proposes instead a *microsimulation* approach. Here, the life histories of individual members of a population are simulated. The population in his model has the demographic make-up of that of England and Wales and its size is governed by two considerations: (i) the computer time involved in microsimulation of very large populations; and (ii) the need for reliable results in a stochastic simulation of relatively rare events.

Each individual is characterized by his or her values for a set of variables which will be used in simulating demographic events, the disease natural history, or screening programs. The values of these variables are updated annually using sets of conditional transition probabilities (e.g. the probability of childbirth given age, marital status, and initial parity). The occurrence of a transition is decided by comparing the relevant probability against a randomly generated number. There is considerable flexibility in modeling screening programs and, since the model follows individuals, it is possible to simulate contacts with the health care system and the "incidental" screening which occurs on such occasions.

Parkin's microsimulation model was developed specifically for cervical cancer screening, but a group working at Erasmus University in the Netherlands has developed a general modeling framework for microsimulation modeling of cancer screening called MIcrosimulation SCreening ANalysis (MISCAN) [33, 61]. Strictly speaking, MISCAN is not itself a model, but rather a model generator – a package that can generate and calculate a variety of these microsimulation models.

The MISCAN approach, like Parkin's model, is based on the actual structure of a population as it develops in a given country at a particular time. The mass screening program under consideration is taken as starting in a particular year and finishing in a particular year. Standard demographic techniques (*see* **Demography**) are used to project the study population to a year well after the nominated end of the program. This allows for both the introduction of the program to be modeled and the effects, after the end of the program, to be followed up.

The basic structure of the cancer model is similar to Knox's earlier model with a detailed classification of clinical and preclinical cancer states, although it uses a smaller number of states. The interaction between the disease model and the screening program is designed to allow projection of screening and treatment costs as well as cancer mortality and morbidity. MISCAN has been widely used to analyze breast and cervical cancer screening programs.

Model Fitting and Validation

Eddy [28] proposed four levels of validation for mathematical models:

1. First-order validation: this requires that the structure of the model makes sense to people who have a good knowledge of the problem.
2. Second-order validation: this involves comparing estimates made by the model with the data that were used to fit the model.
3. Third-order validation: this involves comparing the predictions of the model with data that were available when the model was fitted but that were not used in the estimation of model parameters.
4. Fourth-order validation: this involves comparing the outcomes of the model with observed data when applied to data generated and collected after the model was built (for example, data from a previously unobserved screening program).

In this section we discuss model fitting and validation for cancer screening in the framework of these levels.

First-order validation is generally not difficult to accomplish. The conceptualization of cancer as a series of preclinical and clinical stages is virtually universally accepted as a reasonable characterization of the disease. Problems may arise when the details of the disease stages are specified, but generally a wide variety of model formulations are plausible within the constraints of the limited knowledge of preclinical cancer.

Second-order validation highlights one of the central problems with this sort of deep model. This is the difficulty of directly relating available data to model parameters. The mismatch between the data available, either from screening trials or other sources, and the

model data requirements for parameter estimation has been recognized from the beginning of this type of modeling. Lincoln & Weiss [41, p. 188] note, for example, that

> Here we can do no more than introduce plausible forms for the different functions involved and plausible values for the parameters.

They go on to describe the difficulties in relating available data to the mathematical functions on which their model is based. This is a recurring problem in modeling cancer for screening, and to some extent affects all of the models described in this article.

Some of the analytic models have developed methods of estimating model parameters using standard statistical estimation approaches. Dubin [26], for example, structured his model so that it could directly use the data from screening trials, although as a consequence his model relates less to the disease natural history than do the others. Louis et al. [42] derived nonparametric models for the probability distributions specified in their model and proposed the use of maximum likelihood methods to fit them. Day & Walter [22] used both parametric and nonparametric functions for their preclinical sojourn time and suggested either maximum likelihood methods or least squares criteria to fit them. However, many of the analytic models and all of the simulation models proceed in a more *ad hoc* fashion by varying their disease natural history and model parameters until their models closely reproduce existing data.

Knox [35, pp. 17–18] gives an example of how this *ad hoc* fitting operates, in fitting his earlier model to breast cancer screening data. He describes fitting the natural history data thus:

> A statement of the natural history of the disease process must be provided in the form of a "transition matrix" which gives estimated transfer rates between the various pathological states, modified suitably according to the age of the woman or the duration of the state. This set of values is adjusted iteratively until an output is produced which matches available data on incidence, prevalence and mortality. If, as sometimes happens, more than one natural history statement is capable of mimicking these facts, then the natural history will have to be treated as one of the uncertainties. Subsequent runs will then have to be repeated for a range of natural history alternatives, and each prediction of results will be conditional upon the accuracy of the natural history used.

Parkin [47] provides an example of just such an uncertainty about natural history, with the final model including three different natural histories as alternatives.

This approach to model fitting has the disadvantage that, particularly for models with a large number of unknown parameters, the fit of the predicted values may be close to the observed data whether or not the model is in any sense valid. However, fitting the model to a number of independent data sets simultaneously and validating it against each of these data sets, as was done by van Oortmarssen et al. [61], provides some protection against this possibility.

Third-order validation is usually made difficult by the lack of data. Generally, most available data are used in determining the parameters of the model [56]. Breast cancer models are a good example of this. The only real data sources for fitting models for breast cancer screening are the screening studies, and in particular the RCTs. The first major study was the Health Insurance Plan (HIP) of New York study [53]. This program started screening in 1963. Subsequent studies were not started for another ten years, with the Utrecht Screening Program [18] starting screening in 1974 and the Swedish Two-county Randomized Trial starting in 1977 [58]. This means that many of the models only had access to the HIP data. Screening technology has changed significantly since the HIP program began [61], so when later studies became available they could not be directly compared with the HIP program and, in any case, it is questionable whether models based only on HIP data are directly relevant to modern screening. Because of the long time before mortality benefits from screening are fully apparent, models fitted using solely data from later studies have only appeared relatively recently [61] and, at least in their published form, have generally not addressed the issue of third-order validation. However, as more screening programs are implemented, more data should become available for third-order validation [6].

Eddy [28] recognized that fourth-order validation is only possible in rare cases. However, there are at least two examples of studies which use models in a way that could be called fourth-order validation, coincidentally both using Eddy's own model. Verbeek et al. [62] compare predictions from Eddy's model for breast cancer to data from a mammography screening program in Nijmegen. The authors note that the comparison does not suggest too good a fit.

However, this is only a preliminary study, and further validation work remains to be done. Eddy [29] compares his model for cervical cancer with a later independent analysis of empirical data. In this case the model appears to predict accurately the effect of different cervical cancer screening policies on outcomes that are important for policy decisions.

The best way to see how these models are fitted and used in practice is to examine examples. The following three sections describe an example of fitting a model followed by a description of its application.

An Example of Model Fitting

This section describes the analysis by van Oortmarssen et al. [61] of breast cancer screening based on the MISCAN computer simulation package. This model is designed to reproduce the detection rates and incidence of interval cancers as observed in the screening projects in Utrecht and Nijmegen in the Netherlands.

The basic model structure is shown in Figure 2. The first state is the state of no breast cancer. Women stay in this state until a transition occurs to one of the preclinical states that is detectable by screening (either mammography or clinical examination). The preclinical phase is divided into four states. There is one preinvasive state, intraductal carcinoma *in situ* (dCIS), and three screen detectable invasive states subdivided according to the diameter of the tumor: < 10 mm, $10-19$ mm, and ≥ 20 mm.

The subdivision applied to the preclinical invasive states is also used for the clinical phase and for screen detected tumors. The state "false positives" refers to women with a positive screening examination in whom no breast cancer is found at further assessment. The two end states of the model are "death from breast cancer" and "death from other causes". Transitions into the "death from other causes" state (not shown in the figure) are possible from every other model state and are governed by the Dutch life table, which is corrected for death from breast cancer. The values of the key parameters of the model are summarized in Table 3.

Parameters relating to clinical breast cancer and survival can usually be taken directly from available data. In this case, the preclinical incidence was estimated from the reported Dutch clinical incidence figures shifted to younger ages according to the model's assumptions about the transitions and

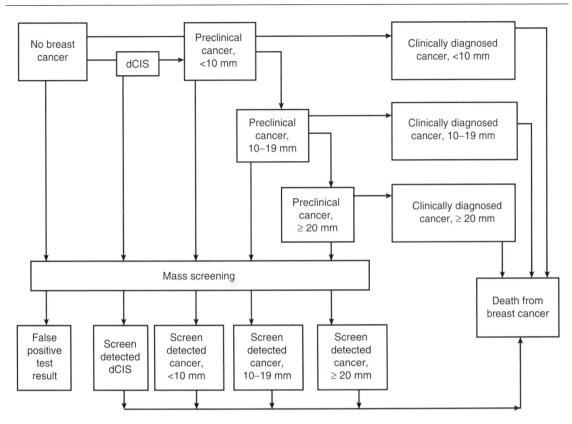

Figure 2 The structure of the disease and screening model for breast cancer developed by van Oortmarssen et al. The state "death from other causes" is not shown. It may be reached from all other states. Source: van Oortmarssen et al. [61]

durations in the preclinical stages. The distribution of the tumor diameters for clinically diagnosed cancers was obtained directly from data on cancers diagnosed outside the screening program in Utrecht and Nijmegen. Survival is described by a fraction cured and a survival time distribution for women who are at risk of dying from breast cancer. The survival time distribution is based on the lognormal, with mean and variance taken from a published analysis of the Swedish Cancer Registry data [52]. The fraction cured was estimated from the Utrecht data on clinically diagnosed cancers and varied with age according to another published analysis of Swedish data on age-specific breast cancer survival [1]. The combination of model assumptions on clinical incidence, stage distribution, and survival result in a good fit for the mortality rate for breast cancer in the Netherlands at all ages.

Parameters relating to the preclinical phase are less easily specified. Parameter estimation was done

by comparing simulated results from the model with data from the Utrecht and Nijmegen projects. An initial set of parameter values, partly taken from an earlier analysis of the HIP screening trial [60], resulted in many discrepancies between the simulated and observed data. The model parameters were systematically varied until a set of model specifications was found which gave an adequate overall fit to the Utrecht and Nijmegen data. Finally, the improvement in prognosis due to screen detection was calculated from the results of the Swedish Two-county screening study [58].

This model passes both first- and second-order validation, in that it is consistent with what is known about the natural history of breast cancer and with previous models developed in the literature, and its results are consistent with the Utrecht and Nijmegen data used in its fitting. Third-order validation is more problematic. As noted above, the HIP data are not directly comparable with those considered here and

Table 3   Key assumptions of the van Oortmarssen et al. breast cancer screening model

Parameter	Assumption
Preclinical incidence	Based on Dutch clinical incidence, 1977–82
Clinical stage distribution	*Independent of age*
<10 mm	10%
10–19 mm	22%
≥ 20 mm	68%
20 year survival of clinically diagnosed breast cancer (*diagnosis at age 55*)	*Age-dependent*
<10 mm	83%
10–19 mm	68%
≥ 20 mm	51%
Duration of preclinical invasive stages	*Average duration (years)*
Age 40 years	1.6
Age 50 years	2.1
Age 60 years	3.0
Age 70 years	4.7
Sensitivity of mammography	*Independent of age*
dCIS	70%
<10 mm	70%
≥10 mm	95%
Impact of early detection	
Mortality reduction for screen detected cancers	52%

Source: van Oortmarssen et al. [61].

the authors used all the other available data in fitting the model. Similarly, fourth-order validation is not possible in this case, since published results from other breast cancer RCTs were not available at the time this analysis was carried out.

An Application of the Model to Breast Cancer Screening

The breast cancer disease model described above was applied to Australian data by Stevenson et al. [57] to simulate the introduction of a breast cancer screening program. Australian breast cancer data and life table data were used to estimate cancer incidence and population **life expectancies**. Pilot testing of screening programs suggested that a screening participation rate of 70% was a reasonable target [6]. All other model parameters were taken from the van Oortmarssen et al. model.

The model was applied to five different screening options defined in terms of the age group offered screening and the interval between successive screens. These are listed in Table 4. Taking 1990 as the nominal starting year, the analysis simulated the introduction of a screening program phased in over five years

Table 4   Breast cancer screening options

Option number	Age group screened (years)	Screening interval (years)
1	50–69	2
2	50–69	3
3	40–49	1
	50–69	2
4	40–49	2
	50–69	3
5	40–69	2

and running for a further 25 years. The simulated total life years lost in the absence of a screening program and the life years saved by screening for each of the screening options are listed in Table 5. These results show a clear benefit in including women aged 40–49 in the screening program and of a two-year interval over a three-year interval. However, they also show that decreasing the interval to one year for women aged 40–49 makes only a marginal improvement.

An analysis of screening should include consideration of costs as well as benefits. A complete discussion of estimating costs is beyond the scope of this

Table 5 Number and proportion of life years saved among Australian women by mammography screening over a 30 year screening period, as estimated from the van Oortmarssen et al. simulation model

Screening option	Total life years lost in the absence of a screening program ('000s)	Number of life years saved as a result of the screening program ('000s)	Life years saved as a percentage of total life years lost
1	3766.6	250.5	6.7
2	3767.0	202.4	5.4
3	3741.2	324.3	8.7
4	3743.1	258.1	6.9
5	3755.6	309.4	8.2

Source: Stevenson et al. [57].

Note. These results are based on the simulation of individual life histories, with the outcomes for each individual being determined randomly by applying the probabilities of developing the disease and of surviving the disease. This means that the outcome for each individual may vary between simulations. This accounts for the small variation in the simulated total life years lost figures.

article, but generally they will be based on both current screening experience (with, for example, screening pilot projects in the location under study) and model based projections. These estimates are usually reported as the present value of the costs. This involves applying an annual discount rate to costs projected for future years. Hence, where costs are compared with benefits, the benefits are usually also presented in present value terms by applying the same annual discount rate.

The estimated total costs and costs per life year saved for the three screening options which include women aged 40–49 are presented in Table 6. This shows that the small increase in life years saved gained by moving to a one year screening interval for women aged 40–49 is offset by a substantial increase in the cost per life year saved.

A Comparison of Two Models for Breast Cancer

Stevenson et al. [57] also simulated the introduction of an Australian breast cancer screening program using Knox's two-state disease model described

above. In Table 7 is presented a comparison between the percentage life years saved for each screening option derived from both this model and the van Oortmarssen et al. model. There are clear differences between the two models, with the Knox model estimates consistently higher for all screening options. Furthermore, the evidence from the Knox model for including women aged 40–49 is more equivocal.

It is tempting to ask which model is right but, while there is some reason for preferring the van Oortmarssen model (because of its more extensive validation), a more relevant question is which model more correctly addresses the issue under study. The Knox model applies to a steady state situation, in which the screening program has been operating for long enough so that no one in the target population is too old to have participated in the full program. The van Oortmarssen et al. model makes allowance for the start of the program excluding some women from fully participating. The effect of this is that the Knox model will overstate the gains in life years saved at the start of the program. The difference in the results

Table 6 Relative cost-effectiveness of screening at different screening intervals for women aged 40–69

Screening option	Net present value of costs to service providers and women ($ million)	Net present value of life years saved ('000s)	Average cost per life year saved ($)
3	1917.8	622.2	3082.3
4	1097.5	628.6	1745.9
5	1374.6	620.6	2215.0

Source: Costs data taken from Australian Health Ministers' Advisory Council report on breast cancer screening [6]. Projected life years saved data taken from Stevenson et al. [57].

Note. Net present value calculated by applying an annual discount rate of 5%.

Table 7 Percentage of total life years saved among Australian women by mammography screening as estimated by two simulation models

Screening option	Life years saved as a percentage of total life years lost – van Oortmarssen et al. model	Life years saved as a percentage of total life years lost – Knox two-stage model
1	6.7	12.6
2	5.4	11.1
3	8.7	12.9
4	6.9	11.1
5	8.2	12.8

Source: Stevenson et al. [57].

for including women aged 40–49 years arise from more realistic assumptions in the van Oortmarssen et al. model about the effect of screening at those ages on subsequent mortality.

Models for Other Diseases

Models for screening can be applied to diseases other than cancer. For example, screening tests exist for diabetes and there is a clear value in its early detection. Undiagnosed diabetes could be considered as a preclinical phase of the disease and modeling techniques applied to investigating its characteristics. Similarly, a disease such as hypertension could be modeled either for its own sake or as a preclinical form of cardiovascular disease.

Some work has been done on simulation modeling for coronary heart disease [38]. This model used **logistic regression** to estimate transition probabilities between risk factor states and heart disease. It focused on the effects of risk factor reduction, but did not address details of screening programs. Hence, it avoided having to model details of the preclinical phase. There have to date been no significant published attempts at modeling the preclinical phase to investigate specific screening programs for chronic diseases other than cancer.

On the other hand, modeling of infectious diseases has a long history in biostatistics (*see* **Communicable Diseases**; **Infectious Disease Models**). Most recently considerable work has been done on disease models of acquired immune deficiency syndrome (AIDS) and human immunodeficiency virus (HIV), although most of this effort has focused on projecting the spread of the disease rather than modeling screening programs (see, for example, Day et al.

[23]). However, there has been some work on modeling screening for infectious diseases.

Lee & Pierskalla's model [40] is a good illustration of the similarities and differences in modeling infectious diseases for mass screening. In this model, the preclinical phase equates to the period during which a disease is infectious but without symptoms and the clinical phase to the period during which symptoms develop, the person seeks treatment, and is isolated or removed from the population. The main quantities used in the modeling are:

1. the number of infected people at a given time;
2. the natural incidence rate of the disease;
3. the rate of transmission of the disease from a contagious unit to a susceptible;
4. the rate of infected units ending the infectious period (i.e. clinical surfacing); and
5. the probability that an infected unit will not be detected by a screening test (i.e. the probability of a false negative).

The crucial difference here is that disease is initiated by spread from one unit to another, as well as by its natural incidence rate. Hence, in addition to the lead time, the main index of benefit is the removal of infected units from the population. Indeed, Lee & Pierskalla show that defining the measure of screening benefit as the average lead time across the population under study is equivalent to defining it as the average number of infected units per time period in the population.

Taking treatment as the endpoint of the model, rather than ultimate mortality, has the advantage of avoiding the necessity of modeling survival in the presence of screening. However, these models still have the difficulty of specifying parameters for an unobserved preclinical phase. For example, Lee &

Pierskalla note that their model is an oversimplification, because it assumes that the sensitivity of the screening test is constant and independent of how long the person has been infected with the disease. They also note that varying this assumption is of little practical use, since data on transmission rates at the various disease states are almost nonexistent.

Current State and Future Directions

The problem of model validation and its effect on the credibility of model based results is still a barrier to their wider use. Nevertheless, there are a number of areas in which modeling can make a uniquely important contribution to our current understanding of screening.

In the absence of specific RCTs, modeling remains the only effective way of evaluating different screening regimes. For example, the inclusion of women aged between 40 and 50 in a mammography screening program is still a contentious issue, with no international consensus on the effectiveness of screening at these ages [6]. While it could be argued that decisions on screening these women should not be made in the absence of reliable evidence on the presence or absence of the benefits, in practice, governments are already developing screening programs and modeling plays an important role in guiding policy-makers.

Modeling also has a crucial role to play in assessing the cost-effectiveness of screening programs. Even for cheap and easily available screening technologies, organized mass screening programs are the best way to insure that the benefits of screening are fully realized [7]. Modeling is not only necessary in order to plan these programs, but funding bodies are unlikely to fund such programs without at least initial cost–effectiveness studies, and modeling is the only practical way to derive the necessary estimates of future benefits and costs.

Miller et al. [44, p. 768] best summarize the current situation when, in discussing some recent models, they say

It is clear that these, and other models already developed or under consideration, may enhance our understanding of the natural history of screen-detected lesions and the process of screening. However, they require validation with the best available data, which is preferably derived from randomised trials, before they could be extrapolated in ways that might guide policy decisions. As such data become

available, assumption-based models need to be modified to incorporate this extra information, in order to improve the extrapolations needed to make policy.

While analytic models have a role in investigating specific facets of the disease and screening process (see, for example, [59]), the more comprehensive simulation models, and particularly the microsimulation models, seem best suited to the overall assessment of costs and effectiveness in screening programs and the investigation of different screening regimes. However, the challenge in using the simulation approach is to derive disease and screening models which are sufficiently complex to model all relevant aspects of screening but sufficiently simple to enable interpretable second-order validation.

References

[1] Adami, H.A., Malker, B., Holmberg, L., Persson, I. & Stone, B. (1986). The relationship between survival and age at diagnosis in breast cancer, *New England Journal of Medicine* **315**, 559–563.

[2] Albert, A. (1981). Estimated cervical cancer disease state incidence and transition rates, *Journal of the National Cancer Institute* **67**, 571–576.

[3] Albert, A., Gertman, P.M. & Louis, T.A. (1978). Screening for the early detection of cancer – I. The temporal natural history of a progressive disease state, *Mathematical Biosciences* **40**, 1–59.

[4] Albert, A., Gertman, P.M., Louis, T.A. & Liu, S.-I. (1978). Screening for the early detection of cancer – II. The impact of the screening on the natural history of the disease, *Mathematical Biosciences* **40**, 61–109.

[5] Alexander, F.E. (1989). Statistical analysis of population screening, *Medical Laboratory Science* **46**, 255–267.

[6] Australian Health Ministers' Advisory Council (1990). *Breast Cancer Screening in Australia: Future Directions*. Australian Institute of Health: Prevention Program Evaluation Series No 1. AGPS, Canberra.

[7] Australian Health Ministers' Advisory Council (1991). *Cervical Cancer Screening in Australia: Options for Change*. Australian Institute of Health: Prevention Program Evaluation Series No 2. AGPS, Canberra.

[8] Australian Institute of Health and Welfare (1992). *Australia's Health 1992: the Third Biennial Report of the Australian Institute of Health and Welfare*. AGPS, Canberra.

[9] Baker, S.G., Connor, R.J. & Prorok, P.C. (1991). Recent developments in cancer screening modeling, in *Cancer Screening*, A.B. Miller, J. Chamberlain, N.E. Day, M. Hakama & P.C. Prorok, eds. Cambridge University Press, Cambridge, pp. 404–418.

[10] Blumenson, L.E. (1976). When is screening effective in reducing the death rate? *Mathematical Biosciences* **30**, 273–303.

[11] Blumenson, L.E. (1977). Compromise screening strategies for chronic disease, *Mathematical Biosciences* **34**, 79–94.

[12] Blumenson, L.E. (1977). Detection of disease with periodic screening: Transient analysis and application to mammography examination, *Mathematical Biosciences* **33**, 73–106.

[13] Brookmeyer, R. & Day, N.E. (1987). Two-stage models for the analysis of cancer screening data, *Biometrics* **43**, 657–669.

[14] Bross, I.D.J., Blumenson, L.E., Slack, N.H. & Priore, R.L. (1968). A two disease model for breast cancer, in *Prognostic Factors in Breast Cancer*, A.P.M. Forrest & P.B. Bunkler, eds. Williams & Wilkins, Baltimore, pp. 288–300.

[15] Chiang, C.L. (1964). A stochastic model of competing risks of illness and competing risks of death, in *Stochastic Models in Medicine and Biology*, J. Gurland, ed. University of Wisconsin Press, Madison, pp. 323–354.

[16] Chiang, C.L. (1980). *An Introduction to Stochastic Processes and their Applications*. Krieger, Huntington, New York.

[17] Chu, K.C. & Connor, R.J. (1991). Analysis of the temporal patterns of benefits in the Health Insurance Plan of Greater New York Trial by stage and age, *American Journal of Epidemiology* **133**, 1039–1049.

[18] Collette, H.J.A., Day, N.E., Rombach, J.J. & de Waard, F. (1984). Evaluation of screening for breast cancer in a non-randomized study (the DOM project) by means of a case control study, *Lancet* **i**, 1224–1226.

[19] Connor, R.J., Chu, K.C. & Smart, C.R. (1989). Stage-shift cancer screening model, *Journal of Clinical Epidemiology* **42**, 1083–1095.

[20] Coppleson, L.W. & Brown, B. (1975). Observations on a model of the biology of carcinoma of the cervix: a poor fit between observations and theory, *American Journal of Obstetrics and Gynecology* **122**, 127–136.

[21] Day, N.E. & Duffy, S.W. (1996). Trial design based on surrogate end points – application to comparison of different breast screening frequencies, *Journal of the Royal Statistical Society, Series A* **159**, 49–60.

[22] Day, N.E. & Walter, S.D. (1984). Simplified models of screening for chronic disease: estimation procedures from mass screening programmes, *Biometrics* **40**, 1–14.

[23] Day, N.E., Gore, S.M. & De Angelis, D. (1995). Acquired immune deficiency syndrome predictions for England and Wales (1992–97): sensitivity analysis, information, decision, *Journal of the Royal Statistical Society, Series A* **158**, 505–524.

[24] Du Pasquier, (1913). Mathematische theorie der Invaliditatsversicherung, *Milt. Verein. Schweiz. Versich.-Math.* **8**, 1–153.

[25] Dubin, N. (1979). Benefits of screening for breast cancer: application of a probabilistic model to a breast cancer detection project, *Journal of Chronic Diseases* **32**, 145–151.

[26] Dubin, N. (1981). Predicting the benefit of screening for disease, *Journal of Applied Probability* **18**, 348–360.

[27] Eddy, D.M. (1980). *Screening for Cancer: Theory, Analysis and Design*. Prentice-Hall, Englewood Cliffs.

[28] Eddy, D.M. (1985). Technology assessment: the role of mathematical modeling, in *Assessing Medical Technologies*, Institute of Medicine, ed. National Academy Press, Washington, pp. 144–153.

[29] Eddy, D.M. (1987). The frequency of cervical cancer screening: comparison of a mathematical model with empirical data, *Cancer* **60**, 1117–1122.

[30] Eddy, D.M. & Shwartz, M. (1982). Mathematical models in screening, in *Cancer Epidemiology and Prevention*, D. Schottenfeld & J.F. Fraumeni, eds. Saunders, Philadelphia, pp. 1075–1090.

[31] Eddy, D.M., Nugent, F.W., Eddy, J.F., Coller, J., Gilbertsen, V., Gottleib, L.S., Rice, R., Sherlock, P. & Winawer, S. (1987). Screening for colorectal cancer in a high-risk population, *Gastroenterology* **92**, 682–692.

[32] Fix, E. & Neyman, J. (1951). A simple stochastic model of recovery, relapse, death and loss of patients, *Human Biology* **23**, 205–241.

[33] Habbema, J.D.F., Lubbe, J.Th.N., van der Maas, P.J. & van Oortmarssen, G.J. (1983). A computer simulation approach to the evaluation of mass screening, in *MEDINFO 83. Proceedings of the 4th World Conference on Medical Informatics*, van Bemmel et al., eds. North-Holland, Amsterdam.

[34] Knox, E.G. (1973). A simulation system for screening procedures, in *Future and Present Indicatives, Problems and Progress in Medical Care, Ninth Series*, G. McLachlan, ed. Nuffield Provincial Hospitals Trust, Oxford, pp. 17–55.

[35] Knox, E.G. (1975). Simulation studies of breast cancer screening programmes, in *Probes for Health*, G. McLachlan, ed. Oxford University Press, London, pp. 13–44.

[36] Knox, E.G. (1988). Evaluation of a proposed breast cancer screening regimen, *British Medical Journal* **297**, 650–654.

[37] Knox, E.G. & Woodman, C.B.J. (1988). Effectiveness of a cancer control programme, *Cancer Surveys* **7**, 379–401.

[38] Kottke, T.E., Gatewood, L.C., Wu, S.C. & Park, H.A. (1988). Preventing heart disease: is treating the high risk sufficient? *Journal of Clinical Epidemiology* **41**, 1083–1093.

[39] Lang, C.A. & Ransohoff, D.F. (1994). Fecal occult blood screening for colorectal cancer – is mortality reduced by chance selection for screening colonoscopy? *Journal of the American Medical Association* **271**, 1011–1013.

[40] Lee, H.L. & Pierskalla, W.P. (1988). Mass screening models for contagious diseases with no latent period, *Operations Research* **36**, 917–928.

[41] Lincoln, T. & Weiss, G.H. (1964). A statistical evaluation of recurrent medical examination, *Operations Research* **12**, 187–205.

[42] Louis, T.A., Albert, A. & Heghinian, S. (1978). Screening for the early detection of cancer – III. Estimation of disease natural history, *Mathematical Biosciences* **40**, 111–144.

[43] Mandel, J.S., Bond, J.H., Church, T.R., Snover, D.C., Bradley, G.M., Schuman, L.M. & Ederer, F. (1993). Reducing mortality from colorectal cancer by screening for fecal occult blood, *New England Journal of Medicine* **328**, 1365–1371.

[44] Miller, A.B., Chamberlain, J., Day, N.E., Hakema, M. & Prorok, P.C. (1990). Report on a workshop of the UICC Project on evaluation of screening for cancer, *International Journal of Cancer* **46**, 761–769.

[45] Morrison, A.S. (1985). *Screening in Chronic Disease*. Oxford University Press, New York.

[46] O'Neill, T.J., Tallis, G.M. & Leppard, P. (1995). A review of the technical features of breast cancer screening illustrated by a specific model using South Australian cancer registry data, *Statistical Methods in Medical Research* **4**, 55–72.

[47] Parkin, D.M. (1985). A computer simulation model for the practical planning of cervical cancer screening programmes, *British Journal of Cancer* **51**, 551–568.

[48] Prorok, P.C. (1976). The theory of periodic screening I: lead time and proportion detected, *Advances in Applied Probability* **8**, 127–143.

[49] Prorok, P.C. (1976). The theory of periodic screening II: doubly bounded recurrence times and mean lead time and detection probability estimation, *Advances in Applied Probability* **8**, 460–476.

[50] Prorok, P.C. (1986). Mathematical models and natural history in cervical cancer screening, in *Screening for Cancer of the Uterine Cervix*, M. Hakama, A.B. Miller & N.E. Day, eds. IARC Scientific Publication, Vol. 76, pp. 185–198.

[51] Prorok, P.C. (1988). Mathematical models of breast cancer screening, in *Screening for Breast Cancer*, N.E. Day & A.B. Miller, eds. Hans Huber, Toronto, pp. 95–109.

[52] Rutqvist, L.E. (1985). On the utility of the lognormal model for analysis of breast cancer survival in Sweden 1961–1973, *British Journal of Cancer* **52**, 875–883.

[53] Shapiro, S., Venet, W., Strax, P., Venet, L. & Roeser, R. (1982). Ten to fourteen year effect of screening on breast cancer mortality, *Journal of the National Cancer Institute* **69**, 349–355.

[54] Shwartz, M. (1978). A mathematical model used to analyse breast cancer screening strategies, *Operations Research* **26**, 937–955.

[55] Shwartz, M. (1978). An analysis of the benefits of serial screening for breast cancer based upon a mathematical model of the disease, *Cancer* **41**, 1550–1564.

[56] Shwartz, M. & Plough, A. (1984). Models to aid in planning cancer screening programs, in *Statistical Methods for Cancer Studies*, R.G. Cornell, ed. Marcel Dekker, New York, pp. 239–416.

[57] Stevenson, C.E., Glasziou, P., Carter, R., Fett, M.J. & van Oortmarssen, G.J. (1990). Using Computer Modelling to Estimate Person Years of Life Saved by Mammography Screening in Australia, Paper presented at the 1990 Annual Conference of the Public Health Association of Australia.

[58] Tabar, L., Fagerberg, G., Duffy, S. & Day, N.E. (1989). The Swedish two county trial of mammography screening for breast cancer: recent results and calculation of benefit, *Journal of Community Health* **43**, 107–114.

[59] van Oortmarssen, G.J. & Habbema, J.D. (1991). Epidemiological evidence for age-dependent regression of pre-invasive cervical cancer, *British Journal of Cancer* **64**, 559–565.

[60] van Oortmarssen, G.J., Habbema, J.D., Lubbe, K.T. & van der Maas, P.J. (1990). A model-based analysis of the HIP project for breast cancer screening, *International Journal of Cancer* **46**, 207–213.

[61] van Oortmarssen, G.J., Habbema, J.D., van der Maas, P.J., de Koning, H.J., Collette, H.J., Verbeek, A.L., Geerts, A.T. & Lubbe, K.T. (1990). A model for breast cancer screening, *Cancer* **66**, 1601–1612.

[62] Verbeek, A.L.M., Straatman, H. & Hendriks, J.H.C.L. (1988). Sensitivity of mammography in Nijmegen women under age 50: some trials with the Eddy model, in *Screening for Breast Cancer*, N.E. Day & A.B. Miller, eds. Hans Huber, Toronto, pp. 29–38.

[63] Walter, S.D. & Day, N.E. (1983). Estimation of the duration of a preclinical state using screening data, *American Journal of Epidemiology* **118**, 865–886.

[64] Walter, S.D. & Stitt, L.W. (1987). Evaluating the survival of cancer cases detected by screening, *Statistics in Medicine* **6**, 885–900.

[65] Zelen, M. & Feinleib, M. (1969). On the theory of screening for chronic diseases, *Biometrika* **56**, 601–614.

(*See also* **Incubation Period of Infectious Diseases**; **Prevalence of Disease, Estimation from Screening Data**)

CHRIS STEVENSON

Screening, Overview

The term "screening" is used to denote a variety of procedures in medicine and epidemiology. "Screening for disease" is mostly used to denote "the examination of asymptomatic people in order to classify them as likely, or unlikely, to have the disease that is the object of screening. People who appear likely to have disease are investigated further to arrive at a final diagnosis. Those people who are found to have the disease are then treated" (Morrison [18]).

This definition describes three distinguishing characteristics of screening for disease. First, screening is targeted at apparently healthy persons who are not aware of symptoms for which medical help would be sought. The **prevalence** of the disease in these persons will in general be (very) low. Secondly, the screening examination will give a crude distinction between persons with a normal test result, who do not receive further special attention, and persons in whom abnormalities are found in the screening test. Different grades of abnormalities may lead to more or less intensive follow-up, ranging from a repeat screening test to immediate treatment. Thirdly, appropriate treatment of disease which is detected early is expected to have a favorable impact on prognosis. The public health goal of screening for disease, "To reduce mortality or morbidity or to improve the quality of life" [12], is achieved by the more favorable outcome of early treatment in the cases identified by the screening test in comparison with similar cases that have been diagnosed on the basis of symptoms.

However, Table 1 shows that this benefit of screening is accrued by a very small proportion (group D+) of the persons screened. Inevitably screening will have a negative impact for other persons (groups C and D−). The small **risks** of some screening tests – for example, the increased risk of miscarriage following amniocentesis as part of antenatal screening, or the radiation risk of mammographic screening – cannot be disregarded completely given the very large number of tests performed (groups ABCD). Participation in screening for a serious disease will lead to anxiety, followed by relief when the result appears to be negative (groups A and B). Although this may sometimes be a relatively small effect, it cannot be neglected given the large number of persons involved.

False positive test results (group C) might lead to a (sometimes serious) burden of follow-up diagnostic tests needed to exclude disease. A true positive test result may still turn out to give adverse effects when early treatment does not improve the prognosis (group D−), but the person has been made aware of the disease for a longer period of time. Lack of improvement may occur when the outcome of early treatment remains unfavorable, but also when a person would have had a very good prognosis without screening.

Several extensions and modifications to the rather strict definition of Morrison are being used; see, for example, Holland & Stewart [13] or Wald [22]. For example, the term screening is also used to describe identification of people at high *risk* of disease (for example, high cholesterol or blood pressure levels) instead of early detection of the disease itself. The public health goal of screening for a disease may also be achieved indirectly, e.g. by preventing morbidity and mortality in other persons than those being screened. For example, specific groups of individuals, such as employees in the food industry, persons applying for a driving licence, or a circumscribed population in which an outbreak of an infectious disease occurred, may be screened to protect the general population.

Table 1 The different outcomes of screening, their usual impact and frequency. Extended version of table given by Morrison [18]

	Outcome	Impact	Proportion of target population
O	Nonparticipation	?	medium–large
A	True negative	anxiety, relief, side-effects of test	large
B	False negative	anxiety, false relief, side-effects of test	very small
C	False positive	moderate adverse effects	(very) small
D−	True positive, serious condition not postponed	adverse	(very) small
D+	True positive, serious condition postponed	large benefit	very small

Performing screening tests in an asymptomatic population can also have a scientific aim, such as to estimate the population prevalence of certain conditions, for example human immunodeficiency virus (HIV) infection (*see* **Prevalence of Disease, Estimation from Screening Data**). This extended usage of the term screening is reflected in the more general definition of McKeown [17]: "A medical investigation which does not arise from a patient's request for advice for a specific complaint".

In medicine and epidemiology, usage of the term screening is not necessarily related to testing of (asymptomatic) individuals, but is often used as a synonym for "testing". In clinical medicine, screening is used to denote testing of symptomatic patients to establish a diagnosis. It is also used in laboratory testing of donor blood for HIV infections, for example, and in medical research (laboratory, epidemiologic surveillance), the term screening is used to denote testing of chemical agents to identify toxic substances.

Discussion of screening for disease in this Section is confined to screening adhering to the strict definition of Morrison, while admitting that it is difficult to draw exact boundaries for this definition. Examples will mostly be derived from cancer screening studies. (See the series *Screening Brief* in the *Journal of Medical Screening* for up-to-date information on screening programs for specific diseases.)

A broad distinction can be made between, on the one hand, genetic screening, and most antenatal and neonatal screening procedures which involve a single screening examination and, on the other hand, screening for chronic diseases, including screening for problems during growth of children and screening for cancer in adults, which typically involve repeated screening tests with intervals between several months to years.

Genetic screening can be done at different times throughout life. It can be performed prior to conception to inform persons of a high risk of conceiving a child with a severe disorder, during pregnancy for early detection and elective termination of pregnancy, shortly after birth to detect treatable disorders, or later in life to enable preventive measures which reduce the risk of developing serious disorders. In antenatal and neonatal screening, optimal timing of the test is important because the gestational age or age of the child determine the **sensitivity** and **specificity** of the test(s) and the possibilities for intervention.

In the case of repeated screening examinations for early detection of diseases such as (breast, cervical, or colorectal) cancer, proper timing of tests is even more complicated because of various time-related factors involved: incidence and prevalence of the detectable preclinical phase (DPCP) varies with age, the sojourn time of the DPCP varies between persons, and test characteristics and the outcome of early treatment vary during the course of the DPCP. The number of factors involved, and the dynamic interrelations between factors, complicate the design, analysis and evaluation of such screening programs (*see* **Screening, Models of**).

Important questions in analysis and evaluation of screening for disease are:

1. Will screening indeed reduce the mortality and/or morbidity in the population and, if so, what is the estimated magnitude of the reduction?
2. What are the favorable and adverse effects and costs of different screening policies, and what will be the impact on existing health care? A policy is characterized by the recommended age(-range) to be screened, the screening test(s) used, the intervals between examinations in the case of repeated screening, and the diagnostic follow-up and subsequent treatment to be applied.
3. What are efficient policies, and is screening worthwhile?
4. Does the screening program, when implemented as part of routine care, perform adequately?

These issues are discussed in turn in the following sections.

Establishing the Effectiveness of Screening

The effect of a certain screening policy on mortality and morbidity depends on several factors, such as the screening test, the natural history of the disease, the diagnostic and treatment options for the disease, the improvement in prognosis resulting from early treatment, and, at the level of the population, the degree of participation in the screening program, including possible selective participation of high risk groups. Figure 1 shows these factors for a single screening examination, one screening test, and a disease with a fixed duration for the DPCP.

Together, these factors determine not only the positive health effect of screening, but also its negative

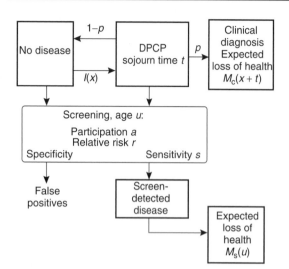

Figure 1 A single screening examination for a disease with a DPCP starting at age x. Without screening, the disease will remain unnoticed until progressive cases are diagnosed clinically at age $z = x + t$. Screening at age u will lead to false positive test results, but also to early detection and treatment for part of the prevalent cases at age u, i.e. in participants for which $x < u < x + t$ and the test result is correct. These true positive cases will include persons with nonprogressive disease that would never have been diagnosed in the absence of screening

$$
\begin{aligned}
x &= \text{age at onset of the DPCP} \\
I(x) &= \text{incidence density of the DPCP} \\
t &= \text{sojourn time in the DPCP, probability density} \\
 &\quad f(t) \\
p &= \text{proportion with progressive disease among} \\
 &\quad \text{incidence } I(x) \\
a &= \text{proportion participating in screening at age } u \\
r &= \text{relative risk of participants} \\
s &= \text{sensitivity of the screening test} \\
M_s(u) &= \text{expected loss of health following detection by} \\
 &\quad \text{screening at age } u \\
M_c(z) &= \text{expected loss of health following clinical} \\
 &\quad \text{diagnosis at age } z = x + t
\end{aligned}
$$

effects and its costs. Figure 2 shows examples of disease histories, starting from the onset of the DPCP, for which screening has favorable or adverse effects. In these examples it is assumed that the main goal of screening is to prevent death from the disease, such as, for example, in cancer screening. A cure point is indicated, denoting a hypothetical point in the history where treatment ceases to be effective [9].

In history (a), the disease is detected by a true positive screening test result, and death from the disease is to be prevented by screening since detection

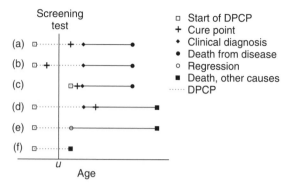

Figure 2 Example disease histories that are missed, diagnosed without benefit, or diagnosed with favorable effect, by a single screening examination at age u. The cure point indicates a hypothetical moment in the disease history where treatment ceases to be effective. The thick line indicates the DPCP

occurs before the cure point. Death from the disease will not be prevented in the case of a false negative test result or inadequate follow-up in this history. Screening will also be ineffective and have merely adverse effects when it is too late (history (b)), or when the DPCP has a short sojourn time and is missed by the screen (history (c)). Screening has no impact on mortality and clear negative effects in history (d), where clinical diagnosis would also have occurred before the cure point, in history (e) of regressive disease where the DPCP would never have been detected in the absence of screening, and in history (f) where the person dies from other causes before the disease would have been diagnosed clinically. The increasing likelihood of the last type of history at older ages should be kept in mind in evaluating screening for diseases such as cancer of the prostate that mainly occur in the elderly.

The lead time is the length of the time interval between the moments of detection by screening and clinical diagnosis without screening. The average lead time is indicative of the potential positive effect of screening, since a longer average lead time means that more cases can be detected before the cure point is reached. But in histories (b) and (d), the lead time only represents a negative effect: the person is merely aware of having serious disease for a longer period of time. Histories (a) and (c) illustrate the **length-biased** sampling phenomenon, which means that screening tends to pick up histories with long sojourn times selectively. Zelen & Feinleib [26] have pointed out the consequences for the mean lead time ($\bar{L}$) of screen-detected cases at a single screening examination:

$$\bar{L} = \frac{1}{2}\left(\bar{t} + \frac{\sigma_t^2}{\bar{t}}\right), \qquad (1)$$

indicating that the mean lead time is longer than the mean sojourn time $\bar{t}$ when the variance σ_t^2 of the sojourn time distribution exceeds its mean value.

For the simplified situation of Figure 1 with a single screening test at age u, the true prevalence $D(u)$ of preclinical disease is given by

$$D(u) = \int_{x=0}^{u}\int_{t=u-x}^{\infty} I(x)f(t)\mathrm{d}t\mathrm{d}x, \qquad (2)$$

where $I(x)$ denotes the incidence density of the DPCP and $f(t)$ the probability density function of the sojourn time t in the DPCP.

The expected health effects $G(u)$ for the population in which this single screening examination is taking place accrue to the screen-detected cases. This is a subset of the prevalent cases, including persons who participate in screening and have a certain associated **relative risk**, and for whom the test has a true positive result. The health effect for these cases is obtained by subtracting the loss of health M_c in a situation without screening for the fraction p of progressive cases, which would have been diagnosed clinically at age $x + t$, from the loss of health M_s in all screen-detected cases at age u in the situation with screening:

$$G(u) = \int_{x=0}^{u}\int_{t=u-x}^{\infty} I(x)f(t)ars$$
$$\times\, [M_s(u) - pM_c(x + t)]\mathrm{d}t\mathrm{d}x, \qquad (3)$$

where $I(x)$ denotes the **incidence density** of the DPCP, $f(t)$ the probability density of the sojourn time t in the DPCP, a the proportion participating in screening at age u, r the relative risk of participants, and s the sensitivity of the screening test.

In (3), the lead time for screen-detected progressive cases is $x + t - u$, the time interval between detection at screening and clinical diagnosis in the absence of screening. In the example of a potentially lethal disease as presented in Figure 2, the measures M_c and M_s for the loss of health might be taken to represent the lethality from the disease following diagnosis and treatment. Comparison of M_c and

M_s on the individual level is, of course, impossible, because the exact clinically diagnosed counterparts of screen-detected cases will always remain unknown.

In general it will be difficult to obtain direct estimates of the components of (3), except for $M_c(\cdot)$ and $M_s(\cdot)$, which may be based on follow-up registries (*see* **Disease Registers**) of clinically diagnosed and screen-detected patients. Although it is tempting to compare $M_c(\cdot)$ and $M_s(\cdot)$ directly, this will give rise to incorrect conclusions because of four sources of sampling **bias** that all tend to lead to a too favorable estimate for the effect of screening.

If not all preclinical stages progress ($p < 1.0$), then the comparison will yield a too optimistic estimate because of overdiagnosis bias (see history (e) in Figure 2.) Self-selection bias (*see* **Selection Bias**) with respect to survival occurs when participants in screening would have had a better prognosis anyhow, for example because of self-selection of health-conscious persons. Self-selection may also be related to the risk of developing the disease. Participants have been observed to have a higher than average risk in breast cancer screening [23], but the opposite has been observed in cervical cancer screening [1]. Lead time bias occurs when cumulative lethality is compared for equal durations of follow-up after diagnosis, giving screen-detected cases an advantage equal to the duration of the lead time even in the absence of a real effect of screening. Length-biased sampling will also lead to biased comparisons if the sojourn time and M_c are correlated, for example when slowly developing preclinical disease also has a better-than-average prognosis.

Lead time bias and length biased sampling are specific for screening, and different approaches have been proposed to correct these biases [24]. However, these correction methods are always based on assumptions about the sojourn time distribution, and will not lead to unambiguous evidence about the effect of screening.

The four biases can only be avoided by conducting a randomized controlled trial (RCT). In its basic form, a population involved in an RCT is randomly divided in a study group in which persons are invited to be screened, and a **control** group in which no screening is offered. The endpoint to be compared between the two groups is the condition that is to be prevented by early detection and treatment, for example mortality in cancer screening. Use of other endpoints – for example, diagnosis of malignancy in cervical cancer screening – might lead to biased estimates of the effect of screening when, on average, screen-detected cases are less severe than clinically diagnosed cases. A huge population will be needed to obtain sufficient power, and several design variants have been proposed to limit trial costs [9]. The impact of trials has been considerable, both in diminishing the use of screening for lung cancer, and in speeding up implementation of breast cancer screening program in several countries. Screening for lung cancer did not turn out to be effective according to RCT results, despite clear differences in survival between screen-detected and clinically diagnosed patients [10]. In most RCTs conducted thus far, screening for breast cancer has been found to reduce breast cancer mortality in women above age 50, but results for women below age 50 are still not conclusive [5, 21].

Use of disease-specific outcome measures in an RCT is controversial. Critics state that the beneficial effect should be checked from overall mortality and morbidity. But this would require an enormous trial size. Even the combined results of four Swedish breast cancer trials, with a relative risk for breast cancer death of 0.80 (95% confidence interval (CI) 0.70–0.92) did not show a discernible effect on overall mortality in the trial population [20].

Some screening tests that are widely used have never been rigorously tested in an RCT. One example is cervical cancer screening, for which a very large RCT would be required. In such a situation, estimates of the effectiveness of screening can only be obtained from nonexperimental designs, such as **cohort studies, case–control studies**, and **ecologic studies**.

In cohort studies, a comparison of morbidity and mortality is made between persons with different screening experience in the cohort. Case–control studies for testing the effectiveness of screening have become increasingly popular, but the outcomes are highly sensitive to several kinds of bias such as overdiagnosis bias, self-selection bias, and healthy screenee bias (see Morrison [18] or Weiss [25]). This has been demonstrated empirically by performing a case–control study on data from an RCT [11].

In ecologic studies, an investigation is made into the association between the morbidity or mortality and the screening intensity in different populations. Cervical cancer screening is now generally considered to be effective on the basis

of the findings of many **observational studies:** cohort studies and case–control studies (International Agency for Research against Cancer (IARC) Working Group [14]) and ecologic analyses (see, for example, Läärä et al. [16]).

The Favorable and Adverse Effects and Costs of Alternative Policies

When screening is being considered in a country or region, usually different screening policies are being considered which might differ in their effects and costs. Only a limited number of policies have been rigorously tested in RCTs, which are typically carried out in countries or regions with marked differences with respect to, for example, incidence or mortality rate, participation in screening, and specific characteristics and quality of the screening procedures. Furthermore, the long follow-up in many screening trials implies that their results typically pertain to screening technology from the past. These observations complicate both combined analysis of trial results, and extrapolation of these results to other situations such as the near future in a new country in which screening is being considered. Also, RCTs tend to focus on the serious health effects to be prevented by screening (category D+ in Table 1), paying less attention to the adverse effects of screening.

Two methods are used to resolve (partially) these problems – modeling and use of surrogate endpoint measures.

In building a model, assumptions have to be made about the factors listed in Figure 1. These assumptions can be checked by fitting the model to available data from RCTs and to data from nonexperimental screening studies. For example, outcomes of cancer screening models are compared with observed detection rates at successive screening rounds, incidence of clinical disease in the interval between screening exams, and with the stage-distribution of these different types of cases. Characteristics of, and trends in, background variables can be taken into account explicitly in a model. In this way, known differences between trials can be incorporated in combined analyses of RCT results (see [5]). Models are increasingly being used to make predictions about other screening policies than those tested in trials, and to transfer outcomes from trials to specific characteristics in other areas (see, for example, [6]).

Introducing screening for a disease in a population will change the type and amount of diagnostic and treatment procedures for this disease. In a first screening round, a relatively large pool of prevalent cases will have a positive test result, leading to a temporary increase in demand for assessment and treatment, followed by a decrease in later screening rounds. Models can make quite detailed predictions of these changes, which is useful in planning of equipment, recruitment, and training of personnel, and in anticipation of changes in clinical procedures [4].

The number of assumptions used in screening models may easily become quite large, and some of these assumptions lack a thorough foundation. Use of surrogate outcome measures can be regarded as an attempt to obtain a more direct empirical basis in comparing different policies, without the lengthy follow-up period needed in large RCTs [2]. A surrogate outcome measure is a short-term observed result of a screening program that is known (or suspected) to be closely associated with the long-term impact on morbidity and mortality. Such a relation can be estimated from RCT data. For example, mortality reduction after breast cancer screening has been shown to be closely associated with particular changes in the stage distribution of diagnosed cancer cases.

Surrogate outcome measures can be used to evaluate various small adaptations of policies that have already been proven to be effective. The surrogate outcome measures of the policy variants can be compared directly, and the observed differences can also be translated into predicted differences in reduction of mortality and morbidity.

Efficient Policies

In deciding about screening policies an important criterion is the ratio of the health effects of a screening program and its incremental costs, i.e. the difference in (medical) costs between the situation with and without screening. The incremental costs of a screening policy are directly related to the cost of administering and assessing the screening test, but may also be influenced by the impact of screening on the demand for diagnostic and treatment procedures. For each level of the incremental costs, an optimal screening policy exists which gives the highest effectiveness (net health benefit) or the best cost-effectiveness

ratio. Figure 3 shows a typical intensity–response relationship which emerges when different numbers of screenings are compared. The net health benefit is relatively high for a single screening test. The extra benefit decreases for each additional screening examination. When the number of screening tests per person increases, the adverse effects of screening might well become larger than the favorable effects. For example, extending screening to older ages will increasingly lead to detection of cases that would not have been diagnosed in the absence of screening, leading to reduction in quality of life that is no longer compensated for by a decrease in mortality.

Although the top of the curve in Figure 3 represents the policy with the maximum effectiveness, the marginal cost-effectiveness of this policy is very poor. If the x-axis of Figure 3 represents costs, the curve can be interpreted as the efficient frontier, i.e. the set of all Pareto-optimal screening policies – policies for which no alternative can be found that give both higher health benefits and lower costs [8]. A good policy on this frontier would be the one which still shows an acceptable marginal cost-effectiveness ratio.

Simulation models have been applied to derive the efficient frontier of screening policies [7, 8, 15].

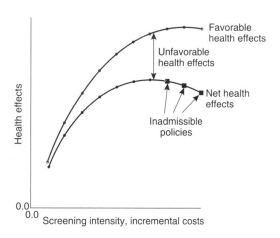

Figure 3 Relation between intensity of screening and its favorable and unfavorable health effects (intensity–response curve) or similarly between the incremental costs of screening and health effects (efficient frontier). The net health benefit summarizes the favorable and adverse effects of screening

Monitoring of Screening Program

If screening is not conducted properly, effectiveness and cost-effectiveness can easily be impaired. A well-known example is the cervical cancer screening program in the UK, which has not been able to prevent increasing mortality rates in young women [19]. Each of the stages in the screening process could give rise to loss of potential benefits, and sometimes also to excessive negative effects. Sufficient coverage of the population at risk, adequate administration of the test and interpretation of test results, compliance with follow-up in the case of suspicious results, and proper treatment of early stages of the disease are all necessary to achieve the health benefits at a reasonable cost. Quality assurance and monitoring are important in this respect.

Measures of performance can be defined for each component of a screening program – e.g. the participation rate and **predictive value** of a positive test result – and should encompass diagnostic and treatment procedures applied to screen-detected disease. Target values for the short-term results of a screening program (such as detection rates and incidence of interval cases) can be specified on the basis of experience from randomized trials and pilot projects [3]. Regular evaluation of the screening results and of the costs of the screening program may than lead to timely revision of the screening policy.

References

[1]   Boyes, D.A., Morrison, B., Knox, E.G., Draper, G.J. & Miller, A.B. (1982). A cohort study of cervical cancer screening in British Columbia, *Clinical Investigations in Medicine* **5**, 1–29.

[2]   Day, N.E. (1991). Surrogate measures in the design of breast cancer screening trials, in *Cancer Screening*, A.B. Miller, J. Chamberlain, N.E. Day, M. Hakama & P.C. Prorok, eds. Cambridge University Press, Cambridge, pp. 392–403.

[3]   Day, N.E., Williams, D.R.R. & Khaw, K.T. (1989). Breast cancer screening programmes: the development of a monitoring and evaluation system, *British Journal of Cancer* **59**, 954–958.

[4]   De Koning, H.J., Van Oortmarssen, G.J., Van Ineveld, B.M. & Van der Maas, P.J. (1990). Breast cancer screening: its impact on clinical medicine, *British Journal of Cancer* **61**, 292–297.

[5]   De Koning, H.J., Boer, R., Warmerdam, P.G., Beemsterboer, P.M.M. & Van der Maas, P.J. (1995). Quantitative interpretation of age-specific mortality reductions

from the Swedish breast cancer screening trials, *Journal of the National Cancer Institute* **87**, 1217–1223.

[6]   Eddy, D.M. (1980). *Screening for Cancer: Theory, Analysis and Design*. Prentice-Hall, Englewood Cliffs.

[7]   Eddy, D.M. (1990). Screening for cervical cancer, *Annals of Internal Medicine* **113**, 214–226.

[8]   Eddy, D.M. (1990). Screening for colorectal cancer, *Annals of Internal Medicine* **113**, 373–384.

[9]   Etzioni, R.D., Connor, R.J., Prorok, P.C. & Self, S.G. (1995). Design and analysis of cancer screening trials, *Statistical Methods in Medical Research* **4**, 3–17.

[10]   Flehinger, B.J., Kimmel, M., Polyak, T. & Melamed, M.R. (1993). Screening for lung cancer, *Cancer* **72**, 1573–1580.

[11]   Gullberg, B., Andersson, I., Janzon, L. & Ranstam, J. (1991). Screening mammography, *Lancet* **337**, 244.

[12]   Hakama, M. (1991). Screening, in *Oxford Textbook of Public Health*, Vol. 3. Oxford University Press, Oxford.

[13]   Holland, W.W. & Stewart, S. (1990). *Screening in Health Care – Benefit or Bane?* The Nuffield Provincial Hospitals Trust, London.

[14]   IARC Working Group on Evaluation of Cervical Cancer Screening Programmes (1986). Screening for squamous cervical cancer: duration of low risk after negative results of cervical cytology and its implication for screening policies, *British Medical Journal* **293**, 659–664.

[15]   Koopmanschap M.A., Lubbe J.Th.N., Van Oortmarssen G.J., Van Agt, H.M.E., Van Ballegooijen, M. & Habbema, J.D.F. (1990). Economic aspects of cervical cancer screening. *Social Science and Medicine* **30**, 1081–1087.

[16]   Läärä, E., Day, N.E. & Hakama, M. (1987). Trends in mortality from cervical cancer in the Nordic countries: association with organized screening programmes, *Lancet* **i**, 1247–1249.

[17]   McKeown, T. (1968). Validation of screening procedures, in *Screening in Medical Care: Reviewing the Evidence*. The Nuffield Provincial Hospitals Trust, Oxford.

[18]   Morrison, A.S. (1992). *Screening in Chronic Disease*, 2nd Ed. Oxford University Press, New York.

[19]   Murphy, M.F.G., Campbell, M.J. & Goldblatt, P.O. (1988). Twenty years' screening for cervical cancer of the uterine cervix in Great Britain, 1964–84: further evidence for its ineffectiveness, *Journal of Epidemiology and Community Health* **42**, 49–53.

[20]   Nyström, L., Larsson, L.-G., Wall, S., Rutqvist, L.E., Andersson, I., Bjurstam, N., Fagerberg, G., Frisell, J. & Tabár, L. (1996). An overview of the Swedish randomized mammography trials: total mortality pattern and the representativity of the study cohorts, *Journal of Medical Screening* **3**, 85–87.

[21]   Nyström, L., Rutqvist, L.E., Wall, S., Lindgren, A., Lindqvist, M., Rydén, S., Andersson, I., Bjurstam, N., Fagerberg, G., Frisell, J., Tabár, L., & Larsson, L-G. (1993). Breast cancer screening with mammography: overview of Swedish randomized trials, *Lancet* **341**, 973–978.

[22] Wald, N.J. (1994). Guidance on Terminology, *Journal of Medical Screening* **1**, 76.

[23] Walter, S.D. & Day, N.E. (1983). Estimation of the duration of the pre-clinical state using screening data, *American Journal of Epidemiology* **118**, 865–886.

[24] Walter, S.D. & Stitt, L.W. (1987). Evaluating the survival of cancer cases detected by screening, *Statistics in Medicine* **6**, 885–900.

[25] Weiss, N.S. (1994). Application of the case–control method in the evaluation of screening, *Epidemiologic Reviews* **16**, 102–108.

[26] Zelen, M. & Feinleib, M. (1969). On the theory of screening for chronic diseases, *Biometrika* **56**, 601–613.

(*See also* **Diagnostic Tests, Evaluation of**)

GERRIT J. VAN OORTMARSSEN

Secondary Base Case–Control Study *see* Case–Control Study

SEIR Model *see* Infectious Disease Models

Selection Bias

Selection bias is a **bias** that arises when individuals included in a study are not representative of the **target population** for the study. Selection bias can arise because an inappropriate sampling frame is used, because inappropriate sampling methods are applied, or because some of those sampled refuse to participate in the study (*see* **Bias from Nonresponse**). In studies relying on samples of convenience, such as **hospital-based case–control studies** or clinical trials in which patients volunteer for particular treatments, it is difficult to rule out the possibility of selection bias (*see* **Bias in Case–Control Studies; Bias in Cohort Studies; Bias in Observational Studies; Bias, Overview; Missing Data in Epidemiologic Studies; Validity and Generalizability in Epidemiologic Studies**).

M.H. GAIL

Self-Selection Bias *see* Validity and Generalizability in Epidemiologic Studies

Sensitivity

In the context of diagnostic testing or disease **screening**, sensitivity refers to the proportion of individuals with the target disease who have a positive test result. In other words, it is the probability that an actual case of disease will be correctly diagnosed by the test. In probability terms, sensitivity is Pr(positive test|disease). Consider Table 1 for the general relationship between the test results and the true disease state. Then, the sensitivity is given by $a/(a + c)$. A synonym is the *true positive rate*, invoking the proportion of positive test results among the denominator of true disease cases.

Achievement of high sensitivity is important when case detection is important, specifically where the implied costs of missing disease cases (i.e. giving false negative test results to cases) are high relative to the costs of incorrectly assigning positive test results to individuals without the disease (the so-called false positive results). Typically, if the test is designed for high sensitivity, the false positive rate $b/(b + d)$ will also be high and the test **specificity** $d/(b + d)$ will be low.

A test with high sensitivity is useful clinically for the purpose of ruling out possible disease; a negative result from such a test implies a relatively high chance of not having the disease.

Therapeutic decisions are often considered using a likelihood ratio calculation. The likelihood ratio, LR, here is

$$LR = \frac{\text{Pr(positive test|disease)}}{\text{Pr(positive test|no disease)}}$$

Table 1

	Disease present	Disease absent
Test positive	a	b
Test negative	c	d

or, equivalently the ratio of sensitivity to $(1 -$ specificity). The positive and negative **predictive values** are also relevant.

In simple formulations, sensitivity and specificity are often assumed to be independent of the **prevalence** of disease in the population. In practice, these test characteristics may actually depend on prevalence, for a variety of reasons. For instance, if testing is carried out in a population in which the prevalence is higher because of a greater proportion of mild disease, one would expect sensitivity to be lower. Such effects may occur artifactually on occasion; for instance, because of different clinical definitions of disease operative in various populations.

A second meaning of sensitivity is used in the context of describing the measurement properties of a device. The sensitivity here refers to the smallest stimulus that the device can detect, or the smallest input required so that the device can provide an appropriate output. This idea is commonly used to describe electronic components, but is also used to characterize the lowest concentration or amount of a substance that is detectable by the device, such as in clinical chemistry testing. A similar interpretation pertains to the sensitivity of an individual, organism or biological system, depending on the context.

In the context of data analysis, sensitivity may refer to the degree of dependence of the results to assumptions invoked by the particular techniques employed (e.g. an assumption of normality in a regression calculation), or to features in the data (e.g. the presence and position of an outlier observation). Lack of sensitivity to such characteristics is known as robustness. For further details of methods to examine sensitivity (in this sense), see sensitivity analysis.

Bibliography

Altman, D.G. (1991). *Practical Statistics for Medical Research*. Chapman & Hall, London, Chapter 14.

Sackett, D.L., Haynes, R.B., Guyatt, G.H. & Tugwell, P. (1991). *Clinical Epidemiology: A Basic Science for Clinical Medicine*, 2nd Ed. Little, Brown, & Company Boston, Chapter 4.

(*See also* **Clinical Epidemiology, Overview**; **Diagnostic Tests, Evaluation of**)

S.D. WALTER

Sex Ratio at Birth

Most human populations contain approximately equal numbers of males and females. This apparent equality can clearly be only approximate, since the mortality and migration rates of the two sexes vary in different ways with age and with time. In most communities the males slightly outnumber the females at birth, a ratio of about 1.05 being typical, but are subject to higher mortality rates, so that females are in excess at higher ages and have the higher expectations of life. Studies of the variation in the sex ratio are predominantly concerned with the sex ratio at birth, conventionally expressed as the ratio of males to females (sometimes multiplied by 100 or 1000). In some research studies it is more convenient to use the proportion of males, denoted here by p. More formally, the ratio at birth is the *secondary sex ratio*, the *primary sex ratio* being the ratio at conception. Reference is sometimes made to the less well-defined *tertiary sex ratio*, the ratio of males to females at an age at which children become independent of their parents, or perhaps at the onset of reproductive capacity.

The primary sex ratio is especially difficult to estimate, since many early spontaneous abortions are not observed. The equiprobability of X- and Y-bearing sperm might lead one to expect a ratio of unity. However, some workers have suggested that the ratio is very high, sperm bearing the Y-chromosome perhaps being more successful in achieving fertilization. Conversely, Hytten [20] argues that in spontaneous abortions during the first trimester females considerably outnumber males, suggesting that the primary sex ratio is quite low. Later in pregnancy there are more male than female fetuses, but more males than females miscarry or are stillborn. McKeown & Lowe [31] reported that sex ratios in early stillbirths (after 28 weeks' gestation) were not greatly in excess of unity, but that they increased slightly with gestational age.

The secondary sex ratio (for which we shall use merely the term "sex ratio") has been a topic of statistical interest for over 200 years. Statisticians and probabilists in the eighteenth and nineteenth centuries seized on the data emerging from birth registers to exemplify the developing theory of binary events; we summarize their work below. During the twentieth century most studies have been motivated by demographic, epidemiologic or genetic considerations. From the demographic point of view, the sex ratio contributes to an understanding of the age–sex composition of a population, although its effect is very limited because it varies between populations to such a small extent. The epidemiologist is interested in even small differences in the sex ratio between population groups, or in trends over time, because they may point to the possible effects of environmental agents or differing lifestyles.

Much interest has focused on surveys of the sex distributions in families of various sizes. These studies are interesting from a general point of view, and in relation to the effects of family limitation. Perhaps a more important purpose is to examine the evidence for variability in the sex ratio, in order to shed light on the heritability of the sex ratio [9]. If the tendency to produce an excess of offspring of one or the other sex is genetically determined, then it will be subject to natural selection. Fisher [13] and others [22, 23] have offered theories as to how such a mechanism might act. It is therefore of some interest to see whether distributions of the sex composition in different families provide any evidence for such variation. As we shall note later, such evidence is hard to find.

Early Studies

The following summaries rely heavily on the much fuller accounts given by Hald [18, 19]. The earliest statistical study appears to be that of Graunt [17], who noted the slight excess of males at both christenings and burials, in both London and Romsey. Graunt regarded the near equality as a justification for the practice of monogamy rather than polygamy.

Arbuthnot's study [1] is celebrated as the first recorded example of a statistical significance test. Arbuthnot noted that, for each of the 82 years between 1629 and 1710, there were more male than female christenings in London. A sign test gives a p-value of $(1/2)^{82}$. Arbuthnot regarded the excess of male christenings (and hence, presumably, of births) as evidence of divine providence in compensating for the higher mortality risks encountered by males. The calculations of Nicholas Bernoulli [3] showed that the 82 proportions of males are over-dispersed relative to the binomial distribution, although Bernoulli himself appears to have accepted the hypothesis of homogeneity, the mean proportion of males being 0.516.

Daniel Bernoulli [2] used the normal approximation to the binomial to study a related data set, i.e. of christenings in London between 1664 and 1758. He noted that the overall estimate of p was 0.513, but that the value fell to 0.510 during the decade 1721–1730. Taking the 10 values during that decade, he showed that they agreed with normal variation for $p = 0.510$ (as judged by the number of years for which the value fell within probable error limits), but less satisfactorily for $p = 0.513$. The demographers Struyck (1687–1769) and Süssmilch (1707–1767), in the meantime, had extended Graunt's descriptive work to cover data sets from various regions, but avoiding any probabilistic analyses.

Laplace [26] used the numbers of male and female births in Paris during the period 1745–1770 to illustrate the calculation of a posterior probability using the normal approximation to the binomial, finding, of course, that the probability of a ratio favoring females was extremely low. Cournot [4] used a similar approach to compare sex ratios in different subgroups, showing an awareness of the danger of multiple comparisons. Poisson [33] examined births in France for 1817–1826, and found no evidence for over-dispersion between these 10 values, again using the normal approximation. He then examined the yearly figures for different administrative areas, and found too high a frequency of instances where female births were in excess, suggesting that variation between years and between areas had been obscured in the overall picture.

Recent Epidemiologic Work

Although the eighteenth- and nineteenth-century workers were mainly concerned to illustrate theoretical results by using conveniently extensive sets of binary data, many of them were interested in variations in p between different population groups. Explanations of these differences were less easy to find.

Modern workers have access to even more extensive data sets, and publications exploring group differences abound. Yet, explanations remain contentious, and different studies often seem contradictory.

Time trends in national data sets are easily established. Between 1838 and 1997 the sex ratio for live births in England and Wales showed a roughly sinusoidal curve, with smoothed values falling from about 1.05 to 1.04 around 1895, rising to about 1.06 between 1945 and 1975, and falling to a little over 1.05 in 1995 [29, Figure 6.5]. A similar trend in Japan between 1900 and 1995, with a peak at about 1.07 around 1970 and a subsequent fall to about 1.05 in 1995, is reported by Ohmi et al. [32]. Similar recent falls have been reported for other countries [5].

Many other associations have been reported. Black populations have frequently been shown to have low ratios, but extensive ethnic comparisons are hampered by the lack of reliable data in many developing countries. The sex ratio tends to decline with maternal age [28]. A negative relationship with the sex ratio has been reported for a very wide range of factors, including maternal smoking, maternal schizophrenia, fathers who fly extensively, births in late autumn and winter, and multiple births, with a complex effect of parents' hormonal levels and time of conception during the menstrual cycle [20, 29]. The sex ratio tends to decline with increases in the stillbirth rate, a natural consequence of the higher ratio for stillbirths.

Claims for associations need to be replicated with sufficiently large studies to eliminate random variation and serendipitous selection. However, there seems to be a general finding that low sex ratios are associated with deprivation of some sort. Unexpected changes in the sex ratio may therefore provide a form of monitoring to detect adverse environmental effects. This must, however, be a rather blunt instrument, as the change in sex ratio may not become evident for some time after the causative event, and the effect will be nonspecific. In 1978 the sex ratio in Northern Ireland (and in three adjacent countries of the Republic of Ireland) was unusually low (about 1.01), but no explanation has been found.

Family Studies

Geissler [14] published data on the distributions of boys and girls in families of various sizes, for about four million births in Saxony for 1876–1885. The data have various deficiencies, being derived from statements by parents at the time of birth registration, recording the numbers of previous children of each sex. They have, nevertheless, been the subject of extensive analyses by, among others, Gini [15, 16], Fisher [12], Lancaster [24] and Edwards [6]. Much of the research has been concerned with

possible deviations from the binomial distributions to be expected from purely random sampling with constant p. One difficulty here is that parents may be less likely to stop having children if the current sex distribution is unbalanced, so the sex distributions of completed families of any given size above two might be expected to show excess frequencies for the extreme categories. However, this effect of family limitation may have been less pronounced in Geissler's data than in some later data sets of this type.

Lancaster's [24] doubts about the reliability of Geissler's data were dismissed by Gini [16] and Edwards [6], but have been reiterated by Lancaster [25]. Edwards [6] concluded that the data showed excess variability of p between families, which he represented by the beta-binomial distribution, and Lindsey & Altham [27] fitted a variety of models for over-dispersion, suggesting that the effect increased with family size.

Edwards and Fraccaro have analyzed several later data sets in which the sequence of boys and girls in each family is recorded: 14 230 French families [7], 5477 Swedish families [10, 11], and 60 334 Finnish families [8]. The Swedish data show no evidence of any form of heterogeneity. The French and Finnish data support the hypothesis of a positive correlation between the sexes of adjacent births, as distinct from the fixed correlation between *all* members of the family that would be expected if there were merely a between-family variance component.

The possible effect of family limitation on these data sets is unclear. As Edwards & Fraccaro observe, the effect may be mitigated by considering the frequencies of different ordered sex combinations in the first N children in families with N or more, but this is not a complete solution to the problem. An alternative approach is to estimate p directly from observations of the Nth birth, separately for each ordered combination of outcomes for the first $N - 1$. Maconochie & Roman [30] examined in this way a large collection of 549 048 singleton births in Scotland from 1975 to 1988, derived from linked records of maternity discharges. They found no evidence of heterogeneity between families, or for the effect of birth order, maternal age, maternal height, paternal or maternal social class, year of delivery, or season of birth, the estimated sex ratio being 1.06.

The evidence for heterogeneity between families is thus, at best, equivocal. If heterogeneity were to be clearly established, it would remain to be shown that this was genetic rather than environmental. As Edwards [9] remarks, "... if genetic variability exists, it is of a very low order of magnitude".

The articles by Edwards [9] and James [21] provide more extensive reviews of the literature on the sex ratio.

Acknowledgments

I am grateful to Drs Anthony Edwards and Alison Macfarlane for suggesting many of the references used in this article.

References

[1]   Arbuthnot, J. (1712). An argument for Divine Providence, taken from the constant regularity observ'd in the births of both sexes, *Philosophical Transactions of the Royal Society of London* **27**, 186–190. Reprinted in *Studies in the History of Statistics and Probability*, Vol.2, M.G. Kendall & R.L. Plackett, eds. Griffin, London, 1977.

[2]   Bernoulli, D. (1770–1771). Mensura sortis ad fortuitam successionem rerum naturaliter contingentium applicata, *Novi Comment. Acad. Sci. Imp. Petrop.* **14**, 26–45; **15**, 3–28.

[3]   Bernoulli, N. (1713). Letter to P.R. de Montmort, in *Essay d'Analyse sur les Jeux de Hazard*, 2nd Ed., by P.R. de Montmort, Quillau, Paris, reprinted by Chelsea, New York, 1980.

[4]   Cournot, A.A. (1843). *Exposition de la Théorie des Chances et des Probabilités*. Hachette, Paris.

[5]   Davis, D.L., Gottlieb, M.B. & Stampnitzky, J.R. (1998). Reduced ratio of male to female births in several industrial countries: a sentinel health indicator?, *Journal of the American Medical Association* **279**, 1018–1023.

[6]   Edwards, A.W.F. (1958). An analysis of Geissler's data on the human sex ratio, *Annals of Human Genetics* **23**, 6–15.

[7]   Edwards, A.W.F. (1959). Some comments on Schützenberger's analysis of data on the human sex ratio, *Annals of Human Genetics* **23**, 233–238.

[8]   Edwards, A.W.F. (1961). A factorial analysis of sex ratio data, *Annals of Human Genetics* **25**, 117–121.

[9]   Edwards, A.W.F. (1962). Genetics and the human sex ratio, *Advances in Genetics* **11**, 239–272.

[10] Edwards, A.W.F. & Fraccaro, M. (1958). The sex distribution in the offspring of 5,477 Swedish ministers of religion, 1585–1920, *Separat ur Hereditas* **44**, 447–450.

[11] Edwards, A.W.F. & Fraccaro, M. (1960). Distribution and sequences of sexes in a selected sample of Swedish families, *Annals of Human Genetics* **24**, 245–252.

[12] Fisher, R.A. (1925). *Statistical Methods for Research Workers*. Oliver & Boyd, Edinburgh.

[13] Fisher, R.A. (1930). *The Genetical Theory of Natural Selection*. Oxford University Press, London and New York.

[14] Geissler, A. (1889). Beiträge zur Frage des Geschlechtsverhältnisses der Geborenen, *Zeitschrift des Königlichen Sächsischen Statistichen Bureaus* **35**, 1–24, 56.

[15] Gini, C. (1908). *Il Sesso dal Punto di Vista Statistico*. Sandron, Milan.

[16] Gini, C. (1951). Combinations and sequences of sexes in human families and mammal litters, *Acta Genetica et Statistica Medica* **2**, 220–244.

[17] Graunt, J. (1662). *Natural and Political Observations Mentioned in a Following Index, and Made upon the Bills of Mortality*. Martin, Allestry & Dicas, London.

[18] Hald, A. (1990). *A History of Probability and Statistics and their Applications before 1750*. Wiley, New York.

[19] Hald, A. (1998). *A History of Mathematical Statistics from 1750 to 1930*. Wiley, New York.

[20] Hytten, F.E. (1982). Boys and girls, *British Journal of Obstetrics and Gynaecology* **89**, 97–99.

[21] James, W.H. (1987). The human sex ratio. Part I: a review of the literature, *Human Biology* **59**, 721–752.

[22] Kalmus, H. & Smith, C.A.B. (1960). Evolutionary origin of sexual differentiation and the sex ratio, *Nature* **186**, 1004–1006.

[23] Karlin, S. (1986). *Theoretical Studies on Sex Ratio Evolution*. Princeton University Press, Princeton.

[24] Lancaster, H.O. (1950). The sex ratio in sibships, with special reference to Geissler's data, *Annals of Eugenics* **15**, 153–158.

[25] Lancaster, H.O. (1994). *Quantitative Methods in Biological and Medical Sciences: A Historical Essay*. Springer-Verlag, New York.

[26] Laplace, P.S. (1781). Mémoire sur les probabilités, *Mémoires de l'Académie Royale des Sciences de Paris* **1778**, 227–332.

[27] Lindsey, J.K. & Altham, P.M.E. (1998). Analysis of the sex ratio by using overdispersion models, *Applied Statistics* **47**, 149–157.

[28] Lowe, C.R. & McKeown, T. (1950). The sex ratio of human births related to maternal age, *British Journal of Preventive and Social Medicine* **4**, 75–85.

[29] Macfarlane, A.J. & Mugford, M. (1999). *Birth Counts: Statistics of Pregnancy and Childbirth, Vol.1, Text*, 2nd Ed. Stationery Office, London.

[30] Maconochie, N. & Roman, E. (1997). Sex ratios: are there natural variations within the human population?, *British Journal of Obstetrics and Gynaecology* **104**, 1050–1053.

[31] McKeown, T. & Lowe, C.R. (1951). The sex ratio of stillbirths related to cause and duration of gestation. An investigation of 7,066 stillbirths, *Human Biology* **23**, 41–60.

[32] Ohmi, H., Hirooka, K. & Mochizuki, Y. (1999). Reduced ratio of male to female births in Japan, *International Journal of Epidemiology* **28**, 597–598.

[33]   Poisson, S.D. (1830). Mémoire sur la proportion des naissances des filles et des garçons, *Mém. R. Acad. Sci. Inst. Fr.* **9**, 239–308.

P. ARMITAGE

Simple Epidemic *see* Epidemic Models, Stochastic

Simpson's Paradox

Simpson's paradox can be illustrated with an example, as Simpson did in his 1951 paper [8]. In that example, 40 patients are treated for a certain disease, whereas the control group consisted of 12 people. The results are given in the following $2 \times 2 \times 2$ contingency table, which shows the relationship between treatment and response (whether alive or dead) separately for males and females. Table 1 also shows the marginal table obtained by collapsing over the sex variable.

The odds ratios (*see* **Odds Ratio**) for the first two 2×2 tables (male/female) are both 5/6, which implies that the treatment is effective for both males and females. However, the odds ratio of the combined table is 1.0, which means the treatment is not effective. This phenomenon is called Simpson's paradox, which states that the direction of association between variables X (untreated/treated) and Y (alive/dead) may reverse after pooling over a covariate Z (male/female). The paradox can occur because pooling can lead to inappropriate weighting of the different subgroups [2].

Yule [11] first discovered this phenomenon, and it is also called the Yule–Simpson paradox. Numerous real-life examples of Simpson's paradox have been reported in many areas, including epidemiology,

physics, social science, psychology, and sports. For example, Cohen et al. [3] compared tuberculosis deaths in New York City and Richmond, Virginia, in 1910. If the population was divided into racial groups, then Richmond had a lower death rate in both white and nonwhite categories, but the overall death rate was lower in New York.

In the context of contingency tables, Simpson's paradox is restricted neither to one association measure – the odds ratio, nor to $2 \times 2 \times 2$ tables. Let $[a_i, b_i; c_i, d_i]$, $i = 1, \ldots, K$, denote cell counts in a $2 \times 2 \times K$ table, and let $[a = \sum a_i, b = \sum b_i; c = \sum c_i, d = \sum d_i]$ be the corresponding marginal table. Let $\alpha(a_i, b_i; c_i, d_i)$ represent a measure of the association, such as the odds ratio $\alpha(a_i, b_i; c_i, d_i) = (a_i d_i)/(b_i c_i)$. *Simpson's paradox* occurs if $(a_i d_i)/(b_i c_i) > 1 (< 1)$ for all i, and $(ad)/(bc) \leq 1 (\geq 1)$. The paradox is also called *association reversal* by Samuels [7]. Good et al. [6] extended Simpson's paradox to an *amalgamation paradox*, which is defined as follows:

$$\alpha(a, b; c, d) > \max \alpha(a_i, b_i; c_i, d_i) \quad \text{or}$$

$$\alpha(a, b; c, d) < \min \alpha(a_i, b_i; c_i, d_i),$$

where the measure of association α can be the odds ratio or some other measure, such as the relative risk.

It is frequently helpful to collapse high-dimensional contingency tables, since the collapsed table has larger cell frequencies, fewer parameters, and is easier to interpret (*see* **Collapsibility**). It is then of interest to know when a table can be safely collapsed, avoiding the paradox. Let $X \perp Y$ and $X \perp Y|Z$ denote the independence and conditional independence of X and Y, respectively. Wermuth [9] showed that for a $2 \times 2 \times 2$ table we can meaningfully pool over a covariate Z and expect to find the same odds ratio in the marginal table and the partial tables (*strict collapsibility*) if and only if $X \perp Z|Y$ or $Y \perp Z|X$ (see also Bishop et al. [1]). Strict collapsibility implies that Simpson's paradox does not occur. A similar result was obtained for

Table 1   Survival by treatment among males and among females

	Male		Female		Combined	
	Untreated	Treated	Untreated	Treated	Untreated	Treated
Alive	4	8	2	12	6	20
Dead	3	5	3	15	6	20

the relative risk [9]. Whittemore [10] showed that an $I \times J \times 2$ table is strictly collapsible if and only if at least one of the two-factor interactions of Z with X or Y in a loglinear model is zero. A table is called *strongly collapsible* (Ducharme et al. [5]) if it remains strictly collapsible no matter how it is partially collapsed (the definition was generalized to n-dimensional contingency tables by Whittemore). In this case, the odds ratio is totally independent of the level of the covariate. Ducharme et al. [5] provided a necessary and sufficient condition for a table to be strongly collapsible.

The paradox can also be avoided by a carefully designed experiment. For a $2 \times 2 \times K$ table, if the ratio of the sums of the two rows of each of the 2×2 partial tables remains constant, the design is called *row-uniform*. A *column-uniform* design can be similarly defined. If a design is both row-uniform and column-uniform, then the odds ratio of the combined table falls between the maximum and minimum of that of the individual tables [6], so the amalgamation paradox is avoided. Samuels [7] gave a necessary and sufficient condition to avoid association reversal, and also obtained a similar result in a regression setting.

When Simpson's paradox does occur in practice, what will the appropriate conclusion be? For example, if a disease is unrelated to a genotype for both whites and nonwhites but they are related when the two racial groups are combined, one is interested in knowing whether the disease is related to the genotype. Suppose X takes value G (genotype A) or $\overline{G}$ (other than genotype A), Y takes value D (disease) or $\overline{D}$ (no disease), and Z is a covariate indexing race. If $X \perp Y|Z$ without $X \perp Y$, Simpson's paradox occurs. Dawid [4] defined Z as a sufficient set of covariates if $Y \perp I|(X, Z)$, where I contains the labels of individual units of the population. In the above example, race is a sufficient covariate if given a person's race and genotype; whether the disease occurs does not depend on an individual person. If Z is sufficient and $X \perp Y|Z$, then the disease is unrelated to the genotype even though they look related when the tables are collapsed over Z.

References

[1] Bishop, Y.M.M., Fienberg, S.E. & Holland, P.W. (1975). *Discrete Multivariate Analysis: Theory and Practice*. MIT Press, Cambridge, Mass.

[2] Blyth, C.R. (1972). On Simpson's paradox and the sure-thing principle, *Journal of the American Statistical Association* **67**, 364–366.

[3] Cohen, M.R. & Nagel, E. (1934). *An Introduction to Logic and Scientific Method*. Harcourt Brace, New York.

[4] Dawid, A.P. (1979). Conditional independence in statistical theory (with discussion), *Journal of the Royal Statistical Society, Series B* **41**, 1–31.

[5] Ducharme, G.R. & Lepage, Y. (1986). Testing collapsibility in contingency tables, *Journal of the Royal Statistical Society, Series B* **48**, 197–205.

[6] Good, I.J. & Mittal, Y. (1987). The amalgamation and geometry of two-by-two contingency tables, *Annals of Statistics* **15**, 694–711.

[7] Samuels, M.L. (1993). Simpson's paradox and related phenomena, *Journal of the American Statistical Association* **88**, 81–88.

[8] Simpson, E.H. (1951). The interpretation of interaction in contingency tables, *Journal of the Royal Statistical Society, Series B* **13**, 238–241.

[9] Wermuth, N. (1987). Parametric collapsibility and the lack of moderating effects in contingency tables with a dichotomous response variable, *Journal of the Royal Statistical Society, Series B* **49**, 353–364.

[10] Whittemore, A.S. (1978). Collapsibility of multidimensional contingency tables, *Journal of the Royal Statistical Society, Series B* **40**, 328–340.

[11] Yule, G.U. (1903). Notes on the theory of association of attributes in statistics, *Biometrika* **2**, 121–134 (Reprinted in *Statistical Papers of George Udny Yule*, Griffin, London, pp. 71–84).

JIANPING DONG

Simulation Extrapolation (SIMEX) *see* Measurement Error in Epidemiologic Studies

Single Imputation Methods *see* Missing Data in Epidemiologic Studies

Social Desirability Bias *see* Bias in Observational Studies

Software, Biostatistical

Biostatisticians, and applied researchers using statistics, started to use statistical computer packages (by which I mean pre-written and compiled instructions to the computer for performing some form of statistical analysis) for data analysis during the 1950s. Almost immediately changes occurred in what data were analyzed and in how they were analyzed. Changes in computer hardware have brought changes in the type and quantity of software available. The advent of micro-computers in the late 1970s and early 1980s increased the rate of change and the amount of new software packages. There are currently well over 1000 statistical software packages available on a range of computer hardware platforms.

A database of citations to published reviews of statistical software is available [8]. A good review should tell potential users what the package does, how well it does it, how easy the package is to learn and to use, and how flexible the package is. Also available is information on how certain extendable packages make both vendor-written and user-written extensions available to users; information about the cost, and example contributions, have been presented in the "Editor's notes" of the Statistical Computing Section of *The American Statistician* (see, for example, [8]).

Some Historical Notes

The 1950s saw the first occurrence of statistical software, usually specialized single purpose programs that would run on one type of machine only. Some of these were written by users, but hardware vendors were the first important source (for example, SSP from IBM). The appearance of FORTRAN in the late 1950s saw the first real surge of software and the first occurrence, to my knowledge, of generally useful software not written by a hardware vendor; this was "BIMED", later called BMD, then Biomedical Data Processing Program (BMDP), which was started at the University of California at Los Angeles about 1960. By the mid-1960s several other packages had appeared, including PSTAT, SPSS, and SAS in the US and Genstat from England and Australia. All of these packages still exist. A number of other packages also appeared during the 1960s (e.g. OSIRIS, Datatext), but most of these, as far as I know, are no longer available.

These packages were neither well integrated nor comprehensive in coverage by the standards of today. They often used unacceptable algorithms or were prone to coding mistakes which gave wrong, or inaccurate, answers. (For example, Longley [17], using a multicollinear data set, showed problems in a number of packages.) However, prior to the availability of packages such as these, days could be spent, using a mechanical calculator or pencil and paper, to estimate, say, one regression with two covariates on a relatively small data set.

The late 1960s and early 1970s not only saw the appearance of additional software packages, some highly specialized (e.g. just for sample-size calculations) rather than general purpose, but also witnessed the setting up of committees by statistical associations to work on evaluating and designing software: GLIM originated under the auspices of a Royal Statistical Society(RSS) Committee; the American Statistical Association (ASA) set up a Committee on Statistical Program Packages in 1973 to help in evaluating software [3, 4]. The RSS committee, now called the "GLIM Working Party" still exists, as does the software, and the RSS receives a royalty on each version of GLIM sold. The ASA, however, no longer has any such committee.

A Categorization Scheme for Biostatistical Software

The range of software currently available makes any categorization scheme somewhat problematic. The categorization presented here is limited to one dimension: the type of user to whom the vendor expects to sell (and is further limited to software aimed at professionals); a broader categorization scheme can be found in [9]. It is impossible to include all existing packages. I primarily included packages well known to me; within each category the packages are listed alphabetically. Owing to space limitations, only contact information and a brief overview of the package are given. Contact information is for the headquarters of the company; many companies have sales and support offices in other countries.

General Purpose, Useful for Biostatistics

1. Integrated packages, including:

    (a) BMDP, SPSS Inc., 444 N. Michigan Ave., Chicago, IL 60611, USA; (312) 329-4000;

its original design was aimed squarely at biostatistical goals; it is available for several computer platforms (disk operating system (DOS)); a version with a Windows front-end is available from Statistical Solutions, Stonehill Corporate Center, Suite 104, 999 Broadway, Saugus, MA 01906, USA.

(b) Data Desk, Data Description, Inc., P.O. Box 4555, Ithaca, NY 14852, USA; (607) 257-1000; it is available on both Macintosh and Windows platforms.

(c) Genstat, Numerical Algorithms Group, Ltd, Wilkinson House, Jordan Hill Road, Oxford OX2 8DR, UK; (+44) 1865-511245; runs under Windows and several workstation operating systems, including UNIX, VMS and SunOS.

(d) GLIM, Numerical Algorithms Group, Ltd, Wilkinson House, Jordan Hill Road, Oxford OX2 8DR, UK; (+44) 1865-511245; runs under DOS and several workstation operating systems (e.g. UNIX, VMS, SunOS).

(e) JMP, SAS Institute, Inc., SAS Campus Drive, Cary, NC 27513, USA; (919) 677-8000; it is available for both the Macintosh and Windows platforms.

(f) Minitab, Minitab Inc., 3081 Enterprise Drive, State College, PA 16801, USA; (814) 238-3280; has been widely used in educational environments; it is available for several computer platforms (Macintosh, Windows, UNIX and mainframes).

(g) NCSS, 329 North 1000 East, Kaysville, UT 84037, USA; (801) 546-0445; runs under Windows.

(h) SAS, SAS Institute, Inc., SAS Campus Drive, Cary, NC 27513, USA; (919) 677-8000; runs under several platforms (Windows, UNIX, mainframes).

(i) SPSS, SPSS Inc., 444 N. Michigan Ave., Chicago, IL 60611, USA; (312) 329-4000; originally designed for use by social scientists; runs under several platforms (Macintosh, Windows, UNIX, mainframes).

(j) Stata, Stata Corp., 702 University Drive East, College Station, TX 77840, USA; (800) 782-8272; runs under several platforms (Macintosh, Windows, UNIX).

(k) Statistica, Statsoft, Inc., 2325 East 13th St., Tulsa, OK 74104, USA; (918) 749-1119; runs under Macintosh and Windows operating systems.

(l) Systat, SPSS Inc., 444 N. Michigan Ave., Chicago, IL 60611, USA; (312) 329-4000; runs under Macintosh, Windows and UNIX operating systems.

2. Packages based on programming languages; many of these, as well as at least some of the extensible packages mentioned elsewhere, can use subroutine libraries:

(a) Gauss, Aptech Systems, Inc., 23804 SE Kent-Kangley Road, Maple Valley, WA 98038, USA, (206) 432-7855; runs under Windows and UNIX; contains numerous statistical routines; there are also several "packages" (sets of Gauss routines) written in Gauss and relevant to biostatistical users.

(b) Matlab, The Mathworks, Inc., 24 Prime Park Way, Natick, MA 01760, USA; (508) 647-7000; runs under Windows, UNIX; although most early routines were aimed at engineers, there are now a sizable number of statistical routines.

(c) R, a public domain near-clone of S-Plus; this can be found on Statlib (www address: `http://lib.stat.cmu.edu/`).

(d) SC, Mole Software, 34 Greenville Road, Bloomfield, Belfast BT5 5EP, N. Ireland; (+44) (0) 1232 454640; runs under DOS and UNIX.

(e) S-plus, StatSci Division of MathSoft, 1700 Westlake Avenue North, Suite 500, Seattle, WA 98109, USA, (206) 283-8802; based on the AT & T product "S"; S-Plus runs under Windows and UNIX; many new forms of analysis first appear as S (or S-Plus) programs.

(f) XLISP-STAT, available for free by anonymous ftp from umnstat.stat.umn.edu; there are versions for the Macintosh, UNIX, and Microsoft Windows; there are at least four research groups that have written packages based on XLISP-STAT; an introduction to this package can be found in [22, 23]; introductions to three of the packages can be found in [21], [25], and [26].

Aimed Specifically at Biostatistical Users

1. General purpose:

    (a) Egret, Cytel Software Corp., 675 Massachusetts Avenue, Cambridge, MA 02139, USA, (617) 661-2011; runs under Windows.
    (b) Epicure, HiroSoft International Corp., 1463 E. Republican Ave., Suite 103, Seattle, WA 98112, USA, (206) 328-5301; runs under DOS and UNIX.
    (c) EpiInfo, originated at the US Centers for Disease Control (CDC) and since then the result of collaboration between the CDC and the World Health Organization; it is available for free on the Internet (ftp site: ftp.cdc.gov); can also be purchased with a printed manual of over 500 pages, from USD, Inc., 2075-A West Park Place, Stone Mountain, GA 30087, USA, (770) 469-4098; runs under DOS.
    (d) Epilog Plus, Epicenter Software, P.O. Box 90073, Pasadena, CA 91109, USA; (818) 304-9487; runs under Windows.
    (e) True Epistat, Epistat Services, 2011 Cap Rock Circle, Richardson, TX 75080, USA; (214) 680-1376; runs under DOS.

2. Special purpose:

    (a) EAST, Cytel Software Corp., 675 Massachusetts Avenue, Cambridge, MA 02139, USA; (617) 661-2011; for design of sequential trials; runs under DOS.
    (b) PEST, The MPS Research Unit, The University of Reading, Earley Gate, Reading RG6 6FN, UK; for design and analysis of sequential trials; runs under DOS.

Special Purpose Software that is Often Relevant to Biostatisticians

1. Randomization software:

    (a) RT, B.F.J. Manly, The Centre for Applications of Statistics and Mathematics, University of Otago, PO Box 56, Dunedin, New Zealand; 64-3-479-7774; randomization procedures for a number of parametric

procedures, including anova, linear regression, spatial data, time series; runs on DOS.

    (b) StatXact, LogXact, CyTel Software Corp., 675 Massachusetts Avenue, Cambridge, MA 02139, USA; (617) 661-2011; StatXact includes randomization versions of a large number of nonparametric analyses; LogXact performs exact logistic regression; each runs under Windows.
    (c) Testimate, idv-Datenanalyse und Versuchsplanung, Wessobrunner Strasse 6, D-82131 Gauting/München, Germany; 089/8 50 80 01; includes randomization versions of a large number of nonparametric analyses;

2. Software for estimating sample sizes when designing studies. The following have specific biostatistical orientations:

    (a) Egret, Cytel Software Corp., 675 Massachusetts Avenue, Cambridge, MA 02139, USA, (617) 661-2011; runs under Windows.
    (b) N and NSURV, idv-Datenanalyse und Versuchsplanung, Wessobrunner Strasse 6, D-82131 Gauting/München, Germany; 089/8 50 80 01; runs under DOS.
    (c) PASS, 329 North 1000 East, Kaysville, UT 84037, USA; (801) 546-0445; runs under Windows.

3. Software for correlated data, including longitudinal studies:

    (a) standard software: several of the packages included elsewhere in this list, including BMDP, LIMDEP SAS, S-Plus and Stata, include special routines for this type of analysis.
    (b) software for analyzing surveys; only one package above has adequate routines for dealing with weighted survey data: Stata; there are specialized packages, also:
    (i) SUDAAN, Research Triangle Institute, 3040 Cornwallis Road, P.O. Box 12194, Research Triangle Park, NC 27709, USA; (919) 541-6602; runs under Windows, UNIX and mainframes;
    (ii) WESVAR, Westat, Inc., 1650 Research Blvd., Rockville, MD 20850; available for

free over the Internet (can start at WesVar @ Westat.com).

(c) software for hierarchical models:
(i) HLM, Scientific Software International, 1525 East 53rd St., Suite 530, Chicago, IL 60615, USA; (312) 684-4920; runs under Windows or DOS;
(ii) MLn, The Multilevel Models Project, Mathematical Sciences, Institute of Education, University of London, 20 Bedford Way, London WC1H 0AL, UK; +44(0)171 612 6682; runs under Windows.

4. Software from other disciplines: econometric software such as LIMDEP; Econometric Software, Inc., 15 Gloria Place, Plainview, NY 11803, USA; (516) 938-5254; runs under DOS. Many of its routines are of the same type as biostatisticians use and it has some unique features, e.g. the survival analysis routines include left-truncated data and "cure" models.

5. Software for a specific form of analysis:

(a) Survival; see [10] and [12].
(b) Spatial; some of the above packages, especially Epilog Plus, Genstat, RT and S-Plus have some routines; there are some very specialized packages but they tend to be oriented to geostatistics and use very different jargon.
(c) Circular; Oriana, Kovach Computing Services, 85 Nant-y-Felin, Pentraeth, Anglesey LL75 8UY, Wales, UK; (+44) (0) 1248-450414; specifically oriented to analysis of data in degrees (e.g. angular data such as might be used in a study of spinal injuries) or time (used in health services research); runs under Windows; the only other software I know of are some user-written routines in Stata.

6. Bayesian software; while there are a number of Bayesian software packages, most have never been reviewed anywhere; overviews appear in [5], [6], and [20]. Newer packages have started to appear, including

(a) Bayesian inference Using Gibbs Sampling (BUGS); World Wide Web address: http://www.mrcbsu.cam.ac.uk/bugs; versions for Windows and UNIX; "carries out Bayesian inference on complex statistical problems for which there is no exact analytic solution".

(b) B/D: World Wide Web address: http://fourier.dur.ac.uk:8000/stats/bd; runs under Windows; "an interactive programming language which allows complete a priori and diagnostic analyses of Bayesian linear statistical problems".

Some Assessment Criteria

The following issues are of particular importance in assessing any statistical software package, regardless of whether it is specifically aimed at biostatistical users: the quality of the manual, the ease of learning and the ease of use of the package, and the accuracy of its computations.

Although some vendors would have purchasers believe that their package is usable without a manual, there are reasons for users to examine the manual carefully. Information in the manual should include:

1. Information on what is available (though each user must decide whether what is available is what is wanted, and, more importantly, whether it works in the way wanted and whether all the options desired are present).
2. At least one index; if it there is at least one, how good is it?
3. Examples of using the software; are the examples complete? That is to say, do the examples only display how the new commands (menu choices, etc.) work or is everything shown that one would actually need to complete an analysis?
4. Information on other sources of help, including courses, books, web sites, etc.
5. Information on how to interface this package with the operating system and/or with other types of software packages (such as word processing software).
6. Technical information relating to the algorithm used and how the vendor tested the software; there should be citations to the professional literature as well. Note that, as yet, very few vendors

actually provide this (for a discussion in the context of a comparative review, see [2]).

7. A list, and explanation, of error messages; these should be clear to someone who does not have a PhD in computer science and should also be given at the same level as the statistical text.

Manuals can also be used to discover whether the package appears to be aimed at the right type of user; for this, you should examine the manual(s) with the following in mind:

1. What type of language is used in describing and explaining the package? Jargon is rampant and differs dramatically across different disciplines.
2. What level of statistical language is used (e.g. beginner or professional)?
3. What types of graphical output are available and how integrated are the graphics and the statistical routines?
4. What types of checks and diagnostic information are available to help decide whether there are problems with the results of an estimation procedure?
5. How flexible is the software with respect to:

   (a) nonstandard problems, e.g. are there choices of algorithms for standard routines such as linear regression?
   (b) output; can the user affect the output of the package to ensure that it is in the most usable format for that particular use?

For a discussion of some criteria useful in assessing manuals, see [1], [18], the accompanying discussion of these articles, and the rejoinders by the authors.

A criterion often mentioned is ease of learning of the package. My experience, however, has been that this is really only important for people who will be infrequent users of the software, as these people will essentially be learning the package over again each time they use it. However, for others, the cost of learning is easily overshadowed by ease of use considerations, especially since, for even the hardest-to-learn packages, it rarely takes more than a few hours to learn at least enough to obtain some output.

Ease of use is sometimes, mistakenly, listed with ease of learning as a criterion. It is however both different and much more important. It is also, generally, harder to assess since the determination of whether something is easy to use is heavily dependent on both

the level of the user and what the user is trying to do, as well as on the structure of the program. Program structure affects ease of use in many ways; a simple example relates to the difference between typing a command and clicking on a menu item. How this affects a given user depends on whether the menu defaults are what is primarily wanted and how easy it is to choose different options. Of course, at the other extreme, some users want so much of what they choose to do to be dependent on the situation, that no menu-driven program could possibly be considered "easy to use". Furthermore, there are many issues that vendors have never considered and these cannot, of course, be present in a menu. Whether they are available in a command system depends on the amount of thought the vendor put into making the package flexible (a detailed example is provided in [9]). Ease of use can also be aided by the availability of books about the packages, user groups, including e-mail lists and Usenet news groups, vendor newsletters, etc. Integration and ease of recall of various parts of the numerical and graphical output, and integration of the packages to the operating system and to other software (e.g. word processors), are also important here.

Earlier, I mentioned the issue of whether the language used in the manual was appropriate to the statistical expertise of the user. A related issue has to do with the ease with which one can assess one's analytic output. This is affected by numerous factors, including the quality of the error messages, the presence of statistics that can be used to assess assumptions underlying the technique used, and the quality and integration with the statistics of the graphics.

The final criterion to be discussed here is the quality of the numerical algorithms, which affects not only the accuracy of the result, but whether the package provides an answer, and, if it does, the efficiency with which it arrives at the answer.

1. Try the examples in the manual (the vendor should supply all example data sets on the disk with the program). If the examples cannot be reproduced, then immediately contact the vendor. While this appears to be a very simple test that no vendor should ever fail, some packages do fail this test.
2. Check reviews, especially those by reputable statisticians (e.g. reviews in *The American Statistician* or in *Applied Statistics*) (unfortunately, this

latter journal is dropping its review section). A good review will supply much more information than just that related to accuracy; in particular, information should be included on the level of user targeted and on the ease of learning and using the package. Furthermore, I believe that comparative reviews are much more useful than reviews of individual packages.

3. Look in the literature for test data sets. Many "tests" are so well known that no vendor fails them anymore (this is true, for example, of the Longley [17] data). Furthermore, some tests are not relevant to the work that any particular user does. However, there are valuable benchmarks and tests in the literature (see for example, [7], [14], [15], [19], and [24]) that will help users and vendors test (a) whether the algorithms are appropriate, (b) what happens at the boundaries of either allowed data or standard language, and (c) the quality of the algorithms being used.

4. Build your own library of test data sets that are important in your own work and for which problems have previously been found. Try this library on every new package, and every upgrade received.

5. Examine the "validation" or "certification" section of the documentation, if it exists; unfortunately, most vendors do not yet provide such a section. If such a section exists, look for information regarding the algorithms used and the range and type of issues and of data used to test the software. The documentation should also discuss carefully the issue of how the vendor decided that the test result was acceptable. Also, note whether the vendor says that all tests are re-run after making any change to the software; this "regression testing" is necessary since fixing a bug in software often introduces one or more new bugs and this possibility must be checked.

6. Finally, run the analysis in at least one other software package and carefully compare the results. For this final check, the importance of having algorithm information in the manual is highlighted because for many analyses different algorithms should produce different results. This is especially true in many nonparametric analyses where the treatment of ties greatly affects the results.

Where to Go for More Information

There are no good general sources of information on what software is available. Eventually, there will probably be a source on the Internet which can be added to frequently. The number of software packages, particularly for educational uses, is growing rapidly. Some information, of course, is already available: numerous journals print reviews and a database of citations to these reviews is available [8]; numerous data sets useful for testing exist at statlib (at Carnegie Mellon University; WWW address: `http://lib.stat.cmu.edu/`) and other places on the internet. A "Statistical Software Guide" is produced approximately every two-three years. The most recent appearance of this guide, in print, was [16], but information is currently being gathered for an update report. However, none of this information is either well organized or complete. There is one commercial source of information, SciTech International, which publishes *Software for Science*; however, even their list (almost 2000 products, but including non-analysis packages such as word-processing software) is incomplete; they are especially weak, obviously, regarding shareware and freeware, which is often specialized and is often available on the Internet. Many of the vendors mentioned above have Internet World Wide Web sites; the best source for finding these in general is via a competitor: Stata, at its site (`http://www.stata.com`) maintains links to the sites of other vendors, including several suppliers of free software.

The Future – Maybe

Statistical software has been changing rapidly in recent years. The main changes, as of 1996, relate to (a) the existence of numerous specialized software packages; (b) the movement, slowly, of these specialized routines into general purpose packages; and (c) a heavy emphasis on graphical analysis, especially new types of graphics and new ways of integrating graphics into standard analysis.

While these are valuable, necessary, and will continue, there are two other changes that would be very valuable to the profession. The first relates to a better integration of what we already know about statistical assumptions with our analysis. For example, we know that the two-sample t test is somewhat affected by different variances (the amount depending on the ratio of the groups' sample sizes); many would find it helpful if, along with requested result, the software gave some information about the validity of this, and other, assumptions, for the data used. This might also help guard against the "misuse" of statistical software by those who are not well trained in statistics. This issue has been discussed in numerous articles dating back to at least the 1970s [11]. Though noting a number of potential problems, Goodnight clearly favored this type of "offensive validity checking". Haux [13] provides a number of citations on this issue and then gives a detailed example for the Mann–Whitney test and notes that BMDP, SAS and SPSS are each unsatisfactory. Note that the software should not stop the user from doing an analysis. Rather, a user should just want be provided with some additional information without making a number of other requests to the software (e.g. a separate request for equal variances, for symmetry, for heterogeneity, etc.).

A large part of any project relates to data management and data manipulation. Much, and in many projects all, of this is done with the same statistical software used for analysis. However, no current program keeps a reversible history of what the user does to the data and many do not even keep any history (or log or journal) of what was done. The unfortunate result is that often even the analyst cannot reproduce certain results. Thus, another desirable change is the implementation of some form of reversible history of data management and data manipulation so that any particular state of the data could be re-created. Some type of coding scheme should be attached to both this history and to each analysis so that for any given output it would be clear which state of the data was used in its production. The current reliance on *ad hoc*, individual, schemes is inefficient, ineffective, and unnecessary. Version control software, as used in software development, database management and even some word-processing software should be generalizable to statistical software.

References

[1]   Berk, K.N. & Francis, I.S. (1978). A review of the manuals for BMDP and SPSS (with comments and rejoinders), *Journal of the American Statistical Association* **73**, 65–70.

[2]   Boomsma, A. & Molenaar, I.W. (1993). Four electronic tables for probability distributions, *American Statistician* **48**, 153–162.

[3]   Francis, I. & Heiberger, R.M. (1975). The evaluation of statistical program packages – the beginning, in *Proceedings of the Computer Science and Statistics Eighth Annual Symposium on the Interface*, J.W. Frane, ed. Los Angeles, pp. 106–109.

[4]   Francis, I., Heiberger, R.M. & Velleman, P.F. (1975). Criteria and considerations in the evaluation of statistical program packages, *American Statistician* **29**, 52–56.

[5]   Goel, P.K. (1988). Software for Bayesian analysis: current status and additional needs, in *Bayesian Statistics*, Vol. 3, J.M. Bernardo, M.H. DeGroot, D.V. Lindley & A.F.M. Smith, eds. Oxford University Press, Oxford.

[6]   Goel, P.K. (1988). Software for Bayesian analysis: current status and additional needs – II, in *Computing Science and Statistics: Proceedings of the 20th Symposium on the Interface*, E.J. Wegman, D.T. Gantz & J.J. Miller, eds. American Statistical Association, Alexandria.

[7]   Goldstein, R. (1987). Linear regression on IBM PC/XT/ AT's, in *Computer Science and Statistics: Proceedings of the 19th Symposium on the Interface* R.M. Heiberger & M.T. Martin, eds. American Statistical Association, Alexandria, pp. 219–228.

[8]   Goldstein, R. (1994). Editor's notes, *American Statistician* **48**, 254–255.

[9]   Goldstein, R. (1997). Computer packages, *Encyclopedia of Statistical Sciences, Update Volume*. Wiley, New York, to appear.

[10]   Goldstein, R. Anderson, J., Ash, A., Craig, B., Harrington, D. & Pagano, M. (1989). Survival analysis software on MS/PC-DOS computers, *Journal of Applied Econometrics* **4**, 393–414.

[11]   Goodnight, J.H. (1975). Validity checking: how far should we go? in *Proceedings of the Computer Science and Statistics Eighth Annual Symposium on the Interface*, J.W. Frane, ed. Los Angeles, pp. 146–148.

[12]   Harrell, F.E., Jr & Goldstein, R. (1997). A survey of microcomputer survival analysis software: the need for an integrated framework, *American Statistician* **51**, 360–373.

[13]   Haux, R. (1983). How to detect and prevent errors in computer-supported statistical analysis: an example, *Methods of Information in Medicine* **22**, 87–92.

[14]   Heiberger, R.M., Velleman, P.F. & Ypelaar, M.A. (1983). Generating test data with independently controllable features for multivariate general linear forms, *Journal of the American Statistical Association* **78**, 585–595.

[15]   Knuth, D.E. (1981). *The Art of Computing*, Vol. 2: *Seminumerical Algorithms*, 2nd Ed. Addison-Wesley, Reading.

[16]   Koch, A. & Haag, U. (1995). The statistical software guide '94/95, in *Statistical Software Newsletter, Computational Statistics & Data Analysis* **19**, 237–261.

[17]   Longley, J.W. (1967). An appraisal of least-squares programs for the electronic computer from the point of view of the user, *Journal of the American Statistical Association* **62**, 819–841.

[18] Muller, M.E. (1978). A review of the manuals for BMDP and SPSS (with comments and rejoinders), *Journal of the American Statistical Association* **73**, 71–80.

[19] Nash, J.C. (1990). *Compact Numerical Methods for Computers: Linear Algebra and Function Minimization*, 2nd Ed. Adam Hilger, Bristol.

[20] Press, S.J. (1989). *Bayesian Statistics*. Wiley, New York.

[21] Stine, R. (1997). AXIS: an extensible graphical user interface, in *Statistical Computing Environments for Social Research*, R. Stine & J. Fox, eds. Sage, Thousand Oaks, pp. 175–192.

[22] Tierney, L. (1990). *LISP-STAT: An Object-Oriented Environment for Statistical Computing and Dynamic Graphics*. Wiley, New York.

[23] Tierney, L. (1997). Data analysis using LISP-STAT, in *Statistical Computing Environments for Social Research*, R. Stine & J. Fox, eds. Sage, Thousand Oaks, pp. 66–88.

[24] Velleman, P.F. & Ypelaar, M.A. (1980). Constructing regressions with controlled features: a method of probing regression performance, *Journal of the American Statistical Association* **75**, 839–844.

[25] Weisberg, S. (1997). The R-code: a graphical paradigm for regression analysis, in *Statistical Computing Environments for Social Research*, R. Stine & J. Fox, eds. Sage, Thousand Oaks, pp. 193–206.

[26] Young, F.W. & Bann, C.M. (1997). ViSta: a visual statistics system, in *Statistical Computing Environments for Social Research*, R. Stine & J. Fox, eds. Sage, Thousand Oaks, pp. 207–235.

RICHARD GOLDSTEIN

Software, Epidemiological

Historically, many specialized intellectual domains have had data analysis software specifically designed for that domain, including such areas as economics, geology, chemistry and epidemiology. Other domains, including sociology, astronomy and political science, have seen little of this specialization. Furthermore, in those areas, such as epidemiology, that have had numerous specialized packages, some of the packages have fallen by the wayside while others have grown and still others have appeared. In some areas, such as economics, the major specialized packages, for example, Limdep, have become more like standard general-purpose packages. However, this has generally not happened with the epidemiologic packages. Finally, at least one general-purpose package, Stata,

has incorporated a number of epidemiologic analytic routines, jargon and all.

In this article I review some of the specialized epidemiologic software, whether related to the design of studies or to their analysis. I also discuss some of the advantages and disadvantages of having specialized software for a discipline. Both issues are clarified by the presence of a general-purpose analytic package that contains a set of epidemiologic analysis routines. Other general-purpose packages will generally be ignored (*see* **Software, Biostatistical**).

Why Epidemiologic Software?

To write about epidemiologic software, one must locate it, one must define it (or at least its boundaries), and one must have at least some idea regarding what distinguishes epidemiologic software from other data analysis software. While I have undoubtedly missed some small epidemiologic software packages, I hope that I have included all major packages and at least a representative selection of the smaller packages. The following, in alphabet order, is a list of the packages I will be emphasizing in this article:

- Cluster, version 3.1 (free from the Centers for Disease Control (CDC)): this DOS-based package has 12 different techniques to help in disease clustering. It is fairly straightforward to use, but is certainly not elegant.

- Egret for Windows, version 1 (commercial; other packages from the same company include StatXact and LogXact): this package is primarily for fairly specialized modeling of epidemiologic and biomedical data. It includes **additive** and **multiplicative** versions of several models (e.g. logistic and Poisson) as well as random-effects logistic regression. It is very easy to use, much easier than when it was a DOS package. This is its first appearance as a Windows package. The same vendor sells Egret SIZ, a DOS package for determining sample size or power for nonlinear regressions, StatXact, a package for the exact analysis of tabular data, and including a power module for data to be analyzed via tables, and LogXact, a package for exact **logistic** or **Poisson regression**. LogXact also contains a Monte Carlo option for data sets for which maximum-likelihood estimates do not converge, but that are too large for exact analysis. `Egret SIZ` is the only package of these that is not easy to use. Furthermore, it requires the user to collapse continuous predictor variables into categorical variables, which can be difficult to do without biasing one's result (*see* **Bias**). The material in `Egret SIZ` is based on Self & Mauritsen [11].

- `Epicalc`, version 1.02 (free): this simple Windows package is just for analyzing epidemiologic tables. It is very easy to use when you already have summary data.

- `Epicure`, version 2.10 (commercial): this package is primarily for specialized modeling of epidemiologic and biomedical data. A wide range of models are included. This package is DOS-based and is fairly easy to use, but not as easy as, say, `Egret`.

- `EpiInfo`, version 6.04, and `EpiMap`, version 2 (free from the CDC): `EpiInfo` has extensive capabilities regarding questionnaires, data entry and data checking, but modest analytic capacity. Taking full advantage requires some programming skill. `EpiMap` has extensive mapping abilities and uses `EpiInfo` data directly. If one only wants a little from these packages, they are easy to use. However, using their full power requires some work by the user.

- `Epilog Windows`, version 1 (commercial): this package is easier to use as a Windows package than it was as a DOS package. It is very modular, which I am not a fan of, but it is also the most complete of the specialized packages.

- `EpiMeta`, version 1 (free from the CDC): relatively easy to use for its quite limited purpose of simple meta-analyses.

- `PEPI`, version 3.01 (free): this DOS package is slowly being made into a Windows package. It is comprised of a large number of separate modules, which can make it a pain to use. This pain is somewhat ameliorated in DOS by an integrated menu that accesses all modules and by a Windows help file that tells the user which module to use. The preliminary parts of the new Windows version go some way to solving the problems caused by separate modules. `PEPI` is primarily for use on summary data and has no data management facilities of its own.

- `Stata`, version 6 (commercial; general purpose): this large, general-purpose, Windows/Macintosh/UNIX package is the most complete of all considered here. It is included because it has specialized routines for epidemiologists. It is very easy to use, even at a fairly advanced level. If the user requires, the program is extensible and there is a wide-ranging user community that is actively extending this program. The Windows version was used in writing this article.

- `True Epistat`, version 5.3 (commercial): this is a DOS package and is very modular. I find the data management facilities awkward to use, though this version is an improvement over earlier versions.

- `Win Episcope`, version 2.0 and `WinEpi Ratios`, version 1.0 (free): these simple packages are easy to use for tables when you already have summary data.

Note that several major, general-purpose packages are not included here as they have no specialized epidemiologic routines, including the Biomedical Data Processing Program (BMDP), `SAS`, `SPSS`, `S-Plus` and `Systat`. The last four, at least, are under active development and are used by many epidemiologists. Each of these has many of the elements discussed below and/or listed in one of the two tables. However, because they do not use epidemiologic jargon, I have not included them in this article (*see* **Software, Biostatistical**).

As part of my preparation, I invited the producers of each of the above packages (except for `Cluster` and `EpiMeta`) to tell me why they thought there should, or should not, be specialized epidemiological software. I received responses from all except the `WinEpi` series (note: the `WinEpi` series is aimed at veterinary epidemiology). As one would expect, the providers of specialized epidemiologic software provided reasons for having such specialized software, while the people from `Stata`, a general-purpose package with some specialized epidemiologic routines included, provided reasons why one would not want specialized software. I received a total of seven responses from different software providers; since there was a lot of overlap in their responses, I just summarize the major issues raised:

1. *The output produced is the type of output used by epidemiologists*. Three vendors said this, with

one adding that it was desirable to exclude the "statistical clutter" that general-purpose packages added even when they also produced the type of output desired by epidemiologists. This issue seems best exemplified by tables where many epidemiologists expect specific output (e.g. **odds ratio** (OR) and a confidence interval for this ratio). An example of the added clutter produced by some packages might be, I suppose, statistics such as lambda or Cramer's V. Note, however, some problems with this.

(a) There are cases where one should want the additional statistics; that is, what one person might call "statistical clutter" might be desirable to other people or even to that person if the person learned about that statistic. (Lambda is an example of a proportional reduction in the error statistic; if one uses it in models, as epidemiologists do, might not one also want to use it for tables?)

(b) One trend that has clearly increased over the last 20 years is for analysts in one area to read, and contribute to, the literature in other areas. If every discipline used its own specialized software, this would be a harder task. Certain choices by software providers already make this harder; for example, Stata, in its epidemiologic tables routine (epitab), includes McNemar's test for matched case–control data. Their output tables even use standard epidemiologic language (e.g. the rows and columns are labeled exposed and unexposed). One problem arises here because other disciplines, including various social sciences, call **case–control studies** by other names and do not use the words "exposed" and "unexposed". A related issue, which ties this to the first point above, is that Quinn McNemar was not an epidemiologist – he was a social psychologist, and when he designed this test he was not using data that were related to health in any way. Rather, he was interested in those who changed preferences regarding presidential candidates according to consecutive public opinion polls (McNemar [6]). When general-purpose packages bend a statistic like this, they endanger their general use (note: Stata has another, not specifically epidemiologic,

procedure that also produces McNemar's test, this time without the epidemiologic jargon). When specialized users refuse to acknowledge other uses, and other users, they risk becoming dead ends.

(c) While I agree that cluttered output is undesirable, I see no problem with software producers giving users the option to choose which output is to be shown. At the extreme, asking for a table would show only the table with no inference procedures shown unless specifically requested, and each type of inferential procedure desired would have to be specifically requested. Software that includes macros could include example macros showing, for example, the output that an epidemiologist might want, while a second macro might show the output that a psychologist would want.

2. *Ease of use, particularly via epidemiologic jargon.* At least four software providers mentioned this. Several providers specifically mentioned the desirability of this for users who were not full-time epidemiologists. I certainly agree that extreme ease of use, accompanied by standard epidemiologic jargon (to the extent it exists) makes misuse of the software less likely by these people and is therefore a good thing. Inclusion of this jargon in general-purpose statistical software is, by the same token, dangerous (unless one feels that the only possible misusers are the epidemiologists, something I strongly doubt). Related to this was the idea that single-purpose packages (i.e. software that only does one type of analysis, or that is useful with respect to a certain design issue) are generally easier to use than are general-purpose packages. Similarly, certain support issues are clearly part of this, including manuals that give fully worked out epidemiologic examples, textbooks that use a particular software package, and the presence of Usenet news groups and/or e-mail list-servers related to the package. Only the manual examples seem to argue against general-purpose packages (since all the others can, and do, easily co-exist with general-purpose packages) and even this can be handled, though some ways of attempting this may work better than others.

3. *Hard-to-find statistical procedures and tests.* This was mentioned by at least five providers. An

example is disease **clustering**. There is no question that in epidemiology, as in other disciplines, specialized software packages that include useful analytic routines not available in most general-purpose packages are highly desirable. Some of these might be added to an extensible general-purpose package by a user, or by the provider, but some are so unusual, and difficult to program, that a specialized package might be the only realistic alternative.

4. *Epidemiology has unique demands for data entry and for data manipulation.* One provider argued this. The examples provided (double entry and verification, changing the ordering of categories in a table) are not convincing since users from many disciplines need all of these and more.

My conclusion is that there is a place, and a need, for specialized epidemiologic software, primarily for routines that are not included, or only rarely included, in general-purpose statistical software packages. However, many of the other reasons for specialized software packages are unconvincing at best. Worse, specialized packages that offer only "simple" routines are dangerous. For example, use of tables without the ability to generalize to a model allows too much chance of misleading the researcher. Many epidemiologic tables provide exactly the same result that one would receive from a simple **logistic regression** or **Poisson regression**. The general-purpose package that provides both tables and

models allows one to test assumptions and to use covariates – the specialized tool that only has the tables, no matter how perfectly epidemiologic they are, is dangerous.

Software for Designing and Implementing Studies

Historically, the primary emphasis in software has been on analyzing data. Specialized packages, outside of epidemiology, exist for sample size determination and for the assignment of subjects to groups. Some of the epidemiologic software discussed here has the capability of helping a researcher to design or implement a study and those capabilities are discussed in this section. The capabilities of nonepidemiologic specialized software and of other general-purpose software are not discussed here. Software for determination of power, or sample size, have been reviewed elsewhere (e.g. Goldstein [3], Thomas & Krebs [12]) (*see* **Software, Biostatistical**). Software for subject assignment, including matching, has unfortunately not been generally reviewed, to my knowledge.

Several of the packages included here have routines for sample size determination. For the most part, only fairly simple situations are covered. Many statisticians will use simulation for complicated studies, but most of the specialized epidemiologic software has no simulation ability. Table 1 shows what is available for those packages that have any capability for

Table 1 Type of sample size determination

Software	Means	Proportions	Other models[a]	Simulation
Egret SIZ/StatXact		StatXact	nonlinear reg.	Egret SIZ
Epicalc[b]	Yes	Yes	cc	
EpiInfo		Yes	cc, cohort	
Epilog (Power)[c]	Yes	Yes		
PEPI	Yes	Yes	OLS	
Win Episcope	Yes	Yes	cc, cohort	
Stata	Yes	Yes	rm	Yes
True Epistat	Yes	Yes	survival	

[a]Nonlinear reg. refers to `Egret SIZ`, which will calculate sample sizes for several types of nonlinear regression: logistic, conditional logistic, Poisson, Cox proportional hazards. cc = case–control study, cohort = cohort study, rm = repeated measures study, survival = comparison of two survival curves.
[b]Mark Myatt, the provider of `Epicalc`, also provides some specialized packages for calculating sample size for simple surveys and for "LQAS triage-style surveys".
[c]Epicenter Software, the vendor of `Epilog`, also sells a program called "`Power`" specifically for sample size determination. This was reviewed in Goldstein [3] and in Thomas & Krebs [12], but was not re-reviewed for this article.

either sample size determination or for simulation. In addition, some of the developers of `Epicure` have produced a separate, and free, power program that is unique in that it can easily be used for tests of interactions. This program, "`Power`", is currently included as a module in the package "Epitome" and is being turned into a stand-alone Windows-based program. Note that there is little in any of the packages with respect to calculating power and/or determining sample size for any type of regression model.

None of the specialized packages includes any routines, or simulation capability, to allow for the determination of sample size for research studies involving complex samples. Furthermore, only `Egret SIZ`, a separate product requiring that it be separately purchased, has extensive regression capabilities and the requirement for categorizing any continuous predictor reduces the usefulness of this package. On the other hand, several of the specialized packages include the ability to calculate the needed sample size for simple **case–control** or for simple **cohort studies**, both of which are important in epidemiology. On the face of it, the above table is depressing – specialized packages should be, at least through simulation, capable of much more than they are. The simple studies that are currently covered are, in my opinion, mostly useful for beginners and students.

What other aspects of study design, particularly of the design of epidemiologic studies, are available? There are at least three other areas in which software can help: the design of data collection instruments (e.g. questionnaires); the assignment or allocation of study subjects (e.g. **matching** or blocked randomization); and data editing (i.e. data checking and correction). Unfortunately, in these aspects also, the various packages are fairly weak. This is not, however, to say that there is nothing available or that what is available is weak – it is just that too little is available, even though what is available is generally pretty good. With respect to data collection, the EPED module in `EpiInfo` can be very helpful, particularly regarding questionnaires. When combined with the CHECK module for data checking and verification, `EpiInfo` can be very helpful to researchers. Some other packages have provided less useful routines for data checking including `Epilog` (`Proc Check`) and `Stata` (`assert`, `inspect`, etc.). Any reasonable analytic package will provide some ability to check one's data for problems through standard descriptive statistics. `Epilog`'s `Proc Check` allows one to go a little

further by allowing user input to flag, in different ways, any problem records as they are found. With some programming on the part of the user, `Stata`'s relevant commands can also provide additional help.

Although many authors have pointed out problems with matching, it can still be useful in epidemiologic studies. The biggest problem, for many, is how to find the matches. Of the packages examined, only `Epilog` (`Proc Control`) provides help here: for example, caliper matching (i.e. matching within limits, such as ± 5 years of age) is fairly easy to set up and the user can select the number of matches to select per case. A related issue is the ability to set up blocked randomization; `PEPI`, `Stata` and `True Epistat` have routines for this.

One can easily imagine other tasks that would be useful. For example, in longitudinal studies, software that helped with the tracing process, either through helping to find people via hooks to internet databases, or that helped determine which of several people found was the correct one, would be very useful. `Stata`'s extensibility could be used here, though it has not been. Another possibility relates to the presence of multiple control groups – none of the packages has anything, either on the data management end or in analysis (except for relatively simple tables and hypothesis tests) related to this potentially very useful procedure.

Data Management Issues

Some data management issues (e.g. data entry and verification) were discussed above. A few others are mentioned here. However, because of the wide variety of possible issues, I cannot hope to cover everything. I believe that there is a certain minimum that each package (except the simplest special-purpose analysis packages) should contain, including:

- merging files (adding new variables to the same cases), including many-to-one merges
- appending files (adding new cases to the data set)
- recoding variables
- transformations of variables, including a wide variety of built-in mathematical, statistical and string functions; some, at least, should be usable "on the fly" when estimating models (e.g. $\log(y) = f(x_1, x_2,$ etc.)
- splitting files
- generating random numbers/samples

- changing files from wide format (repeated measures as part of the same case) to long format (each measure as a separate case) and back again; this is often necessary for different kinds of longitudinal analysis
- an extensive ability to deal with character data, especially names, addresses and, at least to some extent, free text
- the ability to override any automatic decisions made by the software (e.g. one should be able to change easily the way data, or results, are displayed)
- date functions, both so that, e.g. calculation of age at any given time point is easy, and so that graphs and other output can easily be labeled in an appropriate way
- time-series, including seasonal effects
- automatic generation of appropriate indicator variables from a categorical variable, including user choice of reference group when estimating models
- easy ways to find any duplicate cases in the data
- multiple indicators for missing values (to indicate different reasons for being missing), and correct handling of missing values during transformations and the generation of new variables (e.g. when forming a new indicator variable that is coded as 1 when either $x > 5$ or $y > 3$, the new variable should be equal to 1 if x is equal to 6 even if y is missing)
- dealing with runs, or spells, or series of events (particularly those that do not fit into standard time-series formats).

None of the packages here is ideal in this respect and most of them are pretty weak with relatively short lists of built-in abilities. Stata is the strongest in this regard, even if one excludes user-added capabilities. With the addition of user-written routines, Stata is much stronger than any of the other packages with respect to data management. Stata even has the ability to add notes to the data, or to individual variables in the data, that will be permanently saved with the data and can be edited.

Data Analysis

The heart of any of these packages is its analytic capabilities. Unfortunately, this is also the heart of one of the major disputes between some statisticians

and some epidemiologists: whether to emphasize OR or **relative risk** (RR). It appears that many epidemiologists prefer measures of RR while many statisticians prefer the OR. In fact, a major strand of epidemiologic literature deals with the question of when an event is rare enough so that the OR is a good approximation of the RR! For many statisticians, the dependence of RR on the rate in the control group makes it a poor choice for any use. A cross-cutting, and more meaningful, dispute is whether to emphasize absolute or relative measures of effect. In a sense, the answer to both issues is the inclusion of multiple measures of effect, or at least the ability to obtain any effect measure the user desires. For tables, the software could offer options that the user could pick from; for models, different effects result naturally from different models. Thus, offering numerous models, especially when they are closely related, seems the obvious answer. For example, generalized linear models (GLMs) offer, through different choices of link functions, the ability to obtain different measures of effect. A simple example involves models based on the binomial distribution: using a logit link results in **logistic regression** with an OR effect; using a log link gives an RR effect, while using an identity link gives an effect measured in rate differences.

Another difference appears to be the dependence of many users on tables. However, ignoring potential **confounders**, or other relevant covariates, can be dangerous, since their inclusion could mean very different results. Again, a package that includes both tables and models should solve this problem. If the documentation of the package discusses which models appropriately build on which tables, as does Stata's, the user is in the best possible situation.

Table 2 presents a simple checklist of various relevant forms of analysis for the major packages. Those packages that only include tables (Epicalc and Win Episcope/WinEpi Ratios) are not included in the table. Also, the column for EpiInfo includes the other CDC packages (EpiMeta and Cluster). The danger of such a table, of course, is that it can be misleading for certain specialized issues and packages. There is little doubt that Epicure, for example, looks weaker than it actually is in such a table because it has a number of unique models that are not included but should be considered. In particular, it is the only included package that has models that are neither additive nor

Table 2 Data analysis routines

Analysis	Egret	Epicure	EpiInfo	Epilog	PEPI	Stata	True Epistat
Standardization	Y		Y	Y	Y	Y	Y
SMR		Y		Y	Y	Y	Y
Multidimensional tables				Y			
Complex surveys			Y			Y	
Disease clustering			Cluster	Y			
Meta-analysis			EpiMeta	Y	Y	Y	Y
Linear models	Y	Y		Y	Simple	Y	Y
Censored linear models				Y		Y	
Logistic regression	Y	Y		Y	Y	Y	Y
Additive logistic regression	Y	Y				Y	
Exact logistic	LogXact			Y			
Ordinal logistic				Y		Y	
Polytomous logistic				Y		Y	
Conditional logistic	Y	Y		Y	Y	Y	Y
Poisson regression	Y	Y		Y	Y	Y	
Cox models	Y	Y		Y		Y	Y
Parametric survival models	Y	Y		Y		Y	
Kaplan–Meier analysis	Y	Y		Y	Y	Y	Y
Extensive nonlinear models		Y		Y		Y	
Recursive partitioning (trees)				Y			
Simulations	Y	Y				Y	
Bootstrap						Y	
Multilevel models	Y			Y		Y	
Seasonality				Y	Y		
Maps			EpiMap	Y			

Note: Entries in the table, other than "Y", refer to other packages from the same provider (counting the CDC as one provider).

multiplicative (*see* **Additive Model**; **Multiplicative Model**). Egret also suffers in this way, though to a lesser extent. Even Stata suffers as it is the only package with a full GLM (though Epicure has aspects of GLM), which I have not included in the table.

The items in Table 2 were largely selected on the basis of three sources: Clayton & Hills [2], Oster [8], and Rothman & Greenland [9]. The table is not complete (an impossible task), but does cover most of the regularly used analytic procedures. Note that I have excluded descriptive statistics and epidemiologic tables, since all packages include these (PEPI does, however, have one interesting unique aspect to its tables: when the user wants kappa, a measure of agreement, PEPI also provides bias-adjusted and prevalence-adjusted bias-adjusted versions; see Byrt et al. [1] and Lantz & Nebenzahl [5]) (*see* **Kappa**). There is little difference in the way that epidemiologic tables are handled by these packages, too little difference to matter to most users. The same is true with respect to tabular analysis of matched

case–control data: all packages offer something, most include some form of exact analysis and some form of **stratification**. I have also left out nonparametric statistics since this would require either a simple, misleading row on whether there are any, or an additional table. Instead, note that Egret, EpiInfo and PEPI have some nonparametric techniques, while Epilog, Stata and True Epistat have quite a lot of nonparametric statistical routines. All of the named packages have some exact procedures, but here I mean the more traditional nonparametric (e.g. Mann–Whitney rank sum, sign test) techniques.

The following are brief descriptions of those routines that might not be obvious from their row title.

- *Multidimensional tables, often called loglinear analysis*: this refers to tables with three or more variables. Note that most such tables are relatively easy to estimate in packages with **Poisson regression**. Some people might expect stub-and-banner tables here, but I have not included them since only Stata has anything like such tables and its version is quite limited. "Stub-and-banner" tables can have multiple variables as the rows and/or as the columns. They are often used when summarizing the study population in one table (e.g. showing the distribution by group and by gender, showing the mean ages of each group, and the mean time since exposure).

- *Complex surveys*: this refers to analysis of data gathered via a nonsimple random sample (e.g. a clustered random sample). Note that EpiInfo can only analyze means and rates, while Stata can also estimate a number of regression models on these samples.
- *PEPI*: this provides simple, but not multiple, linear and nonparametric regression.
- *Censored linear models*: the Buckley–James model in Epilog appears to be superior to the Tobit model in Stata (Moon [7]).
- *Parametric survival models*: these include, for example, exponential or Weibull models for survival analysis. More on various forms of survival analysis and software can be found in Goldstein et al. [4] (*see* **Survival Analysis, Overview**).
- *Extensive nonlinear models*: with the recent interest in neural networks, there has been a corresponding increase in statistical models with extensive nonlinearities among the predictor variables in a model. Epilog has a neural network routine. Stata, instead, has more statistical procedures, including generalized additive models (GAMs), cubic splines and fractional polynomials. Stata also has a more traditional nonlinear least squares routine.
- *Simulations and bootstrap*: as we learn more about the weaknesses of traditional models, and as computers become more powerful, many researchers are turning to computer-intensive methods. The row for "exact logistic regression" is one type of computer-intensive routine, a specific use of randomization of the data. Simulation and bootstrap are two other computer-intensive methods. Their implementation in Stata calls on the user to write some code for their specific use, but supplies all the front-end and back-end and housekeeping work so that actually doing a simulation to see the effect of errors in the predictor variables, for example, is very little work. The work required in Epicure is, however, considerable. Egret has especially easy-to-use Monte Carlo routines. However, the user can only use

Monte Carlo where offered in the package and thus there is no flexibility. If it is offered and what it simulates is what you want (e.g. a *p*-value or confidence interval) then it is very easy to use; if it is not offered, then it cannot be used. Note that for small samples, either exact or simulated results will usually provide more accurate results than will use of the bootstrap.

- *Multilevel models, sometime called random coefficient or hierarchic models*: these are relatively limited in epidemiologic software as yet, but some packages have at least some capabilities (e.g. random effects logistic regression).
- *Seasonality*: the reference here is to epidemiologic uses for, for example, the detection of seasonal or secular trends in disease incidence (as compared, for example, with the use of traditional time-series techniques, which usually need more data).

Note that those packages that have extensive regression routines (Egret, Epicure, Epilog, Stata and True Epistat) also have extensive diagnostics for these regressions, including goodness-of-fit statistics and procedures. While there are minor differences in the offered routines, I believe that any of them would be sufficient for most users.

There are two other important analytic techniques that I think should be included: errors-in-variables (or misclassification) and multiple imputation. It is surprising, and disturbing, that of all the epidemiologic literature dealing with **misclassification**, only PEPI and Stata have anything of relevance, and neither is very good, though Stata's simulation abilities can be of great help. Multiple imputation (Rubin [10], Vach & Blettner [13]) is of importance when there are **missing data**, as, in my experience, there always are. Stata has an impute command, but it is for single imputation and will often give a result that is misleadingly precise – no other package has anything. I believe that these are major failures of all the included software.

None of the packages has excellent graphics, either analytic or publication. All could benefit from more effort in this area. On the other hand, the analytic graphics in most of the packages are sufficient for everyday use by a data analyst. Many of the graphic procedures would have been considered excellent as recently as 10 years ago – but now they are all behind the times. In addition, as noted above, many of these packages are still DOS-based; many of the Windows graphics adapters do not work well in DOS, further impairing the value of the graphics offered by these packages.

I have not specifically commented on importing or exporting data as a general matter (although a few comments are scattered above). In general, the presence of two specialized file-format transfer packages (DBMS/COPY and StatTransfer) makes this issue relatively unimportant. Either of these packages can be used for file import or export. DBMS/COPY can also be used to summarize data either for input into one of the summary-data-only packages (e.g. Epi-Calc or PEPI) or for making stub-and-banner tables for inclusion in a report or publication. Both of these programs can import from, and export to, many other packages, including DBMS programs (e.g. ACCESS), spreadsheets (e.g. QuattroPro), statistical packages such as Stata, SAS or SPSS, and even some specialized graphics packages.

Finally, no matter how much thought a software provider puts into the output from their data management and analysis routines, not everyone will be happy. This presents another advantage of an extensible package – users, or the provider, can provide alternative ways to analyze the data or to present results. While several software providers mentioned output and reporting as one of the reasons for having specialized epidemiologic software, the examples they cited are unimpressive – in almost all cases users will want to change the presentation of results for publication purposes; in almost all cases, this will be very difficult, requiring users to type in the results anew. The only exception is Stata, where user-written routines have added important output flexibility.

The importance of having an extensible package is, I hope, clear, even for those who do not expect ever to extend a package themselves. After all, if there are easy ways to share extensions, all can benefit from the extensions of a few. For example, Stata, the only extensible package here, has several ways to share additions to the package: there is a bimonthly publication, the *Stata Technical Bulletin* (STB) that is filled with new routines from both users and the vendor (and the software is available over the Internet); there is an active user community that both supplements the company's technical support and is a source of additions, primarily from users, to the package – this e-mail listserv can be joined via the company's web site (see below).

Documentation

Over the years, I have examined dozens, if not hundreds, of statistical software packages. The packages discussed here have particularly strong manuals – a very pleasant surprise. All the commercial packages, as well as those from the CDC, have extensive documentation, with extensive professional citations and fully worked examples of the use of the software. Furthermore, in general, the free packages, such as PEPI, at least have extensive help files, which are unusually good, in my opinion (note that PEPI also has a complete manual, as does EpiInfo). Several of the packages even include references to their manual in their online help, something I like and find helpful. The major weakness of most of the packages is in their indexes: only Egret's is as extensive and well-organized as I like (Epicure's is almost as good; its major weakness is that one has to remember to go to the index in the Release 2.0 manual to obtain coverage for all three manuals).

Conclusion

My answer to whether there should be specialized epidemiologic software is a qualified yes: there is always a place (1) for relatively limited specialized software that is primarily useful for quick calculations on tables and provides output that is almost exactly what an epidemiologist is expecting, and (2) for analytic techniques that are primarily useful for particular disciplines, and that have not, yet, made it into general-purpose packages. However, it is a mistake to think that specialized software is all that is needed: no discipline is entirely self-sufficient – there are techniques from other disciplines that are useful and important for epidemiologists. It would be prohibitively expensive for a provider of epidemiologic software to try to match Stata, SAS or S-Plus; it would also be a terrible waste of resources. There is also an important place, in my opinion, for both free and shareware analytic software and I am glad to find that there are several healthy free epidemiologic software packages.

In addition, there is great value to having free packages available (particularly for students and for those who are really part-time epidemiologists), especially if they are very easy to use and include unique features. Several of the free packages discussed here are very easy to use and both `EpiInfo` and `PEPI` have unique features. I hope that the commercial vendors pay attention to these, and other, free packages. However, there is a danger with these packages. Too little attention has been paid to the biasing effects of using simple statistical models, such as $2 \times K$ tables. When combined with the tendency to ignore misclassification and the effects of **missing data**, we can see, I think, one major need in the field: easy to use packages that allow users to build from tables to regression models of various kinds and that allow, and adjust, for misclassification and other types of errors in variables.

Software Sources

Cluster: `http://www.atsdr.cdc.gov/HS/cluster.html`

Egret for Windows: CYTEL Software Corp., 675 Massachusetts Avenue, Cambridge, MA 02139, USA; (617) 661–2011; `http://www.cytel.com` Epicalc: `http://www.myatt.demon.co.uk/index.htm`

Epicure: HiroSoft International Corp., 1463 E. Republican Ave., Suite 103, Seattle, WA 98112, USA; (206) 328–5301; `http://www.hirosoft.com`

EpiInfo: `ftp://ftp.cdc.gov`; directory for Epi-Info: `/pub/software/epi/epiinfo`; directory for EpiMap (not discussed here): `/pub/software/epi/epimap`

Epilog Windows: Epicenter Software, P.O. Box 90073, Pasadena, CA 91109, USA; (818) 304–9487; `http://icarus2.hsc.usc.edu/epicenter`

EpiMeta: `http://www.cdc.gov/epo/dpram/epimeta/epimeta.htm`

PEPI: `http://www.brixtonbooks.demon.co.uk/otherbks.htm#PEPI`: PEPI for Windows, test version: `http://www.myatt.demon.co.uk/index.htm`

Stata: Stata Corp., 702 University Drive East, College Station, TX 77840, USA; (409) 696–4600; `http://www.stata.com`

True Epistat: Epistat Services, 2813 Clearmeadow Drive, Mesquite, TX 75181, USA; (972) 222–3904

Win Episcope and WinEpi Ratios: `http://infecipi.unizar.es/pages/ratio/soft_uk.htm`

References

[1] Byrt, T., Bishop, J. & Carlin, J.B. (1993). Bias, prevalence and kappa, *Journal of Clinical Epidemiology* **46**, 423–429.

[2] Clayton, D. & Hills, M. (1993). *Statistical Models in Epidemiology*. Oxford University Press, Oxford.

[3] Goldstein, R. (1989). Power and sample size via MS/PC-DOS computers, *The American Statistician* **43**, 253–260 (Correction: **44**, 264).

[4] Goldstein, R., Anderson, J., Ash, A., Craig, B., Harrington, D. & Pagano, M. (1989). Survival analysis software on MS/PC-DOS computers, *Journal of Applied Econometrics* **4**, 393–414.

[5] Lantz, C.A. & Nebenzahl, E. (1996). Behavior and interpretation of the kappa statistic: resolution of the two paradoxes, *Journal of Clinical Epidemiology* **49**, 431–434.

[6] McNemar, Q. (1947). Note on the sampling of the difference between correlated proportions or percentages, *Psychometrika* **12**, 153–157.

[7] Moon, C.-G. (1989). A Monte Carlo comparison of semiparametric tobit estimators, *Journal of Applied Econometrics* **4**, 361–382.

[8] Oster, R.A. (1998). An examination of five statistical software packages for epidemiologists, *American Statistician* **52**, 267–280.

[9] Rothman, K.J. & Greenland, S. (1998). *Modern Epidemiology*, 2nd Ed. Lippincott-Raven Publishers, Philadelphia.

[10] Rubin, D.B. (1996). Multiple imputation after 18+ years, *Journal of the American Statistical Association* **91**, 473–489.

[11] Self, S.G. & Mauritsen, R.H. (1988). Power/sample size calculations for generalized linear models, *Biometrics* **44**, 79–86.

[12] Thomas, L. & Krebs, C.J. (1997). A review of statistical power analysis software, *Bulletin of the Ecological Society of America* **78**, 128–139 (or, `http://sustain.forestry.ucb.ca/cacb/power`).

[13] Vach, W. & Blettner, M. (1998). Missing data in epidemiologic studies, in *Encyclopedia of Biostatistics*, Vol. 4, P. Armitage & T. Colton, eds. Wiley, Chichester, pp. 2641–2654.

(*See also* **Software, Biostatistical**)

RICHARD GOLDSTEIN

Sojourn Time *see* Length Bias

Source Population *see* Target Population

Space–Time Interaction *see* Communicable Diseases

Spatial Autocorrelation *see* Geographical Analysis

Specificity

For diagnostic or **screening** tests, the specificity is the probability that an individual without the disease will receive a correct, negative test result. A synonym is the true negative rate, this being the proportion of negative results assigned among the denominator of true noncases of disease. In the table for the entry on **sensitivity**, the specificity is $d/(b + d)$. The false positive rate $b/(b + d)$ is the complement of specificity; in other words, it is the probability that an individual without disease will get a positive test result.

A test with high specificity is useful clinically for ruling in potential disease; a positive result from such a test implies a relatively high chance of having the disease. Typically, if a test is designed to have high specificity, its false negative rate $c/(a + c)$ will also be high and the test sensitivity $a/(a + c)$ will be correspondingly low.

Achievement of high specificity is important when the implied costs of giving false positive test results to noncases are high relative to the costs of incorrectly assigning negative test results to individuals with the disease (the so-called false-negative results). For instance, in population screening programs for rare diseases such as cancer, high specificity is desirable to avoid large numbers of false positive test results that would require clinical follow-up to determine their true, nondisease status.

A second meaning of specificity refers to the capability of a measuring device (e.g. in the clinical chemistry laboratory) to detect a particular target substance in a sample of material, as opposed to giving a false positive reading with other substances.

In multivariate analysis, particularly in factor analysis, specificity refers to the proportion of total variation that is associated with a factor.

(See also **Clinical Epidemiology, Overview**; **Diagnostic Tests, Evaluation of**)

S.D. WALTER

SPSS *see* Software, Biostatistical

Standard Population *see* Standardization Methods

Standardization Methods

Standardization methods are used to adjust for the effects of age and sex, and possibly other factors, in the comparison of disease **rates** between two or more populations. In what follows, adjustment for age will be described, but all the methods can be extended to adjust for other factors, such as sex.

Standardization methods have a long history, and rank among the earliest statistical tools developed. Keiding [22] has traced their origins to eighteenth century actuarial mathematicians, though they were re-invented a century later by Neison and Farr. Neison was a famous statistician of his day, writing regularly in the *Journal of the Statistical Society* on a wide variety of subjects. Farr was a government official who worked as the "compiler of abstracts" in the Office of the Registrar General for England and Wales from 1839 to 1880. These two eminent men recognized that the comparisons of crude death rates (*see* **Vital Statistics, Overview**) were not sufficient for examining mortality patterns over time (*see* **Morbidity and Mortality, Changing Patterns in the Twentieth Century**), or between geographic areas (*see* **Geographic Patterns of Disease**; **Mortality, International Comparisons**). They also showed that the average age at death was not an appropriate index for assessing differences in mortality [26].

In 1841, Farr published age-specific death rates and compared them to rates for the previous three years to show how the pattern of mortality had changed (Registrar General 1841; see [38]). Examination of age-specific rates (usually stratified by sex as well) is widely considered to be the most comprehensive way of comparing disease rates across populations. However, when many populations and types of disease are to be studied, the number of individual rates requiring scrutiny, rapidly becomes awkwardly large. A further summarization of the data is therefore required.

Farr introduced the idea of an external standard population, against which other populations could be compared (Registrar General, 1853; see [38]). His standard was the so-called "healthy counties" in England and Wales. He calculated a set of standard death rates for these counties against which those for other counties could be compared. He then took each of the age-specific rates in the "healthy counties" and multiplied them by the numbers of people of comparable age in the county of interest. In this way he derived an **expected number of deaths** in each age group.

This was not an entirely new method, as Neison had performed similar calculations on rates from two areas of London to prove that the method of comparing average ages at death was flawed [26]. Farr, however, went on to sum the age-specific expected deaths to give the total number of deaths in each county that would be expected if the mortality was the same as in the "healthy counties". The expected number could be compared with the observed number to assess how each county's mortality differed from that in the standard (*see* **Excess Mortality**). Multiplying the ratio of observed to expected deaths by the crude rate in the standard population provided a standardized rate for each county (Registrar General 1857; see [38]). This method is now known as *indirect standardization* and it has remained in widespread use to this day. Since then, other methods have been

suggested, but indirect standardization is possibly still the most popular.

Rates and Ratios

Standardized rates, such as those produced by Farr, are expressed as the number of deaths (or cases of disease) per head of population. These can be compared with crude rates in the standard population and are expressed in the same units as normally used for the presentation of rates (e.g. number of deaths per 100 000 population). Possibly more often, however, standardized ratios are quoted. These compare the disease burden (*see* **Burden of Disease**) in the population of interest with that in the standard population. A ratio of 1 therefore indicates that the populations are similar in terms of the disease in question. Often, ratios are presented as percentages by multiplying them by 100, although this convention will not be used here. Some of the methods that will be described do not provide standardized rates *per se*, but multiplying the ratio by the crude rate in the standard population is a way of obtaining an adjusted rate.

Choice of Standard Population

Most methods of standardization require a standard population against which the population of interest (index population) is to be compared. Usually, the choice of standard is fairly obvious. Thus, for example, in trying to summarize age-specific rates for geographic regions within a country, the national population could be used as a standard. When examining rates for a variety of countries, a world population or the population of the appropriate continent would be suitable standards. Frequently, however, the sum of the set of index populations to be examined is used as the standard.

A variety of standard populations have been used in the successive volumes of *Cancer Incidence in Five Continents*, [32]. These have included estimated African and European and world populations, and a truncated world population that only includes the ages 35–64 in five year age bands. The reason behind the choice of this unusual population was to avoid the examination of rates being dominated by cancers occurring at older ages; cancers at younger ages may give more clues to etiology than those occurring later in life. The most recent volume on cancer incidence [36] has, however, used only the approximate world population.

The important point to note is that different choices of standard population can give rise to different results. Thus identifying a suitable standard is a prerequisite for applying standardization methods. All standardized measures represent a comparison with a chosen standard population.

Notation

The notation used for the formulas for standardized rates and ratios varies widely. The notation used here is given in Table 1.

Indirect and Direct Standardization

Indirect and direct standardization are the two most widely used methods for standardizing rates. Other methods have been proposed, but have not achieved the same popularity.

Indirect Standardization

The information required for use of the indirect method is as follows:

1. age-specific rates in a standard population;
2. the size of the index population in each age group; and
3. the total number of deaths (or cases of disease) in the index population.

The formula for the indirectly standardized ratio is

$$d \bigg/ \sum n_i R_i.$$

Such ratios are widely known as Standardized Mortality Ratios (SMRs) when deaths have been studied. Similar names are adopted for morbidity, such as Standardized Incidence Ratios for cancer **incidence rates**. An alternate way of considering an indirectly standardized ratio is as a ratio of the observed number of events to the number expected in the index population on the basis of standard rates; in other words,

$$\text{SMR} = d/e, \quad \text{where } e = \sum n_i R_i.$$

One can then obtain the indirectly standardized rate by multiplying the ratio by the crude rate in the standard population:

$$dR \bigg/ \sum n_i R_i.$$

Table 1 Notation

Description	Index population	Standard population
Population in age group i	n_i	N_i
Total population	$n = \sum n_i$	$N = \sum N_i$
Deaths/events in age group i[a]	d_i	D_i
Total number of deaths/events	$d = \sum d_i$	$D = \sum D_i$
Death/event rate in age group i	$r_i = d_i/n_i$	$R_i = D_i/N_i$
Crude death/event rate	$r = d/n$	$R = D/N$
Number of deaths from all causes in age group i	a_i	A_i
Proportion of all deaths due to cause of interest in age group i	$p_i = d_i/a_i$	$P_i = D_i/A_i$
Number of deaths from all causes other than the specific cause of interest in age group i	$s_i = a_i - d_i$	$S_i = A_i - D_i$
Odds of death from specific cause compared to other causes	$m_i = d_i/s_i$	$M_i = D_i/S_i$
Number of years in age group i	y_i	
Mid-point of ith age group	h_i	

[a]For proportional analyses, this is the numbers of deaths/events from a specific cause in age group i. For all other indices, this can refer to deaths/events from all causes or a specific cause.

Direct Standardization

A challenge to the indirect method of standardization came in 1883 from within the Registrar General's Office (Registrar General, 1883; see [38]). Ogle proposed the use of what is now known as the *direct method of standardization*. The method can be considered as the opposite of indirect standardization. The type of information required on the standard population for the indirect method is required for the index population in the direct method and vice versa. Thus the information needed for calculating a directly standardized ratio is:

1. age-specific rates in the index population;
2. the size of the standard population in each age group; and
3. the total number of deaths (or cases of disease) in the standard population.

The formula for the directly standardized ratio, usually termed the Comparative Mortality Figure (CMF) when deaths are being considered, is as follows:

$$\sum N_i r_i \bigg/ D.$$

Analogous to the formula for the SMR, the CMF can be expressed as a ratio of the expected deaths in the standard population on the basis of index rates to the total number of deaths in the standard population; in other words,

$$\text{CMF} = E/D, \quad \text{where } E = \sum N_i r_i.$$

Multiplying by the crude rate in the standard population gives the standardized rate as follows:

$$R \sum N_i r_i \bigg/ D = \sum N_i r_i \bigg/ N,$$

since $D/R = N$.

Discussion of Direct and Indirect Methods

The direct method is often advocated as the ideal, because it preserves consistency between different index populations. Thus if each age-specific rate in one index population is greater than the rate for the same age group in another index population, then the standardized rate in the former should be greater than in the latter. This is not necessarily true for indirect standardization. When a large number of index populations are compared to the same standard, the consistency property is important. Often, the standardized rates will be compared between index populations to make statements about differences between their disease rates. A method that may fail to preserve consistency could give rise to misleading conclusions about the disease burdens in different populations. However, it is hard to find examples in practice in which serious problems of this nature have arisen.

Direct standardization can be useful in a situation in which disease rates in the appropriate standard population are unavailable. For example, the *Cancer Incidence in Five Continents* volumes as mentioned above [32, 36]) have used approximate world, African, and European populations. Since cancer registration is patchy worldwide, world cancer incidence rates are unknown. Estimating world rates by summing the numbers of cancers and population sizes in those countries with data would under-represent the cancer burden in Africa, for example. It is much easier to derive an approximate population distribution by age for the world than to estimate world cancer rates. The actual numbers in each age group need not be world figures as long as the ratios between different age groups are approximately correct. Once standard population numbers are available, directly standardized rates can be produced from the age-specific rates from the countries of interest.

Conversely, if age-specific rates in the index population are unavailable, the direct method cannot be used. It is rare to know the total number of cases of disease but not their ages. However, in such a situation, provided that the age distribution of the population is known, then the indirect method could be used.

One might wonder why the indirect method is used so widely, and indeed this question is still a subject of debate. The argument for the indirect method is that it is more stable when studying rates based on small numbers of deaths. If the age-specific rates in the index population are zero for a number of age groups, then the directly standardized rate or ratio is poorly estimated and can have a large standard error. Indeed, the SMR generally has a lower standard error than the CMF, no doubt in part because it is the first approximation to the maximum likelihood estimate of the index under the assumption that the number of deaths follows a Poisson distribution. These factors have led to the indirect method being widely used, particularly in Britain, for analyses of small geographic areas or occupational groups (see, for example, Office of Population Censuses and Surveys, 1986, 1990 [33, 34]; and *see* **Geographic Patterns of Disease**; **Occupational Mortality**). Breslow & Day [2] have pointed out that the SMR is preferred for the analysis of **cross-sectional** data according to **birth cohort** rather than calendar period. This is because the age intervals for which age-specific rates are available tend to vary for different generations, which precludes calculation of the CMF.

SMRs are widely used in analyses of **cohort studies**. The members of the study (index) population are followed through time, and the numbers of events, such as deaths or cancers, are recorded. **Person-years-at-risk** are calculated for each age group and calendar period, which provide the n_i to be multiplied by the age- and calendar period-specific rates R_i from the standard population (usually national rates). We thus obtain an expected number of events, which is compared with the observed number in the study population. The ratio of the observed to expected numbers gives the SMR. When many different causes of death or cancer sites are to be studied, many of the age-specific rates in the study population are zero and so the direct method is rarely used. Only in very large cohort studies does the use of CMFs become

feasible and, even then, only for major **causes of death**.

Other Methods

A wide variety of other methods has been proposed since 1883, when the direct method was advocated. Many have been suggested for the analysis of mortality rates and thus have the word "mortality" in their name. There is no reason, though, why other forms of disease rates should not be summarized using these methods. The formulas for the various rates and ratios are given in Table 2; some methods only provide a standardized rate and no ratio, or vice versa. The origins of these methods and the reasons for them have been reviewed by Inskip et al. [20]. Most of the methods have been suggested in an attempt to circumvent problems identified in the two main methods. Sadly, nothing can circumvent the difficulty that the only reliable way of comparing disease rates is by examining age-specific data.

Few of these methods have become widely used and so they are not discussed in detail here. One that is used regularly, however, is Day's cumulative rate [8]. This has been used in the *Cancer Incidence* volumes since its proposal. It is one of the few methods ever suggested which does not require a standard population, and therefore, perhaps should

Table 2 Formulas for standardized rates and ratios

Rate		Ratio	
Name	Formula	Name	Formula
Comparative mortality rate	$\frac{1}{2}\sum\left(\frac{n_i}{n}+\frac{N_i}{N}\right)r_i$	Comparative mortality index [40]	$\dfrac{\sum(n_i/n+N_i/N)r_i}{\sum(n_i/n+N_i/N)R_i}$
Equivalent average death rate [44]	$\dfrac{\sum y_i r_i}{\sum y_i}$	Yule's index [44]	$\dfrac{\sum y_i r_i}{\sum y_i R_i}$
Cumulative rate [8]	$\sum y_i r_i$	Yerushalmy's relative mortality index [43]	$\dfrac{\sum y_i r_i/R_i}{\sum y_i}$
		Liddell's relative mortality index [25]	$\sum(N_i r_i/NR_i)$
		Relative risk index [27]	$\sum\dfrac{N_i n_i r_i}{(N_i+n_i)R_i}\bigg/\sum\dfrac{N_i n_i}{N_i+n_i}$
		Kerridge's inverse method [23]	$\sum(d_i/nR_i)$
		Fisher's Ideal Index [12]	$\left(\dfrac{d}{\sum R_i n_i}\times\dfrac{\sum r_i N_i}{D}\right)^{1/2}$

not be counted as a "standardization" procedure *per se*. The principle is simple, in that it is the sum of the age-specific rates for each year to age 74. Usually, rates are only available in age bands comprising a number of years. The cumulative rate is then obtained by multiplying each age-specific rate by the number of years it spans, before summing them. The resulting rate is an approximation to the cumulative risk of acquiring the disease from birth to age 74. This gives a useful measure of the disease burden in the population and comparisons can readily be made between two populations of interest. The method does, however, assume that there is no other cause of death to be considered, and this would argue against its use for comparing two populations with widely differing all-cause mortality rates (such as comparing rates in Africa with those in Europe). No ratio is usually derived from this method, although, intuitively, two groups can be compared by taking the ratios of their cumulative rates.

Proportional Methods

Problems arise when no reliable estimates of the population at risk are available. Routine occupational mortality analyses usually suffer from this problem. This is because there are differences in the questions asked about a person's occupation in censuses and those asked of informants of a death. Indeed, the person notifying the death may be unable to give as accurate a description of the occupation as the deceased would have provided on a census form. While SMRs have been widely used for occupational mortality analyses, their weaknesses have to be acknowledged, and they are often **biased** (*see* **Occupational Epidemiology**; **Occupational Health and Medicine**).

A different approach has been adopted in many analyses of this type. In each age group, the population size in each age group is replaced by the number of all-cause deaths. Thus the rates are replaced by the proportions of all deaths due to the cause of interest. A method analogous to that for the SMR is then used to provide a **Proportional Mortality Ratio (PMR)**:

$$d \Big/ \sum a_i P_i.$$

Analyses of proportional mortality (although not as ratios) have a longer history than other standardization methods. As far back as 1662, John Graunt [17] considered the proportion of deaths due to different causes in order to assess the importance of different diseases in leading to death. However, it was not until the twentieth century that proportional methods became popular in a variety of contexts, particularly occupational analyses. The analysis of occupational mortality in England and Wales for 1931 (Registrar General, 1938; see [39]) gave some proportions of deaths due to the cause of interest, but it was not until the comparable report for 1961 (Registrar General, 1971; see [39]) that the ratios were given. They have been used ever since in the analysis of occupational mortality for England and Wales, but it was only in the latest report that they have been used exclusively (Office of Population Censuses and Surveys, 1995 [35]). Indeed, the latest volume also describes cancer incidence data by occupation, again using proportional measures, but these are Proportional Incidence Ratios (PIRs), with all types of incident cancer forming the denominator of the proportions, rather than all deaths.

When suitable populations at risk are unavailable, proportional methods have to be used. Analysis of all-cause mortality does, however, become impossible, as the ratios take the value of unity. Criticisms of the method focus on the problems of bias. If the PMR is used as a proxy for the SMR, it will be biased upward when the all-cause SMR is low (and vice versa). Kupper et al. [24] and Decouflé et al. [9] have discussed the relationship between the PMR and the SMR; the PMR is approximately equal to the ratio of the cause-specific SMR to the all-cause SMR. Kupper et al. [24] termed this ratio the relative SMR (RSMR). In the absence of standardization for any factors, the RSMR and PMR are identical. Since the aim is to standardize, this is unhelpful, but empirical studies have shown that the PMR is a useful proxy for the RSMR [41]. If one is only interested in disease rates in comparison with the standard population, this presents problems for the analysis of groups with very low or high all-cause mortality. However, changes in the distribution of disease within groups should not be ignored, and so the PMR is of value in its own right. PMRs may well lead to useful etiologic clues, particularly in occupational groups with low overall mortality. In such groups, diseases with rates comparable to those in the standard population would be missed by an SMR analysis but would be identified by an elevated PMR.

PMRs can also be biased by abnormally low or high mortality from causes other than that of interest. This problem has been examined by McDowall [30]. He pointed out that it is only the largest causes that seriously influence the PMR for other causes. This led him to suggest re-calculations of the PMR, successively excluding the major causes of death from both the standard and index proportions.

The method of calculation of the PMR is similar to that for the SMR, as it employs an indirect standardization approach, albeit of proportions instead of rates. In 1983, Zeighami & Morris [45] proposed an alternative to the PMR which is analogous to a direct standardization method, the formula being

$$\sum A_i p_i \Big/ D,$$

but this does not appear to have been widely used.

Mortality Odds Ratio

A different approach to proportional mortality analyses was proposed by Miettinen & Wang [31]. Their ratio is equivalent to the **odds ratio** used in the analysis of **case–control studies**. The "cases" are deaths from the cause of interest and the "controls" are deaths from all other causes. "Exposure" is then membership of the study group of interest (e.g. a particular occupational group, or residence in a specific geographic area), and the "unexposed" are all those not in the group of interest and form the "standard" for this method. The formula for the Mortality Odds Ratio (MOR) is

$$d \Big/ \sum s_i M_i.$$

This index is attractive, as it can be interpreted in a similar way to a case–control study, although the choice of other deaths as controls is not necessarily ideal. It is straightforward to show that the unadjusted PMR is always more conservative than the MOR. When such methods are being used for screening large amounts of data, such as in routine occupational mortality statistics, many false positives are identified. The use of a more conservative index may be an advantage. With the current speed of computers, the fact that the PMR is simpler to calculate is a minor point, but may still be a consideration if large data sets are to be analyzed (*see* **Proportional Mortality Study**).

Person-Years-of-Life Lost

One concern about most standardization methods is that they give most weight to the age groups that contain the largest numbers of events. In most mortality or morbidity analyses, the elderly therefore receive most emphasis. Restriction of the age groups under study can help, and indeed Yule's method [44] (see Table 2) and Day's cumulative rate [8] require an upper age limit for their calculation. However, for certain analyses, deaths occurring at younger ages may be of greatest interest.

In the early 1950s, there was considerable discussion about this problem [11, 18, 28, 29]. Whether examining changes in mortality over time, or comparing occupational groups, it is often of interest to know whether there are differences at younger ages that are missed by analyses dominated by many events among the elderly. Haenszel [18] loosely defined person–years of life lost as "the total number of years lost through the failure of individuals to live some allotted life span", and pointed out that working-years lost "refer to those falling between the productive ages between 20 and 65". He went on to point out that "it has long been recognized that a count of deaths alone did not give a complete picture of mortality, and measures have been sought which would make some allowance for the widely held intuitive idea that a death at age 70, for example, does not represent as great a loss to society as death at age 35".

While standardized rates of years of life lost can be calculated and used for comparison of groups, ratios are usually more readily understood. To obtain either rates or ratios, the deaths in each age group in the index and standard population are multiplied by the years of life lost in each age group.

Two different forms of years of life lost factors have been suggested. The first is simply to choose an upper age limit of interest and subtract from it the mid-age of each age group. Thus, if years to age 70 were of interest, the years-of-life lost in age group 35–39 would be 33. The formula for the standardized ratio is therefore

$$\frac{\sum d_i(70 - h_i)}{\sum n_i R_i(70 - h_i)}$$

This is equivalent to a weighted indirectly standardized ratio, and by analogy the directly standardized form is

$$\frac{\sum N_i r_i (70 - h_i)}{\sum D_i (70 - h_i)}.$$

Upper age limits other than 70 can be used and, indeed, a lower age limit such as 15 or 20 for occupational mortality can be incorporated by ignoring deaths in childhood.

The other form of weights to represent years of life lost are obtained from **life table** estimates of **life expectancy**. The number of years that a person at the mid-age of each age group can be expected to live is estimated from life tables derived from death rates for the standard population. These weights can then be used in the above formulas replacing $70 - h_i$.

Variances and Standard Errors

In estimating standard errors, we usually assume that the standard rates and populations are stable and their sampling errors can be ignored. This is not always true, but, rightly or wrongly, the assumption is usually made. We also assume that the populations in the index population are fixed. Therefore, the only random variables to consider are the age-specific rates in the index population, or, more simply, the numbers of events in each age group in the index population. The events in each age group are also assumed to be independent of each other.

It is worth noting that almost all the formulas for standardized rates and ratios can be written as a weighted sum of the age-specific rates in the index population:

$$\sum w_i r_i,$$

where the w_i are the weights.

Thus, for the directly standardized rate, the weights are

$$w_i = N_i / N,$$

while for the indirect method they are

$$w_i = n_i R \Big/ \sum n_i R_i.$$

Similar formulas exist for the ratios. Most of the ratios can be written as a weighted average of the age-specific ratios in the form

$$\frac{\sum (w_i r_i / R_i)}{\sum w_i}$$

or, sometimes more conveniently, as a ratio of the weighted age-specific rates:

$$\frac{\sum w_i r_i}{\sum w_i R_i}.$$

Using the first form, the weights for the CMF (directly standardized ratio) are D_i and for SMR (indirectly standardized ratio) are $n_i R_i$. All the other rates and ratios in Table 2 can be written in this form with differing values of w_i, the only exception being Fisher's Ideal Index [12].

The next step is therefore to consider the standard error of the r_i (or d_i). There are two approaches to this.

Use of the Binomial Distribution

Chiang [6] developed an approach based on the binomial distribution. He noted that rates r_i are not proportions, but derived a formula for each rate as a function of the proportions of deaths d_i in the hypothetical population from which the deaths were drawn. This requires knowing the distribution of the ages of the events within each age group. As an approximation it is reasonable to assume that all events occur in the middle of the age range. Chiang's formula for the variance of the r_i then becomes

$$\frac{r_i(2 - y_i r_i)}{n_i(2 + y_i r_i)}.$$

This leads to the variance of the standardized rate being

$$\sum w_i^2 \, \text{var}(r_i),$$

and that of the ratio being

$$\frac{\sum \left[\dfrac{w_i^2}{R_i^2} \, \text{var}(r_i) \right]}{\left(\sum w_i \right)^2}.$$

The standard errors are then the square roots of the variances.

Use of the Poisson Distribution

The alternative approach to estimating the standard errors is to assume that the numbers of events in each age group follow a Poisson distribution. (It is worth nothing, however, that this assumption may not be valid and that extra-Poisson variability may need to be investigated [3]. The variance of a Poisson variable is equal to its expectation, for which the observed number of events is the best approximation available. The denominators of the rates (the n_i) can be absorbed into the weights and so the formulas for the variances of the rates and ratios become

$$\sum w_i^2 r_i \Big/ n_i$$

and

$$\frac{\displaystyle\sum \frac{w_i^2 r_i}{R_i^2 n_i}}{\left(\sum w_i\right)^2},$$

respectively.

These formulas reduce to fairly simple forms for direct and indirect standardization, and these are given in Table 3.

The formulas for the standard errors of the PMR (indirectly and directly obtained) are similar to those in Table 3. The numbers in the populations are replaced by the numbers of all-cause deaths, and the rates are replaced by the proportions of deaths. However, it is worth noting that the proportions of deaths due to the cause of interest are true proportions, unlike rates, and so the binomial distribution could be used in the derivation of the standard errors.

Table 3 Variances of directly and indirectly standardized rates and ratios

Method	Rate	Ratio
Direct	$\sum(N_i^2 r_i/N^2 n_i)$	$\sum(N_i^2 r_i/D^2 n_i)$
Indirect	$\dfrac{\sum R_i^2 d_i}{\left(\sum n_i R_i\right)^2}$	$\dfrac{d}{\left(\sum n_i R_i\right)^2} = \dfrac{d}{e^2}$

Note that when SMRs are under discussion alone, the variance is usually given as O/E^2, although the use of upper case letters and O for the total number of (observed) deaths is not consistent with the notation used here for index and standard populations.

Confidence Intervals

In deriving confidence intervals for rates and ratios, similar assumptions are made as for the estimation of standard errors (se). Again, we have to make assumptions about the distribution of the rates and ratios.

Confidence Intervals for Rates

Confidence intervals for rates can be derived by assuming that the rates follow a normal distribution. The method, therefore, is to add and subtract 1.96 times the standard error from the rate. If rates are small, this leads to problems, as negative values can occur. In such cases, it is preferable to consider the standard error of the logarithm of the rate. Using the standard approximation

$$\operatorname{var}(\log x) = \operatorname{var} x/x^2,$$

the standard error of the logarithm of a standardized rate can be obtained as

$$\operatorname{se}\,(\log(\text{rate})) = (\operatorname{se}\,(\text{rate}))/\text{rate}.$$

Using this, a 95% confidence for the logarithm of the rate can be obtained, and taking exponentials gives the 95% confidence interval for the rate itself.

Such estimates of confidence intervals rely on the adequacy of the normal assumption, either for the rate or its logarithm. The assumption tends to be poor when the rates are low. This is particularly a problem when we are calculating weighted sums of the age-specific rates, each of which may be small. Dobson et al. [10] have addressed this issue. They have discussed a number of alternate methods for estimating the confidence interval for a Poisson parameter, and derived an improved estimate for the confidence interval for a weighted sum of the events in each age group.

The lower point and upper point of the interval are

$$\text{standardized rate} + (V/d)^{1/2}(d_{\mathrm{L}} - d)$$

and

$$\text{standardized rate} + (V/d)^{1/2}(d_{\mathrm{U}} - d),$$

where

$$V = \sum w_i^2 r_i,$$

and d_L and d_U are the lower and upper confidence interval for the total number of observed deaths, d. Various tables of confidence intervals for Poisson variables exist, usually for a number of levels of confidence. Those given by Gardner [15] provide 90%, 95%, and 99% confidence intervals. Alternatively, Dobson et al. [10] provide a list of approximate methods for obtaining d_L and d_U.

Recently, there has been considerable research into improved methods for obtaining confidence intervals for standardized rates. As Swift [42] has noted, most of these have been computer intensive methods, and none appears to have been used routinely. Swift himself suggested an approximate bootstrap method which he compared with other methods using simulation studies. It appears that the debate on calculation of confidence intervals has not yet run its course. Since all methods are approximate, a sensible approach might be to produce a number of confidence intervals calculated in different ways to see how they vary.

Confidence Intervals for Ratios

Similar considerations apply to the confidence interval for a ratio. Ratios are decidedly nonnormal and often the logarithm is considered, with its approximate standard error being calculated as described above. The formula for standard error of the logarithm of the directly standardized ratio (CMF) is

$$\left(\sum N_i^2 r_i/n_i\right)^{1/2} \bigg/ \sum N_i r_i,$$

whereas that for the logarithm of the indirectly standardized ratio (SMR) reduces to

$$1/\sqrt{d}.$$

An alternative method for the calculation of confidence intervals for the SMR (and for the indirectly standardized PMR) requires us to assume that the total number of observed deaths in the index population, d, is a Poisson variable. d_L and d_U, the lower and upper points of the confidence interval for d, are first obtained from tables or approximations and then the corresponding confidence interval for the SMR is

$$d_L/E - d_U/E.$$

These formulas are now widely used for the calculation of confidence intervals, and it is unusual to

derive confidence intervals for SMRs using the standard errors. Computationally intensive methods could also be used, but the above formula is considered appropriate for most needs.

Regression Models

Increasingly, mortality rates are being modeled using regression techniques. Keiding [22] discusses some of these approaches at the end of his historical review paper. Generalized linear modeling can be used to analyze rates, and a number of papers have explored the issues relating to such analyses [13, 14]. More recently, there has been increasing interest in Bayesian approaches using Monte Carlo methods [1] and generalized estimating equations.

Recurrent Outcomes

An important new development in the standardization of rates is the consideration of recurrent outcomes. Most of the methods described above have been developed with a single outcome per person in mind, notably death. Even when cancer has been of interest, the number of people with multiple cancers is so small that the cancers have been assumed to be independent. Epidemiology has moved on from there, to deal with outcomes that can occur more than once within an individual. Examples are admission to hospital, episodes of back pain, and attacks of asthma.

Although the standardized rates can be calculated as for nonrecurrent events, the standard errors are larger because of the lack of independence of recurrent events. Glynn et al. [16] used the negative binomial distribution to account for departures from the assumption, inherent in the use of the Poisson distribution, that the recurrent events occur randomly. The variance of each age-specific rate in the index population is then

$$(r_i + r_i^2/k)/n_i,$$

where k is an index of extra-Poisson variation in the rate, with smaller values of k indicating larger departures from the Poisson distribution. k has to be estimated from the data and Glynn et al. suggest use of the method of moments estimator.

The variance of the standardized rate is then

$$\sum (w_i^2) \, \mathrm{var}(r_i),$$

from which the standard error can be obtained by taking the square root. Again, to obtain confidence intervals, taking logarithms as described above is recommended.

Often one wishes to compare a number of standardized rates (for recurrent or single events). Carriere & Roos [5] have developed a simple test for the comparison of H standardized rates against a standard rate that can be compared with the chi-square distribution on H degrees of freedom. If S_h is the standardized rate in the hth index population, and R is the crude rate in the standard population, then the test statistic is

$$\sum (S_h - R)^2 / \text{var}(S_h),$$

where the summation is over the H populations of interest. If the standard rate is simply the overall rate obtained from the combined index populations, then the test statistic should be compared with the chi-square distribution on $H - 1$ degrees of freedom.

More complex approaches are recommended when the data are available for each individual followed up over time. In this way, the events occurring for each person are known. The analysis of such outcomes requires approaches used for the analysis of longitudinal data. Methods mentioned above such as generalized estimating equations, Bayesian approaches using Markov chain Monte Carlo methods, and other methods for multilevel modeling could be applied. These are, however, computationally intensive and analysis of large data sets can be very time-consuming.

Computation

Despite the long history of standardization methods, standard statistical packages rarely allow for their use. Most users have to write their own procedures, and link their data to the standard rates. Routines or macros within standard packages have been written by individuals and some have been published recently for use by others. Immonen-Räihä et al. [19] published a macro for use in SAS (*see* **Software, Biostatistical**) which they developed to analyze data on hospitalization and death from coronary heart disease. Clayton & Hills [7] have produced a suite of routines for use in STATA for the analysis of case–control and prevalence studies, and these can be used for deriving standardized rates. For users of other packages, specific programs for analysis of individual data sets

are usually written by the user. Spreadsheets containing the standard rates, population, and numbers of events, and comparable information for the index, population, can also be used to derive the standardized rates/ratios.

For modeling approaches to the analysis of rates, many packages are available and will not be outlined here.

Discussion of Methods

Over the years, many methods of standardization have been proposed. No single method has emerged on top and a variety are in use. Direct and indirect standardization are undoubtedly the most popular, but other methods such as PMRs have to be employed in certain circumstances. A recent report of occupational mortality in Italy [21] gave a table summarizing occupational mortality analyses from many countries worldwide in recent years. The method used for obtaining standardized ratios in each analysis was listed, and four different methods had been employed. None used a direct method, whereas this is commonly used in cancer studies (see, for example, Parkin et al. [36]) and in many geographic analyses (see, for example, Pickle et al. [37]).

Estimating standard errors and deriving confidence intervals are not straightforward, and many methods are in widespread use. The final verdict has not yet been reached as to which methods are best, and the debate is likely to continue for many years.

As a final note, and to return to where we began, we must be aware that in any standardization procedure we lose something. Much of the debate about which methods to use is due to the fact that no standardized measure can replace the analysis of the age-specific rates themselves. We should understand that summaries can be distorted by patterns in particular age groups. Before one employs any standardization, one should scrutinize the individual age groups. Burack et al. [4] have argued forcibly for examining the age-specific rates, but it has to be acknowledged that in large-scale studies of routine data, even examining the standardized rates or ratios for each subset of the population (such as each occupational group) is an unwieldy task. Scrutiny of the age-specific rates for every group would be impossible. However, perhaps we should take the advice of Burack et al., at least in part, and before commenting on any particular standardized rate or ratio as being particularly high or low we should be more prepared to examine the original age-specific data.

References

[1] Bean, J.A., Wiltse, C.G. & Woolson, R.E. (1987). Small sample behaviour of hypothesis tests related to indirect standardized rates: a Monte Carlo study, *Statistics in Medicine* **6**, 61–70.

[2] Breslow, N.E. & Day, N.E. (1987). *Statistical Methods in Cancer Research, II, The Design and Analysis of Cohort Studies.* International Association for Research in Cancer, Lyon.

[3] Brillinger, D.R. (1986). The natural variability of vital rates and associated statistics, *Biometrics* **42**, 693–734.

[4] Burack, T.S., Burack, W.R. & Knowlden, N.F. (1983). Cancer II: distortions in standardized rates, *Journal of Occupational Medicine* **25**, 737–744.

[5] Carriere, K.C. & Roos, L.L. (1994). Comparing standardized rates of events, *American Journal of Epidemiology* **140**, 472–482.

[6] Chiang, C.L.C. (1961). Standard error of the age-adjusted death rate, *US Department of Health Education and Welfare, Vital Statistics Special Reports*, Vol. 47, 271–285.

[7] Clayton, D. & Hills, M. (1995). Analysis of follow-up studies, *Stata Technical Bulletin* **27**, 19–26.

[8] Day, N.E. (1976). Cumulative rate and cumulative risk, in *Cancer Incidence in Five Continents*, Vol. III. J. Waterhouse, C. Muir, P. Correa & J. Powell, eds. International Association for Research in Cancer, Lyon.

[9] Decouflé, P., Thomas, T.L. & Pickle, L.W. (1980). Comparison of the proportionate mortality ratio and standardized mortality ratio risk measures, *American Journal of Epidemiology* **111**, 263–269.

[10] Dobson, A.J., Kuulasmaa, K., Eberle, E. & Scherer, J. (1991). Confidence intervals for weighted sums of Poisson parameters, *Statistics in Medicine* **10**, 457–462.

[11] Doughty, J.H. (1951). Mortality in terms of lost years of life, *Canadian Journal of Public Health* **42**, 134–141.

[12] Fisher, I. (1927). *The Making of Index Numbers.* Houghton Mifflin, Boston.

[13] Frome, E.L. (1983). The analysis of rates using Poisson regression models, *Biometrics* **39**, 665–674.

[14] Gail, M. (1978). The analysis of heterogeneity for indirect standardized mortality ratios, *Journal of the Royal Statistical Society, Series A* **141**, 224–234.

[15] Gardner, M.J. (1989). Tables for the calculation of confidence intervals, in *Statistics with Confidence*, M.J. Gardner & D.G. Altman, eds. BMJ, London, pp. 116–118.

[16] Glynn, R.J., Stukel, T.A., Sharp, S.M., Bubolz, T.S., Freeman, J.L. & Fisher, E.S. (1993). Estimating the variance of standardized rates of recurrent events, with application to hospitalizations among the elderly in New England, *American Journal of Epidemiology* **137**, 776–786.

[17] Graunt, J. (1662). *Natural and Political Observations made upon the Bills of Mortality.* London: re-published by the Johns Hopkins Press, Baltimore (1939).

[18] Haenszel, W. (1950). A standardized rate for mortality defined in units of lost years of life, *American Journal of Public Health* **40**, 17–26.

[19] Immonen-Räihä, P., Hätönen, S., Torppa, J. & Toivanen, A. (1994). A statistical analysis system macro for age-standardized incidence rates, *Computer Methods and Programs in Biomedicine* **44**, 79–83.

[20] Inskip, H., Beral, V. & Fraser, P. (1983). Methods for age-adjustment of rates, *Statistics in Medicine* **2**, 455–466.

[21] Instituto Superiore per la Prevenzione e la Sicurezza del Lavoro (1995). *Mortalità per Professioni in Italia negli Anni '80.* Collana Quaderni ISPESL, Rome.

[22] Keiding, N. (1987). The method of expected number of deaths 1786–1886–1986, *International Statistical Review* **55**, 1–20.

[23] Kerridge, D. (1958). A new method of standardizing death rates, *British Journal of Preventive and Social Medicine* **12**, 154–155.

[24] Kupper, L.L., McMichael, A.J., Symons, M.J. & Most, B.M. (1978). On the utility of proportional mortality analysis, *Journal of Chronic Diseases* **31**, 15–22.

[25] Liddell, F.D.K. (1960). The measurement of occupational mortality, *British Journal of Industrial Medicine* **17**, 228–233.

[26] Lilienfeld, D.E. (1978). "The greening of epidemiology": sanitary physicians and the London epidemiological society (1830–1870), *Bulletin of the History of Medicine* **52**, 503–528.

[27] Lilienfeld, D.E. & Pyne, D.A. (1979). On indices of mortality: deficiencies, validity and alternatives, *Journal of Chronic Diseases* **32**, 463–468.

[28] Logan, W.P.D. & Benjamin, B. (1953). Loss of expected years of life – a perspective view of changes between 1848–72 and 1952, *Monthly Bulletin of the Ministry of Health and the Public Health Laboratory Service* **12**, 244–252.

[29] Martin, W.J. (1951). Life table mortality as a measure of hygiene, *The Medical Officer* **86**, 151–153.

[30] McDowall, M. (1983). Adjusting proportional mortality ratios for the influence of extraneous causes of death, *Statistics in Medicine* **2**, 467–475.

[31] Miettinen, O. & Wang, J.D. (1981). An alternative to the proportionate mortality ratio, *American Journal of Epidemiology* **114**, 144–148.

[32] Muir, C., Waterhouse, J., Mack, T., Powell, J. & Whelan, S., eds (1987). *Cancer Incidence in Five Continents*, Vol. V. International Association for Research in Cancer, Lyon.

[33] Office of Population Censuses and Surveys (1986). *Occupational Mortality 1979–80, 1982–83. Decennial Supplement.* HMSO, London.

[34] Office of Population Censuses and Surveys (1990). *Mortality and Geography.* HMSO, London.

[35] Office of Population Censuses and Surveys and Health and Safety Executive, (1995). *Occupational Health, Decennial Supplement.* HMSO, London.

[36] Parkin, D.M., Muir, C.S., Whelan, S.L., Gao, Y.T., Ferlay, J. & Powell, J., eds (1992). *Cancer Incidence in Five Continents*, Vol. VI. International Association for Research in Cancer, Lyon.

[37] Pickle, L.W., Mason, T.J., Howard, N., Hoover, R. & Fraumeni, J.F. (1987). *Atlas of U.S. Cancer Mortality among Whites: 1950–1980.* US Department of Health and Human Services (DHSS Publication no. (NIH) 87-2900), Washington, D.C.

[38] Registrar General (1841, 1853, 1857, 1883). *Annual Report of the Registrar General for England and Wales.* HMSO, London.

[39] Registrar General (1938, 1971). *Registrar General's Decennial Supplement on Occupational Mortality, 1931, 1961.* HMSO, London.

[40] Registrar General (1941). *Registrar General's Statistical Review of England and Wales.* HMSO, London.

[41] Roman, E., Beral, V., Inskip, H., McDowall, M. & Adelstein, A. (1984). A comparison of standardized and proportional mortality ratios, *Statistics in Medicine* **3**, 7–14.

[42] Swift, M.B. (1995). Simple confidence intervals for standardized rates based on the approximate bootstrap method, *Statistics in Medicine* **14**, 1875–1888.

[43] Yerushalmy, J. (1951). A mortality index for use in place of the age-adjusted death rate, *American Journal of Public Health* **41**, 907–922.

[44] Yule, G.U. (1934). On some points relating to vital statistics, more especially statistics of occupational mortality, *Journal of the Royal Statistical Society* **97**, 1–84.

[45] Zeighami, E.A. & Morris, M.D. (1983). The measurement and interpretation of proportionate mortality, *American Journal of Epidemiology* **117**, 90–97.

Bibliography

A list of further reading is given below. This consists of articles and books which have not been referenced above but may be of interest to those who want further information. They include some references which date back many years, but which have contributed to the development of current views on standardized methods.

Benjamin, B. (1968). *Health and Vital Statistics.* George Allen & Unwin, London.

Berry, G. (1983). The analysis of mortality by the subject–years method, *Biometrics* **39**, 173–184.

Breslow, N.E. & Day, N.E. (1975). Indirect standardization and multiplicative models for rates, with reference to the age adjustment of cancer incidence and relative frequency data, *Journal of Chronic Diseases* **28**, 289–303.

Fox, A.J. & Adelstein, A.M. (1978). Occupational mortality: work or way of life?, *Journal of Epidemiology and Community Health* **32**, 73–78.

Gaffey, W.R. (1976). A critique of the standardized mortality ratio, *Journal of Occupational Medicine* **18**, 157–160.

Hanley, J. & Liddell, D. (1985). Fitting relationships between exposure and standardized mortality ratios, *Journal of Occupational Medicine* **27**, 555–560.

Hickey, R.J., Clelland, R.C. & Clelland, A.B. (1980). Epidemiological studies of chronic disease: maladjustment of observed mortality rates, *American Journal of Public Health* **70**, 142–150.

Keiding, N. (1991). Age-specific incidence and prevalence: a statistical perspective, *Journal of the Royal Statistical Society, Series A* **154**, 371–412.

Kilpatrick, S.J. (1962). Occupational mortality indices, *Population Studies* **16**, 175–187.

Kleinman, J.C. (1977). Age-adjusted mortality indexes for small areas: applications to health planning, *American Journal of Public Health* **67**, 834–840.

Liddell, F.D.K. (1979). Excess PYLL for occupational mortality comparisons, *International Journal of Epidemiology* **8**, 185–186.

Liddell, F.D.K. (1984). Simple exact analysis of the standardised mortality ratio, *Journal of Epidemiology and Community Health* **38**, 85–88.

McDowall, M. (1983). William Farr and the study of occupational mortality, *Population Trends* **31**, 12–19.

McMichael, A.J. (1976). Standardized mortality ratios and the "Healthy Worker Effect": scratching beneath the surface, *Journal of Occupational Medicine* **18**, 165–168.

Miettinen, O.S. (1972). Standardization of risk ratios, *American Journal of Hygiene* **6**, 383–388.

Milham, S. (1975). Methods in occupational mortality studies, *Journal of Occupational Medicine* **17**, 581–585.

Milham, S. (1985). Improving occupational standardized proportionate mortality ratio analysis by social class stratification, *American Journal of Epidemiology* **121**, 472–475.

Morris, J.A. & Gardner, M.J. (1988). Calculating confidence intervals for relative risks (odds ratios) and standardised ratios and rates, *British Medical Journal* **296**, 1313–1316.

Osborn, J. (1975). A multiplicative model for the analysis of vital statistics rates, *Applied Statistics* **24**, 75–84.

Redmond, C. & Breslin, P.P. (1975). Comparison of methods for assessing occupational hazards, *Journal of Occupational Medicine* **17**, 313–317.

Rockette, H.E. & Arena, V.C. (1987). Evaluation of the proportionate mortality index in the presence of multiple comparisons, *Statistics in Medicine* **6**, 71–77.

Romeder, J.M. & McWhinnie, J.R. (1977). Potential years of life lost between ages 1 and 70: an indicator of premature mortality for health planning, *International Journal of Epidemiology*, **6**, 143–151.

Stukel, T.A., Glynn, R.J., Fisher, E.S., Sharp, S.M., Lu-Yao, G. & Wennberg, J.E. (1994). Standardized rates of recurrent outcomes, *Statistics in Medicine* **13**, 1781–1791.

Tsai, S.P. & Wen, C.P. (1986). A review of methodological issues of the standardized mortality ratio (SMR) in occupational cohort studies, *International Journal of Epidemiology* **15**, 8–21.

Tsai, S.P., Hardy, R.J. & Wen, C.P. (1992). The standardized mortality ratio and life expectancy, *American Journal of Epidemiology* **135**, 824–831.

Wong, O. (1977). Further criticisms on epidemiological methodology in occupational studies, *Journal of Occupational Medicine* **19**, 220–222.

Wong, O. & Decouflé, P. (1982). Methodological issues involving the standardized mortality ratio and proportionate mortality ratio in occupational studies, *Journal of Occupational Medicine* **24**, 299–304.

HAZEL INSKIP

Standardized Incidence Ratio (SIR) *see* Standardization Methods

Standardized Mortality Odds Ratio (SMOR) *see* Proportional Mortality Study

Standardized Mortality Ratio (SMR)

The standardized mortality ratio (SMR) is the ratio of the number of deaths observed in a given (index) population to the number of deaths expected. The number of expected deaths is calculated as $\sum_i n_i R_i$, where n_i is the number of persons in category i of the index population and R_i is the corresponding category-specific event rate in a standard population. Categories are usually defined by age, gender and race or ethnicity. Sometimes one will categorize only on age and study a single gender and racial group. For example, one could create an age-adjusted SMR for white males. The SMR is sometimes multiplied by 100. The SMR is called an indirect standardized rate

and is distinguished from directly standardized rates, which are weighted averages of the category-specific rates in the index population (*see* **Standardization Methods** for a comparison of these two types of standardization).

The SMR, like other forms of standardization, is used to create summary mortality statistics that can be used to compare populations with differing distributions of individuals in age, gender and race categories. Indirect standardization is also used to create the standardized incidence ratio (SIR) for comparing disease incidence rates.

Like any summary statistic, the SMR can be misleading and can obscure important differences in category-specific rates among populations. When, however, ratios of category-specific rates comparing one index population with the next are constant across categories and when the rates are small so that the numbers of events are approximately Poisson distributed, SMRs are ideal summary statistics [1]. Indeed, SMRs are maximum likelihood estimates of the parameter θ_j in a Poisson regression model with expectation $\theta_j R_i$ in category i of population j, where R_i is assumed known. If R_i is not known, then it can also be estimated via **Poisson Regression** [1]. Formal methods for comparing SMRs and analyzing heterogeneity among groups of SMRs are given in Gail [2].

References

[1] Breslow, N.E. & Day, N.E. (1985). The standardized mortality ratio, in *Biostatistics: Statistics in Biomedical, Public Health and Environmental Sciences*, P.K. Sen, ed. Elsevier, New York, pp. 55–74.

[2] Gail, M. (1978). The analysis of heterogeneity for indirect standardized mortality ratios, *Journal of the Royal Statistical Society, Series A* **141**, 224–234.

M.H. GAIL

Standardized Mortality Ratio (SMR) Regression *see* Poisson Regression for Survival Data in Epidemiology

Standardized Proportional Mortality Ratio (SPMR) *see* Proportional Mortality Study

Stones' Maximum Likelihood Ratio Test *see* Geographical Analysis

Stratification

Stratification refers in epidemiology to a design that improves the efficiency of analytical procedures to control for **confounding** by causing **controls** to have the same distribution over strata defined by levels of potential **confounders** as cases in a **case–control study** or as the exposed cohort in a **cohort study** (*see* **Matching**; **Frequency Matching**). Stratification (or stratified analysis) also refers to the analytical strategy that controls for confounding by estimating the association between exposure and disease status within strata defined by categorized levels of potential confounders and then combining stratum-specific results to obtain an overall estimate of exposure effect (*see* **Mantel–Haenszel Methods**; **Matched Analysis**).

In the context of survey sampling, stratification is an efficient design that usually allocates larger samples to strata of the population within which the estimate has a large variance (*see* **Sample Surveys**).

M.H. GAIL

Structural Modeling *see* Measurement Error in Epidemiologic Studies

Study Base *see* Case–Control Study

Study Population

The term *study population* is often used to refer to the population from which observations are drawn; that is, the sampled population (*see* **Target Population**). In other writings, it has been used to refer to the study sample [1].

Reference

[1]   Kleinbaum, D.G., Kupper, L.L. & Morgenstern, H. (1984). *Epidemiologic Research: Principles and Quantitative Methods*. Van Nostrand, New York.

(*See also* **Validity and Generalizability in Epidemiologic Studies**)

SANDER GREENLAND

Subject-Years Method *see* Expected Number of Deaths

SUDAAN *see* Random Digit Dialing Sampling for Case–Control Studies

Sufficient-Component Cause (SCC) Model *see* Causation

Surface Models for Screening *see* Screening, Overview

Surveillance of Diseases

Modern public health surveillance of disease has been defined by Langmuir [14] as "the continued

Table 1 Distinctions between public health surveillance and epidemiologic research (adapted from Thacker & Berkelman [24])

	Surveillance	Epidemiologic research
Main purpose	Problem detection Problem description Trigger either investigation or intervention Suggest hypotheses	Hypothesis testing Problem description
Data collection		
Frequency	Ongoing	Time-limited
Methods	Normally routine systems	Specially tailored for study
Volume of data	Minimal	Considerable
Completeness of data	Often incomplete	Usually complete
Data analyses	Usually simple and descriptive	Often complex

Dissemination of information	Timely, regular, targeted to
	   public health agencies
		Not timely, sporadic, targeted
		   to academics and clinical
		   audience

watchfulness over the distribution and trends of incidence through the systematic collection, consolidation and evaluation of morbidity and mortality reports and other relevant data". It is now usual to add to this definition the final link of applying these data to prevention and control [26]. But this public health activity is not new. One of the earliest examples of population surveillance was that developed in the City of London in the sixteenth and seventeeth centuries to detect plague, so that the City Fathers could decide when to close theaters and limit the assembly of crowds, and the Royal Court could leave for the countryside [31]. Data on plague deaths were collected by parish clerks, summated each week and reported in the "Bills of Mortality". The system neatly illustrates the steps in surveillance, which are the systematic collection of data, analyses to produce statistics, interpretation to provide information—which is then reported fast enough so that action can be taken—followed by continuing surveillance to evaluate the success of the action.

The concept of surveillance is simple, but in practice there is a tendency for surveillance systems to drift from their original objectives and too easily lose their focus on public health action—"Reporting does not equal surveillance". It is therefore important that surveillance as a dynamic public health activity is distinguished from managing registries (*see* **Disease Registers**) and other health information systems such as registrations of births and deaths (*see* **Vital Statistics, Overview**), though these may be useful

data sources for surveillance. It is also important to recognize that public health surveillance differs from epidemiologic research in a number of important ways [24] (Table 1). The need for ongoing reporting (which distinguishes surveillance from occasional surveys) to provide information for action requires that surveillance systems are simple in construction, place minimal demands on data providers, and report accurate, readily understood, and timely information. Systems have often degenerated because data requirements have not been agreed with data providers and have become overburdened with secondary objectives. Consequent failure to report in a timely way had led to the loss of credibility with data providers. Recent successful infectious disease surveillance systems have used electronic reporting to minimize the burden on data providers and provide high-quality, rapid reporting [11, 29].

Guidelines on the evaluation of surveillance systems have been proposed by the Centers for Disease Control (CDC) [13], although few national systems appear to have been audited as recommended. The criteria include:

1. a description of the *public health importance* of the health event, including incidence and **prevalence**, severity of disease as measured by mortality rates and **case fatality** rates, and preventability;
2. a description of *the system*, including the objectives, the population under surveillance, case definitions, a flowchart of data collection, details of

data transfer, data analyses, and dissemination of information;

3. a measure of the *usefulness* of the surveillance system, including decisions and actions taken as a result of the information generated;
4. evaluation of *key attributes* of the system, including simplicity, flexibility, acceptability, **sensitivity, positive predictive value**, representativeness, and timeliness;
5. the *cost* of the system.

Surveillance Systems

Up until the 1960s, public health surveillance activities were developed mainly for infectious disease control (*see* **Communicable Diseases**). Since then surveillance has been applied to many diseases, including congenital malformations (*see* **Teratology**), injuries, occupational illness (*see* **Occupational Epidemiology**), and adverse drug reactions, principally through the work of Langmuir at the CDC [25]. Similar approaches have been taken to the surveillance of uptake of vaccines, and the surveillance of hazards, such as chemical accidents and the surveillance of behavioral risk factors [9]. Surveillance systems for chronic diseases have been less well developed [26]. Specific objectives of surveillance include:

1. early detection of changes in disease or risk factor prevalence and incidence to trigger rapid investigation and control;
2. measuring trends in disease, hazards, microbial agents, and risk factors to set priorities for interventions, and to evaluate disease-control programs;
3. to describe the basic epidemiology and natural history of disease in order to develop hypotheses about **causation** which can be tested by separate research studies (*see* **Descriptive Epidemiology**).

Data Collection

Surveillance data may be sought actively or acquired passively by making use of routinely generated data such as death registrations (*see* **Death Certification**) or hospital admissions. A common weakness of surveillance systems is the lack of agreed case definitions. This applies to most laboratory reporting and notifiable diseases in the UK. In the US, the CDC have published surveillance case definitions for infectious diseases [30].

Statistical Analysis

Usually, the routine analysis of surveillance data is simply the presentation of **incidence rates** by time, place, and person, using graphs, histograms, and maps. However, more sophisticated methods are increasingly being used [23]. Particular statistical issues include the use of time series analysis to model epidemics (*see* **Epidemic Models, Stochastic**), the early recognition of unusual events in routine data against a variable baseline rate [4], small area analysis of **clustering**, adjustment for delays and incompleteness of reporting, the use of surveillance data to predict the course of epidemics (e.g. acquired immune deficiency syndrome (AIDS)).

Reporting

Timely reporting to those responsible for public health action is an essential part of a *bona fide* surveillance system. Timeliness is defined by the objectives of the surveillance. For infectious disease, timely reporting may need to be measured in hours, a target which can now be achieved globally through the Internet [7]. For chronic diseases, annual and quarterly reporting may be sufficient. Typically, surveillance reports appear either as specifically produced publications (e.g. *Communicable Disease Report, Office of National Statistics Monitor, Morbidity and Mortality Weekly Report*, and *Weekly Epidemiological Record*, or as electronic bulletins, such as EPINET [19]).

Infectious Diseases Surveillance

The best recent example of the power of surveillance is the case of AIDS. Following the first reports of a new clinical disease, surveillance based on a complex case definition quickly established the risk groups of AIDS and thereby the probable routes of transmission, so enabling preventive advice to be promulgated, even before the human immunodeficiency virus (HIV) was discovered.

Subsequent surveillance using clinical reports of AIDS and laboratory reporting of HIV infection has been important in confirming the risk groups, reassuring the population about the absence of risk from casual contact and identifying localities of high incidence so that services can be targeted. Mathematical modeling using surveillance data has enabled prediction of the epidemic and has identified key transmission factors (e.g. number of sexual partners) in the maintenance of the disease [20].

Statutory Notification

In England and Wales, mandatory notification of infectious disease was introduced nationally in 1899. The current list of diseases is shown in Table 2. Notifications are made by registered medical practitioners. In England and Wales, weekly summaries of these data are now published in the Public Health Laboratory Service (PHLS) *Communicable Disease Report (CDR)*. The data are

later corrected and published quarterly and annually by the Office for National Statistics (ONS). The chief advantages of these data are that they are available quickly, and they relate to defined populations so that rates by age and sex can be calculated. The defects of the data are lack of case definitions and variable under-notification. Interestingly, the fee to medical practitioners to notify did not improve notification rates [18].

Laboratory Reporting of Microbiological Data

The PHLS developed laboratory reporting in the 1940s and 1950s [8]. Data are analyzed within a week of receipt by the Communicable Disease Surveillance Center to produce tables and line lists which are used in compiling narrative reports for publication in the *CDR*. The recent introduction of CoSurv [11] has substantially replaced manual with electronic reporting. The main benefits of laboratory reports are that they are highly specific since they

Table 2   Statutorily notifiable diseases in England and Wales

Under the Public Health (Control of Disease) Act 1984

Cholera	Relapsing fever
Food poisoning	Smallpox
Plague	Typhus

Under the Public Health (Infectious Diseases) Regulations 1988

Acute encephalitis	Ophthalmia neonatorum
Acute poliomyelitis	Paratyphoid fever
Anthrax	Rabies
Diphtheria	Rubella
Dysentery (amoebic and bacillary)	Scarlet fever
Leprosy	Tetanus
Leptospirosis	Tuberculosis
Malaria	Typhoid fever
Measles	Viral hemorrhagic fever
Meningitis	Viral hepatitis
Meningococcal septicemia (without meningitis)	Whooping cough
Mumps	Yellow fever

Notes

"Viral hemorrhagic fever" means Argentine hemorrhagic fever (Junin), Bolivian hemorrhagic fever (Machupo), Chikungunya fever, Congo/Crimean hemorrhagic fever, Dengue fever, Ebola virus disease, hemorrhagic fever with renal syndrome (Hantaan), Kyasanur forest disease, Lassa fever, Marburg disease, Omsk hemorrhagic fever, and Rift valley disease.

There are minor differences in notifiable diseases in Scotland and Northern Ireland. Some diseases are notifiable locally; for example, psittacosis in Cambridge.

AIDS is *not* statutorily notifiable, but clinicians report cases voluntarily, in strict confidence, to the directors of the Communicable Disease Surveillance Center (CDSC) in England and Wales and of the SCIEH in Scotland. Advice about reporting is available from these centres and from genito-urinary medicine physicians.

are based on laboratory-diagnosed infections and the fine typing of the infecting organisms [27], they often include clinical and epidemiologic details, and they allow for free-text comment. The reporting system is flexible, and unusual or new infections can be reported, even though they were not included in the original reporting instructions. However, the reports are limited to infections for which there is a suitable laboratory test.

General Practice Reporting of Clinical Data

The Royal College of General Practitioners (RCGP) set up a reporting system in 1966 based on first consultations to a limited number of volunteer practices [6]. In 1996 there were 367 participating general practitioners in 93 practices, serving a population of about 70 000 people; similar systems exist in Wales, Scotland, and the European countries [22]. They act primarily as early warning systems, particularly for influenza epidemics, providing data rapidly, and they have the advantages that the data are related to defined practice populations; they are useful for some common diseases which are not notifiable and for which laboratory tests are not usually performed, such as chickenpox.

Serological Surveillance

In 1990 in the UK, a serologic study to measure the spread of HIV infection in the population was begun; it has continued since and become a routine surveillance system [21]. Samples from sera collected for clinical purposes are unlinked from personal identifiers but remain linked to epidemiologic information (*see* **Record Linkage**); sera remaining unused are then tested for HIV infection.

Surveillance of Vaccine Preventable Diseases, Vaccine Uptake, and Vaccine Reactions

A comprehensive system of surveillance of vaccine-preventable diseases has been developed using the notification system, laboratory reporting, and regular serologic surveys of antibody levels in stored sera taken for other purposes [1]. Vaccine uptake is followed by the Cover of Vaccination Evaluated Rapidly (COVER) [2] system in the UK, which uses the national child health system in which all children in the UK are registered by a health authority.

Successive cohorts of children born within three-month periods are identified and their vaccination status at predefined target dates determined. Quarterly reports are published by the CDSC and the comparative uptake rates are known by Districts within a few months. Health authorities have used the data to study and remedy reasons for low uptake. Surveillance of vaccine safety has used the Yellow Card Scheme, but record linkage of district health authority child health records and computerized hospital admissions records is a promising new method of postmarketing surveillance of vaccine safety [5]. Vaccine efficacy can also be the subject of surveillance if population rates of disease and the proportion of cases vaccinated (PCV) and the proportion of the population vaccinated (PPV) can be routinely measured [3]. Vaccine efficacy is calculated by the following expression:

$$1 - \frac{PCV}{1 - PCV} \times \frac{1 - PPV}{PPV}.$$

Injury Surveillance

Particularly in Australia [10], hospital-based Emergency Room data have been used successfully to follow trends in injuries and identify etiologic risk factors. In the UK, injury surveillance currently relies on mortality data and hospital admissions, which will miss most common injuries such as fractures. Locally developed population-based schemes have illustrated the potential benefit of using Emergency Room databases [16]. In the US, systems have been developed to monitor spinal cord, firearm, and sports injuries [24].

Surveillance of Birth Defects

Following the thalidomide disaster, registries of congenital malformations were set up in several countries for the early detection of malformations in order to investigate causes. However, incompleteness and inaccuracy of reports has reduced their potential effectiveness. Monitoring etiologically linked groups of malformations rather than single defects has been recommended [12]. In Europe, the European Registration of Congenital Anomalies (EURO-CAT) concerted action project of the European Union collates standardized data from national and regional registries.

Occupational Illness and Injury Surveillance

In the UK, occupational illness and injuries are reportable by law under the Reporting of Injuries Diseases and Dangerous Occurrences Regulations (RIDDOR) Act, which came into force on 1 April 1986. The Health and Safety Executive are the responsible agency who will investigate incidents and develop guidelines and regulations for prevention.

Pharmacosurveillance

In many countries voluntary reporting systems for adverse reactions to drugs and vaccines have been developed. In the UK, the Yellow Card Scheme is run by the Committee on Safety of Medicines. In the US, the Food and Drug Administration (FDA) collects data from physicians and reports findings in the *FDA Drug Bulletin*. The World Health Organization has set up an international registry linked to national centers (*see* **Pharmacoepidemiology, Overview**).

Chronic Disease Surveillance

The use of mortality data for surveillance was the basis of the pioneering work of William Farr, who, as Compiler of Abstracts at the General Register Office from 1839 to 1879, used vital statistics to alert government and the public to health problems [15]. He developed a classification of diseases that eventually led to the **International Classification of Diseases**. The routine, timely analysis and reporting of cause and age-specific death rates continued today by the Office of National Statistics can legitimately be considered as chronic disease surveillance, as is illustrated by the London smog epidemic in 1952 [17]. Publication of the death registration totals for the week ending December 13 in London identified considerable **excess mortality**, leading to a government enquiry and eventually to the Clean Air Act. Another example is the identification of excess deaths during heat waves in the US, which has resulted in development of advice for prevention. In Russia and Eastern Europe, a sudden increase in death rates in men has been observed since 1991 [28], which highlights the

utility of monitoring crude death rates in identifying chronic disease problems, and emphasizes the need for chronic disease surveillance.

References

[1]   Begg, N.T. & Miller, E. (1990). Role of epidemiology in vaccine policy, *Vaccine*, **8**, 180–189.

[2]   Begg, N.T., Gill, O.N. & White, J.M. (1989). COVER (Cover of Vaccination Evaluated Rapidly): description of the England and Wales schemes, *Public Health* **103**, 81–89.

[3]   Farrington, C.P. (1993). Estimation of vaccine effectiveness using the screening method, *International Journal of Epidemiology* **22**, 742–746.

[4]   Farrington, C.P. & Beale, A.D. (1993). Computer-aided detection of temporal clusters of organisms reported to the Communicable Disease Surveillance Centre, *Communicable Disease Report* **3**, R78–R82.

[5]   Farrington, P., Pugh, S., Colville, A., Flower, A., Nash, J., Morgan-Capner, P., Rush, M. & Miller, E. (1995). A new method for active surveillance of adverse events from diphtheria/tetanus/pertussis and measles/mumps/rubella vaccines, *Lancet* **345**, 567–569.

[6]   Fleming, D.M., & Crombie, D.L. (1985). The incidence of common infectious diseases: the weekly returns service of the Royal College of General Practitioners, *Health Trends* **17**, 13–16.

[7]   Giesecke, J. (1995). The fine web of surveillance, *Lancet* **346**, 196.

[8]   Grant, A.D. & Eke, B. (1993). Application of information technology to the laboratory reporting of communicable disease in England and Wales, *Communicable Disease Report* **3**, R75–R78.

[9]   Haperin, W. & Baker, E.L. Jr (1992). *Public Health Surveillance*. Van Nostrand Reinhold, New York.

[10]   Harrison, J. & Tyson, D. (1993). National injuries surveillance in Australia, *Acta Paediatrica Japonica* **35**, 171–178.

[11]   Henry, R. & Palmer, S. (1996). Evaluation of a public health electronic surveillance network, *Health Trends* **28**, 22–25.

[12]   Khoury, M.J., Botto, L., Mastioiacovo, P., Skjaerven, R., Castilla, E. & Erickson, J.D. (1994). Monitoring for multiple congenital anomalies: an international perspective, *Epidemiologic Reviews* **16**, 335–350.

[13]   Klauke, D.N., Buehler, J.W., Thacker, S.B., Gibson Parrish, R., Trowbridge, F.L., Berkelman, R.L. & the Surveillance Coordination Group (1988). Guidelines for evaluating surveillance systems, *Morbidity and Mortality Weekly Report* **37**, (SS-5), 1–8.

[14]   Langmuir, A.D. (1963). The surveillance of communicable diseases of national importance, *New England Journal of Medicine* **268**, 182–192.

[15] Langmuir, A.D. (1976). William Farr: founder of modern concepts of surveillance, *International Journal of Epidemiology* **5**, 13–18.

[16] Lyons, R.A., Lo, S.V., Heaven, M. & Littlepage, B.N.C. (1995). Injury surveillance in children–usefulness of a centralised database of accident and emergency attendances, *Injury Prevention* **1**, 173–176.

[17] Macfarlane, A. (1906). Daily mortality and environment in English conurbations. Air pollution, low temperature, and influenza in Greater London, *British Journal of Preventive and Social Medicine* **31**, 54–61.

[18] McCormick, A. (1987). Notification of infectious diseases: the effect of increasing the fee paid, *Health Trends* **19**, 7–8.

[19] Palmer, S.R. & Henry, R. (1992). Epinet in Wales: PHLS Cadwyn Cymru: development of a public health information system, *PHLS Microbiology Digest* **9**, 107–109.

[20] Report (1996). The incidence and prevalence of AIDS and prevalence of other severe HIV disease in England and Wales from 1995 to 1999: projections using data to the end of 1994, *Communicable Disease Report* **6**, R1–R24.

[21] Report (1996). *Unlinked Anonymous HIV Prevalence Monitoring Programme, England and Wales*. Department of Health, London.

[22] Salmon, R.L. & Bartlett, C.L.R. (1995). European surveillance systems, *Review of Medical Microbiology* **6**, 267–276.

[23] Stroup, D.F. (1994). Special analytic issues, in *Principles and Practice of Public Health Surveillance*, S.M. Tentich & R.E. Churchill, eds. Oxford University Press, Oxford, pp. 136–149.

[24] Thacker, S.B. & Berkelman, R.L. (1988). Public health surveillance in the United States, *Epidemiologic Reviews* **10**, 164–190.

[25] Thacker, S.B. & Gregg, M.B. (1996). Implementing the concepts of William Farr: the contributions of Alexander D. Langmuir to public health surveillance and communications, *American Journal of Epidemiology* **144** (supplement), S23–S28.

[26] Thacker, S.B. & Stroup, D.F. (1994). Future directions for comprehensive public health surveillance and health information systems in the United States 1994, *American Journal of Epidemiology* **140**, 383–397.

[27] Threlfall, E., Frost, J., Ward, L. & Rowe, B. (1996). Increasing spectrum of resistance in multiresistant *Salmonella typhirmurium, Lancet* **347**, 1053–1054.

[28] Tillinghast, S.J. & Tchernjavskii, V.E. (1996). Building health promotion into health care reform in Russia, *Journal of Public Health Medicine* **18**, 472–473.

[29] Valleron, A.J. & Garnerin, P. (1993). Computerised surveillance of communicable diseases in France, *CDR Review* **3**, R82–R87.

[30] Wharton, M., Chorba, T.L., Vogt, R.L., Morse, D.L. & Buehler, J.W. (1990). Casexsxs definitions for public health surveillance, *Morbidity and Mortality Weekly Report* **39**, RR13–RR43.

[31] Wilson, F.P. (1927). *The Plague in Shakespeare's London*. Clarendon Press, London.

Bibliography

Berkelman, R.L., Stromp, D.F. & Buehler, J.W. (1997). *Public Health Surveillance*, 3rd Ed. Oxford Textbook of Public Health, Oxford University Press, Oxford.

Detels, R., Holland, W.W., McEwan, J. & Omenn, G.S. eds. (1997). *The Methods of Public Health*, Vol. 2. Oxford University Press, New York.

Eylenbosch, W.J. & Noah, N.D. (1988). *Surveillance in Health and Disease*. Oxford University Press, Oxford.

Stroup, D.F., Wharton, M., Kafadar, K. & Dean, A.G. (1993). Evaluation of a method for detecting aberrations in public health surveillance data, *American Journal of Epidemiology* **137**, 373–380.

White, J.M., Fairley, C.K., Owen, D., Matthews, R.C. & Miller, E. (1996). The effect of an accelerated immunization schedule on pertussis in England and Wales, *Communicable Disease Report* **6**, R86–R91.

S. PALMER

Survival Analysis, Overview

Survival analysis is the study of the distribution of life times, i.e. the times from an initiating event (birth, start of treatment, employment in a given job) to some terminal event (death, relapse, disability pension). A distinguishing feature of survival data is the inevitable presence of incomplete observations, particularly when the terminal event for some individuals is not observed; instead, it is only known that this event is at least later than a given point in time. This is *right-censoring*.

The aims of this article are to provide a brief historical sketch of the long development of survival analysis and to survey what we have found to be central issues in the current methodology of survival analysis.

History

The Prehistory of Survival Analysis in Demography and Actuarial Science

Survival analysis is one of the oldest statistical disciplines, with roots in **demography** and actuarial science in the seventeenth century; see Westergaard [45, Chapter 2; 47] for general accounts of the history of **vital statistics** and Hald [24] for specific accounts of the work before 1750.

The basic **life table** methodology in modern terminology amounts to the estimation of a survival function (one minus distribution function) from life times with delayed entry (or left truncation, see below) and right censoring. This was known before 1700, and explicit parametric models at least since the linear approximation of de Moivre [14] (see, for example, [24, p. 517], later examples being due to Lambert [33, p. 483],

$$\left(1 - \frac{x}{96}\right)^2 - 0.6176 \left[\exp\left(-\frac{x}{31.682}\right)\right.$$
$$\left. - \exp\left(-\frac{x}{2.43114}\right)\right],$$

and the influential nineteenth century proposals by Gompertz [21] and Makeham [37], who modeled the **hazard** function as bc^x and $a + bc^x$, respectively.

Motivated by the controversy over smallpox inoculation, D. Bernoulli [5] laid the foundation of the theory of **competing risks**; see Seal [42] for a historical account. The calculation of expected number of deaths (how many deaths would there have been in a study population if a given standard set of death rates applied) also dates back to the eighteenth century; see Keiding [30] and the article on **Expected Number of Deaths**.

Among the important methodologic advances in the nineteenth century was, in addition to the parametric survival analysis models mentioned above, the graphical simultaneous handling of calendar time and age in the **Lexis diagram** [35]; cf. [31].

Two very important themes of modern survival analysis may be traced to early twentieth century actuarial mathematics: multistate modeling in the particular case of disability insurance (see, for example, [15]); and nonparametric estimation in continuous time of the survival function in the competing risk problem under delayed entry and right censoring (Böhmer [7]).

At this time, survival analysis was not an integrated component of theoretic statistics. A characteristic scepticism about "the value of life-tables in statistical research" was voiced by Greenwood [22] in the *Journal of the Royal Statistical Society*, and Westergaard's [46] guest appearance in *Biometrika* on "Modern problems in vital statistics" had no reference to sampling variability. This was despite the fact that these two authors were actually statistical pioneers in survival analysis: Westergaard [44] by deriving what we would call the standard error of the standardized mortality ratio (re-derived by Yule [48]; see Keiding [30] (*see* **Standardization Methods**); and Greenwood [23] with his famous expression for "the "errors of sampling" of the survivorship tables" (see below).

The "Actuarial" Life Table and the Kaplan–Meier Estimator

At the mid-twentieth century, these well-established demographic and actuarial techniques were presented to the medical–statistical community in influential surveys such as those by Berkson & Gage [4] and Cutler & Ederer [13]. In this approach, time is grouped into discrete units (e.g., one-year intervals) and the chain of survival frequencies from one interval to the next are multiplied together to form an estimate of the survival probability across several time periods. The difficulty is in the development of the necessary approximations due to the discrete grouping of the intrinsically continuous time and the possibly somewhat oblique observation fields in cohort studies and more complicated demographic situations. The penetrating study by Kaplan & Meier [29], the fascinating genesis of which was chronicled by Breslow [8], in principle eliminated the need for these approximations in the common situation in medical statistics in which all survival and censoring times are known precisely. Kaplan & Meier's tool (which they traced back to Böhmer [7]) was to shrink the observation intervals to include at most one observation per interval. Although overlooked by many later authors, Kaplan & Meier also formalized the age-old handling of delayed entry (actually also covered by Böhmer) through the necessary adjustment for the "risk set", the set of individuals alive and under observation at a particular value of the relevant time variable.

Among the variations on the actuarial model, we will mention two.

Harris et al. [25] anticipated much recent work, in, for example, acquired immune deficiency syndrome (AIDS) survival studies, in their generalization of the usual life-table estimator to the situation in which the death and censoring times are known only in large, irregular intervals.

Ederer et al. [16] developed a "relative survival rate ... as the ratio of the observed survival rate in a group of patients to the survival rate expected in a group similar to the patients ...", thereby connecting to the long tradition of comparing observed with expected (see, for example, [30]).

Parametric Survival Models

Parametric survival models were well-established in actuarial science and demography, but have never dominated medical uses of survival analysis. However, in the 1950s and 1960s important contributions to the statistical theory of survival analysis were based on simple parametric models. One example is the maximum likelihood approach by Boag [6] to a "cure" model assuming eternal life with probability c and lognormally distributed survival times otherwise. The exponential distribution was assumed by Littell [36], when he compared the "actuarial" and the maximum likelihood approach to the "T-year survival rate", by Armitage [3] in his comparative study of two-sample tests for clinical trials with staggered entry, and by Feigl & Zelen [18] in their model for (uncensored) lifetimes, the expectations of which were allowed to depend linearly on covariates, generalized to censored data by Zippin & Armitage [49].

Cox [11] revolutionized survival analysis by his semiparametric regression model for the hazard, depending arbitrarily ("nonparametrically") on time and parametrically on covariates. For details on the genesis of Cox's paper, see Prentice [40] and Reid [41].

Multistate Models

Traditional actuarial and demographic ways of modeling several life events simultaneously may be formalized within the probabilistic area of finite-state Markov processes in continuous time. An important and influential documentation of this was by Fix & Neyman [19], who studied recovery, relapse,

and death (and censoring) in what is now commonly termed an illness–death model allowing for competing risks. Chiang, for example in his 1968 monograph [9], extensively documented the relevant stochastic models, and Sverdrup [43], in an important paper, gave a systematic statistical study. These models have constant transition intensities, although subdivision of time into intervals allows grouped-time methodology of the actuarial life-table type, as carefully documented by Hoem (see, for example, [26]).

Survival Analysis Concepts

The ideal basic independent nonnegative random variables X_i, $i = 1, \ldots, n$, are not always observed directly. For some individuals i the available piece of information is a *right-censoring* time U_i, i.e. a period elapsed in which the event of interest has not occurred (e.g. a patient has survived until U_i). Thus, a generic survival data sample includes $((\tilde{X}_i, D_i), i = 1, \ldots, n)$, where $\tilde{X}_i$ is the smaller of X_i and U_i and D_i is the *indicator*, $I(X_i \leq U_i)$, of not being censored.

Mathematically, the distribution of X_i may be described by the *survival function*

$$S_i(t) = \Pr(X_i > t).$$

If the *hazard function*

$$\alpha_i(t) = \lim_{\Delta t \to 0} \Pr(X_i \leq t + \Delta t | X_i > t)/\Delta t$$

exists, then

$$S_i(t) = \exp(-A_i(t)),$$

where

$$A_i(t) = \int_0^t \alpha_i(u)\mathrm{d}u$$

is the integrated hazard over $[0, t)$. If, more generally, the distribution of the X_i has discrete components, then $S_i(t)$ is given by the product-integral of the cumulative hazard measure. Due to the dynamical nature of survival data, a characterization of the distribution via the hazard function is often convenient. (Note that $\alpha_i(t)\Delta t$ when $\Delta t > 0$ is *small* is approximately the conditional probability of i "dying" just after time t given "survival" until time t.) Also, $\alpha_i(t)$ is the basic quantity in the *counting process approach* to survival analysis (see, for example, [2]).

Nonparametric Estimation and Testing

The simplest situation encountered in survival analysis is the nonparametric estimation of a survival distribution function based on a right-censored sample of observation times $(\tilde{X}_1, \ldots, \tilde{X}_n)$, where the true survival times X_i, $i = 1, \ldots, n$, are assumed to be independent and identically distributed with common survival distribution function $S(t)$, whereas as few assumptions as possible are usually made about the right-censoring times U_i, except for the assumption of *independent censoring*. The concept of independent censoring has the interpretation that the fact that an individual, i, is alive *and uncensored* at time t, say, should not provide more information on the survival time for that individual than $X_i > t$, i.e the right-censoring mechanism should not remove individuals from the study who are at a particularly high or a particularly low risk of dying. Under these assumptions, $S(t)$ is estimated by the Kaplan–Meier estimator [29]. This is given by

$$\widehat{S(t)} = \prod_{\tilde{X}_i \leq t} [1 - D_i / Y(\tilde{X}_i)], \qquad (1)$$

where $Y(t) = \sum I(\tilde{X}_i \geq t)$ is the number of individuals *at risk* just before time t. The Kaplan–Meier estimator is a nonparametric maximum likelihood estimator and, in large samples, $\widehat{S(t)}$ is approximately normally distributed with mean $S(t)$ and a variance which may be estimated by Greenwood's formula

$$\widehat{\sigma^2(t)} = [\widehat{S(t)}]^2 \sum_{\tilde{X}_i \leq t} \frac{D_i}{Y(\tilde{X}_i)[Y(\tilde{X}_i) - 1]}. \qquad (2)$$

From this result, pointwise confidence intervals for $S(t)$ are easily constructed and, since one can also show weak convergence of the entire Kaplan–Meier curve $\{\sqrt{n}[\widehat{S(t)} - S(t)]; 0 \leq t \leq \tau\}$, $\tau \leq \infty$ to a mean zero Gaussian process, simultaneous confidence bands for $S(t)$ on $[0, \tau]$ can also be set up.

As an alternative to estimating the survival distribution function $S(t)$, the *cumulative hazard function* $A(t) = -\log S(t)$ may be studied. Thus, $A(t)$ may be estimated by the Nelson–Aalen estimator

$$\widehat{A(t)} = \sum_{\tilde{X}_i \leq t} D_i / Y(\tilde{X}_i). \qquad (3)$$

The relation between the estimators $\widehat{S(t)}$ and $\widehat{A(t)}$ is given by the *product-integral*, from which it follows that their large sample properties are equivalent. Although the Kaplan–Meier estimator has the advantage that a survival *probability* is easier to interpret than a cumulative hazard function, the Nelson–Aalen estimator is easier to generalize to multistate situations beyond the survival data context. We shall return to this below. To give a nonparametric estimate of the hazard function $\alpha(t)$ itself requires some smoothing techniques to be applied.

Right-censoring is not the only kind of data-incompleteness to be dealt with in survival analysis; in particular, *left-truncation* (or delayed entry), where individuals may not all be followed from time 0 but perhaps from a later entry time V_i conditionally on having survived until V_i, occurs frequently in, for example, epidemiologic applications. Dealing with left-truncation only requires a redefinition of the *risk set* from the set $\{i : \tilde{X}_i \geq t\}$ of individuals still alive and uncensored at time t to the set $\{i : V_i < t \leq \tilde{X}_i\}$ of individuals with entry time $V_i < t$ and who are still alive and uncensored. With $Y(t)$ still denoting the size of the risk set at time t (1), (2), and (3) are all applicable, although one should be aware of the fact that estimates of $S(t)$ and $A(t)$ may be ill-determined for small values of t due to the left-truncation.

When the survival time distributions in a number, k, of homogeneous groups have been estimated nonparametrically, it is often of interest to test the hypothesis H_0 of identical hazards in all groups. Thus, based on censored survival data $((\tilde{X}_{hi}, D_{hi}), i = 1, \ldots, n_h)$ for group $h, h = 1, \ldots, k$, the Nelson–Aalen estimates $\widehat{A_h(t)}$ have been computed, and based on the combined sample of size $n = \sum_h n_h$ with data $((\tilde{X}_i, D_i), i = 1, \ldots, n)$ an estimate of the common cumulative hazard function $A(t)$ under H_0 may be obtained by a Nelson–Aalen estimator $\widehat{A(t)}$. As a general statistic for testing H_0, one may then use a k-vector of sums of weighted differences between the increments of $\widehat{A_h(t)}$ and $\widehat{A(t)}$:

$$Z_h = \sum_{i=1}^{n} K_h(\tilde{X}_i)[\Delta\widehat{A_h}(\tilde{X}_i) - \Delta\hat{A}(\tilde{X}_i)]. \qquad (4)$$

Here, $\Delta\widehat{A_h(t)} = 0$ if t is not among the observed survival times in the hth sample and $K_h(t)$ is 0 whenever $Y_h(t) = 0$; in fact, all weight functions used in practice have the form $K_h(t) = Y_h(t)K(t)$. With this structure for the weight function, the covariance between Z_h and Z_j given by (4) is estimated by

$$\sigma_{hj} = \sum_{i=1}^{n} K^2(\tilde{X}_i) \frac{Y_h(\tilde{X}_i)}{Y(\tilde{X}_i)} \left[\delta_{hj} - \frac{Y_j(\tilde{X}_i)}{Y(\tilde{X}_i)} \right] D_i, \quad (5)$$

and, letting $\mathbf{Z}$ be the k-vector $(Z_1, \ldots, Z_k)'$ and $\boldsymbol{\Sigma}$ the $k \times k$ matrix $(\sigma_{hj}, h, j = 1, \ldots, k)$, the test statistic $X^2 = \mathbf{Z}'\boldsymbol{\Sigma}^- \mathbf{Z}$ is asymptotically chi-square distributed under H$_0$ with $k - 1$ degrees of freedom if all n_h tend to infinity at the same rate. Here, $\boldsymbol{\Sigma}^-$ is a generalized inverse for $\boldsymbol{\Sigma}$.

Special choices for $K(t)$ correspond to test statistics with different properties for particular alternatives to H$_0$. An important such test statistic is the logrank test obtained for $K(t) = I(Y(t) > 0)$. For this test, which has particularly good power for **proportional hazards** alternatives, Z_h given by (4) reduces to $Z_h = O_h - E_h$, with O_h the total number of observed failures in group h and $E_h = \sum D_i Y_h(\tilde{X}_i)/Y(\tilde{X}_i)$ an "expected" number of failures in group h. For the two-sample case $(k = 2)$, one may of course use the square root of X^2 as an asymptotically normal test statistic for the null hypothesis. For the case in which the k groups are *ordered*, and where a score x_h (with $x_1 \leq \cdots \leq x_k$) is attached to group h, a *test for trend* is given by $T^2 = (\mathbf{x}'\mathbf{Z})^2/\mathbf{x}'\boldsymbol{\Sigma}\mathbf{x}$, with $\mathbf{x} = (x_1, \ldots, x_k)'$, and it is asymptotically chi-square with 1 df.

The above linear rank tests have low power against certain important classes of alternatives such as "crossing hazards". Just as for uncensored data, this has motivated the development of test statistics of the Kolmogorov–Smirnov and Cramér–von Mises types, based on maximal deviation or integrated squared deviation between estimated hazards, cumulative hazards, or survival functions.

Parametric Inference

The nonparametric methods outlined in the previous section have become the standard approach to the analysis of simple homogeneous survival data without covariate information. However, parametric survival time distributions are sometimes used for inference, and we shall give a brief review here. Assume again that the true survival times $X_1, \ldots, X_n$ are independent and identically distributed with survival distribution function $S(t; \theta)$ and hazard function $\alpha(t; \theta)$, but that only a right-censored sample $(\tilde{X}_i, D_i)$,

$i = 1, \ldots, n$, is observed. Under independent censoring the likelihood function for the parameter θ is

$$L(\theta) = \prod_{i=1}^{n} (\alpha(\tilde{X}_i; \theta))^{D_i} S(\tilde{X}_i; \theta). \quad (6)$$

The function (6) may be analyzed using standard large-sample theory. Thus, standard tests, i.e. Wald, score, and likelihood ratio tests, are used as inferential tools. Two frequently used parametric survival models are the Weibull distribution with hazard function $\alpha \rho(\alpha t)^{\rho-1}$, and the piecewise exponential distribution with $\alpha(t, \theta) = \alpha_j$ for $t \in I_j$ with $I_j = [t_{j-1}, t_j)$, $0 = t_0 < t_j < \cdots < t_m = \infty$. Both of these distributions contain the very simplest model, the exponential distribution with a constant hazard function as null cases.

Comparison with Expected Survival

As a special case of the nonparametric tests discussed above, a *one-sample* situation may be studied. This may be relevant if one wants to compare the observed survival in the sample with the *expected survival* based on a standard life table. Thus, assume that a hazard function $\alpha^*(t)$ is given and that the hypothesis H$_0 : \alpha = \alpha^*$ is to be tested. One test statistic for H$_0$ is the one-sample logrank test $(O - E^*)/(E^*)^{1/2}$, where E^*, the "expected" number of deaths is given by $E^* = \sum[A^*(X_i) - A^*(V_i)]$ (with A^* the cumulative hazard corresponding to α^*). In this case $\hat{\theta} = O/E^*$, the *standardized mortality ratio*, is the maximum likelihood estimate for the parameter θ in the model $\alpha(t) = \theta \alpha^*(t)$. Thus, the standardized mortality ratio arises from a **multiplicative model** involving the known population hazard $\alpha^*(t)$. Another classical tool for comparing with expected survival, the so-called *expected survival function*, arises from an additive *or excess* hazard model (*see* **Excess Mortality**; **Expected Number of Deaths**).

The Cox Regression Model

In many applications of survival analysis, the interest focuses on how *covariates* may affect the outcome; in clinical trials, adjustment of treatment effects for effects of other explanatory variables may be crucial if the randomized groups are unbalanced with respect to important prognostic factors, and in epidemiologic cohort studies reliable effects of exposure may be obtained only if some adjustment is made for **confounding** variables. In these situations, a *regression model* is useful, and the most important model for survival data is the **Cox** [11] (*proportional hazards*) regression model. In its simplest form it states the hazard function for an individual, i, with covariates $\mathbf{Z}_i = (Z_{i1}, \ldots, Z_{ip})'$ to be

$$\alpha_i(t; \mathbf{Z}_i) = \alpha_0(t) \exp(\boldsymbol{\beta}' \mathbf{Z}_i), \qquad (7)$$

where $\boldsymbol{\beta} = (\beta_1, \ldots, \beta_p)'$ is a vector of unknown regression coefficients and $\alpha_0(t)$, the *baseline hazard*, is the hazard function for individuals with all covariates equal to 0. Thus, the baseline hazard describes the common shape of the survival time distributions for all individuals while the *relative risk* function $\exp(\boldsymbol{\beta}' \mathbf{Z}_i)$ gives the level of each individual's hazard. The interpretation of the parameter, β_j for a dichotomous $Z_{ij} \in \{0, 1\}$ is that $\exp(\beta_j)$ is the relative risk for individuals with $Z_{ij} = 1$ compared to those with $Z_{ij} = 0$, all other covariates being the same for the two individuals. Similar interpretations hold for parameters corresponding to covariates taking more than two values.

The model is *semiparametric* in the sense that the relative risk part is modeled parametrically while the baseline hazard is left unspecified. This semiparametric nature of the model led to a number of inference problems which was discussed in the literature in the years following the publication of Cox's article in 1972. However, these problems were all resolved, and estimation proceeds as follows. The regression coefficients $\boldsymbol{\beta}$ are estimated by maximizing the Cox partial likelihood

$$L(\boldsymbol{\beta}) = \prod_{i=1}^{n} \left[\frac{\exp(\boldsymbol{\beta}' \mathbf{Z}_i)}{\sum_{j \in R_i} \exp(\boldsymbol{\beta}' \mathbf{Z}_j)} \right]^{D_i}, \qquad (8)$$

where $R_i = \{j : \tilde{X}_j \geq \tilde{X}_i\}$, the risk set at time $\tilde{X}_i$, is the set of individuals still alive and uncensored at that time. Furthermore, the cumulative baseline hazard $A_0(t)$ is estimated by the *Breslow estimator*

$$\widehat{A_0(t)} = \sum_{\tilde{X}_i \leq t} D_i \Big/ \sum_{j \in R_i} \exp(\widehat{\boldsymbol{\beta}}' \mathbf{Z}_j), \qquad (9)$$

which is the Nelson–Aalen estimator that one would use if $\boldsymbol{\beta}$ were known and equal to the maximum partial likelihood estimate $\widehat{\boldsymbol{\beta}}$. The estimators based on (8) and (9) also have a nonparametric maximum likelihood interpretation. In large samples, $\widehat{\boldsymbol{\beta}}$ is approximately normally distributed with the proper mean and with a covariance which is estimated by the information matrix based on (8). This means that approximate confidence intervals for the relative risk parameters of interest can be calculated and that the usual large sample test statistics based on (8) are available. Also, the asymptotic distribution of the Breslow estimator is normal; however, this estimate is most often used as a tool for estimating *survival probabilities* for individuals with given covariates, $\mathbf{Z}_0$. Such an estimate may be obtained by the product integral $S(t; \widehat{\mathbf{Z}_0})$ of $\exp(\widehat{\boldsymbol{\beta}}' \mathbf{Z}_0) \widehat{A_0(t)}$. The *joint* asymptotic distribution of $\widehat{\boldsymbol{\beta}}$ and the Breslow estimator then yields an approximate normal distribution for $S(t; \widehat{\mathbf{Z}_0})$ in large samples.

A number of useful extensions of this simple Cox model are available. Thus, in some cases the covariates are time-dependent; for example, a covariate might indicate whether or not a given event had occurred by time t, or a time-dependent covariate might consist of repeated recordings of some measurement likely to affect the prognosis. In such cases the regression coefficients $\boldsymbol{\beta}$ are estimated replacing $\exp(\boldsymbol{\beta}' \mathbf{Z}_j)$ in (8) by $\exp[\boldsymbol{\beta}' \mathbf{Z}_j(\tilde{X}_i)]$.

Also, a simple extension of the Breslow estimator (9) applies in this case. However, the survival function can, in general, no longer be estimated in a simple way because of the extra randomness arising from the covariates, which is not modeled in the Cox model. This has the consequence that the estimates are more difficult to interpret when the model contains time-dependent covariates. Another extension of (7) is the *stratified* Cox model in which individuals are grouped into a number, k, of strata each of which has a separate baseline hazard (*see* **Stratification**). This model has important applications for checking the assumptions of (7). The model assumption of proportional hazards may also be *tested* in a number of ways, the simplest possibility being to add interaction terms of the form $Z_{ij} f(t)$ between Z_{ij} and time, where $f(t)$ is some specified function. Also, various forms of *residuals* as for normal linear models may be used for model checking in (7). In (7) it is finally assumed that a quantitative covariate affects the hazard *loglinearly*. This assumption may also be checked in several ways and alternative models with other relative risk functions $r(\boldsymbol{\beta}'\mathbf{Z}_i)$ may be used.

Other Regression Models for Survival Data

Although the semiparametric Cox model is the regression model for survival data which is applied most frequently, other regression models, for example, *parametric* regression models, also play important roles in practice. Examples include models with a multiplicative structure, i.e. models like (7) but with a parametric specification, $\alpha_0(t) = \alpha_0(t; \boldsymbol{\theta})$, of the baseline hazard, and accelerated failure-time models.

A multiplicative model with important epidemiologic applications is the **Poisson regression** model with a piecewise constant baseline hazard. In large data sets with categoric covariates, this model has the advantage that a sufficiency reduction to the number of failures and the amount of person–time at risk in each *cell* defined by the covariates and the division of time into intervals is possible. This is in contrast to the Cox regression model (7), in which each individual data record is needed to compute (8). The substantial computing time required to maximize (8) in large samples has also led to modifications of this estimation procedure. Thus, in *nested case–control studies*, the risk set R_i in the Cox partial likelihood is replaced by a random sample $\tilde{R}_i$ of R_i (*see* **Case–Control Study, Nested**).

In the accelerated failure time model, the focus is not on the hazard function but on the survival time itself, much like in classical linear models. Thus, this model is given by $\log X_i = \alpha + \boldsymbol{\beta}'\mathbf{Z}_i + \varepsilon_i$ where the error terms are assumed to be independent and identically distributed with expectation 0. Examples include normally distributed ($\varepsilon_i, i = 1, \ldots, n$), and error terms with a logistic or an extreme value distribution, the latter giving rise to a regression model with Weibull distributed life times.

Finally, we shall mention Aalen's nonparametric additive hazard model, where $\alpha_i(t) = \beta_0(t) + \boldsymbol{\beta}(t)'\mathbf{Z}_i(t)$. Here, the regression functions $\beta_0(t), \ldots, \beta_p(t)$ are left completely unspecified and estimated nonparametrically much like the Nelson–Aalen estimator discussed above. This model

provides an attractive alternative to the other regression models discussed in this section.

Multistate Models

Models for survival data may be considered a special case of a *multistate model;* namely, a model with a transient state *alive* (0) and an absorbing state *dead* (1) and where the hazard rate is the force of transition from state 0 to state 1. Multistate models may conveniently be studied in the mathematical framework of *counting processes* with a notation that actually simplifies the notation of the previous sections and, furthermore, unifies the description of survival data and that of more general models like the competing risks model and the illness–death model to be discussed below. We first introduce the counting processes relevant for the study of censored survival data [1]. Define, for $i = 1, \ldots, n$, the stochastic processes

$$N_i(t) = I(\tilde{X}_i \leq t, D_i = 1) \tag{10}$$

and

$$Y_i(t) = I(\tilde{X}_i \geq t). \tag{11}$$

Then (10) is a counting process counting 1 at time $\tilde{X}_i$ if individual i is observed to die; otherwise, $N_i(t) = 0$ throughout. The process (11) indicates whether i is still at risk just before time t. Models for the survival data are then introduced via the *intensity process*, $\lambda_i(t) = \alpha_i(t)Y_i(t)$ for $N_i(t)$, where $\alpha_i(t)$, as before, denotes the hazard function for the distribution of X_i. Letting $N = N_1 + \cdots + N_n$ and $Y = Y_1 + \cdots + Y_n$, the Nelson–Aalen estimator (3) is given by the stochastic integral

$$\widehat{A(t)} = \int_0^t \frac{J(u)}{Y(u)} \mathrm{d}N(u), \tag{12}$$

where $J(t) = I(Y(t) > 0)$. In this simple multistate model, the *transition probability* $P_{00}(0, t)$, i.e. the conditional probability of being in state 0 by time t given state 0 at time 0, is simply the survival probability $S(t)$ which, as described above, may be estimated using the Kaplan–Meier estimator, which is the product-integral of (12). In fact, all of the models and methods for survival data discussed above which are based on the hazard function have immediate generalizations to models based on counting processes. Thus both the nonparametric tests and the

Cox regression model may be applied for counting process (multistate) models.

One important extension of the two-state model for survival data is the *competing risks* model with one transient alive state 0 and a number, k, of absorbing states corresponding to death from cause $h, h = 1, \ldots, k$. In this model the basic parameters are the cause-specific hazard functions $\alpha_h(t), h = 1, \ldots, k$ and the observations for individual i will consist of $[\tilde{X}_i, (D_{hi}, h = 1, \ldots, k)]$, where $D_{hi} = 1$ if individual i is observed to die from cause h, $D_{hi} = 0$ otherwise. Based on these data, k counting processes for each i can be defined by $N_{hi}(t) = I(\tilde{X}_i \le t, D_{hi} = 1)$ and letting $N_h = N_{h1} + \cdots + N_{hn}$, the integrated cause-specific hazard $A_h(t)$ is estimated by the Nelson–Aalen estimator replacing N by N_h in (12). A useful synthesis of the cause-specific hazards is provided by the transition probabilities $P_{0h}(0, t)$ of being dead from cause h by time t. This is frequently called the cumulative incidence function for cause h and is given by

$$P_{0h}(s, t) = \int_s^t S(u)\alpha_h(u)\mathrm{d}u, \qquad (13)$$

and hence it may be estimated from (13) by inserting the Kaplan–Meier estimate for $S(u)$ and the Nelson–Aalen estimate for the integrated cause-specific hazard. In fact, this Aalen–Johansen estimator of the matrix of transition probabilities is exactly the product-integral of the cause-specific hazards.

Another important multistate model is the *illness–death* or *disability* model with two transient states, say *healthy* (0) and *diseased* (1) and one absorbing state *dead* (2). If transitions both from 0 to 1 and from 1 to 0 are possible, the disease is *recurrent*; otherwise, it is *chronic*. Based on such observed transitions between the three states, it is possible to define counting processes for individual i as $N_{hji}(t)$ = number of observed $h \to j$ transitions in the time interval $[0, t]$ for individual i and, furthermore, we may let $Y_{hi}(t) = I$ (i is in state h at time $t-$). With these definitions, we may set up and analyze models for the transition intensities $\alpha_{hji}(t)$ from state h to state j, including nonparametric comparisons and Cox-type regression models. Furthermore, transition probabilities $P_{hj}(s, t)$ may be estimated by product-integration of the intensities.

Other Kinds of Incomplete Observation

A salient feature of survival data is *right-censoring*, which has been referred to throughout in the present overview. However, several other kinds of incomplete observation are important in survival analysis.

Often, particularly when the time variable of interest is age, individuals enter study after time 0. This is called *delayed entry* and may be handled by *left truncation* (conditioning) or *left filtering* ("viewing the observations through a filter"). There are also situations in which only events (such as AIDS cases) that occur *before* a certain time are included (*right truncation*). The phenomenon of *left censoring*, although theoretically possible, is more rarely relevant in survival analysis.

When the event times are only known to lie in an interval, one may use the *grouped time* approach of classical *life tables* (*see* **Life Table**), or (if the intervals are not synchronous) techniques for *interval censoring* may be relevant.

A common framework (coarsening at random) was recently suggested for several of the above types of incomplete observation.

Further Aspects

Survival analysis is a well-established discipline in statistical theory as well as in biostatistics. Several books have appeared, among them the documentation of the actuarial and demographical know-how by Elandt-Johnson & Johnson [17]; the research monograph by Kalbfleisch & Prentice [28], which for a decade maintained its position as main reference on the central theory; the comprehensive text by Lawless [34], also covering parametric models; and the concise text by Cox & Oakes [12], two central contributors to the recent theory. The counting process approach is covered by Fleming & Harrington [20] and by Andersen et al. [2]. Very recently, books intended primarily for the biostatistical user have begun to appear, cf. Collett [10], Marubini & Valsecchi [38], Parmar & Machin [39], Hosmer & Lemeshow [27], and Klein & Moeschberger [32]. Most **software** packages include procedures for handling the basic survival techniques.

Individual heterogeneity may be related to relevant covariates in regression models, but often there is residual heterogeneity, which in other areas of statistics would be captured by the introduction of a random effect. In survival analysis one framework for this is frailty *models*, where a random variable is assumed to multiply the hazard.

For multivariate survival, the innocent looking problem of generalizing the Kaplan–Meier estimator to several dimensions has proved surprisingly intricate. Two other approaches to multivariate survival are important: via marginal models and generalized estimating equations, and via frailty distributions for intraclass correlations.

There have been interesting developments in Bayesian survival analysis and *accelerated life time models* have recently attracted considerable interest and are being generalized to account for dynamic time changes and to the so-called structural nested failure time models.

References

[1] Aalen, O.O. (1978). Nonparametric inference for a family of counting processes, *Annals of Statistics* **6**, 701–726.

[2] Andersen, P.K., Borgan, Ø., Gill, R.D. & Keiding, N. (1993). *Statistical Models Based on Counting Processes*. Springer-Verlag, New York.

[3] Armitage, P. (1959). The comparison of survival curves, *Journal of the Royal Statistical Society, Series A* **122**, 279–300.

[4] Berkson, J. & Gage, R.P. (1950). Calculation of survival rates for cancer, *Proceedings of the Staff Meetings of the Mayo Clinic* **25**, 270–286.

[5] Bernoulli, D. (1766). Essai d'une nouvelle analyse de la mortalité causée par la petite vérole, et des avantages de l'inoculation pour la prévenir, *Histoire de L' Académie Royal des Sciences*, Année MDCCLX, pp. 1–45 of Mémoires.

[6] Boag, J.W. (1949). Maximum likelihood estimates of the proportion of patients cured by cancer therapy, *Journal of the Royal Statistical Society, Series B* **11**, 15–53.

[7] Böhmer, P.E. (1912). Theorie der unabhängigen Wahrscheinlichkeiten, *Rapports, Mémoires et Procés – verbaux du 7e Congrès International d'Actuaires, Amsterdam* **2**, 327–343.

[8] Breslow, N.E. (1991). Introduction to Kaplan & Meier [28]. Nonparametric estimation from incomplete observations, in *Breakthroughs in Statistics II*, S. Kotz & N.L. Johnson, eds. Springer-Verlag, New York, pp. 311–318.

[9] Chiang, C.L. (1968). *Introduction to Stochastic Processes in Biostatistics*. Wiley, New York.

[10] Collett, D. (1994). *Modelling Survival Data in Medical Research*. Chapman & Hall, London.

[11] Cox, D.R. (1972). Regression models and life-tables (with discussion), *Journal of the Royal Statistical Society, Series B* **34**, 187–220.

[12] Cox, D.R. & Oakes, D. (1984). *Analysis of Survival Data*. Chapman & Hall, London.

[13] Cutler, S.J. & Ederer, F. (1958). Maximum utilization of the life table method in analyzing survival, *Journal of Chronic Diseases* **8**, 699–713.

[14] deMoivre, A. (1725). *Annuities upon Lives: or, The Valuation of Annuities upon any Number of Lives; as also, of Reversions. To which is added, An Appendix concerning the Expectations of Life, and Probabilities of Survivorship*. Fayram, Motte & Pearson, London.

[15] du Pasquier, L.G. (1913). Mathematische Theoric der Invaliditätsversicherung, *Mitteilung der Vereinigung der Schweizerische Versicherungs-Mathematiker* **8**, 1–153.

[16] Ederer, F., Axtell, L.M. & Cutler, S.J. (1961). The relative survival rate: a statistical methodology, *National Cancer Institute Monographs* **6**, 101–121.

[17] Elandt-Johnson, R.C. & Johnson, N.L. (1980). *Survival Models and Data Analysis*. Wiley, New York.

[18] Feigl, P. & Zelen, M. (1965). Estimation of exponential survival probabilities with concomitant information, *Biometrics* **21**, 826–838.

[19] Fix, E. & Neyman, J. (1951). A simple stochastic model of recovery, relapse, death and loss of patients, *Human Biology* **23**, 205–241.

[20] Fleming, T.R. & Harrington, D.P. (1991). *Counting Processes and Survival Analysis*. Wiley, New York.

[21] Gompertz, B. (1825). On the nature of the function expressive of the law of human mortality, *Philosophical Transactions of the Royal Society of London, Series A* **115**, 513–580.

[22] Greenwood, M. (1922). Discussion on the value of life-tables in statistical research, *Journal of the Royal Statistical Society* **85**, 537–560.

[23] Greenwood, M. (1926). The natural duration of cancer, *Reports on Public Health and Medical Subjects* **33**, 1–26. HMSO, London.

[24] Hald, A. (1990). *A History of Probability and Statistics and Their Applications before 1750*. Wiley, New York.

[25] Harris, T.E., Meier, P. & Tukey, J.W. (1950). The timing of the distribution of events between observations, *Human Biology* **22**, 249–270.

[26] Hoem, J.M. (1976). The statistical theory of demographic rates: a review of current developments (with discussion), *Scandinavian Journal of Statistics* **3**, 169–185.

[27] Hosmer, D.W. & Lemeshow, S. (1999). *Applied Survival Analysis*. Wiley, New York.

[28] Kalbfleisch, J.D. & Prentice, R.L. (1980). *The Statistical Analysis of Failure Time Data*. Wiley, New York.

[29] Kaplan, E.L. & Meier, P. (1958). Non-parametric estimation from incomplete observations, *Journal of the American Statistical Association* **53**, 457–481, 562–563.

[30] Keiding, N. (1987). The method of expected number of deaths 1786–1886–1986, *International Statistical Review* **55**, 1–20.

[31] Keiding, N. (1990). Statistical inference in the Lexis diagram, *Philosophical Transactions of the Royal Society London A* **332**, 487–509.

[32] Klein, J.P. & Moeschberger, M.L. (1997). *Survival Analysis. Techniques for Censored and Truncated Data*. Springer-Verlag, New York.

[33] Lambert, J.H. (1772). *Beyträge zum Gebrauche der Mathematik und deren Anwendung*, Vol. III. Berlin.

[34] Lawless, J.F. (1982). *Statistical Models and Methods for Lifetime Data*. Wiley, New York.

[35] Lexis, W. (1875). *Einleitung in die Theorie der Bevölkerungsstatistik*. Trübner, Strassburg.

[36] Littell, A.S. (1952). Estimation of the *T*-year survival rate from follow-up studies over a limited period of time, *Human Biology* **24**, 87–116.

[37] Makeham, W.M. (1860). On the law of mortality, and the construction of mortality tables, *Journal of the Institute of Actuaries* **8**, 301–310.

[38] Marubini, E. & Valsecchi, M.G. (1995). *Analysing Survival Data from Clinical Trials and Observational Studies*. Wiley, Chichester.

[39] Parmar, M.K.B. & Machin, D. (1995). *Survival Analysis: a Practical Approach*. Wiley, Chichester.

[40] Prentice, R.L. (1991). Introduction to Cox [11]. Regression models and life-tables, in *Breakthroughs in Statistics II*, S. Kotz & N.L. Johnson, eds. Springer-Verlag, New York, pp. 519–526.

[41] Reid, N. (1994). A conversation with Sir David Cox, *Statistical Science* **9**, 439–455.

[42] Seal, H.L. (1977). Studies in the history of probability and statistics, XXXV: multiple decrements or competing risks, *Biometrika* **64**, 429–439.

[43] Sverdrup, E. (1965). Estimates and test procedures in connection with stochastic models for deaths, recoveries and transfers between different states of health, *Skandinavisk Aktuarietidskrift* **48**, 184–211.

[44] Westergaard, H. (1882). *Die Lehre von der Mortalität und Morbilität*. Fischer, Jena.

[45] Westergaard, H. (1901). *Die Lehre von der Mortalität und Morbilität*, 2nd Ed. Fischer, Jena.

[46] Westergaard, H. (1925). Modern problems in vital statistics, *Biometrika* **17**, 355–364.

[47] Westergaard, H. (1932). *Contributions to the History of Statistics*. King, London.

[48] Yule, G. (1934). On some points relating to vital statistics, more especially statistics of occupational mortality (with discussion), *Journal of the Royal Statistical Society* **97**, 1–84.

[49] Zippin, C. & Armitage, P. (1966). Use of concomitant variables and incomplete survival information with estimation of an exponential survival parameter, *Biometrics* **22**, 655–672.

PER KRAGH ANDERSEN & NIELS KEIDING

Survival Bias in Prevalent Case–Control Studies *see* Bias from Survival in Prevalent Case–Control Studies

Susceptible Infectious-Recovered (SIR) Model *see* Communicable Diseases

Synergy of Exposure Effects

Although environmental regulation of chemical exposures is typically based on laboratory studies in which animals are dosed to single agents, humans are invariably exposed to mixtures. People who drink may smoke as well. Cigarette smoke itself is an example of a mixture. Modeling and predicting the effects of combined exposures, or of exposures experienced in a particular temporal sequence, remain challenges to toxicologists and epidemiologists.

The effect associated with several exposures in combination sometimes far exceeds what would have been expected on the basis of their separate effects, a phenomenon known as "synergism" (or "synergy"). One example is the occurrence of lung cancer in relation to exposure to cigarette smoking and arsenic, where the risk in those exposed to both is high [6]. While the etiologic basis for this particular mutual enhancement of effect is not well understood, the demonstration of synergism of exposures can provide important insight into causal mechanisms and can suggest strategies for intervention. For example, mental retardation invariably ensues when a child has the metabolic disorder phenylketonuria and also consumes the amino acid phenylalanine in his or her diet; removal of dietary phenylalanine prevents the adverse effect. Negative synergism, known as "antagonism", can also arise, as when exposure to the polio virus follows exposure to the polio vaccine. Examples of more subtle forms of antagonism include scenarios where two different chemical exposures compete for the same population of receptor sites or when one interferes with the absorption or metabolism of the other.

While most would agree that epidemiologic synergism among exposures exists, defining it is problematic. Usually "synergism" is said to be present when the effect of exposure to a combination of factors exceeds the sum of the separate, factor-specific effects. We must then define what it means to "sum" effects. Such a definition would establish a model for independence, compared with which positive departures could be considered synergistic, and negative departures, antagonistic. Synergism and antagonism cannot be defined except in relation to some definition for independence of effect, except in rare scenarios where only one of the two factors has an effect when experienced without the other, and the effect of the combined exposures exceeds that of the one factor alone. The phenylketonuria example and the polio vaccine example were both of the latter, unambiguous type.

Most instances of mutual enhancement of effect are not of that simple, pure form, so a more general definition is needed. When the outcome of interest is binary, e.g. the occurrence of a particular disease, the exposure–response formulation often includes specification of a function to serve as a "link" between the risk of disease and the exposures. If the risk of disease, r, is first subjected to a "logit" transformation, by taking the logarithm of the "odds", $r/(1 - r)$, then effect additivity on this inherently multiplicative scale is very different from additivity on the untransformed, "absolute", i.e. additive scale (*see* **Additive Model**). Thus, for example, if two factors each increase the risk of disease, and their combined effect can be correctly represented by a **logistic** model with no **interaction** ("product") term, then an additive formulation *would* require a positive interaction term. Conversely, the adequacy of an additive model for the combined effects would mean that a **multiplicative model** would require an interaction term. The distinction between this kind of statistical interaction, which corresponds simply to departure from additivity on some mathematically convenient scale, and biologic interaction, which corresponds to true biologic mutual enhancement of a causal mechanism, has long been appreciated by biostatisticians and epidemiologists [7, 16], who have searched for a formulation with biologic interpretability. The notion of synergism or "biologic interaction" can be defined as

"the inter-dependent operation of two or more causes to produce disease" [15]. A related concept is that of independence of two factors (say, A and B) in a public health sense, which is said to occur "when the number of cases of disease that would occur in the population does not depend on the extent to which A and B occur together in the same individuals" [15].

While synergism or antagonism can involve causative factors or protective factors, the choice of null model can be different for the joint effect of protective factors [2, 23]; or for the joint effect of a protective and a causative factor. The discussion that follows will apply only to the combined effect of causative factors, i.e. factors that each can increase the risk of the disease under study.

Rothman [14] proposes a conceptual framework for disease causality, where several "component" causes act together to form in their aggregate a "sufficient" cause, for which each component cause is necessary to its completion. (This conceptual model can be extended to continuous exposures by supposing that exceedence of a particular level of exposure is required for each sufficient cause in which the continuous exposure participates.) A single exposure may participate in (i.e. be a necessary component in) several different sufficient causes if there are several distinct pathways that involve it and can lead to the disease. If two exposures participate in the same sufficient cause, then that cause can only produce the disease when both are present, and such a pathway would imply synergism between the two exposures in a biologic sense [14] (*see* **Causation**).

For a single exposure, the difference between the incidence of the disease among those with the factor and among those without the factor can be interpreted as the **incidence rate** of completion for those sufficient causes that require that factor. By extension, the incidence rate for those with two factors, say A and B, minus those with neither is the sum of the incidence rate for completion of those sufficient causes involving A and not B and the incidence rate for completion of those sufficient causes involving B and not A, unless there exist one or more sufficient causes that require both A and B. In this way, the "causal pies" model proposed by Rothman leads naturally to the following model for independence based on incidence rates:

$$I_{AB} - I_{\overline{AB}} = I_{A\overline{B}} - I_{\overline{AB}} + I_{\overline{A}B} - I_{\overline{AB}}, \qquad (1)$$

where the overbar indicates the absence of the factor. This can be seen as additivity on the "risk difference" or absolute scale, and Rothman argues that absolute additivity is the only proper epidemiologic null model for "independent" effects. (Notice, however, that unless the lifetime risks are very small, model (1) does not imply the independence of A and B in the public health sense defined above: to the extent that A and B co-occur, the A-dependent and B-dependent pathways will compete for the same victims.) Such a model can easily be fitted to cohort data using standard statistical packages, such as SAS (the GENMOD procedure) and GLIM [19] (*see* **Software, Biostatistical**). The data are considered to provide evidence for synergism if the fit is significantly improved by inclusion of an interaction term, i.e. a nonzero γ, in the following model:

$$R[D|A, B \text{ status}] = \mu + \alpha(A \text{ present}) + \beta(B \text{ present})$$
$$+ \gamma(\text{ both } A \text{ and } B \text{ present}),$$

where R denotes the incidence of the disease. For multilevel exposures, d_1 and d_2, to two exposures that now are not simply present or absent, the above zero-γ null formation generalizes to linearity in $f(d_1)$ and $g(d_2)$, for exposure-specific exposure–response functions $f(\cdot)$ and $g(\cdot)$.

It is instructive to think about what self-independence would mean for a single exposure. Exposure to 40 units of an exposure can be thought of as a combined exposure to two doses of 20 units each, or to 30 units, together with 10 units, and so on. For these separate exposures to combine independently, one can show that the exposure–response must be linear. Low-level alpha radiation provides an example where self-independence is plausible. Irreparable chromosomal damage at the cellular level caused by bombardment by a passing alpha particle is random, rare, and heritable, providing radiobiologists with a strong theoretical justification for a linear exposure–response.

Returning to the binary exposure scenario, when a **case–control** design is used to study the etiology of a rare disease, the incidence rates in (1) cannot be estimated. However, dividing through by the background incidence, and letting RR_{AB} denote the **relative risk** for the combined exposure, relative to the background risk, leads to the approximate relation:

$$RR_{AB} = RR_{A\overline{B}} + RR_{\overline{A}B} - 1.0, \qquad (2)$$

and thus independence can be assessed using case–control data. Wacholder & Weinberg [20] provide methods for evaluating the fit of the additive model to case–control data, under various designs.

We have thus far considered effects of two exposures on disease risk, presuming that the unexposed state is unambiguously defined, whereas Greenland & Poole [4] point out that the choice of coding of one level as "unexposed" can be arbitrary. One example is sex, where males could be considered unexposed (to being female) or females could be considered unexposed (to being male). This raises the question as to how such factors should be incorporated in evaluations of synergistic effects. One can use algebra to show, however, that the above additivity criterion for independence is invariant under recoding of such a variable.

Under the usual understanding of the sufficient causes model, the disease invariably occurs once all components of a particular sufficient cause have been assembled, and in this sense Rothman's conceptual model is deterministic. Others have preferred to begin with a more stochastic conceptual approach and have nonetheless arrived at the same null model (1) for independence. In this way, divergent approaches to conceptualizing independence converge to a common mathematical formulation for the null model.

The stochastic approach has its roots in toxicology. Bliss [1] defines "independent joint action" between "poisons" as meaning that "the poisons or drugs act independently and have different modes of toxic action". Finney [3] provides mathematical rigor by specifying that "simple independent action" between two factors obtains if the outcomes are probabilistically independent. For one exposed to levels d_1 and d_2 of two different factors, the probability of avoiding the outcome (1 minus the risk) can be denoted $Q(d_1, d_2)$, so that the background "spontaneous" probability of nonoccurrence is $Q(0, 0)$. Probabilistic independence implies the following relationship:

$$Q(d_1, d_2) = \frac{Q(d_1, 0)Q(0, d_2)}{Q(0, 0)}. \qquad (3)$$

This reflects a scenario where the two causal mechanisms are completely separate and unrelated and where each of the exposure-dependent causal processes is independent of the background causal processes, i.e. those mechanisms that can produce the disease in the absence of either exposure.

Weinberg [23] describes a paradigm for this idealized model (3) in relation to two hunters, unaware of each other's presence, but shooting at the same ducks. To survive, a duck must stay clear of both. Under this independence scenario, the probability that the duck will survive some interval of time is the product of the probabilities that it escapes both hunters and also does not die of causes unrelated to being shot. This is the simplest probability-based notion of independence, corresponding to the situation where the exposures have completely separate biological modes of action.

This model, which can be written in generalized linear model form as additive in the log of the non-response, $\ln[Q(d_1, d_2)]$, has been applied to assessing synergism in animal experiments [21] and Korn & Liu [9] proposed a **Mantel–Haenszel**-type statistic for synergism based on follow-up with continuous failure times.

Mathematically, models (1) and (3) are equivalent. If one integrates risk over any fixed length of time, then the additive formulation (1) can be seen (replacing the factor A by the continuous d_1 and B by d_2) as equivalent to model (3), where the function $Q(d_1, d_2)$ is interpreted as the probability of survival without the disease over the specified follow-up interval for those with rates as given by (1). Conversely, the model given by (3) can be shown to imply model (1), because the negative of $\ln[Q(d_1, d_2)]$ converges in the limit, as the interval of time (hence the associated risk) becomes small, to the incidence rate associated with the combined exposure (d_1, d_2).

In the context of a rare disease, either formulation leads naturally to the case–control-based index for synergism proposed by Rothman [13]:

$$ S = \frac{RR_{AB} - 1}{RR_{A\overline{B}} + RR_{\overline{A}B} - 2}, $$

who also defines a synergism index for cohort data and provides standard error formulas for computing confidence intervals. Another index for synergism, resembling the usual interaction term in analysis of variance, provides a direct estimate for the **excess risk** associated with synergistic effects among those with both exposures: $T = R_{AB} - R_{\overline{A}B} - R_{A\overline{B}} + R_{\overline{A}\overline{B}}$ has certain advantages but can only be estimated in the context of a **cohort study** [7]. Wahrendorf et al. [21] propose a different index that can be used in

cohort studies:

$$ W = \frac{Q(A, B)Q(0, 0)}{A(\overline{A}B)Q(A, \overline{B})}, $$

which, for a rare outcome, is approximately $\exp(-T)$, and should, in general, be one under independence. Weinberg [23] refers to W as a "health ratio" similar to a risk ratio (*see* **Relative Risk**), but interpretable as the proportion *avoiding* the disease divided by the expected (based on independence) proportion avoiding disease, among those with both exposures. Simulations comparing W, T, and a third index, G, proposed by Korn & Liu [9], revealed that tests based on $\ln(W)$ had close-to-nominal size and relatively good power [12].

Statistics representing the fractional excess in the disease rate that is attributable to the synergistic effects of two factors have been developed, based on this model for independence. Hamilton [5] defines the "proportion of disease attributable to synergism" by taking the difference between the observed and expected risk among those with both divided by the overall risk and multiplying by the **prevalence** in the population of the combined exposure. Walker [22] later defines the "proportion of disease attributable to the combined effect of two factors" differently, by subtracting the expected from the observed rate of disease in those exposed to both factors and dividing by the observed rate. The difference between the indices proposed by Hamilton, and Walker, is that the Hamilton index divides by the overall population rate, while that of Walker divides by the disease rate among those with both exposures. Thus, the latter is more focused on etiology and the former on public health.

Darroch & Borkent [2] have recently revisited the question of how to assess the proportion of disease attributable to synergistic effects, within the context of a deterministic paradigm described by Hamilton [5]. They begin with the presumption that there are six types of people in the population: those who will get the disease regardless of their exposure to A and/or B; those who will *not* get the disease regardless of their exposure to A and/or B; those who will get the disease with A but will not with B or with neither; those who will get the disease with B but will not with A or with neither; those who will get the disease with A or with B but will not with neither; and those who will only get the disease in the presence of both A and B. Because only four parameters are estimable on the basis of relating the combined exposure to the observable risk of the disease, the fraction in the synergistic category, who would only get the disease with both exposures, cannot be directly estimated. Darroch & Borkent [2] propose an estimate based on maximum entropy, and illustrate its application to the problem of partitioning the cases of lung cancer among those exposed to both smoking and radiation into four parts: the fraction caused by smoking alone; the fraction caused by radiation alone; the fraction that would have developed even with neither exposure; and the fraction that developed as a result of the combined exposure. Extensions of this approach to multilevel exposures remain to be developed.

Both conceptualizations, the deterministic one championed by Rothman and Hamilton, and the probabilistic one preferred by toxicologists, are useful for clarifying our thinking about causality, but both have limitations. Suppose there are two distinct sufficient causes for the disease of interest, one requiring A and one requiring B. Koopman [8] points out that if they have a component cause in common, say C, then A and B will compete for the same pool of susceptibles, i.e. those with C, and this competition can produce apparent antagonism. This will be true even if we presume that the two sufficient causes are independent among those with C. Such shared causes may be common. Genetic factors, for example, can interact with exposures to produce disease; the existence of genetically based contributory causes, while usually unknown to the investigator, may be the rule rather than the exception.

Seen in the hunter paradigm for probabilistic independence, some ducks, depending on their size and coloring, are easier to see (hence to shoot) than others. Such variation among individuals in inherent susceptibility can produce apparent nonindependence, even when the causal processes (the two hunters) are truly functioning independently at the level of each individual at risk. Darroch & Borkent allow for the resulting inherent nonidentifiability of parameters within a deterministic conceptual framework by proposing a maximum entropy approach, while others [10, 23] compute upper and lower bounds for synergism indices that allow for covarying susceptibilities to A and to B across individuals in the population.

Whenever the epidemiologist begins with parameter relationships observed in the data and draws inferences regarding the likelihood that causal mechanisms for two different exposures are biologically linked, warning bells should sound: the same epidemiologic data can be consistent with very different underlying biologic scenarios, as discussed at length by Thompson [18]. Nevertheless, epidemiology can provide important clues regarding interdependent causal mechanisms.

A related set of issues not discussed here involves the epidemiologic identification of "initiator/promoter" relationships among pairs of exposures, where their temporal ordering can have an effect on risk [11] and [17] (*see* **Effect Modification**).

References

[1]   Bliss, C.I. (1939). The toxicity of poisons applied jointly, *Annals of Applied Biology* **26**, 585–615.

[2]   Darroch, J. & Borkent, M. (1994). Synergism, attributable risk and interaction for two binary exposure factors, *Biometrika* **81**, 259–270.

[3]   Finney, D.J. (1971). *Probit Analysis*, 3rd Ed. Cambridge University Press, New York.

[4]   Greenland, S. & Poole, C. (1988). Invariants and noninvariants in the concept of interdependent effects, *Scandinavian Journal of Work Environment and Health* **14**, 125–129.

[5]   Hamilton, M.A. (1979). Choosing the parameter for a 2×2 table or a $2 \times 2 \times 2$ table analysis, *American Journal of Epidemiology* **109**, 362–375.

[6]   Hertz-Picciotto, I., Smith, A.H., Holtzman, D., Lipsett, M. & Alexeeff, G. (1992). Synergism between occupational arsenic exposure and smoking in the induction of lung cancer, *Epidemiology* **3**, 23–31.

[7]   Hogan, M., Kupper, L., Most, B. & Haseman, J. (1978). Alternatives to Rothman's approach for assessing synergism (or antagonism) in cohort studies, *American Journal of Epidemiology* **108**, 60–67.

[8]   Koopman, J.S. (1977). Causal models and sources of interaction, *American Journal of Epidemiology* **106**, 439–444.

[9]   Korn, E. & Liu, P.-Y. (1983). Interactive effects of mixtures of stimuli in life table analysis, *Biometrika* **70**, 103–110.

[10]   Miettinen, O.S. (1982). Causal and preventive interdependence, *Scandinavian Journal of Work Environment and Health* **8**, 159–168.

[11]   Moolgavkar, S., Luebeck, E., Krewski, D. & Zielinski, J. (1993). Radon, cigarette smoke, and lung cancer: a re-analysis of the Colorado Plateau uranium miners' data, *Epidemiology* **4**, 204–217.

[12]   Piegorsch, W., Weinberg, C. & Haseman, J. (1986). Testing for simple independent action between two factors for dichotomous response data, *Biometrics* **42**, 413–419.

[13] Rothman, K. (1976). The estimation of synergy or antagonism, *American Journal of Epidemiology* **103**, 506–511.

[14] Rothman, K.J. (1986). *Modern Epidemiology*. Little, Brown, & Company Boston.

[15] Rothman, K., Greenland, S. & Walker, A. (1980). Concepts of interaction, *American Journal of Epidemiology* **112**, 467–470.

[16] Saracci, R. (1980). Interaction and synergism, *American Journal of Epidemiology* **112**, 465–466.

[17] Thomas, D., Pogoda, J., Langholz, B. & Mack, W. (1994). Temporal modifiers of the radon – smoking interaction, *Health Physics* **66**, 257–262.

[18] Thompson, W. (1991). Effect modification and the limits of biological inference from epidemiologic data, *Journal of Clinical Epidemiology* **44**, 221–232.

[19] Wacholder, S. (1986). Binomial regression in GLIM: estimating risk ratios and risk differences, *American Journal of Epidemiology* **123**, 174–184.

[20] Wacholder, S. & Weinberg, C. (1994). Flexible maximum likelihood methods for assessing joint effects in case–control studies with complex sampling, *Biometrics* **50**, 350–357.

[21] Wahrendorf, J., Zentgraf, R. & Brown, C.C. (1981). Optimal designs for the analysis of interactive effects of two carcinogens or other toxicants, *Biometrics* **37**, 45–54.

[22] Walker, A. (1981). Proportion of disease attributable to the combined effect of two factors, *International Journal of Epidemiology* **10**, 81–85.

[23] Weinberg, C.R. (1986). Applicability of the simple independent action model to epidemiologic studies involving two factors and a dichotomous outcome, *American Journal of Epidemiology* **123**, 162–173.

CLARICE R. WEINBERG

Systematic Error

Systematic error is the **bias** that results when a data-gathering process or method of analysis leads to results expected to deviate from the true quantity to be estimated. Unlike **random error**, systematic error is not ameliorated by increasing sample size, which only serves to obtain more precise **biased** estimates of the desired quantity (*see* **Random Error** for a simple example of systematic error.) Specific types of systematic errors in epidemiologic studies are discussed in several articles (*see* **Bias in Case–Control Studies**; **Bias in Cohort Studies**; **Bias in Observational Studies**; **Bias, Overview**; **Confounding**; **Validity and Generalizability in Epidemiologic Studies**).

M.H. GAIL

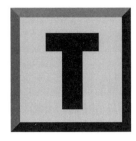

Target Population

The concept of a *target population* is an informal one, sometimes defined as "the population about which information is wanted" [1] or the "totality of elements which are under discussion and about which information is desired" [4]. Often, the word "population" refers to this concept; see, for example, Kendall & Stuart [3] or Freedman et al. [2]. The word "target" emphasizes, however, that this population is not necessarily the same as the one that we end up sampling. The latter population is sometimes called the *sampled population* [1, 4] or (in epidemiology) the *source population* [6]. Ideally, in **descriptive epidemiologic** studies, the two populations would be identical, but practical concerns usually lead to large discrepancies. For example, when a poll of the entire US population is desired but, for cost reasons, only a telephone survey of four cities is done, the sampled population comprises persons who have a telephone and live in those cities, rather than the target (US) population.

In studies of causal effects (*see* **Causation**) it may be helpful or even essential for the sampled population to extend beyond or even exclude the target population. Consider a target population comprising five persons who were exposed to high asbestos levels during a job assignment, one of whom later developed mesothelioma (a very rare form of cancer). The question of whether this high rate of the disease was caused by the asbestos could not be approached by sampling the target. Only by comparison to a much larger reference experience (namely, the extensive prior data on the rate of mesothelioma in workers exposed and not exposed to asbestos) can we make any meaningful inference about the target. In settings such as this example, in which inferences about structural relations in the target are inferred from observations on other populations, it has been proposed to refer to the latter as *evidentiary populations* [5]. Such evidentiary populations are typically larger and sometimes more accurately measured than the target, although they may not be comparable to the target population in all important respects (*see* **Confounding**).

Issues of inferences from the sampled population to the target are sometimes classified as problems of generalizability or external validity. These issues are distinct from the issues that arise in making inferences about the sampled population from a sample (*see* **Validity and Generalizability in Epidemiologic Studies**).

References

[1] Cochran, W.G. (1977). *Sampling Techniques*, 3rd Ed. Wiley, New York.
[2] Freedman, D., Pisani, R. & Purves, R. (1978). *Statistics*. Norton, New York.
[3] Kendall, M. & Stuart, A. (1977). *The Advanced Theory of Statistics*, 4th Ed., Vol. 1: *Distribution Theory*. Macmillan, New York.
[4] Mood, A.M., Graybill, F.A. & Boes, D.C. (1974). *Introduction to the Theory of Statistics*. McGraw-Hill, New York.
[5] Poole, C. (1987). Evidence, targets, and proportional attribution (letter), *American Journal of Epidemiology* **125**, 1095–1096.
[6] Rothman, K.J. & Greenland, S. (1998). *Modern Epidemiology*, 2nd Ed. Lippincott, Philadelphia.

SANDER GREENLAND

Telephone Sampling

The use of the telephone for **sample survey** data collection requires the selection of samples of telephone numbers to identify sampling units for interviewing. The sampling techniques employed to make these selections are those used for many other problems where samples must be selected. However, several unique features of the sampling frames, the sets of materials useful for sample selection, have stimulated the development of sample designs specific to telephone surveys.

The available frames vary from one country to the next as telephone system characteristics vary. Since our own experience has been limited to telephone sampling frames available in the US, the discussion here concerns frames and sampling methods to select telephone households in the US. Frames and sampling methods in other countries will have similar features to those described here, although specific aspects of the frames and methods may require modification to improve the efficiency or other properties of survey operations.

Telephone sampling methods have largely developed and been applied in the context of household surveys. The methods can and have been adapted to other populations such as establishments. The present discussion is restricted, though, to sampling methods for household populations.

The presentation is divided into four major sections. Background on frames and basic telephone sampling methods are described in the next section. The following section addresses specific telephone sample designs, while the subsequent section presents estimators for the principal telephone sampling methods. The final section is a comparison of designs based on cost, variance, implementation, and **bias** considerations.

Frames and Basic Telephone Sampling Methods

The Telephone Household Population

Often the population of interest is broader than telephone households, seeking to include all households regardless of whether they have a telephone. To reduce the costs of data collection through the use of the telephone, investigators decide to compromise on the **target population**, defining a survey population of telephone households when in fact they seek to make inferences about all households. The disjuncture between target and survey population for many telephone surveys raises several important issues concerning noncoverage of households without telephones and the appropriateness of inference to a population other than the survey population.

Noncoverage of households without telephones can introduce **bias** into sample estimates. The bias depends both on the proportion of households that are not covered and the differences between telephone and nontelephone households on the characteristics of interest. Approximately 5% of US households do not have a telephone, and the percentage of persons who live in such households is even smaller. While the overall rate of noncoverage is small, and may be reassuring to some investigators, noncoverage varies substantially with a number of characteristics that may be related to variables being measured in a survey. For example, nontelephone households tend to have younger and more mobile populations and to be located in rural areas of the South of the US and in central cities. Noncoverage rates can rise to 15% or higher for some subpopulations, a level that is considered unacceptable to those who need to produce estimates for many small subgroups of the US population from the survey data.

The characteristics of nontelephone households have been examined in several reviews (see, for example, [15]). Nontelephone households tend to have higher rates of unemployment, have higher rates of smokers, and experience higher rates of crime victimization. Telephone surveys could produce biased estimates of employment, health, or social characteristics. Adjustments to telephone survey data to attempt to compensate for noncoverage may reduce the bias. The use of poststratification, or population control adjustments, for this purpose are discussed later.

Telephone Systems

Telephone systems vary from country to country, but there are features of the systems that are similar despite the variation. Telephone numbers are grouped into geographical areas. For example, in the US, telephone numbers consist of three parts: a three-digit area code, a three-digit prefix (or central office code), and a four-digit suffix. The area code and prefix are established as part of an international system that extends across the US, Canada, Mexico, and the Caribbean. These numbers are not, of course, assigned at random across the entire geographic area covered by the phone system. Area codes are assigned to specific geographic regions that in the US do not, for the most part, cross state boundaries but otherwise do not correspond to political boundaries. Thus, there is a one-to-one correspondence between an area code and a geographic area. For instance, area code 313 is assigned to a region of southeast Michigan including a sizable portion of Detroit.

Prefixes are repeated across area codes, and within area codes are not generally geographically defined. However, prefixes are grouped into geographic areas called exchanges which are defined for the purposes of providing public service and maintaining the phone service. For example, the Ann Arbor exchange within the 313 area code is a geographic area roughly approximating the city of Ann Arbor and surrounding areas and is assigned more than 20 different prefixes. Households and businesses requesting a telephone service within the geographic area defined as the Ann Arbor exchange must be assigned a telephone number whose prefix is one of 20 serviced by the exchange. No other exchange within the same area code can use the prefixes assigned to the Ann Arbor exchange. There is little further geographic differentiation within most exchanges with respect to prefixes. Some exchanges with large numbers of prefixes will be divided into wire centers responsible for a subdivision of the area covered by the exchange and containing a subset of the prefixes assigned to the entire exchange.

The majority of the exchanges in the US are assigned only a single prefix. Exchanges have been until the recent past areas designated by public service commissions within which companies were able to obtain exclusive rights to provide a phone service. Service requirements are such that the land area covered by an exchange is limited, yet population density for a given exchange can vary enormously. Thus, some exchanges have very few customers, and enough numbers are available in a single prefix to assign to all customers. Other exchanges have large numbers of customers, and multiple prefixes are assigned to the exchange.

Suffixes are grouped in sets of 10 000. They are typically assigned by local telephone service personnel based on existing assignment patterns. There does

not appear to be any particular system by which new customer requests for services are assigned suffixes within a prefix.

However, patterns of the assignment of suffixes within prefixes do emerge when the entire system is examined. In exchanges with multiple prefixes and larger numbers of customers, prefixes and suffixes are assigned haphazardly, depending on the availability of unassigned numbers within a prefix at the time of assignment. But in exchanges with a single prefix and a small number of customers, suffixes have been assigned in groupings to reduce the cost of assignment and to make telephone assignment easier. Older electromechanical switching equipment allowed smaller companies to assign all numbers in a single "1000-bank" of consecutive numbers all beginning with the same first digit of the four digit suffix. A company would only have to purchase a single bank of 1000 switches for its customers, thereby reducing costs. Telephone numbers in the more numerous single-prefix exchanges are thus effectively clustered, often at the 1000-bank level, as well as at the 100-bank level. Several telephone sampling methods described subsequently take advantage of this clustered assignment of numbers to improve the efficiency of identifying telephone numbers assigned to residential units.

Sampling Frames

There are four types of frame problems that arise in telephone sampling: listings on the frame that are not elements of the population (referred to as *blanks*); elements in the population for which there is no corresponding listing (*noncoverage*); listings on the frame which yield multiple elements in the population (*clustering*); and elements in the population which have two or more listings on the frame (*duplicates*). Each of these deficiencies can lead to bias in survey estimates or inefficiency in survey operations. Sampling statisticians develop selection procedures which try to reduce or eliminate bias due to these deficiencies. They also have been instrumental in finding selection procedures which reduce the inefficiencies associated with some of these deficiencies.

Three principal frames are used for telephone sampling: telephone numbers, directories, and commercial lists. The frame of telephone numbers can be created through a combination of a list of area code and prefix combinations with randomly generated suffixes. The area code prefix combinations can be obtained for local studies from examination of local telephone directories, which are fairly up to date at the prefix level. For surveys covering larger areas than a local community, area code prefix combinations can be obtained in the US from Bell Core Research (BCR), Inc. The BCR frame is updated monthly and contains all area code and prefix combinations for the US, as well as for Canada, Mexico, and the Caribbean. The area codes and prefixes must be subset to the US to reduce the amount of screening of generated numbers for US telephone household surveys.

While the BCR frame affords virtually complete coverage of telephone households, it suffers from a substantial number of blank listings. Less than 25% of the generated numbers are assigned to residential units. It is operationally inefficient to use a simple **random digit dialing** scheme of area code, prefix, and randomly generated suffix. Other methods have been developed to take advantage of the inherent clustering of residential numbers in 1000 banks that increase the proportion of generated numbers assigned to residential units to more than 60%.

The BCR frame with randomly generated suffixes also has the disadvantage of duplicate listings. Households with more than one telephone number used for residential purposes are represented on the frame multiple times. Probability sampling methods require that the number of telephone numbers in a household be acquired and used to develop a compensatory weight for estimation.

Directories have been widely used as a frame for local studies. They are inexpensive to acquire for a local area, and simple list sampling methods can be used to select samples quickly, although not necessarily easily. Directory frames are difficult to assemble for wider geographic areas, with more than 5000 directories published across the US each year. Their popularity as a sampling frame is due to cost and convenience and to the lower proportion of blank listings in the directory compared to the telephone number frame: approximately 10%–15% of listings in a residential directory in the US are no longer residential.

On the other hand, directory frames suffer from noncoverage of the telephone household population due to unlisted numbers and changes in the telephone status of households. The percentage of telephone households which do not appear in directories exceeds 35% in the US, varying from low percentages (10%) in suburban and rural areas to more than 60% in some urban locations in the West such as Los Angeles. Survey designers generally do not ignore these high proportions of unlisted or out-of-date listings, and choose to use random digit dialing methods or other schemes that afford higher coverage.

Further, directories have higher levels of duplicate listings because subscribers can purchase additional listings. For example, a married couple at the same address with different surnames may choose for a small fee to appear in the directory under both names. The duplicate listing increases the chance of their telephone household being selected, which must, from a probability sampling point of view, be compensated through a weight for the household. Thus, a telephone directory has duplicate listings both because of multiple telephone numbers per household and multiple listings of the same telephone number in the directory.

Commercial firms now assemble electronic files in the US based on directories collected from across the country. Directory entries (name, address, and phone number) are either keyed or added to the file when an electronic format is available. Lists based on directories are supplemented by lists of automobile registrations obtained from approximately 30 states that release such data publicly. The combined file is subjected to processing to assign a zip code to each entry for the purposes of mailing. Several firms have taken advantage of the availability of telephone numbers in such files to create national directories and to draw and sell samples of telephone numbers from them. The commercial frames suffer from a small proportion of blank listings as well as the failure to cover unlisted numbers as well as duplicate listings described for directory frames.

Each of the three frames described here have generated different sampling methods that attempt to take advantage of strengths of the frame and reduce the impact of weaknesses in the frame. The methods are often classified as one of three types: simple list frame sampling methods suitable for directories; random digit dialing methods based on the telephone number frame; and list-assisted methods based on directories or commercial lists generating samples that include unlisted numbers as well. We do not discuss the sampling methods as applied to directories here, but do examine the random digit dialing and list-assisted methods in the next section.

Telephone Sample Designs

All of the sampling designs discussed in this section assume the availability of a frame of telephone numbers which includes all possible telephone numbers in the target population. Very limited auxiliary information is available for the telephone numbers in the BCR frame: exchange name, geographic coordinates for the center of the exchange, and time zone. Importantly, though, the BCR frame does include new area code–prefix combinations approximately 3 months before they are added to the telephone system. Thus, in principle, the BCR-generated frame will provide complete coverage of the telephone household population but with little auxiliary information for the purposes of **stratification** or other design efficiencies.

The primary problem with commercial list frames is incomplete coverage of the telephone household population. Conversely, the primary problem with the BCR-generated frame is the inclusion of many telephone numbers which are not assigned to a household. The development of telephone sampling designs has been motivated almost entirely by a desire to develop an efficient methodology for sampling from the BCR frame.

Sample Designs Using the BCR Frame

The sample designs in this section document statistical sampling methodology for sampling residential households using only the BCR frame. Since approximately 95% of all residential households (and not only telephone households) can be linked to this frame, the researcher must give careful consideration to the question of how well the telephone population represents the target population with respect to the variables of primary interest.

Simple Random Digit Dialing (RDD). The simplest and most direct approach to utilizing the BCR frame is to select telephone numbers from the frame randomly, call the selected numbers and conduct the requisite interview for each number that is found to be connected to an in-scope household. Numbers are selected and called until the desired sample size, say n, of in-scope households is attained. As noted earlier, only about 20%–25% of the sample telephone numbers will be assigned to households, so the number of calls required, say n', will be considerably larger than n. The expected number of required

calls is n/p, where p is the proportion of telephone numbers assigned to residential households. Thus, in order to account for the ineligible listing, the sample of telephone numbers from the BCR frame must be four to five times as large as the desired sample of n telephone households.

In general, the determination of the status of a telephone number is a costly matter, especially for telephone numbers not assigned to households. Frequently, a number must be dialed several times in order to determine its status. Since procedures must be specified for each type of dialing outcome, the use of the BCR list (or any list with a high proportion of spurious listing) will greatly increase the administrative and operational costs of telephone survey operations. This general subject is discussed in detail by Lepkowski [9]. For the purpose of constructing a simple cost model, let c_0 be the cost of determining the status of a number not assigned to an in-scope household, c_1 the cost of determining the status of a number assigned to an in-scope household, and c_2 the cost of conducting the survey interview. The total cost of the survey is then given by $C = n(c_1 + c_2) + (n' - n)c_0$ and the expected total cost of a simple random digit dialing survey is given by $E(C) = n[(c_1 + c_2) + c_0(1 - p)/p]$. Obviously, for p in the neighborhood of 0.20–0.25, the component of expected cost due to unproductive calls, i.e. $nc_0(1 - p)/p$, will be a substantial proportion of total expected cost. The telephone designs described in the following sections were all motivated by a desire to reduce the proportion of cost due to unproductive calls.

The Mitofsky–Waksberg Design. The two-stage random digit dialing design proposed by Mitofsky [10] and more fully developed by Waksberg [17] has been so widely employed in telephone surveys that it has become nearly synonymous with RDD telephone surveys. The method capitalizes on the clustering of telephone numbers assigned to residential households within banks of consecutive telephone numbers. As noted above, only about 20%–25% of the numbers in the BCR frame are assigned to households; however, among banks of 100 consecutive numbers with at least one number assigned to a household, over 60% of the numbers are assigned to residential households. Clearly, if the 100-banks with one or more residential numbers could be identified and if sampling were restricted to those banks, then the proportion of unproductive calls could be substantially reduced.

The Mitofsky–Waksberg technique starts by grouping the numbers in the BCR frame into 100-banks by using the area code, the three-digit prefix, and first two digits of the suffix to specify each bank. In the first stage 100-banks are selected at random, with replacement, and a telephone number within the bank is selected at random and dialed. If the selected number is found to be eligible, then the bank is retained for second-stage sampling. The process is continued until a specified sample of m 100-banks is attained. Within each retained 100-bank, telephone numbers are selected at random, without replacement, until a total of k eligible numbers (including the original number used to retain the 100-bank) have been identified.

Thus, the Mitofsky–Waksberg technique utilizes a two-stage design where 100-banks are selected – with probability proportional to number of eligible telephone numbers – in the first stage and a fixed-size sample of eligible households is selected in the second stage. Thus, the sample of $n = mk$ eligible households is selected with equal (but unknown) probability. The efficiency of the Mitofsky–Waksberg technique derives from the fact that the eligible telephone numbers are concentrated in a relatively small proportion of the 100-banks. Letting t be the proportion of 100-banks with no eligible numbers, then the total expected number of calls is $n[1 - t(k - 1)/k]/p$ and the expected total cost is

$$\mathrm{E}(C) = n\{(c_1 + c_2) + c_0[1 - p - t(k - 1)/k]/p\}.$$

Clearly both the expected number of calls and the expected cost decrease as k increases. Nationally, t is in the neighborhood of 0.65, so even modest values of k can lead to substantial cost savings.

Although the Mitofsky–Waksberg technique offers an elegant method to improve telephone survey efficiency, there are practical problems. The most obvious is that some 100-banks may have fewer than the requisite k eligible households, in which case all numbers in the bank will, of necessity, be called. Even then, compensatory weighting will be required. Another problem is that it is not always possible to determine accurately the eligibility status of a selected number. In the first stage this may lead to the incorrect inclusion or exclusion of 100-banks. In the second stage, some numbers may still be unresolved at the end of the survey period, so that fewer than k eligible households are identified for the bank. Another more subtle, problem is intrabank correlation, which is discussed in more detail in a later section.

The Potthoff Design.   The design suggested by Potthoff [11] is similar to the Mitofsky–Waksberg design, except that eligibility is extended to a broader, larger class of telephone number which he termed *auspicious* numbers. Typically the auspicious numbers include not only the residential household numbers, but also ring-without-answer numbers and other results for which the residential status is unknown. This broader definition reduces the amount of screening needed for the first stage and the amount of replacement required at the second stage. Another innovative development by Potthoff [11, 12] specifies that $c \geq 2$ numbers be selected per bank in the first stage. Sampling in the second stage depends on the number of auspicious numbers observed in the first stage, but this is not discussed in detail here.

The Potthoff sampling design yields an equal probability sample of eligible numbers. Replacement is required for only a small number of selected prefix areas and it reduces ambiguities about the status of numbers dialed at the first stage. Also, as c increases, the chances of obtaining a bank that will be exhausted in the second stage are reduced.

Implementation of the Potthoff design requires knowledge about the proportion of auspicious numbers that are actually eligible numbers in order to determine the appropriate sample size. The administrative structure is more complex and the training requirements are increased for this procedure relative to the Mitofsky–Waksberg.

Sample Designs Utilizing Published Residential Telephone Numbers

As discussed in the first section, lists of published residential telephone numbers for the entire US are available from several vendors. Since 85%–90% of the telephone numbers on these lists are connected to residential households, a straightforward random or systematic selection of numbers from such a list would be much more efficient than the designs used for sampling the BCR list. Unfortunately, the typical directory-based list only includes about 70% of the residential telephone households. Comparisons of telephone households with and without published numbers indicates that substantial bias may result if households without published numbers are omitted from the sampling frame [2]. The designs discussed in this section attempt to capitalize on the efficiency inherent in directory-based sampling while extending the coverage of the design to include the entire residential telephone population.

Designs Based on Plus Digit Dialing. Plus digit dialing is a directory-assisted procedure in which a sample of telephone numbers is selected from the directory and an integer is added to the suffix of the selected number. For instance, in plus-one dialing the integer "one" is added to the suffix of each number selected from the directory. The resulting sample of telephone numbers generally includes both listed and unlisted numbers; in addition, it yields a higher proportion of productive numbers than does the simple RDD design. Unfortunately this procedure has a number of theoretical problems. In general, the numbers in the target population have unequal and unknown probabilities of selection. In fact, some of the unlisted numbers may have a zero probability of selection unless the unlisted numbers are evenly mixed among the listed numbers. Such a mixing phenomena is, at best, difficult to verify. Generalizations of this design in which the last d digits (two or more) are replaced by a randomly generated d digit number have been suggested.

A closely related design, based on half-open intervals of telephone numbers, was suggested by Frankel & Frankel [5]. In numeric-order directories a cluster is defined to consist of a listed telephone number together with all numbers up to, but not including, the next listed number. A sample of clusters is selected from the directory by simply selecting a simple random sample of telephone numbers from the directory. This method achieves known, nonzero, probabilities of selection for all telephone households; however, the potentially large variation in cluster size can introduce formidable operational problems. Furthermore, this method is subject to estimation difficulties as cluster size and sample are both random variables. This basic design can be modified for use with alphabetical-order directories, but in this case the theoretical and operational problems are compounded by reporting error problems.

A Design Based on Two-Stage Sampling. A two-stage sampling design, utilizing a directory list, was proposed by Sudman [14]. This procedure, which was originally suggested by Stock [13], uses 1000-banks of telephone numbers (which are identified by the first six digits of the telephone number) as the first-stage sampling unit. The selection of 1000-banks is similar to the first-stage selection in the Mitofsky–Waksberg method except that the directory of listed numbers is used to select the first-stage sample. Thus, the probability of selection in the first stage is proportional to the number of listed numbers in the 1000-bank. In the second stage, numbers are selected until a predetermined fixed number of listed numbers are selected, and interviews are attempted for households with both listed and unlisted numbers. It should be noted that unlisted numbers in 1000-banks with no listed number have zero probability of selection, but in most cases this is not a serious problem. Of more concern is the fact that the determination of listing status often depends on a respondent report which can be in error; however, use of a directory in reverse telephone number order can eliminate this source of error.

Unlike the Mitofsky–Waksberg method, the Sudman procedure will produce unequal-size clusters of sample telephone households, although the variation in cluster size is usually not very large. Also, the potential for exhausted clusters exists, but with 1000 numbers (instead of 100 numbers, as in the Mitofsky–Waksberg method) this is of minor concern.

Designs Using Both the BCR Frame and Published Telephone Numbers

It should be noted that the designs discussed earlier require only the BCR frame, while those just discussed require only a published list of residential telephone numbers. The designs discussed in this Section require both. The basic idea behind these designs is to unite directly the desirable coverage properties of the BCR frame with the relatively high sampling efficiency of a frame of listed telephone numbers.

Dual Frame Designs. An RDD sample of n_B telephone households is selected from the BCR frame and simultaneously a sample of n_D telephone households is selected from the directory list frame. Letting n'_B and n'_D be the respective number of calls required to achieve the desired sample sizes, the cost of the dual frame design is given by

$$C = (n_B + n_D)(c_1 + c_2) + c_0(n'_B + n'_D - n_B - n_D).$$

The expected cost of a dual-frame survey is given by

$$E(C) = n\{c_1 + c_2 + c_0[\lambda(1 - p_B)/p_B$$
$$+ (1 - \lambda)(1 - p_D)/p_D]\},$$

where $n = n_B + n_D$ is the total sample size, $\lambda = n_B/n$ is the proportion of the total sample allocated to the BCR frame, p_B is the proportion of telephone numbers in the BCR frame assigned to residential households, and p_D is the proportion of telephone numbers in the directory frame assigned to residential households. As p_B is in the neighborhood of 0.20–0.25 and p_D is usually in the neighborhood of 0.80–0.85, the expected cost (for a fixed total sample size n) will decrease as λ decreases.

There are several possible ways to combine the data from the two frames for estimation. In general, dual-frame estimators are more complicated than the estimators for the previously discussed designs. Groves & Lepkowski [6] provide a detailed discussion of the issue of dual-frame estimation and the problem of sample allocation to the two frames so as to attain the minimum cost for a specified variance.

To implement dual-frame methodology, the directory status (i.e. listed or unlisted) of each residential household from the BCR sample must be known. To avoid using potentially unreliable respondent reports regarding their listing status, numbers selected from the BCR frame can be matched to the directory list at the time of sample selection. If the directory frame contains addresses for the listed numbers, then it is possible to send advance letters for the purpose of improving response rates. In general, the dual-frame design requires a sophisticated administrative operation; also, costs may be increased by the need to match the BCD sample to the directory frame and by the use of a more complicated estimator. The benefits of a higher response rate should more than offset the costs of advance letters.

Directory-Based Stratification.   For this design the directory list is used for the purpose of stratifying the BCR frame so as to improve sampling efficiency. In a typical application, the directory list is used to identify all 100-banks in the BCR frame with one or more directory listed telephone numbers. The BCR frame is then partitioned into two strata; one stratum contains all telephone numbers in 100-banks with one or more listed numbers and the other stratum contains all other numbers. The first stratum is often referred to as the high-density stratum, while the second is referred to as the residual stratum. Simple RDD samples are then selected from each stratum, with a much larger sample selected from the high-density stratum. The basic strategy behind this design is the same as

for the Mitofsky–Waksberg method, i.e. telephone numbers for residential households tend to be highly clustered within 100-banks with listed numbers, so if banks containing such telephone numbers can be identified and sampled at a higher rate, then sampling efficiency can be greatly improved. Casady & Lepkowski [3] found that at the national level the proportion of the BCR frame assigned to the high-density stratum would be approximately 0.38 but it would contain about 95% of the numbers assigned to residential households. Thus, the proportion of numbers in the high-density stratum assigned to households is approximately 0.55, while the proportion of numbers assigned to households in the residual stratum is only about 0.02.

Assume that an RDD sample of n_1 telephone households is selected from the high-density stratum and that a sample of n_2 telephone households is selected from the residual stratum. Then, the cost for the stratified design is given by

$$C = (n_1 + n_2)(c_1 + c_2) + c_0(n_1' + n_2' - n_1 - n_2),$$

where n_1' and n_2' are the respective numbers of calls required to achieve the desired sample sizes. The expected cost of the stratified sample is

$$E(C) = n\{c_1 + c_2 + c_0[\gamma(1 - p_1)/p_1$$
$$+ (1 - \gamma)(1 - p_2)/p_2]\},$$

where n is the total sample size, $\gamma = n_1/n$ is the proportion of the total sample allocated to the high-density stratum, p_1 is the proportion of telephone numbers in the high-density stratum assigned to residential households, and p_2 is the proportion of telephone numbers in the residual stratum assigned to residential households. As p_1 is in the neighborhood of 0.55 and p_2 is usually in the neighborhood of 0.02, the expected cost (for a fixed total sample size n) will decrease as γ increases. The allocation of the sample to the strata to minimize the cost for a fixed variance (or minimize the variance for a fixed cost) is discussed in detail in [3].

The probability of selection is known, positive, and equal within a stratum, so the estimation of population totals is straightforward. The estimation of a population mean at the stratum level is also straightforward, but the estimation of the overall population mean requires that the total residential telephone population be estimated and then a ratio estimator be used to estimate the population mean. A more detailed discussion of estimated means and variances is given later.

Under the relatively simple cost model given above, this design compares favorably with the Mitofsky–Waksberg design. In practice, directory-based stratification with simple RDD sampling within stratum has proven to have an advantage with respect to implementation and administration. There are two costs associated with this design that are not included in the simple model: the cost of the commercial list itself and the cost of stratifying the BCR frame. The cost of the commercial list will vary with vendor and with time, but for any large-scale, continuing survey operation this should be a relatively minor cost component. Both the costs cited above are fixed costs and can be amortized over multiple studies to reduce greatly the impact on any single study.

Directory-Based Truncation. This approach is really a special case of the preceding one in that no sample is allocated to the residual stratum, i.e. the BCR frame is truncated by removing the residual stratum. The greatly increased hit rate, together with the other advantages of the directory-based stratification design, make this an extremely attractive approach. The obvious disadvantage is that not all of the target population is accessible when the frame is truncated. In the example given above, approximately 5% of the telephone population will not be covered by the truncated frame. However, experience has indicated [1] that for many variables the out-of-scope population is very similar to the target population, so that very little bias results from truncation. As previously noted, approximately 5%–7% of the household population is not included in the telephone population, and any additional bias due to truncation of the BCR frame is probably minimal.

Estimation

The probability features of these designs must be taken into account in the computation of estimates from the samples. The basic principles of such estimation are described briefly here for means (and by implication, for proportions) and their sampling variances. In addition, poststratification, or population control adjustment, is in some cases applied to telephone survey data to attempt to adjust the telephone household sample to the distribution of all households.

Estimating Means

For the simple RDD design, let $\overline{Y}_{\mathrm{RDD}}$ be the simple mean of the n observations of the household variable y. Similarly, let $\overline{Y}_{\mathrm{MW}}$ be the simple mean of the mk observations under the Mitofsky–Waksberg design. Both $\overline{Y}_{\mathrm{RDD}}$ and $\overline{Y}_{\mathrm{MW}}$ are design-unbiased for the population mean μ; furthermore, $\mathrm{var}(\overline{Y}_{\mathrm{RDD}}) = \sigma^2/n$ and $\mathrm{var}(\overline{Y}_{\mathrm{MW}}) \cong (\sigma^2/mk)[1 + \rho(k-1)]$, where σ^2 is the population variance and ρ is the intra-100-bank correlation for the variable y.

The estimation of the population mean for the directory-based stratified designs is somewhat more complicated. Sampling within stratum is RDD, so $\overline{Y}_h$ (the simple mean of the n_h observations from the hth stratum) is unbiased for the stratum population mean μ_h. It follows that $Y_t' = \sum_{h=1}^{H} N_h(n_h/n_h')\overline{Y}_h$ is approximately unbiased for the population aggregate of the y values for telephone households and $N_t' = \sum_{h=1}^{H} N_h(n_h/n_h')$ is approximately unbiased for the total number of telephone households, say N_t. Thus, the ratio estimator, $\overline{Y}_{\mathrm{Strat}} = Y_t'/N_t'$, is approximately unbiased for the population mean and

$$\mathrm{var}(\overline{Y}_{\mathrm{Strat}}) \cong \sum_{h=1}^{H} \frac{z_h^2 \sigma_h^2 [1 + (1 - p_h)\lambda_h]}{n_h},$$

where p_h is the proportion of telephone numbers in the hth stratum assigned to residential households, z_h is the proportion of the telephone household population included in the hth stratum and $\lambda_h = (\mu_h - \mu)^2/\sigma_h^2$.

Several other statistical issues should be kept in mind when utilizing telephone designs:

1. In general, ratio estimators are required for estimating subclass means, in which case the relatively simple variance expressions above are not applicable.
2. The designs above yield samples of households, not persons. If persons are selected within households then additional weighting and more complex estimators are required.
3. To have unbiased estimators, the weights of households with multiple telephones must be adjusted to account for their higher probability of selection.
4. The estimators above are based on the use of random digit dialing to achieve fixed sample size. This requires that the status of all numbers selected be determined, which, in turn, requires

careful record keeping and close supervision. Because fixed sample sizes are required for each retained 100-bank, the Mitofsky–Waksberg method is more complex and thus the need for tight control is even more important.

Estimating Sampling Variance

For the purpose of estimating var($\overline{Y}_{RDD}$), we let Y_i be the value of the variable y for the ith household selected. An unbiased estimator for var($\overline{Y}_{RDD}$) is given by $\widehat{var}(\overline{Y}_{RDD}) = \hat{\sigma}^2/n$, where

$$\hat{\sigma}^2 = \frac{\sum_{i=1}^{n}(Y_i - \overline{Y}_{RDD})^2}{n-1}.$$

For the Mitofsky–Waksberg sampling we let Y_{ij} be the value of the variable y for the jth selected household in the ith retained 100-bank. An unbiased estimator for var($\overline{Y}_{MW}$) is given by

$$\widehat{var}(\overline{Y}_{MW}) = \frac{1}{m}\frac{\sum_{i=1}^{m}(\overline{Y}_i - \overline{Y}_{MW})^2}{m-1},$$

where

$$\overline{Y}_i = \left(\sum_{j=1}^{k}Y_{ij}\right)\bigg/ k.$$

For the stratified design we let Y_{hi} be the value of the variable y for the ith household selected in the hth stratum. Applying the linearization technique to the ratio estimator $\overline{Y}_{Strat}$ yields the variance estimator

$$\widehat{var}(\overline{Y}_{Strat}) = \sum_{h=1}^{H} \frac{\hat{z}_h^2\hat{\sigma}_h^2[1 + (1 - \hat{p}_h)\hat{\lambda}_h]}{n_h},$$

where

$$\hat{p}_h = \frac{n_h}{n_h'},$$

$$\hat{z}_h = \frac{N_h\hat{p}_h}{N_t'},$$

$$\hat{\sigma}_h^2 = \frac{\sum_{i=1}^{n_h}(Y_{hi} - \overline{Y}_h)^2}{n_h - 1},$$

and

$$\hat{\lambda}_h = (\overline{Y}_h - \overline{Y}_{Strat})^2/\hat{\sigma}_h^2.$$

Although results are not given in detail, the linearization technique can also be used to derive estimators for the variance of the ratio estimators required for subclass means.

Poststratification

In traditional sampling theory, poststratification arises when the variables to be used to create strata are not available at the time of selection. That is, one may be interested in partitioning the population into G post-strata using variables collected during the survey. As under proportionately allocated stratified sampling, improvements in precision are possible with suitable modification to variance estimation. Poststratification requires that for each sample element the poststrata be known and that poststratum weights, say W_g, are available for each poststratum. The poststratum weights must come from an outside source such as a census, census projections, or administrative records. For example, poststrata based on age and gender may be created for the respondents if suitable population counts or proportions W_g can be found for age and gender groups in the population. In telephone sampling, poststratification often adjusts not to the population residing in telephone households, but rather to the population residing in all households. This form of poststratification is applied to obtain estimates that have, in a certain sense, been adjusted to the distribution of the population in all households and not just telephone households.

In summary, poststratification is applied as follows:

1. Sort the sample into G poststrata based on some observed characteristic(s).
2. Obtain sample weights W_g for the population, typically from an outside source such as a larger survey, census or census projection data, or administrative records.
3. Compute the means $\overline{Y}_g$ for the characteristic of interest separately for each poststratum and compute the overall mean $\overline{Y}_{ps} = \sum_{g=1}^{G} W_g\overline{Y}_g$.
4. For variance estimators, use

$$\widehat{var}(\overline{Y}_{ps}) \cong \frac{1}{n}\left[\sum_{g=1}^{G} W_gS_g^2 + \sum_{g=1}^{G} W_g(1 - W_g)\frac{S_g^2}{N_g}\right]$$

or, alternatively,

$$\widehat{\text{var}}(\overline{Y}_{\text{ps}}) \cong \frac{1}{n} \sum_{g=1}^{G} W_g S_g^2 \left[1 + \frac{1 - W_g}{N_g} \right],$$

where S_g^2 is an estimator for the within-poststratum element variance, and N_g is the population size for poststratum g. The form of the estimators S_g^2 will depend on the sample design.

In almost all practical situations the poststratified estimate $\overline{Y}_{\text{ps}}$ will have smaller variances than the estimated mean without the poststratification.

Poststratification is also often referred to as population-control adjustment. Generally, poststratified weights are applied at the element level, and weighted estimates computed using the poststratified weights are "adjusted" to the outside distribution represented by the W_g. In the case of the RDD design the effects of this adjustment can be seen more clearly if we reexpress the poststratified estimate of the mean as follows. Let r denote the number of respondents in the sample and r_g denote the number of respondents in the gth poststratum. In addition, let Y_{gi} denote the value of characteristic Y for the ith respondent in the gth poststratum. Then the poststratified mean can be written in terms of element weights w_{gi} as follows:

$$\overline{Y}_{\text{ps}} = \sum_{g=1}^{G} W_g \overline{Y}_g = \sum_{g=1}^{G} N_g \overline{Y}_g \Big/ N$$

$$= \frac{\sum_{g=1}^{G} \left(\dfrac{r}{N} \right) \left(\dfrac{N_g}{r_g} \right) \sum_{i=1}^{r_g} Y_{gi}}{\sum_{g=1}^{G} \left(\dfrac{r}{N} \right) N_g}$$

$$= \frac{\sum_{g=1}^{G} \sum_{i=1}^{r_g} w_{gi} Y_{gi}}{\sum_{g=1}^{G} \dfrac{N_g/N}{1/r}}$$

$$= \frac{\sum_{g=1}^{G} \sum_{i=1}^{r_g} w_{gi} Y_{gi}}{\sum_{g=1}^{G} \sum_{i=1}^{r_g} \left(\dfrac{1}{r_g} \right) \dfrac{N_g/N}{1/r}} = \frac{\sum_{g=1}^{G} \sum_{i=1}^{r_g} w_{gi} Y_{gi}}{\sum_{g=1}^{G} \sum_{i=1}^{r_g} w_{gi}}.$$

That is, the weight w_{gi} is the ratio of the proportion in the population in the gth poststratum to the proportion in the sample in the gth stratum: $w_{gi} = (N_g/N)/(r_g/r)$. Thus, poststratification of a telephone household sample of respondents to a distribution based on all households provides a simultaneous adjustment for nonresponse and noncoverage of the households without telephones.

There are several features of poststratification for telephone samples that are important to observe. Typically, the W_g are census or other related data for all households, not just telephone households. Secondly, while the poststratification adjustment may be viewed as an adjustment for both **nonresponse** and noncoverage (*see* **Nonsampling Errors**) it is often applied in practice after some form of nonresponse compensation through weighting. Thirdly, it may not be possible to obtain population weights W_g across a full cross-classification of characteristics for the population, but marginal distributions may be available. Raking ratio adjustment procedures can be used to generate a complete distribution of the cross-classification based on the marginal distributions. For example, population weights may be available for age and education, but not their cross-classification. Raking ratio estimation can be used to generate the cross-classification based on a "main effects" model for age and education. The raked cross-classification weights for the population are then applied to the respondent distribution to generate element-level weights as indicated above.

Comparison of Designs

Cost–Variance Tradeoffs

The cost function, together with the variance of the estimator of the population mean given before, can be used to determine the size of the within-100-bank sample size k that will minimize that expected cost for a fixed variance (or minimize the variance for a fixed cost) for the Mitofsky–Waksberg design. An explicit expression for the optimal value of k can be found in [17]. Similarly, the cost function, together with the variance of the estimator of the population mean given before, can be used to determine the sample allocation to the strata that will minimize the expected cost for a fixed variance (or minimize the variance for a fixed cost) for directory-based stratification. Explicit expressions for sample allocation can be found in [3].

Using generally accepted values of cost factors and population parameters for the simple cost models and the variance expressions cited above, Casady & Lepkowski concluded that both the Mitofsky–Waksberg design and directory-based stratification offer considerable improvement over the simple RDD design. They also concluded that on the basis of the simple cost model alone there was little difference in efficiency between the two approaches; however, if the possibility of additional bias could be tolerated, then the truncated design was by far the most efficient.

Implementation Considerations for Telephone Samples

There are a host of features of the telephone system that affect the implementation of the designs described in the preceding section. We discuss here several of the more important ones briefly.

The identification of the residential status of each telephone number generated in RDD or list-assisted samples is not always an easy process. Numbers that are answered must be checked for residential use, and those used for mixed residential and business purposes must be suitably classified (usually any residential use is sufficient to classify a number as residential). Some numbers are readily identified as nonresidential because they are not in service, and a recording clearly indicates that status. Many numbers that are not in service are not connected to a recording to indicate their status, but are connected to a "ringing machine". Thus, interviewers screening telephone numbers to determine residential status cannot distinguish residential numbers where no one is at home from numbers not currently in service.

This latter problem of numbers that repeatedly ring without answer is an important consideration in the implementation of some designs. It is difficult to manage the ring-without-answer numbers in two-stage RDD designs that require the replacement of nonresidential numbers, particularly in time-limited survey data collection periods. Many survey organizations treat ring-without-answer numbers that have been called at varying times of day and days of the week as nonresidential. If the nonresidential classification is made late in the study period, then the replacement number has a relatively short period during which it can be called. Replacements often do not get the same variation in time of day and day of week calling that can be applied to original numbers. Thus,

many survey organizations now prefer sampling procedures that give them a fixed sample of telephone numbers rather than one that may generate new telephone numbers late in the survey period.

At the end of the study period, ring-without-answer numbers that have been called repeatedly must be classified as residential or not in order to close out the study. If a number has been called at a variety of times and days, then it may be arbitrarily classified as nonresidential. It thus does not count against the response rate for the survey because it has been classified as nonsample. On the other hand, ring-without-answer numbers that have not been called enough times are typically classified as residential and nonresponding, leading to a conservative calculation of the response rate.

To overcome these difficulties, and to reduce the costs of screening telephone numbers for residential status, automated screening systems have been developed to identify at a minimum telephone numbers that are connected to recordings indicating whether they are in service. The typical recording is preceded by a "tri-tone" without any ringing of a telephone number. Proprietary hardware and software has been developed which dials telephone numbers and detects the tri-tone recording. Numbers with a tri-tone recording are dropped from further sampling. Numbers without the tri-tone will often have a "ring splash" in which the telephone will ring momentarily while the hardware disconnects the call.

Surveys that are statewide or national in scope have geographic boundaries for the population that correspond to area code boundaries. Sample numbers generated within the sample area codes will be assigned to residences within the target geographic area. Many surveys target geographically defined populations whose boundaries do not match area code and exchange boundaries. In these cases, one may redefine the population, limiting it to that residing in specified exchanges, or one may select a sample from a set of exchanges that covers the entire geographic area but includes areas outside the target. Telephone numbers must then be screened not only for residential status but also for location of residence, based on respondent self-reporting. The classification of ring-without-answer numbers is even more problematic in these screening surveys.

Identification of duplicates in each of the frames also typically involves a respondent self-report. Responding households are asked if they have more than one telephone number assigned to the household, and, if so, the number of such numbers assigned. This self-reported number of telephone numbers through which a household may be reached is subsequently used to generate a weight for estimation. Many survey organizations also check for wrong connections and operator misdialing. Misdialed numbers are discarded, as are wrong connections, to avoid further complications in the weighting process for duplicate listings of a household.

Social science and health surveys also frequently select a single eligible person in a household for more interviewing. For example, on a survey involving marital satisfaction, a single adult will be selected to avoid contamination of responses among adults who converse about the content of the survey between interviews. Respondent selection must be done at an early stage in the interview. The procedure for objective respondent selection described by Kish [7] has been widely used in telephone surveys for this purpose, but it leads to an undesirable consequence – increased nonresponse rates. Households are reluctant to participate in a survey when the first questions are designed to obtain a roster of eligible persons living in the household. Alternative methods include a procedure described by Troldahl & Carter [16] and the nearest-birthday method (see [8] for a description). These latter procedures have been shown to be biased, but they continue to be used because they are easy to apply and avoid concerns about increased nonresponse rates.

Finally, answering machines and cellular telephones are posing increasing problems for telephone sampling operations. Answering machines do allow, for the most part, ready identification of residential units. Messages can be left asking that the household call a toll-free number, and calling of households with answering machines can be scheduled at a variety of times of day and days of week to try to reach the household at a time when a person will answer the phone. Cellular telephones pose a different problem. Are such telephone numbers residential or business? Further, the subscriber incurs a charge when they receive such calls. Cellular telephone numbers may be mixed in with other numbers with the same prefix, making identification difficult. Yet they are more readily answered than telephones at a residence. In addition, a well-trained interviewer can make arrangements to call a household at another number, thus reducing the cost to the telephone subscriber.

Bias

A critical issue in the use of the truncated frame is the magnitude of the bias introduced by dropping the low-density stratum. Various studies have shown that an average of less than 5% of the US household population are in the low-density stratum [1, 4]. Thus it is likely that the additional coverage bias will not be substantial for many characteristics of the total population. Connor & Heeringa [4] show that the coverage bias associated with the truncated frame is negligible for economic attitude measurements. Brick et al. [1] show that the coverage bias for the sociodemographic measure is also small, although for some characteristics and for some subgroups of the population, the additional coverage bias may be large enough to be of concern. Generally, though, the empirical investigations have confirmed the speculation that the additional coverage bias associate with the truncated frame can be safely ignored.

Choice Among Alternative Designs

As indicated previously, the choice among alternative designs is largely based on a consideration of cost and error properties of each design. Typically, three basic cost factors are considered: the cost of generating the sample of telephone numbers, the cost of screening the sample, and the "convenience" of working with the sampling procedure in implementation (a cost consideration that is often difficult to quantify). On the error side, there are two principal concerns: coverage of the telephone household population and sampling variance.

If we examine three main competitors on these characteristics, we can see why organizations are today making particular choices among alternative designs. For example, it is inexpensive to generate telephone numbers in the Mitofsky–Waksberg two-stage RDD sample design. Screening is efficient in the second stage since nearly 65% of the telephone numbers are residential. The Mitofsky–Waksberg design presents a number of difficulties in implementation, including replacement of nonresidential numbers and exhausted clusters. These can be substantial inconveniences for some survey operations, and alternative methods that avoid these problems have substantial attraction. On the error side, the Mitofsky–Waksberg design does provide complete coverage of the telephone household population. Sampling variances are larger than for element sample designs because of the cluster sample selection and well-known increases in variance due to within-cluster homogeneity among sample elements. That is, design effects for Mitofsky–Waksberg samples are greater than one.

The stratified design has a somewhat different set of characteristics. The sample-generation costs can be high. The listed stratum sample can be purchased from a commercial sampling firm at a reasonably low cost per sample number, but the unlisted stratum sample requires further stratification of numbers and two-stage RDD samples drawn from each unlisted stratum. Screening costs are also higher than for the Mitofsky–Waksberg design since approximately 50% of the sample telephone numbers in the listed stratum are residential, and an even lower percentage are residential in the unlisted stratum. Given that different sampling methods are used across strata, sample selection is less convenient for the stratified design than for the Mitofsky–Waksberg design. However, the stratified design does eliminate the need to replace numbers in the listed stratum, and there will be no exhausted clusters in that stratum either. In terms of error, the stratified design does cover the entire telephone household population. Sampling variances will be smaller for the stratified design than for the Mitofsky–Waksberg design because it is element sampling, and some improvements in precision due to stratification can be expected.

The truncated design has the disadvantage relative to the Mitofsky–Waksberg and stratified designs of noncoverage of telephone households in 100-banks with no listed numbers. The level of noncoverage is low, and empirical investigations have shown that the difference for many characteristics between the covered and noncovered populations is small. Samples drawn using the truncated design are inexpensive when obtained from commercial sampling firms. The screening costs of the truncated design are intermediate to those of the Mitofsky–Waksberg and the stratified designs since approximately 50% of the generated telephone numbers will be residential. The truncated design is the most convenient among the three designs considered here since no replacement numbers are needed, and the sample is drawn only from the listed stratum; no two-stage sampling is needed for the unlisted stratum. The sampling variances of estimates should be the smallest for the truncated design since it is a stratified element sample with no cluster sampling.

The sampling practitioner is faced with a choice between designs which provide complete coverage but a number of inconveniences in selection and a design with less complete coverage but a number of conveniences in selection. Given the empirical evidence on the size of the bias due to the noncoverage of telephone households in 100-banks without listed numbers, current practice favors the latter truncated design. That is, practitioners are choosing truncated sampling methods for telephone surveys based on a classic, although informal, cost–error tradeoff.

References

[1]   Brick, J.M., Waksberg, J., Kulp, D. & Starer, A. (1995). Bias in list assisted telephone samples, *Public Opinion Quarterly* **59**, 218–235.

[2]   Brunner, J.A. & Brunner, G.A. (1971). Are voluntarily unlisted telephone subscribers really different?, *Journal of Marketing Research* **8**, 121–124.

[3]   Casady, R.J. & Lepkowski, J.M. (1993). Stratified telephone sampling designs, *Survey Methodology* **19**, 103–113.

[4]   Connor, J. & Heeringa, S. (1992). Evaluation of Two Cost-Efficient RDD Designs. Paper presented at the Annual Meeting of the American Association for Public Opinion Research, St Petersburg, May 18, 1992.

[5]   Frankel, M.R. & Frankel, L. (1977). Some recent developments in sample survey design, *Journal of Marketing Research* **14**, 280–293.

[6]   Groves, R.M. & Lepkowski, J.M. (1985). Dual frame mixed mode survey designs, *Journal of Official Statistics* **1**, 263–286.

[7]   Kish, L. (1965). *Survey Sampling*. Wiley, New York.

[8]   Lavrakas, P.J. (1987). *Telephone Survey Methods: Sampling, Selection, and Supervision*. Sage, Newbury Park.

[9]   Lepkowski, J.M. (1988). Telephone Sampling Methods in the United States, in *Telephone Survey Methodology*, R.M. Groves, P.P. Biemer, L.E. Lyberg, J.T. Massey, W.L. Nicholls, II & J. Waksberg, eds. Wiley, New York, pp. 73–98.

[10] Mitofsky, W. (1970). Sampling of Telephone Households, *CBS News Memorandum*, Unpublished.

[11] Potthoff, R.F. (1987). Some generalizations of the Mitofsky-Waksberg techniques for random digit dialing, *Journal of the American Statistical Association* **82**, 409–418.

[12] Potthoff, R.F. (1987). Generalizations of the Mitofsky–Waksberg technique for random digit dialing: some added topics, in *American Statistical Association 1987 Proceedings of Survey Research Methods Section*. American Statistical Association, Alexandria, pp. 615–620.

[13] Stock, J.S. (1962). How to improve samples based on telephone listings, *Journal of Marketing Research* **2**, 50–51.

[14] Sudman, S. (1973). The uses of telephone directories for survey sampling, *Journal of Marketing Research* **10**, 204–207.

[15] Thornberry, O.T. & Massey, J.T. (1988). Trends in U.S. telephone coverage across time and subgroups, in *Telephone Survey Methodology*, R.M. Groves, P.P. Biemer, L.E. Lyberg, J.T. Massey, W.L. Nicholls, II & J. Waksberg, eds. Wiley, New York, pp. 25–50.

[16] Troldahl, V.C. & Carter, R.E., Jr (1964). Random selection of respondents within households in phone surveys, *Journal of Marketing Research* **1**, 71–76.

[17] Waksberg, J. (1978). Sampling methods for random digit dialing, *Journal of the American Statistical Association* **19**, 103–113.

Robert J. Casady & James M. Lepkowski

Teratology

Aristotle used *terata* to mean monsters, which he interpreted as the result of forces upsetting reproduction from its normal natural development. Thus teratology (derived from Greek *terata*, meaning monster/prodigy, + logy) became the term used in medicine and biology for the study of monstrosities and abnormal forms in man, animals, or plants as described by Warkany [17].

This article is restricted to the occurrence of these abnormal births in man. Literature on birth defects in laboratory animals exposed to pharmaceutical substances in the search for new treatments is described by Shepard [14] and Schardein [13].

The first use of the term, teratology, is generally attributed to Isidore Geoffroy Saint-Hilaire of Paris, son of Etienne, a distinguished teratologist. Teratology encompasses what are now known to be genetically inherited conditions, developmental conditions, e.g. Down syndrome, which are not inherited by any Mendelian or other mechanisms, and the common birth defects or congenital malformations whose etiology is largely unknown. This very heterogeneous collection of defects affecting the newborn and children comes within the health services remit of the medical or clinical geneticist.

Historical Development

Historically, abnormal births were viewed with a mixture of curiosity and superstition and were generally regarded as a portent of ill luck. The Chaldeans used their occurrence to predict the future, as documented on clay tablets in the Royal Library of Nineveh in the reign of Asshurbanipal, King of Assyria in 700 BC. Likewise, the Romans used monstrous births for divination and also developed the concept of maternal impression whereby mental modification of expectant mothers was thought to influence their offspring. The Spartans passed a law requiring pregnant women to look at statues of Castor and Pollux so that their babies might be born perfect and strong. An ancient Egyptian anencephalic mummy was found in a sepulchre used for animals, monkeys, and sacred ibises, in the catacombs of Hermopolis. In Paris it was unwrapped by Etienne Saint-Hilaire and his assistants who found it not to be a monkey but an eighth month of gestation human fetus with anencephalus. The specimen joined the collection of the King of Prussia in Berlin. During bombing of that city in World War II the museum was hit, the collection destroyed, and this specimen disappeared.

From the time of the Renaissance onwards collections of descriptions of abnormal births were published including a text by the famous French surgeon, Ambroise Paré, an eight-volume treatise in Italian by Taruffi, German texts by Förster and Ahfeld, and Ballantyne's works in English together with the journal *Teratologia* which he set up and edited. By the beginning of this century a large number of birth defects were known, statistical methods of measuring the degree of likeness between relatives by correlation (co-relation) analysis had been discovered by Galton and the study of Mendelian and other types of inheritance was under way. From the 1950s onwards studies were made of early abortions, human cells and chromosomes, and birth defect registers (*see* **Disease Registers**) and monitoring systems (*see* **Surveillance of Diseases**) were set up.

Types of Study

Teratological investigations in humans can be classified as **descriptive epidemiological** studies, **analytic epidemiological** studies, and case reports (*see* **Case Series, Case Reports**). Descriptive epidemiological studies describe the frequency (usually the **prevalence** at birth) of congenital anomalies in a particular community and how this frequency varies by geographic area, year and month of birth, or with characteristics of person such as socioeconomic status, maternal age, and parity. This type of study usually is based on information available from existing sources such as birth certificates, **death certificates**, or hospital records.

Broadly classified, analytic epidemiologic studies include case–control and cohort studies, and clinical trials. In **case–control studies** in the field of teratology, a group of index cases (births/fetuses with anomalies, other adverse reproductive outcomes such as miscarriages) is identified and information is sought about prior exposures, often during a reference period such as periconception. A **control** series is identified on whom similar information is obtained. The purpose of the control series is to provide information on the distribution of exposure in the population at risk of the adverse reproductive outcome under consideration. Information on the distribution of exposure is compared between cases and controls, and a measure of association, the **odds ratio**, may be calculated which closely approximates the **relative risk**. Important issues in evaluating the validity of data from case–control studies include the appropriateness of the control group or control groups chosen, and the similarity in the degree of accuracy of the data on exposures for cases and controls.

In a **cohort study** as applied to teratology, a group of women is classified in terms of exposure status at some defined point in time prior to the occurrence of the outcome of interest and are followed up to determine reproductive outcome. Exposure status may refer to the fact of exposure vs. nonexposure, e.g. work with video display units during pregnancy or with the husband or partner working in a specific occupation during pregnancy, or it may relate to degree of exposure, for example the reported intake of specific dietary factors per week. The frequency of adverse reproductive outcomes is compared between the groups, and on this basis the relative risk associated with the exposure may be calculated. Fewer cohort studies than case–control studies have been carried out because, for comparable statistical power, substantially greater numbers of subjects need to be studied. Another potentially important problem of cohort studies in this context is that ascertainment may be influenced by knowledge of the exposure status of the mother of the infant being examined. Studies of familial aggregation may

be classified as a special type of cohort study in which the "exposure" is having an affected relative. Special techniques of analysis have been applied in some of these studies, such as segregation analysis and linkage analysis.

Another special type of cohort study is the clinical trial. In trials, assignment to exposure is determined by the investigator. The randomized control trial is the definitive method of evaluating interventions. If the trial is of adequate size, then the randomization ensures comparability of the group assigned to receive the intervention and the control group for potentially **confounding** factors, both known and unknown. A further refinement is to make both the woman receiving the intervention and those responsible for her care and that of the child unaware of whether or not she has received the intervention. This minimizes the chance that the women will change their behavior in a way that is related to the intervention and also the possible effect of knowledge of exposure status on the ascertainment of reproductive outcome. The only randomized trials carried out to date in the field of teratology have related to vitamin supplementation during the periconceptional period. Nonrandomized trials have been carried out regarding the possible preventive effect of multivitamin supplementation against recurrent neural tube defects (NTDs) and orofacial clefts.

In teratology, the number of analytic epidemiologic studies carried out is small compared with the fields of cancer or heart disease in adults.

Classification and Frequency

Classification and how this relates to morphology is fundamental to any understanding of teratology. However, this subject is complex. Unlike plant taxonomy, no Linnaeus has appeared to embrace the whole field of diverse birth defects and classify them according to any universally agreed order. The modern-day equivalents of the collections of the last century are McKusick's catalog [10] and the *Birth Defects Encyclopedia* [2]. The former is mainly concerned with genetically inherited conditions although it does include a large number of birth defects and associated syndromes. Other useful reference sources are those made by the March of Dimes Birth Defects Foundation in the US and the International Clearinghouse for Birth Defects Monitoring Systems [8].

The usual definition of an **incidence rate** is the number of occurrences of a disease that manifest in a unit of time in a known population of individuals at risk. This definition is not easy to apply to congenital anomalies, as it implies a process occurring regularly over the period of time chosen. In embryonic development, the frequency of an event in one week is unlikely to be the same as in the next week. It is more natural to think of prevalence, that is the proportion of living embryos with the condition, at a point in time or at the time of an event, such as birth. Prevalence is more simple because the denominator changes rapidly as a result of pregnancy loss, and because many congenital anomalies represent not so much something that occurs, but something that does not occur, such as fusion of the palatal shelves (cleft palate) or neural tube closure (NTDs). If it were possible to obtain complete information, then the progress over time of a cohort of embryos could be followed, documenting depletion as a result of miscarriage and the events relating to organogenesis in the survivors.

The **cumulative incidence rate** is the total frequency of an event in a cohort of at-risk subjects up to a relevant time. There are theoretical and practical problems of estimating both the numerator and the denominator of this incidence rate. Theoretical problems concern the manifestation of anomalies throughout development. There is evidence that the mammalian embryo is capable of regeneration and of repairing itself. If these findings were applicable to man, then an apparently normal child may have shown defects at an early stage of intrauterine development, leading to underestimation of cumulative incidence. The practical problems of estimating incidence rates include pregnancy termination, undetected abortion, and problems of ascertainment. Antenatal diagnosis with selective termination of pregnancy has had a substantial impact on the numbers of births with certain types of congenital anomalies diagnosed at the time of delivery. Only the cases from pregnancies which went to term are eligible to be notified to the national birth defects monitoring scheme. Failure to include fetuses from terminated pregnancies may greatly distort the epidemiologic information, so it is now accepted practice to include fetuses with anomalies detected by antenatal diagnosis with subsequent termination of pregnancy in the estimation of the "prevalence at birth" of congenital anomalies.

Landmark Studies

Frequency and Types of Birth Defects

One of the first studies to address this lack of information about the frequency and types of birth defects throughout the world was that by the World Health Organization (WHO) in 1958 and later discussed at an informal meeting at Ann Arbor, Michigan, in April 1959. Stevenson and colleagues conducted a WHO supported prospective study of births in 24 centers in 16 countries and described the occurrence and types of birth defects found in stillborn and liveborn infants [16]. Outcomes relating to 421 781 pregnancies were traced based on 416 695 single births, 5022 sets of twins, 63 sets of triplets, and one set of quadruplets. A 400 page book containing basic tables for each center was published. The group recognized biases in the data, particularly in the centers which recorded hospital births only. This research demonstrated the large impact of NTDs on fetal wastage and a correlation between these defects and dizygous twinning. Consanguinity between parents increased stillbirth rates and early **infant mortality** rates, these being highest where parents are most closely related.

Vitamin A Deficiency

Why do birth defects occur? For the majority and wide spectrum of abnormalities observed, environmental factors have been identified in only a few instances. Hale observed a Duroc–Jersey sow, who received a ration deficient in vitamin A, at the Texas Agricultural Experimental Station. She gave birth on March 29, 1932, to 11 pigs, all of which were born without eyeballs [7]. Ten were alive at birth, one lived 4 days, one lived 3 hours, while all the others died within 5 minutes after birth. He postulated that the abnormalities were caused by vitamin A deficiency. The study marked the beginning of experimental teratology and led to many future studies using animal models for the experimental investigation of birth defects. The pharmaceutical industry built on this work extensively to investigate nutritional imbalances, drugs, chemicals, irradiation, and many other postulated teratogenic substances. Some 60 years later the Chief Medical Officer of the UK issued a warning that women who were pregnant or might become pregnant must not take excessive quantities of vitamin A. While this message relates to overprovision rather than underprovision, the origin of this work goes back to Hale's key paper.

German Measles

In the first 6 months of 1941 in Sydney, Australia, there were an unusual number of cases of congenital cataract. Gregg, an ophthalmologist, personally saw 13 cases [6]. He noted that as well as these babies being born with bilateral cataract, they were of small size, ill-nourished, and difficult to feed. Many had congenital heart defects. There were a few with monocular cataract which in two-thirds of cases was associated with microphthalmia. Close questioning of the mothers revealed that they had German measles during early pregnancy. There had been a widespread and severe epidemic in Australia in 1940. Altogether 78 children with congenital cataract were ascertained and of these 68 were associated with a definite history of maternal rubella infection.

Thalidomide

At a meeting of the German Paediatric Society at Kassel in October, 1960, Kosenow and Pfeiffer presented photographs and X-rays of two infants with aplasia of the extremities and various other defects. Within a few months another doctor, Wiedemann, reported similar cases. At the Paediatric Society meeting on November 18, 1961, Lenz suggested that the drug, thalidomide, might be the cause, as it appeared in 17 out of the 20 maternal records that he had investigated [9]. The manufacturers withdrew thalidomide (trade names Contergan, Distaval, Softenon) and all other preparations containing this substance from the market on November 25, 1961. However, the damage was done. Some 129 cases were studied by Lenz at the University of Hamburg. Another 203 cases were reported to him by letter from the rest of West Germany and also isolated cases from Belgium, Brazil, England, Egypt, Israel, Sweden, Switzerland, and a few cases from the US. The much more strict enforcement of food and drugs legislation in the US ensured that many fewer births were affected in North America than in Europe.

Thalidomide is a derivative of glutamic acid, discovered in Germany, and first marketed in 1956. It was well tolerated, considered safe, and used as an analgesic, sedative, and hypnotic agent. By the time of the papers by Lenz & Knapp in 1962 [9], at least 2000 children with drug-induced abnormalities had been born in West Germany. Worldwide it is thought at least 8000 children had been affected by thalidomide.

Identification of the Relationship between Diet and NTDs as a Paradigm of Teratological Investigation

Several features of the descriptive epidemiology of NTDs led to a dietary hypothesis for their etiology. Details are contained in [5]. There was an increased prevalence at birth of NTDs in the offspring of women of lower socioeconomic status compared with the offspring of other women. In the British Isles, and some other areas, the highest rates of anencephalus were amongst babies conceived in the spring and early summer, possibly linked to a lack of fresh vegetables in the winter. Body stores of certain nutrients are low in the spring. Improved all-year availability of various nutrients might in part explain the recent changes in seasonal pattern. It was known from the 1950s that therapeutic abortions could be induced by giving a folic acid antagonist 4-aminopteroylglutamic acid taken orally. This was interpreted to indicate that folic acid deficiency could induce abortion and possibly malformations.

A Case–Control Study

In western Australia, Bower & Stanley, using notifications to the local malformation registry in the period 1982–84 ascertained 77 infants with NTDs [1]. They were compared with two control groups each matched by date of last menstrual period: a group of 77 infants with other malformations registered in the same way, and a group of 154 normal infants. A telephone interview was conducted to obtain details of demographic and other factors. A three-part questionnaire was mailed to each mother, comprising a section on food frequencies during the period from 9 months before to 9 months after the last menstrual period, a section on illness and drugs taken for nausea in pregnancy, cooking methods, changes in diet and other factors over the same period, and a 24-hour dietary record to be completed on a specified day after receipt. These data were used to assess the daily dietary intake of folate, including that provided by supplementation, and intakes of a number of other nutrients. Participation rates were very high: 93% for mothers of cases, 88% for mothers of infants with other malformations, and 84% for mothers of normal infants. A statistically significant association of reduced NTD risks with increased reported intake of total folate was observed.

A Cohort Study

Milunsky et al. [12] reported a cohort study based on information collected on women undergoing prenatal testing by maternal serum α-fetoprotein screening or amniocentesis in Massachusetts. Information on diet in the first 8 weeks of pregnancy was obtained using a food frequency questionnaire, and on vitamin supplementation in the 3 months before and 3 months after conception, was collected by telephone interview. A total of 22 715 study subjects was available for analysis, of whom 49 had an infant with a neural tube defect. There was a statistically significant protective effect of taking multivitamins at least once a week before conception and during the first trimester, with a relative risk of 0.36 (95% confidence interval 0.15–0.83). The effect was almost entirely restricted to preparations containing folic acid. The relative risk associated with folic acid supplementation in the first 6 weeks of pregnancy was 0.29 (95% confidence interval 0.15–0.55). Amongst women who did not use supplements containing folic acid, the relative risk of NTDs associated with a dietary intake of more than 100 micrograms daily was 0.42 (95% confidence interval 0.16–1.15).

A Nonrandomized Clinical Trial

Smithells and colleagues carried out a multicenter nonrandomized prospective trial of periconceptional multivitamin supplementation in the prevention of NTDs [15]. They selected mothers who already had had one affected offspring. The oral tablets taken (Pregnavite Forte-F, made by Bencard) consisted of a mixture of folic acid, numerous vitamins, and a mineral supplement containing iron, calcium, and phosphorus. There were three groups. The fully supplemented group of 185 mothers, who took one tablet three times a day for at least 28 days prior to conception until the date of the second missed period, produced 178 infants or fetuses, of whom one (0.6%) had an NTD. This compared with 13 births with an NTD (5.0%) out of 260 infants or fetuses of unsupplemented mothers; a significant difference (relative risk 0.12, $p < 0.01$). There was also a third group of partially supplemented mothers defined as those conceiving

within 28 days of beginning supplementation or commencing supplementation after conception but known to have missed tablets for more than one day. These results produced immediate and widespread interest.

An early and sustained criticism was why a randomized design had not been used. Smithells et al. eventually stated that they originally intended to use a double-blind randomized design but that this protocol was rejected by three separate hospital research ethics committees. Owing to the absence of randomization, women therefore selected themselves into the supplemented and nonsupplemented groups (*see* **Selection Bias**). There were other criticisms. There was no true placebo group; which preparation might be effective, multivitamin or folic acid, was not clear.

A Randomized Clinical Trial

The debate for and against the need and ethical justification for a larger and valid randomized trial of folic acid supplementation continued. By September 1982 the UK Government had approved funding for 3 years and asked the Medical Research Council (MRC) to carry out such a study.

The MRC vitamin study [11] was a randomized double-blind prevention trial with a factorial design conducted at 33 centers in seven countries to determine whether supplementation with folic acid or a mixture of seven other vitamins (A, D, B1, B2, B6, C, and nicotinamide) around the time of conception can prevent NTDs (anencephalus, spina bifida, encephalocele). Some 1817 women who had at least one previous affected pregnancy with an NTD were allocated at random to one of four groups (see Table 1).

Some 1195 had a completed pregnancy in which the status of the fetus or infant was ascertained with respect to having or not having an NTD. A known abnormality occurred in 27: six in the folic acid groups

Table 1 The 2×2 factorial design used in the UK MRC randomized trial of folic acid and other dietary supplementation in high-risk pregnancies

Group		Folic acid	
		Yes	No
Multivitamins	No	A	C
	Yes	B	D

Note: All women had a previous offspring with NTD and all received minerals supplement.

and 21 in the other two groups. This is a 72% protective effect (relative risk 0.28, 95% confidence interval 0.12–0.71). No significant protection effect was found with respect to the other vitamins (relative risk 0.80, 95% confidence interval 0.32–1.72). Of the centers, 17 were in the UK, seven were in Hungary, three in Australia, three in Canada, and one each in Israel, Moscow, USSR, and Lyon, France. The randomization was carried out by the Clinical Trials Service Unit at Oxford. Women took one capsule a day from the date of randomization until 12 weeks of pregnancy, estimated from the first day of the last menstrual period. The folic acid capsules contained 4 mg of the substance. The multivitamin groups contained various amounts of the various vitamins. The control substance consisting of minerals contained dried ferrous sulphate and calcium phosphate. There was an independent data monitoring committee which reviewed progress every 6 months. The trial was double-blind with neither patients nor their medical attendants knowing which regime had been allocated.

There was a 2 × 2 factorial design:

A Folic acid and minerals.   C Minerals only.
B Folic acid, minerals and   D Minerals and other
   other vitamins.   vitamins.

In this design the effect of folic acid is determined by comparing groups A and B together vs. groups C and D together. The effect of multivitamins is determined by comparing groups B and D together vs. groups A and C together. If it is thought that there might be a synergistic action between folic acid and multivitamins then only group B would benefit. This factorial design with 2000 participants would give a statistical power of 80% to detect a reduction in recurrence from 4% to 2% using a one-sided significance level of 0.05. This degree of difference is similar to that observed by Smithells et al., who reported a reduction of recurrence risk from 4.7% to 0.7%. About one woman was being recruited each working day and it was thought that the trial would continue until around 1993. However, in April 1991 the data monitoring committee recommended that the trial be stopped. The results of the trial had been kept under review and assessed by sequential analysis for which the cumulative difference between the number of NTDs occurring in the folic acid and nonfolic acid groups was plotted against the total number of NTDs occurring in the study.

By April 12, 1991, results showed that this difference had passed the preset lower boundary in the sequential analysis. At this point 1817 women had been randomized and findings were known on 1195 informative pregnancies. The findings were very clear and showed a significant beneficial effect specific to folic acid supplementation. This important trial was based on measuring the reduction in recurrence risk. Roughly, only 5% of mothers who produce offspring with NTDs have previously had at least one affected birth. The great majority, about 95% of mothers who produce NTD births have only one such occurrence.

This key question of whether a periconceptional vitamin supplementation with folic acid or multivitamins would prevent the first occurrence of NTDs in a similar fashion was studied by Czeizel & Dudás in Hungary and reported in 1992 [3]. They randomized women in two groups. Some 2104 women received the folic acid and vitamin supplement and 2052 women received a trace element supplement which contained copper, manganese, zinc, and vitamin C. Birth defects were significantly more prevalent in the group receiving the trace element supplement compared with the folic acid and vitamin supplement group (22.9 per 1000 and 13.3 per 1000 births, respectively; $P = 0.02$).

The mechanism whereby folic acid supplementation in the periconceptional period reduced the occurrence and recurrence risk of NTDs has not been determined. It is clear that supplementation does not act to correct a simple nutritional deficiency, because most pregnant women carrying an affected fetus have levels of folate above the deficient range. Therefore, the possibility that an abnormality in folate metabolism is responsible for a large proportion of NTDs is being investigated. Functional variants in some of the enzymes involved in folate metabolism can be identified by demonstrating differences in the genes encoding them. Three studies have suggested that homozygosity for the V677T mutation in the gene coding for 5,10-methylenetetrahydrofolate reductase (MTHFR), which results in a thermolabile variant of the MTHFR enzyme, is a risk factor for spina bifida.

Particular Statistical Concepts, Problems, and Techniques

It is useful to compare progress in teratology with research in another field such as cancer. In the latter, descriptive studies have led to case–control studies of each of the common cancers, possible treatments have been identified and tested using clinical trials. In teratology these developments have not happened. There is the difficulty of direct observation, and the major problem of assessing exposure. However, compared with cancer, the interval between exposure and outcome in a fetus or newborn is relatively short and new cohorts of births are formed by the natural process of conception, gestation, and birth.

Another key problem relates to the frequency of birth defects. For example a case–control study would need at least 750 cases and a similar number of controls to detect an exposure factor which changed the incidence of any of the most common birth defects, e.g. NTDs, by a factor of 50%. In turn this would require a population of around 750 000 births corresponding to a total population of at least 50 million persons. This corresponds to an entire year of births in France or England and Wales and at least 2 years of births in Australia or Canada. In the MRC trial of folic acid we have noted that this required collaboration between 33 centers drawn from 14 countries. It follows that there is a great need for international collaboration.

Fundamental problems exist relating to classification. The debate is summarized by the phrase "lumpers and splitters". Birth defects rarely, if ever, occur as an all or nothing phenomenon. Taxonomy is crucial. Further difficulties arise due to the observation of more than one defect occurring in the same individual and the large number of complex syndromes that have now been described. A systematic study of each of the major common birth defects using rigorous case–control studies has not yet been completed. Once the selection of subjects for study has been made there may be errors and **bias** in observations (*see* **Measurement Error in Epidemiologic Studies**). One of the most difficult to assess is logical and not statistical, and relates to the definition of affected individuals. Errors of measurement may occur. Bias is common, most frequently due to incomplete ascertainment.

Solutions to These Problems

Classification problems may be clarified by new and better observations and techniques. Detailed biochemical studies and possible genetic defects have been identified using deoxyribonucleic acid (DNA) methods in the case of NTDs. The human genome project will undoubtedly provide a great deal of knowledge relating to teratology. Progress could be made by extending existing malformation registers. These should contain more accurate observations, preferably verified by experienced clinicians, more complete ascertainment of birth defects in a defined community, and in due course larger data sets. Analysis specifically of cases with malformations of more than one system may have greater statistical power to detect associations with putative teratogens if the exposure of interest is primarily associated with a pattern of multiple defects of unknown cause rather than with isolated defects.

Monitoring

Several surveillance systems for births with malformations were established after the thalidomide tragedy of 1961. Tests for statistically significant increases in observed numbers of cases as compared with baseline expected numbers are made on a monthly basis in England and Wales and Norway, on a 1, 2, 3, 6 and 12 monthly basis in Atlanta, and on a quarterly basis in the Birth Defects Monitoring Programme in the US. Many of the surveillance schemes participate in the International Clearinghouse for Birth Defects Monitoring Systems. Most of these are based solely on malformations recorded in the neonatal period. There are also systems in which malformations are recorded irrespective of the age at detection. In Europe, a number of this type are included in a concerted action project on the registration of congenital abnormalities and twins in the European Community (EUROCAT).

The statistical methods used have been of the following types: (i) graphical display of frequencies; (ii) chi-square linear trend analysis; (iii) comparison of observed numbers of cases of specific types of congenital anomalies with the numbers expected according to the Poisson distribution; (iv) "self-reinforcing" techniques, notably the cumulative sum ("cusum") technique and the sets method; and (v) scan analysis (*see* **Scan Statistics for Disease Surveillance**). Some comparisons of these techniques have been carried out. In applications with small denominator populations, the Poisson technique was found to be inefficient compared with the sets method and the cusum technique. In applications with larger denominator populations, the cusum technique is somewhat more efficient than the Poisson and sets techniques. In simulation analysis for four specific groups of malformations, the cusum technique showed greater **sensitivity**, **specificity**, and accuracy than the sets method. One obvious limitation of these techniques, which applies to certain types of malformations only, is the difficulty of obtaining data on terminations of pregnancy in which fetuses with certain types of anomalies have been detected by antenatal diagnosis. The size of the population surveyed is a crucial issue in view of the fact that most teratogens identified to date have had a low prevalence of exposure, and the background rate of specific anomalies is low.

Clustering in Time and Space

The recognition and investigation of clusters of congenital anomalies, and particularly the assessment of whether the occurrence of **clustering** or a particular cluster is purely a chance phenomenon, leads to considerable methodological and practical difficulties. The available studies can be classified into one of three groups based on the motivation for the investigation: (i) studies carried out to test if clustering exists within a predefined population of births, in the absence of specific spontaneous reporting of clusters or a specific hypothesis concerning an environmental agent; (ii) studies carried out when the existence of the cluster has been suspected and spontaneously reported, usually either by clinicians or local inhabitants; and (iii) studies initiated because of concern about specific environmental exposures. In the 1970s, recognition of the problems of investigating spatial clustering led to investigation being focused more on the identification of time space clustering using the methods of Ederer et al. [4]. All of these approaches have been used in investigations of neural tube defects; no clear-cut evidence of clustering was found in any study.

Anticipated Developments and Unresolved Problems

Progress in teratology, as in other fields, requires accurate and perceptive observation which in turn relates to the power and sophistication of techniques and instruments available at the time. It is likely that this will be revolutionized by the new work in genome research, the identification of chromosomal differences between mothers of affected and nonaffected offspring, and in due course by the detection of how these differences are manifest via biochemical

pathways or other means. The definition and identification of clusters of birth defects is unresolved and continues to be of concern. Such outbreaks are notified from time to time usually accompanied by requests for investigation. These are difficult, expensive and time-consuming and the majority so far have rarely led to finding any new cause.

The etiology of most types of congenital anomalies remains unknown. For many types of anomaly there is an elevated recurrence risk, probably due to a combination of genetic and environmental factors. Advances in molecular genetics have made it possible to genotype large numbers of individuals by polymerase chain reaction (PCR) techniques. This greatly simplifies the investigation of genotype–environment interaction. For example, research has identified an increased risk of orofacial clefts among individuals with the uncommon allele for transforming growth factor alpha (TGFα).

Progress is being made at finding reasons why some rare defects occur, but this has had a small effect to date on the overall burden of the common teratological defects (*see* **Burden of Disease**), which remain a major public health problem.

References and Annotated Bibliography

[1]   Bower, C. & Stanley, F.J. (1989). Dietary folate as a risk factor for neural-tube defects: evidence from a case–control study in Western Australia, *Medical Journal of Australia* **150**, 613–619.

[2]   Buyse, M.L., ed. in chief. (1991). *Birth Defects Encyclopedia*. The Centre for Birth Defects Information Services, Inc., Dover, Mass., and Blackwell Scientific, Oxford. (A reference source describing known defects in detail.)

[3]   Czeizel, A.E. & Dudás, I. (1992). Prevention of the first occurrence of neural-tube defects by periconceptional vitamin supplementation, *New England Journal of Medicine* **327**, 1832–1835.

[4]   Ederer, H.B., Myers, M.H. & Mantel, N. (1964). A statistical problem in time and space: do leukaemia cases come in clusters?, *Biometrics* **20**, 626–638.

[5]   Elwood, J.M., Little, J. & Elwood, J.H. (1992). *Epidemiology and Control of Neural Tube Defects*. Oxford University Press, Oxford. (A monograph detailing research and methodological issues relating to these malformations.)

[6]   Gregg, N.M. (1941). Congenital cataract following German measles in the mother, *Transactions of the Ophthalmological Society of Australia* **3**, 35–46.

[7]   Hale, F. (1933). Pigs born without eye balls, *Journal of Heredity* **24**, 105–106.

[8]   International Clearinghouse for Birth Defects Monitoring Systems (1991). *Congenital Malformations Worldwide*. Elsevier, Amsterdam. (A description of the work of this nongovernmental organization of the World Health Organization and the participating centers who joined during 1974–88.)

[9]   Lenz, W. & Knapp, K. (1962). Foetal malformations due to Thalidomide, *German Medical Monthly (English language edition of the Deutsche Medizinische Wochenschrift)* **7**, 253–358.

[10]   McKusick, V.A., with the assistance of Francomano, C.A., Antonarakis, S.E. & Pearson P.L. (1994). *Mendelian Inheritance in Man. A Catalog of Human Genes and Genetic Disorders*, 11th Ed. 2 Vols. Johns Hopkins University Press, Baltimore. (A comprehensive computerized listing of all reports in the literature relating to known and possible genetic diseases and syndromes, including many congenital malformations. Each brief entry has an identification number, description, author, and literature citation. The catalog is continuously updated and republished periodically.)

[11]   Medical Research Council (MRC) Vitamin Study Research Group (1991). Prevention of neural tube defects: Results of the Medical Research Council vitamin study, *Lancet* **338**, 131–137.

[12]   Milunsky, A., Jick, S.S., Bruell, C.L., MacLaughlin, D.S., Rothman, K.J. & Willett, W. (1989). Multivitamin/folic acid supplementation in early pregnancy reduces the prevalence of neural tube defects, *Journal of the American Medical Association* **262**, 2847–2852.

[13]   Schardein, J.L. (1993). *Chemically Induced Birth Defects*, 2nd Ed. Marcel Dekker, New York. (A catalog relating to these teratogenic agents.)

[14]   Shepard, T.H. (1995). *Catalog of Teratogenic Agents*, 8th Ed. Johns Hopkins University Press, Baltimore. (A useful computer-maintained reference file relating to this aspect of birth defect causation.)

[15]   Smithells, R.W., Sheppard, S., Schorah, C.J., Seller, M.J., Nevin, N.C., Harris, R., Read, A.P. & Fielding, D.W. (1980). Possible prevention of neural-tube defects by periconceptional vitamin supplementation, *Lancet* **i**, 339–340.

[16]   Stevenson, A.C., Johnston, H.A., Stewart, M.I.P. & Golding, D.R. (1966). Congenital malformations: a report of a study of series of consecutive births in 24 centres, *Bulletin of the World Health Organization* **34**, Supplement, 9–127.

[17]   Warkany, J. (1971). *Congenital Malformations. Notes and Comments*. Year Book Medical Publishers, Chicago. (A large wide-ranging text based on a lifetime experience of this pediatrician and teratologist based at Cincinnati.)

(*See also* **Birth Defects Registries**)

J.H. ELWOOD & J. LITTLE

Test–Retest Reliability *see* Agreement, Measurement of

Time Lag Effect

The term *time lag effect* refers to the delay between the time of an intervention or exposure onset, such as the date on which a person begins smoking cigarettes, and the subsequent development of a health outcome, such as the diagnosis of lung cancer. A variety of such time lag effects are described in the article, **Latent Period**. To design and to analyze prevention trials efficiently, one must account for the sometimes considerable time lag between the onset of intervention and subsequent beneficial health effects.

M.H. GAIL

Time-Related Exposure *see* Occupational Health and Medicine

Transmission Models *see* Communicable Diseases

Transportability *see* Measurement Error in Epidemiologic Studies

Truncation; Truncation Product-Limit Estimator *see* Biased Sampling of Cohorts in Epidemiology

Two-by-Two Tables, Series of *see* Mantel–Haenszel Methods

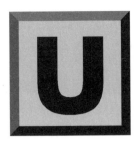

Unhealthy Migrant Effect *see* Migrant Studies

Unmasking Bias *see* Detection Bias

Vaccine Efficacy *see* Communicable Diseases

Validation Data *see* Measurement Error in Epidemiologic Studies

Validation Study

Validation studies obtain information on **measurement errors** in exposures and other covariates used in epidemiologic studies by comparing the conventional exposure measurements with "gold standard" measurements. Reliability studies, unlike validation studies, provide information on the measurement error process by replicating the conventional exposure measurements. Validation studies can be applied to study a broader range of error processes than reliability studies, which are based on a special error model. Data from validation studies or reliability studies are needed to correct relative **risk** estimates for **bias** and to obtain valid inference in the presence of measurement error (*see* **Misclassification Error**).

To define these ideas more precisely, let **Y** be the response variable, and let **X** be the true value(s) of the covariate. In some cases, **X** can never be observed and can be thought of as a *latent* variable. In other cases, **X** is a "gold standard" method of covariate assessment which is infeasible and/or expensive to

administer to large numbers of study participants. Usually, instead of observing **X**, an error-prone measurement **W** is observed. Finally, there may be covariates $\mathbf{Z_1}$ upon which the model for response depends that are never misclassified or measured with error. In main study/validation study designs, the main study yields the data $(\mathbf{Y}_i, \mathbf{W}_i, \mathbf{Z}_i), i = 1, \dots, n_1$. If the validation study is *internal*, it yields the observations $(\mathbf{Y}_i, \mathbf{W}_i, \mathbf{X}_i, \mathbf{Z}_i), i = n_1 + 1, \dots, n_1 + n_2$. If the validation study is *external*, it produces observations $(\mathbf{W}_i, \mathbf{X}_i, \mathbf{Z}_{2i}), i = n_1 + 1, \dots, n_1 + n_2$ observations. There may be covariates, denoted $\mathbf{Z}_2$, upon which the measurement error and/or misclassification model depend but of which the model for response is independent; we denote the unique elements of $\mathbf{Z}_1$ and $\mathbf{Z}_2$ by **Z**. An external validation study is a useful option only when there are a priori reasons to believe that measurement error/misclassification is **nondifferential**, i.e. that $f(\mathbf{Y}|\mathbf{W}, \mathbf{X}, \mathbf{Z}) = f(\mathbf{Y}|\mathbf{X}, \mathbf{Z})$. This definition can be rewritten as $f(\mathbf{W}|\mathbf{Y}, \mathbf{X}, \mathbf{Z}) = f(\mathbf{W}|\mathbf{X}, \mathbf{Z})$, in which form the nondifferential error feature is more apparent.

Without validation or reliability data, it is possible only to perform sensitivity analyses under hypothesized scenarios for measurement error and/or misclassification. Without information about the nature and extent of the measurement error and/or misclassification, sensitivity analyses yield wide ranges of the parameter(s) estimates, and cannot assess the true uncertainty of the estimates. It is possible in certain instances to test hypotheses about **X**, however, even in the absence of validation data. For generalized linear models with $\dim(\mathbf{X}) = \dim(\mathbf{W}) = 1$, the usual score test, based upon the main study data alone, will have the correct size, although its power will be reduced unless $\mathbf{X}$ is linearly related to $\mathbf{W}$ and $\mathbf{Z}$ [16]. The same results apply for the global null hypothesis about $\mathbf{X}$. Validation and/or reliability data are required for valid estimation and inference in nearly all other circumstances. An exception occurs when the model for $\mathbf{Y}$ given $(\mathbf{X}, \mathbf{Z}_1)$ is **logistic** and the model for $\mathbf{X}$ given $(\mathbf{W}, \mathbf{Z}_2)$ is Gaussian. In this case, when $\dim(\mathbf{X}) = \dim(\mathbf{W}) = 1$, the parameters of both models are identifiable from the main study alone [10], although as yet unpublished work by Spiegelman & Rosner indicates that estimates of these parameters are difficult to obtain, and when obtained, are usually very imprecise.

A reliability study can be used to estimate variance components in the classic, random within-person, measurement error model

$$\mathbf{W} = \mathbf{X} + \mathbf{U}, \qquad (1)$$

where $\mathbf{U}$ is a mean zero error term with variance–covariance Σ. It is only when (1) applies that replicate data, as would be obtained in a reliability study, can be used for valid estimation and inference in the presence of covariate measurement error. Eq. (1) has been applied to the assessment of measurements of blood pressure, serum hormones, and other serum biomarkers such as vitamin concentrations.

A validation study can be used for a wide range of error models. A validation study may be expensive or infeasible because it requires that the true value $\mathbf{X}$ be observable, at least in some small sample of n_2 study participants. That is, a "gold standard" technique for measuring the quantity of interest without error must be available. In most situations, it is impossible to measure exposure perfectly. If measurement error/misclassification methods are used with an "alloyed" or imperfect gold standard, $\mathbf{X}'$, the results of the analysis can be misleading. If $\mathbf{X}'$ and $\mathbf{Z}$ are uncorrelated, however, the results may be interpreted as those which would have been obtained had the (imperfect) gold standard measurements $\mathbf{X}'$ been available for all study participants, rather than just those in the validation study. Under certain circumstances, if the errors in $\mathbf{X}'$ and $\mathbf{W}$ are uncorrelated, the regression calibration estimate will provide unbiased measurement error correction for the gold standard, $\mathbf{X}$ [14, 18]. In some realistic examples, the bias in regression calibration estimates is small even when the errors are moderately correlated.

In this article it is assumed, unless stated otherwise, that the validation study is sampled completely at random. That is, if V is a random variable which equals 1 if a participant is in the validation study and 0 otherwise, we assume $\Pr(V = 1 | \mathbf{Y}, \mathbf{X}, \mathbf{W}, \mathbf{Z}) = \pi$, independent of $\mathbf{Y}, \mathbf{X}, \mathbf{W}$, and $\mathbf{Z}$.

Two-stage designs (*see* **Case–Control Study, Two-Phase**) allow V to depend upon $\mathbf{Y}, \mathbf{W}$ and $\mathbf{Z}$. Two-stage designs allow one to control the selection of validation study participants so as to increase statistical efficiency or reduce cost. These options require the validation study to be *internal*. Two-stage designs have several limitations. Many validation studies yield data on numerous covariates. For example, in a prospective **cohort study** yielding information on cancer and cardiovascular endpoints, it may be necessary to validate many nutrient measures simultaneously. An optimal design for one response/covariate pair may be inefficient for another. Although some authors have found that the optimal sampling probability function, π depends on $\mathbf{Y}$ ([17] and as yet unpublished work by Holcroft & Spiegelman) in cohort studies and many **nested case–control** studies, it will not be possible to identify the optimal π as a function of $\mathbf{Y}$, since covariate status is best ascertained before observing $\mathbf{Y}$.

The remainder of this article will discuss strategies for optimizing (n_1, n_2), assuming that the validation sample is taken completely at random. Solutions to this problem are mathematically complex, and software is not widely available. In a two-stage design, $(n_1 + n_2, \pi)$ must be optimized, which poses an even more difficult theoretical and computational problem. Nevertheless, further research on two-stage designs may lead to improvements on the designs presented below.

The valid use of an external validation study requires that the measurement error model $f(\mathbf{X}|\mathbf{W}, \mathbf{Z}_2)$ is the same in the external population as in the main study. This assumption is necessarily true for an internal validation study, supplied completely at random. By Bayes' Theorem $f(\mathbf{X}|\mathbf{W}, \mathbf{Z}_2) = f(\mathbf{W}|\mathbf{X}, \mathbf{Z}_2) f(\mathbf{X}, \mathbf{Z}_2) / f(\mathbf{W}, \mathbf{Z}_2)$. Although in many instances it may be reasonable to assume that $f(\mathbf{W}|\mathbf{X}, \mathbf{Z}_2)$ may be "transportable" from one population to the next, provided the instruments used to measure $\mathbf{X}$ and $\mathbf{W}$ are identical, it is less reasonable to assume that the unobservable marginal density $f(\mathbf{X}, \mathbf{Z}_2)$ in the main study population is the same as that in an external validation population. Thus, an internal validation study is more convincing than an external validation study.

Two recent epidemiologic textbooks devote a chapter to the design and analysis of validation and reliability studies. Armstrong et al. [1, Chapter 4] focus primarily on the design and analysis of reliability studies, but there is some consideration of validation studies as well. Willett [19] discusses validation study design for dietary intake questionnaires. Willett gives a simple formula for calculating the sample size of a validation study, based on the criterion of testing $H_0 : \rho = \rho_0$ vs. $H_a : \rho = \rho_A$ with prespecified power $1 - \beta$ and nominal size α, where ρ is the correlation between the usual exposure method (**W**) and the gold standard (**X**):

$$n = 3 + \frac{(Z_\alpha + Z_\beta)^2}{|\rho_A - \rho_0|},$$

where Z_α and Z_β are the standard normal deviates for α and β, respectively. This criterion for validation study sample size is not designed to ensure adequate sample size for measurement error correction, and is strictly useful only when the estimation of the correlation between **X** and **W** is the end goal. Willett reports some otherwise unpublished data which examined the influence of validation study sample size on the precision of **odds ratio** corrected for measurement error by regression calibration, where it had been found that for "realistic conditions" ($0.5 < \rho < 0.7$), validation studies with more than 150–200 subjects provide little additional precision.

Design of Main Study/Validation Studies

Choice of the Optimization Criterion for Efficient Study Designs

In the biomedical research setting, research proposals will usually not be approved for funding unless the proposed study has power of 80% or more to test the central scientific hypothesis. The study design process seeks to minimize the proposed budget while assuring adequate statistical power. Because the unit cost of measuring **X** can be 100 or more times that of measuring **W**, validation studies can be expensive, and efficient main study/validation study designs are essential. Incorporating these design features is important, because it is seldom possible to collect

validation data after the main study has been completed. Calculation of a point estimate, typically an odds ratio or hazard ratio, and the construction of confidence intervals around this estimate are often primary analytic goals in observational biomedical research, where measurement error and misclassification frequently arise. Greenland proposed the *discriminatory power* criterion [5] for these settings. One specifies the two sample sizes needed, respectively, to test the null hypothesis, $H_0 : \beta = \beta_L$ against the alternative, $H_a : \beta = \beta_U$, each with prescribed size and power. According to the discriminatory power criterion, the required sample size is the maximum of these two sample sizes. In **relative risk models**, because the variance of the estimate of the parameter of interest, $\hat{\beta}$, depends on the value of the parameter of interest, β, typically the log odds ratio or log hazard ratio, the discriminatory power criterion will usually produce optimal sample sizes larger than those produced by the traditional power criterion. An alternative criterion is to specify the expected confidence interval width at a specified relative risk, but this criterion may produce designs with unknown, possibly subnominal confidence levels for different, equally plausible values of the relative risk.

Given unit costs r_Y, r_W, and r_X for a single measurement of **Y**, **W**, and **X**, respectively, the optimization criterion we prefer minimizes the total study cost, C, with respect to (n_1, n_2), subject to minimum discriminatory power requirements. In a main study/external validation study design,

$$C(n_1, n_2) = (r_D + r_W)n_1 + (r_W + r_X)n_2$$

and maximization over (n_1, n_2) is subject to the constraints

$$1 - \Phi \left[\frac{Z_{1-\alpha/2}[V_L(n_1, n_2)]^{1/2} - \beta_U + \beta_L}{[V_U(n_1, n_2)]^{1/2}} \right] \geq \Pi,$$

and

$$\Phi \left[\frac{-Z_{1-\alpha/2}[V_U(n_1, n_2)]^{1/2} - \beta_L + \beta_U}{[V_L(n_1, n_2)]^{1/2}} \right] \geq \Pi.$$

Here $V_L(n_1, n_2)$ and $V_U(n_1, n_2)$ are the expected values of the variances of $\hat{\beta}$ evaluated at β_L and β_U, respectively, over the distribution of (**D**, **X**, **W**) for the study population to be investigated, Π is the minimal acceptable discriminatory power, and z_γ is

γth quantile of the standard normal distribution. For a main study/internal validation study design, the cost function

$$C(n_1, n_2) = \min[(r_{\mathbf{D}} + r_{\mathbf{W}})n_1 + (r_{\mathbf{W}} + r_{\mathbf{X}} + r_{\mathbf{D}})n_2,$$
$$(r_{\mathbf{D}} + r_{\mathbf{X}})n_2^*]$$

is used, since there may be a discontinuity point in the main study/internal validation study design optimization equations at which the fully validated design, consisting only of observations $(\mathbf{Y}_i, \mathbf{W}, \mathbf{Z}_{1i})$, $i = 1, \ldots, n_2$, is optimal.

Within this framework, one must supply the necessary design specifications, which will vary from one setting to another, and substitute the appropriate formulas for V_L and V_U to obtain the optimal values of n_1 and n_2. Even with a simple formula for var $\hat{\beta}$, the solution cannot be written in closed form because the constraints are complex. Numerical solutions can be found using a nonlinear multiparameter optimization subroutine such as DNCONF in IMSL [8], with a call to an application-specific subroutine implementing the appropriate variance formula.

Although the design criteria discussed above are all functions of the variance of $\hat{\beta}$ as well as other parameters, the expected confidence interval width criterion is simply proportional to the square root of this variance. A limitation of most of the papers on validation study design is that they investigate design issues only by the criterion of expected confidence interval width.

Optimal Study Design for Misclassified Binary Exposure Variables

When binary exposure variables are subject to misclassification, the simplest misclassification model, $f_2(\mathbf{X}|\mathbf{W}; \theta)$, can be completely described with two parameters, $\theta = (\omega, \varphi)$, namely the **sensitivity**

$$\omega = \Pr(\mathbf{W} = 1 | \mathbf{X} = 1),$$

and the **specificity**

$$\varphi = \Pr(\mathbf{W} = 0 | \mathbf{X} = 0).$$

This model is less restrictive than the measurement error model (1), since the error distribution depends on $\mathbf{X}$, except in the special case when $\omega = 1 - \varphi$. Further complexity in the misclassification model can be introduced by allowing that ω and/or φ vary with $\mathbf{Y}$, as in the case of **recall bias** in a **case–control**

study, or allowing ω and/or φ to vary with some other covariate(s), $\mathbf{Z}$. In most instances, optimal study designs will depend on the underlying true exposure **prevalence**, $\Pr(\mathbf{X} = 1)$.

Palmgren [11] studied internal validation designs for case–control studies and with the same proportions of the sample allocated to validation for cases and controls. Palmgren found the optimal allocation proportion, $n_2/(n_1 + n_2)$, to minimize the null variance of the estimated log odds ratio, $\hat{\beta}$, subject to fixed cost. She also determined the optimal allocation proportion to minimize the variance of $\hat{\beta}$ subject to fixed cost. She did not base her designs on a classical power criterion nor on the discriminatory power criterion.

To use Palmgren's formulation, the investigator must specify the odds ratio, the sensitivity and specificity for measuring exposure, the exposure prevalences in cases and controls, and the costs of measuring $\mathbf{W}$ and $\mathbf{X}$. When $\beta = 0$ and the sensitivity and specificity are assumed to be the same for cases and controls, the optimal design for minimizing the variance of $\hat{\beta}$ is the fully validated design, $(n_1 = 0)$, unless the square of the correlation between $\mathbf{W}$ and $\mathbf{X}$ is greater than the cost ratio $r_{\mathbf{W}}/r_{\mathbf{X}}$, in which case the optimal design is the main study only $(n_2 = 0)$. When sensitivity and specificity are allowed to depend upon case status, the optimal allocation ranges between 0 and 1, depending on the other design parameters. Palmgren also provided some results for minimizing the variance of the maximum likelihood estimator of β, for $\beta \neq 0$, subject to fixed cost, under the assumptions that the sensitivity and specificity are equivalent for cases and controls and for a one-to-one case–control ratio. It is shown that for small β, case–control ratios near one-to-one and in most cases when the cost ratio, $r_{\mathbf{X}}/r_{\mathbf{W}}, \geq 4$, the main study/internal validation study design is more efficient than the fully validated design. When the exposure is rare, the optimal design depends more heavily on the value of the specificity parameter, and when the exposure is common, the optimal design depends more heavily on the sensitivity parameter.

A useful contribution of [11] are equations (A1) and (A2), which give the nonnull and null formulas for the variance of the maximum likelihood estimator of β.

Greenland [6] also minimized the variance of $\hat{\beta}$ subject to fixed cost, but he used the matrix method for estimating β [2, 7, 12], rather than maximum likelihood. Greenland found that the optimal proportion allocated to the validation study increases dramatically when **differential** misclassification is assumed. He concluded that the fully validated design is optimal or near optimal in many cases and has the additional advantages of permitting standard methods of data analysis and of assuring representativeness of the validation sample. Although Greenland's recommendations are clearly appropriate for low cost ratios (r_X/r_W ranging between 3 and 12) and high case–control ratios (e.g. where $Pr(\mathbf{Y}) \approx 0.50$), it is not clear at what point this recommendation no longer applies. For cost ratios, r_X/r_W, above 100, or lower case–control ratios, the main study/validation study design is likely to be preferable.

Chernoff & Haitovsky [4] and Zelen & Haitovsky [20] considered optimal design in the estimation and testing settings, respectively. They admitted as the class of optimal designs a linear combination of the eight designs derived from four possibilities for case and controls: (i) main study only; (ii) validate all subjects with $\mathbf{W} = 1$; (iii) validate all subjects with $\mathbf{W} = 0$; and (iv) validation study only. Designs were optimized by minimizing the variance of the estimate of $Pr(\mathbf{X} = 1|\mathbf{Y} = 1) - Pr(\mathbf{X} = 1|\mathbf{Y} = 0)$, for fixed cost, and differential misclassification was assumed at known misclassification rates. They found that the optimal design was a combination of two of the eight sampling plans, one for cases and the other for controls. As long as the sensitivity, specificity, and costs of collecting the data are the same for cases and controls, the same type and sample size of design for cases and controls is optimal.

Optimal Study Designs for a Continuous Covariate Measured with Error

Buonaccorsi [3] provided optimal allocation formulas for minimizing the variance of the estimate of the odds ratio subject to specified cost, when $\dim(\mathbf{X}) = \dim(\mathbf{W}) = 1$, $\dim(\mathbf{Z})$ is arbitrary, and $\mathbf{Y}$ is a binary outcome. These formulas apply when $(\mathbf{X}, \mathbf{W}, \mathbf{Z})$ are jointly multivariate normal given $\mathbf{Y}$ but where the measurement error model, $f_2(\mathbf{X}|\mathbf{W})$, may be a function of $\mathbf{Y}$ or dependent on other covariates $\mathbf{Z}_2$. Under these assumptions, the odds ratio can be validly and efficiently estimated through the normal discriminant analysis model instead of the **logistic regression** model. Buonaccorsi derived a closed-form expression for the optimal proportion of study subjects validated under the main study/internal validation study design,

$n_2/(n_1 + n_2)$, as a function of six quantities: (i) unit costs for $\mathbf{Y}$, $(\mathbf{W}, \mathbf{Z})$ and $\mathbf{X}$ (r_Y, r_W, and r_X); (ii) total cost for the study (C); (iii) value for the log odds ratio of $\mathbf{Y}$ from a unit change in $\mathbf{X}$ (β); (iv) multiple correlation between $\mathbf{X}$ and $(\mathbf{W}, \mathbf{Z})$ (this quantity can be taken to represent the extent of measurement error resulting from failure to observe $\mathbf{X}$); (v) the variance of $\mathbf{X}$ (σ_x^2); and (vi) the marginal probability of $\mathbf{Y}$ [$Pr(\mathbf{Y})$]. With the exception of the measurement error parameter and the quantities relating to cost, all of these quantities would be required for study design calculations even when $\mathbf{X}$ were perfectly measured. Buonaccorsi gave a simple formula for the variance of the measurement-error corrected estimate of β.

Spiegelman & Gray [13] also investigated optimal study design for binary regression in the case of a single continuous covariate measured with error but, unlike Buonaccorsi, they relied on the discriminatory power criterion. In addition to considering the main study/internal validation study design paradigm, they also considered the main study/external validation study designs. Since external validation study data will often be obtained as an afterthought at the end of a prospective study, choosing the optimal sample sizes, n_1 and n_2, is of less practical importance. However, it is instructive to compare cost, power, and sampling ratios as given by optimal internal and external validation study settings. From efficiency considerations, it was shown that an internal validation study is optimal. However, as $Pr(\mathbf{Y})$ becomes small, the efficiency advantage of the main study/internal validation study design virtually disappears relative to the main study/external validation study design.

Rather than assuming that $(\mathbf{W}, \mathbf{X}, \mathbf{Z})$ are jointly normal given $\mathbf{Y}$, Spiegelman & Gray assume that $\mathbf{X}|\mathbf{W}$ is multivariate normal. Unlike Buonaccorsi, they did not consider the presence of additional perfectly measured exposure variables $\mathbf{Z}$, and they require that $E(\mathbf{X}|\mathbf{W})$ is linear. Without the joint multivariate normality assumption, the normal discriminant model cannot be used to obtain an unbiased estimate of β. Instead, the logistic regression model must be used. This is the model upon which Spiegelman & Gray based their sample size calculations. Iterative methods must be used to find optimal main study and validation study sample sizes when $f_2(\mathbf{X}|\mathbf{W})$ is normal and $f_1(\mathbf{Y}|\mathbf{X})$, the model for the outcome conditional on the true exposure, is logistic. In order to find the optimal design in this framework, the investigator needs to identify six quantities: (i) r_Y, r_X, and r_W; (ii) $\Pr(Y)$; (iii) β_L and β_U, the two values of the log odds ratio between which the study is designed to discriminate; (iv) the mean and variance of W; (v) the parameters for the conditional mean of X given W, α', and γ, where $E(X|W) = \alpha' + \gamma W$, and $\text{var}(X|W)$; and (vi) the desired confidence level, α, and the required discriminatory power, Π.

Spiegelman & Gray found that the fully validated design is optimal only when r_X/r_W is small, $\Pr(Y = 1)$ is large, and the magnitudes of β_U and β_L are relatively far from the null but close together. They found that the optimal percent allocation to the validation study increased as the unit cost of Y increased. Figure 1 shows the cost of the optimal main study/internal validation study designs for sample disease frequencies [$\Pr(Y)$] equal to 0.005. In this figure RY, RX, and RW are the unit costs for measuring Y, X, and W, respectively, and, when X and W are standardized, γ corresponds to the correlation between X and W. Designs are optimized to discriminate with 95% power between two hypothesized values of the odds ratios, and the scenarios considered are given in the legend. Cost increases dramatically as the distance between the two hypothesized odds ratios decreases, and as measurement error increases.

In the context of **nutritional epidemiology**, two additional papers on validation study design have appeared. Stram et al. [15] considered validation study design for minimizing the variance of the regression calibration estimate of the odds ratio, under the constraint of fixed total cost for an external validation study. They derived equations for the optimal choice of the number of subjects and the number of days per subject of diet records or diet recalls (X') when the food frequency questionnaire (W) is used to assess diet in the main study. It is assumed that the relationship between X and X' is given by the assumption of random within-person variation, following (1). They found that the optimal validation study size and number of replicates per subject depend on the ratio between the costs of the initial and subsequent 1-day diet records, and on the ratio of the variance in a single replicate of X' to the variance of the true underlying diet. The authors concluded that, in most settings, the optimal study design will rarely require more than five 1-day diet records per validation study participant. Kaaks et al. [9] derived a closed-form expression for the increase due to measurement error in the number of cases needed in a main study/external study design using regression calibration, as a function of the validation study sample size, the correlation between X and W, the odds ratio, and the conditional variance of X given W. They inverted this expression to optimize n_2 as a function of these other parameters, subject to a specified degree of precision in the regression calibration estimate of β per subject.

Conclusion

In main study/validation study design, the criterion used for design optimization should be carefully chosen. For both validity and efficiency considerations, internal validation studies are preferred over external ones. Particularly when the sample disease frequency is not rare and when the cost of the gold standard is not prohibitive, completely validated designs may be optimal. Owing to the lack of user-friendly software, it does not appear that explicitly optimized main study/validation study designs have been used by scientific investigators. Further work could involve making the identification of optimal designs more accessible in the field.

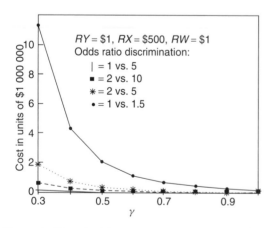

Figure 1 Plot of minimized cost to discriminate between two hypothesized odds ratios, against γ, where $E(X|W) = \alpha' + \gamma W$. When X and W are standardized, γ is corr (W, X)

Acknowledgment

This work was supported by National Cancer Institute grants CA50587 and CA03416.

References

[1]   Armstrong, B.K., White, E. & Saracci, R. (1992). *Principles of Exposure Measurement in Epidemiology.* Oxford University Press, Oxford, Chapter 4.

[2]   Barron, B.A. (1977). The effects of misclassification on the estimation of relative risk, *Biometrics* **33**, 414–418.

[3]   Buonaccorsi, J.P. (1990). Doubling sampling for exact values in the normal discriminant model with application to binary regression, *Communications in Statistics – Theory and Methods* **19**, 4569–4586.

[4]   Chernoff, H. & Haitovsky, Y. (1990). Locally optimal designs for comparing two probabilities from binomial data subject to misclassification, *Biometrika* **77**, 797–806.

[5]   Greenland, S. (1988). On sample size and power calculations for studies using confidence intervals, *American Journal of Epidemiology* **128**, 231–236.

[6]   Greenland, S. (1988). Statistical uncertainty due to misclassification: implications for validation substudies, *Journal of Clinical Epidemiology* **41**, 1167–1174.

[7]   Greenland, S. (1988). Variance estimation for epidemiologic effect estimates under misclassification, *Statistics in Medicine* **7**, 745–757.

[8]   IMSL (1987). *User's Manual: Math Library.* IMSL, Houston.

[9]   Kaaks, R., Riboli, E. & van Staveren, W. (1995). Sample size requirements for calibration studies of dietary intake measurements in prospective cohort investigations, *American Journal of Epidemiology* **142**, 557–565.

[10] Küchenhoff, H. (1990). *Logit- und Probitregression mit Fehlen in den Variabeln.* Anton Hain, Frankfurt am Main.

[11] Palmgren, J. (1987). Precision of double sampling estimators for comparing two probabilities, *Biometrika* **74**, 687–694.

[12] Selen, J. (1986). Adjusting for errors in classification and measurement in the analysis of partly and purely categorical data, *Journal of the American Statistical Association*, **81**, 75–81.

[13] Spiegelman, D. & Gray, R. (1991). Cost-efficient study designs for binary response data with Gaussian covariate measurement error, *Biometrics* **47**, 851–869.

[14] Spiegelman, D., Schneeweiss, S. & McDermott, A. (1997). Measurement error correction for logistic regression models with an "alloyed gold standard", *American Journal of Epidemiology* **145**, 184–196.

[15] Stram, D.O., Longnecker, M.P., Shames, L., Kolonel, L.N., Wildens, L.R., Pike, M.C. & Henderson, B.E. (1995). Cost-efficient design of a diet validation study, *American Journal of Epidemiology* **142**, 353–362.

[16] Tosteson, T. & Tsiatis, A. (1988). The asymptotic relative efficiency of score tests in a generalized linear model with surrogate covariates, *Biometrika* **77**, 11–20.

[17] Tosteson, T.D. & Ware, J.H. (1990). Designing a logistic regression study using surrogate measures for exposure and outcome, *Biometrika* **77**, 11–21.

[18] Wacholder, S., Armstrong, B. & Hartge, P. (1993). Validation studies using an alloyed gold standard, *American Journal of Epidemiology* **137**, 1251–1258.

[19] Willett, W.C. (1990). *Nutritional Epidemiology.* Oxford University Press, New York, pp. 115–118.

[20] Zelen, M. & Haitovsky, Y. (1991). Testing hypotheses with binary data subject to misclassification errors: analysis and experimental design, *Biometrika* **78**, 857–865.

(*See also* **Measurement Error in Epidemiologic Studies**)

DONNA SPIEGELMAN

Validity and Generalizability in Epidemiologic Studies

The validity of a study of human subjects is often separated into two components: the validity of the inferences drawn as they pertain to members of the source population (*internal validity*), and the validity of the inferences as they pertain to people outside that population (*external validity* or *generalizability*). Internal validity parallels the statistical concept of generalizing from sample to source population, while generalizability involves more informal inference beyond a source population to **target populations**.

Scientific generalization extends beyond statistical generalization of study results to the formulation of abstract concepts relating the study factors. The concepts are abstract in the sense that they are not tied to specific populations; instead they amount to the specification of a more general scientific theory. Internal validity is a prerequisite for the study to contribute usefully to this process of abstraction, but the generalization process is otherwise separate from the concerns of internal validity and the mechanics of the study design.

Validity

Internal validity implies validity of inference for the study subjects themselves. Specifically, it implies an accurate measurement apart from **random errors**. Numerous types of **biases** can detract from internal validity; for examples, see [19]. The distinction among these biases is occasionally difficult to make, but three general types can be identified: **selection bias, confounding**, and information bias. These categories are not always clearly demarcated; factors that appear to be responsible for a selection bias can also be viewed, under some circumstances, as confounding factors. Occasionally, certain information biases can also be construed as confounding.

Selection Bias

Most epidemiologic studies involve a comparison of two or more groups with regard to either disease or exposure frequency. Bias is a distortion of the effect that is measured. Selection biases are distortions that result from procedures used to select subjects, and from factors that influence study participation.

Self-Selection Bias.   One form of such bias is *self-selection* bias. When the Centers for Disease Control (CDC) investigated subsequent leukemia incidence among troops who had been present at the Smoky Atomic Test in Nevada [3], 76% of the troops identified as members of that cohort (*see* **Cohort Study**) had known outcomes. Of this 76%, 82% were traced by the investigators, but the other 18% contacted the investigators on their own initiative in response to publicity about the investigation. This self-referral of subjects is ordinarily considered a threat to validity, since the reasons for self-referral may be associated with the outcome under study [6]. In the Smoky study, there were four leukemia cases among the $0.18 \times 0.76 = 15\%$ of cohort members who referred themselves and four among the $0.82 \times 0.76 = 62\%$ of cohort members traced by the investigators, for a total of eight cases among the 76% of the cohort with known outcomes. These data indicate that self-selection bias was a small but real problem in the Smoky study. If the 24% of the cohort with unknown outcomes had a leukemia incidence like that of the subjects traced by the investigators, then we should expect that only $4(24/62) = 1.5$ or about one or two cases occurred among this 24%, for a total of only nine or 10 cases in the entire cohort. If, however, we assumed that the 24% with unknown outcomes had a leukemia incidence like that of subjects with known outcomes, then we would calculate that $8(24/76) = 2.5$ or about two or three cases occurred among this 24%, for a total of 10 or 11 cases in the entire cohort.

Self-selection can also occur before subjects are identified for study. For example, it is routine to find that the mortality of active workers is less than

that of the population as a whole [9, 15]. This "healthy-worker effect" presumably derives from a screening process, perhaps largely self-selection, that allows relatively healthy people to become or remain workers, whereas those who remain unemployed, retired, disabled, or otherwise out of the active worker population are as a group less healthy [23] (*see* **Occupational Epidemiology**).

Diagnostic Bias.   Another type of selection bias occurring before subjects are identified for study is *diagnostic bias* [19]. When the relation between oral contraceptives and venous thromboembolism was first investigated with **case–control studies of hospitalized patients**, there was concern that some of the women had been hospitalized with a diagnosis of venous thromboembolism because their physicians suspected a relation between this disease and oral contraceptives and had known about oral contraceptive use in patients who presented with suggestive symptoms [20]. A study of hospitalized patients with thromboembolism could lead to an exaggerated estimate of the effect of oral contraceptives on thromboembolism if the hospitalization and determination of the diagnosis were influenced by the history of oral contraceptive use.

Many varieties of selection bias could be described. The common element of such biases is that the relation between exposure and disease is different for those who participate and those who should be theoretically eligible for study, including those who do not participate. The result is that associations observed in the study represent a mix of forces determining participation as well as forces determining disease. It is sometimes (but not always) possible to disentangle the effects of participation determinants from those of disease determinants using analytic methods for the control of confounding.

Confounding.   The term **confounding** has been used for several different concepts, which are contrasted in confounding. In the context of validity, confounding is a bias. Although this bias can occur in experiments, it is a considerably more important issue in nonexperimental research.

On the simplest level, confounding may be considered a confusion of effects. Specifically, the apparent effect of the exposure of interest (which may be null) is distorted because the effect of an extraneous factor is mistaken for or mixed with the actual exposure effect (which may be null). The distortion introduced by a confounding factor can be large, and it can lead to overestimation or underestimation of an effect depending on the direction of the associations that the confounding factor has with exposure and disease. Confounding can even change the apparent direction of an effect.

A more precise definition of confounding begins by considering the manner in which effects are estimated. Let us assume that we wish to estimate the degree to which exposure has changed the frequency of disease in an exposed cohort. To do so, we must estimate what the frequency of disease would have been in this cohort had exposure been absent. To accomplish this task, we observe the disease frequency in an unexposed cohort. But rarely could we take this unexposed frequency as fairly representing what the frequency would have been in the exposed cohort had exposure been absent, because the unexposed cohort would differ from the exposed cohort on many factors that affect disease frequency besides exposure. To express this problem, we say that the comparison of the exposed and unexposed is *confounded*, because the difference in disease frequency between the exposed and unexposed results from a mixture of several effects, including (but not limited to) any exposure effect.

The extraneous factors responsible for difference in disease frequency between the exposed and unexposed are called **confounders**. In addition, factors associated with these extraneous causal factors that can serve as surrogates for these factors are also commonly called confounders. The most extreme example of such a surrogate is chronologic age. Increasing age is strongly associated with *aging* – the accumulation of cell mutations and tissue damage that lead to disease – but increasing age does not itself cause such pathogenic changes, for it is just a measure of how much time has passed since birth.

Regardless of whether a confounder is a cause of the study disease or merely a surrogate for such a cause, its chief characteristic is that it would be predictive of disease frequency within the unexposed (reference) cohort – otherwise it could not explain why the unexposed cohort fails to represent properly what the exposed cohort would experience in the absence of exposure. For example, suppose all the exposed were men and all the unexposed women. If unexposed men would have the same incidence as unexposed women, then the fact that all the unexposed were women rather than men could not account for any confounding that is present.

Information Bias

Once the subjects to be compared have been identified, the information to be compared must be obtained. Bias in evaluating an effect can occur from errors in obtaining the needed information. Information bias can occur whenever there are errors in the measurement of subjects, but the consequences of the errors are different depending on whether the distribution of errors for one variable (for example, exposure or disease) depends on the actual value of other variables.

For discrete variables, **measurement error** is usually called classification error or **misclassification**. Classification error that depends on the values of other variables is referred to as *differential misclassification* (*see* **Differential Error**). Classification error that does not depend on the values of other variables is referred to as *nondifferential misclassification* (*see* **Nondifferential Error**).

Differential Misclassification. Suppose a cohort study were undertaken to compare incidence rates of emphysema among smokers and nonsmokers. Emphysema is a disease that may go undiagnosed without unusual medical attention. If smokers, because of concern about health-related effects of smoking or as a consequence of other health effects of smoking (such as bronchitis), seek medical attention to a greater degree than nonsmokers, then emphysema might be diagnosed more frequently among smokers than among nonsmokers simply as a consequence of the greater medical attention. Unless steps were taken to ensure comparable follow-up, an information bias would result: a spurious excess of emphysema incidence would be found among smokers compared with nonsmokers that is unrelated to any biologic effect of smoking. This is an example of differential misclassification, since the underdiagnosis of emphysema, a classification error, occurs more frequently for nonsmokers than for smokers. Unlike the diagnostic bias in the studies of oral contraceptives and thromboembolism described earlier, it is not a selection bias, since it occurs among subjects already included in the study. Nevertheless, the similarities between some selection biases and differential misclassification biases are worth noting.

In case–control studies of congenital malformations, the etiologic information may be obtained at interview from mothers. The case mothers have recently given birth to a malformed baby, whereas the vast majority of control mothers have recently given birth to an apparently healthy baby. Another variety of differential misclassification, referred to as **recall bias**, can result if the mothers of malformed infants recall exposures more thoroughly than mothers of healthy infants. It is supposed that the birth of a malformed infant serves as a stimulus to a mother to recall all events that might have played some role in the unfortunate outcome. Presumably such women will remember exposures such as infectious disease, trauma, and drugs more accurately than mothers of healthy infants, who have not had a comparable stimulus. Consequently, information on such exposures will be ascertained more frequently from mothers of malformed babies, and an apparent effect, unrelated to any biologic effect, will result from this recall bias. Recall bias is a possibility in any case–control study that uses an anamnestic response, since the cases and controls by definition are people who differ with respect to their disease experience, and this difference may affect recall.

The bias that is caused by differential misclassification can either exaggerate or underestimate an effect. In each of the examples above, the misclassification serves to exaggerate the effects under study, but examples to the contrary can also be found. Because of the relatively unpredictable effects of differential misclassification, some investigators go through elaborate procedures to ensure that the misclassification will be nondifferential, such as blinding of exposure evaluations with respect to outcome status. Unfortunately, even in situations when blinding is accomplished or in cohort studies in which disease outcomes have not yet occurred, collapsing continuous or categorical exposure data into fewer categories can induce differential misclassification [8, 21].

Nondifferential Misclassification. Nondifferential exposure or disease misclassification occurs when the proportion of subjects misclassified on exposure does not depend on disease status, or when the proportion of subjects misclassified on disease does not depend on exposure. When the misclassification is independent of other errors, bias introduced by such nondifferential misclassification of a binary exposure or disease is predictable in direction, namely toward the null value [5, 11, 12, 17] (*see* **Bias Toward the Null**). Contrary to popular misconceptions, however, nondifferential exposure or disease misclassification can sometimes produce bias away from the null [4, 7, 13, 22]. If the misclassification is extreme, the misclassification can go beyond the null value and reverse direction.

When the exposure is polytomous (that is, has more than two categories) and there is nondifferential misclassification between two of the categories and no others, the effect estimates for those two categories will be biased toward one another [1, 22]. In particular, the effect estimate for the lower exposure category will be shifted toward that of the higher exposure category, and away from the null value. It is also possible for independent nondifferential misclassification to bias trend estimates away from the null or reverse a trend [7]. Such examples are unusual, however, because trend reversal cannot occur if the mean exposure measurement increases with true exposure [24].

Nondifferential Misclassification of Disease.   The effects of nondifferential misclassification of disease resemble those of nondifferential misclassification of exposure. In most situations, nondifferential misclassification of a binary disease outcome will produce bias toward the null, provided that the misclassification is independent of other errors. There are, however, some useful special cases in which such misclassification produces no bias in the risk ratio (*see* **Relative Risk**); in addition, the bias in the risk difference is a simple function of the **sensitivity** and **specificity**. For a discussion, see Rothman & Greenland [18].

Pervasiveness of Nondifferential Misclassification.
Since the bias from independent nondifferential misclassification of a dichotomous exposure is always in the direction of the null value, historically it has not been a great source of concern to epidemiologists, who have generally considered it more acceptable to underestimate effects than to overestimate effects. Nevertheless, such misclassification is a serious problem: the bias it introduces may account for certain discrepancies among epidemiologic studies. Many studies ascertain information in a way that guarantees substantial misclassification, and many studies use classification schemes that can mask effects in a manner identical to nondifferential misclassification.

Suppose aspirin transiently reduces risk of myocardial infarction. The word *transiently* implies a brief induction period. Any study that considered as exposure aspirin use outside of a narrow time interval before the occurrence of a myocardial infarction would be misclassifying aspirin use: there is relevant use of aspirin, and there is use of aspirin that is irrelevant because it does not allow the exposure to act causally under the causal hypothesis with its specified induction period. Many studies ask about "ever use" (use at any time during an individual's life) of drugs or other exposures. Such cumulative indices over an individual's lifetime inevitably augment possibly relevant exposure with irrelevant exposure, and can thus introduce a bias toward the null value through nondifferential misclassification.

In cohort studies in which there are disease categories with few subjects, investigators are occasionally tempted to combine outcome categories to increase the number of subjects in each analysis, thereby gaining precision. This collapsing of categories can obscure effects on more narrowly defined disease categories.

Nondifferential exposure and disease misclassification is a greater concern in interpreting studies that seem to indicate the absence of an effect. Consequently, in studies that indicate little or no effect, it is crucial for the researchers to consider the problem of nondifferential misclassification to determine to what extent a real effect might have been obscured. On the other hand, in studies that describe a strong nonzero effect, preoccupation with nondifferential exposure and disease misclassification is rarely warranted, provided that the errors are independent. Occasionally, critics of a study will argue that poor exposure data or a poor disease classification invalidate the results. This argument is incorrect, however, if the results indicate a nonzero effect and one can be sure that the classification errors produced bias towards the null, since the bias will be in the direction of underestimating the effect.

Generally speaking, it is incorrect to dismiss a study reporting an effect simply because there is substantial nondifferential misclassification of exposure, since an estimate of effect without the misclassification could be even greater, provided that the misclassification probabilities apply uniformly to all subjects. Thus, the implications of nondifferential misclassification depend heavily on whether the study is perceived as "positive" or "negative". Emphasis on

measurement instead of on a qualitative description of study results lessens the likelihood for misinterpretation, but even so it is important to bear in mind the direction and likely magnitude of a bias.

Misclassification of Confounders.   If a confounding variable is misclassified, the ability to control confounding in the analysis is hampered [2, 10, 14]. While independent nondifferential misclassification of exposure or disease usually biases study results in the direction of the null hypothesis, independent nondifferential misclassification of a confounding variable will usually reduce the degree to which confounding can be controlled and thus can cause a bias in either direction, depending on the direction of the confounding. For this reason, misclassification of confounding factors can be a serious problem.

If the confounding is strong and the exposure–disease relation is weak or zero, misclassification of the confounding factor can lead to extremely misleading results. For example, a strong causal relation between smoking and bladder cancer, coupled with a strong association between smoking and coffee drinking, makes smoking a strong confounder of any possible relation between coffee drinking and bladder cancer. Since the control of confounding by smoking depends on accurate smoking information, and since some misclassification of the relevant smoking information is inevitable no matter how smoking is measured, some residual confounding is inevitable [16]. The problem of residual confounding would be even worse if the only available information on smoking were a simple dichotomy such as "ever smoked" vs. "never smoked", since the lack of detailed specification of smoking prohibits adequate control of confounding. The resulting confounding is especially troublesome because to many investigators and readers it may appear that confounding by smoking has been controlled.

Generalizability

Many epidemiologists and statisticians have taught that generalization from a study group depends on the study group being a representative subgroup of the target population, in the sense of a sample. If scientific generalization were simply a matter of statistical generalization, however, it would be limited literally to those individuals who might have been included, through sampling, as study subjects. If this notion were correct, there would be no application to humans of any results obtained from animal research. In addition, every population would require its own set of studies, and these studies would have to be repeated for every new generation.

The tendency to use "representative" study groups probably derives from early experience with surveys for which the inferential goal was only description of the surveyed population. Social scientists often rely on statistical inference because decisions about what is relevant for generalization are more difficult in the social sciences, and populations are considerably more diverse in sociologic phenomena than in biologic phenomena. In the biologic sciences, however, investigators conduct experiments using animals with characteristics selected to enhance the validity of the experimental work rather than to represent the target population. Epidemiologic study designs are usually stronger if subject selection is guided by the need to make a valid comparison, which may call for severe restriction of admissible subjects to a narrow range of characteristics, rather than by an attempt to make the subjects representative, in a sampling sense, of the potential target populations.

Ultimately, the goal of a purely scientific study is to contribute to scientific knowledge. The process of synthesizing knowledge from observations is, after centuries of examination, not yet well understood. In most sciences, however, the process involves moving from the particulars of a set of observations to the abstraction of a scientific hypothesis or theory that is more or less divorced from time and place: the abstractions apply to a broader domain of experience than that observed or sampled from. Such scientific generalization amounts to moving from time- and place-specific observations to an abstract "universal" hypothesis, such as "cigarette smoking causes lung cancer". This process is neither mechanical nor statistical, nor does it involve specific target populations (although the hypothesis may be limited to certain biological subgroups, such as a specific genotype). In this sense, the term external validity is a misnomer, and the term generalization must be interpreted as abstraction. Selection of study groups that are representative of larger populations in the statistical sense will generally not enhance the ability to abstract universal statements from observations, but selection of study groups for characteristics that enable a study to

distinguish effectively between competing scientific hypotheses will do so.

In addition to scientific goals, some studies also have a goal of measuring effects and predicting the impact of interventions in a specific target population. In contrast to scientific inference, these pragmatic goals may depend more closely on the representativeness of study subjects with respect to the target population. For example, if a clinical trial is conducted using patients with a good prognosis, the results from the trial may not predict well the results when the new intervention is applied to patients with a poor prognosis. Thus, some effort may be needed in the study design to ensure that enough subjects are included from each of several major subgroups of the target, such as males and females. Even in this situation, complete representativeness is not always desirable, for a more efficient study might be obtained by oversampling some subgroups and then standardizing the study estimate to the target population.

Acknowledgment

Adapted from Rothman, K.J. & Greenland, S. (1998). *Modern Epidemiology*, 2nd Ed. Lippincott, Philadelphia, Chapter 8, with permission.

References

[1]   Birkett, N.J. (1992). Effect of nondifferential misclassification of estimates of odds ratios with multiple levels of exposure, *American Journal of Epidemiology* **136**, 356–362.

[2]   Brenner, H. (1993). Bias due to non-differential misclassification of polytomous confounders, *Journal of Clinical Epidemiology* **46**, 57–63.

[3]   Caldwell, G.G., Kelley, D.B. & Heath, C.W. Jr (1980). Leukemia among participants in military maneuvers at a nuclear bomb test: a preliminary report, *Journal of the American Medical Association* **244**, 1575–1578.

[4]   Chavance, M., Dellatolas, G. & Lellouch, J. (1992). Correlated nondifferential misclassifications of disease and exposure, *International Journal of Epidemiology* **21**, 537–546.

[5]   Copeland, K.T., Checkoway, H., Holbrook, R.H. & McMichael, A.J. (1977). Bias due to misclassification in the estimate of relative risk, *American Journal of Epidemiology* **105**, 488–495.

[6]   Criqui, M.H., Austin, M. & Barrett-Connor, E. (1979). The effect of non-response on risk ratios in a cardiovascular disease study, *Journal of Chronic Diseases* **32**, 633–638.

[7]   Dosemeci, M., Wacholder, S. & Lubin, J. (1990). Does nondifferential misclassification of exposure always bias

a true effect toward the null value?, *American Journal of Epidemiology* **132**, 746–749.

[8] Flegal, K.M., Keyl, P.M. & Nieto, F.J. (1991). Differential misclassification arising from nondifferential errors in exposure measurement, *American Journal of Epidemiology* **134**, 1233–1244.

[9] Fox, A.J. & Collier, P.F. (1976). Low mortality rates in industrial cohort studies due to selection for work and survival in the industry, *British Journal of Preventive and Social Medicine* **30**, 225–230.

[10] Greenland, S. (1980). The effect of misclassification in the presence of covariates, *American Journal of Epidemiology* **112**, 564–569.

[11] Gullen, W.H., Berman, J.E. & Johnson, E.A. (1968). Effects of misclassification in epidemiologic studies, *Public Health Reports* **53**, 1956–1965.

[12] Keys, A. & Kihlberg, J.K. (1963). The effect of misclassification on the estimated relative prevalence of a characteristic, *American Journal of Public Health* **53**, 1656–1665.

[13] Kristensen, P. (1992). Bias from nondifferential but dependent misclassification of exposure and outcome, *Epidemiology* **3**, 210–215.

[14] Marshall, J.R. & Hastrup, J.L. (1996). Mismeasurement and the resonance of strong confounders: uncorrelated errors, *American Journal of Epidemiology* **143**, 1069–1078.

[15] McMichael, A.J. (1976). Standardized mortality ratios and the "healthy worker effect": scratching beneath the surface, *Journal of Occupational Medicine* **18**, 165–168.

[16] Morrison, A.S., Buring, J.E., Verhoek, W.G., Aoki, K., Leck, I., Ohno, Y. & Obata, K. (1982). Coffee drinking and cancer of the lower urinary tract, *Journal of the National Cancer Institute* **68**, 91–94.

[17] Newell, D.J. (1962). Errors in interpretation of errors in epidemiology, *American Journal of Public Health* **52**, 1925–1928.

[18] Rothman, K.J. & Greenland, S. (1998). *Modern Epidemiology*, 2nd Ed. Lippincott, Philadelphia, Chapter 8.

[19] Sackett, D.L. (1979). Bias in analytic research, *Journal of Chronic Diseases* **32**, 51–63.

[20] Sartwell, P.E., Masi, A.T., Arthes, F.G., Greene, G.R. & Smith, H.E. (1969). Thromboembolism and oral contraceptives: an epidemiologic case–control study, *American Journal of Epidemiology* **90**, 365–380.

[21] Wacholder, S., Dosemeci, M. & Lubin, J.H. (1991). Blind assignment of exposure does not prevent differential misclassification, *American Journal of Epidemiology* **134**, 433–437.

[22] Walker, A.M. & Blettner, M. (1985). Comparing imperfect measures of exposure, *American Journal of Epidemiology* **121**, 783–790.

[23] Wang, J.D. & Miettinen, O.S. (1982). Occupational mortality studies: principles of validity, *Scandinavian Journal of Environmental Health* **8**, 153–158.

[24] Weinberg, C.R., Umbach, D.M. & Greenland, S. (1994). When will nondifferential misclassification preserve the direction of a trend?, *American Journal of Epidemiology* **140**, 565–571.

(*See also* **Bias in Case–Control Studies; Bias in Cohort Studies; Bias in Observational Studies; Bias, Overview**)

KENNETH J. ROTHMAN & SANDER GREENLAND

van Elteren Test *see* Mantel–Haenszel Methods

Verbal Autopsy *see* Morbidity and Mortality, Changing Patterns in the Twentieth Century

Vital Statistics, Overview

Vital statistics, as a scientific discipline, is a subdomain of **demography**, the study of the characteristics of human populations. Vital statistics comprises a number of important events in human life including birth, death, fetal death, marriage, divorce, annulment, judicial separation, adoption, legitimation, and recognition. The term "vital statistics" is also applied to individual measures of these vital events. Thus, a birth rate is an example of a vital statistic and an analysis of trends in birth rates is an example of an application in the field of vital statistics. A vital statistics system is the total process of collecting by civil registration, enumeration, or indirect estimation, information on the frequency of occurrence of vital events, selected characteristics of the events and the persons concerned, and the compilation, analysis, evaluation, and dissemination of these data in summarized statistical form. Other life events of demographic importance such as change of place of residence (migration), change of citizenship (naturalization), and change of name are not included, mainly because information on these is usually derived from other statistical systems such as population registers [1].

Systems for Collecting Vital Statistics

It is generally accepted that the preferred method for individual countries to collect vital statistics is through a civil registration system. This is recognized by the United Nations (UN) and other international organizations, as well as by the many countries that have had civil registration laws and regulations in place and in operation for many years [1, 2]. Nevertheless, a number of newly emergent and developing nations, facing the difficulties and length of time it takes to create a satisfactory civil registration system, have instituted alternative procedures to acquire statistical data to describe the levels and trends for key vital events, particularly for fertility and mortality measurements. The UN recognizes the importance of a civil registration system for each country as the preferred source of vital statistics data for the long run. However, use of an alternative data collection system is recommended as an interim measure for meeting needs for essential information where a civil registration system of acceptable quality does not yet exist. Other systems include, for example, probability area samples, purposeful area samples, records-based surveys, and **record linkage**. Furthermore, the UN recommends a priority order for the types of vital statistics data to be collected. The highest need is given to data on births and deaths, followed in order by marriages, divorces, fetal deaths, annulments, judicial separations, adoptions, legitimations, and recognitions [1].

Uses of Vital Records and Vital Statistics

Vital records created through a civil registration system have two classes of use. They have value individually as legal documents for the persons named thereon; they also constitute the input, when aggregated, for the various vital statistics measures that are used to study the demographics and health of populations and population subgroups.

For the individual, a birth record is a legal document establishing name, parentage, birth data, order of birth for multiple births, legitimacy, and

citizenship, nationality, or geographic place of birth. A wide variety of individual rights and civil entitlements depends on these facts, including proof of age for school entrance, motor vehicle drivers' licenses, military service and other age-related activities, establishment of eligibility for family allowances, insurance benefits, tax benefits, inheritance rights, issuance of passports, etc. The death record provides documentary proof of the facts of death needed for social security and insurance purposes such as time and place of death and the medical cause of death. Proof of death and the associated facts are also used for property inheritance rights, for remarriage rights of surviving spouses, etc. Marriage and divorce records serve to document rights to special social and economic programs and benefits for the married, including tax privileges for couples, alimony, change of nationality based on marriage, and the right to remarry. Many rights of children, their parents, and their guardians are dependent on records of adoption, legitimation, and recognition.

Individual vital records may also be used administratively as the basis for initiating maternal and child health services, including child immunization programs, or for epidemiologic investigations into disease outbreaks or assessments of causes of accidents and injuries. Another important administrative use of individual vital records especially of death records (*see* **Death Certification**), is for the updating or clearing of files such as electoral rolls, social security files, **disease registers**, cohort follow-up studies, tax registers, etc.

In aggregated form, vital records become a collection of vital statistics, most often in the form of means, medians, and various ratios such as proportions and **rates**. Whether collected by civil registration or by other means, vital statistics serve as key demographic variables in the analysis of population size, growth and geographic distribution, especially when used in conjunction with periodic population censuses. When census data are used as a base, current intercensal estimates of population size can be made, and projections into the future can be prepared using estimates of future trends in fertility, natality, and mortality linked with estimates of net migration. In addition to the importance of vital statistics to the study of population size and growth trends, other national and subnational economic and social concerns such as health, welfare, education, occupation, housing, urbanization, family structure, and income are also affected by these measures. In the fields of public health and medicine, for example, levels and trends of **infant and perinatal mortality** are often used as surrogate measures of levels and trends in the overall health and well-being of nations. **Life expectancy** at birth is also frequently used to compare the overall effects of mortality and its determinants. **Cause of death** information provides a foundation upon which much research into diseases and disease prevention is based.

Differentials in mortality by sex, age, racial groups, and other variables are often the basis for the planning of health and medical intervention programs. In addition, the planning and provision of public and private housing, educational facilities, social security and private insurance plans, medical facilities, and consumer goods of all kinds are examples of activities dependent on vital statistics data. At the international level, vital statistics provide a basis for comparing important demographic, social, and economic differences and trends over time among countries or regions of the world.

Definitions of Selected Vital Events

Standard statistical definitions of vital events have been promulgated by international agencies [1, 5]. In some cases, legal definitions may differ from the international standards in varying degrees, but, in many cases, national vital statistics reports are either based on the standard statistical definitions or do not differ in principle. In cases where comparability among countries is compromised because of the use of nonstandard definitions, international agencies and others presenting national comparisons of tabular, graphical or descriptive vital statistics usually provide appropriate cautions to users. Nevertheless, users of vital statistics data need to ascertain the comparability of the data before drawing reliable conclusions about national differences. The World Health Organization (WHO) promulgates a number of vital statistics definitions as part of the **International Classification of Diseases (ICD)**. These definitions are incorporated in regulations adopted by the World Health Assembly and which each WHO member country has agreed to follow [4]. Nevertheless, it is still necessary to ensure that the standard definitions have been followed for a given data set. The international standard definitions for selected vital events are given below.

Live Birth. This is the complete expulsion or extraction from its mother of a product of conception, irrespective of the duration of the pregnancy, which, after such separation, breathes or shows any other evidence of life, such as beating of the heart, pulsation of the umbilical cord, or definite movement of voluntary muscles, whether or not the umbilical cord has been cut or the placenta is attached; each product of such a birth is considered liveborn [5].

Fetal Death. This is death prior to the complete expulsion or extraction from its mother of a product of conception, irrespective of the duration of pregnancy; the death is indicated by the fact that after such separation the fetus does not breathe or show any other evidence of life, such as beating of the heart, pulsation of the umbilical cord, or definite movement of voluntary muscles [5].

Maternal Death. This is the death of a woman while pregnant or within 42 days of termination of pregnancy, irrespective of the duration and the site of the pregnancy, from any cause related to or aggravated by the pregnancy or its management, but not from accidental or incidental causes. Maternal deaths may be subdivided into two groups: direct obstetric deaths which are the result of obstetric complications of the pregnant state (pregnancy, labor, and the puerperium), from interventions, omissions, incorrect treatment, or from a chain of events resulting from any of these; and indirect obstetric deaths which are the result of previously existing disease or disease that developed during pregnancy and which was not due to direct obstetric causes, but which was aggravated by physiologic effects of pregnancy [5].

Infant Death. This is the death of a liveborn infant who dies before completing its first year of life.

Neonatal Death. This is the death of a liveborn infant who dies during the first 28 completed days of life. These may be subdivided into early neonatal deaths, occurring during the first seven days of life, and late neonatal deaths, occurring after the completion of the seventh day but before the completion of 28 days [5].

Perinatal Death. This is the death of a fetus or newborn infant occurring after 22 completed weeks

(154 days) of gestation (the time when fetal weight is normally about 500 g), but prior to the completion of seven days after birth [5].

Marriage. This is the act, ceremony or process by which the legal relationship of husband and wife is constituted. The legality of the union may be established by civil, religious, or other means recognized by the laws of each country [1].

Divorce. This is a final legal dissolution of a marriage which confers on the parties the right to remarriage under civil, religious, or other provisions, according to the laws of each country [1].

Definitions of Selected Vital Statistics Measures

Raw vital statistics most often are comprised of counts of how often a specified vital event has occurred, rather than on measurements of continuous variables such as height, weight, or blood pressure. The analysis of vital data depends mainly on the conversion of observed frequencies into indices, ratios, and probabilities. Counts of vital events often do have utility, but, for the majority of uses, absolute frequencies are not sufficient and it becomes necessary to compute relative numbers, including crude rates, various types of specific rates, percentages, probabilities, and other ratios.

Some of the more commonly encountered vital statistics relative numbers are defined and calculated as follows.

Crude Death Rate

The most common form of mortality measurement is the crude death rate. It is computed from the following formula [3]:

$$m_{cd} = (D/P)k,$$

where m_{cd} is the crude death rate, D is the total number of deaths for a given area and time period, usually a calendar year, P is the size of population at risk of dying, usually taken as the estimated population at the midpoint of the calendar year, and k is a constant, usually taken as 1000.

The crude rate is so named to differentiate it from various specific and adjusted rates and represents the total or overall death rate without regard to the various component elements which combine to produce the total figure. The crude death rate is usually expressed as "the number of deaths per 1000 persons" for a specified place (country, city, state, etc.) for a given year.

Specific Death Rate

Detailed analyses of vital statistics frequently go beyond the overall risk of death in the population as a whole. Many studies deal with subsets of the population or with particular classes of deaths. Epidemiologists often focus on deaths from a particular disease or class of diseases. Actuaries and demographers are concerned with differences in mortality by sex and in different age groups within the population. Environmental and **occupational health** specialists are interested in the differential risks of dying in selected occupations, and in different geographic subdivisions such as urban and rural areas. To meet these kinds of needs, various specific death rates are calculated. Specific rates for different age groups are called *age-specific death rates*; rates for males and females are called *sex-specific death rates*, rates for particular causes of death are called *cause-specific death rates*. Rates may be specific for combinations of characteristics. For example, age–sex–race-specific death rates are computed separately for each age group by race and sex. Specific death rates are approximations of true probabilities. That is, the denominator of the ratio is an estimate of the total number of events of a particular type that could happen, while the numerator is a count of those that did happen.

Specific death rates are computed as follows [3]:

$$m_{sd} = (d_i/p_i)k,$$

where m_{sd} is the specific rate for any defined ith class, d_i is the number of deaths occurring in the ith class for a given area and time, p_i is the number of persons in the ith class of the population for the same area and time, and k is a constant, usually 100 000.

For cause-specific death rates, the denominator, p_i, in the above formula is replaced by P, the total population exposed to the risk of death. Therefore, a cause-specific death rate measures the risk in the total population of dying from a specified cause of death.

Infant Mortality Rate

The infant mortality rate is considered by many as one of the important indicators of the overall level of health and social well-being of a country or other geopolitical area. This is, in part, because a large proportion of deaths in the first year of life are considered to be preventable through adequate prenatal care, good nutrition for women and infants, and improved control of the environment, including injury prevention.

The infant mortality rate is computed as follows [3]:

$$m_i = (d_{<1}/B)k,$$

where m_i is the infant mortality rate, $d_{<1}$ is the number of deaths to liveborn infants under one year of age during a specified time period, usually one year, B is the total number of live births during the same time period, and k is a constant, usually 1000.

The infant mortality rate is a proxy for the age-specific death rate for the "under one year of age group" and is intended to be a measure of the risk of dying during the first year of life. The numerators of the infant mortality rate and the "under one year of age" age-specific death rate are the same. For a denominator, however, a reliable estimate of the size of the population under one year of age for a given time period is hard to obtain, even in a census year. As a proxy measure, the denominator may be considered to be the number of births occurring during the period. For either of these choices of denominator, there is some mismatch with the numerator in terms of a true probability number. Not all events in the numerator arise from the events in the denominator. For example, in the infant mortality rate, some of the deaths under one year of age in a given year and counted in the numerator were actually born in the previous year and are not represented in the denominator, while some of the births represented in the denominator will die before their first birthday but the deaths will occur in the next year and are not included in the numerator. However, when the birth rate is fairly stable from one year to the next, calculation of the infant mortality rate results in a ratio that closely approximates the probability of a live-born infant dying within the first year of life. When the birth rate is not stable from year to year, a more accurate mortality rate may be computed by following each live birth occurring during a one year period and measuring how many of them die before their first birthday.

Neonatal, Early Neonatal and Postneonatal Mortality Rates

The *neonatal mortality rate* is defined as follows [5]:

$$m_n = (d_{<1\ mo}/B)k,$$

where m_n is the neonatal mortality rate, $d_{<1\ mo}$ is the number of deaths of infants under 1 month of age during a specified time period, B is the number of live births occurring during the same time period, and, k is a constant, usually 1000.

The neonatal mortality rate, like the infant mortality rate, is a proxy for an age-specific death rate. It approximates the risk of dying in the first month of life. The relative importance of an infant mortality rate compared with the corresponding neonatal mortality rate depends on the proportionate age distribution of the deaths under one year of age. Generally, when the infant mortality rate is low, a large proportion of infant deaths occur during the first month of life. The neonatal mortality rate then reflects an important measure of the mortality risk for infants. Conversely, when the infant mortality rate is high, larger proportions of deaths fall into the older age groups under a year. Often it is useful to partition the deaths of infants under one year of age into two groups: those dying before one month of age, and those dying between one month and their first birthday. The former comprise the numerator, $d_{<1\ mo}$, of the neonatal mortality rate, while the latter can be used to calculate the *postneonatal mortality rate*:

$$m_{pn} = (d_{1\ mo-1\ yr}/B)k,$$

where m_{pn} is the postneonatal mortality rate, $d_{1\ mo-1\ yr}$ is the number of deaths occurring between 1 month and 1 year of age during a specified time period, B is the number of live births occurring during the same time period, and k is the same constant used in the neonatal mortality rate, usually 1000.

In similar fashion, the neonatal deaths may be partitioned into those dying within the first week of life and the remainder that survive the first seven days but die before one month of age. The risk of dying in the first week of life is measured by the *early neonatal mortality rate*, m_{en}, as follows [5]:

$$m_{en} = (d_{<7\ days}/B)k,$$

where the components of the calculation are the same as in the neonatal and postneonatal mortality rates, except that the numerator contains only those deaths to infants occurring during the first week of life.

Perinatal Mortality Rate

The perinatal period, as defined earlier, is the period of time surrounding the event of birth. It includes the time that a fetus spends in utero after it has reached 22 weeks of gestation and continues through the birth process until the end of the first week of life after birth. The perinatal mortality rate measures mortality occurring during this period. The rate, therefore, combines deaths of fetuses of specified gestational age with deaths of liveborn infants who die in their first week of life. The determination of whether a fetus is born dead or whether it shows any sign of life before expiring is not always clear-cut; social, economic, and cultural factors, as well as medical and biological considerations, tend to push the fetal death rate in one direction or the other in different societies, thus making comparisons of neonatal or infant mortality among countries difficult. By using the perinatal mortality rate for comparisons, this difficulty is minimized since fetuses dying just before or during the birth process as well as those born alive but dying shortly thereafter are all included in the calculation [5]:

$$m_{peri} = [d_{peri}/(F + B)]k,$$

where m_{peri} is the perinatal mortality rate, d_{peri} is the number of deaths of fetuses of 22 or more weeks of gestation plus deaths of liveborn infants of less than 7 days of age during a specified period, usually a calendar year, F is the number of fetal deaths of 22 or more weeks of gestation during the same period, B is the number of live births during the same period, and, k is a constant, usually 1000.

Note that, unlike the infant and neonatal mortality rates, the denominator of the perinatal mortality rate combines both the number of live births and the number of fetal deaths of 22 or more weeks of gestation. This denominator is called "total births" and better approximates the population from which the numerator could arise than would a denominator restricted to only live births. On the other hand, it is recognized that it is easier to collect reliable counts of live births than of fetal deaths, thus introducing another source of error into the calculation of the perinatal mortality rate.

Maternal Mortality Rate

The maternal mortality rate is calculated as follows [5]:

$$m_m = [(d_{md} + d_{mi})/B]k,$$

where m_m is the maternal mortality rate, d_{md} is the number of direct maternal deaths in a specified time period, usually 1 year, d_{mi} is the number of indirect maternal deaths in the same period, B is the number of live births in the same period, and k is a constant, usually 10 000 or 100 000.

A related measure, the *direct obstetric mortality ratio*, may be calculated from the above formula but using in the numerator only the direct maternal deaths, d_{md}.

Proportionate Mortality

Proportionate mortality, sometimes known as the death ratio (*see* **Proportional Mortality Ratio (PMR)**), is defined as [3]:

$$p_d = (d_i/D)k,$$

where p_d is the proportionate mortality, d_i is the number of deaths in a specified class during a stated time period, D is the total number of deaths in the same time period, and k is a constant, usually 100 or 1000.

Proportionate mortality ratios may be calculated for any class of deaths, but their most common uses are for given causes or group of causes of death expressed as percentages of deaths from all causes, or for deaths at a specified age expressed as percentages of deaths at all ages.

Crude Birth Rate

The crude birth rate is the most frequently used overall measure of the reproduction of a population. Like its counterpart, the crude death rate, it is influenced by many factors and represents a proxy for more specific fertility measurements. It is calculated as follows [3]:

$$m_{cb} = (B/P)k,$$

where m_{cb} is the crude birth rate, B is the total number of live births for a given area and time period, P is the total population at the midpoint of the time period, and, k is a constant, usually 1000.

Comparing Vital Statistics Data

Aggregated vital statistics data, whether in tabular or graphical form, often appear as time trends for particular variables such as causes or groups of causes of death, or for age and sex groups of the population. They also appear frequently as comparisons between countries or other geographical entities for a point in time, usually a particular year. In either case, great care must be taken to ensure that the quality of the data in the groups being compared warrants making the comparisons. In registration based systems, measures or estimates of completeness of reporting of vital events should be known. In sample based systems, the representativeness of the sample and the **nonresponse** rate is important. In the comparison of data between two or more geographic places, it is important to ascertain if common definitions and procedures were used to collect, process, analyze, and present the data; in looking at time trends, it is essential to know if the definitions of the events and the procedures for classifying the data remained constant over the entire time period being studied. This latter point is particularly important when looking at trends in causes of death since the instrument for grouping diseases into categories for study, the ICD, is revised approximately every 10 years (*see* **Morbidity and Mortality, Changing Patterns in the Twentieth Century**; **Mortality, International Comparisons**). Vital statistics data are often presented in statistical compendia published by official national and international organizations that attempt to include important notes for interpretation of the data in headnotes and footnotes to tables, appendices, etc. The user is cautioned to pay careful attention to such explanatory or cautionary notes.

References

[1]   United Nations (1973). Principles and Recommendations for a Vital Statistics System. *Statistical Papers, Series M, No. 19, Rev. 1*. United Nations, New York.

[2]   United States Bureau of the Census (1971). *The Methods and Materials of Demography*, H. Shryock, J. Siegel et al., eds. US Government Printing Office, Washington.

[3]   United States Department of Health, Education, and Welfare (1965). Techniques of Vital Statistics. Reprint of Chapters I–IV, *Vital Statistics Rates in the United States, 1900–1940*. National Center for Health Statistics, Washington.

[4]   World Health Organization (1967). *WHO Nomenclature Regulations*. World Health Organization, Geneva.

[5]   World Health Organization (1992). *International Statistical Classification of Diseases and Related Health Problems: 10th revision*, 3 vols. World Health Organization, Geneva.

R.A. Israel

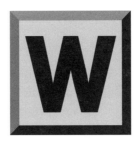

WESVAR *see* Random Digit Dialing Sampling for Case–Control Studies

Woolf's Statistic and Heterogeneity Test *see* Mantel–Haenszel Methods

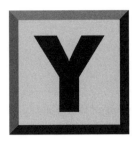

Yule's Q *see* Agreement, Measurement of

Author Index

Subject Index